OXIDATIVE STRESS AND DISEASES

Edited by **Volodymyr Lushchak**
and **Dmytro V. Gospodaryov**

Oxidative Stress and Diseases
Edited by Volodymyr Lushchak and Dmytro V. Gospodaryov

Published by InTech
Janeza Trdine 9, 51000 Rijeka, Croatia

Publishing Process Manager Sasa Leporic

Technical Editor Teodora Smiljanic

Cover Designer InTech Design Team

Additional hard copies can be obtained from orders@intechopen.com

Oxidative Stress and Diseases, Edited by Volodymyr Lushchak and Dmytro V. Gospodaryov
p. cm.
ISBN 978-953-51-0552-7

For EU product safety concerns:
IN TECH d.o.o., Prolaz Marije Krucifikse Kozulić 3, 51000 Rijeka, Croatia,
info@intechopen.com or visit our website at intechopen.com.

Meet the editors

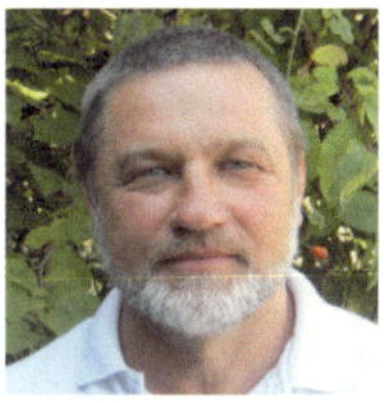

Dr. Volodymyr I. Lushchak graduated from the Lomonosov Moscow State University (Soviet Union) in 1982. In 1986 he defended his Ph.D. Theisis and in 2002 his D.Sc. Dissertation. He obtained his full professor title in 2004. From 1987 to 1998 he worked in Southern Seas Biology Institute of Academy of Sciences of Ukraine. In 1998 Dr. Lushchak joined Vassyl Stefanyk Precarpathian National University in Ivano-Frankivsk,Ukraine) where he currently works as the head of the Department of Biochemistry and Biotechnology. He also worked at Universities of Canada, Brazil, United Kingdom, Finland, Poland, Sweden and Germany. Dr. Lushchak's scientific interests are related to effects of environmental conditions and molecular aspects of adaptive responses in bacteria, fungi, plants and animals. Although interested in general aspects of metabolism regulation, his interests are mainly focused on the homeostasis of reactive species of oxygen, nitrogen and carbon.

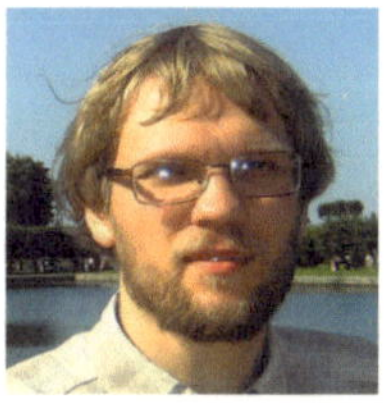

Dr. Dmytro V. Gospodaryov graduated from the Chernivtsi National University named after Yuriy Fedkovych (Ukraine) in 2001. In 2005, he defended Ph.D. thesis "Protein And Lipid Oxidation In The Yeast Saccharomyces Cerevisiae And The Role Of Catalases In Its Prevention" supervised by Prof. V. Lushchak. Since 2004, Dmytro Gospodaryov has been working as an Assistant Professor at Department of Biochemistry and Biotechnology of Stefanyk Precarpathian National University in Ivano-Frankivsk. Dr. Gospodaryov's scientific interests of are related to metabolic conditions which can induce and aggravate oxidative stress (e.g., deficiencies in antioxidant or related enzymes). He is also interested in oxidative stress induced by abnormalities in transition metal metabolism or by influence of high concentrations of transition metals.

Contents

Preface

The increased level of reactive oxygen species (ROS) in living organisms over 60 years ago was implicated in the development of diseases and aging (Harman, 1956; 1983). This book is a collective scientific monograph presenting several important aspects related to ROS role in human and animal pathologies. In 1985, German scientist Helmut Sies first denoted oxidative stress concept, which immediately attracted attention of researchers in diverse basic fields. Several discoveries substantially stimulated the interest to ROS as ones related to many diseases. They were descriptions of catalytic function of superoxide dismutase (erythrocuprein or hemocuprein) by McCord and Fridovich (1969) and role of superoxide anion in host defense against pathogens (Babior et al., 1973; McCord, 1974). The knowledge on ROS roles in diverse biological processes in living organisms was summarized in an excellent book by Halliwell and Gutteridge (1999). An obvious question arises during the accumulation of data on the ROS involvement in diseases: is oxidative stress their reason or consequence? In most cases, we cannot directly answer the question, but it is absolutely clear that reactive species accompany many pathologies. And even more – in some cases antioxidants were able to attenuate the symptoms, but in most cases the expectations on antioxidants as a panacea for many diseases was not confirmed what finally led to understanding that suppression of free radical processes also may have negative consequences for the organisms. In 1980, Arthur Hailey described the miracle drug saving many lives in a novel "Strong Medicine". That was a rather efficient antioxidant, but side effects were related to suppression of immune system and weakening defense against infections, the effects well known now. More and more recent data reflect the situation that ROS are involved in many living processes, and organisms delicately control their levels. The question on low specificity of ROS effects has also been clarified to some extent. Really, being chemically highly reactive, the processes with ROS participation are determined first of all by their species and forms, temporary-spatial generation and elimination, presence of available sensors and targets. So we are really dealing with a complicated net that is an integral part of living organisms and is usually under strict control, but if not properly controlled may result in injuries of diverse nature. Our understanding of ROS role in biological systems has evolved from recognizing of them as clearly damaging side-products of cellular metabolism changing normal physiological processes, through appreciation of their roles as critically important elements of host defense against pathogens, to recognition of their role as regulators of many physiological processes.

On December 16, 2011, a Google Scholar search for "oxidative stress" and "disease" yielded about 1,430,000 publication hits, whereas in Scopus and Pubmed databases it yielded 135,381 and 94,195 hits, respectively. Enormous interest to the ROS roles has been indirectly confirmed by the project by InTech Publisher, with the book on oxidative stress. We initially planned to publish one book, but when the project was started, more than 90 propositions were received. Therefore, recognizing the popularity of the field and interest of many scientists to share their knowledge with a broad auditory, we decided to divide the propositions and publish three books.

The Introduction section (V. I. Lushchak & D.V. Gospodaryov), that briefly covers the general aspects of oxidative stress theory, shows the potential cellular targets for ROS attacks, and via understanding of key aspects along with the details of ROS roles in biological systems, describes potential benefits from this understanding and its use to prevent or cure certain diseases. The detailed knowledge of the mechanisms with participation of reactive species may provide interesting targets for general and directed therapy or prophylactics of many diseases.

The book is divided into six sections. The first section, entitled "General Aspects" is the smallest one and contains only one chapter "Oxidative stress: cause and consequence of diseases" by D. V. Gospodaryov & V. I. Lushchak, It provides the readers with information on genetic polymorphism or deficiency of antioxidant and related enzymes which, not always, but in some cases may realize predisposition to develop certain pathologies. The enzymes analyzed in this chapter include antioxidant and associated ones such as glucose-6-phosphate dehydrogenase, catalase, cytosolic (Cu,Zn-containing), mitochondrial (Mn-containing) and extracellular superoxide dismutases, glutathione peroxidase, reparation and detoxification enzymes 8-hydroxy-2′-deoxyguanosine glycosylase, glutathione-S-transferases, etc. The last parts of the chapter are devoted to model organisms used to reveal the role of oxidative modifications of antioxidant and related enzymes in disease progression and model organisms, such as mice, fish, fruit flies, nematodes, plants, cell cultures, budding yeast, or even bacteria, broadly used to study different aspects concerning relationships between oxidative stress and diseases.

Cardiovascular diseases (CVD) are the number one killer in developed countries. Therefore, the second part of the book, entitled "Cardiovascular Diseases" and containing seven chapters, is supposed to disclose the relationships between ROS and these pathologies. The first chapter of this section "Reactive Oxygen Species and Cardiovascular Diseases" by V. E. Valenti describes animal models to study ROS-induced cardiovascular diseases, sources of ROS in cells with particular interest to heart, oxidative damage to vessels and kidney and is finalized by the role of nervous system in ROS-induced CVD. R. Iturriaga and R. Del Rio cover the role of carotid body in cardioventilatory alterations induced by obstructive sleep apnea. The factors of risk of CVD, including metabolic complications of obesity, frequently referred as a metabolic syndrome, and diabetes are connected with adipocytokine homeostasis and may lead to cardiovascular pathologies, are covered in the chapter authored by A. B. Z. Gómez et al. The team from the USA, M. Garelnabi, S. Kakumanu, and D. Litvinov, demonstrates the role of oxidized lipids in development of atherosclerosis, one of the most common CVDs. There is no doubt that animal models may help to identify key aspects of disease development, and therefore the chapter by J. C. Fantinelli et al. clearly shows some peculiarities of oxidative damage to cardiac tissue in normotensive and spontaneously hypertensive rats, with substantial attention to aging, which is one of the risk factors of CVD. Mitochondria are well known to be the main cellular ROS source and physiological processes in this organella are tightly related to ROS production, elimination, and their involvement in apoptosis and necrosis in connection with CVD, which is highlighted by S. Hernández-Reséndiz et al. Early diagnostics of CVD is the key to successful and proper treatment, and their identification is a very attractive aspect of all studies in the field. S. Kumphune compares different products of oxidative modification of biomolecules such as lipids, proteins and nucleic acids with the focus on ones related to CVD to some extent.

In the next section, entitled "Diabetes Mellitus", we present different aspects of relationships between diabetes and ROS. In most cases, diabetes is not a directly damaging fast killer, but affects patients via diverse complications such as cardiovascular, nephrological and neurological diseases, etc. O. O. Erejuwa from Malaysia systematically describes the relationships between operation of ROS generation and elimination systems, development of oxidative stress and diabetes mellitus. That led the author to the conclusion that if antioxidants alone may not be useful to reduce diabetes-induced damages to cellular components, they may be efficient when combined with hypoglicemic drugs. However, even then they cannot prevent the development of certain diabetic complications. S. M. Tan et al. extend the previous chapter underlining that antioxidants may reduce diabetic complications such as diabetes-associated atherosclerosis, cardiomyopathy, nephropathy with the use of endogenic and externally added antioxidants like ebselen (mimetic of glutathione peroxidase), different mimetics of superoxide dismutase, inhibitors of NADPH oxidase, mitochondrially-targeted antioxidants and augmentation, enhancers of activities of antioxidant enzymes via activation of transcription factor Nrf2. Since it is widely believed that antioxidants may reduce diabetes-induced damage to organisms, one more chapter, written by N.-N. Enikő, presents data on effectiveness of antioxidants, especially of natural origin from fruits and vegetables, in treatment of diabetes and its complications. This book section is finalized by the chapter of N. H. Al-Rawi, describing a rather unusual approach to evaluate certain saliva parameters for diagnostics of diabetes.

The section "Systemic, Neuronal and Hormonal Pathologies" includes chapters related to relationship between ROS metabolism and diverse systems. The section is opened by the L. Lázár review on the role of oxidative stress in female reproduction and pregnancy, where the author highlights the information on the ROS role in normal and pathological pregnancies, embryo and fetal malformation, pregnancy-related pathologies and potential of supplementation with antioxidants. An experimental work presented by Z. Jovanović describes the effects of oxidants, cumene hydroperoxide and hydrogen peroxide on electrophysiological parameters such as spontaneous spike potential and Ca^{2+}-activated K^+ current in leech Retzius nerve cells and clearly demonstrates the regulatory ROS role and potential benefits of glutathione in maintaining of cell functions, which can be used to understand fundamental pathogenic mechanisms in the mammalian brain during normal aging, as well as in neurodegenerative diseases such as Alzheimer's and Parkinson's. The Polish team led by J. Zuwala-Jagiello presents an experimental material on circulation of advanced oxidation protein products, Nε-(carboxymethyl) lysine and pro-inflammatory cytokines in patients with liver cirrhosis and postulate that the advanced oxidation protein products such as modified albumin can be used as a marker of oxidative stress in healthy people and liver cirrhosis patients. The relationship between oxidative stress and neurodegenerative diseases attracted the attention of not only basic scientists, but also clinicians, and the chapter written by A. Norazit et al. provides readers with the information on this aspect in the case of Parkinson’s disease and compares the model studies with cell cultures, experimental animal models and humans. E. Cano-Europa wt al. describe the operation of the system of thyroid hormones under normal conditions, at hypo- and hyperthyroidism in detail, followed by the relationship between alterations of thyroid hormone status and ROS-steady state levels, with special interest to the role of glutathione in operation of the system. M. Škurlová presents interesting materials on the ROS role in functioning of joints and after general introduction discloses potential ROS roles in the development of human autoimmune joint diseases, particularly rheumatoid arthritis and systemic lupus erythematosus, which was logically finalized by the question if antioxidants can be beneficial at autoimmune joint diseases. T. Shimosawa et al. logically state that supplementation with vitamins C and E, either alone or in combination with each other or with other antioxidant vitamins, does not appear to be efficient in treatment of cardiovascular diseases and they therefore investigated a role of oxidative stress in consequences of multiple organ damages in mice and possible new therapeutic agents such as adrenomedullin (a 52-amino-acid peptide), platinum nanoparticles and bardoxolone methyl. A. H. Yang and W. Huang nicely cover a topic connected to the operation of our eyes and its relationship with ROS. They described the functioning of blood-retinal barrier in detail, how it is impacted by ROS and retinal vein occlusion induced by the inhibitor of a mitogen-activated protein kinase kinase.

The section entitled “Cancer” consists of only two chapters, what does not reflect an enormous attention of basic and clinic scientists to the problem. This attention to the problem is related to clearly enhanced level of ROS in transformed cells due to which antioxidants are expected to be beneficial in this case (Steinbrenner & Sies, 2009). Probably, survival of cancer cells possessing higher steady-state ROS levels than normal cells is provided by efficient antioxidant systems. At least two approaches may be used to kill cancer cells – increase in ROS steady-state levels and the use of antioxidants to prevent progression of diseases, which is covered by M. de Miguel and M. D. Cordero in their chapter on oxidative therapy against cancer. The authors describe the use of amitriptyline, a commonly prescribed tricyclic antidepressant drug that is well known to death investigators, forensic pathologists, and toxicologists, but in cancer cases it causes mitochondrial dysfunction, increasing mitochondrial ROS production. An experimental chapter submitted by a Finnish group led by K. Ketola clearly shows that monensin, an ionophore related to the crown ethers, induces oxidative stress and reduces prostate cancer cell migration and cancer stem cell population probably via decrease of NF-κB pathway activity.

The final section, "Antioxidants as Therapeutics" includes two chapters devoted to analysis of potential benefits of antioxidants. Immediately after the discovery of free radicals in biological systems and their harmful effects, it was logically predicted that antioxidants could be beneficial to health protecting cellular structures against ROS-induced modifications. However, the problem was not so straightforward – in many cases antioxidants were found to be non-effective, and in some cases they were even harmful. The issue is described in detail by P. Pérez-Matute et al. They list diets containing antioxidants with recognized benefits to health, but further show that not everything with antioxidants is positive and provide examples of side effects of antioxidants, their neutral or even deleterious effects and propose some explanations. V. Blas-Valdivia and colleagues provide the information on health benefits of diverse nutraceuticals such as polyphenols, terpenes, chlorophylls, polyunsaturated fatty acids and vitamins, and other vitamins with the focus on the micro-algal sources of these compounds. The Chlorophyceae class is rich in these nutraceuticals and genus Chlorella, Chlamydomonas, Haematococcus, and Dunaliella are extensively studied from this point of view.

The book is expected to be interesting to researchers in the field of basic investigations interested in the involvement of reactive oxygen species and oxidative stress in diverse pathologies, medical scientists and practical physicians wishing to perform first of all prophilactics and further cure different pathologies.

Prof. Dr. Volodymyr I. Lushchak
PhD, DSc, Department of Biochemistry and Biotechnology,
Vassyl Stefanyk Precarpathian National University, Ivano-Frankivsk,
Ukraine

Dr. Dmytro V. Gospodaryov
Senior Research Fellow, Ph.D., Department of Biochemistry,
Vassyl Stefanyk Precarpathian National University, Postdoctoral Fellow,
Institute of Biomedical Technology, University of Tampere, Tampere,
Finland

Section 1

Introduction

1

Introductory Chapter

Volodymyr I. Lushchak and Dmytro V. Gospodaryov
Precarpathian National University, Ivano-Frankivsk, Ukraine

1. Introduction

The term "oxidative stress" was first defined by Helmut Sies (1985) as "Oxidative stress" came to denote a disturbance in the prooxidant-antioxidant balance in favor of the former". In order to reflect the findings of last 25 years in the field, such as plural ROS roles and dynamics of their levels we recently proposed one more definition such as "Oxidative stress is a situation when steady-state ROS concentration is transiently or chronically enhanced, disturbing cellular metabolism and its regulation and damaging cellular constituents" (Lushchak, 2011b). Understanding of mechanisms of reactive oxygen species (ROS) formation and operation of the systems responsible for ROS elimination were necessary prerequisites for such formulation. Fenton reaction, enzymatic systems like cytochromes P450, xanthine oxidase or respiratory chains were identified as ROS producers. Studies on catalase and peroxidase since the beginning of 20th century (Loew, 1900; Popov & Zvyagilskaya, 2007), and discovery of superoxide dismutase by McCord and Fridovich (1969), lead to suggestion, that cells have specialized systems for conversion of ROS to less reactive compounds. After introduction, the term "oxidative stress" has been accreting with medical issues. Today, one could find in literature connection of oxidative stress to almost all of well-known diseases. The most important of them are cardiovascular and neurodegenerative ones, diabetes, cancer, viral and bacterial infections, taking millions of lives every year.

In the simplest case, pathology originates from the perturbations in either reactive species formation, their elimination or in both simultaneously. Many of real situations are much more complicated, that is difficult to determine the crucial event for disease origin. In some cases, gene mutations can be responsible for the imbalance in ROS metabolism. In other ones, a range of environmental influences would produce metabolic changes. Antioxidant therapy seems to be useful in both cases. It is often important to know, if oxidative stress was a primary event leading to the disease or it was developed during the disease.

Diseases caused by gene polymorphism are curable hard, and here only really emerging gene therapy could be the best solution. In addition, environment can be changed easier. We need to understand how environmental changes may induce oxidative stress and perturb redox processes. This field is rather broad. Food toxins or even some of usual meals supposed to be safe, cigarette smoke or polluted air, car exhaust fumes or pesticides can be prerequisites for enhanced oxidant formation or impairment in antioxidant defence system.

Evidences for connection of oxidative stress with the stresses induced by other factors are promptly gained. The potency of transition metals, some herbicides and carbohydrates to promote oxidative stress was recently showed (Lushchak et al., 2009a; Lushchak et al., 2009b; Lushchak, 2011; Semchyshyn et al., 2011). The same thing is concerned to many physical factors like heat, sound or ionizing irradiations. After all, inflammation induced by traumatic event or pathogenic agent like viral, bacterial or protist infections can result in oxidative stress. Disturbances in ROS metabolism, caused by multiple external factors or by DNA mutations, lead, eventually, to progressive tissue damage and subsequent degeneration.

Identification of specific targets for ROS is one more thing important for the development of appropriate therapy. Moreover, place of ROS formation and their targets determine often particular connection with certain pathology. Proteins, nucleic acids and lipids are the most critical targets for ROS and their derivatives. Important enzymes, standing on crossroads of metabolic pathways, are frequently inactivated at excessive ROS formation not counterbalanced by antioxidants. Glyceraldehyde-3-phosphate dehydrogenase, aconitase, glucose-6-phosphate dehydrogenase and superoxide dismutase are the most studied examples (Bagnyukova et al., 2005; Lushchak, 2007; Grant, 2008; Di Domenico et al., 2010; Avery, 2011). The list is indeed much longer including representatives for almost all metabolic pathways in different tissues, as well as ion transporters (Unlap et al., 2002), receptors (Anzai et al., 2000), and other proteins. Polyunsaturated fatty acid residues of diverse lipids are mainly subjected to oxidation by ROS in this class of compounds. Protein oxidation results in formation of carbonylated or glutathionylated derivates, whilst non-enzymatic lipid oxidation yields 4-hydroxy-2-nonenal, isoprostanes, malondialdehyde and diene conjugates (Hermes-Lima, 2004b). Reactive species, particularly hydroxyl radical, are also involved in carbohydrate oxidation, what is especially harmful for nucleic acid pentose backbones (Gutteridge & Halliwell, 1988; Hermes-Lima, 2004b). Nucleotides are not any exception. Mutagenesis resulted from guanosine oxidation is widely described (reviewed in Hermes-Lima, 2004b). Cells may possess even special receptors for some products of oxidation, e.g. receptors for F_2-isoprostanes and advanced glycation end products (Fukunaga et al., 1997) or scavenger receptors for oxidized low-density lipoproteins (Ashraf & Gupta, 2011). Increase in ROS production was found to be also regulated via specific receptors (Thannickal & Fanburg, 2000). Production of ROS driven by transforming growth factor-β1, by receptors for endothelial or platelet-derived growth factors, as well as for angiotensin II or advanced glycation end-products (Thannickal & Fanburg, 2000) are among the most discussed examples. These facts suggest robust cellular control for ROS metabolism.

Oxidized derivatives of proteins and lipids may also damage other molecules exacerbating consequences of oxidative stress. For instance, 4-hydroxy-2-nonenal was shown to modify proteins through the interaction with amino group of lysine, cysteine or histidine residues. That results in the formation of Michael adducts. The formed adducts can impair considerable number of metabolically important proteins like transporters of glucose and glutamate, GTP-binding proteins, ion-motive ATPases and so forth (reviewed in (Mattson, 2009)). Ability to initiate protein carbonylation was also demonstrated for MDA (Burcham & Kuhan, 1996).

Nowadays, the knowledge about important signalling role for some ROS has gained in addition to their known deleterious roles (Thannickal & Fanburg, 2000; Dröge, 2002). It is known that ROS, namely hydrogen peroxide, can regulate c-Jun N-terminal kinase pathway, apoptosis initiation, tumour suppression by means of p53, ion channels and G-protein-coupled receptors (Thannickal & Fanburg, 2000; Dröge, 2002; Ushio-Fukai, 2009).

The term "reactive oxygen species" has itself seems become insufficient. It would be difficult to speak today about oxidant metabolism considering only ROS. In many contemporary studies, ROS are examined along with reactive nitrogen species (RNS), reactive carbon species (RCS), reactive chlorine species (RChS), and reactive sulphur species (RSS) (Hermes-Lima, 2004b; Ferreri et al., 2005). Formation for most of them is driven by specialized systems and is finely controlled (Dröge, 2002). It suggests a bunch of important roles for these highly reactive molecules. Some of these roles may even not be discovered. More and more interactions between ROS, RNS, RCS and RSS are found from study to study. The formation of peroxinitrite, a powerful oxidant and RNS, in reaction between nitric oxide and superoxide anion radical is a commonly known example in this case. Similarly, thiyl radicals, which are considered to be RSS, can be formed under the interaction of peroxyl or hydroxyl radical with thiol-containing compounds (Ferreri et al., 2005). Thus, once the formation of ROS has overwhelmed cellular detoxifying capacity, there is a big potential for generation of other highly reactive molecules with different properties and targets.

Ischemia, atherosclerosis, stroke and different types of inflammation were, probably, the first recognized pathological states closely connected with oxidative stress. The strong association between ROS and pathological states were disclosed here. At all these states, probability of ROS formation is much higher than in normal physiological state. For instance, mitochondria of ischemic cells increase the steady-state level of electrons which may escape electron carriers under reperfusion leading to one-electron reduction of oxygen (Hermes-Lima, 2004a). During inflammatory processes, ROS are produced purposely by NADPH oxidases (Lassègue & Griendling, 2010). In both these cases ROS seem to accompany disease flow, but are not the cause. A relation between oxidative stress and commonly known neurodegenerative disorders and diabetes was also found. These diseases are believed to be caused by ROS. It is known that alloxan, a compound broadly used for experimental diabetes induction, is a redox-cycling compound damaging insulin-producing pancreatic β-cells (Lenzen, 2008). Alzheimer's and Parkinson's diseases are connected with impairment of mitochondrial function resulting in enhanced ROS generation (Henchcliffe & Beal, 2008). The key proteins composing protein aggregates in Parkinson's and Alzheimer's diseases, α-synuclein and β-amyloid, respectively, were found to be capable to produce ROS themselves (Atwood et al., 2003; Wang et al., 2010). Diabetic complications are found to be induced by the formation of advanced glycation end products which interact with specialized receptors and promote ROS production (Forbes et al., 2008).

The term "human disease" has been defined as a condition worsening usual human being and working capacity, and in some cases leading to death. Illness state is also a disorder of homeostasis connected with impairment of important parts of either whole organism, or specific proteins, whole cells, and even whole tissues and organs. In this context, ROS role as damaging agents would seem to be evident in disease origin. Despite that ROS in many works are described in their halo of harmfulness, especially in concern with diseases, there is also a complementary view on beneficial role of ROS in adaptation to stress (Ristow & Schmeisser, 2011; Lushchak, 2011a). Protein oxidation may also not always be harmful. Particularly, reversible oxidation of some key enzymes may respond to metabolic reorganization promoting to some extent cell adaptation to enhanced ROS production (Grant, 2008). Even protein carbonylation may have signalling role in vascular system (Wong et al., 2010) and in some examples activates proteins (Lee & Helmann, 2006). These findings should also be taken into account at analysis of association between oxidative stress and particular diseases. Participation of ROS in signaling, their roles in regulation of apoptosis and cell adaptation significantly complicate our view on them as a cause of diseases. Consequently, the view on oxidative stress should also be altered. Now, it is emerging impression that oxidative stress is not only the state when oxidation prevails. It is more resemble to the state of disturbance redox control mechanisms when "harmful" and undesirable for cell survival oxidation is prevailing, and physiological functions of ROS are altered or reprogrammed to promot cell death (Jones, 2006). Using this approach, one can suggest that cell death may result not only from several dozens of oxidized proteins and lipids. If we would not have any oxidation events, disturbance of physiological ROS metabolism might turn several dozens of processes in wrong direction. It may have more systemic effects, spread on whole organism, rather than causing cell death in particular tissue.

In the current book, the most topical issues of connection between oxidative stress and broadly known pathologies are examined. They include presumably cardiovascular diseases, hypertension and diabetes. Some attention is paid to well-known neurological diseases and cancer. Issues like reproduction, immunity, hormonal disorders are also affected. Some chapters are devoted to discussion on antioxidant therapy, though antioxidant clue goes through all other chapters as well. It is worth noting, knowledge highlighted in this book is collected all over the world. It implies the topic is long ago out of particular laboratories and elaborated by medical scientists in many countries. In some points concerns of the authors coincide, in other ones they are unique. Thus, the book mirrors many different aspects of pathological roles of ROS. We did not aim to make it comprehensive as much as possible. It is rather impossible taking into account that oxidative stress today has many faces. If someone would like to get specific knowledge on this topic from the beginning, the best advice would be to choose firstly the branch among incomprehensive canopy of oxidative stress studies. The book aimed to show how the field is studied in different countries and what is common for all investigations.

The connection between oxidative stress and diseases is mentioned in introduction of almost every article in the field. However, there is a difference between *in vitro* studies, studies on cell cultures, laboratory animals and clinical studies with humans. The last ones are most complicated for perception, but they provide a picture of reality. In this context, it is a pleasure to realize that some of the authors of this book are physicians whose studies are conducted on patients. The results from these studies are always more difficult for interpretation than those from model experiments carried out at cultivated cells. Nevertheless, clinical studies are highly complicated for understanding of ROS contribution in illness state. Once the implication of ROS in particular disease found, it suggests possibility of antioxidant therapy. However, how it is mentioned in one of the chapters, under some conditions antioxidants may act also as pro-oxidants. Following redox pioneers, John Gutteridge and Barry Halliwell, here one could say "pro-oxidants can be better for you in some circumstances" (Gutteridge & Halliwell, 2010). Moreover, modulation of signalling pathways linked with ROS may be more effective than simple antioxidant therapy. Most of known antioxidants can act also as signalling molecules, but there are also many compounds important for signaling that are not antioxidants. Other crucial thing is prophylactics. Cardiovascular diseases, diabetes, obesity, metabolic syndrome, neurological and hormonal disorders, impairment in kidney and liver functioning, mentioned in the book and described in terms of free radical biology, are not always strictly genetically conditioned. They are lifestyle and life condition pathologies often with onset in late age. So, they can be prevented. It is, probably, the most important conclusion that can be drawn from the generalized data. Even genetically caused pathologies could be attenuated by wisely arranged prophylactics if the defect is not too serious. That is also the reason for the accumulation, generalization and systematization knowledge obtained at different levels, with different models and clinical studies. We hope that this book will disclose, at least partially, the state of the problem worldwide and the current directions of laboratories focused on studies for implication of ROS in different pathologies. We also believe that it will help researchers to find weak places in current understanding and advise them quite novel and non-standard approaches to find and decipher mechanisms of diseases.

Finally, we would like to thank all authors for their contributions and hard work to match and unify the "philosophy" of this book. We also thank to our colleagues from Precarpathian National University and University of Tampere who supported us and helped us in preparation and edition of the chapters, especially to those who raised complex questions and promoted us to answer them. We are also grateful to the "In-Tech" Publisher personnel, especially Ms. Sasa Leporic, who assisted us in the arrangement of the book and scheduling our activities.

2. References

Anzai, K., Ogawa, K., Ozawa, T., Yamamoto, A. (2000). Oxidative modification of ion channel activity of ryanodine receptor, *Antioxidants & Redox Signaling*, Vol. 2, No. 1, pp. 35-40.

Ashraf, M.Z. & Gupta, N. (2011). Scavenger receptors: implication atherothrombotic disorders, *The International Journal of Biochemistry & Cell Biology*, Vol. 43, No. 5, pp. 697-700.

Atwood, C.S., Obrenovich, M.E., Liu, T., Chan, H., Perry, G., Smith, M.A. & Martins, R.A. (2003). Amyloid-β: a chameleon walking in two worlds: a review of the trophic and toxic properties of amyloid-β, *Brain Research. Brain Research Reviews*, Vol. 43, No. 1, pp. 1-16.

Avery, S.V. (2011). Molecular targets of oxidative stress, *The Biochemical Journal*, Vol. 434, No. 2, pp. 201-210.

Bagnyukova, T.V., Vasylkiv, O.Y., Storey, K.B. & Lushchak, V.I. (2005). Catalase inhibition by amino triazole induces oxidative stress in goldfish brain, *Brain Research*, Vol. 1052, No. 2, pp. 180-186.

Burcham, P.C. & Kuhan, Y.T. (1996). Introduction of carbonyl groups into proteins by the lipid peroxidation product, malondialdehyde, *Biochemical & Biophysical Research Communications*, Vol. 220, No. 3, pp. 996-1001.

Cadenas, E. & Sies, H. (1985). Oxidative stress: excited oxygen species and enzyme activity, *Advances in Enzyme Regulation*, Vol. 23, pp. 217-237.

Di Domenico, F., Perluigi, M., Butterfield, D.A., Cornelius, C. & Calabrese, V. (2010). Oxidative damage in rat brain during aging: interplay between energy and metabolic key target protein, *Neurochemical Research*, Vol. 35, No. 12, pp. 2184-2192.

Dröge, W. (2002). Free radicals in the physiological control of cell function, *Physiological Reviews*, Vol. 82, No. 1, pp. 47-95.

Ferreri, C., Kratzsch, S., Landi, L. & Brede, O. (2005). Thiyl radicals in biosystems: effects on lipid structures and metabolisms, *Cellular & Molecular Life Sciences*, Vol. 62, No. 7-8, pp. 834-847.

Forbes, J.M., Coughlan, M.T. & Cooper, M.E. (2008). Oxidative stress as a major culprit in kidney disease in diabetes, *Diabetes*, Vol. 57, No. 6, pp. 1446-1454.

Fukunaga, M., Yura, T., Grygorczyk, R. & Badr, K.F. (1997). Evidence for the distinct nature of F_2-isoprostane receptors from those of tromboxane A2, *American Journal of Physiology*, Vol. 272, No. 4, Part 2, pp. F477-F483.

Grant, C.M. (2008). Metabolic reconfiguration is a regulated response to oxidative stress, *Journal of Biology*, Vol. 7, No. 1. doi:10.1186/jbiol63

Gutteridge, J.M.C. & Halliwell, B. (1988). The deoxyribose assay: an assay both for "free" hydroxyl radical and for site-specific hydroxyl radical production, *The Biochemical Journal*, Vol. 253, No. 3, pp. 932-933.

Gutteridge, J.M.C. & Halliwell, B. (2010). Antioxidants: molecules, medicines and myths, *Biochemical & Biophysical Research Communications*, Vol. 393, No. 4, pp. 561-564.

Henchcliffe, C. & Beal, M.F. (2008). Mitochondrial biology and oxidative stress in Parkinson disease pathogenesis, *Nature Clinical Practice. Neurology*, Vol. 4, No. 11, pp. 600-609.

Hermes-Lima, M. (2004a) Oxidative stress and medical sciences, In: *Functional Metabolism: Regulation and Adaptation*, Kenneth B. Storey, pp. 369-382, Wiley-Liss, NY.

Hermes-Lima, M. (2004b) Oxygen in biology and biochemistry: role of free radicals, In: *Functional Metabolism: Regulation and Adaptation*, Kenneth B. Storey, pp. 319-368, Wiley-Liss, NY.

Jones, D.P. (2006). Redefining oxidative stress, *Antioxidants & Redox Signaling*, Vol. 8, No. 9-10, pp. 1865-1879.

Lassègue, B. & Griendling, K.K. (2010). NADPH oxidases: functions and pathologies in the vasculature, *Arteriosclerosis, Thrombosis & Vascular Biology*, Vol. 30, No4, pp. 653-661.

Lee, J.R. & Helmann, J.D. (2006). The PerR transcription factor senses H_2O_2 by metal-catalized histidine oxidation, *Nature*, Vol. 440, No. 7082, pp. 363-367.

Lenzen, S. (2008). The mechanisms of alloxan- and streptozotocin-induced diabetes, *Diabetologia*, Vol. 51, No. 2, pp. 216-226.

Loew, O. (1900). A new enzyme of general occurrence in organisms. A preliminary note, *Science*, Vol. 11, No. 279, pp. 701-702.

Lushchak, O.V., Kubrak, O.I., Lozinsky, O.V., Storey, J.M., Storey, K.B. & Lushchak V.I. (2009a). Chromium (III) induces oxidative stress in goldfish liver and kidney, *Aquatic Toxicology*, Vol. 93, No. 1, pp. 45-52.

Lushchak, O.V., Kubrak, O.I., Storey, J.M., Storey, K.B. & Lushchak, V.I. (2009b). Low toxic herbicide Roundup induces mild oxidative stress in goldfish tissues, *Chemosphere*, Vol. 76, No. 7, pp. 932-937.

Lushchak, V.I. (2007). Free radical oxidation of proteins and its relationship with functional state of organisms, *Biochemistry (Moscow)*, Vol. 72, No. 8, pp. 809-827.

Lushchak, V.I. (2011a) Adaptive response to oxidative stress: Bacteria, fungi, plants and animals. *Comparative Biochemistry and Physiology C* Vol. 153, pp.175-190.

Lushchak, V.I. (2011b). Environmentally induced oxidative stress in aquatic animals, *Aquatic Toxicology*, Vol. 101, No. 1, pp. 13-30.

Mattson, M.P. (2009). Roles of the lipid peroxidation product 4-hydroxynonenal in obesity, the metabolic syndrome, and associated vascular and neurodegenerative disorders, *Experimental Gerontology*, Vol. 44, No. 10, pp. 625-633.

McCord, J.M. & Fridovich, I. (1969). Superoxide dismutase: an enzymic function for erythrocuprein (hemocuprein), *The Journal of Biological Chemistry*, Vol. 244, No. 22, pp. 6049-6055.

Popov, V.O. & Zvyagilskaya, R.A. (2007). A.N. Bach – a revolutionary in politics and science (commemorating the 150th anniversary of academician A.N. Bach), *Biochemistry (Moscow)*, Vol. 72, No. 10, pp. 1029-1038.

Ristow, M. & Schmeisser, S. (2011). Extending lifespan by increasing oxidative stress, *Free Radical Biology and Medicine*, Vol. 51, No. 2, pp. 327-336.

Semchyshyn, H.M., Lozinska, L.M., Miedzobrodzki J. & Lushchak, V. (2011). Fructose and glucose differentially affect aging and carbonyl/oxidative stress parameters in *Saccharomyces cerevisiae* cells, *Carbohydrate Research*, Vol. 346, No. 7, pp. 933-938.

Sies, H. (1985). Oxidative stress: Introductory remarks, In: *Oxidative stress*, Helmut Sies, pp. 1-8. Academic Press, London.

Thannickal, V.J. & Fanburg, B.L. (2000). Reactive oxygen species in cell signalling, *American Journal of Physiology*, Vol. 279, No. 6, pp. L1005-L1028.

Unlap, T., Hwang, E.H., Siroky, B.J., Peti-Peterdi, J., Kovacs, G., Williams, I. & Bell, P.D. (2002). Enhanced susceptibility of a Na^+/Ca^{2+} exchanger isoform from mesangial cells of salt-sensitive Dahl/Rapp rat to oxidative stress inactivation, *Annals of the New York Academy of Sciences*, Vol. 976, pp. 342-344.

Ushio-Fukai, M. (2009). Vascular signaling through G protein coupled receptors – new concepts, *Current Opinion in Nephrology and Hypertension*, Vol. 18, No. 2, pp. 153-159.

Wang, C., Liu, L., Zhang, L., Peng, Y. & Zhou, F. (2010). Redox reactions of the α-synuclein-Cu^{2+} complex and their effects on neuronal cell viability. *Biochemistry*, Vol. 49, No. 37, pp. 8134-8142.

Wong, C.M., Marcocci L., Liu, L. & Suzuki, Y.J. (2010). Cell signaling by protein carbonylation and decarbonylation, *Antioxidants & Redox Signaling*, Vol. 12, No. 3, pp. 393-404.

Section 2

General Aspects

2

Oxidative Stress: Cause and Consequence of Diseases

Dmytro Gospodaryov and Volodymyr Lushchak
Precarpathian National University,
Ivano-Frankivsk,
Ukraine

1. Introduction

Oxidative stress, termed as an imbalance between production and elimination of reactive oxygen species (ROS) leading to plural oxidative modifications of basic and regulatory processes, can be caused in different ways. Increased steady-state ROS levels can be promoted by drug metabolism, overexpression of ROS-producing enzymes, or ionizing radiation, as well as due to deficiency of antioxidant enzymes. The plethora of ways leading eventually to oxidative stress is depicted in Figure 1. This chapter has several aims. The main aim is to show examples which mirror our knowledge on the role of oxidative stress in origin of diseases as well as its significance in disease complications. It was it that oxidative stress is described over developed pathology and nothing is told, if it was initial, triggering event or it was a consequence of the metabolic shift caused by other factors. Virtually, it would be important to develop a cure for specific diseases. The other aim of this chapter is to spotlight the role of enzyme deficiencies in promotion of oxidative stress during pathological conditions. These deficiencies are often caused by mutations in genes coding antioxidant or related enzymes, i.e. by genetic polymorphism. Mutations are preconditions for many diseases, which cannot be prevented in most cases. Nevertheless, complete understanding of the ways from the gene to disease symptoms is necessary condition for successful therapy. Attention should be paid also to full or partial loss of the enzyme activity via exogenous factors or via other indirect reasons. Many connections can be drawn between certain pathologies and oxidative modification of proteins. Most antioxidant and related enzymes are targets for oxidative modification. Hence, if oxidative stress was primary event, possible oxidative modifications of antioxidant enzymes may exacerbate diseases and define cell destiny. Finally, it is worth mentioning advantages and disadvantages of diverse models which serve for disclosing of mechanisms underlying ROS contribution to diseases. Predominant number of studies is conducted on mice and cell cultures. Significant insights were received with use of lower organisms like budding yeast, nematodes and fruit flies. All model organisms and cell cultures have certain limitations and disadvantages. So far, the largest benefit can be brought out from complex studies, involving many model systems and investigating phenomena from different points of view.

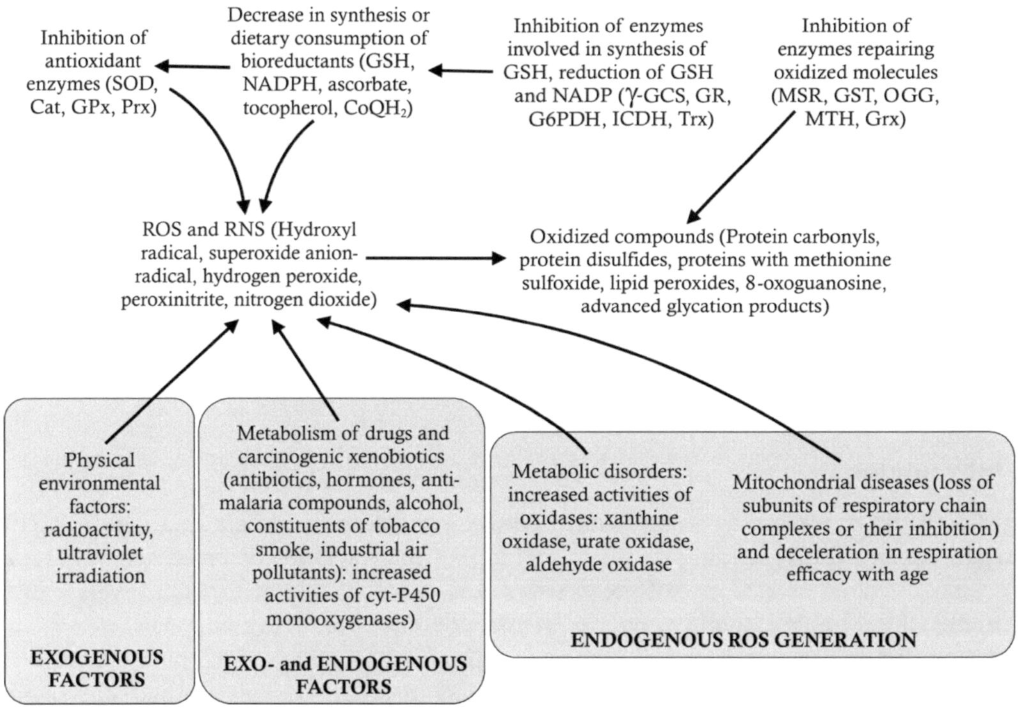

Fig. 1. Ways leading to oxidative stress. Reactive oxygen species are constantly produced in cells by electron transport chains and some enzymes, like xanthine oxidase, aldehyde oxidase, cytochrome-P450 monooxygenases, etc. Increased ROS production may be promoted by exogenous factors (temperature variation, radioactivity, ultraviolet irradiation, xenobiotics), metabolic disorders or inherited diseases affecting electron transport chain. Deficiencies in antioxidant enzymes or impaired metabolism of low-molecular-mass antioxidants will also lead to elevation of ROS concentration over steady-state level. Negative consequences of elevated ROS level can be alleviated by repair enzymes. Abbreviations: SOD – superoxide dismutase, Cat – catalase, GPx – glutathione-dependent peroxidase, Prx – peroxyredoxin, GSH – reduced glutathione, $CoQH_2$ – ubiquinol, γ-GCS – γ-glutamylcysteine synthetase, GR – glutathione reductase, G6PDH – glucose-6-phosphate dehydrogenase, ICDH – isocitrate dehydrogenase, Trx – thioredoxin, MSR – methionine sulfoxide reductase, GST – glutathione S-transferase, OGG – 8-hydroxy-2′-deoxyguanosine glycosylase, MTH – oxidized purine nucleotide triphosphatase, Grx – glutaredoxin.

2. Genetic polymorphism of antioxidant and related enzymes

Genetic polymorphism is frequently related to large number of pathologies. Enzymes involved in defence against ROS are not an exception. All enzymes contributing to antioxidant defence can be classified to really antioxidant ones, dealing directly with ROS as substrates, and auxiliary ones (we will call them also related to or associated antioxidant enzymes). The latter enzymes respond for reparation or degradation of oxidatively modified molecules, maturation and posttranslational modification of antioxidant enzymes, metabolism of low molecular mass antioxidants, etc. As a rule, genetic polymorphisms of enzymes of these two big groups may lead to oxidative stress and consequent diseases, among which cancer, neurodegeneration, cardiovascular disorders, and diabetes are most frequently mentioned. Some of them, like diabetes, cardiovascular and neurodegenerative diseases, are connected with cell death. On the other hand, cancer presents opposite side, and is marked by abnormal cell proliferation. Indeed, ROS guide to cell death when their targets are proteins or lipids. Cell proliferation can be promoted, at least partially, by oxidative modification of nucleic acids and subsequent mutations. Nevertheless, several exceptions from this "rationale" have already been described. For example, it is known that nitration of transcription factor p53 by peroxynitrite, one of the reactive nitrogen species, is associated with human glioblastoma (Halliwell, 2007). In many other cases, oxidative modification of proteins leads to cell damage. Examples which confirm this are reviewed elsewhere (Nyström, 2005) and some of them will be described below. The functions and cellular roles of antioxidant or associated enzymes will define the consequences which happen in case of polymorphism of the genes coding these enzymes.

2.1 Glucose-6-phosphate dehydrogenase deficiency

The most striking example among polymorphisms of genes coding enzymes related to antioxidant defence is well-known deficiency in glucose-6-phosphate dehydrogenase (G6PDH) which leads to favism. In this case, there is no very strong phenotype; only additional exogenous factors, like drugs or certain types of food, tolerated by unaffected individuals, can reveal the pathology. Lifestyle, diet or adventitious diseases may exacerbate consequences of decreased enzyme activity. Opposite situation is also possible: deficiencies in antioxidant and related enzymes may exacerbate other pathologies, namely infectious and neurodegenerative diseases, as well as cancer. Glucose-6-phosphate deficiency was one of the first known to mankind deficiencies of auxiliary antioxidant enzymes. Favism caused by this enzymopathy is known from ancient times and is exhibited as haemolytic anaemia induced by consumption of broad beans (*Vicia faba*) (Beutler, 2008). First report, discovering contribution of G6PDH deficiency to sensitivity to an anti-malaria drug, primaquine, was published more than half century ago (Alving et al., 1956). Association of G6PDH deficiency with favism was drawn soon after that, when several independent studies found that this disorder is attributed only to individuals with low G6PDH activity (Sansone & Segni, 1958; Zinkham et al., 1958). The mechanism for the haemolytic anaemia, which develops in response to ingestion of *V. faba* beans at G6PDH deficiency, is consistent with several observations. *V. faba* contains polyhydroxypyrimidine compounds, prone to redox-cycling, like glycoside vicine and its aglycone divicine, as well as isouramil (Fig. 2). It was shown that they were involved in production of superoxide anion radical and hydrogen peroxide (Baker et al., 1984). Primary product is likely superoxide anion radical, because it was shown that all three compounds could promote release of iron from ferritin (Monteiro & Winterbourn, 1989). Oxidation of iron ion in iron-sulphur clusters was found to be related to the effect of superoxide anion radical (Avery, 2011). Indeed, iron ion release was inhibited by superoxide dismutase for divicine and isouramil, while combination each of the three compounds with ferritin promoted lipid peroxidation in liposomes (Monteiro & Winterbourn, 1989). Interestingly, alloxan, compound chemically related to divicine and isouramil, is widely known as a superoxide generator, and is used for experimental induction of diabetes (Lenzen, 2008).

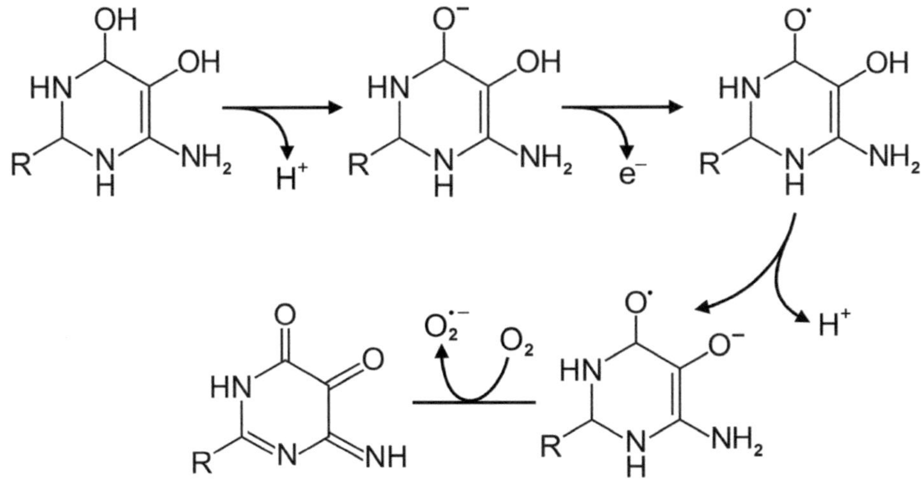

Fig. 2. Redox modifications of compounds from broad beans (*Vicia faba*). R is amino group for divicine and hydroxyl-group for isouramyl. Modified from (Chevion et al., 1982).

Formation of NADPH, catalyzed by G6PDH and 6-phosphogluconate dehydrogenase in pentose phosphate pathway, is thought to serve for a general antioxidant defence, and is frequently described by scheme shown in Fig. 3.

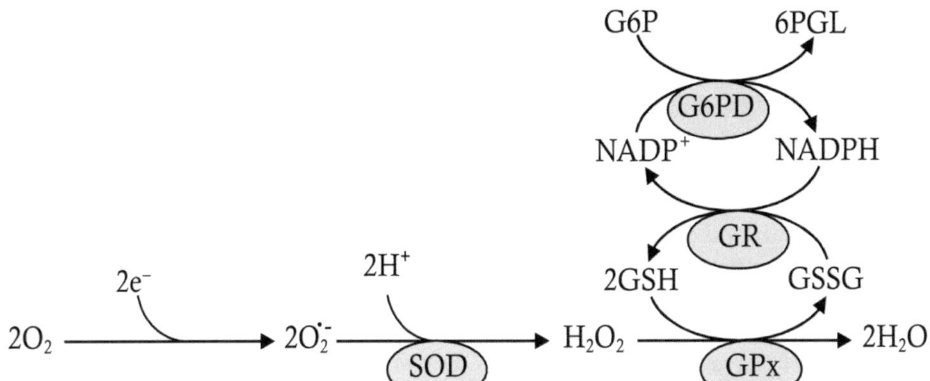

Fig. 3. Functional cooperation between G6PDH and GPx, explaining importance of G6PDH for erythrocyte survival. Abbreviations: SOD, superoxide dismutase; GPx, glutathione peroxidase; GR, glutathione reductase; G6PDH, glucose-6-phosphate dehydrogenase; GSH, reduced glutathione; GSSG, oxidized glutathione; $NADP^+$, oxidized nicotineamide adenine dinucleotide phosphate; NADPH, reduced nicotineamide adenine dinucleotide phosphate; G6P, glucose-6-phosphate; 6PGL, 6-phosphogluconolactone. Indeed, SOD produces one molecule of oxygen and one molecule of hydrogen peroxide. This reaction is more complex than it is represented on the figure and goes in two subsequent stages. One NADPH molecule is produced in reaction catalyzed by G6PDH per G6P molecule, and one more at the next step of the pentose phosphate pathway catalysed by 6-phosphogluconate dehydrogenase.

According to Fig. 3, superoxide dismutase produces hydrogen peroxide, which, in turn, is reduced in glutathione peroxidase reaction to water with concomitant oxidation of glutathione. This reaction needs reduced glutathione which acts as a reductant. Glutathione reductase maintains concentration of reduced glutathione using NADPH as an electron and proton donor. Hence, oxidative stress, caused by redox-cycling compounds, and advanced oxidation of haemoglobin and other proteins in erythrocytes is seemed to underlie the anaemia. It is believed that NADPH may be also needed for catalase operation (Kirkman & Gaetani, 2007). There are also indirect hints that G6PDH may play a role in assembly of iron-sulphur clusters, the main cellular target for superoxide anion radical attack. In particular, in bacteria *Escherichia coli*, G6PDH and SOD belong to the same regulon, namely SoxRS (Demple, 1996; Lushchak, 2001). It is known that NADPH may be absolutely necessary for iron-sulfur cluster formation (Fig. 4) as well as for haem synthesis (Wingert et al., 2005).

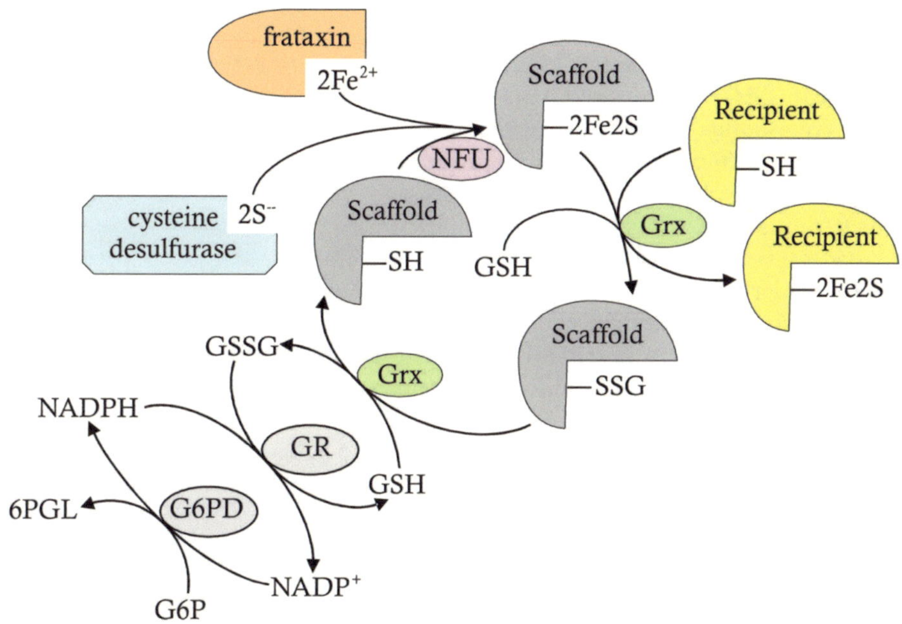

Fig. 4. Role of NADPH in iron-sulfur cluster assembly. Frataxin and cysteine desulfurase provide iron and sulfur for the clusters. NFU - alternative scaffold protein involved in assembly of iron-sulfur clusters. The clusters are assembled on other scaffold proteins and transferred to acceptor proteins like aconitase, succinate dehydrogenase, and ferredoxin. Glutaredoxins (e.g., Grx5) are supposed to be responsible for delivery of the clusters to recipient proteins using GSH. NADPH is spent for reduction of glutathione. Modified from (Bandyopadhyay et al., 2008) and (Tamarit et al., 2003).

In this case, produced NADPH is used also to maintain pool of reduced glutathione, while the latter goes for assembly of iron-sulfur clusters. It was demonstrated that glutaredoxin 5 is particularly responsible for the assembly of iron-sulfur clusters and haem synthesis (Wingert et al., 2005), where it takes part in iron-sulfur cluster delivery to proteins (Lill & Muhlenhoff, 2006). Other enzymes involved in the assembly of the clusters, ferredoxins, may also depend on NADPH (Pain et al., 2010).

Deficiency in G6PDH is widespread among people in tropical countries where a high risk of malaria is concomitantly observed (Cappellini & Fiorelli, 2008). It is believed that the G6PDH-deficient phenotype gives an adaptive advantage to survive under malaria threat (Cappellini & Fiorelli, 2008; Nkhoma et al., 2009). Indeed, progression of protist *Plasmodium falciparum*, causing malaria, is impossible in G6PDH-deficient erythrocytes because of cell "suicide" (Föller et al., 2009). In this context, it was shown that *P. falciparum* propagation in normal erythrocytes needs 5'-phosphoribosyl-1-pyrophosphate (PRPP) synthetase activity. On the other hand, PRPP synthetase was shown to be strongly dependent on the level of reduced glutathione (GSH). Since G6PDH-deficient erythrocytes possess low GSH level, the activity of PRPP synthetase is low in these cells and restricts parasite growth rate (Roth et al., 1986).

Some other pathologies are also associated with G6PDH deficiency. They are diabetes (Niazi, 1991; Gaskin et al., 2001; Carette et al. 2011), vascular diseases (Gaskin et al., 2001), and cancer (Ho et al., 2005). It is possible that induced oxidative stress in particular cells can be a ground for these phenotypes. It was shown that GSH may react with superoxide anion radical (Winterbourn & Metodiewa, 1994) providing partial defence against this ROS. In this case, decreased GSH pool in G6PDH-deficient individuals enhances their sensitivity to redox-active compounds, producing superoxide. Superoxide is able to react also with nitric oxide, leading to the formation of rather harmful oxidant peroxynitrite (Lubos et al., 2008). However, relation of this reaction to diabetes and vascular diseases is not because of peroxynitrite production and subsequent oxidative damage, but rather because of decrease in nitric oxide level. The latter is an important second messenger in certain signalling pathways particularly related to vasodilation (Förstermann, 2010). There is some probability also that individuals with G6PDH-deficiency may fail to regulate properly blood pressure (Matsui et al., 2005). Despite possible impairment in nitric oxide production, there is also other way to connect G6PDH deficiency with vascular diseases. It is known, that development of vascular diseases depends on the levels of homocysteine and folate, intermediates in metabolism of sulfur-containing amino acids (Stipanuk, 2004; Joseph et al., 2009; Rimm & Stampfer, 2011). Production of two these metabolites depends on GSH and NADPH levels in cells (Leopold & Loscalzo, 2005).

Data regarding association of G6PDH deficiency with cancer are controversial, because some studies demonstrated that G6PDH-deficient patients may additionally suffer from cancer (Pavel et al., 2003), while others state opposite (Cocco et al., 1989, 2007). Nevertheless, both situations are possible. In particular, there is a large data body indicating that different cancer types are developed at increased DNA damage. It often happens under polymorphism in enzymes contributing to DNA repair, what will be discussed below. Under conditions which would promote oxidative DNA damage, antioxidant function of could prevent cancer. On the other hand, NADPH supply at certain conditions may be even harmful leading to enhanced oxidative damage and cancer development. Indeed, it was shown that G6PDH was particularly responsible for cell growth and frequently correlated with cell growth (Ho et al., 2005). Tian and colleagues (1998) found that cancer cells possessed several times higher G6PDH activity. The positive correlation between tumour progression and G6PDH activity was found also for humans (Batetta et al., 1999).

Increased NADPH supply resulting from G6PDH overexpression can lead to so-called "reductive stress" (Rajasekaran et al., 2007; Lushchak, 2011). Enhanced activity of G6PDH, a lipogenic enzyme, was found at diabetes and obesity (Gupte, 2010). In humans, G6PDH is regulated by many transcription factors, in particular, SREBP-1a (sterol regulatory element binding protein) (Amemiya-Kudo et al., 2002), AP-1 (Kletzien et al., 1994) and Sp1 (Franzè et al., 1998). It was shown that elevation of G6PDH activity might lead to enhanced lipid synthesis (Salati et al., 2001; Park et al., 2005; Lee et al., 2011) and to possible reductive stress (Dimmeler & Zeiher, 2007; Rajasekaran et al., 2007; Ralser & Benjamin, 2008).

Despite intensive investigations, information on lifespan and adventitious diseases of G6PDH-deficient patients remains scarce. It is complicated to understand compensatory mechanisms for a loss of the enzyme important for the production of NADPH and pentose phosphates, and to anticipate all possible sides, both negative and positive ones and, therefore, further studies are needed.

2.2 Catalase deficiency

At 1947, Japanese otolaryngologist Shigeo Takahara firstly described catalase deficiency, called acatalasemia, for a child with oral ulcer (Kirkman & Gaetani, 2007). Since that time, many studies on acatalasemia were performed. It was noted, that some patients with acatalasemia, namely those with Japanese and Peruvian types, suffer from progressive oral ulcers known as Takahara's disease. The cause is considered to consist in ability of oral Streptococci to produce hydrogen peroxide which may promote death of mouth mucosa cells in acatalasemic patients (Ogata et al., 2008). In fact, several pathogenic bacteria, like *Streptococcus pneumoniae* or *Mycoplasma pneumoniae* may produce hydrogen peroxide by means of their oxidase systems and therefore might be rather dangerous to acatalasemic patients. Nevertheless, Brennan and Feinstein (1969) on the model of acatalatic mice demonstrated that *Mycoplasma pulmonis*, a pathogenic H_2O_2-producing mollicute, may cause fast development of the disease in the animals (Brennan & Feinstein, 1969). Interestingly, acatalatic mice faster recovered after disease, probably because of bacterial autointoxication by high hydrogen peroxide concentrations.

Catalase deficiency is also associated with diabetes mellitus (Góth, 2008). This association is attributed for Hungarian hypocatalasemic patients. They were shown to possess higher levels of homocysteine and lower levels of folate (Leopold & Loscalzo, 2005). It hints, on one hand, to abnormalities of sulfur metabolism, but on the other hand, it is commonly known that higher homocysteine levels are related to cardiovascular diseases (Lubos et al., 2007), the fact we mentioned above in the context of G6PDH deficiency.

Despite high importance of antioxidant enzymes for cell survival, their loss is usually not characterized by severe phenotype. That is probably because cells have many counterparts of antioxidant enzymes. For example, in addition to G6PDH, NADPH can also be produced by NADPH-dependent isocitrate dehydrogenase, malic enzymes or $NAD(P)^+$-transhydrogenase. Catalase can be substituted by other hydrogen peroxide utilizing enzymes, namely glutathione peroxidase, cytochrome c peroxidase, thioredoxin peroxidase, etc. Superoxide dismutase deficiency can be compensated to some extent by ions of transition metals (Batinic-Haberle et al., 2010) or other proteins which may exhibit weak superoxide dismutase activity, e.g. ceruloplasmin (Goldstein et al., 1982). Nevertheless, it should also be taken into account that often whole deletion of some enzymes leads to the lethal phenotypes in mice models. Particularly, knockout on manganese-containing superoxide dismutase (Mn-SOD) causes early lethality of experimental mice (Halliwell, 2007). It is also supposed that complete lack of G6PDH activity leads to prenatal death. Almost all mutations on G6PDH present mutations of single nucleotide or several nucleotide deletions without frameshift in the coding region (Ho et al., 2005). Notably, knockouts on whole gene, causing full loss of the activity, can also be investigated with experimental models, like mice (see also below), but are rarely found in reality.

2.3 Polymorphism of Cu,Zn-SOD and protein aggregation

Special attention should be paid to polymorphism of genes coding SOD. More than 100 nucleotide substitutions for the gene SOD1 coding human cytosolic copper- and zinc-containing SOD (Cu,Zn-SOD) were described (Valentine et al., 2005). Point mutations in SOD1 gene lead often to the pathologies by the mechanism different of that for other antioxidant or related enzymes, like described above catalase and G6PDH. It is known that several mutations in SOD1 gene are associated with cases of familial amyotrophic lateral sclerosis (ALS), a neurodegenerative disease which is characterized by paralysis and subsequent death (Vucic & Kiernan, 2009). Mutations in SOD1 can also be found in individuals with sporadic ALS. Moreover, it was proposed that Cu,Zn-SOD may account for all cases of ALS (Kabashi et al., 2007). Mechanisms of the disease development are still unknown, but there are many evidences that oxidative stress, developed in neurons, is rather caused by unexpected pro-oxidative activity of SOD than by the loss of the activity at all (Liochev & Fridovich, 2003). To the present knowledge, molecules of mutated SOD are also assembled into insoluble, amyloid-like proteinaceous aggregates (Valentine & Hart, 2003). It was found that the aggregates cause harm to the cells not only via oxidative stress, but also via inhibition of glutamate receptors (Sala et al., 2005; Tortarolo et al., 2006) and induction of apoptosis (Beckman et al., 2001). A pioneer in SOD studies, Irwin Fridovich, presented some examples of unusual activities of SOD, such as oxidase-like or reductase-like ones (Liochev & Fridovich, 2000). His works and data of other authors suggest that SOD, being mutated or placed in specific conditions, may produce more harmful ROS than hydrogen peroxide, i.e. hydroxyl radical (Yim et al., 1990; Kim et al., 2002). Some studies suggested that SOD aggregation can be triggered by higher susceptibility to oxidation of mutated protein (Rakhit et al., 2002; Poon et al., 2005). Indeed, Cu,Zn-SOD is considered to be rather stable, resistant to many, deleterious to other proteins, compounds (Valentine et al., 2005). Though it was also found that Cu,Zn-SOD is susceptible to oxidative modification (Avery, 2011). Moreover, some mutations may convert the enzyme into the form more susceptible to oxidation. Many substitutions of amino acids in polymorphic Cu,Zn-SOD variants do not present change from less susceptible to oxidation amino acid residues to more susceptible ones. For example, one of the most common substitutions, A4V, is a change from one nonpolar side chain to the other one at N-terminus (Schmidlin et al., 2009). However, even such substitutions may result in conformational changes which, in turn, can lead to unmasking of easily oxidizible amino acid gropus and exposure them to protein surface. Regarding A4V mutation, it is known that alanine at N-terminus of Cu,Zn-SOD is acetylated (Hallewell et al., 1987). In some cases, this posttranslational modification may prevent protein from oxidation (Seo et al., 2009) or ubiquitination (Arnesen, 2011). Mutations can also make the enzyme more vulnerable to oxidation in view of that Cu,Zn-

SOD is bearing ions of transition metal. Latter case suggests possibility of metal catalyzed oxidation, and it was shown in some studies that SOD is prone to oxidation (Kabashi et al., 2007). The other group of the noted amino acid substitutions in Cu,Zn-SOD, like valine to methionine, glutamate to lysine, aspartate to tyrosine, glycine to arginine (Orrell, 2000) establishes direct change to more oxidizible side chain. So far, it is still not clear if oxidative modification of mutated SOD takes place in ALS development.

In this context, it would be relevant to mention other pathologies connected with accumulation of amyloid-like aggregates. They include Alzheimer (properly β-amyloid accumulation), Huntington (accumulation of mutated huntingtin particles), and Parkinson (accumulation of α-synuclein) diseases. Some proteins can also be components of the aggregates under all of aforementioned diseases, but they are out of scope of this chapter. Many links with oxidative stress have been discovered for these pathologies since time their molecular mechanisms were disclosed. However, most studies are concentrated mainly on the development of oxidative stress during the course of a disease. It is still unclear, if oxidative stress could be the cause of the pathology or, at least, be responsible for its progression and general symptoms. To date, there is no direct evidence if some kind of oxidative modifications of protein is involved in the aggregate formation. Nevertheless, some hints collected from different studies afford to assume that oxidative stress might be the cause of these diseases (Norris & Giasson, 2005).

In some cases, the brain trauma precedes the disease (McKee et al., 2009; Knight & Verkhratsky, 2010). This traumatic event may become a predisposition to further pathology, and triggering signal for oxidative stress, developed during inflammation. A chronic traumatic encephalopathy, found often in American football players, is the distinguishable example for this event (Omalu et al., 2010). This tauopathy is characterized by accumulation of tau protein aggregates. The similar causes, like initial traumatic event, are described for several cases of Parkinson disease (Uryu et al., 2003).

Human amyloid precursor protein and matured human β-amyloid possess rather high affinity to ions of transition metals (Kong et al., 2008). Moreover, this metal binding capacity confers it both, antioxidant and prooxidant, properties (Atwood et al., 2003) what depends on the intracellular environment and type of the metal ion bound. In the case of mutations or at certain cell milieu, affected by external factors, this protein can also be easily oxidized. The ability to bind metals dependently on conditions provide both, antioxidant and prooxidant, properties which was shown for α-synuclein (Zhu et al., 2006) and prion PrP (Brown et al., 2001; Nadal et al., 2007).

Notably, G6PDH and Cu,Zn-SOD provide examples of the enzymes which become unstable after single amino acid change throughout the whole primary sequence. In G6PDH case, single amino acid substitution may lead to severe loss of activity, while in Cu,Zn-SOD case amino acid substitution may not lead to the loss of activity, but frequently causes considerable alteration of the protein properties. It would be important to decipher not only the mechanisms for the development of particular pathology, but the reasons of high mutability of the genetic loci, coding G6PDH and Cu,Zn-SOD. There is also a sense to understand why these enzymes are so susceptible to mutations.

2.4 Polymorphism of Mn-SOD, extracellular SOD and glutathione peroxidase

Unlike Cu,Zn-SOD, less mutations were found in the gene coding human manganese-containing superoxide dismutase (SOD2). Substitution of alanine-16 to valine (so called "Ala variant") is the most known mutation (Lightfoot et al., 2006). This mutation has recently been associated with cancers of breast, prostate, ovaries and bladder, as well as non-Hodgkin lymphoma, mesothelioma and hepatic carcinoma (Lightfoot et al., 2006). A16V substitution affects N-terminus of the protein, particularly, leading sequence responsible for the mitochondrial targeting (Sutton et al., 2003, 2005). It was shown that mice homozygous in SOD2 knock-out died after birth due to lung damage (Halliwell, 2007). Heterozygotes, in turn, demonstrated increased appearance of malignant tumours developed with age.

Mammals possess also extracellular Cu,Zn-SOD (EC-SOD) encoded in humans by gene SOD3. The enzyme is a homotetramer presenting in plasma, lymph, and synovial fluid (Forsberg et al., 2001). Extracellular SOD is abundant particularly in the lung, blood vessels, and the heart. In blood vessels EC-SOD activity can reach up to 50% of total SOD activity (Gongora & Harrison, 2008). Consequently, polymorphism of SOD3 gene is associated with pulmonary and cardiovascular diseases. It was shown, that mice lacking EC-SOD were more susceptible to hyperoxia, had vascular dysfunctions and were predisposed to hypertension (Carlsson et al., 1995). The ability to bind extracellular matrix proteoglycans containing heparan and hyaluronan sulfates is a distinguishable property of EC-SOD (Dahl et al., 2008). Additionally, this enzyme can associate with collagen type I and fibrillin 5 (Gongora & Harrison, 2008). Due to this binding capacity, EC-SOD can operate locally on the surface of endothelial cells. The most known polymorphism came from C-to-G transversion in the second exon of SOD3 gene, leading to the substitution of arginine-213 by glycine (R213G) (Chu et al., 2005). The substitution is located closer to C-terminal end of the protein (whole enzyme consists of 251 amino acid residues) and affects heparin-binding domain. Hence, the mutated enzyme maintains the activity, but fails to attach the surfaces of endothelial cells and also possesses higher resistance to trypsin-type proteinases. The 8-10-fold increase in heterozygotes, and up to 30-fold increase in homozygotes in serum SOD activity are reported for the persons with the R213G polymorphism (Fukai et al., 2002). Studies *in vitro* showed that EC-SOD with R213G substitution lost approximately one third of capacity to bind type I collagen. Nevertheless, binding to the endothelial cell surface was dramatically decreased (Dahl et al., 2008), whereas only tissue-bound EC-SOD can be vasoprotective (Chu et al., 2005). Different studies found association between R213G substitution in EC-SOD with increased risk of ischemic cardiovascular and cerebrovascular diseases for diabetic patients or individuals with renal failure on hemodialysis (Nakamura et al., 2005).

Polymorphism of glutathione peroxidase (GPx) was found to be associated with some cancers. Four GPx isoforms have been described in humans. It was found that mutations in exon 1 of human GPx-1 gene lead to appearance of polyalanine tract at N-terminus of the protein (Forsberg et al., 2001). These tracts themselves are not connected with diminished enzyme activity. Another polymorphism, substitution of proline-198 to leucine, was found in Japanese diabetic patients and associated with intima-media thickness of carotid arteries (Hamanishi et al., 2004). The same substitution for adjacent proline-197 was associated with lung and breast cancers, as well as with cardiovascular diseases (Forsberg et al., 2001). Mice knockouted in GPx-1 and GPx-2 developed intestinal cancers (Halliwell, 2007).

2.5 Polymorphism of enzymes involved in reparation of oxidized molecules

Mutations may also affect enzymes involved in DNA reparation. The enzyme 8-hydroxy-2′-deoxyguanosine glycosylase (hOGG) encoded in human genome by the gene hOGG1 is probably the most known example. Recent studies associate mutations in hOGG1 with different cancer types, such as lung, stomach and bladder cancers (Sun et al., 2010). Most of the mutations in this gene affect exon 7 and cause serine-to-cysteine substitution. It was demonstrated that substitution S326C in hOGG1 protein confers susceptibility to oxidation and makes the enzyme prone to form disulfide bond between different polypeptide chains (Bravard et al. 2009). The possibility to form disulfide bonds in the mutated hOGG1 is additionally supported by the fact that serine-326 in the protein is flanked by positively charged amino acid residues, lysine and arginine, from N-terminus and arginine and histidine from C-terminus (Bravard et al. 2009). Such amino acid cluster is thought to increase possibility for disulfide bond formation in the case of serine-to-cysteine substitution. Some studies showed that hOGG1 overexpression lead to inhibition of H_2O_2-induced apoptosis in human fibroblasts (Youn et al., 2007).

Hydrolase MTH1 is other important enzyme preventing incorporation of oxidized purine nucleotide triphosphates in DNA (Nakabeppu et al., 2006). Knockout of this enzyme in mice resulted in increased frequency of lung, stomach and liver tumours with age (Halliwell, 2007).

Glutathione S-transferases (GSTs) are recognised as important antioxidant enzymes. However, they have broader function consisted in conjugation of different electrophilic compounds with glutathione (Hayes et al., 2005). Oxidatively modified compounds as well as lipid oxidation products, like 4-hydroxy-2-nonenal, are subjected to conjugation with glutathione. In general, GSTs are belong to xenobiotic-elimitating system. Some of them, namely GSTs of μ class, are known well by their ability to eliminate polycyclic aromatic hydrocarbons, oxidized previously by cytochrome P450 monooxygenases. To date, eight classes of GSTs have been described: α, κ, μ, σ, ζ, π, θ and ω. Cytosolic enzymes belong to classes α, μ, π and θ (Konig-Greger, 2004). The gene coding GSTM1 (GST of μ class, isoform 1) is appeared to be highly polymorphic and found inactivated in half of human population. Several studies associate polymorphism of GSTM1 with lung cancer (Ford et al., 2000; Forsberg et al., 2001; Mohr et al., 2003), although reports are controversial. For example, meta-analysis conducted by Benhamou *et al.* (2002) found no association of GSTM1 null genotype with lung cancers as well as with smoking. Other authors found such association and reported increased susceptibility to cancerogens among Caucasian and African-American populations (Cote et al., 2005). Polymorphism of GSTM1 was also found to be associated with head and neck carcinomas (Konig-Greger, 2004). The need in GSTM1 and its role in prevention of lung cancer are explained by the ability of the enzyme to detoxify constituents of cigarette smoke, such as mentioned above polycyclic aromatic hydrocarbons. Some studies also associate lung cancer with polymorphism of GSTT1 (GST of θ class) which participates in catabolism of tobacco smoke constituents, such as halomethanes and butadione (Cote et al., 2005). Similar association was found for GSTP1 (GST of π class) (Wenzlaff et al., 2005). Substitution of isoleucine-105 to valine, resulting from a single nucleotide polymorphism at exon 5 of GSTP1 gene, lead to considerably decreased activity of the enzyme. Moreover, it was shown earlier that polymorphism of glutathione S-transferase P1 confers susceptibility to chemotherapy-induced leukaemia (Allan et al., 2001).

Mechanism for regulation of GSTs by carcinogenic events was described recently (McIlwain et al., 2006), and involves GSTs of different classes in signalling pathways. It was shown that GSTPs can associate with c-Jun N-terminal kinase (JNK) preventing its phosphorylation. Oxidation of GSTPs under oxidative stress causes dissociation of the enzyme from JNK and allows phosphorylation of the latter. Thus, phosphorylated JNK triggers signalling pathways promoting either proliferation, or apoptosis (McIlwain et al., 2006). Similar mechanism was proposed for GSTM which can interact with apoptosis signalling kinase-1 (ASK1) preventing its autophosphorylation. In both cases, GSTPs and GSTMs, oxidative modification of the proteins plays a central role.

3. Role of oxidative modifications of antioxidant and related enzymes in disease progression

From examples, ascribed above, it was seen that sometimes genetic polymorphism of genes coding antioxidant enzymes may result in serious consequences to health, while in other cases, like ALS, it leads to lethality. It is very important to understand how oxidative stress is developed under full or partial loss of activity of certain antioxidant enzyme, how it can be replaced by cellular resources, and what leads to development of certain disease. It is important that in some cases antioxidant enzymes themselves can be targets for ROS attack. Moreover, operation of many antioxidant enzymes depends on the availability of cofactors and prosthetic groups listed in Table 1.

Enzyme	Prosthetic group or cofactor
Cu,Zn-Superoxide dismutase	Ions of copper and zinc
Mn-Superoxide dismutase	Manganese ions
Catalase	Haem, iron, NADPH
Glutathione peroxidase	Reduced glutathione
Glutathione reductase	Flavin adenine dinucleotide

Table 1. Requirements of antioxidant enzymes in cofactors and prosthetic groups

Many disorders related to the metabolism of transition metals, amino acids or low molecular mass reductants are known to be connected with activities of antioxidant enzymes. Particularly, impairement in selenium uptake or synthesis of selenocysteine needed for glutathione peroxidases may lead to GPx deficiency and subsequent disorders such as cardiovascular ones (Lubos et al., 2007). Disruption of iron-sulfur clusters by superoxide anion radicals or peroxynitrite leads frequently to impairment of many metabolic pathways. Indeed, aconitase, NADH-ubiquinone-oxidoreductase (complex I of mitochondrial electron transport chain), ubiquinol-cytochrome c oxidoreductase (complex III), ribonucleotide reductase, ferredoxins possess iron-sulfur clusters, susceptible to oxidation. Owing to this, aconitase is used as one of oxidative stress markers (Lushchak, 2010). On the other hand, iron is a component of haem, a prosthetic group in catalase holoenzyme. Susceptibility to oxidative modification is described for catalase, glutathione peroxidase, Cu,Zn-SOD (Pigeolet et al., 1990; Tabatabaie & Floyd, 1994; Avery, 2011), and G6PDH (Lushchak & Gospodaryov, 2005). The latter is believed to be one of the most susceptible to oxidation enzymes (Lushchak, 2010). Thus, oxidative stress induced by exogenous factors, like carcinogens, certain drugs, ions of transition metals, etc., or by metabolic disorders, like diabetes, can be exacerbated by oxidative modification of antioxidant enzymes. These assumptions demonstrate the potential of antioxidant therapy in particular cases.

At some pathological states, whatever the cause of the disease, oxidative stress is seen to be a powerful exacerbating factor. Type II diabetes, cardiovascular diseases and neurodegenerative diseases, associated with protein aggregation are among such pathologies. Indeed, enhanced level of glucose results in higher probability of protein glycation (Wautier & Schmidt, 2004). Products of amino acid glycation, like N^{ε}-carboxymethyllysine, pyralline, pentosidine can activate receptors to advanced glycation end products (Huebschmann et al., 2006). In turn, these receptors can activate endothelial NADPH oxidase, the enzyme which produces superoxide radicals (Sangle et al., 2010). The ability of β-amyloid to produce reactive oxygen species has been described in many studies (reviewed in Sultana & Butterfield, 2010). Enhanced ROS production was also found in neurons at ALS (Liu et al., 1999). Loss or inhibition of mitochondrial respiratory chain complex I in dopaminergic neurons is described for Parkinson's disease (Marella et al., 2009). Such inhibition of complex I intensifies production of superoxide anion radical by mitochondrial respiratory chain (Adam-Vizi, 2005). It would be important to mention that most of the mitochondrial diseases are caused by loss of complex I subunits (Scacco et al., 2006). Thus, oxidative stress can be crucial factor promoting cell death at mitochondrial diseases.

4. Model organisms for study oxidative stress involvement in diseases

Model organisms, such as mice, fishes, fruit flies, nematodes, plants, cell cultures, budding yeast, or even bacteria, are broadly used to study different aspects concerning connection between oxidative stress and diseases. The necessity of these model studies is linked with relative rarity of some diseases, like ALS or Huntington disease, as well as with well known difficulties of studying humans. Clinical studies or case analyses give raw material for further investigation of mechanisms using lower organisms or cell cultures. Disclosing of function for protein encoded by the gene *TTC19* provides the example of such studies (Ghezzi et al., 2011). The works started from the analysis of several clinical cases, followed by studies with cell cultures and fruit flies to get mechanistic explanation for function of the mutated protein. Usage of mice or rats, as mammallian models, lower organisms and cell cultures is beneficial in view of relative easiness of specific knockout production. However several caveats exist regarding possible artifacts which could be obtained with model studies. Possible sources of artefacts resulting from cell culture studies were reviewed by Halliwell (2007). The main point here is that widely used conditions for cell culture growth may confer mild oxidative stress itself, because of high oxygen partial pressure and lack of antioxidants in cultural media. The examples described above, demonstrate relatively easy ways to produce transgenic mice with knockout on the whole gene. Nevertheless, some cases require expression of properly mutated gene than no expression at all, like in the case with mutated Cu,Zn-SOD at ALS. In the situation with ALS, only mutated gene induces pathology, while mice with Cu,Zn-SOD knockout are viable (Sentman et al. 2006). However, it is known that polymorphism of Mn-SOD in humans, e.g. A16V substitution, is not characterized by severe phenotype (Ma et al., 2010), while mice with Mn-SOD knockout are not viable (Halliwell, 2007). Fish, fruit flies, worms, plants and yeasts have even more disadvantages because of larger difference between their and human metabolism. However, usage of these model organisms affords to study particular mechanisms of the phenomena.

Whole genome sequences for most of the lower organisms were obtained during last two decades, what is also beneficial

Elucidation of molecular mechanisms of Friedreich's ataxia, a progressive hereditary neurological disorder (Kaplan, 1999; Knight et al., 1999), and discovery of chaperon for Cu,Zn-SOD (Culotta et al., 2006) are the most striking examples, proving merits of studies on model organisms. Moreover, all genes responsible for transport and utilization of iron in humans are mapped against yeast homologs (Rouault & Tong, 2008). It is also worth mentioning that details of copper transport, underlying Wilson and Menke diseases, were also discovered on the budding yeast model (Van Ho et al., 2002). This organism was used also for uncovering mechanisms of amyotrophic lateral sclerosis and allowed to find many details of posttranslational maturation of apo-Sod1 protein (Furukawa et al., 2004).

Budding yeasts were also used for advancement in understanding of redox-sensor capabilities for several regulatory proteins. One of them is AP-1 (activator protein 1) which in yeast is presented by YAP1 ortholog and is the central regulator of expression of the genes coding antioxidant enzymes (Lushchak, 2010). In yeast, but not in mammal cells, AP-1 operation is regulated by reversible oxidation of cysteine residues with subsequent translocation of the protein from cytoplasm into nucleus (Lushchak, 2011). It was also shown that reactive nitrogen species can activate YAP1 also (Lushchak et al., 2010). There are also several studies on budding yeasts revealed changes in gene expression and protein synthesis in response to oxidants (Godon et al., 1998; Thorpe et al., 2004; Temple et al., 2005). Experiments conducted in our laboratory with acatalatic budding yeast had shown that the loss of mitochondrial catalase is not crucial for yeast surviving, while loss of the cytosolic enzyme or both isoenzymes lead to serious growth retardation and is accompanied by inhibition of other enzymes (Lushchak & Gospodaryov, 2005). Interestingly, like in some cases with antioxidant enzyme deficiencies in humans, only special conditions revealed catalase deficiency in the yeast, e.g. ethanol consumption. The similar data were obtained with yeast strains deficient in either Cu,Zn-SOD or Mn-SOD, or both isoenzymes (Lushchak et al., 2005b). Glycerol as a carbon source was an exacerbating factor, which forced cells to perform respiratory metabolism instead more common for *Saccharomyces cerevisiae* fermentation. As in the case with catalase, loss of SOD lead to decreased activities of whole bunch of important enzymes, including antioxidant ones. Surprisingly, the cells deficient in Cu,Zn-SOD demonstrated more dramatic decrease in the activity of isocitrate dehydrogenase than the cells deficient in both SOD isoenzymes (Lushchak et al., 2005b). On the other hand, inhibition of Cu,Zn-SOD by *N,N'*-diethyldithiocarbamate increased the activity of NADPH-producing enzymes and glutathione reductase while decreased catalase activity (Lushchak et al., 2005a). The latter work clearly showed that the highest content of protein carbonyls was associated with moderate SOD activities. The situation is somewhat reminiscent to ALS pathology where oxidative damage results from the aggregates of mutated SOD.

Fruit fly *Drosophila melanogaster* is emerging model to study mechanisms of commonly known neurological diseases and diabetes (Pandey & Nichols, 2011) and diabetes (Kühnlein, 2010; Pandey & Nichols, 2011). However, despite advances in these fields done on *D. melanogaster*, it seems that fruit fly is the also good organism to investigate regulatory mechanisms underlying development of oxidative stress at neurological diseases. Fruit flies, unlike budding yeast, share more properties of signalling machinery with that for humans. Hence, Drosophila seems very convenient model organism to investigate ways of ROS production connected with numerous signalling pathways, like those involved c-Jun N-terminal kinase or transcription regulators NF-κB, p53, FoxO, TOR or AP-1.

5. Conclusions and perspectives

Oxidative stress can be induced in different ways, some of which are connected with known pathologies. Deficiencies in antioxidant or related enzymes are the factors which can result in oxidative stress. Genetic polymorphism is the most common cause of these deficiencies. Despite importance of such enzymes as catalase and glucose-6-phosphate dehydrogenase, deficiencies in them are rarely characterized by severe phenotype and become obvious often under special conditions. For glucose-6-phosphate dehydrogenase deficiency, consumption of redox-active compounds with food or drug treatment are risk factors. Polymorphism of copper and zinc-containing superoxide dismutase may lead to the development of amyotrophic lateral sclerosis, a severe neurodegenerative disorder. Polymorphism of genes coding glutathione peroxidases and enzymes involved in repair of oxidative injuries are frequently associated with carcinogenesis. Many antioxidant and related enzymes are themselves susceptible to oxidative modification. At enhanced ROS steady-state levels in some pathological states, like diabetes and cardiovascular or neurodegenerative diseases, oxidative modification of antioxidant enzymes may exacerbate the disease. It was found that antioxidant enzymes like Cu,Zn-SOD, catalase, glutathione peroxidase and others are susceptible to oxidative modification. Thus, oxidative stress caused initially by environmental factors and conditions, like hypoxia, drug metabolism, metal ions (e.g., chromium, cobalt, nickel, high concentrations of iron and copper) in particular situations could be enhanced and exacerbated by the following deficiency of antioxidant enzyme activity. And, vice versa, deficiency in particular antioxidant enzyme can be revealed by specific environmental conditions like drug metabolism at G6PDH deficiency, hyperoxia in case of lack of mitochondrial superoxide dismutase, or tobacco smoke in case of glutathione S-transferase. Regardless, whether primary or secondary role oxidative stress plays in disease progression, antioxidant therapy looks promising approach especially in combination with specific drugs. Nevertheless, it should be applied cautiously taking into account that antioxidants may acquire prooxidant properties dependently on conditions. Moreover, excess of reductants like glutathione may lead to the development of reductive stress and make cells insensitive to apoptotic signals, consequently converting them into neoplastic, prone to form tumours.

To date, there is quite large collection of data indicating the association of polymorphism of certain enzymes with cancers, neurodegenerative, cardiovascular diseases, diabetes, etc. Unfortunately, the roles of antioxidant and related enzymes in disease progression are still poorly understood. The huge work has been done to disclose the role of Cu,Zn-SOD in amyotrophic lateral sclerosis, and although many aspects are still obscure, it seems to be the issue attracting high attention. On the other hand, association of Mn-SOD and GPx deficiencies with certain diseases remains controversial. In all cases, oxidative modification of essential compounds, like proteins, lipids, carbohydrates and nucleic acids, is underestimated. For instance, changes in susceptibility of amyloid precursor or tau protein to oxidation may be a cause of their aggregation, similarly to Cu,Zn-SOD. However, information on this issue is scarce up to now; simply because of investigations do not go in this direction. More attention is paid to consequences, and reports on development of oxidative stress under cardiovascular diseases, diabetes, and neurodegeneration, are widely spread. It is difficult to catch conception of the disease; however properties of proteins and critical events leading to the disease could be modelled or studied *in vitro*. Despite significant limitations, a great impact from application of lower organism models, like budding yeast, nematodes and fruit flies, is appeared today. Turn to view on oxidative stress as a cause of the diseases due to damage of important molecules might considerably change therapeutic approaches. Such knowledge on oxidative stress as a trigger of the disease might also suggest necessary changes in human lifestyle and nutrition strategies for the prophylactics.

6. References

Adam-Vizi, V. (2005). Production of reactive oxygen species in brain mitochondria: contribution by electron transport chain and non-electron transport chain sources, *Antioxidants & Redox Signaling*, Vol. 7, No. 9-10, pp. 1140-1149.

Allan, J. M., Wild, C. P., Rollinson, S., Willett, E. V., Moorman, A. V., Dovey, G. J., Roddam, P. L., Roman, E., Cartwright, R. A., & Morgan, G. J. (2001). Polymorphism in glutathione S-transferase P1 is associated with susceptibility to chemotherapy-induced leukemia, *Proceedings of the National Academy of Sciences of the United States of America*, Vol. 98, No. 20, pp. 11592-11597.

Alving, A. S., Carson, P. E., Flanagan, C. L., & Ickes, C. E. (1956). Enzymatic deficiency in primaquine-sensitive erythrocytes, *Science (New York, N.Y.)*, Vol. 124, No. 3220, pp. 484-485.

Amemiya-Kudo, M., Shimano, H., Hasty, A. H., Yahagi, N., Yoshikawa, T., Matsuzaka, T., Okazaki, H., Tamura, Y., Iizuka, Y., Ohashi, K., Osuga, J.-ichi, Harada, K., Gotoda, T., Sato, R., Kimura, S., Ishibashi, S., & Yamada, N. (2002). Transcriptional activities of nuclear SREBP-1a, -1c, and -2 to different target promoters of lipogenic and cholesterogenic genes, *Journal of Lipid Research*, Vol. 43, No. 8, pp. 1220-1235.

Arnesen, T. (2011). Towards a functional understanding of protein N-terminal acetylation, *PLoS Biology*, Vol. 9, No. 5.

Atwood, C.S., Obrenovich, M.E., Liu, T., Chan, H., Perry, G., Smith, M.A. & Martins, R.N. (2003). Amyloid-β: a chameleon walking in two worlds: a review of the trophic and toxic properties of amyloid-β, *Brain Research Reviews*, Vol. 43, pp. 1-16.

Avery, S.V. (2011). Molecular targets of oxidative stress, *Biochemical Journal*, Vol. 434, pp. 201-210.

Baker, M. A., Bosia, A., Pescarmona, G., Turrini, F.& Arese, P. (1984). Mechanism of action of divicine in a cell-free system and in glucose-6-phosphate dehydrogenase-deficient red cells. *Toxicologic Pathology*, Vol. 12, No. 4, pp. 331-336.

Bandyopadhyay, S., Gama, F., Molina-Navarro, M. M., Gualberto, J. M., Claxton, R., Naik, S. G., Huynh, B. H., Herrero, E., Jacquot, J. P., Johnson, M. K., & Rouhier, N. (2008). Chloroplast monothiol glutaredoxins as scaffold proteins for the assembly and delivery of [2Fe-2S] clusters, *The EMBO Journal*, Vol. 27, No. 7, pp. 1122-1133.

Batetta, B., Pulisci, D., Bonatesta, R. R., Sanna, F., Piras, S., Mulas, M. F., Spano, O., Putzolu, M., Broccia, G. & Dessì, S. (1999). G6PDH activity and gene expression in leukemic cells from G6PDH-deficient subjects. *Cancer Letters*, Vol. 140, No. 1-2, pp. 53-58.

Beckman, J. S., Estévez, A. G., Crow, J. P., & Barbeito, L. (2001). Superoxide dismutase and the death of motoneurons in ALS, *Trends in Neurosciences*, Vol. 24, No. 11 Suppl, pp. S15-20.

Benhamou, S., Lee, W. J., Alexandrie, A.-K., Boffetta, P., Bouchardy, C., Butkiewicz, D., Brockmöller, J., Clapper, M. L., Daly, A., Dolzan, V., Ford, J., Gaspari, L., Haugen, A., Hirvonen, A., Husgafvel-Pursiainen, K., Ingelman-Sundberg, M., Kalina, I., Kihara, M., Kremers, P., Le Marchand, L., London, S. J., Nazar-Stewart, V., Onon-Kihara, M., Rannug, A., Romkes, M., Ryberg, D., Seidegard, J., Shields, P., Strange, R. C., Stücker, I., To-Figueras, J., Brennan, P., & Taioli, E. (2002). Meta- and pooled analyses of the effects of glutathione S-transferase M1 polymorphisms and smoking on lung cancer risk, *Carcinogenesis*, Vol. 23, No. 8, pp. 1343-1350.

Beutler, E. (2008). Glucose-6-phosphate dehydrogenase deficiency: a historical perspective, *Blood*, Vol. 111, No.1, pp. 16-24.

Bravard, A., Vacher, M., Moritz, E., Vaslin, L., Hall, J., Epe, B. & Radicella, J.P. (2009) Oxidative status of human *OGG1*-S326C polymorphic variant determines cellular DNA repair capacity. *Cancer Research*, Vol. 69, pp. 3642-3649.

Brennan, P. C. & Feinstein, R. N. (1969). Relationship of hydrogen peroxide production by Mycoplasma pulmonis to virulence for catalase-deficient mice, *Journal of Bacteriology*, Vol. 98, No. 3, pp. 1036-1040.

Brown, D. R, Clive, C. & Haswell, S. J. (2001). Antioxidant activity related to copper binding of native prion protein, *Journal of Neurochemistry*, Vol. 76, No.1, pp. 69-76.

Cappellini, M. D. & Fiorelli, G. (2008). Glucose-6-phosphate dehydrogenase deficiency, *Lancet*, Vol. 371, No. 9606, pp. 64-74.

Carette, C., Dubois-Laforgue, D., Gautier, J.-F. & Timsit, J. (2011). Diabetes mellitus and glucose-6-phosphate dehydrogenase deficiency: from one crisis to another, *Diabetes & Metabolism*, Vol. 37, No. 1, pp. 79-82.

Carlsson, L. M., Jonsson, J., Edlund, T., & Marklund, S L. (1995). Mice lacking extracellular superoxide dismutase are more sensitive to hyperoxia, *Proceedings of the National Academy of Sciences of the United States of America*, Vol. 92, No. 14, pp. 6264-6268.

Chevion, M., Navok, T., Glaser, G. & Mager, J. (1982). The chemistry of favism-inducing compounds. The properties of isouramil and divicine and their reaction with glutathione, *European Journal of Biochemistry*, Vol. 127, No. 2, pp. 405-409.

Chu, Y., Alwahdani, A., Iida, S., Lund, D.D., Faraci, F.M., & Heistad, D.D. (2005). Vascular effects of the human extracellular superoxide dismutase R213G variant, *Circulation*, Vol. 112, No. 7, pp. 1047-1053.

Cocco, P., Dessí, S., Avataneo, G., Picchiri, G. & Heinemann, E. (1989). Glucose-6-phosphate dehydrogenase deficiency and cancer in a Sardinian male population: a case-control study, *Carcinogenesis*, Vol. 10, No. 5, pp. 813-816.

Cocco, P., Ennas, M.G., Melis, M. A., Sollaino, C., Collu, S., Fadda, D., Gabbas, A., Massarelli, G., Rais, M., Todde, P. & Angelucci, E. (2007). Glucose-6-phosphate dehydrogenase polymorphism and lymphoma risk, *Tumori*, Vol. 93, No. 2, pp. 121-123.

Cote, M.L., Kardia, S.L.R., Wenzlaff, A.S., Land, S.J., & Schwartz, A.G. (2005). Combinations of glutathione S-transferase genotypes and risk of early-onset lung cancer in Caucasians and African Americans: a population-based study, *Carcinogenesis*, Vol. 26, No. 4, pp 811-819.

Culotta, V.C., Yang, M. & O'Halloran, T.V. (2006). Activation of superoxide dismutases: putting the metal to the pedal, *Biochimica et Biophysica Acta*, Vol. 1763, No. 7, pp. 747-758.

Dahl, M., Bowler, R.P., Juul, K., Crapo, J.D., Levy, S. & Nordestgaard, B.G. (2008). Superoxide dismutase 3 polymorphism associated with reduced lung function in two large populations, *American Journal of Respiratory and Critical Care Medicine*, Vol. 178, No. 9, pp. 906-912.

Demple, B. (1996). Redox signaling and gene control in the *Escherichia coli* soxRS oxidative stress regulon - a review, *Gene*, Vol. 179, No. 1, pp. 53-57.

Dimmeler, S., & Zeiher, A.M. (2007). A «reductionist» view of cardiomyopathy, *Cell*, Vol. 130, No. 3, pp. 401-402.

Föller, M., Bobbala, D., Koka, S., Huber, S., Gubbins, E. & Lang, F. (2009). Suicide for survival - death of infected erythrocytes as host mechanism to survive malaria, *Cell Physiology and Biochemistry*, Vol. 24, 133-140.

Ford, J.G., Li, Y., O'Sullivan, M.M., Demopoulos, R., Carte, S., Taioli, E. & Brand-Rauf, P.W. (2000). Glutathione S-transferase M1 polymorphism and lung cancer risk in African-Americans, *Carcinogenesis*, Vol. 21, No. 11, pp. 1971-1975.

Forsberg, L., de Faire, U. & Morgenstern, R. (2001). Oxidative stress, human genetic variation, disease, *Archives of Biochemistry and Biophysics*, Vol. 389, No. 1, pp. 84-93.

Förstermann, U. (2010). Nitric oxide and oxidative stress in vascular disease, *Pflügers Archiv: European Journal of Physiology*, Vol. 459, No. 6, pp. 923-939.

Franzè, A., Ferrante, M.I., Fusco, F., Santoro, A., Sanzari, E., Martini, G., & Ursini, M.V. (1998). Molecular anatomy of the human glucose 6-phosphate dehydrogenase core promoter, *FEBS Letters*, Vol. 437, No. 3, pp. 313-318.

Fukai, T., Folz, R.J., Landmesser, U., & Harrison, D.G. (2002). Extracellular superoxide dismutase and cardiovascular disease, *Cardiovascular Research*, Vol. 55, No.2, pp 239-249.

Furukawa, Y., Torres, A.S., & O'Halloran, T.V. (2004). Oxygen-induced maturation of SOD1: a key role for disulfide formation by the copper chaperone CCS, *The EMBO Journal*, Vol. 23, No. 14, pp. 2872-2881.

Gaskin, R. S., Estwick, D. & Peddi, R. (2001). G6PDH deficiency: its role in the high prevalence of hypertension and diabetes mellitus, *Ethnicity & Disease*, Vol. 11, No. 4, pp. 749-754.

Ghezzi, D., Arzuffi, P., Zordan, M., Da Re, C., Lamperti, C., Benna, C., D'Adamo, P., Diodato, D., Costa, R., Mariotti, C., Uziel, G., Smiderle, C. & Zeviani, M. (2011). Mutations in TTC19 cause mitochondrial complex III deficiency and neurological impairment in humans and flies, *Nature Genetics*, Vol. 43, No. 3, pp. 259-263.

Godon, C., Lagniel, G., Lee, J., Buhler, J.M., Kieffer, S., Perrot, M., Boucherie, H., Toledano, M. B., & Labarre, J. (1998). The H_2O_2 stimulon in *Saccharomyces cerevisiae*, *The Journal of Biological Chemistry*, Vol. 273, No. 35, pp. 22480-22489.

Goldstein, I. M., Kaplan, H. B., Edelson, H. S. & Weissmann, G. (1982). Ceruloplasmin: an acute phase reactant that scavenges oxygen-derived free radicals, *Annals of the New York Academy of Sciences*, Vol. 389, pp. 368-379.

Gongora, M.C. & Harrison, D.G. (2008). Sad heart from no SOD, *Hypertension*, Vol. 51, pp. 28-30.

Góth, L. (2008). Catalase deficiency and type 2 diabetes, *Diabetes Care*, Vol. 31, No. 12, p. e93.

Gupte, S.A. (2010). Targeting the Pentose Phosphate Pathway in Syndrome X-related Cardiovascular Complications, *Drug Development Research*, Vol. 71, No. 3, pp. 161-167.

Hallewell, R.A., Mills, R., Tekamp-Olson, P., Blacher, R., Rosenberg, S., Ötting, F., Masiarz, F.R. & Scandella, C.J. (1987). Amino terminal acetylation of authentic human Cu,Zn superoxide dismutase produced in yeast, *Biotechnology*, Vol. 5, pp. 363-366.

Halliwell, B. (2007). Oxidative stress and cancer: have we moved forward? *Biochemical Journal*, Vol. 401, pp. 1-11.

Hamanishi, T., Furuta, H., Kato, H., Doi, A., Tamai, M., Shimomura, H., Sakagashira, S., Nishi, M., Sasaki, H., Sanke, T. & Nanjo, K. (2004). Functional variants in the glutathione peroxidase-1 (GPx-1) gene are associated with increased intima-media thickness of carotid arteries and risk of macrovascular diseases in japanese type 2 diabetic patients, *Diabetes*, Vol. 53, No. 9, pp. 2455-2460.

Hayes, J.D., Flanagan, J.U., & Jowsey, I.R. (2005). Glutathione transferases, *Annual Review of Pharmacology and Toxicology*, Vol. 45, pp. 51-88.

Ho, H.-Y., Cheng, M.-L. & Chiu, D. T.-Y. (2005). G6PDH - an old bottle with new wine, *Chang Gung Medical Journal*, Vol. 28, No. 9, pp. 606-612.

Huebschmann, A.G., Regensteiner, J.G., Vlassara, H., & Reusch, J.E.B. (2006). Diabetes and advanced glycoxidation end products, *Diabetes Care*, Vol. 29, No. 6, pp. 1420-1432.

Imlay, J.A. (2008). Cellular defenses against superoxide and hydrogen peroxide, *Annual Review of Biochemistry*, Vol. 77, pp. 755-776.

Joseph, J., Handy, D.E. & Loscalzo, J. (2009). *Quo vadis*: whither homocysteine research?, *Cardiovascular Toxicology*, Vol. 9, No. 2, pp. 53-63.

Kabashi, E., Valdmanis, P.N., Dion, P. & Rouleau, G.A. (2007). Oxidized/misfolded superoxide dismutase-1: the cause of all amyotrophic lateral sclerosis? *Annals of Neurology*, Vol. 62, No. 6, pp. 553-559.

Kaplan, J. (1999). Friedreich's ataxia is a mitochondrial disorder, *Proceedings of the National Academy of Sciences of the United States of America*, Vol. 96, No. 20, pp. 10948-10949.

Kim, K.S., Choi, S.Y., Kwon, H.Y., Won, M. H., Kang, T.C., & Kang, J.H. (2002). Aggregation of alpha-synuclein induced by the Cu,Zn-superoxide dismutase and hydrogen peroxide system, *Free Radical Biology & Medicine*, Vol. 32, No. 6, pp. 544-550.

Kirkman, H.N. & Gaetani, G.F. (2007). Mammalian catalase: a venerable enzyme with new mysteries, *Trends in Biochemical Sciences*, Vol. 32, No. 1, pp. 44-50.

Kletzien, R.F., Harris, P.K., & Foellmi, L.A. (1994). Glucose-6-phosphate dehydrogenase: a «housekeeping» enzyme subject to tissue-specific regulation by hormones, nutrients, and oxidant stress, *The FASEB Journal: Official Publication of the Federation of American Societies for Experimental Biology*, Vol. 8, No. 2, pp. 174-181.

Knight, R. A. & Verkhratsky, A. (2010). Neurodegenerative diseases: failures in brain connectivity? *Cell Death and Differentiation*, Vol. 17, pp. 1069-1070.

Knight, S. A., Kim, R., Pain, D.& Dancis, A. (1999). The yeast connection to Friedreich ataxia, *American Journal of Human Genetics*, Vol. 64, No. 2, pp. 365-371.

Kong, G.K.-W., Miles, L.A., Crespi, G.A.N., Morton, C.J., Ng, H.L., Barnham, K.J., McKinstry, W.J., Cappai, R., & Parker, M.W. (2008). Copper binding to the Alzheimer's disease amyloid precursor protein, *European Biophysics Journal: EBJ*, Vol. 37, No. 3, pp. 269-279.

Konig-Greger, D., Riechelmann, H., Wittich, U., & Gronau, S. (2004). Genotype and phenotype of glutathione-S-transferase in patients with head and neck carcinoma, *Otolaryngology – Head and Neck Surgery: Official Journal of American Academy of Otolaryngology-Head and Neck Surgery*, Vol. 130, No. 6, pp. 718-725.

Kühnlein, R.P. (2010). Drosophila as a lipotoxicity model organism--more than a promise? *Biochimica et Biophysica Acta*, Vol. 1801, No. 3, pp. 215-221.

Lee, J.-W., Choi, A.H., Ham, M., Kim, J.-W., Choe, S.S., Park, J., Lee, G.Y., Yoon, K.-H., & Kim, J.B. (2011). G6PDH up-regulation promotes pancreatic beta-cell dysfunction, *Endocrinology*, Vol. 152, No. 3, pp. 793-803.

Lenzen, S. (2008). The mechanisms of alloxan- and streptozotocin-induced diabetes, *Diabetologia*, Vol. 51, No. 2, pp. 216-226.

Leopold, J.A. & Loscalzo, J. (2005). Oxidative enzymopathies and vascular disease. *Arteriosclerosis, Thrombosis, and Vascular Biology*, Vol. 25, No. 7, pp. 1332-1340.

Lightfoot, T.J., Skibola, C.F., Smith, A.G., Forrest, M.S., Adamson, P.J., Morgan, G.J., Bracci, P.M., Roman, E., Smith, M.T. & Holly, E.A. (2006). Polymorphisms in the oxidative stress genes superoxide dismutase, glutathione peroxidase and catalase and risk of non-Hodgkin's lymphoma, *Haematologica*, Vol. 91, No. 9, pp. 1222-1227.

Lill, R. & Mühlenhoff, U. (2006). Iron-sulfur protein biogenesis in eukaryotes: components and mechanisms, *Annual Review of Cell and Developmental Biology*, Vol. 22, pp. 457-486.

Liochev, S.I. & Fridovich, I. (2000). Copper- and zinc-containing superoxide dismutase can act as a superoxide reductase and a superoxide oxidase, *The Journal of Biological Chemistry*, Vol. 275, No. 49, pp. 38482-38485.

Liochev, S.I. & Fridovich, I. (2003). Mutant Cu,Zn superoxide dismutases and familial amyotrophic lateral sclerosis: evaluation of oxidative hypotheses, *Free Radical Biology & Medicine*, Vol. 34, No. 11, pp. 1383-1389.

Liu, D., Wen, J., Liu, J., & Li, L. (1999). The roles of free radicals in amyotrophic lateral sclerosis: reactive oxygen species and elevated oxidation of protein, DNA, and membrane phospholipids, *The FASEB Journal: Official Publication of the Federation of American Societies for Experimental Biology*, Vol. 13, No. 15, pp. 2318-2328.

Lubos, E., Handy, D.E. & Loscalzo, J. (2008). Role of oxidative stress and nitric oxide in atherothrombosis, *Frontiers in Bioscience*, Vol. 13, pp. 5323-5344.

Lubos, E., Loscalzo, J. & Handy, D.E. (2007). Homocysteine and glutathione peroxidase-1, *Antioxidants & Redox Signaling*, Vol. 9, No. 11, pp. 1923-1940.

Lushchak, V.I. (2001) Oxidative stress and mechanisms of protection against it in bacteria, *Biochemistry (Moscow)*. Vol. 66, No. 5, pp. 592-609.

Lushchak, V.I. (2010). Oxidative stress in yeast, *Biochemistry (Moscow)*, Vol. 75, No. 3, pp. 281-296.

Lushchak, V.I. (2011). Adaptive response to oxidative stress: Bacteria, fungi, plants and animals, *Comparative Biochemistry and Physiology. Toxicology & Pharmacology: CBP*, Vol. 153, No. 2, pp. 175-190.

Lushchak, O.V., Inoue, Y., & Lushchak, V.I. (2010). Regulatory protein Yap1 is involved in response of yeast *Saccharomyces cerevisiae* to nitrosative stress, *Biochemistry (Moscow)*. Vol. 75, No. 5, pp. 629-664.

Lushchak, V.I. & Gospodaryov, D.V. (2005). Catalases protect cellular proteins from oxidative modification in *Saccharomyces cerevisiae*, *Cell Biology International*, Vol. 29, No. 3, pp. 187-192.

Lushchak, V., Semchyshyn, H., Lushchak, O. & Mandryk, S. (2005a). Diethyldithiocarbamate inhibits in vivo Cu,Zn-superoxide dismutase and perturbs free radical processes in the yeast *Saccharomyces cerevisiae* cells, *Biochemical and Biophysical Research Communications*, Vol. 338, No. 4, pp. 1739-1744.

Lushchak, V., Semchyshyn, H., Mandryk, S. & Lushchak, O. (2005b). Possible role of superoxide dismutases in the yeast *Saccharomyces cerevisiae* under respiratory conditions, *Archives of Biochemistry and Biophysics*, Vol. 441, No. 1, pp. 35-40.

Ma, X., Chen, C., Xiong, H., Fan, J., Li, Y., Lin, H., Xu, R., Huang, G., & Xu, B. (2010). No association between SOD2 Val16Ala polymorphism and breast cancer susceptibility: a meta-analysis based on 9,710 cases and 11,041 controls, *Breast Cancer Research and Treatment*, Vol. 122, No. 2, pp. 509-514.

Marella, M., Seo, B.B., Yagi, T., & Matsuno-Yagi, A. (2009). Parkinson's disease and mitochondrial complex I: a perspective on the Ndi1 therapy, *Journal of Bioenergetics and Biomembranes*, Vol. 41, No. 6, pp. 493-497.

Matsui, R., Xu, S., Maitland, K.A., Hayes, A., Leopold, J.A., Handy, D. E., Loscalzo, J., & Cohen, R. A. (2005). Glucose-6 phosphate dehydrogenase deficiency decreases the vascular response to angiotensin II, *Circulation*, Vol. 112, No. 2, pp. 257-263.

McIlwain, C.C., Townsend, D.M. & Tew, K.D. (2006). Glutathione S-transferase polymorphisms: cancer incidence and therapy, *Oncogene*, Vol. 25, pp. 1639-1648.

McKee, A. C., Cantu, R. C., Nowinski, C. J., Hedley-Whyte, E. T., Gavett, B. E., Budson, A. E., Santini, V. E., Lee, H.-S., Kubilus, C. A. & Stern, R. A. (2009). Chronic traumatic encephalopathy in athletes: progressive tauopathy after repetitive head injury, *Journal of Neuropathology and Experimental Neurology*, Vol. 68, No. 7, pp. 709-735.

Mohr, L.C., Rodgers, J.K., & Silvestri, G.A. (2003). Glutathione S-transferase M1 polymorphism and the risk of lung cancer, *Anticancer Research*, Vol. 23, No. 3A, pp. 2111-2124.

Monteiro, H.P. & Winterbourn, C.C. (1989). Release of iron from ferritin by divicine, isouramil, acid-hydrolyzed vicine, and dialuric acid and initiation of lipid peroxidation, *Archives of Biochemistry and Biophysics*, Vol. 271, No. 2, pp. 536-545.

Nadal, R. C., Abdelraheim, S. R., Brazier, M. W., Rigby, S. E. J., Brown, David R. & Viles, J. H. (2007). Prion protein does not redox-silence Cu^{2+}, but is a sacrificial quencher of hydroxyl radicals, *Free Radical Biology & Medicine*, Vol. 42, No. 1, pp. 79-89.

Nakabeppu, Y., Kajitani, K., Sakamoto, K., Yamaguchi, H. & Tsuchimoto, D. (2006). *MTH1*, an oxidized purine nucleoside triphosphatase, prevents the cytotoxicity and neurotoxicity of oxidized purine nucleotides, *DNA Repair*, Vol. 5, No. 7, pp. 761-772.

Nakamura, M., Ando, Y., Sasada, K., Haraoka, K., Ueda, M., Okabe, H., & Motomiya, Y. (2005). Role of extracellular superoxide dismutase in patients under maintenance hemodialysis, *Nephron. Clinical Practice*, Vol. 101, No. 3, pp. c109-115.

Niazi, G.A. (1991). Glucose-6-phosphate dehydrogenase deficiency and diabetes mellitus, *International Journal of Hematology*, Vol. 54, No. 4, pp. 295-298.

Nkhoma, E.T., Poole, C., Vannappagari, V., Hall, S.A. & Beutler, E. (2009). The global prevalence of glucose-6-phosphate dehydrogenase deficiency: a systematic review and meta-analysis, *Blood Cells, Molecules & Diseases*, Vol. 42, No. 3, pp. 267-278.

Norris, E.H. & Giasson, B.I. (2005). Role of oxidative damage in protein aggregation associated with Parkinson's disease and related disorders, *Antioxidants & Redox Signaling*, Vol. 7, No. 5-6, pp. 672-684.

Nyström, T. (2005). Role of oxidative carbonylation in protein quality control and senescence, *The EMBO Journal*, Vol. 24, No. 7, pp. 1311-1317.

Ogata, M., Wang, D.-H. & Ogino, K. (2008). Mammalian acatalasemia: the perspectives of bioinformatics and genetic toxicology, *Acta Medica Okayama*, Vol. 62, No. 6, pp. 345-361.

Omalu, B.I., Hamilton, R.L., Kamboh, M.I., DeKosky, S.T. & Bailes, J. (2010). Chronic traumatic encephalopathy (CTE) in a National Football League Player: Case report and emerging medicolegal practice questions, *Journal of Forensic Nursing*, Vol. 6, No. 1, pp. 40-46.

Orrell, R.W. (2000). Amyotrophic lateral sclerosis: copper/zinc superoxide dismutase (SOD1) gene mutations, *Neuromuscular Disorders: NMD*, Vol. 10, No. 1, pp. 63-68.

Pain, J., Balamurali, M.M., Dancis, A., & Pain, D. (2010). Mitochondrial NADH kinase, Pos5p, is required for efficient iron-sulfur cluster biogenesis in *Saccharomyces cerevisiae*, *The Journal of Biological Chemistry*, Vol. 285, No. 50, pp. 39409-39424.

Pandey, U.B., & Nichols, C.D. (2011). Human disease models in *Drosophila melanogaster* and the role of the fly in therapeutic drug discovery, *Pharmacological Reviews*, Vol. 63, No. 2, pp. 411-436.

Park, J., Rho, H.K., Kim, K.H., Choe, S.S., Lee, Y.S., & Kim, J.B. (2005). Overexpression of glucose-6-phosphate dehydrogenase is associated with lipid dysregulation and insulin resistance in obesity, *Molecular and Cellular Biology*, Vol. 25, No. 12, pp. 5146-5157.

Pavel, S., Smit, N.P., van der Meulen, H., Kolb, R.M., de Groot, A.J., van der Velden, P.A., Gruis, N.A., & Bergman, W. (2003). Homozygous germline mutation of CDKN2A/p16 and glucose-6-phosphate dehydrogenase deficiency in a multiple melanoma case, *Melanoma Research*, Vol. 13, No. 2, pp. 171-178.

Pigeolet, E., Corbisier, P., Houbion, A., Lambert, D., Michiels, C., Raes, M., Zachary, M.D., & Remacle, J. (1990). Glutathione peroxidase, superoxide dismutase, and catalase inactivation by peroxides and oxygen derived free radicals, *Mechanisms of Ageing and Development*, Vol. 51, No. 3, pp. 283-297.

Poon, H.F., Hensley, K., Thongboonkerd, V., Merchant, M.L., Lynn, B.C., Pierce, W.M., Klein, J. B., Calabrese, V. & Butterfield, D.A. (2005). Redox proteomics analysis of oxidatively modified proteins in G93A-SOD1 transgenic mice - a model of familial amyotrophic lateral sclerosis, *Free Radical Biology & Medicine*, Vol. 39, No. 4, pp. 453-462.

Rajasekaran, N.S., Connell, P., Christians, E.S., Yan, L.-J., Taylor, R.P., Orosz, A., Zhang, X. Q., Stevenson, T. J., Peshock, R.M., Leopold, J.A., Barry, W.H., Loscalzo, J., Odelberg, S.J., & Benjamin, I.J. (2007). Human αB-crystallin mutation causes oxido-reductive stress and protein aggregation cardiomyopathy in mice, *Cell*, Vol. 130, No. 3, pp. 427-439.

Rakhit, R., Cunningham, P., Furtos-Matei, A., Dahan, S., Qi, X.-F., Crow, J.P., Cashman, N. R., Kondejewski, L.H. & Chakrabartty, A. (2002). Oxidation-induced misfolding and aggregation of superoxide dismutase and its implications for amyotrophic lateral sclerosis, *The Journal of Biological Chemistry*, Vol. 277, No. 49, pp. 47551-47556.

Ralser, M., & Benjamin, I.J. (2008). Reductive stress on life span extension in *C. elegans*, *BMC Research Notes*, Vol. 1, p. 19.

Rimm, E.B. & Stampfer, M.J. (2011). Folate and cardiovascular disease: one size does not fit all, *Lancet*, Vol. 378, No. 9791, pp. 544-546.

Roth, E.F. Jr., Ruprecht, R.M., Schulman, S., Vandersberg, J. & Olson, J.A. (1986). Ribose metabolism and nucleic acid synthesis in normal and glucose-6-phosphate deficient human erythrocytes infected with *Plasmodium falciparum*, *Journal of Clinical Investigation*, Vol. 77, No. 4, pp. 1129-1235.

Rouault, T.A., & Tong, W.H. (2008). Iron-sulfur cluster biogenesis and human disease, *Trends in Genetics: TIG*, Vol. 24, No. 8, pp. 398-407.

Sala, G., Beretta, S., Ceresa, C., Mattavelli, L., Zoia, C., Tremolizzo, L., Ferri, A., Carrì, M.T., & Ferrarese, C. (2005). Impairment of glutamate transport and increased vulnerability to oxidative stress in neuroblastoma SH-SY5Y cells expressing a Cu,Zn superoxide dismutase typical of familial amyotrophic lateral sclerosis, *Neurochemistry International*, Vol. 46, No. 3, pp. 227-234.

Salati, L.M., & Amir-Ahmady, B. (2001). Dietary regulation of expression of glucose-6-phosphate dehydrogenase, *Annual Review of Nutrition*, Vol. 21, pp. 121-140.

Sangle, G.V., Zhao, R., Mizuno, T.M., & Shen, G.X. (2010). Involvement of RAGE, NADPH oxidase, and Ras/Raf-1 pathway in glycated LDL-induced expression of heat shock factor-1 and plasminogen activator inhibitor-1 in vascular endothelial cells, *Endocrinology*, Vol. 151, No. 9, pp. 4455-4466.

Sansone, G. & Segni, G. (1958). Nuovi aspetti dell'alterato biochimismo degli eritrociti di favici: assenza pressochè completa della glucoso-6-P deldrogenasi, *Bollettino Della Società Italiana Di Biologia Sperimentale*, Vol. 34, No. 7, pp. 327-329.

Scacco, S., Petruzzella, V., Bertini, E., Luso, A., Papa, F., Bellomo, F., Signorile, A., Torraco, A., & Papa, S. (2006). Mutations in structural genes of complex I associated with neurological diseases, *The Italian Journal of Biochemistry*, Vol. 55, No. 3-4, pp. 254-262.

Schmidlin, T., Kennedy, B. K. & Daggett, V. (2009). Structural changes to monomeric CuZn superoxide dismutase caused by the familial amyotrophic lateral sclerosis-associated mutation A4V, *Biophysical Journal*, Vol. 97, pp. 1709-1718.

Sentman, M.-L., Granström, M., Jakobson, H., Reaume, A., Basu, S., & Marklund, Stefan L. (2006). Phenotypes of mice lacking extracellular superoxide dismutase and copper- and zinc-containing superoxide dismutase, *The Journal of Biological Chemistry*, Vol. 281, No. 11, pp. 6904-6909.

Seo, J.H., Lim, J.C., Lee, D.-Y., Kim, K.S., Piszczek, G., Nam, H.W., Kim, Y.S., Ahn, T., Yun, C.-H., Kim, K., Chock, P.B., & Chae, H.Z. (2009). Novel protective mechanism against irreversible hyperoxidation of peroxiredoxin: Nα-terminal acetylation of human peroxiredoxin II, *The Journal of Biological Chemistry*, Vol. 284, No.20, pp. 13455-13465.

Stipanuk, M.H. (2004). Sulfur amino acid metabolism: pathways for production and removal of homocysteine and cysteine, *Annual Review of Nutrition*, Vol. 24, pp. 539-577.

Sultana, R., & Butterfield, D.A. (2010). Role of oxidative stress in the progression of Alzheimer's disease, *Journal of Alzheimer's Disease: JAD*, Vol. 19, No. 1, pp. 341-353.

Sun, L.-M., Shang, Y., Zeng, Y.-M., Deng, Y.-Y., & Cheng, J.-F. (2010). hOGG1 polymorphism in atrophic gastritis and gastric cancer after *Helicobacter pylori* eradication, *World Journal of Gastroenterology: WJG*, Vol. 16, No. 35, pp. 4476-4482.

Sutton, A., Imbert, A., Igoudjil, A., Descatoire, V., Cazanave, S., Pessayre, D. & Degoul, F. (2005). The manganese superoxide dismutase Ala16Val dimorphism modulates both mitochondrial import and mRNA stability, *Pharmacogenetics & Genomics*, Vol. 15, No. 5, pp. 311-319.

Sutton, A., Khoury, H., Prip-Buus, C., Cepanec, C., Pessayre, D. & Degoul, F. (2003). The Ala16Val genetic dimorphism modulates the import of human manganese superoxide dismutase into rat liver mitochondria, *Pharmacogenetics*, Vol. 13, No. 3, pp. 145-157.

Tabatabaie, T., & Floyd, R.A. (1994). Susceptibility of glutathione peroxidase and glutathione reductase to oxidative damage and the protective effect of spin trapping agents, *Archives of Biochemistry and Biophysics*, Vol. 314, No. 1, pp. 112-119.

Tamarit, J., Belli, G., Cabiscol, E., Herrero, E., & Ros, J. (2003). Biochemical characterization of yeast mitochondrial Grx5 monothiol glutaredoxin, *The Journal of Biological Chemistry*, Vol. 278, No. 28, pp. 25745-25751.

Temple, M.D., Perrone, G.G., & Dawes, I.W. (2005). Complex cellular responses to reactive oxygen species, *Trends in Cell Biology*, Vol. 15, No. 6, pp. 319-326.

Thorpe, G.W., Fong, C.S., Alic, N., Higgins, V.J., & Dawes, I.W. (2004). Cells have distinct mechanisms to maintain protection against different reactive oxygen species: oxidative-stress-response genes, *Proceedings of the National Academy of Sciences of the United States of America*, Vol. 101, No. 17, pp. 6564-6569.

Tian, W.N., Braunstein, L.D., Pang, J., Stuhlmeier, K.M., Xi, Q.C., Tian, X. & Stanton, R C. (1998). Importance of glucose-6-phosphate dehydrogenase activity for cell growth, *The Journal of Biological Chemistry*, Vol. 273, No. 17, pp. 10609-10617.

Tortarolo, M., Grignaschi, G., Calvaresi, N., Zennaro, E., Spaltro, G., Colovic, M., Fracasso, C., Guiso, G., Elger, B., Schneider, H., Seilheimer, B., Caccia, S., & Bendotti, C. (2006). Glutamate AMPA receptors change in motor neurons of SOD1 G93A transgenic mice and their inhibition by a noncompetitive antagonist ameliorates the progression of amytrophic lateral sclerosis-like disease, *Journal of Neuroscience Research*, Vol. 83, No. 1, pp. 134-146.

Uryu, K., Giasson, B.I., Longhi, L., Martinez, D., Murray, I., Conte, V., Nakamura, M., Saatman, K., Talbot, K., Horiguchi, T., McIntosh, T., Lee, V.M.-Y. & Trojanowski, J. Q. (2003). Age-dependent synuclein pathology following traumatic brain injury in mice, *Experimental Neurology*, Vol. 184, No. 1, pp. 214-224.

Valentine, J.S. & Hart, P.J. (2003). Misfolded CuZnSOD and amyotrophic lateral sclerosis, *Proceedings of the National Academy of Sciences of the United States of America*, Vol. 100, No. 7, pp. 3617-3622.

Valentine, J.S., Doucette, P.A., & Zittin Potter, S. (2005). Copper-zinc superoxide dismutase and amyotrophic lateral sclerosis, *Annual Review of Biochemistry*, Vol. 74, pp. 563-593.

Van Ho, A., Ward, D.M. & Kaplan, J. (2002). Transition metal transport in yeast, *Annual Review of Microbiology*, Vol. 56, pp. 237-261.

Vucic, S. & Kiernan, M.C. (2009). Pathophysiology of neurodegeneration in familial amyotrophic lateral sclerosis, *Current Molecular Medicine*, Vol. 9, No. 3, pp. 255-272.

Wautier, J.-L., & Schmidt, Ann Marie. (2004). Protein glycation: a firm link to endothelial cell dysfunction, *Circulation Research*, Vol. 95, No. 3, pp. 233-238.

Wenzlaff, A.S., Cote, M.L., Bock, C.H., Land, S.J., & Schwartz, A.G. (2005). GSTM1, GSTT1 and GSTP1 polymorphisms, environmental tobacco smoke exposure and risk of lung cancer among never smokers: a population-based study, *Carcinogenesis*, Vol. 26, No. 2, pp. 395-401.

Wingert, R.A., Galloway, J.L., Barut, B., Foott, H., Fraenkel, P., Axe, J.L., Weber, G.J., Dooley, K., Davidson, A.J., Schmid, B., Schmidt, B., Paw, B.H., Shaw, G.C., Kingsley, P., Palis, J., Schubert, H., Chen, O.S., Kaplan, J. & Zon, L.I. (2005). Deficiency of glutaredoxin 5 reveals Fe-S clusters are required for vertebrate haem synthesis, *Nature*, Vol. 436, No. 7053, pp. 1035-1039.

Winterbourn, C.C. & Metodiewa, D. (1994). The reaction of superoxide with reduced glutathione, *Archives of Biochemistry and Biophysics*, Vol. 314, No. 2, pp. 284-290.

Yim, M.B., Chock, P.B, & Stadtman, E.R. (1990). Copper, zinc superoxide dismutase catalyzes hydroxyl radical production from hydrogen peroxide, *Proceedings of the National Academy of Sciences of the United States of America*, Vol. 87, No. 13, pp. 5006-5010.

Youn, C.-K., Song, P.I., Kim, M.-H., Kim, J.S., Hyun, J.-W., Choi, S.-J., Yoon, S.P., Chung, M.H., Chang, I.-Y., & You, H.J. (2007). Human 8-oxoguanine DNA glycosylase suppresses the oxidative stress induced apoptosis through a p53-mediated signaling pathway in human fibroblasts, *Molecular Cancer Research: MCR*, Vol. 5, No. 10, pp. 1083-1098.

Zhu, M., Qin, Z.-J., Hu, D., Munishkina, L.A. & Fink, A.L. (2006). α-Synuclein can function as an antioxidant preventing oxidation of unsaturated lipid in vesicles, *Biochemistry*, Vol. 45, pp. 8135-8142.

Zinkham, W.H., Lenhard, R.E., Jr. & Childs, B. (1958). A deficiency of glucose-6-phosphate dehydrogenase activity in erythrocytes from patients with favism, *Bulletin of the Johns Hopkins Hospital*, Vol. 102, No. 4, pp. 169-175.

Section 3

Cardiovascular Diseases

3

Reactive Oxygen Species and Cardiovascular Diseases

Vitor Engrácia Valenti[1,2], Luiz Carlos de Abreu[2], Celso Ferreira[2] and Paulo H. N. Saldiva[1]
[1]*Faculdade de Medicina da Universidade de São Paulo,*
[2]*Faculdade de Medicina do ABC,*
Brazil

1. Introduction

Reduction or oxidation caused by addition or loss of any electron is responsible for alterations in functional and structural profile of molecules, hence, changing signaling mechanism. Reactive free radicals play a crucial role in different physiological mechanisms ranging from the immune defense to cell signaling and inflammation (Elahi & Matata, 2006). There is increasing evidence that irregular production of free radicals lead to enhanced stress on cellular structures and causes changes in molecular pathways that underpins the pathogenesis of several relevant human disorders, such as cancer, heart diseases, the process of physiological ageing and neurological diseases (Pacher & Szabo, 2008; Lushchak, 2011a; Lushchak, 2011b). Comprehending the involvement of free radical stress in the pathogenesis of disease will allow us to investigate the development of oxidative stress; a condition that occurs due to an imbalance between cellular production of oxidant molecules and the availability of appropriate antioxidants species that defend against them. It is hoped that this knowledge will subsequently lead to the development of effective therapeutic interventions against oxidative stress.

The main molecules that are involved in redox signaling are called as reactive oxygen species (ROS), in which we may include hydrogen peroxide (H_2O_2), nitric oxide (NO), hydroxyl radical, superoxide ($O^{2\bullet-}$) and peroxynitrite. Current redox signaling investigations indicate that all the vascular constituents, including vascular smooth muscle cells (VSMCs), endothelial and adventitial cells and macrophages, produce ROS (Papaharalambus & Griendling, 2007). ROS are involved in signal transduction which is related to relaxation and contraction of blood vessels, migration, growth and death of vascular cells, and also extracellular matrix (ECM) alterations.

It is known that vascular diseases such as peripheral vascular disease, coronary artery disease and cerebrovascular diseases are the largest cause of morbidity and mortality in industrialized countries. Some common risk factors for vascular disease, including diabetes and hypertension are still prevalent in Western and other populations, indicating that vascular disease will possible continue to impose a substantial burden on health care resources throughout the next generation. The earliest detectable changes in vascular disease states are irregularities of the endothelium, resulting in loss of the endothelium's normal homeostatic functions that normally act to inhibit disease-related mechanisms such as thrombosis and inflammation. Particularly, it was previously demonstrated that nitric oxide (NO) produced by NO synthase (eNOS) in the vascular endothelium modulates blood flow and pressure and presents important antiatherogenic effects on platelets, vascular smooth muscle and endothelial cells (Umans and Levi, 1995).

Many previous studies have already demonstrated the effects of oxidative stress on the cardiovascular system. Superoxide dismutase (SOD), an enzyme that catalyze the dismutation of $O^{2\bullet-}$ into oxygen and H_2O_2, injected into brainstem areas involved in cardiovascular regulation decreased sympathetic nerve activity and decreased blood pressure in swine (Zanzinger and Czachurski, 2009). According to Campese et al. (2004) the lack of low-density lipoprotein (LDL) receptor-enhanced cholesterol blood levels enhanced ROS and impared baroceptor reflex function. Monahan et al (2004) indicated that oxidative stress collaborates to age-associated decreases in cardiovagal baroreflex sensitivity in healthy subjects. Conversely, it was indicated in male smokers that circulating antioxidants had no effect on baroceptor reflex, and minor effects on the cardiovascular system were seen following acute fat and vitamin ingestion (Wright et al, 2009). Overall, comprehending the process which redox signaling modulates cardiovascular system will provide further precise ROS regulation as a therapy for cardiovascular disorders. In this chapter we summarize concepts regarding oxidative stress related to cardiovascular disorders.

2. Models of ROS-induced cardiovascular diseases

Basic science applied in animal is indispensable to comprehend the pathogenesis, mechanisms involved in therapeutic agents, molecular process, and environmental or genetic factors that increases the risks of disease development. The species of animal studied are influenced by numerous aspects. Usually, animals with small size are preferred because they are more manageable and experiments are less expensive. According to the guide of the principles of animal research, we should use the lowest possible animal and, nowadays, permission would not be granted for using larger animals unless a similar experiment could not be performed on rodent. Nevertheless, a major criticism of using rodents is that they may not adequately correspond to the human situation and this fact occasionally justifies the use of larger animals such as pigs and monkeys (Rees & Alcolado, 2005). In this topic we described the main animal models used in the literature to investigate the mechanisms involved in ROS-induced cardiovascular disorders.

The relationship between enhanced ROS and hypertension is well established in many studies involving diet or endocrine-induced and surgically-induced hypertensive animals (Banday et al, 2007). A variety of evidence suggests that ROS collaborate to impaired endothelial function in several forms of hypertension and that there is enhanced ROS in the microvessels of spontaneously hypertensive rats (SHR) and Dahl salt-sensitive hypertensive rats (Manning et al, 2003). An interesting study by Lenda et al (2000) suggested that ROS can also collaborate to a decreased endothelium-dependent dilation in normotensive rats under an enhanced salt diet. Although the latent level of ROS in contributing to damaged endothelium-dependent vasodilation and decreased NO production during increased dietary salt intake, the nature and mechanisms of the impaired vascular relaxation with the high-salt diet and the role of enhanced ROS in contributing to salt-induced changes in vascular function and hypertension are not completely understood (Cai & Harrison, 2000).

Hypertension is a result of enhanced ROS, however, data regarding the most potent cause of ROS-induced hypertension is controversial. In fact, oxidative stress does not elucidate the cause of every kind of hypertension, which develops through many processes. A small number of clinical investigations indicated the protective property of antioxidants (Ceriello et al, 1991; Galley et al, 1997). Nevertheless, it is known that not all animal models of hypertension are related to ROS (Rajagopalan et al, 1996). Additionally, clinical studies demonstrated negative correlation between arterial pressure and oxidative stress markers in subjects with mild to moderate hypertension (Cracowski et al, 2003). It is hard to find a cause–effect association between hypertension and oxidative stress in clinical studies, however, some studies indicated that increased ROS is a risk factor for human hypertension (Adbilla et al, 2007).

Animal models are important to support the link between hypertension and oxidative stress. Some procedures performed in animal models helped to comprehend the mechanisms involved in ROS-induced hypertension (Rajagopalan et al, 1996; Puzserova et al, 2010; Valenti et al, 2011a).

The group of Zucker and coworkers from Nebraska have used a model based on heart failure in rabbits (Mousa et al, 2008). According to their method, a platinum wire pacing electrode is sutured to the epicardium of the left ventricle in the rabbits. A ground electrode is secured to the left atrium. All wires are tunneled beneath the skin and exited in the midscapular area. The chest is closed and evacuated; in the same setting, a radiotelemetry unit is implanted into the right femoral artery with the tip of its catheter in the descending aorta to monitor blood pressure and heart rate in the conscious state. Rabbits were allowed to recover from surgery for two weeks before they were used in the study. They developed a rapid pacing model of chronic heart failure. After recovery from surgery, animals are paced at a rate of 360–380 beats/min with the use of a small, light-weight pacing unit of their own design. The pacing rate is adjusted and monitored by frequent echocardiograms. In general, each rabbit is paced at 360 beats/minute for the first week to determine whether it would tolerate this protocol. After the first week, the pacing rate is enhanced to 380 beats/minute and continued at this rate for the remainder of the protocol. The rabbits are continuously paced for 3 weeks. Cardiac dimensions (left ventricular end-diastolic diameter, left ventricular end-systolic diameter, fractional shortening, and ejection fraction) and other hemodynamic parameters are monitored on a weekly basis. Additionally, to left ventricular dimension changes, clinical signs of chronic heart failure such as ascites, pulmonary congestion, and cachexia are appreciated as symptoms of this chronic heart failure model. This model is well accepted in the literature and it was observed enhanced production of ROS in the heart and in the brainstem. Furthermore, they measured two of the three major SOD isoforms (Cu,Zn-SOD and Mn-SOD) and the catalytic subunit of NAD(P)H oxidase, gp91phox into the brainstem. They reported that protein expression of both CuZn SOD and Mn SOD was significantly downregulated in the chronic heart failure condition. The gp91phox protein was significantly enhanced in chronic heart failure rabbits (Gao et al, 2007). The more affected area was the rostroventrolateral area of the medulla oblongata.

The renovascular model of hypertension is a model which presented enhanced level of ROS (Campos et al, 2011). In this model, rats are anesthetized with ketamine and xylazine (40 mg and 10 mg/kg, respectively, ip); the left renal artery is exposed through an abdominal incision, and the renal artery and renal vein are dissected free from the adherent tissues. The left renal artery is partially obstructed with a silver clip of 0.2-mm width. No clip obstruction is applied to the sham-operated group (n = 15). Animals are submitted to the final experimental procedures 3 or 6 weeks after the surgical procedure. Systolic blood pressure is measured in conscious rats using a pneumatic tail-cuff method.

The role of ROS has been shown in this model of ROS-induced cardiovascular injury, in which the chronic administration of a SOD mimetic, tempol, to reduce ROS was shown to reduce blood pressure (Welch et al, 2003). Moreover, tempol was more effective than AT1 antagonist (candesartan) in reducing blood pressure and in improving renal function in renovascular hypertensive rats, suggesting that ROS plays an important role in mediating of renovascular hypertension (Palm et al, 2010). However, besides the actions of ROS on many tissues, the brain is one of the Ang II targets most affected by ROS. Even when an increase in plasma renin activity is modest after moderate renal artery stenosis, ROS remains increased and collaborates to hypertension (Lerman et al, 1991).Therefore, the involvement of Ang II is believed to decline, whereas ROS increases, during the progression of the 2K1C model. Our hypothesis is that even with a modest increase in circulating Ang II, this peptide acting in the CNS through AT1 receptors might collaborate to NADPH activation, which leads to an increase in local ROS production, causing sympathoexcitation and arterial hypertension.

The central regulation of the sympathetic nervous system (SNS) involved in cardiovascular regulation is complex, involving multiple reflex pathways and neural connections with a large number of neurotransmitters and neuromodulators acting in specific groups of neurons in the CNS involved in the tonic and reflex control of the cardiovascular system. In the CNS, Ang II is able to increase sympathetic vasomotor tone and blood pressure, and is involved in the pathogenesis of many experimental models of hypertension (Campos, 2009). Therefore, the close functional association between NADPH oxidase and the Ang II is of particular relevance in linking oxidative stress in the brain to sympathoexcitation and hypertension. For instance, intracerebroventricular infusion of NADPH oxidase inhibitor antagonizes the pressor response induced by centrally mediated Ang II actions (Gao et al, 2007). In the brain, the overexpression of SOD, an enzyme responsible for $O^{2\bullet-}$ breakdown, also abolishes the central pressor effect of the octapeptide, suggesting that in the CNS there is a positive correlation between the increase in ROS and the central pressor response mediated by Ang II (Zimmerman et al, 2004). Considering that the paraventricular nucleus of the hypothalamus (PVN) and the rostroventrolateral medulla (RVLM) contain critically important neurons involved in the control of sympathetic vasomotor tone and arterial pressure (Valenti et al, 2011a), in the studies reviewed in this article it was examined an increase in AT1 receptor expression and oxidative stress markers within these two nuclei in renovascular hypertension. NAD(P)H oxidase subunits (p47phox and gp91phox) and anti-oxidant enzyme CuZnSOD mRNA expression were quantified in the RVLM and PVN of renovascular hypertensive rats. It was hypothesized that the overactivity of NADPH oxidase-derived ROS associated with a reduction in the activity of CuZnSOD within the RVLM and PVN could collaborate to renovascular hypertension, particularly in the renin-dependent phase of hypertension.

In hypertensive renovascular rats, there is a significant increase in systemic ROS, estimated by the thiobarbituric acid reactive substance (TBARS) level in plasma, compared with control rats. Administration of tempol or Vitamin C systemically decreased blood pressure and RSNA only in renovascular hypertensive rats, indicating that the depressor effect in response to the anti-oxidant administration is mediated by a reduction in sympathetic vasomotor activity (Oliveira-Sales et al, 2008).

Some studies evaluated the effects of ROS on vascular properties in rat aorta (Toba et al, 2010; Olukman et al, 2010). Others tried to reveal the mechanisms involved in ROS-induced cardiovascular disease inside the brainstem (Zanzinger et al, 2009; Valenti et al, 2011a; Campos et al, 2011).

The SHR is a model which has been well investigated (He et al, 2011). SHR and stroke-prone SHR (SPSHR), genetic models that develop hypertension spontaneously, exhibit enhanced NAD(P)H driven $O^{2\bullet-}$ generation in resistance (mesenteric) and conduit (aortic) vessels (Rodriguez-Iturbe et al, 2003). This is associated with NAD(P)H oxidase subunit overexpression and enhanced oxidase activity (Kishi et al, 2004). Several polymorphisms in the promoter region of the p22phox gene have been identified in SHR (Zalba et al, 2001). This has clinical relevance because an association between a p22phox gene polymorphism and NAD(P)H oxidase-mediated $O^{2\bullet-}$ production in the vascular wall of patients with hypertension and atherosclerosis has been described (Moreno et al, 2003).

Enhanced expression of p47phox has been reported in the renal vasculature, macula densa, and distal nephron from young SHR, suggesting that renal NAD(P)H oxidase upregulation precedes development of hypertension (Kishi et al, 2004). Diminished nitric oxide bioavailability as a consequence of enhanced vascular $O^{2\bullet-}$ generation and downregulation of the thioredoxin system may also collaborate to oxidative stress in SHR and SPSHR (Touyz 2003). Treatment with antioxidant vitamins, NAD(P)H oxidase inhibitors, SOD mimetics, and BH_4 and Ang II type-1 (AT1) receptor blockers decrease vascular $O^{2\bullet-}$ production and attenuate development of hypertension in these models (Rodriguez-Iturbe et al, 2003; Shokoji et al, 2003). Taken together, these findings suggest that oxidative stress in genetic hypertension involves enhanced NAD(P)H oxidase activity and dysfunctional endothelial nitric oxide synthase (uncoupled NOS) and is regulated, in part, by AT1 receptors. Figure 1 presents a surgical procedure to record mean arterial pressure and heart rate, while Figure 2 shows recordings from one normotensive Wistar Kyoto and one SHR rat illustrating reflex bradycardia (top) in response to blood pressure increases. In this Figure we may observe the enhanced mean arterial pressure of the SHR compared to the control animal.

In animal models of diabetes, several functional and structural alterations of the heart or in cardiac muscle have been documented (Russel et al, 2006). In most studies of type 1 diabetes mellitus, diabetes are induced after administration of the pancreatic beta-cell toxin streptozotocin, and most studies of type 2 diabetes mellitus have been performed in genetic models of obesity and insulin resistance such as the Zucker fatty rat or db/db mice, both of which have mutations that impair leptin receptor signaling, or ob/ob mice, which lacks leptin. Furthermore, because diabetes mellitus develops at varying tempos in these models, it is important to bear in mind that studies performed in animals before the onset of diabetes may reflect changes that are secondary to the underlying obesity and insulin resistance, and

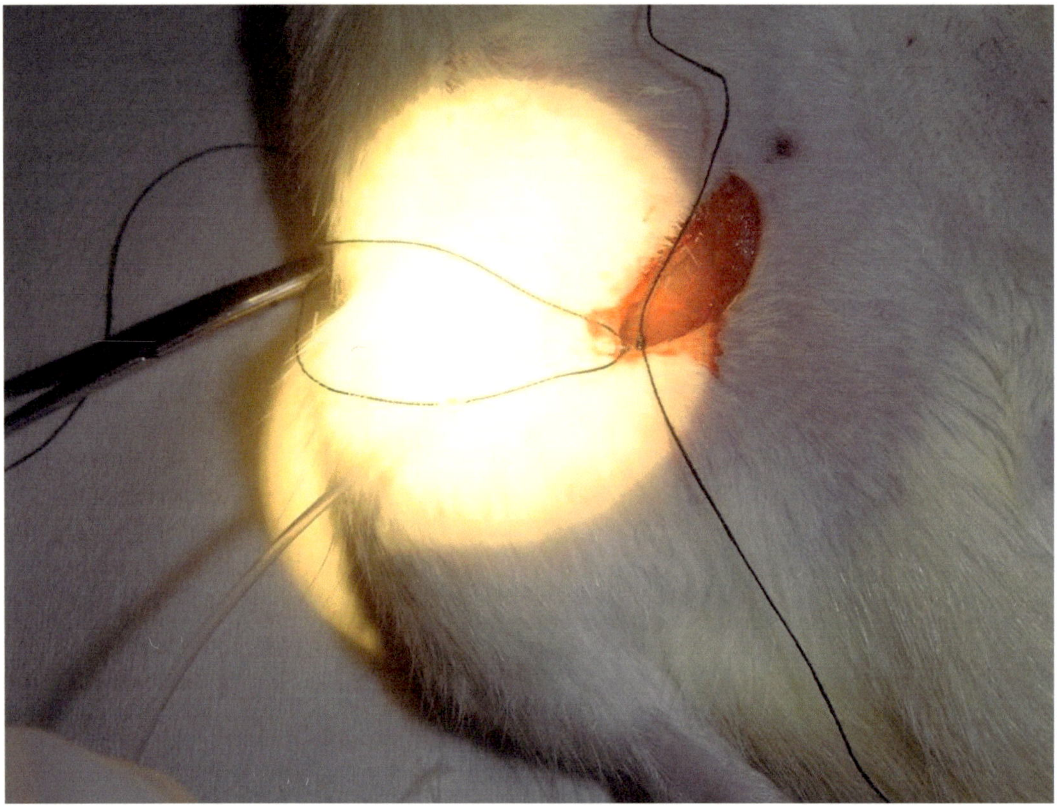

Fig. 1. Surgical procedure to record basal mean arterial pressure and heart rate in one spontaneously hypertensive rat.

studies performed after the onset of diabetes may reflect the added effects of hyperglycemia of various durations. Most studies have been performed in isolated perfused hearts and reveal depressed cardiac function (Aasum et al, 2002; Aasum et al, 2003). In vivo studies in these rodent models have provided evidence for systolic and diastolic dysfunction by echocardiography (Christoffersen et al, 2003) but in some studies using invasive left ventricle catheterization in mouse models of obesity and diabetes mellitus, left ventricle contractility as determined by developed pressure/developed tension was initially enhanced and may reflect the impact of the enhanced plasma volume and perhaps sympathetic activation associated in part with the underlying obesity (Buchanan et al, 2005). These first observations were additionally clarified later (Van den Bergh et al, 2006). It was assessed the hemodynamic changes in db/db mouse hearts in vivo using a pressure–volume instrument. It was reported decreased contractility using load-independent variables such as preload recruitable stroke work, but steady-state measurements of cardiac output and other load-dependent parameters were increased in db/db mice compared with control mice because of favorable loading conditions, specifically enhanced preload and decreased afterload.

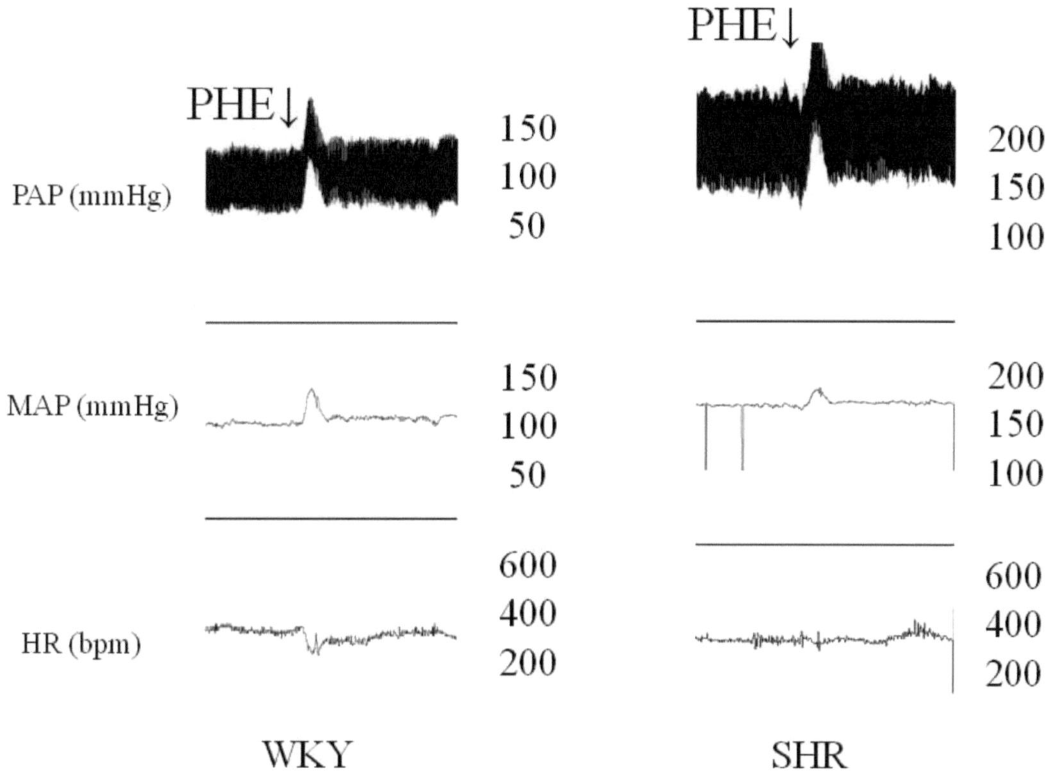

Fig. 2. Recordings from one Wistar Kyoto control rat and one spontaneously hypertensive rat illustrating reflex bradycardia (top) in response to blood pressure increases. Infusions were given in bolus. MAP: mean arterial pressure; PAP: pulsatile arterial pressure; HR: heart rate; PHE: phenylephrine.

Enhanced ROS production in the diabetic heart is a contributing matter to the progression and the development of diabetic cardiomyopathy (Cai et al, 2006). Cumulative superoxide-mediated damage or cellular dysfunction results when an imbalance exists in ROS generation and ROS-degrading pathways. Enhanced ROS generation and impaired antioxidant defenses could both collaborate to oxidative stress in diabetic hearts. Several groups have shown that ROS is overproduced in both type 1 and type 2 diabetes (Cai et al, 2006). Under physiological states, most of the ROS generated within cells arises from mitochondria. Whereas enhanced mitochondrial ROS generation has been shown in various tissues such as endothelial cells that are exposed to hyperglycemia (Brownlee, 1995), relatively few studies to date have directly measured mitochondrial ROS production in mitochondria obtained from diabetic hearts. However, overexpression of mitochondrial superoxide dismutase (SOD2) in the heart of a mouse model of type 1 diabetes mellitus reversed altered mitochondrial morphology and function and maintained cardiomyocyte function (Shen et al, 2006). Evidence also exists for enhanced production of ROS from non mitochondrial sources such as NADPH oxidase or decreased neuronal nitric oxide synthase (NOS1) activity coupled with enhanced activation of xanthine oxidoreductase (Saraiva et al, 2006). Whereas evidence for enhanced ROS production in diabetes mellitus is reasonably strong, the effect of diabetes on antioxidant defenses in the heart is controversial. Thus, the activities/expression levels of glutathione peroxidase, copper/zinc SOD, or catalase were either enhanced (Li et al, 2006) or decreased (Matkovics et al, 1997). Enhanced ROS generation may activate maladaptive signaling pathways, which may lead to cell death, which could collaborate to the pathogenesis of diabetic cardiomyopathy. Enhanced ROS production was associated with enhanced apoptosis, as evidenced by enhanced in situ nick end-labeling (TUNEL) staining and caspase 3 activation in ob/ob and db/db hearts (Barouch et al, 2003). In the same study, enhanced ROS was also associated with enhanced DNA impairment and loss of activity of DNA repair pathways that declined more rapidly with age in diabetic versus control animals.

Therefore, enhanced ROS-modulated cell death is able to promote irregular cardiac remodeling, which ultimately may collaborate to the morphological characteristic and functional abnormalities that are associated with diabetic cardiomyopathy. In addition to causing cellular injury, enhanced ROS production might lead to cardiac dysfunction via other mechanisms. For instance, enhanced ROS has been proposed to amplify hyperglycemia-induced activation of protein kinase C isoforms, enhanced formation of glucose-derived advanced glycation end products, and enhanced glucose flux through the aldose reductase pathways (Brownlee et al, 1995), which may all collaborate to various ways to the development of cardiac complications in diabetes mellitus. Enhanced ROS also might collaborate to mitochondrial uncoupling, which could impair myocardial energetic metabolism in diabetes.

Strategies that enhance mitochondrial ROS scavenging systems have been demonstrate to be effective in decreasing diabetes-induced cardiac dysfunction. Overexpression of metallothionein, catalase, and manganese SOD (Shen et al, 2006) in the heart reversed diabetic cardiomyopathy in animal models of both type 1 and type 2 diabetes. Therefore, strategies that either reduce ROS or augment myocardial antioxidant defense mechanisms might have therapeutic efficacy in improving myocardial function in diabetes mellitus.

In summary, experimental protocols applied in animals are necessary to understand the pathological events involved in cardiovascular diseases development. However, there are differences between human and animals like rat and mouse. Thus, we should be careful when interpreting data aiming to apply in humans regarding processes related to therapeutic agents, molecular process, and environmental or genetic factors that enhances the risks for cardiovascular disorders development.

3. Sources of ROS in cells

The literature indicated that vascular cells, as well as cardiomyocytes and neurons, produce ROS, contributing to the development of disorders related to the cardiovascular system. Although several enzyme systems produce ROS, many of them are prevalent in pathologic processes. Among the main ROS generators we may include cytochrome P450, the mitochondrial respiratory chain, xanthine oxidase (XO), uncoupled endothelial nitric oxide synthase (eNOS), heme oxygenase, myeloperoxidase, lipoxygenase, cyclooxygenase and NADPH oxidases. Some of these systems have been proven to be relevant to hypertension (Lee & Griendling, 2008).

Others mechanisms involved in ROS production are better described in the chapters from this book. Thus, we will only briefly describe the main sources in this topic.

Based on the literature, the NOX family includes seven members, which are NOX1-5 and DUOX1-2. NOX2 NADPH oxidase is the predominant source of ROS production in humans (Nauseef, 2004). The main sources of ROS are phagocytic cells—neutrophils and macrophages. NOX2-NADPH oxidase is formed by functional transmembrane heterodimers, gp91 phox and p22 phox (also known collectively as the cytochrome b558), and four regulatory cytosolic subunits—p40 phox , p47 phox , p67 phox , and the small GTPase, Rac2. In the dormant state, cytochrome b558 resides in intracellular vesicles, while cytosolic Rac2 remains inactive in the guanosine diphosphate (GDP) bound state via interaction with RhoGDI (Ando et al, 1992). Upon the initiation of phagocytosis, GDP-Rac2 is converted to GTP-Rac2 through the activity of a Rac guanine nucleotide exchange factor. This allows for Rac2 translocation to the plasma or phagosomal membrane, thereby allowing the subsequent transit of cytochrome b558 from the vesicle to the membrane (Diebold and Bokoch, 2001). Concurrently, p47 phox is phosphorylated and undergoes a conformational change that now exposes two SRC-homology 3 regions to interact with the proline rich motif on p22 phox (Dusi et al, 1993). Furthermore, Phox homology domains on p47 phox allow for binding to phosphatidylinositol 3-phosphate (PI(3)P) and PI(3,4)P2, transient phosphoinositides that are generated only at the plasma membrane upon phagocytosis, thus, further stabilizing p47 phox localization to cytochrome b558 (Nauseef, 2004).

Among ROS sources, the NADPH oxidases are considered unique because from those components it is generated ROS in a highly regulated mode whereas ROS are generated as a by-product of enzymatic activity for all the other sources (Cave et al, 2006). Moreover, NADPH oxidases can stimulate further ROS production from one or more of the above enzymes, thereby being able to act as initiating sources of ROS. $O^{2\bullet-}$radical is the first moiety that is generated by NADPH oxidases (or most of the other sources) and can be rapidly dismutated to H_2O_2. The biological effects of ROS are expected to depend on the specific moiety generated, its localization and the relative balance between levels generated and the activity of antioxidant mechanisms; most signaling effects of ROS are considered to be mediated by H_2O_2 which is more stable and diffusible than $O^{2\bullet-}$.

XO is another potential source for ROS in vasculature. XO is a form of xanthine oxidoreductase that occurs in two different forms. The predominant form, xanthine dehydrogenase (XDH), can be converted into XO reversibly by direct oxidation of critical cysteine residues or irreversibly by proteolysis (Harris et al, 1999). XO is expressed mainly in the endothelium, and its expression and activity are enhanced by Ang II or oscillatory shear in a NADPH oxidase-dependent manner (Landmesser et al, 2007).

Mitochondrial electron transport generates $SO^{2\bullet-}$ as a side product of electron transport during oxidative phosphorylation. Most superoxide never escapes the highly reducing state of the mitochondrial matrix. If the $SO^{2\bullet-}$ generation is excessive, however, superoxide can escape to the intermembraneous space and cytosol via anion channels (Aon et al, 2004).

In summary, the investigation of the sources of reactive oxygen species is essential to describe new pathways involved in the pathogenesis of cardiovascular diseases as well as to develop new therapies to treat those disorders.

4. ROS in the heart

It is already known in the literature some mechanisms regarding the role of antioxidants during oxidative stress caused by ROS in the heart tissue. Among the enzymatic and non-enzymatic antioxidants involved in ROS-induced heart tissue injury we may include catalase, glutathione, SOD, ascorbid acid, melatonin, Vitamin C and E, among others. The antioxidant system in SHR cardiomyopathic hearts is induced, possibly due to events of enhanced ROS. This conditioning of the antioxidant system may help to overcome acute stress situations caused by ROS in the failing myocardium (Takimoto & Kass, 2007).

There are several potential sources of ROS in the heart with chronic heart failure (CHF). Excessive ROS derived from mitochondria have been shown in cardiomyocytes from experimental models of myocardial infarction and rapid pacing-induced heart failure (Ide et al, 2001). The enzyme xanthine oxidase produces $O^{2\bullet-}$ as a byproduct of the terminal steps of purine catabolism and recent studies suggest that it collaborates to oxidative stress in CHF. Xanthine oxidase expression and activity are enhanced in experimental models of CHF as well as in human end-stage CHF.

Nitric oxide synthase enzymes normally generate nitric oxide, but may instead generate $O^{2\bullet-}$ if this molecule becomes "uncoupled", a state that is mainly observed likely in the setting of lack of the BH4, which is a NOS cofactor or the NOS substrate l-arginine. NOS uncoupling and subsequent $O^{2\bullet-}$ production are implicated in the genesis of vascular endothelial dysfunction in patients with heart failure (Dixon et al, 2003).

In this context, infiltrating inflammatory cells are also an important source of ROS, mainly in conditions such as myocarditis and in the early stages after myocardial infarction. Recent evidence suggests that complex enzymes called NADPH oxidases are mainly important with regard to redox signalling in CHF and its antecedent conditions (Li et al, 2002). These enzymes catalyse electron transfer from NADPH to molecular oxygen, resulting in the formation of $O^{2\bullet-}$. NADPH oxidase activity has been found to be enhanced in experimental models of left ventricle hypertrophy and CHF as well as in end-stage failing human myocardium (Li et al, 2002).

Interestingly, ROS produced by NADPH oxidases can promote ROS generation by other sources, thereby increasing total levels of ROS. For instance, $O^{2\bullet-}$ from NADPH oxidase may oxidize and degrade BH4, thereby leading to NOS uncoupling, and this mechanism has been shown in diabetes and experimental hypertension (Verhaar et al, 2004). Similarly, NADPH oxidase-derived ROS may also activate xanthine oxidase (Li and Shah, 2004).

Previous studies have already investigated the relationship between the regulation of myocardial growth and death by NADPH oxidase. The classical phagocyte oxidase (gp91phox or Nox2) is also expressed in non-phagocytic cells in the heart, such as cardiomyocytes and fibroblasts (Bendall et al, 2002; Zhang et al, 2006). Activation of Nox2 requires stimulus-induced membrane translocation of cytosolic regulatory subunits, including p47phox, p67phox, p40phox, and Rac1, a small GTPase (Uhlinger et al, 1994). In resting cells, p47phox, p67phox, and p40phox form a ternary complex in the cytoplasm, whereas Rac associates with Rho-GDP dissociation inhibitor. When cells are stimulated with agonists for G protein-coupled receptors, such as angiotensin II (Ang II) type 1 receptors, p47phox is phosphorylated by protein kinase C, which in turn undergoes conformational changes and allows the phox homology (PX) domain and the SH3 domain in p47phox to interact with phosphoinositides and p22phox in the membrane, respectively (Ago et al, 2004). As p67phox and p40phox interact with p47phox, this process leads to membrane translocation of p67phox and p40phox. Rac1 translocates to the membrane independently of p47phox and p67phox, where they form a functional complex with the Nox2-p22phox heterodimer, followed by a transfer of electrons to molecular oxygen (Quinn et al, 1993). Therefore, the activity of Nox2 is subjected to regulation through multiple mechanisms.

In relation to myocardial damage and NADPH oxidase, the loss of cardiomyocytes through apoptosis or necrosis causes impairment in cardiac function in the heart submitted to chronic myocardial infarction (Wencker et al, 2003). Oxidative stress is involved in the pathogenesis of apoptosis through various pathways, in which it is included activation of enzymes involved in pro-apoptotic signaling, for example, JNK, p38, ASK-1, and CaMKII (Matsuzawa and Ichijo, 2005), effects on the cellular anti-apoptotic signaling and direct effects of ROS on mitochondria, leading to cytochrome-c release.

Although excessive production of ROS by Noxs is detrimental, local and modest production of H_2O_2 and $O^{2\bullet-}$ by Noxs allows those component to function as signaling molecules, thereby mediating physiological responses. For instance, since Noxs are functional at low pO_2, Noxs may function as a sensor, and ROS generated by Noxs as a transducer, for hypoxia (Shiose et al, 2001). Erythropoietin (EPO) synthesis occurs in the renal tubular cells, where Nox4 is abundantly expressed (Lacombe et al., 1988). Since DPI, an antioxidant drug, not only blocks oxygen sensing but also inhibits Nox4 in renal tubular cells, it has been proposed that Nox4 is an O_2 sensor in the kidney and may regulate EPO production. The causative role of Nox4 in mediating EPO synthesis through its function as an O_2 sensor remains to be shown. Recently, a role of Nox4 in mediating angiogenesis during cardiac hypertrophy was reported. Pathological hypertrophy induces upregulation/activation of Nox4, which in turn causes stabilization of HIF-1α, upregulation of VEGF, and increases in angiogenesis (Zhang et al, 2006). It appears that the protective effect of Nox4 prevails under the authors' experimental conditions. It remains unknown, however, whether such a mechanism is sufficient to overcome increases in cell death and mitochondrial dysfunction directly caused by upregulation of Nox4 in response to hypertrophic stimuli (Ago et al, 2003).

In addition, the regulation of Ca^{2+} level in cardiac myocytes is centrally important not only in excitation–contraction coupling but also in many other processes such as the regulation of gene expression and cellular energetics. ROS are recognized to be capable of influencing cellular Ca^{2+} regulation at several levels, notably via redox alterations of key amino acid residues involved in the function and gating properties of intracellular and plasma membrane ion channels and transporters — e.g., L-type channels, the Na^+/Ca^{2+} exchanger, the sarcoplasmic reticulum (SR) ATPase (SERCA) and the ryanodine receptor (Hool and Corry, 2007). Recent studies have started to address the role of NADPH oxidase-derived ROS in these effects.

It has been reported that ryanodine receptor-mediated Ca^{2+}-induced Ca^{2+} release in rat cardiac myocytes is inhibited by an endogenous NADH oxidase activity in the SR, although the molecular nature of this oxidase was not established (Cherednichenko et al, 2004). In contrast to this study, Sanchez et al. (2008) reported the presence of Nox2 NADPH oxidase activity in canine cardiac SR and showed that oxidase activation enhanced S-glutathionylation of ryanodine receptors and hence SR Ca^{2+} release – effects which were abrogated by apocynin (a purported Nox inhibitor, but which may act as a non-selective antioxidant). The same group also showed that oxidase activity and the effects on SR Ca^{2+} release were augmented by tachycardia (Sanchez et al, 2008). $O^{2\bullet-}$-radical production by NADPH oxidase on the SR of bovine coronary artery smooth muscle cells has also been shown to regulate calcium-induced calcium release (Yi et al, 2006). In isolated cardiac myocytes, plasma L-type Ca^{2+} channel open-state probability was reportedly enhanced by endothelin-1 together with enhanced NADPH oxidase activity, effects which were abolished in cardiomyocytes pre-treated with a specific NADPH oxidase inhibitor, gp91ds-tat (Zeng et al, 2008). These studies suggest that NADPH oxidases may acutely regulate at least two channels directly involved in intracellular Ca^{2+} homeostasis, i.e. the L-type Ca^{2+} channel and the ryanodine receptor.

In summary, Figure 3 presents the main mechanisms involved in ROS-induced cardiovascular disorders. Many studies implicate ROS-generating NADPH oxidases in redox signaling in cardiovascular cells and involvement in pathological processes such as cardiac hypertrophy, fibrosis, apoptosis and ventricular remodeling.

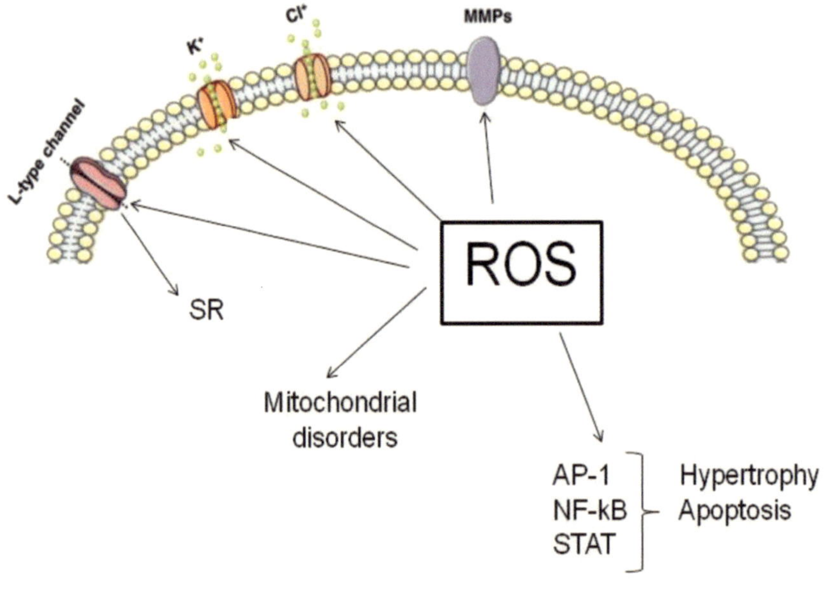

Fig. 3. Main mechanisms involved in the potential effects of NADPH oxidase-derived ROS in the cardiac myocyte. SR: sarcoplasmic reticulum; MMPs: matrix metalloproteinases; CICR: calcium-induced calcium release.

5. ROS-Induced vascular damage

ROS are involved in pathological and physiological processes in the vasculature. Enhanced arterial pressure is partially caused by enhanced total peripheral vascular resistance, which is due to disorders of structural remodeling of blood vessels and vasomotor function. Vascular diseases including coronary artery disease, cerebrovascular and peripheral vascular diseases are the largest cause of mortality and morbidity in industrialized countries. Many common risk factors for vascular disease, such as hypertension and diabetes, remain prevalent in Western and other populations, suggesting that vascular disease will continue to impose a substantial burden on health care resources throughout the next generation. The earliest detectable changes in vascular disease states are irregularities of the endothelium, resulting in loss of the endothelium normal homeostatic functions that normally act to inhibit disease-related processes such as inflammation and thrombosis. In particular, nitric oxide (NO) produced by NO synthase (eNOS) in the vascular endothelium modulates blood flow and pressure (Umans & Levi, 1995) and has important antiatherogenic effects on platelets, vascular smooth muscle and endothelial cells.

It is known that ROS causes vascular tone increase, because it influences endothelium regulatory role and also due to its effects on vascular smooth muscle contractility. By influencing phenotype regulation of vascular smooth muscle cells, death of vascular cells, cell migration, atypical growth, and extracellular matrix (ECM) reorganization, ROS collaborate to vascular remodeling (Lee & Griendling, 2008).

The fact that nitric oxide (NO) is scavenged by superoxide suggests that superoxide production may in part underlie endothelial dysfunction in human atherosclerosis, as it does in some experimental models of vascular disease.

In vitro (Lambeth et al, 2000) and in vivo (Vita et al, 1990) studies indicate that ACh-mediated vasorelaxations in human vessels are inversely related to the number of atherosclerotic risks factors present. Nonetheless, functional studies of human vascular superoxide production have been more limited (Lambeth et al, 2000). It was found large variability in both NO mediated vascular relaxations and basal superoxide production in internal mammary arteries (Huraux et al. (1999), however, there was no consistent associations between these two parameters or with clinical risk factors (Lambeth et al, 2000).

It was investigated superoxide production by NAD(P)H oxidase in human vessels and the relationships between superoxide production, atherosclerotic risk factor profile and endothelial dysfunction. It was reported the expected inverse correlation between risk factor profile and NO-mediated endothelium-dependent relaxations in vessel ring isometric tension studies. However, it was also found that superoxide production by NAD(P)H oxidases progressively enhanced with increasing risk factor profile (Guzik et al, 2000). Furthermore, NAD(P)H oxidase-mediated superoxide production was inversely correlated with NO-mediated vasorelaxations in individual patients, such that patients with the highest superoxide production had the most deficient endothelial function.

The association between enhanced vascular NAD(P)H oxidase activity and impaired endothelial vasorelaxations may be due to direct scavenging of NO by superoxide, as has been demonstrated in animal model systems. However, the both could result independently from increasing exposure of endothelium, media and adventitia to factors acting through different signaling pathways. Alternatively, superoxide may directly modulate NO-mediated vascular signaling, for instance by peroxynitrite-induced nitration of G proteins or other membrane components (Feron et al, 1999). Previous data suggest that G protein-coupled receptor function is deficient in atherosclerosis (Liao & Clark, 1995). Previous observation that vasorelaxations to ACh were significantly lower than maximal relaxations to the calcium ionophore A23187 is consistent with this hypothesis, and with observations in human internal mammary arteries (Hurax et al, 1999). Nevertheless, the significant correlation between ACh and A23187 - induced relaxations, and the association of NADH-dependent superoxide production with both ACh and A231287- stimulated vasorelaxations suggest that a change in G protein-coupled receptor signaling is unlikely to be the sole mechanism underlying decreased NO-mediated vasorelaxations, as A23187 activates endothelial NO synthase independently of any receptor mediated pathway. Alternatively, superoxide may impair endothelial function by direct effects on endothelial NO synthase activity, (Peterson et al, 1999), possibly mediated through oxidation of the NOS cofactor, tetrahydrobiopterin (BH4).

Many studies have focused on the potential role of BH4 oxidation different oxidized biopterin species in reducing BH4 bioavailability for eNOS (Figure 4).

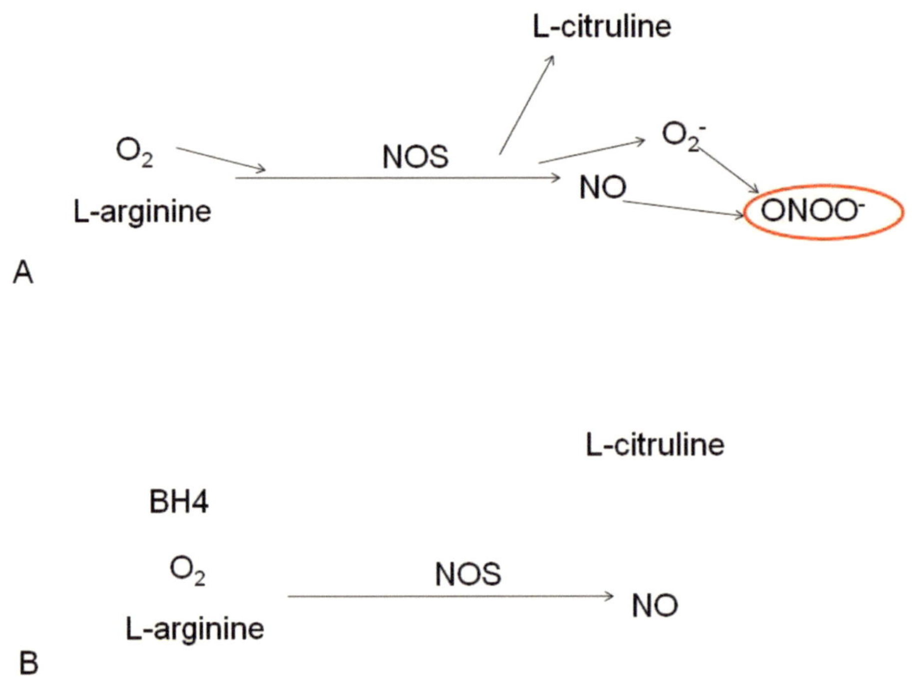

Fig. 4. Schematic representation of nitric oxide synthase (NO synthase) reaction leading to l-citrulline and nitric oxide (NO) from l-arginine and oxygen (O_2) without (A) and with BH4 (B). It is important to note that this reaction without BH4 increases ROS.

Although superoxide can indeed react directly with BH4, the rate constant of this reaction is many orders of magnitude lower than that for NO with superoxide (Vasquez-Vivar et al, 2002). A more likely mechanism for BH4 oxidation is the interaction with peroxynitrite (generated from the interaction between NO and superoxide). It was indicated that peroxynitrite can oxidize BH4 within minutes at physiologically relevant concentrations (Crabtree et al, 2011). EPR (electron paramagnetic resonance) spectroscopy experiments have demonstrated that peroxynitrite oxidizes BH4 to the (non-protonated) BH3 (trihydrobiopterin) radical, and then to BH2, with a rate constant estimated to be 6 × 103 M−1 s−1, several-fold higher than reactions between peroxynitrite and ascorbate, glutathione or thiol groups (Gao et al, 2009). Oxidation not only directly reduces BH4 bioavailability, but the oxidation products themselves (such as BH2), which have no cofactor activity, may compete with BH4 for binding to endothelial NOS (eNOS) (Crabtree et al, 2008).

ROS are also involved in vascular remodeling. Vascular remodeling is defined as alteration of structure leading to alteration in wall thickness and lumen diameter. It can be induced through passive adaptation to chronic changes in hemodynamics and/or through neurohumoral factors including Ang II and ROS. The progression of hypertension involves two different types of vascular remodeling: inward eutrophic remodeling and hypertrophic remodeling (Schiffrin, 2004). Eutrophic remodeling is characterized by decreased lumen size, thickening of the media, enhanced media:lumen ratio and, usually, little change in medial cross-sectional area. In this case, the change in vascular smooth muscle (VSMC) size is negligible (Korsgaard et al, 1993), and medial growth toward the lumen is mainly mediated by reorganization of cellular and non cellular material of the existing vascular wall, accompanied by enhanced apoptosis in the periphery of the blood vessel (166). This is common in small resistance arteries of essential hypertensive patients and SHR (Korsgaard et al, 1993).

On the other hand, hypertrophic remodeling characterized by an increase in wall cross-sectional area predominates in conduit arteries of secondary hypertension, such as those of renovascular hypertensive patients or Ang II-infused hypertensive rats. An increase in cell size and enhanced accumulation of ECM proteins such as collagen and fibronectin are specific features of hypertrophic remodeling (Rizzoni et al, 2000). Hence, VSMC hypertrophy and ECM synthesis are required for hypertrophic remodeling. Both mechanical wall stress and humoral mediators such as Ang II collaborate to hypertrophic remodeling (Rizzoni et al, 2000).

The both forms of remodeling frequently coexist in different vascular beds and at different stages of hypertension, which occurs even in the same subject. Even though the determinants of each type of remodeling have not been clearly described, the reorganization of media mediated by phenotype modulation of VSMCs, migration, cellular growth, apoptosis, and ECM production and rearrangement is thought to be common to both processes. These events occur cooperatively and simultaneously.

Thus, it is not easy to distinguish contributions of each component in vivo. Vascular remodeling is improved by treatment with tempol, antioxidant vitamins (Chen et al, 2011), Ang II receptor antagonists, or NADPH oxidase inhibitors in animal experimental models, as well as in clinical trials (Zhou et al, 2005), emphasizing the role of ROS.

Recent studies with improved forms of ROS scavenging enzymes, specific inhibitors for different ROS generating enzymes, and redox signaling pathway blocking agents allow subtle modulation of redox signaling and may overcome the redundancy of general antioxidant treatments. Therefore, the spatial and temporal aspects of redox signaling in the vasculature are of much importance to understand the etiological role of ROS and to develop better strategies to treat hypertension.

6. Oxidative stress in the kidney

Renal artery obstruction can cause arterial hypertension, which is followed by impaired renal function and renal atrophy. Cardiovascular disorders caused by kidney injury are in part regulated by renin release from the stenotic kidney, with a subsequent increase in angiotensin II (Ang II) synthesis (Trinquart et al, 2010). Ang II results in the activation of $O^{2\bullet-}$ generation through nicotinamide adenine dinucleotide phosphate (NADPH) oxidase, a multi-subunit enzyme, which is one of the enzymatic sources of $O^{2\bullet-}$ (Chabrashvili et al, 2002).

The mechanism(s) by which ANG II produces superoxide is not entirely elucidated yet. However, Mollnau et al. (2002) found that ANG II infusion during seven days enhanced expression of nox 1, gp91(phox), and p22(phox) subunits of NADPH oxidase via a PKC system. The mechanism which involves ANG II-mediated increase in the release of superoxide locates into activity a series of events that may play relevant functions in increased blood pressure.

Previous studies were conducted in attempt to clarify the specific components of ROS that are involved in the development of ANG II-induced hypertension. Haas et al. (1999) are among the first to demonstrate that the slow hypertensive response to ANG II was accompanied by a significant elevation of ROS as estimated indirectly by increases in plasma F2-isoprostanes, an oxidative metabolite of arachidonic acid (Morrow et al, 1990). Nishiyama et al. (2002) also demonstrated that a prolonged infusion of ANG II in rats stimulates ROS production. In this study, the administration of tempol, a SOD mimetic, reversed the vasoconstriction and produced vasodilation via an NO-dependent mechanism.

Ortiz et al. (2011) found in rats that the development of slow pressor responses to ANG II could be inhibited by the administration by antioxidants such as tempol and vitamin E. As a result of antioxidant treatment, there was a fall in renal blood flow and glomerular flow rate, whereas the indexes of oxidative stress, TBARS, and isoprostanes were found to be decreased in peripheral circulation as well as the renal vein.

Some investigations suggest that the decrease in the NO concentration due to interaction with superoxide anon radical constitutes a major component in the development of the observed vasoconstriction. Supporting the assumption that inhibition of NO synthesis enhances the vasoconstrictor effect of ANG II are the studies of Kitamoto et al. (2000). These investigators found that the continuous administration of l-NAME (a NOS inhibitor) to Sprague-Dawley rats for seven days induced ROS production, which was dependent on ANG II, because the effect was blocked by the administration of ANG II receptor blockers. Relevant to these findings are the studies of Usui et al. (1999), who also found an increase in ROS produced byl-NAME, which was blocked by the administration of antioxidants. In this study, l-NAME blockade was associated with an increase in angiotensin converting enzyme activity in the aorta. The studies of Kitamoto et al. (2000) and Usui et al. (199) reveal an interesting aspect of ANG II, NO, and oxidative stress. They suggest that a simple decrease in NO synthesis leaves unbalanced ANG II, which induces ROS release. This situation will be further stimulated by the increase in converting enzyme activity, which can accelerate the production of ANG II causing a positive feedback for oxidative stress.

The question of whether NO inhibition alone can cause ROS production without the participation of ANG II should be further explored. As mentioned previously, NOS can produce superoxide when BH4 is oxidized to BH4, leading to an increase in ROS and a reduction in NO (Figure 4). This could set up a vicious cycle that accentuates NO dysfunction and tends to perpetuate oxidative stress. These alterations may constitute an important mechanism of dysregulation that produces hypertension and renal dysfunction (see later). An example of this alteration is the SHR in which blood pressure can be normalized by the administration of BH4 (McIntyre et al, 1997).

Researches performed in the renovascular model of hypertension in rats have shown relevant data regarding the relationship between oxidative stress and hypertension. The central regulation of the sympathetic nervous system (SNS)

involved in cardiovascular regulation is complex, involving multiple reflex pathways and neural connections with a large number of neurotransmitters and neuromodulators acting in specific groups of neurons in the central nervous sysem (CNS) involved in the tonic and reflex control of the cardiovascular system. In the CNS, Ang II is able to increase sympathetic vasomotor tone and blood pressure, and is involved in the pathogenesis of many experimental models of hypertension. Thus, the close functional association between NADPH oxidase and the Ang II is of particular relevance in linking oxidative stress in the brain to sympathoexcitation and hypertension (Campos, 2009). For instance, intracerebroventricular infusion of NADPH oxidase inhibitor antagonizes the pressor response induced by centrally mediated Ang II actions (Gao et al, 2004).

In the brain, the overexpression of SOD, an enzyme responsible for O_2 breakdown, also abolishes the central pressor effect of the octapeptide (Zimmerman et al, 2004) suggesting that in the CNS there is a positive correlation between the increase in ROS and the central pressor response mediated by Ang II. Considering that the paraventricular nucleus of the hypothalamus (PVN) and the rostroventrolateral medulla (RVLM) contain critically important neurons involved in the control of sympathetic vasomotor tone and arterial pressure (Colombari et al, 2001).

Previous studies reviewed and examined whether there was an increase in AT1 receptor expression and oxidative stress markers within these two nuclei in 2K1C hypertension. NAD(P)H oxidase subunits (p47phox and gp91phox) and antioxidant enzyme CuZnSOD mRNA expression were quantified in the RVLM and PVN of 2K1C hypertensive rats. It was hypothesized that the overactivity of NADPH oxidase-derived ROS associated with a reduction in the activity of CuZnSOD within the RVLM and PVN could collaborate to 2K1C hypertension, particularly in the renin-dependent phase of hypertension.

In summary, the recent studies support the idea that an increase in ROS in the kidney is involved in the development of cardiovascular disorders, playing a major role in maintaining high arterial pressure and sympathetic drive under conditions of renovascular hypertension.

7. The involvement of the nervous system in ROS-induced cardiovascular disease

Neurons in the brain present increased density of polyunsaturated fatty acids in its cell membranes. Fatty acids are targets of free radicals. An indirect marker of ROS, TBARS is enhanced in the brainstem of SPSHR compared to age-matched control (Hirooka, 2008). Others reported enhanced ROS in the brainstem of rabbits with heart failure (Gao et al, 2007).

The activity of sympathetic and parasympathetic systems, which are both involved in cardiopulmonary reflex, as well as the cardiovascular regulation, is under the control of a medullary circuitry comprising the nucleus of the solitary tract (NTS), rostral (RVLM) and caudal ventrolateral medulla (CVLM) and the nucleus ambiguous. Drugs injection into the fourth cerebral ventricle (4th V) may easily reach structures surrounding the ventricular system like the area postrema and the dorsal motor nucleus of the vagus (Colombari et al, 2001) (Figure 5). Those areas are also involved in cardiovascular reflex responses, in which we may include baroreflex (Valenti et al, 2009a; Valenti et al, 2009b; Cisternas et al, 2010).

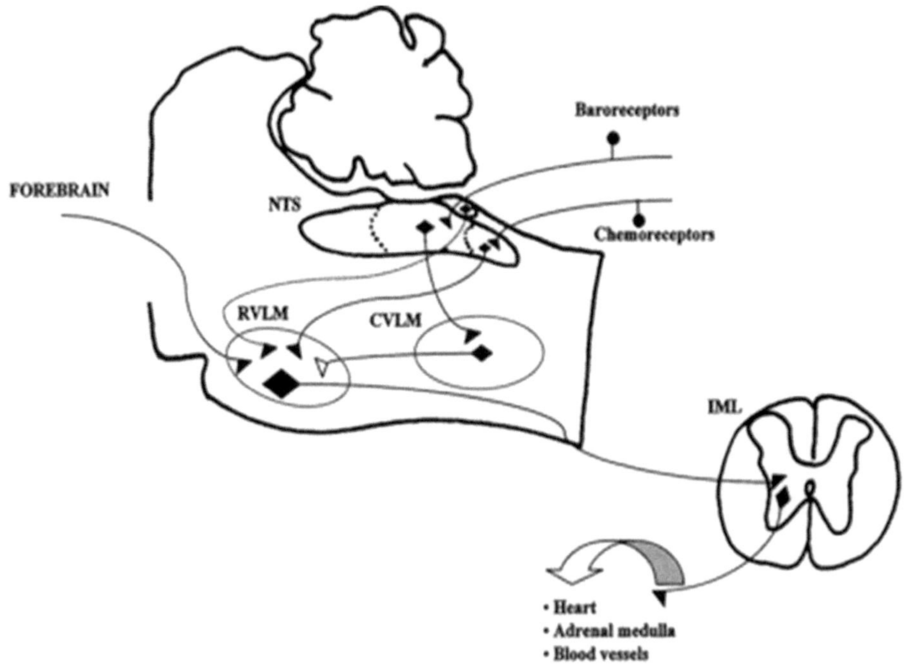

Fig. 5. Schematic sagittal view of the medulla oblongata showing brain pathways implicated in neurogenic hypertension. Premotor neurons from the RVLM send excitatory synapses to preganglionic neurons situated in the intermediolateral cell column (IML), providing sympathetic efference to target organs. The RVLM is the group of neurons that receive excitatory afference from the commissural nucleus of the solitary tract (NTS) and area postrema. It also receives inhibitory afferences from the caudoventrolateral medulla (CVLM). Adapted from Valenti et al, 2007.

A previous investigation suggested that brain ROS is associated with enhanced sympathetic activity (Gao et al, 2007) and systemic ROS is also related to impaired baroreflex (Bertagnolli et al, 2006). In addition, it was reported increase of NAD(P)H oxidase activity and expression into the RVLM, the primary central site for the maintenance of sympathetic nerve activity, in CHF rabbits. In the same sequence of procedures, the same authors observed that a reduction of brain $O^{2\bullet -}$ by tempol, a SOD mimetic, decreased the sympathetic outflow in chronic heart failure rabbits. Conversely, an increase of central $O^{2\bullet -}$ due to administration of the SOD inhibitor diethyldithiocarbamic acid enhanced the sympathetic outflow in both normal and chronic heart failure rabbits (Gao et al, 2007). Taken together, those data suggest that antioxidant enzymes, i.e., SOD and catalase, into the brainstem are involved in baroceptor reflex regulation, since baroreflex is modulated by sympathetic and parasympathetic activity (Valenti et al, 2009a).

Recent studies from our laboratory have investigated the effects of ROS into the fourth cerebral ventricle (4th V) on cardiovascular responses.

In one study (Valenti et al, 2011a) it was evaluated the effects of 3-amino-1,2,4-triazole (ATZ), a catalase inhibitor, into the 4th V on baroreflex components in conscious rats. It was revealed that this drug significantly attenuated bradycardic and tachycardic reflex, bradycardic peak and it also decreased heart rate range 30 minutes after its injection. While in Wistar rats treated with vehicle (saline 0.9%) there were no significant changes regarding baseline mean arterial pressure (MAP) and heart rate (HR) and baroreflex components. Considering that the tachycardia (tachycardic reflex) in response to SNP is mediated by both sympathetic and parasympathetic activity (Stornetta et al, 1987) and that we reported reduction in the maximal parasympathetic responses to elevation in mean arterial pressure, while there were no changes in tachycardic peak response to decrease in mean arterial pressure (highest sympathetic response), we suggest that ATZ into the 4th V is acutely involved with parasympathetic activity but is not involved in baroreflex changes. The lack of any change in the vehicles groups is consistent with this assumption. In view of the anatomical scope of the 4th V, an action on an only one neuronal cluster is not an easy accomplishment. However, prior researches indicated a preference for parasympathetic system which modulates HR, such as the dorsal motor nucleus of the vagus and nucleus ambiguous, which receive glutamathergic projections from the nucleus of the solitary tract (Colombari et al, 2001).

In another study (Valenti et al, 2011b), it was evaluated the effects of catalase inhibition into the 4th V on cardiopulmonary reflex in conscious Wistar rats. In this method, we used male Wistar rats, which were implanted with a stainless steel guide cannula in the 4th V. The femoral artery and vein were cannulated for MAP and HR measurement and for drug infusion, respectively. After basal mean arterial pressure and heart rate recordings, the cardiopulmonary reflex was tested with a dose of phenylbiguanide (PBG, 8 μg/kg, bolus). Cardiopulmonary reflex was evaluated before and 15 minutes after 1 μl of ATZ (0.01 g/100 μl) injection into the 4th V. Vehicle treatment did not change cardiopulmonary reflex responses. ATZ injected into the 4th V significantly enhanced hypotensive responses without influencing the bradycardic reflex. Taken together, those data suggested that ATZ injected into the 4th V increases sympathetic inhibition but does not change the parasympathetic component of the cardiopulmonary reflex in conscious Wistar rats.

Nevertheless, opposite findings were found in SHR. Another study (Valenti et al, 2011c) was undertaken to evaluate the acute effects of central n-acetylcysteine, an antioxidant drug, on baroreflex in juvenile SHR and age-matched Wistar Kyoto (WKY) rats. It was observed that n-acetylcysteine injection into the 4th V did not significantly change baroreflex gain, bradycardic and tachycardic reflex, bradycardic and tachycardic peak in SHR and WKY rats. Interestingly, n-acetylcysteine caused slight but significant increase in basal heart rate 15 minutes after its injection in conscious WKY rats.

Many previous studies have already demonstrated the effects of oxidative stress in cardiovascular reflex. Zanzinger and

Czachurski (2009) demonstrated that SOD injected into the RVLM decreased sympathetic nerve activity in swine. Several groups have now shown that ROSs stimulate sympathetic outflow (Campese et al, 2004). Campos et al (2011) evidenced that the lack of LDL receptor enhanced cholesterol blood levels, enhanced ROS and impaired baroreflex sentivity. Monahan et al (2007) supported the hypothesis that oxidative stress collaborates to age-associated decreases in cardiovagal baroreflex sensitivity in healthy men. On the other hand, Wright et al (2009) indicated that in male smokers, circulating antioxidants had no effect on baroceptor reflex function and minor effects on the cardiovascular system were seen following acute fat and vitamin ingestion.

In the central nervous system, the complex regulating blood pressure is contained within topographically selective networks characterized at all levels of the neuraxis. Adjustments in this modulation network may lead to labile changes in autonomic function. The development of neurogenic hypertension may involve improper alterations in synaptic function within these networks. Thus, investigations regarding the relationship between the nervous system and the cardiovascular system and its importance to regulation of the physiologic homeostasis are always welcome in the basic and clinical research.

8. Perspectives

At the moment, relevant milestones were achieved with the availability of more overt facts that demonstrates that cardiovascular disorders mechanisms are linked to ROS increase and dysregulation of oxidant-antioxidants systems. The oxidation and nitration of cellular lipids, proteins and nucleic acids, and formation of aggregates of oxidized molecules underlie the loss of cellular function, cellular ageing and the inability of cells to withstand physiological stresses. Moreover, ROS regulate energy metabolism and signal transduction mechanisms in response to situations of nitrosativeor or oxidative stress. Sources of ROS, physiological and pathophysiological conditions, and cellular oxidant targets determine the profile nature of a disease process and resultant outcomes.

In summary, the data presented in this chapter is significant to the literature, because progress in redox signaling provides insight into the function of ROS in the pathological and physiological mechanisms involved in cardiovascular disorders. Nonetheless, the literature raises more questions. Regarding hypertension treatment, there are a few points to be underscored. ROS act as signaling molecules associated with diverse physiological mechanism which are indispensable for normal function of the brainstem. Inappropriate modulation of ROS impairs redox signaling, which is assumed to stimulate pathologic situations, in which we may include hypertension. Moreover, our study reinforces the importance to investigate the integrative neuroscience.

9. Concluding remarks

Advances in ROS signaling provide insight into the role of ROS in the pathological and physiological mechanisms related to cardiovascular disorders. The comprehension of how redox state regulates the cardiovascular system is a relevant step for a best explanation for the mechanism involved in antioxidant species applied in clinical therapies. Therefore, the presentation of data regarding the systems different from the cardiovascular system implicated in ROS-induced cardiovascular diseases is relevant to the integrative physiology and more particularly to control physiology and clinical therapies that aim to prevent cardiovascular disorders such as hypertension and heart failure.

10. References

Aasum, E., Belke, D.D., Severson, D.L., Riemersma, R.A., Cooper, M., Andreassen, M., Larsen, T.S. (2002). Cardiac function and metabolism in type 2 diabetic mice after treatment with BM 17.0744, a novel PPAR-alpha activator. *American Journal of Physiology Heart and Circulatory Physiology,* Vol. 283, No 3 (Septembey), pp. H949–H957, ISSN 0363-6135

Aasum, E., Hafstad, A.D., Severson, D.L., Larsen, T.S. (2003). Age-dependent changes in metabolism, contractile function, and ischemic sensitivity in hearts from db/db mice. *Diabetes, Vol.* 52, No. 2 (February) pp. 434–441, ISSN 1939-327X

Abdilla, N., Tormo, M.C., Fabia, M.J., Chaves, F.J., Saez, G., Redon, J. (2007). Impact of the components of metabolic syndrome on oxidative stress and enzymatic antioxidant activity in essential hypertension. *Journal of Human Hypertension,* V. 21, No.1 (April), pp. 68–75, ISSN 0950-9240

Ago, T., Kuribayashi, F., Hiroaki, H., Takeya, R., Ito, T., Kohda, D. (2003). Phosphorylation of p47phox directs phox homology domain from SH3 domain toward phosphoinositides, leading to phagocyte NADPH oxidase activation. *Proceedings of the National Academic of Science,* USA Vol. 100, No. 8 (April), pp. 4474–4479, ISSN 0027-8424

Ando, S., Kaibuchi, K., Sasaki, T., Hiraoka, K., Nishiyama, T., Mizuno, T., Asada, M., Nunoi, H., Matsuda, I., Matsuura, Y. (1992). Post-translational processing of rac p21s is important both for their interaction with the GDP/GTP exchange proteins and for their activation of NADPH oxidase. *Journal of Biological Chemistry,* Vol. 267, No. 36 (Decembey), pp. 25709–25713, ISSN 0021-9258

Aon, M.A., Cortassa, S., O'Rourke, B. (2004). Percolation and criticality in a mitochondrial network. *Proceedings of the National Academic of Science,* USA Vol. 101, No. 13 (March), pp. 4447–4452, ISSN 0027-8424

Banday, A.A., Muhammad, A.B., Fazili, F.R., Lokhandwala, M. (2007). Mechanisms of oxidative stress-induced increase in salt sensitivity and development of hypertension in Sprague-Dawley rats. *Hypertension,* V. 49, No. 3 (March), pp. 664–671, ISSN 0194-911X

Barouch, L.A., Berkowitz, D.E., Harrison, R.W., O'Donnell, C.P., Hare, J.M. (2003). Disruption of leptin signaling collaborates to cardiac hypertrophy independently of body weight in mice. *Circulation,* Vol. 108, No. 6 (August), pp. 754–759, ISSN 0009-7322

Bendall, J.K., Cave, A.C., Heymes, C., Gall, N., Shah, A.M. (2002). Pivotal role of a gp91(phox)-containing NADPH oxidase in angiotensin II-induced cardiac hypertrophy in mice. *Circulation,* Vol. 105, No. 3 (January) pp. 293–296, ISSN 0009-7322

Bertagnolli, M., Campos, C., Schenkel, P.C., de Oliveira, V.L., De Angelis, K., Belló-Klein, A., Rigatto, K., Irigoyen, M.C. (2006) Baroreflex sensitivity improvement is associated with decreased oxidative stress in trained spontaneously hypertensive rat. Journal of Hypertension, Vol. 24, No. 12 (December), pp. 2437-2443, ISSN 0895-7061

Brownlee, M. (1995). Advanced protein glycosylation in diabetes and aging. *Annual Review of Medicine,* Vol. 46 pp. 223–234, ISSN 0066-4219

Buchanan, J., Mazumder, P.K., Hu, P., Chakrabarti, G., Roberts, M.W., Yun, U.J., Cooksey, R.C., Litwin, S.E., Abel, E.D. (2005). Decreased cardiac efficiency and altered substrate metabolism precedes the onset of hyperglycemia and contractile dysfunction in two mouse models of insulin resistance and obesity. *Endocrinology,* Vol. 146, No. 12 (Decembey), pp. 5341–5349, ISSN 1945-7170

Cai, H., Harrison, D.G. (2000). Endothelial dysfunction in cardiovascular diseases: the role of oxidant stress. *Circulation Research,* V. 87, No. 10 (Novembey), pp. 840–844, ISSN 009-7300

Cai, L., Wang, Y., Zhou, G., Chen, T., Song, Y., Li, X., Kang, Y.J. (2006). Attenuation by metallothionein of early cardiac cell death via suppression of mitochondrial oxidative stress results in a prevention of diabetic cardiomyopathy. *Journal of the American College of Cardiology,* Vol. 48, No. 8 (Octobey), pp. 1688–1697, ISSN 0735-1097

Campese, V.M., Ye, S., Zhong, H., Yanamadala, V., Ye, Z., Chiu, J. (2004). Reactive oxygen species stimulate central and peripheral sympathetic nervous system activity. *American Journal of Physiology Heart and Circulatory Physiology,* V. 287, No.2 (August), pp. H695-H703, ISSN 0363-6135

Campos, R.R. (2009). Oxidative stress in the brain and arterial hypertension. (2009). *Hypertension Research,* V. 32, No. 12 (Decembey), pp. 1047–8, ISSN 0916-9636

Campos, R.R., Oliveira-Sales, E.B., Nishi, E.E., Boim, M.A., Dolnikoff, M.S., Bergamaschi, C.T. (2011). The role of oxidative stress in renovascular hypertension. *Clinical and Experimental Pharmacology and Physiology,* V. 38, No. 2 (February) pp. 144-52, ISSN 1440-1681

Cave, A.C., Brewer, A.C., Narayanapanicker, A., Ray, R., Grieve, D.J., Walker, S. (2006). NADPH oxidases in cardiovascular health and disease. *Antioxidan Redox Signaling,* Vol. 8, No. 5-6 (June), pp. 691–728, ISSN 1523-0864

Ceriello, A., Giugliano, D., Quatraro, A., Lefebvre, P.J. (1991). Antioxidants show an anti-hypertensive effect in diabetic and hypertensive subjects. *Clinical Science,* V. 81, No. 9 (Decembey), pp. 739–742, ISSN 0143-5221

Chabrashvili, T., Tojo, A., Onozato, M.L. (2002). Expression and cellular localization of classic NADPH oxidase subunits in the spontaneously hypertensive rat kidney. *Hypertension,* V. 39, No. 2 (February) pp. 269–74, ISSN 0194-911X

Chen, X., Touyz, R.M., Park, J.B., Schiffrin, E.L. (2001). Antioxidant effects of vitamins C and E are associated with altered activation of vascular NADPH oxidase and superoxide dismutase in strokeprone SHR. *Hypertension,* Vol. 38, No. 3 Pt2 (Septembey), pp. 606–611, ISSN 0950-9240

Cherednichenko, G., Zima, A.V., Feng, W., Schaefer, S., Blatter, L.A., Pessah, I.N. (2004). NADH oxidase activity of rat cardiac sarcoplasmic reticulum regulates calcium-induced calcium release. *Circulation Research,* Vol. 94, No. 4 (March), pp. 478–486, ISSN 009-7300

Christoffersen, C., Bollano, E., Lindegaard, M.L., Bartels, E.D., Goetze, J.P., Andersen, C.B., Nielsen, L.B. (2003). Cardiac lipid accumulation associated with diastolic dysfunction in obese mice. *Endocrinology,* Vol. 144, No. 8 (August), pp. 3483–3490, ISSN 1945-7170

Cisternas, J.R., Valenti, V.E., Alves, T.B., Ferreira, C., Petenusso, M., Breda, J.R., Pires, A.C., Tassi, N., de Abreu, L.C. (2010) Cardiac baroreflex is already blunted in eight weeks old spontaneously hypertensive rats. *International Archives of Medicine,* Vol. 3 (January), pp. 2, ISSN 1755-7682

Colombari, E., Sato, M.A., Cravo, S.L., Bergamaschi, C.T., Campos, R.R. Jr., Lopes, O.U. (2001). Role of the medulla oblongata in hypertension. *Hypertension,* Vol. 38, No. 3 (September), pp. 549-54, ISSN 0950-9240

Crabtree, M.J., Smith, C.L., Lam, G., Goligorsky, M.S., Gross, S.S. 8-Dihydrobiopterin in endothelial cells determines glucose-elicited changes in NO vs superoxide production by eNOS. *American Journal of Physiology Heart and Circulatory Physiology,* V. 294, No. 4 (April), pp. H1530-H1540, ISSN 0363-6135

Crabtree, M.J., Hale, A.B., Channon, K.M. (2011). Dihydrofolate reductase protects endothelial nitric oxide synthase from uncoupling in tetrahydrobiopterin deficiency. *Free Radical Biology & Medicine,* Vol. 50, No. 11 (June), pp. 1639-46, ISSN 0891-5849

Cracowski, J.L., Baguet, J.P., Ormezzano, O., Bessard, J., Stanke–Labesque, F., Bessard, G., Mallion, J.M. (2003). Lipid peroxidation is not enhanced in patients with untreated mild-to-moderate hypertension. *Hypertension,* V. 41, No. 2 (February) pp. 286–288, ISSN 0194-911X

Diebold, B.A., Bokoch, G.M. (2001). Molecular basis for Rac2 regulation of phagocyte NADPH oxidase. *Nature Immunology,* Vol. 2, No. 3 (March), pp. 211–215, ISSN 1529-2908

Dixon, L.J., Morgan, D.R., Hughes, S.M., McGrath, L.T., El-Sherbeeny, N.A., Plumb, R.D., Devine, A., Leahey, W., Johnston, G.D., McVeigh, G.E. (2003). Functional consequences of endothelial nitric oxide synthase uncoupling in congestive cardiac failure. *Circulation,* Vol. 107, No. 13 (April), pp. 1725-8, ISSN 0009-7322

Dusi, S., Della Bianca, V., Grzeskowiak, M., Rossi, F. (1993). Relationship between phosphorylation and translocation to the plasma membrane of p47phox and p67phox and activation of the NADPH oxidase in normal and Ca(2+)-depleted human neutrophils. *Biochemical Journal,* Vol. 290 No. Pt1 (February) pp. 173–178, ISSN 0264-6021

Elahi, M.M., Matata, B.M. (2006). Free radicals in blood: evolving concepts in the mechanism of ischemic heart disease. *Archives of Biochemistry andl Biophysics,* Vol. 450, No. 1 (June), pp. 78-88, ISSN 003-9861

Feron, O., Dessy, C., Moniotte, S., Desager, J.P., Balligand, J.L. (1999). Hypercholesterolemia decreases nitric oxide production by promoting the interaction of caveolin and endothelial nitric oxide synthase. *Journal of Clinical Investigation,* Vol. 103, No. 6 (March), pp. 897-905, ISSN 0021-9738

Galley, H.F., Thornton, J., Howdle, P.D., Walker, B.E., Webster, N.R. (1997). Combination oral antioxidant supplementation reduces blood pressure. *Clinical Science,* Vol. 92, No.4 (April), pp. 361–365, ISSN 0143-5221

Gao, L., Wang,W., Liu, D., Zucker, I.H. (2007). Exercise training normalizes sympathetic outflow by central antioxidant mechanisms in rabbits with pacing-induced chronic heart failure. *Circulation,* Vol. 115, No. 24 (June), pp. 3095-102, ISSN 0009-7322

Gao, L., Pung, Y.F., Zhang, J., Chen, P., Wang, T., Li, M., Meza, M., Toro, L., Cai, H. (2009). Sepiapterin reductase regulation of endothelial tetrahydrobiopterin and nitric oxide bioavailability. *American Journal of Physiology Heart and Circulatory Physiology,* Vol. 297, No. 1 (July) pp. H331-H339, ISSN 0363-6135

Guzik, T.J., West, N.E., Black, E., McDonald, D., Ratnatunga, C., Pillai, R., Channon, K.M. (2000). Vascular superoxide production by NAD(P)H oxidase: association with endothelial dysfunction and clinical risk factors. *Circulation Research,* Vol. 86, No. 9 (May) pp. E85-E90, ISSN 009-7300

Haas JA, Krier JD, Bolterman RJ, Juncos LA, Romero JC. (1999). Low-dose angiotensin II increases free isoprostane levels in plasma. *Hypertension,* Vol. 34, No. 4 Pt2 (Octobey), pp. 983–986, ISSN 0950-9240

Han, Y., Zhang, Y., Wang, H.J., Gao, X.Y., Wang, W., Zhu, G.Q. (2005). Reactive oxygen species in paraventricular nucleus modulates cardiac sympathetic afferent reflex in rats. *Brain Research,* Vol. 1058, No. 1-2 (Octobey), pp. 82-90, ISSN 0006-8993

Harris, C.M., Sanders, S.A., Massey, V. (1999). Role of the flavin midpoint potential and NAD binding in determining NAD versus oxygen reactivity of xanthine oxidoreductase. *Journal of Biological Chemistry,* Vol. 274, No. 8 (February) pp. 4561–4569, ISSN 0021-9258

He, X., Zhang, H.L., Zhao, M., Yang, J.L., Cheng, G., Sun, L., Li, D.L., Jiang, H.K., Zhao, Q., Yu, X.J., Zang, W.J. (2007). Amlodipine ameliorates endothelial dysfunction in mesenteric arteries from spontaneously hypertensive rats. *Clinical and Experimental Pharmacology and Physiology,* Vol. 38, No. 4 (April), pp. 255-61, ISSN 1440-1681

Hirooka, Y. (2008). Role of reactive oxygen species in brainstem in neural mechanisms of hypertension. *Autonomic Neuroscience,* Vol. 142, No. 1-2 (Novembey), pp. 20-4, ISSN 1566-0702

Hool, L.C., Corry, B. (2007). Redox control of calcium channels: from mechanisms to therapeutic opportunities. *Antioxidant and Redox Signal,* Vol., No. 4 (April), pp. 409–435, ISSN 1523-0864

Huraux, C., Makita, T., Kurz, S., Yamaguchi, K., Szlam, F., Tarpey, M.M., Wilcox, J.N., Harrison, D.G., Levy, J.H. (1999). Superoxide production, risk factors, and endotheliumdependent relaxations in human internal mammary arteries. *Circulation,* Vol. 99, No. 1 (January) pp. 53-59, ISSN 0009-7322

Ide, T., Tsutsui, H., Hayashidani, S., Kang, D., Suematsu, N., Nakamura, K., Utsumi, H., Hamasaki, N., Takeshita, A. (2001). Mitochondrial DNA damage and dysfunction associated with oxidative stress in failing hearts after myocardial infarction. *Circulation Research,* Vol. 88, No. 5 (March), pp. 529-35, ISSN 009-7300

Kishi, T., Hirooka, Y., Kimura, Y., Ito, K., Shimokawa, H., Takeshita, A. (2004). Enhanced reactive oxygen species in rostral ventrolateral medulla collaborate to neural mechanisms of hypertension in stroke-prone spontaneously hypertensive rats. *Circulation,* Vol. 109, No. 19 (May) pp: 2357–2362, ISSN 0009-7322

Kitamoto, S., Egashira, K., Kataoka, C., Usui, M., Koyanagi, M., Takemoto, M., Takeshita, A. (2000) Chronic inhibition of nitric oxide synthesis in rats increases aortic superoxide anion production via the action of angiotensin II. *Journal of Hypertension,* Vol. 18, No. 12 (Decembey), pp. 1795–1800 ISSN 0895-7061

Korsgaard, N., Aalkjaer, C., Heagerty, A.M., Izzard, A.S., Mulvany, M.J. (1993). Histology of subcutaneous small arteries from patients with essential hypertension. *Hypertension,* Vol. 22, No. 4 (Octobey), pp. 523–526, ISSN 0950-9240

Lacombe, C., Da Silva, J.L., Bruneval, P., Fournier, J.G., Wendling, F., Casadevall, N. (1988). Peritubular cells are the site of erythropoietin synthesis in the murine hypoxic kidney. *Jounal of Clinical Investigation,* Vol. 81, No. 2 (February) pp. 620–623, ISSN 0021-9738

Lambeth, J.D., Cheng, G., Arnold, R.S., Edens, W.A. (2000). Novel homologs of gp91phox. *Trends in Biochemical Science,* Vol. 25, No. 10 (Octobey), pp. 459-461, ISSN 0968-0004

Landmesser, U., Spiekermann, S., Preuss, C., Sorrentino, S., Fischer, D., Manes, C., Mueller, M., Drexler, H. 2007). Angiotensin II induces endothelial xanthine oxidase activation: role for endothelial dysfunction in patients with coronary disease. *Arteriosclerosis, Thrombosis, and Vascular Biology,* Vol. 27, No. 4 (April), pp. 943-8, ISSN 1524-4636

Lee, M.Y., Griendling, K.K. (2008). Redox signaling, vascular function, and hypertension. *Antioxidants and Redox Signaling,* Vol. 10, No. 6 (June), pp. 1045-59, ISSN 1523-0864

Lenda, D.M., Sauls, B.A., Boegehold, M.A. (2000). Reactive oxygen species may collaborate to decreased endothelium-dependent dilation in rats fed high salt. *American Journal of Physiology,* Vol. 279, No. 1 (July) pp. H7–H14, ISSN 0002-9513

Lerman, L.O., Schwartz, R.S., Grande, J.P., Sheedy, P.J., Romero, J.C. (1990). Noninvasive evaluation of a novel swine model of renal artery stenosis. *Journal of the American Society of Nephrology,* Vol. 10, No 7 (July) pp. 1455–65, ISSN 1555-9041

Li, J.M., Gall, N.P., Grieve, D.J., Chen, M., Shah, A.M. (2002). Activation of NADPH oxidase during progression of cardiac hypertrophy to failure. *Hypertension,* Vol. 40, No. 4 (Octobey), pp. 477-84, ISSN 0950-9240

Li, J.M., Shah, A.M. (2004). Endothelial cell superoxide generation: regulation and relevance for cardiovascular pathophysiology. *American Journal of Physiology,* Vol. 287, No. 5 (Novembey), pp. R1014–R1030.R1030, ISSN 0363-6135

Li, S.Y., Yang, X., Ceylan-Isik, A.F., Du, M., Sreejayan, N., Ren, J. (2006). Cardiac contractile dysfunction in Lep/Lep obesity is accompanied by NADPH oxidase activation, oxidative alteration of sarco(endo)plasmic reticulum Ca2+-ATPase and myosin heavy chain isozyme switch. *Diabetologia,* Vol. 49, No. 6 (June), pp. 1434–1446, ISSN 0012-186X

Liao, J.K., Clark, S.L. (1995). Regulation of G-protein alpha i2 subunit expression by oxidized lowdensity lipoprotein. *Journal of Clinical Investigation,* Vol. 95, No. 4 (April), pp. 1457-1463, ISSN 0021-9738

Lushchak, V.I. (2011). Environmentally induced oxidative stress in aquatic animals. *Aquatic Toxicology,* Vol. 101, No. 1 (January), pp. 13-30, ISSN 0166-445X a

Lushchak, V.I. (2011). Adaptive response to oxidative stress: Bacteria, fungi, plants and animals. *Comparative Biochemistry and Physiology: Toxicology and Pharmacology,* Vol. 153, No. 2 (March), pp. 175-190 ISSN b

Manning, R.D. Jr, Meng, S., Tian, N. (2003). Renal and vascular oxidative stress and salt-sensitivity of arterial pressure. *Acta Physiologica Scandinava,* Vol. 179, No. 3 (Novembey), pp. 243–250, ISSN 0001-6772

Matkovics, B., Sasvari, M., Kotorman, M., Varga, I.S., Hai, D.Q., Varga, C. (1997). Further prove on oxidative stress in alloxan diabetic rat tissues. *Acta Physiologica Hungarica,* Vol. 85, No. 3, pp. 183–192, ISSN 0231-424X

Matsuzawa, A., Ichijo, H. (2005). Stress-responsive protein kinases in redox-regulated apoptosis signaling. *Antioxidants and Redox Signaling,* Vol. 7, No. 3-4 (March-April), pp. 472–481, ISSN 1523-0864

McIntyre M, Hamilton CA, Rees DD, Reid JL, Dominiczak AF. (1997). Sex differences in the abundance of endothelial nitric oxide in a model of genetic hypertension. *Hypertension,* Vol. 30, No. 6 (December), pp. 1517–1524, ISSN 0950-9240

Mollnau, H., Wendt, M., Szocs, K., Lassegue, B., Schulz, E., Oelze, M., Li, H., Bodenschatz, M., August, M., Kleschyov, A.L., Tsilimingas, N., Walter, U., Forstermann, U., Meinertz, T., Griendling, K., Munzel, T. (2002). Effects of angiotensin II infusion on the expression and function of NAD(P)H oxidase and components of nitric oxide/cGMP signaling. *Circulation Research,* Vol. 90, No. 4 (March), pp. E58–E65, ISSN 009-7300

Monahan, K.D., Eskurza, I., Seals, D.R. (2007). Ascorbic acid increases cardiovagal baroreflex sensitivity in healthy older men. *American Journal of Physiology Heart and Circulatory Physiology,* Vol. 3, No. 6 (June), pp. H2113-H2117, ISSN 0363-6135

Moreno, M.U., San Jose, G., Orbe, J., Paramo, J.A., Beloqui, O., Diez, J., Zalba, G. (2003). Preliminary characterisation of the promoter of the human p22(phox) gene: identification of a new polymorphism associated with hypertension. *FEBS Letter,* Vol. 542, No. 1-3 (May) pp. 27–31, ISSN 0014-5793

Morrow, J.D., Harris, T.M., Roberts, L.J. 2nd. (1990). Noncyclooxygenase oxidative formation of a series of novel prostaglandins: analytical ramifications for measurement of eicosanoids. *Analytical Biochemistry,* Vol. 184, No. 1 (January) pp. 1–10, ISSN 0003-2697

Mousa, T.M., Liu, D., Cornish, K.G., Zucker, I.H. (2008). Exercise training enhances baroreflex sensitivity by an angiotensin II-dependent mechanism in chronic heart failure. *Journal of Applied Physiology,* Vol. 104, No. 3 (March), pp. 616:624, ISSN 8750-7587

Nauseef, W.M. (2004). Assembly of the phagocyte NADPH oxidase. *Histochemistry andl Cell Biology,* Vol. 122, No. 4 (Octobey), pp. 277–291, ISSN 1432-119X

Nishiyama, A., Seth, D.M., Navar, L.G. (2002). Renal interstitial fluid concentrations of angiotensins I and II in anesthetized rats. *Hypertension,* Vol. 39, No. 1 (January) pp. 129–134, ISSN 0950-9240

Oliveira-Sales, E.B., Dugaich, A.P., Abreu, N.P. (2009). Oxidative stress supports blood pressure and sympathetic activity in renovascular hypertension. *American Journal of Hypertension,* Vol. 21, No. 5 (May) pp. 98–104, ISSN 0895-7061

Olukman, M., Orhan, C.E., Celenk, F.G., Ulker, S. (2010). Apocynin restores endothelial dysfunction in streptozotocin diabetic rats through regulation of nitric oxide synthase and NADPH oxidase expressions. *Journal of Diabetes and its Complications,* Vol. 24, No. 6 (Novembey), pp. 415-23, ISSN 1056-8727

Ortiz, M.C., Manriquez, M.C., Romero, J.C., Juncos, L.A. (2001). Antioxidants block angiotensin II-induced increases in blood pressure and endothelin. *Hypertension,* Vol. 38, No. 3 Pt 2 (Septembey), pp. 655–659, ISSN 0950-9240

Pacher, P., Szabo, C. Role of the peroxynitritepoly(ADP-ribose), polymerase pathway in human disease. *The American Journal of Pathology,* Vol. 173, No. 1 (July) pp. 2-13, ISSN 0002 9440

Palm, F., Onozato, F., Welch, W.J., Wilcox, C.S. (2010). Blood pressure, blood flow, and oxygenation in the clipped kidney of chronic 2-Kidney, 1-clip rats: Effects of tempol and Angiotensin blockade. *Hypertension,* Vol. 55, No. 2 (February) pp. 298–304, ISSN 0950-9240

Papaharalambus, C.A., Griendling, K.K. (2007). Basic mechanisms of oxidative stress and reactive oxygen species in cardiovascular injury. *Trends in Cardiovascular Medicine,* Vol. 17, No.2, (February), pp. 48 - 54, ISSN 1050-1738

Peterson, T.E., Poppa, V., Ueba, H., Wu, A., Yan, C., Berk, B.C. (1999). Opposing effects of reactive oxygen species and cholesterol on endothelial nitric oxide synthase and endothelial cell caveolae. *Circulation Research,* Vol. 85No. 1 (July) pp. 29-37, ISSN 009-7300

Puzserova, A., Bernatova, I. (2010). Chronic social stress increases nitric oxide-dependent vasorelaxation in normotensive rats. *Interdisciplinary Toxicology,* Vol. 3, No. 4, (Decembey), pp. 109-17, ISSN 1337-9569

Quinn, M.T., Evans, T., Loetterle, L.R., Jesaitis, A.J., Bokoch, G.M. (1993). Translocation of Rac correlates with NADPH oxidase activation. Evidence for equimolar translocation of oxidase components. *Journal of Biological Chemistry,* Vol. 268, No. 28 (Octobey), pp. 20983–20987, ISSN 0021-9258

Rajagopalan, S., Kurz, S., Munzel, T., Tarpey, M., Freeman, B.A., Griendling, K.K., Harrison, D.G. (1996). Angiotensin II-mediated hypertension in the rat increases vascular superoxide production via membrane NADH/NADPH oxidase activation. Contribution to alterations of vasomotor tone. *Journal of Clinical Investigation,* Vol. 97, No. 8 (April), pp. 1916–1923, ISSN 0021-9738

Rees, D.A., Alcolado, J.C. (2005). Animal models of diabetes mellitus. *Diabetic Medicine,* V. 22, No. 4 (April), pp. 359–370, ISSN 0742-3071

Rizzoni, D., Porteri, E., Guefi, D., Piccoli, A., Castellano, M., Pasini, G., Muiesan, M.L., Mulvany, M.J., Rosei, E.A. (2000). Cellular hypertrophy in subcutaneous small arteries of patients with renovascular hypertension. *Hypertension,* Vol. 35, No. 4 (April), pp. 931–935, ISSN 0950-9240

Rodriguez-Iturbe, B., Zhan, C.D., Quiroz, Y., Sindhu, R.K., Vaziri, N.D. (2003). Antioxidant-rich diet relieves hypertension and reduces renal immune infiltration in spontaneously hypertensive rats. *Hypertension,* Vol. 41, No. 2 (February) pp. 341–346, ISSN 0950-9240

Russell, J.C., Proctor, S.D. (2006). Small animal models of cardiovascular disease: tools for the study of the roles of metabolic syndrome, dyslipidemia, and atherosclerosis. *Cardiovascular Pathology,* Vol. 15, No. 6 (Novembey), pp. 318-30, ISSN 1054-8807

Sanchez, G., Escobar, M., Pedrozo, Z., Macho, P., Domenech, R., Hartel, S. (2008). Exercise and tachycardia increase NADPH oxidase and ryanodine receptor-2 activity: possible role in cardioprotection. *Cardiovascular Research,* Vol. 77, No. 2 (January) pp. 380–386, ISSN 1755-3245

Saraiva, R.M., Minhas, K.M., Zheng, M., Pitz, E., Treuer, A., Gonzalez, D., Schuleri, K.H., Vandegaer, K.M., Barouch, L.A., Hare, J.M. (2006). Decreased neuronal nitric oxide synthase expression collaborates to cardiac oxidative stress and nitroso-redox imbalance in ob/ob mice. *Nitric Oxide,* Vol. 16, No. 3 (May) pp. 331–338, ISSN 1089-8603

Shen, X., Zheng, S., Metreveli, N.S., Epstein, P.N. (2006). Protection of cardiac mitochondria by overexpression of MnSOD reduces diabetic cardiomyopathy. *Diabetes,* Vol. 55, No. 3 (March), pp. 798–805, ISSN 1939-327X

Schiffrin, E.L. (2004). Remodeling of resistance arteries in essential hypertension and effects of antihypertensive treatment. *American Journal of Hypertension,* Vol. 17, No. 12 Pt 1 (Decembey), pp. 1192–1200, ISSN 0895-7061

Shiose, A., Kuroda, J., Tsuruya, K., Hirai, M., Hirakata, K., Naito, S. (2001). A novel superoxide-producing NAD(P)H oxidase in kidney. *Journal of Biological Chemistry,* Vol. 276, No. 2 (January) pp. 1417–1423, ISSN 0021-9258

Shokoji, T., Nishiyama, A., Fujisawa, Y., Hitomi, H., Kiyomoto, H., Takahashi, N., Kimura, S., Kohno, M., Abe, Y. (2003). Renal sympathetic nerve responses to tempol in spontaneously hypertensive rats. *Hypertension,* Vol. 41, No. 2 (February) pp. 266–273, ISSN 0950-9240

Stornetta, R.L., Guyenet, P.G., McCarty, R.C. (1987) Autonomic nervous system control of heart rate during baroreceptor activation in conscious and anesthetized rats. *Autonomic Neuroscience: Clinical and Basic,* Vol. 20, No. 2 (August), pp. 121-7, ISSN 1566-0702

Takimoto, E., Kass, D.A. (2007). Role of oxidative stress in cardiac hypertrophy and remodeling. *Hypertension,* Vol. 49, No. 2 (February) pp. 241-8, ISSN 0950-9240

Toba, H., Nakashima, K., Oshima, Y., Kojima, Y., Tojo, C., Nakano, A., Wang, J., Kobara, M., Nakata, T. (2010). Erythropoietin prevents vascular inflammation and oxidative stress in subtotal nephrectomized rat aorta beyond haematopoiesis. *Clinical and Experimental Pharmacology and Physiology,* Vol. 37, No. 12 (Decembey), pp. 1139-46, ISSN 1440-1681

Touyz, R.M. (2003). Reactive oxygen species in vascular biology: role in arterial hypertension. *Expert Review of Cardiovascular Theraphy,* Vol. 1, No. 1 (May) pp. 91–106, ISSN 1477-9072

Trinquart L, Mounier-Vehier C, Sapoval M, Gagnon N, Plouin PF. (2010). Efficacy of revascularization for renal artery stenosis caused by fibromuscular dysplasia: a systematic review and meta-analysis. *Hypertension,* Vol. 56, No. 3 (Septembey), pp. 525-32, ISSN 0950-9240

Uhlinger, D.J., Taylor, D.J., Lambeth, J.D. (1994). p67-phox enhances the binding of p47-phox to the human neutrophil respiratory burst oxidase complex. *Journal of Biological Chemistry,* Vol. 269, No. 35 (Septembey), pp. 22095–22098, ISSN 0021-9258

Umans, J.G., Levi, R. (1995). Nitric oxide in the regulation of blood flow and arterial pressure. *Annual Review of Physiology,* Vol. 57, pp. 771-790, ISSN 0066-4294

Usui M, Egashira K, Kitamoto S, Koyanagi M, Katoh M, Kataoka C, Shimokawa H, Takeshita A. (1999). Pathogenic role of oxidative stress in vascular angiotensin-converting enzyme activation in long-term blockade of nitric oxide synthesis in rats. *Hypertension,* Vol. 34, No. 4 Pt1 (October), p. 546–551 ISSN 0950-9240

Valenti, V. E., Sato, M.A., Ferreira, C., Abreu, L.C. (2007) Neural regulation of the cardiovascular system: Bulbar centers. Revista de Neurociências, Vol. 15, No. 4 (December), pp. 317-320, ISSN 0104-3579

Valenti, V.E., Ferreira, C., Meneghini, A., Ferreira, M., Murad, N., Ferreira Filho, C., Correa, J.A., Abreu, L.C., Colombari, E. (2009) Evaluation of baroreflex function in young spontaneously hypertensive rats. *Arquivos Brasileiros de Cardiologia,* Vol. 92, No. 3 (March), pp. 205-15, ISSN 0066-782X a

Valenti, V.E., Imaizumi, C., de Abreu, L.C., Colombari, E., Sato, M.A., Ferreira, C. (2009) Intra-strain variations of baroreflex sensitivity in young Wistar-Kyoto rats. Clinical and Investive Medicine, Vol. 32, No. 6 (December), pp.E251, ISSN 0147-958X b

Valenti, V.E., de Abreu, L.C., Sato, M.A., Fonseca, F.L., Pérez Riera, A.R., Ferreira, C. (2011). Catalase inhibition into the fourth cerebral ventricle affects bradycardic parasympathetic response to increase in arterial pressure without changing the baroreflex. *Journal of Integrative Neuroscience,* Vol. 10, No. 1 (March), pp. 1-14, ISSN 0219-6352 a

Valenti, V.E., Abreu, L.C., Sato, M.A., Ferreira, C. (2011). ATZ (3-amino-1,2,4-triazole) injected into the fourth cerebral ventricle influences the Bezold-Jarisch reflex in conscious rats. *Clinics,* Vol. 65, No 12 (December), pp. 1339-43, ISSN 807-5932 b

Valenti, V.E., De Abreu, L.C., Sato, M.A., Saldiva, P.H., Fonseca, F.L., Giannocco, G., Riera, A.R., Ferreira, C. (2011). Central N-acetylcysteine effects on baroreflex in juvenile spontaneously hypertensive rats. *Journal of Integrative Neuroscience,* Vol. 10, No. 2 (June), pp. 161-76, ISSN 0219-6352 c

Van den Bergh, A., Flameng, W., Herijgers, P. (2006). Type II diabetic mice exhibit contractile dysfunction but maintain cardiac output by favourable loading conditions. *European Journal of Heart Failure,* Vol. 8 No. 8 (Decembey), pp. 777–783, ISSN 1388-9842

Vasquez-Vivar, J., Duquaine, D., Whitsett, J., Kalyanaraman, B., Rajagopalan, S. (2002). Altered tetrahydrobiopterin metabolism in atherosclerosis: implications for use of oxidized tetrahydrobiopterin analogues and thiol antioxidants, Arteriosclerosis *Arteriosclerosis, Thrombosis, and Vascular Biology,* Vol. 22, No. 10 (Octobey), pp. 1655-1661, ISSN 1524-4636

Verhaar, M.C., Westerweel, P.E., van Zonneveld, A.J., Rabelink, T.J. (2004). Free radical production by dysfunctional eNOS. *Heart,* Vol. 90, No. 5 (May) pp. 494-5, ISSN 1468-201X

Vita, J.A., Treasure, C.B., Nabel, E.G., McLenachan, J.M., Fish, R.D., Yeung, A.C., Vekshtein, V.I., Selwyn, A.P., Ganz, P. (1990). Coronary vasomotor response to acetylcholine relates to risk factors for coronary artery disease. *Circulation,* Vol. 81, No. 2 (February) pp. 491-497, ISSN 0009-7322

Welch, W.J., Mendonca, M., Aslam, S., Wilcox, C.S. (2003). Roles of oxidative stress and AT1 receptors in renal hemodynamics and oxygenation in the postclipped 2K, 1C kidney. *Hypertension,* Vol. 41 No. 3 (March), pp. 692–6, ISSN 0950-9240

Wencker, D., Chandra, M., Nguyen, K., Miao, W., Garantziotis, S., Factor, S.M. (2003). A mechanistic role for cardiac myocyte apoptosis in heart failure, *Journal of Clinical Investigation,* Vol. 111, No. (10 (May) pp. 1497–1504, ISSN 0021-9738

Wright, C.I., Ruediger, H., Kroner, C.I., Janssen, B.J., Draijer, R. (2009). Acute autonomic effects of vitamins and fats in male smokers. *European Journal of Clinical Nutrition,* Vol. 63, No. 2 (February) pp. 246-52, ISSN 0954-3007

Yi, X.Y., Li, V.X., Zhang, F., Yi, F., Matson, D.R., Jiang, M.T. (2006). Characteristics and actions of NAD(P)H oxidase on the sarcoplasmic reticulum of coronary artery smooth muscle. *American Journal of Physiology Heart and Circulatory Physiology,* Vol. 290, No. 3 (March), pp. H1136–H1144, ISSN 0363-6135

Zalba, G., San Jose, G., Beaumont, F.J., Fortuno, M.A., Fortuno, A., Diez, J. (2001). Polymorphisms and promoter overactivity of the p22(phox) gene in vascular smooth muscle cells from spontaneously hypertensive rats. *Circulation Research,* Vol. 88, No. 2 (February) pp. 217–222, ISSN 009-7300

Zanzinger, J., Czachurski, J. (2009). Chronic oxidative stress in the RVLM modulates sympathetic control of circulation in pigs. *Pflugers Archives,* V. 439, No. 4, (Febreuary), pp. 489-494, ISSN 0031-6768

Zeng, Q., Zhou, Q., Yao, F., O'Rourke, S.T., Sun, C. (2006). Endothelin-1 regulates cardiac L-type calcium channels via NAD(P)H oxidase-derived superoxide. *Journal of Pharmacology and Experimental Therapeutics,* Vol. 326, No. 3 (Septembey), pp. 732–738, ISSN 0022-3565

Zhang, M., Kho, A.L., Anilkumar, N., Chibber, R., Pagano, P.J., Shah, A.M. (2006). Glycated proteins stimulate reactive oxygen species production in cardiac myocytes: involvement of Nox2 (gp91phox)-containing NADPH oxidase. *Circulation,* Vol. 113, No. 9 (March), pp. 1235–1243, ISSN 0009-7322

Zhou, M.S., Jaimes, E.A., Raij, L. (2005). Vascular but not cardiac remodeling is associated with superoxide production in angiotensin II hypertension. *Journal of Hypertension,* Vol. 23, No. 9 (Septembey), pp. 1737–1743, ISSN 1473-5598

Zimmerman, M.C., Lazartigues, E., Sharma, R.V., Davisson, R.L. (2004). Hypertension caused by angiotensin II infusion involves enhanced superoxide production in the central nervous system. *Circulation Research,* Vol. 95 No. 2 (July) pp. 210–6, ISSN 009-7300

4

Oxidative Stress in the Carotid Body: Implications for the Cardioventilatory Alterations Induced by Obstructive Sleep Apnea

Rodrigo Iturriaga and Rodrigo Del Rio
Laboratorio de Neurobiología, Departamento de Fisiología, Facultad de Ciencias Biológicas, P. Universidad Católica de Chile, Santiago, Chile

1. Introduction

The obstructive sleep apnea (OSA) syndrome is recognized as an independent risk factor for systemic hypertension. The OSA syndrome is characterized by cyclic episodes of oxygen desaturation due to the partial or complete obstruction of the air flow during sleep. Among the disturbances produced by OSA, the chronic intermittent hypoxia is considered the main factor for developing hypertension. Oxidative stress, inflammation, and sympathetic hyperactivity have been proposed as pathogenic mechanisms involved in the hypertension. However, evidence for a single mechanism has been difficult to establish in OSA patients, because of concomitant comorbidities. Since OSA patients show augmented reflex sympathetic, cardiovascular and ventilatory responses to acute hypoxia, it has been proposed that an enhance carotid body responsiveness to hypoxia is involved in the pathological alterations induced by OSA. This proposal has received further support, since studies performed in animals have shown that intermittent hypoxia selectively enhances the carotid body chemosensory and ventilatory responses to acute hypoxia, producing long-term potentiation of the motor ventilatory and sympathetic discharges. The mechanisms underlying the enhanced carotid body chemosensory reactivity to hypoxia induced by intermittent hypoxia are not completely known. Nevertheless, the available evidence indicates that the repeated episodes of hypoxia-reoxygenation produce local oxidative stress in the carotid body due to the accumulation of reactive oxygen species. In this chapter, we will review and discuss the new evidence supporting the essential role played by the carotid body chemoreceptors, and the contribution of the oxidative stress, endothelin-1 and pro-inflammatory cytokines to the progression of the cardioventilatory alterations induced by chronic intermittent hypoxia.

2. The carotid body chemoreceptors

Most of the mammalian cells respond to hypoxia modifying the expression of genes and proteins, which induce a physiological response to recover the tissue oxygen levels (i.e.

angiogenesis). However, gene expression induction is not fast enough to counteract a rapid drop in systemic oxygen levels. Only the peripheral chemoreceptors located in the carotid and aortic bodies are capable to evoke fast systemic adjustments to overcome a hypoxic episode. The carotid body located in the bifurcation of the carotid arteries is the main arterial chemoreceptor in terms of its contribution to the reflex ventilatory responses to hypoxia (Gonzalez et al., 1994). In humans and mammals, the carotid body initiates the hyperventilatory response induced by hypoxia and activates the sympathetic nervous system. The carotid body is a complex chemoreceptor organ with a high blood flow formed by different types of cells. The glomus cells are considered the oxygen sensors in the carotid body. Glomus cells establish synaptic contacts with the nerve terminals of the primary sensory neurons, whose soma are located in the petrosal ganglion (Gonzalez et al., 1994, Iturriaga & Alcayaga, 2004, Iturriaga et al., 2007). The current model for oxygen chemoreception in the carotid body states that low oxygen induced the inhibition of a voltage-independent potassium TASK-like current, leading to the depolarization of the glomus cells, followed by the entry of Ca^{2+} through L-type Ca^{2+} channels and the subsequent release of one or more excitatory transmitters, which in turn increase the discharges of action potentials in the nerve endings of the chemosensory neurons (Iturriaga & Alcayaga 2004, Iturriaga et al., 2007). The glomus cells contain several molecules proposed as putative excitatory transmitters, such as dopamine, acetylcholine, adenosine nucleotides and peptides. Among these molecules present in glomus cells, acetylcholine and adenosine triphosphate fulfill most of the criteria to be considered as the excitatory transmitters between the glomus cells and petrosal nerve ending (Iturriaga et al., 2007). However, other molecules such as dopamine, histamine, nitric oxide and endothelin-1 acts as modulators of the chemosensory process, acting on the glomus cells or controlling the vasomotor tone of the blood vessel (Iturriaga et al., 2007). More recently, it has been proposed that pro-inflammatory cytokines, such as tumor necrosis factor-α (TNF-α), interleukin 6 (IL-6) and interleukin 1β (IL-1β) are excitatory modulators of the chemoreception process in the rat carotid body (Lam et al., 2008, Liu et al., 2009, Shu et al., 2007).

3. Cardiovascular alterations in patients with obstructive sleep apnea and animals exposed to intermittent hypoxia

The OSA syndrome, a highly prevalent sleep-breathing disorder is now recognized as an independent risk factor for systemic hypertension. Approximately 50% of the OSA patients develop systemic diurnal hypertension and 30% of the hypertensive patients have OSA. The OSA syndrome is also associated with stroke, pulmonary hypertension, coronary artery disease and atrial fibrillation (Garvey et al., 2009, Parati et al., 2007, Somers et al., 2008). The OSA syndrome affect up to 5% worldwide adult population, but according to the report of the American Heart Association in collaboration with the National Heart, Lung, and Blood Institute National Center on Sleep Disorders Research (Somers et al., 2008) "85% of patients with clinically significant and treatable OSA have never been diagnosed, and referral populations of OSA patients represent only the *tip of the iceberg* of OSA prevalence". OSA is characterized by recurrent episodes of partial or complete obstruction of the air flow during sleep produced by the collapse of the pharyngeal airway. The interruption of the air flow produces hypoxia and hypercapnia, negative intrathoraxic pressure, sleep fragmentation and arousal. During the airway occlusion, hypoxia and hypercapnia stimulate the carotid body chemoreceptors increasing the respiratory muscle effort, the vascular sympathetic tone and the arterial blood pressure. Finally, the stimulation of the carotid body chemoreceptors and probably the pulmonary mechanoreceptors elicit arousal and restores the ventilation. Among the disturbances produced by OSA, the exposure to intermittent hypoxia is considered the main factor for developing hypertension. Oxidative stress, inflammation and sympathetic overflow have been proposed as potential pathogenic mechanisms involved in the onset of the hypertension and cardiovascular diseases (Arnardottir et al., 2009, Garvey at al., 2009, Lavie 2003, Somers et al., 2008). However, conclusions from studies performed in humans are conflictive, because of concomitant effects of comorbidities (obesity, cardiovascular diseases, diabetes, etc) associated with OSA (Gozal & Kheirandish-Gozal, 2008, Somer et al., 2008). Thus, animal models of chronic intermittent hypoxia (CIH), which simulate the hypoxic-reoxygenation cycles observed in OSA patients, reproduce several pathologic cardiovascular features of OSA (Fletcher et al., 1992, Pack 2009; Schulz et al., 2008). The hypoxic-reoxygenation episodes in OSA patients enhance the cardiorespiratory and sympathetic responses to acute hypoxia (Carlson et al., 1993; Narkiewicz et al., 1998a, 1998b, 1999); impair the autonomic regulation of the heart rate and the arterial blood pressure (Narkiewicz et al., 1999b, Shiomi et al., 1996) and exacerbate the renin-angiotensin system (Fletcher et al., 2002, Moller et al., 2003). Similarly, animals exposed to intermittent hypoxia show potentiated sympathetic discharges and vascular responses to hypoxia, and develop systemic hypertension (Dick et al., 2007; Fletcher et al., 1992, Greenberg et al., 1999, Zoccal et al., 2008). The autonomic hyperactivity is associated with a reduction of the efficiency of the baroreflex control of heart rate and alterations of heart rate variability in OSA patients (Narkiewicz et al., 1998b, Shiomi et al., 1996) and animals exposed to intermittent hypoxia (Lai et al., 2006; Lin et al., 2007; Rey et al., 2004, 2008). Thus, it is likely that the enhanced sympathetic activity along with the reduction of the baroreflex efficiency would impair the regulation of heart rate and the vasomotor tone of blood vessels eliciting hypertension. Besides that, it has been found that intermittent hypoxia produces parasympathetic withdrawal, attributed in part to neuronal loss in the vagal ambiguous nucleus (Lin et al., 2007, Yan et al., 2008).

4. Contribution of the carotid body to the cardiorespiratory alterations in obstructive sleep apnea and animal exposed to intermittent hypoxia

Patients with recently diagnosed OSA show enhanced ventilatory, sympathetic and vasopressor responses to acute hypoxia, attributed to a potentiated hypoxic chemoreflex (Cistulli & Sullivan, 1994). Narkiewicz et al., (1999) studied the ventilatory, tachycardic and hypertensive responses to acute hypoxia in untreated normotensive OSA patients, and found that the hypoxic stimulation evokes higher ventilatory, tachycardic, and blood pressor responses in OSA patients than control subjects, but the ventilatory and blood pressor responses induced by hypercapnia and by the cold pressor tested in OSA patients were not different from control subjects. Loredo et al., (2001) reported that OSA hypertensive patients present higher basal tidal volumes, suggesting an enhanced carotid body chemosensory drive. Leuenberger et al., (2007) measured changes in sympathetic discharges recorded from the peroneal nerve of normal humans in response to acute hypoxic stimulation before and after the exposure to 30 episodes of apnea. The episodes of apnea do not only increased sympathetic discharges and produced mild increases in arterial blood pressure, but also enhanced the sympathetic neural response to acute hypoxia, indicating that short-term intermittent hypoxia produces a facilitation of the hypoxic chemoreflex in normal humans. Thus, the available evidence supports the proposal that the enhanced oxygen chemoreflex response in OSA patients is produced by the intermittent hypoxia. Similarly, rats and cats exposed to chronic intermittent hypoxia show enhanced hypoxic ventilatory responses to acute hypoxia (Iturriaga et al., 2009, Rey et al., 2004; Reeves et al., 2003) and long-term facilitation of respiratory motor responses (McGuire et al., 2003, Dick et al., 2007, Prahbakar et al., 2005). The long-term potentiated ventilatory responses to acute hypoxia observed in animals exposed to intermittent hypoxia has been attributed to a central facilitation of the serotonin-mediated motor ventilatory output (McGuire et al., 2003). Although, Narkiewicz et al., (1998a, 1998b) found that sympathetic, pressor and ventilatory responses to acute hypoxia were enhanced in OSA patients, and Fletcher et al., (1992) reported that the bilateral carotid body denervation prevents the hypertension in rats exposed to intermittent hypoxia, the idea that carotid body chemoreceptors are involved in the progression of the hypertension did not receive much attention. However, new evidence obtained in the last decade have shown that an abnormal potentiated carotid chemosensory reactivity to hypoxia is crucial to potentiate the sympathetic activity (Iturriaga et al., 2005, 2009, Feng et al., 2008, Garvey at al., 2009; Prabhakar et al., 2005, Rey et al., 2004; Smith & Pacchia, 2007).

5. Intermittent hypoxia enhanced the carotid body chemosensory responses to acute hypoxia

Recording of chemosensory discharges from the carotid sinus nerve have shown that chronic intermittent hypoxia produces long-term potentiation of the carotid body chemosensory responses to acute hypoxia. Indeed, exposure of cats and rats to intermittent hypoxia for 4 to 10 days increases the basal carotid body chemosensory discharges measured in normoxia and enhances the chemosensory responses to acute hypoxia (Peng et al., 2003, Rey et al., 2004, Del Rio et al., 2010). Peng et al., (2003) found that the baseline carotid discharge and the chemosensory responses to acute hypoxia were higher in rats exposed to short cyclic hypoxic episodes followed by normoxia, applied during 8 hrs for 10 days. Similarly, we found that cats exposed to intermittent hypoxia during 8 hrs for 4 days showed enhanced CB chemosensory and ventilatory responses to acute hypoxia (Rey et al., 2004). In rats, we found that intermittent hypoxia for 7 days potentiates the carotid chemosensory responses to acute hypoxia, effect that persisted until 21 days of intermittent hypoxia when animals developed hypertension (Del Rio et al., 2011). Figure 1 illustrates representative recordings of carotid chemosensory responses induced by short hypoxic challenges in a sham rat and in one carotid body from a rat exposed to 5% O_2, 12 times/hr during 8 hrs for 21 days. As is shown in fig. 1, chronic intermittent hypoxia increased the baseline carotid chemosensory discharges measured in normoxia and induced a potentiation of chemosensory responses to acute hypoxia. Since these alterations in the carotid chemosensory function occurred without significant elevation of the arterial blood pressure until 21 days of intermittent hypoxia, the hypertension was preceded by an early potentiation of the carotid body chemosensory and ventilatory responses to hypoxia.

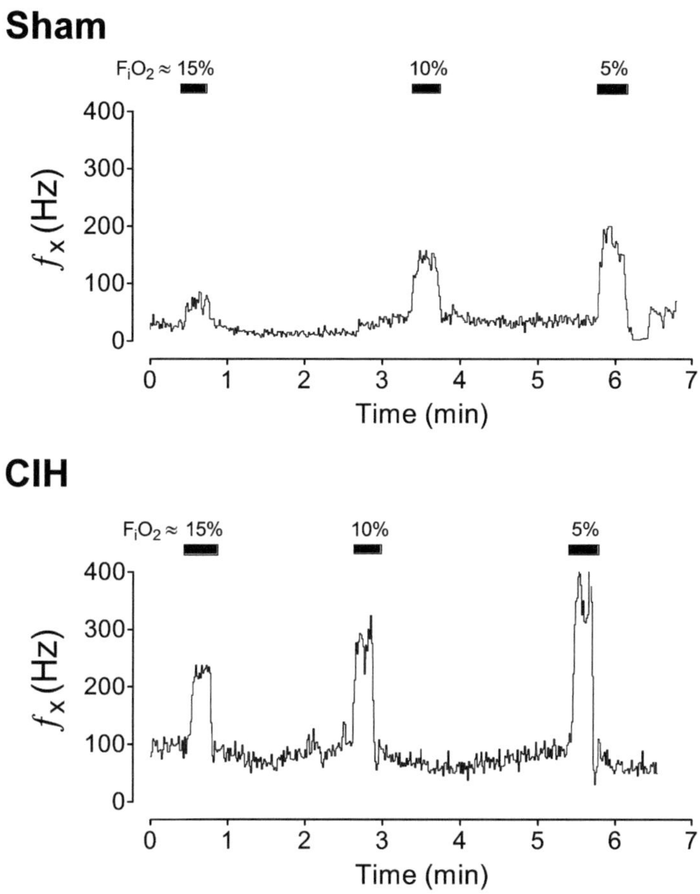

Fig. 1. Carotid body chemosensory potentiation induced by intermittent hypoxia in the rat. The carotid chemosensory discharges in response to various levels of inspired O_2 (FiO_2 ~15 to 5%) were measured from the carotid sinus nerve of a sham rat exposed to air to air cycles and a rat exposed to chronic intermittent hypoxia (CIH) for 21 days. f_X, frequency of carotid chemosensory discharges, expressed in Hz.

6. Mechanisms underlying the potentiation of carotid body chemosensory responses to hypoxia induced by chronic intermittent hypoxia

The enhance carotid chemosensory responses to hypoxia has been associated to increased levels of reactive oxygen species (Peng et al., 2003, Iturriaga et al., 2009, Del Rio et al., 2010) and endothelin-1 within the CB (Rey et al., 2006, Pawar et al., 2009), but it is possible that pro-inflammatory cytokines, which increased in the plasma of OSA patients (Lavie 2003, Jelic et al., 2008) may also contributes to the enhanced carotid body chemosensory responses to acute hypoxia (Iturriaga et al., 2009; Del Rio et al., 2011). Although some studies addressed the effects of intermittent hypoxia on transmitter production and release in the carotid body, very little is known on the functional significance of the role played by the neurotransmitters in the carotid body chemosensory potentiation induced by intermittent hypoxia (See for review Kumar, 2011).

6.1 Reactive oxygen and nitrogen species

Reactive oxygen species (ROS) and reactive nitrogen species (RNS) have been proposed as mediators of the cardiovascular and cognitive morbidities in several diseases including the OSA syndrome (Christou et al., 2003; Gozal & Kheirandish-Gozal, 2008, Lavie 2003) and in pathological consequences of intermittent hypoxia in animal models (Chen et al., 2005, Del Rio et al., 2010, Peng et al., 2003, Peng et al., 2009). Studies performed in OSA patients and animals exposed to chronic intermittent hypoxia have shown that the cyclical episodes of hypoxia-reoxygenation produces systemic oxidative stress due to the accumulation of ROS and RNS, which are well known potential sources of cellular damage. Peng et al., (2003) found evidence that the superoxide radical participates in the potentiation of the rat carotid chemosensory responses to hypoxia induced by intermittent hypoxia. They found that pre-treatment of rats for 10 days before the exposure to intermittent hypoxia with the superoxide dismutase mimetic, manganese (III) tetrakis (1-methyl-4-pyridyl) porphyrin pentachloride (MnTMPyP) prevents the potentiation of the carotid body chemosensory response to hypoxia. In addition, they found that intermittent hypoxia decreases the activity of the ROS sensitive enzyme aconitase in the whole carotid body, as well as the activity of the complex I of the mitochondrial electron transport chain, suggesting that the mitochondria is one of the sources of ROS (Peng & Prabhakar, 2003). More recently, Peng et al., (2009) tested the hypothesis that ROS generated by NADPH oxidase (NOX) mediate the intermittent hypoxia-induced carotid body potentiation. They found that acute hypoxia produced a larger increase in NOX activity in carotid body of rats exposed to intermittent hypoxia for 10 days than that of control carotid bodies. The carotid body chemosensory potentiation was prevented by NOX inhibitors and was not observed in NOX2 deficient mice. On the other hand, MacFarlane and Mitchell (2008) found that application of MnTMPyP into the intrathecal space of the cervical spinal cord abolished the phrenic long-term potentiation induced by acute intermittent hypoxia in rats, suggesting that ROS production is needed for enhancing the phrenic nerve ventilatory discharge. Consequently, ROS formation seems to be necessary for respiratory plasticity induced by intermittent hypoxia, at the level of the carotid body and respiratory motor output. Recently, we tested the hypothesis that oxidative stress contributes to the carotid chemosensory potentiation and the progression of the hypertension in rats exposed to intermittent hypoxia (Del Rio et al., 2010). We hypothesized that oral supplementation of the common antioxidant ascorbic acid (vitamin C) may prevent the carotid chemosensory potentiation and the cardioventilatory alterations including the hypertension induced by the intermittent hypoxic exposure. Accordingly, we studied the effects of ascorbic acid supplementation in the drinking water (1.25 g/l) on plasma lipid peroxidation, arterial blood pressure, and carotid chemosensory responses to acute hypoxia in rats exposed to short hypoxic episodes (5% O_2, 12 times/hr for 8 hrs) for 21 days (Del Rio et al., 2010). We found that exposure of the rats to intermittent hypoxia increased the plasma lipid peroxidation and the formation of 3-nitrotyrosine in the carotid body, the arterial blood pressure and enhanced the carotid chemosensory and ventilatory responses to hypoxia. Ascorbic acid treatment reduced the increased plasma lipid peroxidation and the formation of 3-nitrotyrosine in the carotid body, the potentiation of carotid body chemosensory responses (See Fig. 2), the ventilatory responses to acute hypoxia, as well as the hypertension.

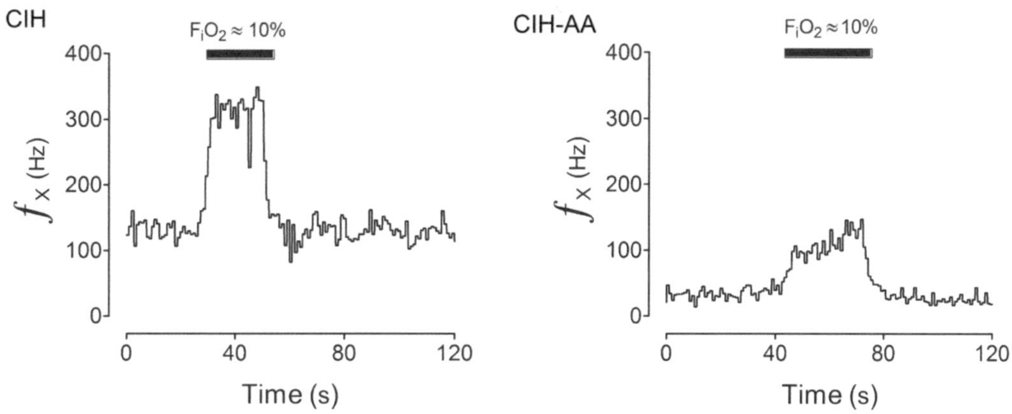

Fig. 2. Effect of ascorbic acid on the potentiated carotid body chemosensory responses to hypoxia induced by intermittent hypoxia. CIH, rat exposed to intermittent hypoxia. CIH-AA, rat exposed to intermittent hypoxia and treated with ascorbic acid. Note that ascorbic acid reduced both the baseline and the chemosensory response to 10% O_2. f_X, frequency of carotid chemosensory discharges, expressed in Hz.

Although the current information suggests that an increased local oxidative stress contributes to the carotid body chemosensory potentiation induced by intermittent hypoxia, the direct participation of ROS on the oxygen chemotransduction process is matter of debate, because no chemosensory excitatory effects of ROS have been observed (Gonzalez et al., 2007). A possible explanation is that an increased level of the superoxide radical in the carotid body may reacts with nitric oxide generating peroxynitrite, a powerful oxidizing agent that nitrates tyrosine residues forming 3-nitrotyrosine. We already found the excessive formation of 3-nitrotyrosine in glomus cells and blood vessels from carotid bodies harvested from rats exposed to intermittent hypoxia (Del Rio et al., 2010, 2011), as is shown in fig. 3. The increased formation of 3-nitrotyrosine indicates that the carotid body tissue is continuously exposed to oxidative stress during the intermittent hypoxic exposure. In addition, we found that a correlation between the marked increase of 3-nitrotyrosine immunoreactivity in the carotid body exposed to intermittent hypoxia and the enhanced carotid chemosensory responses to acute hypoxia (Del Rio et al., 2011), supporting and extending the idea that oxidative-nitrosative stress plays a critical role in the CB chemosensory potentiation (Iturriaga et al., 2009, Peng & Prabhakar, 2003). In OSA patients, Jelic et al., (2008) found that the expression of 3-nitrotyrosine in endothelial cells was greater than controls subjects, indicating that the oxidative stress contributes to the endothelial dysfunction caused by the intermittent hypoxia. In addition to the formation of nitrotyrosine residues, peroxynitrites may also modify iron sulfur clusters, zinc thiolates and other residues. Moreover, peroxynitrites may react with inorganic molecules such as CO_2 producing other free radicals that may modify DNA, lipids or proteins.

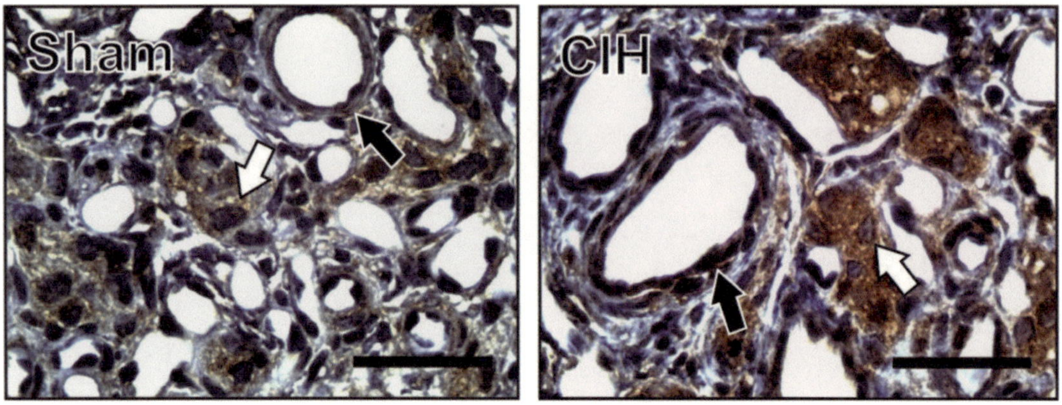

Fig. 3. Exposure to CIH increased 3-nitrotyrosine formation in the glomus cells (white arrows) and endothelial cells (black arrows) from rat carotid bodies. Scale bar, 20 μm.

6.2 Vasoactive molecules

An interesting molecule, which may mediate the carotid body chemosensory potentiation induced by intermittent hypoxia, is endothelin-1 (ET-1). It is known that the plasmatic ET-1 level increases in rats exposed to intermittent hypoxia (Kanagy et al., 2001) and OSA patients (Phillips et al., 1999). This potent vasoconstrictor peptide is expressed in the endothelium, blood vessels and glomus cells of the carotid body (Rey et al., 2007). The application of ET-1 produces chemosensory excitation in both *in situ* and *in vitro* carotid body perfused preparations, but not in the superfused preparation devoid of vascular effects (Rey & Iturriaga, 2004). We found that ET-1 was increased locally in the carotid body of cats exposed to 4 days to intermittent hypoxia by ~10-fold, while ET-1 plasma levels remains unchanged (Rey et al., 2006). The enhanced carotid body chemosensory responses to hypoxia were reduced by the ET receptor blocker bosentan in the intermittent hypoxic - treated cats, but have no effects on the carotid body chemosensory activity in control animals (Rey et al., 2006), indicating that a local increase of ET-1 contributes to enhance the carotid chemosensory responses. Pawar et al., (2009) tested the hypothesis that ET-1 induced by ROS plays a role in intermittent hypoxia induced chemosensory potentiation in the rat neonatal carotid body. They found that intermittent hypoxia enhanced the release of ET-1 and the expression of the ET-A receptor in response to intermittent hypoxia. Systemic administration of MnTMPyP, which prevent the elevation of ROS, reduced the increased basal release of ET-1, the overexpression of ET-A receptor mRNA and the enhanced carotid body chemosensory response to acute hypoxia. These results support the idea that a ROS-induced increase of ET-1 release is involved in the potentiation of carotid body chemosensory response elicited by intermittent hypoxia. Increased plasmatic levels of ROS and ET-1 have been also implicated in the hypertension induced by intermittent hypoxia. Troncoso-Brindeiro et al., (2007) reported that the concurrent treatments of rats exposed to intermittent hypoxia with the SOD mimetic, 4-hydroxy-2,2,6,6-tetramethylpiperidine-*N*-oxyl (TEMPOL), prevents the increased ROS plasmatic level and the hypertension. However, it is worth noting that intermittent hypoxia increases the expression of ET-1 in the rat CB during the first week of hypoxia, and later the ET-1 levels returned back to the control levels (Del

Rio et al., 2011), suggesting that ET-1 may contribute to the enhanced carotid body responsiveness to hypoxia in the early phase of the intermittent hypoxic exposures. In addition to the transient changes in ET-1 expression, we found a significant decrease in the eNOS expression in the rat carotid body at 7 days of intermittent hypoxia (Del Rio et al., 2011), suggesting that chronic intermittent hypoxia may decrease the nitric oxide (NO) levels within the carotid body. Since NO at low concentration is an inhibitory modulator of the carotid chemosensory activity (Iturriaga et al., 2000), a reduced NO level may contribute to enhance the carotid body chemosensitivity, as well as to amplify the vasoconstrictor effect of ET-1. This interpretation is supported by the finding that intermittent hypoxia decreases the expression of the neuronal NO synthase in the rat carotid body (Marcus et al., 2010), suggesting that the removal of the inhibitory NO effects may also contribute to enhance the carotid chemosensory responses to hypoxia. Our results also showed that carotid body iNOS immunorreactive levels increased after 21 days of intermittent hypoxic exposure. Since iNOS produce higher amounts of NO, it is plausible that the NO levels in the carotid body will increase during long-term intermittent hypoxic exposure. It is worth noting that NO has a dual effect on carotid chemosensory discharges. Indeed, Iturriaga et al., (2000) found that at low levels NO is predominantly an inhibitor of the chemosensory discharges, whereas at high concentration NO increases carotid body chemosensory discharges. Thus, it is plausible that high NO levels in the carotid body following long-term intermittent hypoxia may partially contribute to maintain the carotid body chemosensory potentiation.

6.3 Pro-inflammatory cytokines

Endothelial dysfunction has been related to the progression of hypertension in OSA patients and animals exposed to intermittent hypoxia due to the increased plasmatic levels of pro-inflammatory cytokines (Biltagi et al., 2008, Jelic et al., 2008, Jun et al., 2008, Tam et al., 2007, Williams & Scharf, 2007). It is likely that an increased production of ROS induced by the hypoxia-reoxygention cycles may evoke the expression of genes and the synthesis of pro-inflammatory cytokines, mediated by the activation of transcription factors such as the nuclear factor kappa B (NF-κB), the activator protein 1 and HIF-1α (Semenza & Prahbakar, 2007). In response to oxidative stress, HIF-1α induces the expression of several genes including ET-1 and iNOS, but ROS also produces the translocation of NF-κB to the nucleus, increasing the expression of several inflammatory genes such as IL-1β, IL-6, TNF-α, adhesion molecules, iNOS and ET-1 (Janseen-Heininger et al., 2000). Recently, we found that intermittent hypoxia increased the levels of TNF-α and IL-1β in the rat carotid body after 21 days of exposure (Del Rio et al, 2011). We found that glomus cells constitutively expresses TNF-α and IL-1β in the cell bodies and that chronic intermittent hypoxia up-regulates the expression of both TNF-α and IL-1β, without inducing carotid body tissue infiltration with macrophages or changes in TNF-α and IL-1β plasmatic levels (Del Rio et al., 2011). Our results showed that exposure to intermittent hypoxia enhances the rat carotid chemosensory responses to acute hypoxia, and progressively increase the immunorreactive TNF-α and IL-1β expression in the carotid body, suggesting a potential role for this cytokines in modulating the enhanced carotid body chemosensory activity after exposure to intermittent hypoxia.

7. Proposed targets of the effects of ROS in the carotid body

The available evidence indicates that oxidative stress mediated the potentiation of the carotid body chemosensory responses to acute hypoxia, induced by the exposure to intermittent hypoxia. However, the nature of the molecular mechanism by which ROS induced chemosensory potentiation is not known. Based on the presented evidences, we hypothesized that chronic intermittent hypoxia may increase the expression of pro-inflammatory cytokines and other chemosensory modulators, such as ET-1 and NO, which may potentially contribute to enhance the carotid body chemosensory responses to hypoxia. Figure 4 summarized the possible targets of the effects of ROS on oxygen chemoreception in the carotid body. It is plausible that excessive amounts of free radicals may modify the O_2-sensitive K^+ channels, increasing the intracellular Ca^{2+} levels, which in turn evokes the release of excitatory transmitters, but a direct participation of ROS on the O_2 chemotransduction process in the carotid body is not clear (Gonzalez et al., 2007). ROS or other molecules, produced downstream of the ROS signal, which act upon the mitochondria, membrane channels or the gene expression machinery may modify the oxygen sensing in the carotid body. Further studies are required to determine which protein or enzyme complexes involved in the carotid body chemosensory process are affected by ROS or ROS-dependent molecules induced by intermittent hypoxia.

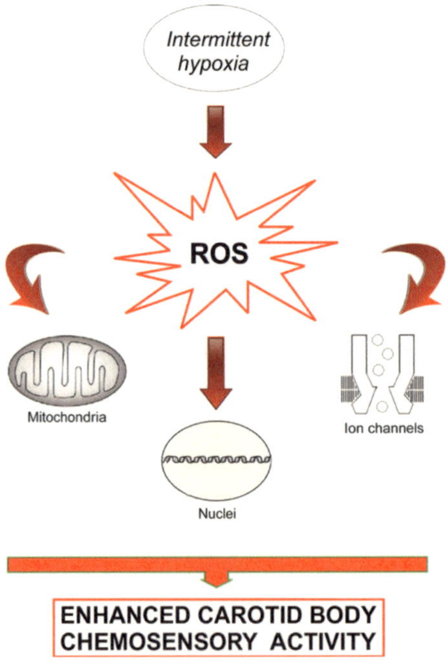

Fig. 4. Proposed targets of the effects of ROS on the potentiation of the carotid body induced by intermittent hypoxia.

8. Integrative model

Figure 5 shown a diagram of the proposed mechanisms involved in the potentiation of the carotid body chemosensory responses to hypoxia induced by intermittent hypoxia, which finally contributes to the development of the hypertension. We postulate that cyclic episodes of hypoxia-reoxygenation enhance the carotid body chemosensitivity to hypoxia, which in turn contributes to elicit a persistent facilitation of the sympathetic neural output. The enhanced sympathetic activity along with a reduction of the baroreflex efficiency should impair the regulation of the heart rate variability and the vasomotor tone of blood vessels, resulting in an elevation of arterial blood pressure. On the other hand, systemic oxidative stress and the inflammation *per se* may contribute to the endothelial dysfunction, leading to the hypertension.

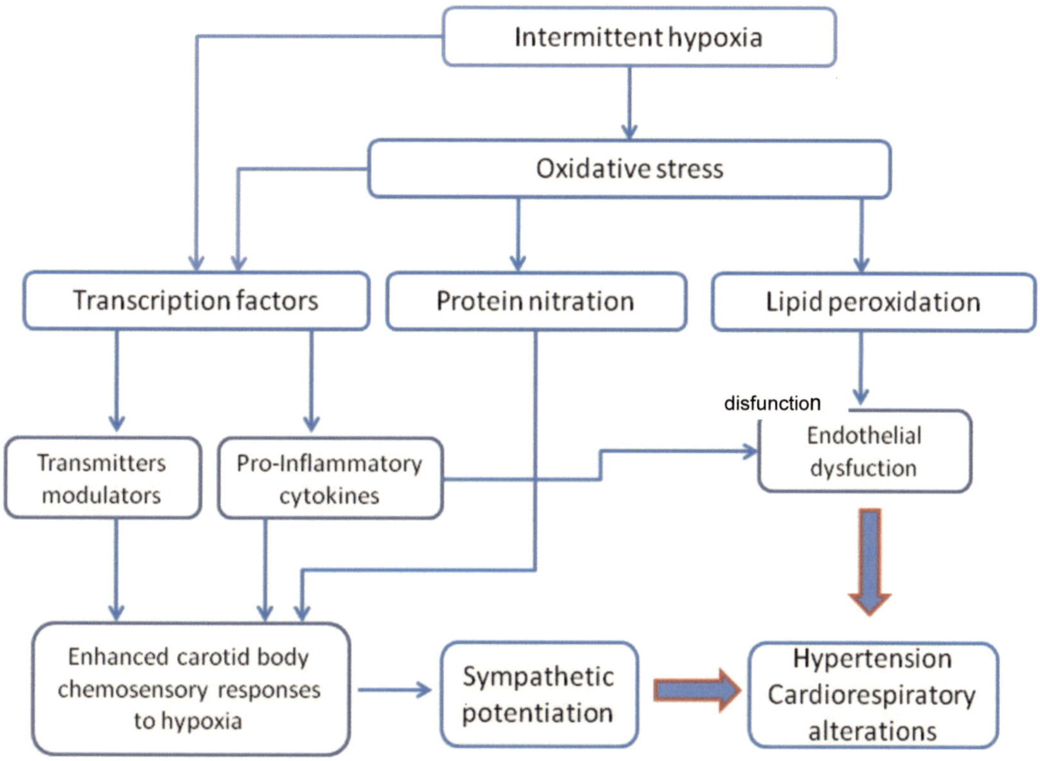

Fig. 5. Proposed mechanisms involved in the hypertension induced by the potentiation of the carotid body chemosensory responses to hypoxia induced by intermittent hypoxia, and the systemic oxidative stress.

9. Conclusion

Autonomic dysfunction has been associated to exposure to chronic intermittent hypoxia in animal models, and is thought to be involved in the increased risk of hypertension and cardiovascular mortality in OSA patients. The cyclic hypoxic episodes in OSA patients potentiate cardiovascular and sympathetic responses induced by hypoxic stimulation of peripheral chemoreceptors, and impair the regulation of arterial blood pressure and the renin–angiotensin system. Intermittent hypoxia enhances the ventilatory and cardiovascular responses to acute hypoxia, suggesting a major role of the carotid body in the pathological cardiorespiratory consequences of intermittent hypoxia. New evidences indicate that intermittent hypoxia induced oxidative stress in the carotid body, which contributes to potentiate the carotid body chemosensory responses to acute hypoxia. Understanding how the oxidative stress interacts with the carotid body chemoreceptor system will provide new insights into the pathophysiological cardiovascular consequences of OSA. Thus, upcoming new knowledge in the field will serve to propose new therapies to moderate the severity of the cardiovascular alterations induced by OSA. We believe that is possible to ameliorate or prevent the hypertension using antioxidants, which will reduced the systemic oxidative stress as well as the carotid body potentiated chemosensitivity to hypoxia.

10. Acknowledgements

Present work was supported by grant 1100405 from the National Fund for Scientific and Technological Development of Chile (FONDECYT). Rodrigo Del Rio was supported by a CONICYT AT-24091043 fellowship.

11. References

Arnardottir, E.S.; Mackiewicz, M.; Gislason, T.; Teff, K.L, & Pack, A.I. (2009). Molecular signatures of obstructive sleep apnea in adults: A review and perspective. Sleep, Vol. 32, pp. 447-470.

Biltagi, M.A.; Maguid, M.A.; Ghafar, M.A.; & Farid, E. (2008). Correlation of 8-isoprostane, interleukin-6 and cardiac functions with clinical score in childhood obstructive sleep apnoea. Acta Paediatr, Vol. 97. pp.1397-1405.

Carlson, J.T.; Hedner, J.; Elam, M.; Ejnell, H.; Sellgren, J. & Wallin, B.G. (1993). Augmented resting sympathetic activity in awake patients with obstructive sleep apnea. Chest, Vol. 103. Pp. 1763–1768.

Chen, L.; Einbinder, E.; Zhang, Q.; Hasday, J.; Balke, C.W. & Scharf, S.M. (2005). Oxidative stress and left ventricular function with chronic intermittent hypoxia in rats. Am J Respir Crit Care Med, Vol. 172. pp. 915-920.

Cistulli, P.A. & Sullivan C.E. (1994). Pathology of sleep apnea. In: Sleep and Breathing. Saunders NA, Sullivan CE (Eds) New York: Marcel Decker.

Christou, I.K.; Moulas, A.N.; Pastaka, C. & Gouroulianis, K.I. (2003). Antioxidant capacity in obstructive sleep apnea patients. Sleep Med, Vol. 4. pp. 225–228.

Del Rio, R.; Moya, E.A. &, Iturriaga R. (2010). Carotid body and cardiorespiratory alterations in intermittent hypoxia: the oxidative link. Eur Respir J, Vol. 36. pp.143-150.

Del Rio, R.; Moya, E.A. &, Iturriaga R. (2011). Differential expression of pro-inflammatory cytokines, endothelin-1 and nitric oxide synthases in the rat carotid body exposed to intermittent hypoxia. Brain Res, Vol. 1395. pp. 74-85.

Dick, T.E.; Hsieh, Y.H.; Wang, N. & Prabhakar, N. (2007). Acute intermittent hypoxia increases both phrenic and sympathetic nerve activities in the rat. Exp Physiol, Vol. 92. pp. 87–97.

Feng, J.; Chen, B.Y. & Cui LY. (2008). Carotid body-mediated changes of sympathetic nerve and their relationships with hypertension. Chin Med J, Vol. 121. pp. 1732-1735.

Fletcher, E,C.; Lesske, J.; Behm, R.; Miller, C,C. & Stauss H, Unger T. (1992). Carotid chemoreceptors, systemic blood pressure, and chronic episodic hypoxia mimicking sleep apnea. J Appl Physiol, Vol. 72. pp.1978-1984.

Fletcher, E.C.; Orolinova, N. & Bader M. (2002). Blood pressure response to chronic episodic hypoxia: the renin-angiotensin system J Appl Physiol, Vol. 92. pp. 627–633.

Garvey, JF.; Taylor, C.T. & McNicholas WT. (2009). Cardiovascular disease in obstructive sleep apnoea syndrome: the role of intermittent hypoxia and inflammation. Eur Respir J, Vol. 33. pp. 1195-1205.

Gonzalez, C.; Almaraz, L.; Obeso, A. & Rigual, R. (1994). Carotid body chemoreceptors: from natural stimuli to sensory discharges. Physiol Rev, Vol. 74. pp. 829-898.

Gonzalez, C.; Agapito, M.T.; Rocher, A.; Gonzalez-Martin, M.C.; Vega-Agapito, V.; Gomez-Niño, A.; Rigual, R.; Castañeda, J. & Obeso, A. (2007). Chemoreception in the context of the general biology of ROS. Respir Physiol Neurobiol, Vol. 157. pp.30-44.

Gozal, D. & Kheirandish-Gozal, L. (2008). Cardiovascular morbidity in obstructive sleep apnea, oxidative stress, inflammation, and much more. Am J Respir Crit Care Med, Vol. 177. pp. 369–375.

Greenberg, HE.; Sica, A.; Batson, D. & Scharf, SM. (1999). Chronic intermittent hypoxia increases sympathetic responsiveness to hypoxia and hypercapnia. J Appl Physiol, Vol. 86. pp. 298-305.

Iturriaga, R.; Villanueva, S.; & Mosqueira, M. (2000). Dual effects of nitric oxide on carotid body chemoreception. J Appl Physiol, Vol. 89. pp. 1005-1012.

Iturriaga, R. & Alcayaga, J. (2004). Neurotransmission in the carotid body: transmitters and modulators between glomus cells and petrosal ganglion nerve terminals. Brain Res Rev, Vol. 47. pp. 46-53.

Iturriaga, R.; Del Rio, R. & Rey, S. (2005). Cardiovascular and ventilatory acclimatization induced by chronic intermittent hypoxia: A role for the carotid body in the pathophysiology of sleep apnea. Biol Res, Vol. 38. pp. 335-340.

Iturriaga, R.; Varas, R.; & Alcayaga, J. (2007). Electrical and pharmacological properties of petrosal ganglion neurons that innervate the carotid body. Respir Physiol Neurobiol, Vol. 157. pp.130-139.

Iturriaga, R.; Moya, E.A. & Del Rio, R. (2009). Carotid body potentiation induced by intermittent hypoxia: implications for cardioventilatory changes induced by sleep apnoea. Clin Exp Pharmacol Physiol, Vol. 36. pp. 1197-1204.

Janssen-Heininger, Y.M.; Poynter, M.E. & Baeuerle, P.A. (2000). Recent advances towards understanding redox mechanisms in the activation of nuclear factor kappaB. Free Radic Biol Med, Vol. 28. pp. 1317-1327.

Jelic, S.; Padeletti, M.; Kawut, S.M.; Higgins, C.; Canfield, S.M.; Onat, D.; Colombo, P.C.; Basner, R.C.; Factor, P. & LeJemtel, T.H. (2008). Oxidative stress, and repair capacity of the vascular endothelium in obstructive sleep apnea. Circulation, Vol. 117. pp. 2270-2278.

Jun, J.; Savransky, V.; Nanayakkara, A.; Bevans, S.; Li, J.; Smith, P.L. & Polotsky, V.Y. (2008). Intermittent hypoxia has organspecific effects on oxidative stress. Am J Physiol Regul Integr Comp Physiol, Vol. 295. pp. 1274 -1281.

Kanagy, N.L.; Walker. B.R. & Nelin, L.D. (2001). Role of endothelin in intermittent hypoxia-induced hypertension. Hypertension, Vol. 37. pp. 511-515.

Kumar, G. (2011). Hypoxia and neurotransmitter synthesis. Am J Physiol Cell Physiol, Vol. 300. pp. 743-751.

Lam, S.Y.; Tipoe, G.L.; Liong, E.C. & Fung M.L. (2008). Chronic hypoxia upregulates the expression and function of proinflammatory cytokines in the rat carotid body. Histochem Cell Biol, Vol. 130. pp. 549-659.

Leuenberger, U.A.; Cynthia, S.; Hogeman, C.S.; Quraishi, S.; Linton-Frazier, L. & Gray, K.S. (2007). Short-term intermittent hypoxia enhances sympathetic responses to continuous hypoxia in humans. J Appl Physiol, Vol. 103. pp. 835-842.

Lavie, L. (2003). Obstructive sleep apnoea syndrome: an oxidative stress disorder. Sleep Med Rev, Vol. 7. pp. 35-51.

Lai, .CJ.; Yang, C.C.H.; Hsu, Y.Y.; Lin, Y.N. & Kuo, T.B.J. (2006). Enhanced sympathetic outflow and decreased baroreflex sensitivity are associated with intermittent hypoxia-induced systemic hypertension in conscious rats. J Appl Physiol, Vol. 100. pp. 1974-1982.

Lin, M.; Liu, R.; Gozal, D.; Wead, W.B.; Chapleau, M.W.; Wurster, R. & Cheng. Z.J. (2007). Chronic intermittent hypoxia impairs baroreflex control of heart rate but enhances heart rate responses to vagal efferent stimulation in anesthetized mice. Am J Physiol Heart Circ Physiol, Vol. 293. pp. 997–1006.

Liu, X.; He, L.; Stensaas, L.; Dinger, B. & Fidone, S.J. (2009). Adaptation to chronic hypoxia involves immune cell invasion and increased expression of inflammatory cytokines in rat carotid body. Am J Physiol Lung Cell Mol Physiol, Vol. 296. pp. 158-166.

Loredo, J.S.; Clausen, J.L.; Nelesen, R.A; Ancoli-Israel, S.; Ziegler, M.G. & Dimsdale, J.E. (2001). Obstructive sleep apnea and hypertension: are peripheral chemoreceptors involved?. Med Hypotheses, Vol. 56. pp. 17-19.

Marcus, N.J.; Li, Y.,L.; Bird, C.E.; Schultz H.D. & Morgan, B.J. (2010). Chronic intermittent hypoxia augments chemoreflex control of sympathetic activity: Role of the angiotensin II type 1 receptor. Respir Physiol Neurobiol, Vol. 171, pp. 36-45.

MacFarlane, P.M. & Mitchell, G.S. (2008). Respiratory long-term facilitation following intermittent hypoxia requires reactive oxygen species formation. Neuroscience, Vol. 152. pp.189-197.

McGuire, M.; Zhang, Y.; White, D.P. & Ling L. (2003). Chronic intermittent hypoxia enhances ventilatory long-term facilitation in awake rats. J Appl Physiol, Vol. 95. pp. 1499-1508.

Moller, D.S.; Lind P.; Strunge B. & Pedersen, E.B. (2003). Abnormal vasoactive hormones and 24-hour blood pressure in obstructive sleep apnea. Am J Hypertens, Vol. 16. pp. 274-280.

Narkiewicz, K.; van de Borne, P.J.; Cooley, R.L.; Dyken, M.E. & Somers, V.K. (1998a). Sympathetic activity in obese subjects with and without obstructive sleep apnea. Circulation, Vol. 98. pp. 772-776.

Narkiewicz, K.; van de Borne, P.J.; Montano, N.; Dyken, M.E.; Phillips, B.G. & Somers V.K. (1998b). Contribution of tonic chemoreflex activation to sympathetic activity and blood pressure in patients with obstructive sleep apnea. Circulation, Vol. 97. pp. 943-945.

Narkiewicz, K.; Montano, N.; Cogliati, C.; van de Borne, P.J.; Dyken, M.E. & Somers, V.K. (1998c). Altered cardiovascular variabilityin obstructive sleep apnea. Circulation, Vol. 98. pp. 1071-1077.

Narkiewicz, K.; van de Borne, P.J.; Pesek, C.A.; Dyken, M.E.; Montano, N. & Somers, V.K. (1999). Selective potentiation of peripheral chemoreflex sensitivity in obstructive sleep apnea. Circulation, Vol. 99. pp. 1183-1189.

Pack, A.I. (2009). Obstructive Sleep Apnea and Cardiovascular Disease: A Perspective and Future Directions. Progress Cardiovasc Dis, Vol. 51. pp. 434-451.

Parati, G.; Lombardi, C. & Narkiewicz, K. (2007). Sleep apnea: epidemiology, pathophysiology, and relation to cardiovascular risk. Am J Physiol Regul Integr Comp Physiol, Vol. 293. pp. 1671-1683.

Pawar, A.; Nanduri, J.; Yuan, G.; Khan, S.A.; Wang, N.; Kumar, G.K. & Prabhakar, N.R. (2009). Reactive oxygen species-dependent endothelin signaling is required for augmented hypoxic sensory response of the neonatal carotid body by intermittent hypoxia. Am J Physiol Regul Integr Comp Physiol, Vol. 296. pp. 735-742.

Peng, Y.J. & Prabhakar N.R. (2003). Reactive oxygen species in the plasticity of breathing elicited by chronic intermittent hypoxia. J Appl Physiol, Vol. 94. pp. 2342-2349.

Peng, Y.J.; Overholt, J.L.; Kline, D.; Kumar, G.K. & Prabhakar, N.R. (2003). Induction of sensory long-term facilitation in the carotid body by intermittent hypoxia: implications for recurrent apneas. Proc Natl Acad Sci U.S.A, Vol. 100. Pp. 10073-10078.

Peng, Y.J.; Nanduri, J.; Yuan, G.; Wang, N.; Deneris, E.; Pendyala, S.; Natarajan, V.; Kumar G.K. & Prabhakar, N.R. (2009). NADPH oxidase is required for the sensory plasticity of the carotid body by chronic intermittent hypoxia. J Neurosci. Vol. 29. pp.4903-4910.

Phillips, B.G.; Narkiewicz, K.; Pesek, C.A.; Haynes, W.G.; Dyken, M.E. & Somers V.K. (1999). Effects of obstructive sleep apnea on endothelin-1 and blood pressure. J Hypertens, Vol. 7. pp. 61-66.

Prabhakar, N.R.; Peng, Y.J.; Jacono, F.J.; Kumar, G.K. & Dick T.E. (2005). Cardiovascular alterations by chronic intermittent hypoxia: importance of carotid body chemoreflexes. Clin Exp Pharmacol Physiol, Vol. 32. pp. 447–449.

Reeves, S.R.; Gozal, E.; Guo, S.Z.; Sachleben, L.R.; Brittian, K.R.; Lipton, A.J. & Gozal D. (2003). Effect of long-term intermittent and sustained hypoxia on hypoxic ventilatory and metabolic responses in the adult rat. J Appl Physiol, Vol. 95. pp. 1767-1774.

Rey, S.; Del Rio, R.; Alcayaga, J. & Iturriaga R. (2004). Chronic intermittent hypoxia enhances cat chemosensory and ventilatory responses to hypoxia. J Physiol London, 560. pp. 577-586.

Rey, S. & Iturriaga, R. (2004). Endothelins and nitric oxide: Vasoactive modulators of carotid body Chemoreception. Curr Neurovasc Res, Vol. 1. pp. 464-473.

Rey, S.; Del Rio, R. & Iturriaga R. (2006). Contribution of endothelin-1 to the enhanced carotid body chemoreception induced by intermittent hypoxia. Brain Res, Vol. 1086. pp. 152-159.

Rey, S.; Corthorn, J.; Chacón, C. & Iturriaga R. (2007). Expression and immunolocalization of endothelin peptides and its receptors, ETA and ETB, in the carotid body exposed to chronic intermittent hypoxia. J Histochem Cytochem, Vol. 55. pp. 167-174.

Rey, S.; Tarvainen, M,P.; Karjalainen, PA. & Iturriaga, R. (2008). Dynamic time-varying analysis of heart rate and blood pressure variability in cats exposed to short-term chronic intermittent hypoxia. Am J Physiol Regul Integr Comp Physiol, Vol. 295. pp. 28-37.

Semenza, G,L. & Prabhakar, N.R. (2007). HIF-1-dependent respiratory, cardiovascular, and redox responses to chronic intermittent hypoxia. Antioxid Redox Signal, Vol. 9. pp. 1391-1396.

Shiomi, T.; Guilleminault, C.; Sasanabe, R.; Hirota, I.; Maekawa, M. & Kobayashi, T. (1996). Augmented very low frequency component of heart rate variability during obstructive sleep apnea. Sleep, Vol. 119. pp. 370-377.

Shu, H.F.; Wang, B.R.; Wang, S.R.; Yao, W.; Huang, H.P.; Zhou, Z.; Wang, X.; Fan, J.; Wang, T. & Ju, G. (2007). IL-1βeta inhibits IK and increases [Ca^{2+}]i in the carotid body glomus cells and increases carotid sinus nerve firings in the rat. Eur J Neurosci, Vol. 25. pp. 3638-3647.

Schulz, R.; Eisele, H.J.; Murzabekova, G. & Weissmann N. (2008). Sleep apnea and cardiovascular disease. Results from animal studies. Pneumologie, Vol. 62. pp.18-22.

Smith, M,L. & Pacchia Ch,F. (2007). Sleep apnoea and hypertension: Role of chemoreflexes in humans. Exp Physiol, Vol. 92. pp. 45-50.

Somers, V.K.; White, D,P.; Amin, R.; Abraham, W.T.; Costa, F.; Culebras, A.; Daniels, S.; Floras, J.S.; Hunt, C,E.; Olson, L.J.; Pickering, T.G.; Russell, R.; Woo, M. & Young, T. (2008). Sleep apnea and cardiovascular disease: An American Heart Association. In collaboration with the National Heart, Lung, and Blood Institute National Center on Sleep Disorders Research. J Am Coll Cardiol, Vol. 52. pp. 686-717.

Tam, C.S.; Wong, M.; Tam, K.; Aouad, L. & Waters K.A. (2007). The effect of acute intermittent hypercapnic hypoxia treatment on IL-6, TNF-alpha, and CRP levels in piglets. Sleep, Vol. 30. pp. 723-727.

Troncoso-Brindeiro, C.M.; Da Silva, A.Q.; Allahdadi, K,J.; Youngblood, V. & Kanagy, N.L. (2007). Reactive oxygen species contribute to sleep apnea-induced hypertension in rats. Am J Physiol Heart Circ Physiol, Vol. 293. pp. 2971-2976.

Williams, A. & Scharf S.M. (2007). Obstructive sleep apnea, cardiovascular disease, and inflammation: is NF-kappaB the key? Sleep Breath, Vol. 11. pp. 69-76.

Yan, B.; Soukhova-O'Hare, G.K.; Li, L.; Lin, Y.; Gozal, D.; Wead, W.B.; Wurster, R.D. & Cheng Z.J. (2008). Attenuation of heart rate control and neural degeneration in nucleus ambiguus following chronic intermittent hypoxia in young adult Fischer 344 rats. Neurocience, Vol. 153. pp. 709-720.

Zoccal, D.B.; Simms, A.E.; Bonagamba, L.G.; Braga, V.A.; Pickering, A.E.; Paton, J.F. & Machado, B.H. (2008). Increased sympathetic outflow in juvenile rats submitted to chronic intermittent hypoxia correlates with enhanced expiratory activity. J Physiol. Vol. 586, 3253-3265.

Adipocytokines, Oxidative Stress and Impaired Cardiovascular Functions

Ana Bertha Zavalza Gómez[1], María Cristina Islas Carbajal[2] and Ana Rosa Rincón Sánchez[3]
[1]*Specialties Hospital, Medical Unit of High Specialty, West National Medical Center, Mexican Institute of Social Security,*
[2]*Cardiovascular Research Unit, Physiology Department, Health Science University Center, University of Guadalajara,*
[3]*Physiology Department, Health Science University Center, University of Guadalajara, Guadalajara, Jalisco, México*

1. Introduction

In spite of the considerable progress in their diagnosis, prevention and treatment, cardiovascular diseases remain the number one cause of death worldwide. This is partially due to the rapidly growing incidence of obesity, which is a well-known independent risk factor for insulin resistance, diabetes, dyslipidaemia, high blood pressure and thrombosis (Lopaschuck et al., 2007).

The metabolic complications of obesity, often referred to as the metabolic syndrome, characterized by a heterogenic complex of symptoms and consist of glucose intolerance, central obesity, dyslipidemia (hypertriglyceridemia, elevated nonesterified fatty acids (NEFAs), and decreased high-density lipoprotein (HDL) cholesterol), and hypertension. These, often culminating in β-cell failure, impaired glucose tolerance and type 2 diabetes (T2D). In addition, dyslipidaemia, coronary heart disease (CHD), systemic hypertension and premature heart failure are pathologies related (Hubert et al., 1983). Abdominal obesity, ectopic lipid accumulation, hepatic steatosis, and sleep apnea can also be included in the metabolic complications of obesity (Parati et al., 2007).

On the other hand, obesity leads to an alteration in the profile of hormones secreted by adipose tissue (adipokines). Secretion of adipocytokines has been shown particularly for visceral fat (Dusserre et al., 2000; Fontana et al., 2007; Yang & Smith, 2007). It is evident that many of these adipokines have the ability to influence other tissues such as the liver, muscle and brain, e.g. the adipokine leptin affects appetite regulation, others have an important impact on the consequences of adipose tissue inflammation (e.g. interleukin 6 (IL), PAI-1, monocyte chemoattractant protein 1 [MCP-1]) and vascular biology (e.g. serum amyloid A [SAA]) (Bastard et al., 2002; Mutch et al., 2001; Sartipy et al., 2003; Stofkova, 2009; Yang et al., 2006). In addition, increased tumor necrosis factor (TNF) and IL-6 expression and secretion from adipose tissue are involved in both whole-body and local insulin resistance at different tissue sites.

The principal purpose of this chapter is to describe how the adipocytokines and oxidative stress interact with insulin signaling in the context of low-grade inflammation related to obesity in order to promote cardiovascular complications.

2. Pathophysiology of cardiovascular morbidity

2.1 Introduction

The pathophysiology of cardiovascular morbidity is complex and multifactorial. Oxidative stress is an important contributory factor to the etiology of many cardiovascular diseases, including atherosclerosis, coronary heart disease (heart attack), cerebrovascular disease (stroke), cardiomyopathies, peripheral vascular disease, diabetes, heart failure, and hypertension (Dusting & Triggle, 2005). Ischemic heart disease and hypertension are the two most important causes of heart failure in the Western world. Other common causes include valvular heart disease (especially aortic stenosis and mitral regurgitation).

Arterial hypertension is the most prevalent cardiovascular risk factor and the leading cause of morbidity and mortality from cardiovascular disease (CVD) worldwide (Gómez-Marcos et al., 2009). Heart failure (HF) is a complex clinical syndrome caused by impaired ventricular performance. It is the final common pathway for a variety of cardiovascular disease processes, leading to potentially disabling symptoms and shortened life expectancy. Currently, 1% of the population aged 50–59 yr, and 10% of those over 80 yr, have HF; is the only major cardiovascular condition that is increasing in prevalence, because of an ageing population and improved survival from other CVD (Kotzé & Howell, 2008). Understanding these profound mechanisms of disease can help clinicians identify and treat CVD, as well as help patients prevent these potentially devastating complications.

2.2 Epidemiology

Cardiovascular diseases are the world's largest killers, claiming 17.1 million lives a year, CVD contributed to a third of global deaths. An estimated 79 400 000 American adults (1 in 3) have 1 or more types of CVD. Of these, 37 500 000 are estimated to be age 65 or older (Rosamond et al., 2007).

Extensive epidemiological research has established diabetes, hyperlipidemia, hypertension, and cigarette smoking, as independent risk factors for CHD. The risk increases 2–3 folds with tobacco smoking, with age and is greater for women than for men. In contrast, cardiac events fall 50% in people who stop smoking and the risk of CVDs, also decreases significantly over the first two years after stopping smoking (Khot, et al., 2003).

The health interview part of the National Health and Nutrition Examination Survey (NHANES) III was used to categorize adults over 50 years of age by presence of metabolic syndrome (National Cholesterol Education Program [NCEP] definition) with or without diabetes. The prevalence of CHD for each group was then determined. Metabolic syndrome (MetS) is very common, with ~44% of the U.S. population over 50 years of age meeting the NCEP criteria. In contrast, diabetes without MetS is uncommon (13% of those with diabetes). Older Americans over 50 years of age without MetS regardless of diabetes status had the lowest CHD prevalence (8.7% without diabetes, 7.5% with diabetes). Those with MetS without diabetes had higher CHD prevalence (13.9%) and, those with both MetS and diabetes had the highest prevalence of CHD (19.2%) compared with those with neither (Alexander et al., 2003).

The Systematic Coronary Risk Evaluation (SCORE) data set comprises data from 12 European cohort studies. The SCORE population was also divided into gender and age strata: under 40, 40–49, 50–59, and over 60. The rate of CVD mortality in each body mass index (BMI) category was calculated, each 5-unit increase in BMI was associated with an increase in CVD mortality of 34% in men and 29% in women. This increases the public health importance of BMI as both a simple indicator and mediator of CVD risk (Dudina et al., 2011).

2.3 Pathologies associated to cardiovascular morbidity

Impaired myocardial diastolic relaxation (e.g., diastolic dysfunction) is the earliest myocardial contractility observed in metabolic conditions such as obesity, insulin resistance, and hypertension. Diastolic dysfunction manifests as a reduction in velocity of myocardial relaxation, as well as decreasing myocardial compliance. Mechanisms that contribute to this selective cardiac dysfunction include decreases in energy production due to reductions in mitochondrial respiration, increased oxidative stress, and defective contractile and intracellular "Ca2+" regulatory proteins. Abnormalities in "Ca2+" signaling/flux and myofilament function contribute to the cardiomyopathic alterations observed in the metabolic syndrome (Ren et al., 2010). Reductions in the oxidative capacity of the mitochondrial electron transport chain are manifested in obese, insulin-resistant persons as well as diabetic patients. Mitochondria in endothelial cells are thought to play an important role in cellular signaling as sensors for local oxygen concentration and regulations of nitric oxide (NO) production. Renin-angiotensin-aldosterone system (RAAS)-mediated increases in nicotinamide-adenine dinucleotide phosphate (NADPH) oxidase activity and generation of reactive oxygen species (ROS) may result in mitochondrial damage and associated decreases in oxidative phosphorylation, Adenosine triphosphate (ATP) production and bioavailable NO (Ren et al., 2010).

The mechanisms underlying ventricular dysfunction are dysfunction of cardiac myocytes and longstanding pressure or volume overload. As myocardial contractility decreases, the stroke volume drops and the end-diastolic volume and pressure increase. If sustained in the long-term, this volume increase leads to what is termed cardiac remodelling. This involves myocardial hypertrophy, chamber enlargement and an increase in ventricular wall stress, and increases oxygen demand. An increase in ventricular stiffness also occurs due to increased collagen deposition in the heart, which impairs filling and exacerbates the situation (Kotzé & Howell, 2008).

The new paradigm of atherosclerosis links oxidative stress, inflammation, thrombosis, and endothelial dysfunction. Growing evidence indicates that chronic and acute overproduction of ROS under pathophysiologic conditions is integral in the development of CVD (Madamanchi et al., 2005). Coronary artery disease (CAD) is one of the most frequent causes of death and disabling symptoms worldwide. Epidemiological studies have indicated the rising prevalence of atherosclerosis globally (Tedgui & Mallat, 2006). Formation of atheromatous plaques in the arteries obstructs the supply of oxygen and nutrients to the myocardium, resulting in CHD (Woods et al., 2000).

2.3.1 Diabetes

Diabetes is a prime risk factor for CVD, the link between diabetes and CVD is complex and multifactorial. The presence of insulin resistance, impaired glucose tolerance, and overt diabetes, are associated with an increased risk of CVD, these conditions are also accompanied by the presence of oxidative stress (Woods et al., 2000). Vascular disorders include retinopathy and nephropathy, peripheral vascular disease (PVD), stroke, and CAD. Diabetes also affects the heart muscle, causing both systolic and diastolic heart failure.

The etiology of this excess cardiovascular morbidity and mortality is not completely clear (Dokken, 2008). Evidence suggests that although hyperglycemia, the hallmark of diabetes, contributes to myocardial damage after ischemic events, it is clearly not the only factor, because both pre-diabetes and the presence of the MetS, even in normoglycemic patients, increase the risk of most types of CVD (Alexander, 2003; Dokken, 2008). In diabetes, where CVD is of particular concern, there are multiple sources of ROS including the auto-oxidation of glucose, increased substrate flux, and decreased levels of NADPH through the polyol pathway. Formation of advanced glycation end products (AGEs) and their interaction with cellular targets, such as endothelial cells, may lead to oxidative stress and promote formation of oxidized LDL (ox-LDL) (Ceriello & Motz, 2004).

The recent explosion of the worldwide epidemic of MetS combining disturbances in glucose and insulin metabolism, excess predominantly abdominally distributed weight, mild dyslipidemia, and hypertension, with the subsequent development of obesity, T2D and CVD, compromises progress made in reducing the morbidity and mortality of CVD in recent years. Cardiovascular risk increases in parallel to insulin resistance (as estimated by the homeostasis model assessment index (HOMA) both patients with diabetes and nondiabetic (Saely et al., 2005).

2.3.2 Metabolic syndrome

The incidence of CVD, coronary heart disease, and T2D has not been well defined in persons with the MetS. Conclusions were that MetS is common and is associated with an increased risk for CVD and T2D in both sexes, according to metabolic syndrome traits. MetS accounts for up to one third of CVD in men and approximately half of new T2D over 8 years of follow-up (Wilson et al., 2005).

A large family study of T2D in Finland and Sweden (the Botnia study) were included in the analysis of cardiovascular risk associated with the MetS. The aim of the study was to assess the prevalence of cardiovascular morbidity and mortality associated with the MetS by applying the WHO definition. In women and men, respectively, the MetS was seen in 10 and 15% of subjects with normal glucose tolerance, 42 and 64% of those with impaired fasting glucose (IFG)/impaired glucose tolerance (IGT), and 78 and 84% of those with T2D. Cardiovascular mortality was markedly increased in subjects with the MetS (12.0 vs. 2.2%, $p < 0.001$). Of the individual components of the MetS, microalbuminuria conferred the strongest risk of cardiovascular death (RR 2.80; $p < 0.002$) (Isomaa et al., 2001).

2.3.3 Obesity

Obesity has been increasing in epidemic proportions in both adults and children. In adults, overweight is defined as a BMI 25 to 29.9 Kg/m^2 and obesity as BMI $\geq$30 Kg/m^2. Other indexes that have been used less commonly but possibly with more predictive power include body fatness, waist circumference (WC), waist-to-hip ratio (WHR), and weight-to-height ratio. A recent study of nearly 360,000 participants from 9 European countries showed that both general obesity and abdominal adiposity are associated with risk of death and support the importance of WC or WHR in addition to BMI for assessing mortality risk. Obesity has many adverse effects on hemodynamics and CV structure and function (Lavie et al., 2009).

Elevated BMI predisposes to congestive heart failure (CHF) by promoting increased blood pressure, diabetes, and CHD. Factors related to obesity and hypertension, include: endothelial dysfunction, insulin resistance, sympathetic nervous system, substances released from adipocytes (IL-6, TNF-α, etc.), and sleep apnea (Poirier et al., 2006).

The role of obesity in the initiation and acceleration of tissue inflammation has been well studied. Excess adipose tissue can contribute to inflammation in two ways: (a) ectopic fat storage induces lipotoxicity, promoting an intracellular inflammatory response and (b) altered adipokine production in obesity contributes to the inflammatory response. It is now recognized that adiponectin has a role in both of these processes. Related to demonstrated association between hypo-adiponectinaemia and metabolic dysfunction (Cnop et al., 2003) the proposal provides that a replacement of adiponectin may function as pharmacological therapy (Chandran et al., 2003).

2.3.4 Endothelial dysfunction

Healthy endothelium regulates blood vessel tone, platelet activation, leukocyte adhesion, thrombogenesis, and inflammation. The net effect of healthy endothelium is vasodilatory, anti-atherogenic, and anti-inflammatory (Dokken, 2008). Endothelial dysfunction has been observed in patients with established coronary artery disease or coronary risk factors, both in the coronary and peripheral vasculature (Heitzer et al., 2001).

As shown in figure 1, endothelial dysfunction a key factor in atherogenesis, is associated with an increased risk of cardiovascular events and highest risk for vascular morbidity and mortality. A major risk for atherosclerotic plaque rupture is aging. One possible mechanism is that aging is associated with endothelial cell senescence, which is a risk factor for endothelial apoptosis and endothelial denudation, rendering the atherosclerotic plaque prone to rupture (Hulsmans et al., 2011).

A primary event in atherogenesis is the infiltration of activated inflammatory cells into the arterial wall. ROS can be produced from both endogenous and exogenous substances. Potential endogenous sources include mitochondria, cytochrome P450 metabolism, peroxisomes, and inflammatory cell activation. In the vascular wall, ROS are generated by several mechanisms, including NADPH oxidases, xanthine oxidase, the mitochondrial respiratory chain, lipoxygenases, and nitric oxide synthases. ROS formation can be stimulated by mechanical forces (e.g., stretch, pressure, shear stress), environmental factors (such as hypoxia), secreted factors coupled to tyrosine kinase receptors (e.g., platelet derived growth factor, PDGF), and secreted factors coupled to G protein-coupled receptors such as angiotensin II (Lehoux et al., 2006; Dokken, 2008; Hulsmans et al., 2011).

The general process of lipid peroxidation consists of three stages: initiation, propagation, and termination (Catalá, 2006). The initiation phase of lipid peroxidation includes hydrogen atom abstraction. Several species can abstract the first hydrogen atom and include the radicals: hydroxyl (−OH), alkoxyl (RO−), peroxyl (ROO−), and possibly HO_2− but not H_2O_2 or O_2−. The membrane lipids, mainly phospholipids, containing polyunsaturated fatty acids are predominantly susceptible to peroxidation because abstraction from a methylene (CH2-) group of a hydrogen atom, which contains only one electron, leaves at the back an unpaired electron on the carbon, CH-. The presence of a double bond in the fatty acid weakens the C–H bonds on the carbon atom nearby to the double bond and thus facilitates H- subtraction. The initial reaction of -OH with polyunsaturated fatty acids produces a lipid radical (L-), which in turn reacts with molecular oxygen to form a lipid peroxyl radical (LOO−).There they secrete ROS and oxidize lipoproteins, inducing foam cell formation and endothelial cell apoptosis, which in turn lead to plaque growth, erosion, and rupture (Hulsmans et al., 2011).

It is now widely recognized that chronic low-grade inflammation and oxidative stress play a key role in the initiation, propagation, and development of metabolic disorders. The aim of Hulsmans et al., (2011), was to review the functional roles of various microRNAs (miRs) in regulating oxidative stress and inflammation in adipose and vascular tissues leading to obesity and atherosclerosis, in order to analyze how these processes can be linked through communication between cells even at a remarkable distance, thus highlighting the communication between inflammatory and endothelial cells. The work of Targonski et al., was performed to evaluate the magnitude of the association between coronary endothelial dysfunction (CED) and cerebrovascular events. Kaplan-Meier analysis indicated that patients with CED had a significantly higher cumulative cerebrovascular event rate than those without CED (P=0.04). Presence of CED in patients without obstructive CAD is independently associated with an increased risk of cerebrovascular events (Targonski et al., 2003).

2.3.5 Dyslipidemia

The major threat to the macrovasculature for patients with and without diabetes is atherosclerosis, and dyslipidemia is highly correlated with atherosclerosis, up to 97% of patients with diabetes are dyslipidemic (Dokken, 2008). Insulin deficiency and insulin resistance promote dyslipidemia accompanied by increased oxidation, glycosylation, and triglyceride enrichment of lipoproteins.

Nonenzymatic glycosylation of HDL shortens its half-life and renders it less protective against atherosclerosis (Duell, 1991). The study of Marsuki et al., was undertaken to evaluate the effect, on macrophage cholesterol efflux, of functional modification of HDL by its glycation. They also investigated the effects of the glycation-inhibitors, metformin (MF) and aminoguanidine (AG), on glycated HDL-mediated cholesterol efflux. The conclusion was that glycated HDL particles are ineffective as acceptors of ATP-binding cassette transporter (ABCG1) mediated cholesterol efflux; and this may explain, at least in part, accelerated atherosclerosis in diabetic patients. Metformin serves as a possible candidate to restore impaired cholesterol efflux and reverse cholesterol transport (Matsuki et al., 2009).

Hypertriglyceridemia can lead to increased production of the small, dense form of LDL and to decrease HDL transport of cholesterol back to the liver (Poirier et al., 2006). In addition to the characteristic pattern of increased triglycerides and decreased HDL cholesterol found in the plasma of patients with diabetes, abnormalities are seen in the structure of the lipoprotein particles, where the predominant form of LDL cholesterol is the small, dense form. Small LDL particles are more atherogenic than large LDL particles because they can more easily penetrate and form stronger attachments to the arterial wall, and they are more susceptible to oxidation (Stocker & Keaney, 2004). In diabetic patients, LDL particles can also become glycated, in a process similar to the glycation of hemoglobin. Glycation of LDL lengthens its half-life and therefore increases the ability of the LDL to promote atherogenesis (Dokken, 2008).

2.3.6 Atherosclerosis

Atherosclerosis is no longer considered a pure lipid disorder. It has become increasingly clear that inflammation is at the root of atherosclerosis and its complications. In addition to playing a causal role in lesion formation, inflammation can yield predictive and prognostic information of considerable clinical utility. In addition to serving as biomarkers of atherosclerotic events, inflammatory mediators directly participate in lesion formation, propagation, and eventual rupture and in this fashion may represent a powerful tool to assess endothelial cell activation. Clearly, understanding the mechanisms and mediators of endothelial dysregulation and inflammation may yield new targets to predict, prevent, and treat cardiovascular disease (Szmitko, 2003).

Many common conditions predisposing to atherosclerosis, such as hypercholesterolemia, hypertension, diabetes, and smoking, are associated with a reduced vascular availability of NO, a free radical that not only produces vasodilation but also has potent antiatherogenic properties, such as inhibition of platelet aggregation, prevention of smooth muscle cell proliferation, reduction of lipid peroxidation, and inhibition of adhesion molecule expression (Landmesser & Harrison, 2001). Impaired endothelium-dependent vasodilation, a surrogate for NO bioavailability, may predict cardiovascular events. Thus, the loss of NO not only alters vascular tone but also may explaining in part why these conditions are risk factors for atherosclerosis.

3. Reactive oxygen species and oxidative stress in cardiovascular diseases

Oxidative stress (OS) is an imbalance between production and degradation of ROS in cells, leading eventually to enhanced oxidative modification of biomolecules. Therefore, is a phenomenon associated with pathogenetic mechanisms of several diseases including atherosclerosis, cancer, diabetes mellitus, heart failure, hypertension, inflammatory diseases, as well as psychological diseases or aging processes (Naito et al., 2010). An increase in ROS and/or a weakening in the antioxidant defense mechanisms can cause OS. Accumulating evidence suggests that OS increases with age, and that therapeutic and life style approaches that reduce oxidative stress likely slow the development of atherosclerotic cardiovascular disease. Increased cellular ROS is an important contributor to the pathophysiology of vascular diseases, including atherosclerosis, restenosis, myocardial infarction and stroke. Additionally, some ROS act as intracellular messengers, and ROS accumulation activates proinflammatory signaling pathways with an increased propensity for the formation of atherosclerotic lesions within the vessel wall (Runge et al., 2010).

The antioxidant enzymes superoxide dismutase (SOD), catalase (CAT) and glutathione peroxidase (GPx) serve as primary line of defense in destroying free radicals. However, there are several human antioxidant genes, classified according to genes whose products are defined as "antioxidant enzymes" the first two groups, and genes whose products are not enzymes, but also deal directly with reactive species. Also, are subclassified into 3 functional groups: peroxidases: catalase, ceruloplasmin (ferroxidase), glutathione peroxidase 1-7, lactoperoxidase, myeloperoxidase, peroxiredoxin 1-6; superoxide dismutases: copper chaperone for superoxide dismutase, superoxide dismutase 1, soluble (amyotrophic lateral sclerosis 1 (adult), superoxide dismutase 2, mitochondrial, superoxide dismutase 3, extracellular and thiol redox proteins: glutaredoxin (thioltransferase), glutaredoxin 2,3,5, glutathione reductase,methionine sulfoxide reductase A, metallothionein 1A, 1B, 1E,1F,1G,1H,1M,1X,2A, protein disulfide isomerase family A, member 6, selenoprotein P, plasma, 1, sulfiredoxin 1 homolog (S. cerevisiae), thioredoxin, thioredoxin 2, thioredoxin domain containing 1,2,3,4,5,6,8,9,10,11,12,13,14,17, thioredoxin interacting protein, thioredoxin-like 1, 4A, 4B, thioredoxin reductase 1,2,3 (Dusting & Triggle, 2005).

An elevation of ROS may cause CVD due the overproduction of superoxide anion (O_2•-). This overproduction is detrimental, because of the rapid interaction of O_2•- with NO, which leads to the loss of NO bioavailability and increase in the production of peroxynitrite (ONOO−). A subsequent reduction in the vascular effects of NO, as well as a reduction in the antiatherogenic effects of NO, as a consequence will compromise cardiovascular function. An elevation of O_2•- will also lead to the oxidation of the important co-factor in the regulation of nitric oxide synthase, tetrahydrobiopterin (BH_4), and this will lead to an "uncoupled eNOS", which will then synthesize O_2•- rather than NO (Dusting & Triggle, 2005).

The term ROS refers to a subset of molecules called "free radicals", however there are some ROS which are not free radicals, such as hydrogen peroxide. This term refers to any molecule that contains an unpaired electron in the outer orbital. This unpaired electron makes the molecule highly reactive that leads to the formation of bonds between the ROS and other compounds (Dokken, 2008). Unpaired electron makes the molecule highly reactive, seeking to either donate an electron to another compound or take up protons from another compound to obtain a stable electron pair. These free radicals include superoxide anion (O_2•-), hydroxyl radical (•OH), and the free radical form of nitric oxide (•NO). Other members of the ROS family include hydrogen peroxide (H_2O_2) and peroxynitrite ($ONOO^-$) (Dusting & Triggle, 2005). On the other hand, several enzyme systems are known to be sources of ROS including the mitochondrial respiratory chain, xanthine oxidase, NADPH oxidase, cyclooxygenase, cytochrome P450, and uncoupled eNOS. Mitochondria are the source of ROS. There is also growing evidence that NADPH-oxidase is a major source of vascular superoxide production.

The high reactivity of free radicals leads to the formation of bonds between the ROS and other compounds, altering the structure and function of the tissue. Because of the reactive propensity of these molecules, ROS can directly damage a number of cell components, such as plasma membranes and organelles (Dokken, 2008). In diabetes, where cardiovascular disease is of particular concern, there are multiple sources of ROS including the autooxidation of glucose, increased substrate flux, and decreased levels of NADPH through the polyol pathway. Formation of AGEs products and their interaction with cellular targets, such as endothelial cells, may lead to oxidative stress and promote formation of oxidized LDL (Ceriello & Motz, 2004).

Increased production of oxygen-derived free radicals such as the superoxide anion has been linked to impaired endothelial vasomotor function in experimental models of atherosclerosis. Accordingly, treatment with antioxidants has been shown to improve coronary and peripheral endothelial function in patients with CAD or coronary risk factors (Heitzer et al., 2001). Mechanisms that contribute to this selective cardiac dysfunction include decreases in energy production due to reductions in mitochondrial respiration, increased oxidative stress, and defective contractile and intracellular "Ca^{2+}" regulatory proteins. Changes in mitochondrial biogenesis and function have been documented in the metabolic syndrome and diabetes. Alterations in mitochondrial biogenesis as well as mitochondrial content and function provoke a heterogeneous group of CVD risk factors that constitute the metabolic syndrome. (Ren et al., 2010). It is increasingly recognized that important aspects of mitochondrial dysfunction that contribute to CVDs are induction of apoptosis and changes in mitochondrial morphology under the influence of oxidative stress. Finally, inefficient mitochondrial oxidative phosphorylation/biogenesis and increases in oxidative stress appear to be overarching abnormalities contributing to cardiac diastolic function, the hallmark of metabolic cardiomyopathy (Ren et al., 2010).

4. Adipocytokines and the metabolic complications of obesity

4.1 Fat depots, adipocitokines and their relation to the human metabolic syndrome

Adipose tissue is composed of adipocytes embedded in a loose connective tissue meshwork containing adipocyte precursors, fibroblasts, immune cells, and various other cell types. Adipose tissue was traditionally considered an energy storage depot with few interesting attributes. However, adipocytes express and secrete a variety of products known as 'adipokines', including leptin, adiponectin, resistin and visfatin, as well as cytokines and chemokines such as TNF-α, IL-6 and monocyte chemoattractant protein (Antuna-Puente et al., 2008) and due to the dramatic rise in obesity and its metabolic sequelae during the past decades, adipose tissue gained tremendous scientific interest. It is now regarded as an active endocrine organ that, in addition to regulating fat mass and nutrient homeostasis, releases a large number of bioactive mediators (adipokines) modulating hemostasis, blood pressure, lipid and glucose metabolism, inflammation, and atherosclerosis (see figure 1).

During positive caloric balance there are two factors important for the development of metabolic disease. First one is a type of the fat accumulation, i.e., due to increase in size (hypertrophy) or in number (hyperplasia) of fat cells. The next factor is a place of fat storage, i.e. subcutaneous (SC) or visceral (Vis) fat (Wajchenberg, 2000; Bays et al., 2008). In humans, white adipose tissue (WAT) produces over 50 'adipokines', including TNF-α which contributes to the low-grade inflammation found in obesity, leptin which has effects on food intake, and a host of other agents with a variety of effects (Lago et al., 2007). In parallel with these proinflammatory events, WAT also produces anti-inflammatory cytokines such as adiponectin (which, paradoxically, tends to be lower in obese individuals) and IL-10 and IL1R1 (IL-1Rα; production of which is proportional to body weight).

4.2 Leptin

Hyperleptinaemia is common in obesity and reflects increased adiposity and leptin resistance. Nevertheless, leptin resistance may not be complete as several actions of leptin, such as cardiovascular sympatho-activation, might be preserved in obese subjects known to be resistant to the metabolic effects of leptin (i.e. selective leptin resistance). Notably, the renal and sympathetic actions of leptin may play an important role in the pathogenesis of hypertension related to obesity and metabolic syndrome. Furthermore, the lipotoxic effect of leptin resistance may cause insulin resistance and β cell dysfunction, increasing the risk of T2D. Leptin has also been shown to possess proliferative, pro-inflammatory, pro-thrombotic, and pro-oxidative actions (Buettner et al., 2006).

4.3 Adiponectin

Adiponectin, referred to as adipocyte complement-related protein of 30 kDa (ACRP30), is a protein secreted from adipocytes (Correia & Rahmouni, 2006), that is abundantly present in plasma (Scherer et al., 1995; Berg et al., 2001). It is now well established that adiponectin has potent salutary actions on peripheral insulin sensitivity, and circulating adiponectin levels are reduced in obesity, insulin resistance and T2D (Scherer et al., 1995; Kern et al., 2003). Mice lacking adiponectin have reduced insulin sensitivity (Weyer et al., 2001; Kubota et al., 2002; Maeda et al., 2002); in contrast, adiponectin overexpression in ob/ob mice, confers dramatic metabolic improvements, e.g., in various mouse models, Holland et al. (2011) show that the insulin-sensitizing and antiapoptotic actions of adiponectin are partly related to its effects on sphingolipid metabolism, providing a new unifying mechanism for the pleiotropic beneficial actions of adiponectin. Adiponectin stimulates the cellular activity of ceramidase, which removes the fatty acyl chain from ceramides. This liberates sphingosine, which can subsequently be phosphorylated by sphingosine kinases to generate the antiapoptotic metabolite sphingosine-1-phosphate (S1P). Furthermore, liver-specific overexpression of the adiponectin receptors, AdipoR1 and AdipoR2, increased hepatic ceramidase activity and, concomitantly, reduced hepatic ceramide content. These *in vivo* models of varying adiponectin expression and AdipoR1 and R2 overexpression demonstrate a strong association between adiponectin levels, hepatic ceramide content and insulin sensitivity (Holland et al., 2011).

In the beta cell model of apoptosis, adiponectin protected against the development of hyperglycemia-a key feature of pancreatic insufficiency-by partially preserving beta cell mass and insulin content. Using mouse primary cardiomyocytes and a pancreatic beta cell line, Holland et al. (2011) showed that adiponectin prevents cell death induced by the saturated fatty acid palmitate and a short chain ceramide analog, C2-ceramide. Mechanistically, the insulin-sensitizing actions of adiponectin, which include enhanced glucose use and fatty acid oxidation (Yamauchi et al., 2003), inhibition of serine kinases that antagonize insulin signaling and enhanced mitochondrial biogenesis, are believed to occur via receptor-dependent activation of the 5′-AMP–activated protein kinase (AMPK). Intriguingly, it is known that adiponectin also exerts potent antiapoptotic effects and prevents myocardial apoptosis in response to ischemia-reperfusion injury (Shibata et al., 2005) and lipid-induced pancreatic beta cell apoptosis (Rakatzi et al., 2004).

Several studies have linked hypoadiponectinemia to diabetes (Kern et al., 2003), hypertension (Kim et al., 2007), atherosclerosis, and endothelial dysfunction (Chow et al., 2007). More recent studies have shown that the high-molecular weight (HMW) oligomer is inversely associated with the risk for diabetes independent of total adiponectin (Kadowaki et al., 2007), and the HMW oligomer is responsible for the association of adiponectin with traits of metabolic syndrome (Heidemann et al., 2008; Lara-Castro et al., 2006). On the other hand, adiponectin improves insulin sensitivity by increasing energy expenditure and fatty acid oxidation through activation of AMPK, and by increasing the expression of PPARα target genes such as CD36, acyl-coenzyme oxidase, and uncoupling protein-2 (Kadowaki et al., 2007). Alternatively, adiponectin may lead to an improved metabolic profile by the expansion of SC adipose tissue with decreased levels of macrophage infiltration (Nawrocki et al., 2006), similar to the actions of peroxisome proliferator-activated receptor (PPAR)-γ agonists; reduction of lipotoxicity and inflammation associated with obesity (Wang et al., 2007), and adiponectin has also had vasculoprotective effects mediated via an increase in endothelial nitric oxide production, or modulation of expression of adhesion molecules and scavenger receptors (Chow et al., 2007; Zhu et al., 2008).

In addition, work in experimental models has shown that adiponectin mediates beneficial actions in cardiovascular and metabolic-associated diseases (Sam & Walsh, 2010). For example, in mouse models, adiponectin modulates hypertrophic signals in the heart and exhibits direct anti-hypertrophic properties; in addition to improving vascular function and pathological remodeling (Antuna-Puente et al., 2008); the hypoadiponectinemia might be observed in subjects with hypertension and other cardiovascular diseases and could be a useful pharmacologic tool to improve membrane microviscosity in hypertension, via the NO dependent mechanisms (Tsuda, 2011).

It has been demonstrated that plasma adiponectin levels increased during weight reduction or blockade of the rennin angiotensin system indicating that adiponectin might be beneficial for preventing the development of atherosclerotic changes. The results of Kurata et al. indicate that blockade of Angiotensin II receptor ameliorates adipocytokine dysregulation and that such action is mediated, at least in part, by targeting oxidative stress in obese adipose tissue.

4.4 Resistin

Resistin is a 12-kDa peptide that was originally discovered as a result of examining differential gene expression of mouse adipose tissue after thiazolidinediones (TZD) treatment (Steppan et al., 2001). The thiazolidinediones a class of drugs that work through PPARγ agonism, are insulin sensitizers and have been shown to improve cardiac risk factors and decrease cardiovascular events; may potentially correct the inflammatory disarray, endothelial dysfunction, dyslipidemia, and plaque vulnerability associated with diabetic cardiovascular disease through their effects on insulin resistance and fat metabolism. Resistin was decreased by TZD treatment of mice and was increased in insulin-resistant mice. Furthermore, treatment with antiresistin antibody improved insulin sensitivity and glucose transport in mice and mouse adipocytes, respectively (Steppan et al., 2001). Additional studies in mice suggest that an important site of action of resistin is on hepatic glucose production (Rajala et al., 2003). Therefore, resistin is clearly an important adipokine that likely plays a role in the development of insulin resistance; however, it appears to be quantitatively less important in humans than other adipokines.

4.5 Visfatin

Visfatin is expressed in many cells and tissues, and was previously identified as a protein involved in B-cell maturation (pre-B colony enhancing factor) (Kitani et al., 2003; Samal et al., 1994). More recently, visfatin was described to be a highly expressed protein with insulin-like functions, and was predominantly found in visceral adipose tissue, from which the name visfatin was derived (Fukuhara et al., 2005). Injection of visfatin in mice lowered blood glucose, and mice with a mutation in visfatin, and nicotinamide adenine dinucleotide (NAD) biosynthetic activity ionotropy, which is essential for β-cell function (Revollo et al., 2007). In human studies, a positive correlation between visceral adipose tissue visfatin gene expression and BMI was noted, along with a negative correlation between BMI and SC fat visfatin (Berndt et al., 2005; Varma et al., 2007), suggesting that visfatin regulation in these different depots is different, and adipose depot ratios are highly dependent on the obesity of the subjects. Variable results were obtained regarding the relationship between visfatin and diabetes or insulin resistance (Varma et al., 2007; Chen et al., 2006; Hammarstedt et al., 2005; Haider et al., 2006). Therefore, there are a number of inconsistencies among the different studies of visfatin, and the role of this adipokine in obesity and insulin resistance is not clear.

4.6 Apelin

Apelin is another short peptide released from adipocytes upon stimulation by e.g. insulin and the endogenous ligand of the human orphan G-protein-coupled APJ receptor. In line with this, plasma apelin levels are increased in obesity associated with insulin resistance and hyperinsulinemia (Beltowski, 2006). In the cardiovascular system, apelin elicits endothelium-dependent, nitric oxide-mediated vasorelaxation and in rodents, apelin also increases cardiac contractility *in vivo* (Ashley et al., 2005; Atluri et al., 2007) and causes a rapid fall in both arterial blood pressure and systemic venous tone (Tatemoto et al., 2001; Lee, 2005) with corresponding reductions in left ventricular afterload and preload (Ashley et al., 2005; Tatemoto et al., 2001).

Apelin-APJ system, expressed in the central nervous system and in a variety of peripheral tissues, is involved in the regulation of the immune response, brain signaling, hemodynamic homeostasis, vasodilatation, inotropy, angiogenesis and glucose metabolism (Sorli et al., 2006; Zhang et al., 2009). In the cardiovascular system, high expression of APJ mRNA has been observed in the heart (Zhang et al., 2009). Apelin expression is restricted to endothelial cells and negligible in cardiomyocytes in normal myocardium, but detectable in failing hearts (Földes et al., 2003). Of all the active fragments identified to date, apelin-13 may represent the most potent biological ligand (Kawamata et al., 2001). Current studies suggest that apelin expression is at least maintained and possibly augmented in mild, compensated chronic heart failure but declines in severe disease (Japp & Newby, 2008). Exogenous apelin administration during myocardial injury can preserve cardiac function (Chandrasekaran, 2008). Some researchers suggested that apelin reduces infarct size and protects myocardial cells against ischemia-reperfusion (I/R) injury by activating the reperfusion injury salvage kinase (RISK) pathway. The RISK pathway incorporates phosphatidylinositol 3-OH kinase (PI3K)/Akt, p44/42 mitogen-activated protein kinase (MAPK) and extracellular signal-regulated MAPK (ERK1/2) (Simpkin, 2007).

5. Inflammatory pathway activation and interactions with endothelial cells

5.1 Endothelial cells

The vascular endothelium, located at the interface of blood and tissue, is able to sense changes in hemodynamic forces and blood borne signals and react by synthesizing and releasing vasoactive substances. Vascular homeostasis is maintained by a balance between endothelium-derived relaxing and contracting factors. With disruption of this balance, mediated by inflammatory and traditional cardiovascular risk factors, the vasculature becomes susceptible to atheroma formation. Inflammatory mediators appear to play a fundamental role in the initiation, progression, and eventual rupture of atherosclerotic plaques.

5.1.1 Endothelial dysfunction

Endothelial dysfunction implies diminished production or availability of NO and/or an imbalance in the relative contribution of endothelium-derived relaxing and contracting factors, those included endothelin-1 (ET-1), angiotensin, and several oxidants. However, endothelial dysfunction, as assessed in terms of vasomotor dysfunction, can occur well before the structural manifestation of atherosclerosis and thus can serve as an independent predictor of future cardiovascular events (Behrendt & Ganz, 2002).

Hypercholesterolemia, traditional cardiovascular risk factor, promotes attachment of blood leukocytes to the endothelium. Oxidized low-density lipoprotein causes endothelial activation and changes its biological characteristics in part by reducing the intracellular concentration of NO (Cominacini, 2001).

On the other hand, angiotensin II can induce the production of ROS, increase the expression of the proinflammatory cytokines as IL-6 and monocyte chemoattractant protein-1 (MCP-1), and upregulate VCAM-1 on ECs. High levels of CRP can also promote endothelial dysfunction by quenching the production of NO and diminishing its bioactivity (Verma, 2002). These endothelial modifications promote inflammation within the vessel wall, setting the stage for the initiation and progression of an atherosclerotic lesion.

5.2 Adiponectin and inflammatory activation

Recent research has focused on the origin of the inflammatory markers in obesity and the extent to which adipose tissue has a direct effect. The production of adipokines by visceral adipose tissue is of particular interest since their local secretion by visceral fat depots may provide a novel mechanistic link between obesity and the associated vascular complications. Under conditions of inflammation associated with cardiovascular disease, as well as an increase in mobilization of fatty acids from adipose tissue, there is increased secretion of pro-atherogenic, pro-inflammatory adipocytokines and chemokines.

The cardiometabolic benefits of adiponectin may be driven largely through improvements in vascular homeostasis, especially through improving endothelial function. Some studies have demonstrated impaired endothelial function in adiponectin-deficient mice (Teoh et al., 2008) demonstrated that adiponectin plays an important role to limit endothelial activation and inflammation in experimental sepsis. On the contrary, in adiponectin-deficient mice exhibit profound reduction in survival following cecal ligation and puncture.

5.3 Mediators of inflammation

The inflammatory processes are mediated by several factors secreted by adipocytes collectively called adipocytokines (adiponectin, leptin, ghrelin, visfatin and resistin) some of which seem to play an important role in obesity-associated insulin resistance and cardiovascular complications. Tissue levels of TNF-α, IL-6, leptin and visfatin were significantly higher in patients with CAD relative to control subjects. Significantly higher tissue levels of these four cytokines from abdominal fat depots were found compared to those from epicardial fat in CAD patients.

IL-6 is secreted by a wide variety of cells such as endothelial cells, adipocytes, β pancreatic cells, monocytes, and macrophages. This cytokine is essential in reducing the inflammatory process by promoting the synthesis of anti-inflammatory cytokines and by negatively regulating inflammatory targets. In humans, higher circulating IL-6 levels have been associated with obesity and visceral fat deposition, increased risk of impaired glucose tolerance, T2D and high blood pressure. IL-6 is a central mediator of the acute-phase response and a primary determinant of hepatic production of CRP. Visceral adipose tissue secretes about two to three times more IL-6 than subcutaneous tissue, secreting also other molecules that stimulate further IL-6 expression (Curti, 2011).

In obesity, the pro-inflammatory effects of cytokines through intracellular signaling pathways involve the NF-κB and JNK systems. Thus, it can be considered that obesity corresponds to a sub-clinical inflammatory condition that promotes the production of pro-inflammatory factors involved in the pathogenesis of insulin resistance (Bastard et al., 2002).

5.4 Vasculature as part of the immune system

Blood vessels are integral components of the immune system; they are important part in lymphocyte circulation and act as portals between tissue and blood compartments. Endothelial cells express toll-like receptors, (Kunjathoor, 2002) whose ligation induces expression of leukocyte adhesion molecules, inducible NO synthase 2, endothelin, IL-1, and other inflammatory molecules. These cells also express the scavenger receptors CD36 and LOX-1, and can internalize ligands such as modified LDL particles. ECs are located at the interface of blood and tissues, and play a pivotal role in the inflammatory response. Their activation causes leukocyte recruitment, increased permeability, edema, and other characteristic features of inflammation. Furthermore, ECs can activate adaptive immunity by presenting foreign antigens to specific T cells.

5.5 Mammalian Target Of Rapamycin (mTOR) signaling pathway

The mammalian target of rapamycin (mTOR) signaling pathway integrates both intracellular and extracellular signals and serves as a central regulator of cell metabolism, growth, proliferation and survival. Discoveries that have been made over the last decade show that the mTOR pathway is activated during various cellular processes (e.g. tumor formation and angiogenesis, insulin resistance, adipogenesis and T-lymphocyte activation) and is deregulated in human diseases such as cancer and T2D (Laplante & Sabatini, 2009). *In vivo* stimulators of adipogenesis have not been clearly identified, but may include insulin, IGF-1, as well as certain fatty acids and/or their metabolites. Insulin/IGF-1 acts on cell surface receptors, activating key intracellular signaling proteins. One of these signaling pathways, mTOR that is binds to, and inhibited by, rapamycin, an immunosuppressant that blocks T cell proliferation. The mTOR protein is a 289-kDa serine-threonine kinase that belongs to the phosphoinositide 3-kinase (PI3K)-related kinase family and is conserved throughout evolution (Laplante & Sabatini, 2009). The role of mTORC1 in regulating lipid synthesis, which is required for cell growth and proliferation, is beginning to be appreciated. It has been demonstrated that mTORC1 positively regulates the activity of sterol regulatory element binding protein 1 (SREBP1) (Porstmann et al., 2008) and of PPAR-γ (Kim & Chen, 2004), two transcription factors that control the expression of genes encoding proteins involved in lipid and cholesterol homeostasis.

The binding of insulin to its cell-surface receptor promotes the tyrosine kinase activity of the insulin receptor, the recruitment of insulin receptor substrate 1 (IRS1), the production of phosphatidylinositol (3,4,5)-triphosphate [PtdIns(3,4,5)P_3] through the activation of PI3K, and the recruitment and activation of AKT at the plasma membrane. In many cell types, activation of mTORC1 strongly represses the PI3K-AKT axis upstream of PI3K. Activation of S6 kinase 1 (S6K1) by mTORC1 promotes the phosphorylation of insulin receptor substrate 1 (IRS-1) and reduces its stability (Harrington et al., 2005). This auto-regulatory pathway, characterized as the S6K1-dependent negative feedback loop, has been shown to have profound implications for both metabolic diseases and tumorigenesis (Manning, 2004) and pro-inflammatory cytokines, such as TNFα, activate IkB kinase-β (IKKβ), which physically interacts with and inactivates tuberous sclerosis complex 1 (TSC1), leading to mTORC1 activation (Lee et al., 2007). This positive relationship between inflammation and mTORC1 activation is thought to be important in tumor angiogenesis and in the development of insulin resistance.

5.6 Adiponectin as anti-inflammatory action

Adiponectin exerts potent anti-inflammatory effects, as documented in experimental studies where authors demonstrate that reduces TNF-α production in response to various stresses in plasma, adipose tissue, vascular wall, heart, and liver (Kojima et al., 2003; Ujiie et al., 2006). In addition, antagonizes several of the inflammatory effects of TNF-α (Ouchi et al., 2003); can facilitate the removal of early apoptotic cells by macrophages and modulate the processes of inflammation and autoimmunity. This activity was mediated by calreticulin expressed on the phagocytic cell surface and not by any of the previously identified adiponectin receptors. Because the accumulation of cell corpses can cause inflammation and immune system dysfunction, these authors suggest a mechanism by which hypoadiponectinemia can contribute to the development of diabetes, atherosclerosis, and other complex diseases in which chronic inflammation is a contributing factor (Takemura et al., 2007). Thus, while AdipoR1 and AdipoR2 may mediate the metabolic properties of adiponectin (Yamauchi et al., 2003), calreticulin controls aspects of adiponectin's antiinflammatory actions (Hug et al., 2004). *In vitro* studies demonstrate that adiponectin adheres to injured vascular endothelium

(Okamoto et al., 2000) and inhibits TNF-α-induced monocyte adhesion to endothelial cells. It also decreases the expression of endothelial cell adhesion molecules (Ouchi et al., 1999) and TNF-α-induced NFkB activation (Ouchi N et al., 2000).

Adiponectin has been shown to have a role in hepatic inflammation and steatosis. Hypo-adiponectinaemia is associated with nonalcoholic steatohepatitis (Targher et al., 2004) and adiponectin has been shown to have beneficial anti-inflammatory effects in liver, reducing steatosis, hepatomegaly and inflammation in mouse models of alcoholic and non-alcoholic fatty liver disease (Xu et al., 2003).

5.7 New mediators of inflammation and endothelial cell activation

5.7.1 Oxidized low-density lipoprotein receptor-1 and LOX-1

Oxidatively modified Ox-LDL and lectin-like oxidized LDL receptor-1 (LOX-1) are contributing factors of endothelial dysfunction, an early cellular event during atherogenesis. The primary receptor for Ox-LDL in endothelial cells is LOX-1. Under physiological conditions, LOX-1 may play a role in host defense (is expressed at low levels), whereas pathological states such as atherosclerosis, diabetes, dyslipedemia, hypertension dramatically and disease states that promote vascular injury, LOX-1 is highly expressed in blood vessels increase (Mattaliano et al., 2010), and may be involved in binding pro-atherogenic materials, such as ox-LDL, that activate the endothelium. With its ability to bind products that induce inflammation and endothelial activation, elevated LOX-1 expression was observed in both initial and advanced atherosclerotic lesions (Li et al., 2002). Induction of LOX-1 expression is mediated by angiotensin II and endothelin-1, both antagonists of NO (Chen et al., 2006). LOX-1 is a type II transmembrane glycoprotein that is known to recognize a wide array of structurally distinct ligands besides Ox-LDL. These include activated platelets, AGEs, apoptotic bodies, bacteria, and CRP. LOX-1 plays a critical role in the development of atherosclerosis. This may suggest that increased LOX-1 transcriptional promoter activity may equal increased LOX-1 gene expression and elevated risk of atherosclerosis. Accordingly, decreased LOX-1 promoter activation may reduce the incidence of atherosclerosis and related diseases (Chen et al., 2006).

5.7.2 Protease-Activated Receptors (PARs)

Protease-Activated Receptors (PARs) are a family of 7-transmembrane–domain, G-protein–coupled receptors that function to link tissue injury to appropriate cellular responses, such as inflammation and tissue repair, which may contribute to disease. Under the influence of the traditional cardiovascular risk factors, the endogenous defenses of the vascular endothelium begin to break down, resulting in endothelial dysfunction and injury (see figure 1). PAR activation is also linked to the secretion of IL–6, the cytokine that promotes CRP synthesis, which itself triggers many of the steps in the inflammatory process. Overall, PAR activation appears to promote the inflammatory response within the intimal tissue, enhancing the initiation and progression of atherosclerotic plaques. Rosiglitazone, a selective PPARγ agonist, exerts anti-inflammatory effects in both obese and T2D individuals by decreasing plasma concentrations of CRP, serum amyloid-A, and matrix metalloproteinase (Stienstra, 2007).

5.7.3 Lipocalin-2

A member of the lipocalin family, lipocalin-2, also known as neutrophil gelatinase-associated lipocalin, modulates inflammation and is another adipokine that is elevated in the adipose tissue of obese mouse models and in the plasma of obese and insulin-resistant humans. *In vitro* studies suggest that lipocalin-2 induces insulin resistance in adipocytes and hepatocytes. The plasma level of another member of the lipocalin family, lipocalin-type prostaglandin D synthase, serves as a biomarker of coronary atherosclerosis (Yan, 2007).

6. Oxidative Stress in conditions and comorbidities that aggregate with cardiovascular disease

Obesity, is associated with inflammation and ROS production, while advanced glycation end-products (AGEs), through their receptor (AGER or RAGE), play an important role on these processes. This is a multiligand receptor of the immunoglobulin superfamily that binds advanced glycation end-products. Thus, increased epicardial, pericardial (EAT), or subcutaneous adipose tissue (SAT) is associated with the presence and severity of coronary artery calcium. The AGE–RAGE engagement is widely related with CVD and ROS generation, mainly mediated by NADPH-oxidase. This enzyme consists in two membrane-bound subunits, the gp91-PHOX protein (NOX2) or some of its homologs (named NOX from 1 to 5) and p22-PHOX protein. Once activated, NADPH-oxidase produces superoxide anions from oxygen and NADPH or NADH. Enhanced ROS production is an important factor associated with some CVD such as CAD. Furthermore, Rodino-Janeiro et al. (2010, 2011) have previously observed that EAT may undergone higher oxidative stress than SAT in patients with CAD because of lower expression of some antioxidant enzymes, like catalase, and higher expression of RAGE in EAT than in SAT. Oxidation of phospholipids in LDL, which infiltrates into the injured vessel wall, results in the formation and accumulation of ox-LDL. These, is pro-atherogenic, produces several abnormal biological responses, such as attracting leukocytes to the intimal of the vessel, improving the ability of the leukocytes to ingest lipids and differentiate into foam cells, and stimulating the proliferation of leukocytes, endothelial cells, and smooth muscle cells, all of which are steps in the formation of atherosclerotic plaque. Furthermore, activated macrophages express scavenger receptors that internalize ox-LDL. However, unregulated uptake of ox-LDL leads to production of lipid-loaded foam cells (Hulsmans et al., 2011).

6.1 Oxidative stress and the beta-cell

Glucotoxicity, lipotoxicity, and glucolipotoxicity are secondary phenomena that are proposed to play a role in all forms of T2D. They are implicated in the pathogenesis of β–cell dysfunction (Poitout & Robertson, 2008). Hyperglycemia and hyperlipidemia follow the primary pathogenesis of diabetes and exert additional toxic effects on β-cells. The concept of toxicity derived because physiologically, it presents a continuous overstimulation of the β-cell by glucose could eventually lead to depletion of insulin stores, worsening of hyperglycemia, and finally deterioration of β-cell function. So, a prolonged *in vitro* exposure of isolated islets or insulin-secreting cells to elevated levels of fatty acids is associated with inhibited glucose-induced insulin secretion, impaired insulin gene expression, and induction of cell death by apoptosis.

6.2 Oxidative stress and diabetic vascular complications

Cardiovascular risk factors promote the production of ROS, excessive generation of ROS and has expression of eNOS been implicated in a variety of pathological events such as diabetes, hypertension, atherosclerosis, ischemia-reperfusion injury, CVD and neurodegenerative disease (Halliwell & Gutteridge, 2007). Results from several studies showed that the increase in ROS levels precedes the hyperglycemia and insulin resistance, suggesting a causal role of ROS in the disease process. Atherosclerosis is considered as the underlying pathology of cardiovascular diseases such as peripheral vascular disease, stroke, and coronary heart disease. The pathology of atherosclerosis is complex and involves structural elements of the arterial wall, platelets, leukocytes, and inflammatory cells such as monocytes and macrophages (Libby et al., 2002; Weber et al., 2008). The endothelium is a dynamic interface between the arterial wall and the circulating cells. Therefore, endothelial dysfunction accounts for one of the primary causes of atherosclerosis. Since the endothelium is the major source of NO in the vasculature, loss of normal cellular function can result in altered NO synthesis. The endothelium provides a constitutive supply of NO from eNOS, and under certain conditions (e.g. inflammation) it can produce excessive NO from the inducible isoform of NOS (iNOS). Therefore, regulation of NOS is central in the development and progression of atherosclerosis.

In particular, increased glucose leads to increased mitochondrial formation of ROS. Superoxide is a ROS that produces peroxynitrite when reacting with NO. Peroxynitrite induces cellular damage through depletion of the co-factor of the eNOS, tetrahydrobiopterin (BH4). Also, it activates the denominated classic pathways of diabetic complications, including: a) the polyol pathway, b) the AGE pathway, c) the protein kinase C (PKC) pathway, and d) the hexosamine pathway. Several studies suggested that intermittent low and high glucose conditions are even more deleterious to endothelial cell function than a steady, constant increase of glucose. These conditions also induce endothelial cells to enter into a proinflammatory state, and this state is associated with the upregulation of various adhesion molecules and proinflammatory cytokines (Piconi et al., 2004).

iNOS is very relevant to diabetic pathophysiology. Recent reports reveal that decreased expression of eNOS accompanies increased expression of iNOS and nitrotyrosine during the progression of diabetes in rats (Nagareddy et al., 2005). This finding suggests that induction of iNOS in cardiovascular tissues is dependent on the duration of diabetes and contributes significantly to depressed responses to vasoactive agents. *In vivo* studies revealed that oxidative stress due to hyperglycemia, occurring before late complications, become clinically evident (Pitocco et al., 2009). This finding suggests that oxidative stress plays a crucial role in the pathogenesis of late diabetic complications. It has also been described in human studies that endothelial cells in diabetes fail to produce sufficient amount of NO and fail to relax in response to endothelium-dependent vasorelaxants e.g. acetylcholine, bradykinin, shear stress, etc (Avogaro et al., 2006).

Further clinical data have demonstrated that rapid glycemic swings are associated with an exacerbated degree of oxidant production in human diabetes (Monnier et al., 2006), and are deleterious to the endothelial function of T2D patients (Ceriello et al., 2008). Overall, these data outline the importance of steady glucose control and the potential involvement of oxidative and nitrosative stress in the pathogenesis of complications due to poorly controlled diabetes. Diabetic subjects have reduced antioxidant capacity which could favor oxidative stress. A decline in important cellular antioxidant defense mechanisms, including the glutathione redox system and vitamin C-vitamin E cycle, significantly increases the susceptibility to oxidative stress. Thus, attempts have been made to reduce oxidative stress-dependent cellular changes in patients with diabetes by supplementation with naturally occurring antioxidants, especially vitamins E and C, lipoic acid levels are reduced in diabetic patients.

It has now been established that measurement of F2-isoprostanes is the most reliable approach to assess oxidative stress status *in vivo*, providing an important tool to explore the role of oxidative stress in the pathogenesis of human disease. In addition, products of the isoprostane (IsoP) pathway have been found to exert potent biological actions and therefore may be pathophysiologic mediators of disease. IsoPs, 8-iso-PGF2α and 8-iso-PGE2 possess potent biological effects in various systems and they also serve as mediators of oxidant stress through their vasoconstrictive and inflammatory properties (Kaviarasan et al., 2009). There exists a significant correlation between blood glucose and urinary IsoPs levels, suggesting that peroxidation is related to glycemic control. In vascular smooth muscle cells, F2-IsoPs formation was found to be induced *in vitro* by high glucose concentrations.

6.3 Cardiovascular disease

The diverse responses of the microvasculature to CVD risk factors include oxidative stress, enhanced leukocyte and platelet-endothelial cell adhesion, impaired endothelial barrier function, altered capillary proliferation, enhanced thrombosis, and vasomotor dysfunction (Granger et al., 2010).

As shown in figure 1, an imbalance between the production and detoxification of ROS in vascular endothelial cells can result in the oxidative modification of cell components, impair cell function and/or can enhance cell death via apoptosis or necrosis. The oxidative activation of enzymes (phospholipase A2) and transcription factors (nuclear factor kB, NFkB) that accompanies excess ROS production can also result in an enhanced biosynthesis of lipids (platelet activating factor, leukotrienes) and proteins (adhesion molecules, cytokines) that promote inflammation. Superoxide, by virtue of its ability to inactivate nitric oxide (an anti-inflammatory molecule), is another link between oxidative stress and the induction of a pro-inflammatory phenotype in the vasculature. This oxidative stress in the vessel wall is often accompanied by an increased production of superoxide anion by circulating immune cells, and there is evidence for a causal link between these two sources of ROS: circulating cells and vessel wall.

Different enzymatic sources have been implicated in the enhanced ROS production, including NADPH oxidase, xanthine oxidase, mitochondrial enzymes, and uncoupled nitric oxide synthase. It remains to clarify whether the pro-hypertensive effects of the superoxide anion relate to its ability to inactivate NO or to indirectly promote the production of endogenous vasoconstrictors, such as endothelin. NADPH-oxidase has received the most attention as a potential source of ROS in hypertension (HTN), followed by xanthine oxidase. Both endothelial cell- and leukocyte-associated NADPH-oxidase have been implicated in HTN-induced superoxide production, and there is evidence linking both cellular sources of the enzyme to activation of the angiotensin II type 1 receptor (AT1r) and to cytokines (TNF-α) derived from circulating immune cells (Crimi et al., 2007; Harrison & Gongora, 2009).

While some adipokines as leptin and adiponectin have been shown to promote the expression of endothelial cell adhesion molecules (CAMs) and leukocyte-endothelial cell adhesion (LECA) are known to exert an inhibitory effect on these responses. The absence of LECA in the microcirculation of obese mice under basal conditions suggests either that the pro- and anti-adhesive adipokines are in balance or that the systemic plasma levels achieved by these mediators do not cause overt inflammation in tissues distant from their source (adipose tissue). The latter possibility is supported by evidence of an increased sensitivity (priming) of endothelial cells and leukocytes in obese animals to inflammatory stimuli.

However, within the microvasculature of adipose tissue, a robust inflammatory response is noted under basal conditions, as reflected by an increased expression of the endothelial cell adhesion molecules ICAM-1 and E- and P-select in, with an accompanying recruitment of rolling and firmly adherent leukocytes, and the formation of platelet-leukocyte aggregates. The reduced LECA may be linked to adiponectin deficiency since the adipokine is a potent inhibitor of LECA and its production/release is diminished during adipogenesis (Singer & Granger, 2007).

6.4 Oxidative stress in aortic valves

Superoxide levels also are increased in stenotic aortic valves from humans. Heistad et al., (2009) found, in stenotic valves removed during surgical replacement of the aortic valve, that superoxide is increased greatly near calcified regions of the valve. Others authors (Miller et al., 2008) also found, in valves obtained at surgery or autopsy, that oxidative stress is increased in stenotic aortic valves. Thus, in calcified stenotic aortic valves as well as in atherosclerotic lesions, oxidative stress is increased. But, there are important differences in mechanisms that account for oxidative stress in aortic valves and in atherosclerotic arteries. In calcific aortic stenosis, increased production of superoxide may be mediated by "uncoupling" of NOS, as NOS primarily produces superoxide instead of nitric oxide NAD(P)H expression and activity do not appear to be increased in aortic valves (Miller et al., 2008). In striking contrast, increased expression and activity of NADPH-oxidase appears to be a major mechanism for oxidative stress in atherosclerotic lesions. Oxidative stress, in addition to contributing to fibrosis, may activate matrix metalloproteinases (MMPs) in the aortic valve and arteries. In the valve, MMPs may play a permissive role in expansion of calcification of the valve, and degraded fragments of collagen and elastin also may increase pro-calcific signaling in valvular interstitial cells. Activation of MMPs in arteries probably is harmful in a different way, by contributing to plaque rupture.

6.5 Atrial fibrillation

Atrial fibrillation (AF) is the most common sustained cardiac arrhythmia in clinical practice and contributes to impaired quality of life, and increased morbidity and mortality. The mechanisms underlying both the initiation and perpetuation of AF are not well established but are thought to involve inflammation and oxidative stress. Furthermore, a number of studies have shown that concentrations of inflammatory mediators or markers, such as IL-6 and high-sensitivity CRP (hs-CRP), are increased in patients with AF. One mechanism that may mediate the effects of inflammation in AF is oxidative stress. Elevated inflammatory biomarkers are strongly associated with AF. Inflammation has important prognostic implications in AF; large prospective studies have shown that elevated hs-CRP levels correlated with risk factors for stroke and overall prognosis. The positive correlation between elevated levels of TNF-α and N-terminal pro-brain natriuretic peptide (NTpBNP) and severity of AF suggests that these biomarkers could be prognostic markers for AF in clinical practice (Li et al., 2010).

6.6 Insulin resistance

A large number of studies have evidenced the pivotal role of oxidative stress in insulin resistance states such as metabolic syndrome, obesity, and T2D (Atabek et al., 2004; Block et al., 2002). Decreased antioxidant capacity, increased production of ROS with oxidation products of lipids, DNA, and proteins have been reported in plasma, urine, and various tissues, suggesting systemic and organ-specific oxidative stress. Recent evidence for systemic oxidative stress includes the detection of increased circulating and urinary levels of the lipid peroxidation product F2-isoprostane (8-epi-prostaglandin F2α) in both T1D and T2D patients (Davi et al., 2003). As described above, ROS and reactive nitrogen species (RNS) are able to directly modify the expression of adiponectin. Secreted almost exclusively from adipocytes, it is inversely correlated with fat mass in obesity and with its associated cardiovascular risk. It should be considered that, plasma and urinary lipid peroxidation markers indicative of systemic OS correlated with lower circulating adiponectin levels.

7. Conclusion

Figure 1 summarizes much of the content of this chapter, because it shows most of the cellular elements and signaling pathways in which highlights the participation of adipocytokines involved in the immune response and oxidative stress on the vascular endothelium. These alterations lead to development of atherosclerosis. And finally this endothelial damage, together with the increase in free radicals can cause multiorgan damage.

In conclusion, abnormal adipocytokine expression with consequent inflammation, oxidative stress itself may result from the inflammatory changes that occur in obesity. Therefore, a vicious cycle that provokes increased oxidative stress in obesity may exist. Reactive oxygen species that lead to increased oxidative stress can be generated in adipocytes and in other cell types such as leukocytes, all of which can be a source of increased oxidative stress in obese humans. Increased oxidative stress is independently associated with obesity measures including body mass index and waist-hip ratio. It is also associated with several CVD risk factors including smoking, blood glucose, and hyperlipidemia. Oxidative stress and increased adipocytokines may also promote endothelial dysfunction, atherogenesis, and coronary heart disease independent of traditional risk factors.

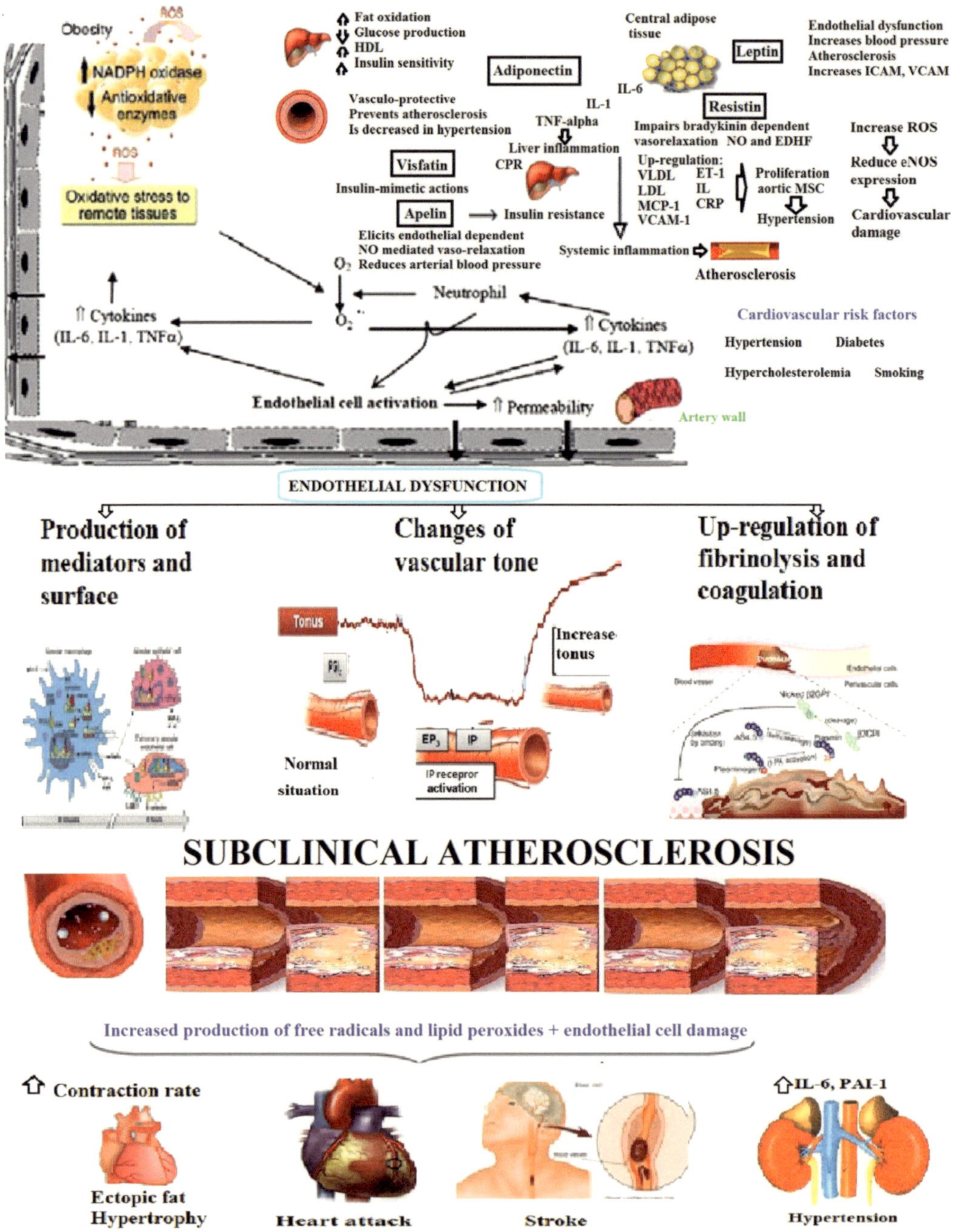

Fig. 1. Impaired cardiovascular functions and adipocytokines actions on oxidative stress. This figure shows the majority of cellular elements and signaling pathways in which highlights the participation of adipocytokines (framed) involved in the immune response and oxidative stress on the vascular endothelium. These alterations lead to development of atherosclerosis. And finally, this endothelial dysfunction can generate harmful free radicals and cause tissue and multiorgan damage.

8. References

Alexander, CM. Landsman, PB. Teutsch SM. & Haffner SM. NCEP. (2003). Defined Metabolic Syndrome, Diabetes, and Prevalence of Coronary Heart Disease Among NHANES III Participants Age 50 Years and Older. *Diabetes*, Vol. 52, No. 5, pp. 1210-1214

Antuna-Puente, B. Feve, B. Fellahi, S. & Bastard, JP. (2008). Adipokines: the missing link between insulin resistance and obesity. *Diabetes Metab*, Vol. 34, No. 1, pp. 2-11

Ashley, EA. Powers, J. Chen, M. Kundu, R. Finsterbach, T. Caffarelli, A. Deng, A. Eichhorn, J. Mahajan, R. Agrawal, R. Greve, J. Robbins, R. Patterson, AJ. Bernstein D. & Quertermous, T. (2005). The endogenous peptide apelin potently improves cardiac contractility and reduces cardiac loading in vivo. Cardiovasc Res, Vol. 65, pp. 73-82

Atabek, ME. Vatansev, H. & Erkul, I. (2004). Oxidative stress in childhood obesity. J Pediatr Endocrinol Metab, Vol. 17, pp. 1063-1068

Atluri, P. Morine, KJ. Liao, GP. Panlilio, CM. Berry, MF. Hsu, VM. Hiesinger, W. Cohen, JE. & Joseph, WY. (2007). Ischemic heart failure enhances endogenous myocardial apelin and APJ receptor expression. Cell Mol Biol Lett, Vol. 12, pp. 127-138

Avogaro, A. Fadini, GP. Gallo, A. Pagnin, E. & de Kreutzenberg, S. (2006). Endothelial dysfunction in type 2 diabetes mellitus. Nutr Metab Cardiovasc Dis, Vol. 16, No. 1, pp. S39-S45

Bastard, JP. Maachi, M. Van Nhieu, JT. Jardel, C. Bruckert, E. Grimaldi, A. Robert, JJ. Capeau, J. & Hainque B. (2002). Adipose tissue IL-6 content correlates with resistance to insulin activation of glucose uptake both in vivo and in vitro. J Clin Endocrinol Metab, Vol. 87, pp. 2084-2089

Behrendt, D. & Ganz, P. (2002). Endothelial function: from vascular biology to clinical applications. Am J Cardiol, Vol. 90, pp. 40L-48L

Beltowski, J. (2006). Apelin and visfatin: unique "beneficial" adipokines upregulated in obesity? Med Sci Monit, Vol. 12, pp. RA112-RA119

Berg, AH. Combs, TP. Du, X. Brownlee, M. & Scherer, PE. (2001). The adipocyte-secreted protein Acrp30 enhances hepatic insulin action. Nat Med, Vol. 7, pp. 947-953

Berndt, J. Klöting, N. Kralisch, S. Kovacs, P. Fasshauer, M. Schön, MR. Stumvoll, M. & Blüher, M. (2005). Plasma visfatin concentrations and fat depot-specific mRNA expression in humans. Diabetes, Vol. 54, No. 10. pp. 2911-2916

Block, G. Dietrich, M. Norkus, EP. Morrow, JD. Hudes, M. Caan, B. & Packer, L. (2002). Factors associated with oxidative stress in human populations. Am J Epidemiol, Vol. 156, pp. 274-285

Buettner, C. Pocai, A. Muse, ED. Etgen, AM. Myers, MG Jr. & Rossetti, L. (2006). Critical role of STAT3 in leptin's metabolic actions. Cell Metab, Vol. 4, No. 1, pp. 49-60

Catalá A. (2006). An overview of lipid peroxidation with emphasis in outer segments of photoreceptors and the chemiluminescence assay. Int J Biochem Cell Biol, Vol. 38, No. 9, pp. 1482-1495

Ceriello, A. & Motz, E. (2004). Is Oxidative Stress the Pathogenic Mechanism Underlying Insulin Resistance, Diabetes, and Cardiovascular Disease? The Common Soil Hypothesis Revisited. Arterioscler Thromb Vasc Biol, Vol. 24, pp. 816-823

Ceriello, A. Esposito, K. Piconi, L. Ihnat, MA. Thorpe, JE. Testa, R. Boemi, M. & Giugliano, D. (2008). Oscillating glucose is more deleterious to endothelial function and oxidative stress than mean glucose in normal and type 2 diabetic patients. Diabetes, Vol. 57, No. 5, pp. 1349-1354

Chandran, M. Phillips, SA. Ciaraldi, T. & Henry, RR. (2003). Adiponectin: more than just another fat cell hormone?. Diabetes Care, Vol. 26, No. 8, pp. 2442-50

Chandrasekaran, B. Dar, O. & McDonagh, T. (2008). The role of apelin in cardiovascular function and heart failure. Eur J Heart Fail, Vol. 10, pp. 725-732

Chen, MP. Chung, FM. Chang, DM. Tsai, JC-R. Huang, HF. Shin, SJ. & Lee, YJ. (2006). ENPP1 K121Q Polymorphism is not Related to Type 2 Diabetes Mellitus, Features of Metabolic Syndrome, and Diabetic Cardiovascular Complications in a Chinese Population. Rev Diabet Stud, Vol. 3, No. 1, pp. 21-30

Chow, WS. Cheung, BM. Tso, AW. Xu, A. Wat, NM. Fong, CH. Ong, LH. Tam, S. Tan, KC. Janus, ED. Lam, TH. & Lam, KS. (2007). Hypoadiponectinemia as a predictor for the development of hypertension: a 5-year prospective study. Hypertension, Vol. 49, No. 6, pp. 1455-1461

Cnop, M. Havel, PJ. Utzschneider, KM. Carr, DB. Sinha, MK. Boyko, EJ. Retzlaff, BM. Knopp, RH. Brunzell, JD. & Kahn, SE. (2003). Relationship of adiponectin to body fat distribution, insulin sensitivity and plasma lipoproteins: evidence for independent roles of age and sex. Diabetologia, Vol. 46, No. 4, pp. 459-69

Cominacini, L. Rigoni, Pasini, AF. Garbin, U. Davoli, A. Campagnola, M. Pastorino, AM. Lo Cascio, V. & Sawamura, T. (2001). The binding of oxidized low-density lipoprotein (ox-LDL) to ox-LDL receptor-1 in endothelial cells reduces the intracellular concentration of nitric oxide through an increased production of superoxide. J Biol Chem, Vol. 276, No. 17, pp. 13750-13755

Correia, ML. & Rahmouni, K. (2006). Role of leptin in the cardiovascular and endocrine complications of metabolic syndrome. Diabetes Obes Metab, Vol. 8, No. 6, 603-610

Crimi, E. Ignarro, LJ. & Napoli, C. (2007). Microcirculation and oxidative stress. Free Radic Res, Vol. 41, No. 12, pp. 1364-1375

Cunningham, JT. Rodgers, JT. Arlow, DH. Vazquez, F. Mootha, VK. & Puigserver, P. (2007). mTOR controls mitochondrial oxidative function through a YY1-PGC-1alpha transcriptional complex. Nature, Vol. 450, No. 7170, pp. 736-740

Curti, MLR. Jacob, P. Borges, MC. Rogero, MM. & Ferreira, SRG. (2011). Studies of Gene Variants Related to Inflammation, Oxidative Stress, Dyslipidemia, and Obesity: Implications for a Nutrigenetic Approach. J Obes, Vol. 2011, pp. 1-30

Davi, G. Chiarelli, F. Santilli, F. Pomilio, M. Vigneri, S. Falco, A. Basili, S. Ciabattoni, G. & Patrono, C. (2003). Enhanced lipid peroxidation and platelet activation in the early phase of type 1 diabetes mellitus: role of interleukin-6 and disease duration. Circulation, Vol. 107, pp. 3199-3203

Dokken, BB. (2008). The Pathophysiology of Cardiovascular Disease and Diabetes: Beyond Blood Pressure and Lipids. Diabetes Spectrum, Vol. 21, No. 3, pp. 160-165

Dudina, A. Cooney, MT. De Bacquer, D. De Backer, G. Ducimetière, P. Jousilahti, P. Keil, U. Menotti, A. Njølstad, I. Oganov, R. Sans, S. Thomsen, T. Tverdal, A. Wedel, H. Whincup, P. Wilhelmsen, L. Conroy, R. Fitzgerald, A. & Graham, I. (2011). Relationships between body mass index, cardiovascular mortality, and risk factors: a report from the SCORE investigators. Eur J Cardiovasc Prev Rehabil, [Epub ahead of print].

Duell, PB. Oram, JF. & Bierman EL. (1991). Nonenzymatic glycosylation of HDL and impaired HDL-receptor-mediated cholesterol efflux. Diabetes, Vol. 40, No. 3, pp. 377-384

Dusserre, E. Moulin, P. & Vidal, H. (2000). Differences in mRNA expression of the proteins secreted by the adipocytes in human subcutaneous and visceral adipose tissues. Biochim Biophys Acta, Vol. 1500:88-96

Dusting, GJ. & Triggle, C. (2005). Are we over oxidized? Oxidative stress, cardiovascular disease, and the future of intervention studies with antioxidants. Vasc Health Risk Manag, Vol. 1, No. 2, pp. 93-97

Evans, JL. & Goldfine, ID. (2000). Alpha-Lipoic acid: a multifunctional antioxidant that improves insulin sensitivity in patients with type 2 diabetes. Diabetes Technol Ther, Vol. 2, No. 3, pp. 401-413

Földes, G. Horkay, F. Szokodi, I. Vuolteenaho, O. Ilves, M. Lindstedt, KA. Mäyränpää, M. Sármán, B. Seres, L. Skoumal, R. Lakó-Futó, Z. deChâtel, R. Ruskoaho, H. & Tóth, M. (2003). Circulating and cardiac levels of apelin, the novel ligand of the orphan receptor APJ, in patients with heart failure. Biochem Biophys Res Commun, Vol. 308, No. 3, pp. 480-485

Fontana, L. Eagon, JC. Trujillo, ME. Scherer, PE. & Klein, S. (2007). Visceral fat adipokine secretion is associated with systemic inflammation in obese humans. Diabetes, Vol. 56, pp. 1010-1013

Fukuhara, A. Matsuda, M. Nishizawa, M. Segawa, K. Tanaka, M. Kishimoto, K. Matsuki, Y. Murakami, M. Ichisaka, T. Murakami, H. Watanabe, E. Takagi, T. Akiyoshi, M. Ohtsubo, T. Kihara, S. Yamashita, S. Makishima, M. Funahashi, T. Yamanaka, S. Hiramatsu, R. Matsuzawa, Y. & Shimomura, I. (2005). Visfatin: a protein secreted by visceral fat that mimics the effects of insulin. Science, Vol. 307, No. 5708, pp. 426-430

Gómez-Marcos, MA. Martínez-Salgado, C. Martin-Cantera, C. Recio-Rodríguez, JI. Castaño-Sánchez, Y. Giné-Garriga, M. Rodriguez-Sanchez, E. & García-Ortiz, L. (2009). Therapeutic implications of selecting the SCORE (European) versus the D'AGOSTINO (American) risk charts for cardiovascular risk assessment in hypertensive patients. BMC Cardiovasc Disord, Vol. 9, pp. 1-17

Granger, DN. Rodrigues, SF. Yildirim, A. & Senchenkova, EY. (2010). Microvascular responses to cardiovascular risk factors. Microcirculation, Vol. 17, No. 3, pp. 192-205

Haider, DG. Leuchten, N. Schaller, G. Gouya, G. Kolodjaschna, J. Schmetterer, L. Kapiotis, S. & Wolzt M. (2006). C-reactive protein is expressed and secreted by peripheral blood mononuclear cells. Clin Exp Immunol, Vol. 146, No. 3, pp. 533-539

Halliwell, R. & Gutteridge, JMC. Free Radicals in Biology and Medicine, 4th edition, Oxford University Press, London, 2007

Hammarstedt, A. Sopasakis, VR. Gogg, S. Jansson, PA. & Smith, U. (2005). Improved insulin sensitivity and adipose tissue dysregulation after short-term treatment with pioglitazone in non-diabetic, insulin-resistant subjects. Diabetologia, Vol. 48, No. 1, pp. 96-104

Harrington, LS. Findlay, GM. & Lamb, RF. (2005). Restraining PI3K: mTOR signalling goes back to the membrane. Trends Biochem Sci Vol, 30, No. 1, pp. 35-42

Harrison, DG. & Gongora, MC. (2009). Oxidative stress and hypertension. Med Clin North Am, Vol. 93:621-635.

Heidemann, CC. Schulze, MB. Franco, OH. van Dam, RM. Mantzoros, CS. & Hu FB. (2008). Dietary Patterns and Risk of Mortality from Cardiovascular Disease, Cancer, and All-Causes in a Prospective Cohort of Women: Heidemann-Dietary Patterns and Mortality. Circulation, Vol. 118, No. 3, pp. 230-237

Heistad, DD. Wakisaka, Y. Miller, J. Chu, Y. & Pena-Silva R. (2009). Novel aspects of oxidative stress in cardiovascular diseases. Circ J, Vol. 73, No. 2, pp. 201-207

Heitzer, T. Schlinzig, T. Krohn, K. Meinertz, T. & Münzel, T. (2001) Endothelial dysfunction, oxidative stress, and risk of cardiovascular events in patients with coronary artery disease. Circulation, Vol. 104, pp. 2673-2678

Holland, WL. Miller, RA. Wang, ZV. Sun, K. Barth, BM. Bui, HH. Davis, KE. Bikman, BT. Halberg, N. Rutkowski, JM. Wade, MR. Tenorio, VM. Kuo, MS. Brozinick, JT. Zhang, BB. Birnbaum, MJ. Summers, SA. & Scherer, PE. (2011). Receptor-mediated activation of ceramidase activity initiates the pleiotropic actions of adiponectin. Nat Med, Vol. 17, pp. 55-63

Hubert, HB. Feinleib, M. McNamara, PM. & Castelli, WP. (1983). Obesity as an independent risk factor for cardiovascular disease: a 26-year follow-up of participants in the Framingham Study. Circulation, Vol. 67, No. 5, pp. 968-977

Hug, C. Wang, J. Ahmad, NS. Bogan, JS. Tsao, TS. & Lodish, HF. (2004). T-cadherin is a receptor for hexameric and high-molecular-weight forms of Acrp30/adiponectin. Proc Natl Acad Sci USA, Vol. 101, No. 28, pp. 10308-10313

Hulsmans, M. De Keyzer, D. & Holvoet, P. (2011). MicroRNAs regulating oxidative stress and inflammationin relation to obesity and atherosclerosis. FASEB J, Vol. 25, No. 8, pp. 2515-2527

Isomaa, B. Almgren, P. Tuomi, T. Forsén, B. Lahti, K. Nissén, M. Taskinen, MR. & Groop, L. (2001). Cardiovascular Morbidity and Mortality Associated With the Metabolic Syndrome. Diabetes Care, Vol. 24, pp. 683-689

Japp, AG. & Newby, DE. (2008). The apelin-APJ system in heart failure: pathophysiologic relevance and therapeutic potential. Biochem Pharmacol, Vol. 75, No. 10, pp. 1882-1892

Chen, J. Liu, Y. Liu, H. Hermonat, PL. & Mehta, JL. (2006). Lectin-like oxidized low-density lipoprotein receptor-1 (LOX-1) transcriptional regulation by Oct-1 in human endothelial cells: implications for atherosclerosis. Biochem J, Vol. 393, No. 1, pp. 255-265

Kadowaki, T. Yamauchi, T. Kubota, N. Hara, K. & Ueki, K. (2007). Adiponectin and adiponectin receptors in obesity-linked insulin resistance. Novartis Found Symp, Vol. 286, pp. 164-176

Kaviarasan, S. Muniandy, S. Qvist, R. & Ismail, IS. (2009). F2-Isoprostanes as Novel Biomarkers for Type 2 Diabetes: a Review. J Clin Biochem Nutr, Vol. 45, No. 1, pp. 1-8

Kawamata, Y. Habata, Y. Fukusumi, S. Hosoya, M. Fujii, R. Hinuma, S. Nishizawa, N. Kitada, C. Onda, H. Nishimura O. & Fujino, M. (2001). Molecular properties of apelin: tissue distribution and receptor binding. BBA Mol Cell Res, Vol. 1538, No. 2-3, pp. 162-171

Kern, PA. Di Gregorio, GB. Lu, T. Rassouli, N. & Ranganathan, G. (2003). Adiponectin expression from human adipose tissue: relation to obesity, insulin resistance, and tumor necrosis factor-alpha expression. Diabetes, Vol. 52, No. 7, pp. 1779-1785

Khot, UN. Khot, MB. Bajzer, CT. Sapp, SK. Ohman, EM. Brener, SJ. Ellis, SG. Lincoff, AM. & Topol, EJ. (2003). Prevalence of Conventional Risk Factors in Patients With Coronary Heart Disease. JAMA, Vol. 290, No. 7, pp. 898-904

Kim, JE. & Chen, J. (2004). Regulation of peroxisome proliferator-activated receptor-gamma activity by mammalian target of rapamycin and amino acids in adipogenesis. Diabetes, Vo. 53, pp. 2748-2756

Kim, JY. van de Wall, E. Laplante, M. Azzara, A. Trujillo, ME. Hofmann, SM. Schraw, T. Durand, JL. Li, H. Li, G. Jelicks, LA. Mehler, MF. Hui, DY. Deshaies, Y. Shulman, GI. Schwartz, GJ. & Scherer, PE. (2007). Obesity-associated improvements in metabolic profile through expansion of adipose tissue. J Clin Invest, Vol. 117, No. 9, pp. 2621-2637

Kitani, T. Okuno, S. & Fujisawa, H. (2003). Growth phase-dependent changes in the subcellular localization of pre-B-cell colony-enhancing factor. FEBS Lett, Vol. 544, No. 1-3, pp. 74-78

Kojima, S. Funahashi, T. Sakamoto, T. Miyamoto, S. Soejima, H. Hokamaki, J. Kajiwara, I. Sugiyama, S. Yoshimura, M. Fujimoto, K. Miyao, Y. Suefuji, H. Kitagawa, A. Ouchi, N. Kihara, S. Matsuzawa, Y. & Ogawa, H. (2003). The variation of plasma concentrations of a novel, adipocyte derived protein, adiponectin, in patients with acute myocardial infarction. Heart, Vol. 89, No. 6, pp. 667-668

Kotzé, Alwyn. & Howell, SJ. (2008). Heart failure: pathophysiology, risk assessment, community management and anaesthesia. Contin Educ Anaesth Crit Care Pain, Vol. 8, No. 5, 161-166

Kubota, N. Terauchi, Y. Yamauchi, T. Kubota, T. Moroi, M. Matsui, J. Eto, K. Yamashita, T. Kamon, J. Satoh, H. Yano, W. Froguel, P. Nagai, R. Kimura, S. Kadowaki, T. & Noda, T. (2002). Disruption of adiponectin causes insulin resistance and neointimal formation. J Biol Chem, Vol. 277, No. 29, pp. 25863-25866

Kunjathoor, VV. Febbraio, M. Podrez, EA. Moore, KJ. Andersson, L. Koehn, S. Rhee, JS. Silverstein, S. Hoff, HF. & Freeman, MW. (2002). Scavenger receptors class A-I/II and CD36 are the principal receptors responsible for the uptake of modified low density lipoprotein leading to lipid loading in macrophages. J Biol Chem, Vol. 277, No. 51, pp. 49982-49988

Kurata, A. Nishizawa, H. Kihara, S. Maeda, N. Sonoda, M. Okada, T. Ohashi, K. Hibuse, T. Fujita, K. Yasui, A. Hiuge, A. Kumada, M. Kuriyama, H. Shimomura, I. & Funahashi, T. (2006). Blockade of Angiotensin II type-1 receptor reduces oxidative stress in adipose tissue and ameliorates adipocytokinedysregulation. Kidney International, Vol. 70, pp. 1717-1724

Lago, F. Dieguez, C. Gómez-Reino, J. & Oreste, G. (2007). Adipokines as emerging mediators of immune response and inflammation. Nat Clin Pract Rheum, Vol. 3, No. 12, pp. 716-724

Landmesser, U. & Harrison, DG. (2001). Oxidant Stress as a Marker for Cardiovascular Events Ox Marks the Spot. Circulation, Vol. 104, pp. 2638-2640

Laplante, M. & Sabatini, DM. (2009). mTOR signaling at a glance. J Cell Science, Vol. 122, pp. 3589-3594

Lara-Castro, C. Luo, N. Wallace, P. Klein, RL. & Garvey, WT. (2006). Adiponectin multimeric complexes and the metabolic syndrome trait cluster. Diabetes, Vol. 55, No. 1, pp. 249-259

Lavie, CJ. Milani, RV. & Ventura, HO. (2009). Obesity and Cardiovascular Disease: Risk Factor, Paradox, and Impact of Weight Loss. J Am Coll Cardiol, Vol. 53, No. 21, pp. 1925-1932

Lee, DK. Saldivia, VR. Nguyen, T. Cheng, R. George, SR. & O'Dowd, BF. (2005). Modification of the terminal residue of apelin-13 antagonizes its hypotensive action. Endocrinology, Vol. 146, No. 1, pp. 231-236

Lee, DF. Kuo, HP. Chen, CT. Hsu, JM. Chou, CK. Wei, Y. Sun, HL. Li, LY. Ping, B. Huang, WC. He, X. Hung, JY. Lai, CC. Ding, Q. Su, JL. Yang, JY. Sahin, AA. Hortobagyi, GN. Tsai, FJ. Tsai, CH. & Hung, MC. (2007). IKK beta suppression of TSC1 links inflammation and tumor angiogenesis via the mTOR pathway. Cell, Vol. 130, No. 3, pp. 440-455

Lee, DF. Kuo, HP. Chen, CT. Wei, Y. Chou, CK. Hung, JY. Yen, CJ. & Hung, MC. (2008). IKKbeta suppression of TSC1 function links the mTOR pathway with insulin resistance. Int J Mol Med, Vol. 22, No. 5, pp. 633-638

Lehoux, S. Castier, Y. Tedgui, A. (2006). Molecular mechanisms of the vascular responses to haemodynamic forces. J Inter Med, Vol. 259, pp. 381-392

Li, DY. Chen, HJ. Staples, ED. Ozaki, K. Annex, B. Singh, BK. Vermani, R. & Mehtat, JL. (2002). Oxidized low-density lipoprotein receptor LOX-1 and apoptosis in human atherosclerotic lesions. J Cardiovasc Pharmacol Ther, Vol. 7, No. 3, pp. 147-153

Li, J. Solus, J. Chen, Q. Rho, YH. Milne, G. Stein, CM. & Darbar, D. (2010). The Role of Inflammation and Oxidative Stress in Atrial Fibrillation. Heart Rhythm, Vol. 7, No. 4, pp. 438-444

Libby, P. Ridker, PM. & Maseri, A. (2002). Inflammation and atherosclerosis. Circulation, Vol. 105, No. 9, pp. 1135-1143

Lopaschuck, GD. Folmes, CDL. & Stanley, WC. (2007). Cardiac energy metabolism in obesity. Circ Res, Vol. 101, No. 4, pp. 335-347

Madamanchi, NR. Vendrov, A. & Runge, MS. (2005). Oxidative Stress and Vascular Disease. Arterioscler Thromb Vasc Biol, Vol. 25, pp. 29-38

Maeda, N. Shimomura, I. Kishida, K. Nishizawa, H. Matsuda, M. Nagaretani, H. Furuyama, N. Kondo, H. Takahashi, M. Arita, Y. Komuro, R. Ouchi1, N. Kihara, S. Tochino, Y. Okutomi, K. Horie, M. Takeda, S. Aoyama, T. Funahashi, T. & Matsuzawa, Y. (2002). Diet-induced insulin resistance in mice lacking adiponectin/aCRP30. Nat Med, Vol. 8, pp. 731-737

Manning, BD. (2004). Balancing Akt with S6K: implications for both metabolic diseases and tumorigenesis. J Cell Biol, Vol. 167, No. 3, pp. 399-403

Mattaliano, MD. Wooters, J. Shih, HH. & Paulsen, JE. (2010). ROCK2 associates with lectin-like oxidized LDL receptor-1 and mediates oxidized LDL-induced IL-8 production. Am J Physiol Cell Physiol, Vol. 298, No. 5, pp. C1180-C1187

Matsuki, K. Tamasawa, N. Yamashita, M. Tanabe, J. Murakami, H. Matsui, J. Imaizumi, T. Satoh, K. & Suda, T. (2009). Metformin restores impaired HDL-mediated cholesterol efflux due to glycation. Atherosclerosis, Vol. 206, No. 2, pp. 434-438

Miller, JD. Chu, Y. Brooks, RM. Richenbacher, WE. Peña-Silva, R. & Heistad, DD. (2008). Dysregulation of antioxidant mechanisms contributes to increased oxidative stress in calcific aortic valvular stenosis in humans. J Am Coll Cardiol, Vol. 52, No. 10, pp. 843-850

Monnier, L. Mas, E. Ginet, C. Michel, F. Villon, L. Cristol, JP. & Colette, C. (2006). Activation of oxidative stress by acute glucose fluctuations compared with sustained chronic hyperglycemia in patients with type 2 diabetes. JAMA, Vol. 295, No. 14, pp. 1681-1687

Mutch, NJ. Wilson, HM. & Booth, NA. (2001). Plasminogen activator inhibitor-1 and haemostasis in obesity. Proc Nutr Soc, Vol. 60, No. 3, pp. 341-347

Nagareddy, PR. Xia, Z. McNeill, JH. & MacLeod, KM. (2005). Increased expression of iNOS is associated with endothelial dysfunction and impaired pressor responsiveness in streptozotocin- induced diabetes. Am J Physiol Heart Circ Physiol, Vol. 289, No. 5, pp. H2144-H2152

Naito, Y. Masaichi-Chang-il, Lee. Kato, Y. Nagai, R. & Yonei, Y. (2010). Oxidative Stress Markers. Anti-Aging Medicine, Vol. 7, No. 5, pp. 36-44

Nawrocki, AR. Rajala, MW. Tomas, E. Pajvani, UB. Saha, AK. Trumbauer, ME. Pang, Z. Chen, AS. Ruderman, NB. Chen, H. Rossetti, L. & Scherer, PE. (2006). Mice lacking adiponectin show decreased hepatic insulin sensitivity and reduced responsiveness to peroxisome proliferator-activated receptor gamma agonists. J Biol Chem, Vol. 281, No. 5, pp. 2654-2660

Okamoto, Y. Arita, Y. Nishida, M. Muraguchi, M. Ouchi, N. Takahashi, M. Igura, T. Inui, Y. Kihara, S. Nakamura, T. Yamashita, S. Miyagawa, J. Funahashi, T. & Matsuzawa, Y. (2000). An adipocytederived plasma protein, adiponectin, adheres to injured vascular walls. Horm Metab Res, Vol. 32, No. 2, pp. 47–50

Ouchi, N. Kihara, S. Arita, Y. Maeda, K. Kuriyama, H. Okamoto, Y. Hotta, K. Nishida, M. Takahashi, M. Nakamura, T. Yamashita, S. Funahashi, T. & Matsuzawa, Y. (1999). Novel modulator for endotelial adhesión molecules: adipocyte-derived plasma protein adiponectin. Circulation, Vol. 100, No. 25, pp. 2473-2476

Ouchi, N. Kihara, S. Arita, Y. Okamoto, Y. Maeda, K. Kuriyama, H. Hotta, K. Nishida, M. Takahashi, M. Muraguchi, M. Ohmoto, Y. Nakamura, T. Yamashita, S. Funahashi, T. & Matsuzawa, Y. (2000). Adiponectin, an adipocyte-derived plasma protein, inhibits endothelial NF-kappaB signaling through a cAMP-dependent pathway. Circulation, Vol. 102, No. 11, pp. 1296-1301

Ouchi, N. Kihara, S. Funahashi, T. Nakamura, T. Nishida, M. Kumada, M. Okamoto, Y. Ohashi, K. Nagaretani, H. Kishida, K. Nishizawa, H. Maeda, N. Kobayashi, H. Hiraoka, H. & Matsuzawa, Y. (2003). Reciprocal association of C-reactive protein with adiponectin in blood stream and adipose tissue. Circulation, Vol. 107, pp. 671-674

Parati, G. Lombardi, C. & Narkiewicz, K. (2007). Sleep apnea: epidemiology, pathophysiology, and relation to cardiovascular risk. Am J Physiol Regul Integr Comp Physiol, Vol. 293, No. 4, pp. R1671-R1683

Piconi, L. Quagliaro, L. Da Ros, R. Assaloni, R. Giugliano, D. Esposito, K. Szabo, C. & Ceriello, A. (2004). Intermittent high glucose enhances ICAM-1, VCAM-1, E-selectin and interleukin-6 expression in human umbilical endothelial cells in culture: the role of poly(ADP-ribose) polymerase. J Thromb Haemost, Vol. 2, No. 8, pp. 1453-1459

Pitocco, D. Zaccardi, F. Di Stasio, E. Romitelli, F. Martini, F. Scaglione, GL. Speranza, D. Santini, S. Zuppi, C. & Ghirlanda, G. (2009). Role of asymmetric-dimethyl-larginine (ADMA) and nitrite/nitrate (NOx) in the pathogenesis of oxidative stress in female subjects with uncomplicated type 1 diabetes mellitus. Diab Res Clin Pract, Vol. 86, No. 3, pp. 173-176

Poirier, P. Giles, TD. Bray, GA. Hong, Y. Stern, JS. Pi-Sunyer, FX & Eckel, RH. (2006). Obesity and Cardiovascular Disease Pathophysiology, Evaluation, and Effect of Weight Loss. Arterioscler Thromb Vasc Biol, Vol. 26, pp. 968-976

Poitout, V. & Robertson, RP. (2008). Glucolipotoxicity: fuel excess and beta-cell dysfunction. Endocr Rev, Vol. 29, No. 3, pp. 351-366

Porstmann, T. Santos, CR. Griffiths, B. Cully, M. Wu, M. Leevers, S. Griffiths, JR. Chung, YL. & Schulze, A. (2008). SREBP activity is regulated by mTORC1 and contributes to Akt-dependent cell growth. Cell Metab, Vol. 8, No. 3, pp. 224-236

Rajala, MW. Obici, S. Scherer, PE. & Rossetti, L. (2003). Adipose-derived resistin and gut-derived resistin-like molecule-β selectively impair insulin action on glucose production. J Clin Invest, Vol. 111, No. 2, pp. 225-230

Rakatzi, I. Mueller, H. Ritzeler, O. Tennagels, N. & Eckel, J. (2004). Adiponectin counteracts cytokine- and fatty acid-induced apoptosis in the pancreatic beta-cell line INS-1. Diabetologia, Vol. 47, No. 2, pp. 249-258

Ren, J. Pulakat, L. Whaley-Connell, A. & Sowers, JR. (2010). Mitochondrial biogenesis in the metabolic syndrome and cardiovascular disease. J Mol Med, Vol. 88, No. 10, pp. 993-1001

Revollo, JR. Körner, A. Mills, KF. Satoh, A. Wang, T. Garten, A. Dasgupta, B. Sasaki, Y. Wolberger, C. Townsend, RR. Milbrandt, J. Kiess, W. & Imai, S. (2007). Nampt/PBEF/visfatin regulates insulin secretion in β cells as a systemic NAD biosynthetic enzyme. Cell Metab, Vol. 6, No. 5, pp. 363-375

Rodino-Janeiro, BK. Salgado-Somoza, A. Teijeira-Fernandez, E. Gonzalez-Juanatey, J R. Alvarez, E. & Eiras, S. (2011). Receptor for advanced glycation end-products expression in subcutaneous adipose tissue is related to coronary artery disease. Eur J Endocrinol, Vol. 164, pp. 529-537

Rosamond, W. Flegal, K. Friday, G. Furie, K. Go, A. Greenlund, K. Haase, N. Ho, M. Howard, V. Kissela, B. Kittner, S, Lloyd, J. McDermott, M. Meigs, J. Moy, C. Nichol, G. O'Donnell, CJ. Roger, V. Rumsfeld, J. Sorlie, P. Steinberger, J. Thom, T. Wasserthiel-Smoller, S. & Hong, Y. (2007). American Heart Association Statistics Committee and Stroke Statistics Subcommittee. Heart Disease and Stroke Statistics-2007 Update: A Report From the American Heart Association Statistics Committee and Stroke Statistics Subcommittee. Circulation, Vol. 115, pp. e69-e171

Runge, MS. Molnar, K. & Madamanchi, NR. (2010). "Old"Hearts and Arteries: The Role of Oxidative Stress. Transactions of the Am Clin and Climat Assoc, Vol. 121, pp. 52-60

Saely, CH. Aczel, S. Marte, T. Langer, P. Hoefle, G. & Drexel, H. (2005). The Metabolic Syndrome, Insulin Resistance, and Cardiovascular Risk in Diabetic and Nondiabetic Patients. J Clin Endocrinol Metab, Vol. 90, pp. 5698-5703

Sam, F. & Walsh, K. (2010). What can adiponectin say about left ventricular function? Heart, Vol. 96, No. 5, 331-332

Samal, B. Sun, Y. Stearns, G. Xie, C. Suggs, S. & McNiece, I. (1994). Cloning and characterization of the cDNA encoding a novel human pre-B-cell colony-enhancing factor. Mol Cell Biol, Vol. 14, No. 2, pp. 1431-1437

Sartipy, P. David, J. & Loskutoff, DJ. (2003). Monocyte chemoattractant protein 1 in obesity and insulin resistance. Proc Natl Acad Sci U S A, Vol. 100, No. 12, pp. 7265-7270

Scherer, PE. Williams, S. Fogliano, M. Baldini, G. & Lodish, HF. (1995). A novel serum protein similar to C1q, produced exclusively in adipocytes. J Biol Chem, Vol. 270, No. 45, pp. 26746-26749

Shibata, R. Sato, K. Pimentel, DR. Takemura, Y. Kihara, S. Ohashi, K. Funahashi, T. Ouchi, N. & Walsh, K. (2005). Adiponectin protects against myocardial ischemia-reperfusion injury through AMPK- and COX-2–dependent mechanisms. Nat Med, Vol. 11, pp. 1096-1103

Simpkin, JC. Yellon, DM. Davidson, SM. Lim, SY. Wynne, AM. & Smith, CCT. (2007). Apelin-13 and apelin-36 exhibit direct cardioprotective activity against ischemia reperfusion injury. Basic Res Cardiol, Vol. 102, No. 6, pp. 518-528

Singer, G. & Granger, DN. (2007). Inflammatory responses underlying the microvascular dysfunction associated with obesity and insulin resistance. Microcirculation, Vol. 14, No. 4-5, pp. 375-387

Sorli, SC. van den Berghe, L. Masri, B. Knibiehler, B. & Audigier, Y. (2006). Therapeutic potential of interfering with apelin signalling. Drug Discov Today, Vol. 11, pp. 1100-1106

Steppan, CM. Brown, EJ. Wright, CM. Bhat, S. Banerjee, RR. Dai, CY. Enders, GH. Silberg, DG. Wen, X. Wu, GD. & Lazar, MA. (2001). A family of tissue-specific resistin-like molecules. Proc Natl Acad Sci U S A, Vol. 98, No. 2, pp. 502-506

Stienstra, R. Duval, C. Müller, M. & Kersten, S. (2007). PPARs, Obesity, and Inflammation. PPAR Res, pp. 95974

Stocker, R. & Keaney, JF Jr. (2004). Role of Oxidative Modifications in Atherosclerosis. Physiol Rev, Vol. 84, pp. 1381-1478

Stofkova, A. (2009). Leptin and adiponectin: from energy and metabolic dysbalance to inflammation and autoimmunity. Endocr Regul, Vol. 43, pp. 157-168

Szmitko, PE. Wang, Chao-Hung. Weisel, RD. Jeffries, GA. Anderson, TJ. & Verma, S. (2003). Biomarkers of Vascular Disease Linking Inflammation to Endothelial Activation: Part II. Circulation, Vol. 108, pp. 2041-2048

Takemura, Y. Ouchi, N. Shibata, R. Aprahamian, T. Kirber, MT. Summer, RS. Kihara, S. & Walsh, K. (2007). Adiponectin modulates inflammatory reactions via calreticulin receptor–dependent clearance of early apoptotic bodies. J Clin Invest, Vol. 117, No. 2, pp. 375-386

Targher, G. Bertolini, L. & Zenari, L. (2004). Hypoadiponectinemia is closely associated with nonalcoholic hepatic steatosis in obese subjects. Diabetes Care, Vol. 27, No. 8, pp. 2085-2086

Targonski, PV. Bonetti, PO. Pumper, GM. Higano, ST. Holmes, DR. & Lerman, A. (2003). Coronary Endothelial Dysfunction Is Associated With an Increased Risk of Cerebrovascular Events. Circulation, Vol. 107, pp. 2805-2809

Tatemoto, K. Takayama, K. Zou, MX. Kumaki I, Zhang, W. Kumano, K. & Fujimiya, M. (2001). The novel peptide apelin lowers blood pressure via a nitric oxide-dependent mechanism. Regul Pept, Vol. 99, No. 2-3, pp. 87-92

Tedgui, A. & Mallat, Z. (2006). Cytokines in atherosclerosis: pathogenic and regulatory pathways. Physiol Rev, Vol. 86, No. 2, pp. 515-581

Teoh, H. Quan, A. Bang, KW. Wang, G. Lovren, F. Vu, V. Haitsma, JJ. Szmitko, PE. Al-Omran, M. Wang, CH. Gupta, M. Peterson, MD. Zhang, H. Chan, L. Freedman, J. Sweeney, G. & Verma, S. (2008). Adiponectin deficiency promotes endothelial activation and profoundly exacerbates sepsis-related mortality. Am J Physiol Endocrinol Metab, Vol. 295, No. 3, pp. E658-664

Torzewski, M. & Lackner, KJ. (2006). Initiation and progression of atherosclerosis-enzymatic or oxidative modification of low-density lipoprotein?. Clin Chem Lab Med, Vol. 44, No. 12, pp. 1389-1394

Tsuda, K. (2011). Roles of Adiponectin and Oxidative Stress in the Regulation of Membrane Microviscosity of Red Blood Cells in Hypertensive Men-An Electron Spin Resonance Study. J Obesity, Article ID548140, 8 pages doi:10.1155/2011/548140

Ujiie, H. Oritani, K. Kato, H. Yokota, T. Takahashi, I. Maeda, T. Masaie, H. Ichii, M. Kamada, Y. Tamura, S. Kihara, S. Funahashi, T. Tomiyama, Y. & Kanakura, Y. (2006). Identification of amino-terminal region of adiponectin as a physiologically functional domain. J Cell Biochem, Vol. 98, pp. 194-207

Varma, V. Yao-Borengasser, A. Rasouli, N. Bodles, AM. Phanavanh, B. Lee, MJ. Starks, T. Kern, LM. Spencer, HJ 3rd, McGehee, RE Jr. Fried, SK. & Kern, PA. (2007). Human Visfatin Expression: Relationship to Insulin Sensitivity, Intramyocellular Lipids, and Inflammation. J Clin Endocrinol Metab, Vol. 92, No. 2, pp. 666-692

Verma, S. Wang, CH. Li, SH. Dumont, AS. Fedak, PWM. Badiwala, MV. Dhillon, B. Weisel, RD. Li, RK. Mickle, DAG. & Stewart, DJ. (2002). A self-fulfilling prophecy: C-reactive protein attenuates nitric oxide production and inhibits angiogenesis. Circulation, Vol. 106, pp. 913-919

Wang, ZV. Schraw, TD. Kim, JY. Khan, T. Rajala, MW. Follenzi, A. & Scherer, PE. (2007). Secretion of the adipocyte-specific secretory protein adiponectin critically depends on thiol-mediated protein retention. Mol Cell Biol, Vol. 27, No. 10, pp. 3716-3731

Weber, C. Zernecke, A. & Libby, P. (2008). The multifaceted contributions of leukocyte subsets to atherosclerosis: lessons from mouse models. Nat Rev Immunol, Vol. 8, No. 10, pp. 802-815

Weyer, C. Funahashi, T. Tanaka, S. Hotta, K. Matsuzawa, Y. Pratley, RE. & Tataranni, PA. (2001). Hypoadiponectinemia in obesity and type 2 diabetes: close association with insulin resistance and hyperinsulinemia. J Clin Endocrinol Metab, Vol. 86, No. 5, pp. 1930-1935

Wilson, PW. D'Agostino, RB. Parise, H. Sullivan, L. James, B. & Meigs, JB. (2005). Metabolic Syndrome as a Precursor of Cardiovascular Disease and Type 2 Diabetes Mellitus. Circulation, Vol. 112, pp. 3066-3072

Woods, A. Brull, DJ. Humphries, SE. & Montgomery, HE. (2000). Genetics of inflammation and risk of coronary artery disease: the central role of interleukin-6. Eur Heart J, Vol. 21, pp. 574-583

Xu, A. Wang, Y. Keshaw, H. Xu, LY. Lam, KS. & Cooper, GJ. (2003). The fat-derived hormone adiponectin alleviates alcoholic and nonalcoholic fatty liver diseases in mice. J Clin Invest, Vol. 112, pp. 91-100

Yamauchi, T. Kamon, J. Minokoshi, Y. Ito, Y. Waki, H. Uchida, S. Yamashita, S. Noda, M. Kita, S. Ueki, K. Eto, K. Akanuma, Y. Froguel, P. Foufelle, F. Ferre, P. Carling, D. Kimura, S. Nagai, R. Kahn, BB. & Kadowaki, T. (2002). Adiponectin stimulates glucose utilization and fatty-acid oxidation by activating AMP-activated protein kinase. Nat Med, Vol. 8, pp. 1288-1295

Yamauchi, T. Kamon, J. Ito, Y. Tsuchida, A. Yokomizo, T. Kita, S. Sugiyama, T. Miyagishi, M. Hara, K. Tsunoda, M. Murakami, K. Ohteki, T. Uchida, S. Takekawa, S. Waki, H. Tsuno, NH. Shibata, Y. Terauchi, Y. Froguel, P. Tobe, K. Koyasu, S. Taira, K. Kitamura, T. Shimizu, T. Nagai, R. & Kadowaki, T. (2003). Cloning of adiponectin receptors that mediate antidiabetic metabolic effects. Nature, Vol. 423, pp. 762-769

Yan, QW. Yang, Q. Mody, N. Graham, TE. Hsu, CH. Xu, Z. Houstis, NE. Kahn, BB. & Rosen, ED. (2007). The adipokine lipocalin 2 is regulated by obesity and promotes insulin resistance. Diabetes, Vol. 56, pp. 2533-2540

Yang, RZ. Lee, MJ. Hu, H. Pollin, TI. Ryan, AS. Nicklas, BJ. Snitker, S. Horenstein, RB. Hull, K. Goldberg, NH. Goldberg, AP. Shuldiner, AR. Fried, SK. & Gong, DW. (2006). Acute-phase serum amyloid A: An inflammatory adipokine and potential link between obesity and its metabolic complications. PLoS Med, Vol. 3, No. 6, pp. 884-894

Yang, X. & Smith, U. (2007). Adipose tissue distribution and risk of metabolic disease: does thiazolidinedione-induced adipose tissue redistribution provide a clue to the answer? Diabetologia, Vol. 50, No. 6, pp. 1127-1139

Zhang, R. Hu, C. Wang, CR. Ma, XJ. Bao, YQ. Xu, J. Lu, JY. Qin, W. Xiang, KS. & Jia, WP. (2009). Association of apelin genetic variants with type 2 diabetes and related clinical features in Chinese Hans. Chin Med J, Vol. 122, No. 11, pp. 1273-1276

Zhu, W. Saddar, S. Seetharam, D. Chambliss, KL. Longoria, C. Silver, DL. Yuhanna, IS. Shaul, PW. & Mineo, C. (2008). The scavenger receptor class B type I adaptor protein PDZK1 maintains endothelial monolayer integrity. Circ Res, Vol. 102, No. 4, pp. 480-487

6

Role of Oxidized Lipids in Atherosclerosis

Mahdi Garelnabi[1],
Srikanth Kakumanu[1] and Dmitry Litvinov[2]
[1]*Department of Clinical Laboratory and Nutritional Sciences,*
School of Health and Environment,
University of Massachusetts Lowell, MA,
[2]*Department of Surgery,*
The Ohio State University, Columbus, OH,
USA

1. Introduction

The role of oxidized lipids in cardiovascular diseases (CVD) has been investigated over the last three decades extensively. A number of studies have been carried out on the mechanisms, and pathways leading to the arterial atherosclerosis. These studies originated from the oxidation hypothesis of the atherosclerosis which was originally proposed more than 25 years ago (Steinberg et al., 1989), and since then experiments were performed by many investigators to further examine and explore the contribution of oxidation and oxidized lipids to cardiovascular diseases. Oxidized fatty acids in the ester and free forms, their decomposition products, cholesterol and its oxidized products, proteins with oxidized amino acid residues and cross-links, and polypeptides with varying extents of covalent modification with lipid oxidation products, and many others substances derived from oxidation have been the subject of detailed studies by many investigators. These products originated *in vivo* from oxidized lipoproteins and lipid membranes were linked to initiation and propagation of atherosclerosis (Zhang & Salomon, 2005; Mitra et al., 2011; Hulsmans et al., 2010). The effect of dietary oxidized fat as a contributor to the oxidative stress was also investigated by several groups including our group (Catapano et al., 2000; Drüeke et al., 2001; Garelnabi et al., 2008; Mitra et al., 2011). While there is a consensus in understanding of initial oxidative steps in the generation of early fatty streak lesions as well as the role of products of peroxidized lipid decomposition such as aldehydes in atherosclerosis, the role of further oxidation into neutral carboxylic acids is still obscure. In this chapter we will review the background of the oxidation theory of lipoproteins and the current state of the knowledge. We will review and summarizes data leading to the current understanding of the role of oxidized lipids in atherosclerosis and some pathways involved in this process. We will also discuss recent studies that elucidate factors leading to oxidative stress including chemical, physical and biological factors. In addition, we will explain the current knowledge of the use of antioxidants; and explain their benefits if any to inhibit oxidation of LDL. This part will discuss in brief some selected clinical data.

1.1 Atherosclerosis

Atherosclerosis is the principal contributor to the pathogenesis of myocardial and cerebral infarction, gangrene, and loss of function in the extremities. The process, which under normal circumstances is a protective response to insults against the endothelium and smooth muscle cells of arterial walls, consists of the formation of fibrofatty and fibrous lesions, and is preceded and accompanied by inflammation. The advanced lesions of atherosclerosis become pathologic, and may cause occlusion of the affected artery, result from an excessive inflammatory-fibroproliferative response to numerous different forms of insult (Ross, 1986).

The earliest recognizable lesion of atherosclerosis is the so-called 'fatty streak', an aggregation of lipid-rich macrophages and T lymphocytes within the innermost layer of the arterial wall, the intima. The ubiquity of the atherosclerotic process is attested by the finding of fatty streaks in the coronary arteries of half of the autopsy specimens from children aged 10 to 14 years (WHO, 1985). Animal observations have shown that fatty streaks precede the development of intermediate lesions, which are composed of layers of macrophages and smooth muscle cells and, in turn, develop into the more advanced, complex, occlusive lesions called fibrous plaques (Fig 1). The fibrous plaques increase in size and, by projecting into the arterial lumen, may impede the flow of blood. They are covered by a dense cap of connective tissue with embedded smooth muscle cells that usually overly a core of lipid and necrotic debris (Garelnabi, 2010).

Most of the sudden deaths from myocardial infarcts are due to ruptures or fissures, particularly in the margins of the fibrous cap where there are more macrophages, resulting in hemorrhage into the plaque, thrombosis, and occlusion of the artery (Ross, 1993). As the process continues, migrating cells reach further beneath the arterial surface, where the monocytes become macrophages, accumulate lipid, become foam cells, and together with the accompanying lymphocytes, become the fatty streak. These often form at sites of pre-existing collections of intimal smooth muscle. Thereafter, continued cell influx and proliferation lead to the more advanced lesions, distinguished by their fibrous character, and ultimately to the fibrous plaque (Ross, 1993).

Studies on animals with artificially induced hypercholesterolemia have confirmed that three processes are involved in the formation of atherosclerotic lesions : (1) The proliferation of smooth muscle cells, macrophages, and possibly lymphocytes; (2) the formation of a connective tissue matrix by smooth muscle cells comprised of elastic fiber proteins, collagen, and proteoglycans; and (3) the accumulation of lipid and mostly free esterified cholesterol in the surrounding matrix and the associate cells (Daley et al., 1994).

There are numerous signals, biochemical in nature, which underlie smooth muscle proliferation. Platelet derived growth factor (PDGF), the first postulated growth factor in atherogenesis is produced by many of the cells involved in the process (i.e., platelets, macrophages, endothelial cells and smooth muscle cells). Activated macrophages can also synthesize fibroblast growth factor (FGF), endothelial derived growth factor (EDGF), and transforming growth factor beta (β-TGF). The combination of these growth factors has been shown to be extremely potent in stimulating the migration and proliferation of fibroblasts and smooth muscle cells, as well as the formation of connective tissue element.

When platelets interact with or adhere to sub-endothelial connective tissue, they are stimulated to release their granule contents. Endothelial cells normally prevent platelet adherence because of the non-thrombogenic character of their surface and their capacity to form antithrombotic substances (e.g., prostacyclin and heparin). When endothelium is injured, platelets are promoted to adhere to its surface and thus, the release of platelet constituents, although it is not clear that platelet adherence to modified endothelium is a common event (Ross, 1986). Several investigators have demonstrated that if platelets are absent from the site of endothelial injury, or if are prevented from the injury sites pharmacologically as in experimental models, then the intimal proliferative lesions that usually accompany such injury will not occur (Friedman et al., 1977; Haker et al., 1983). Oxidized low density lipoproteins (OxLDLs) have been shown to play a key role in the pathogenesis of atherosclerosis, since they are present in atherosclerotic lesions. Indeed, oxidized LDLs inhibit endothelium-dependent relaxation of the rabbit aorta in response to acetylcholine, as well as of porcine coronary artery in response to serotonin and platelets (Tanner et al., 1990).

2. Oxidation of LDL

The major constituents of plaques are lipid-laden foam cells are formed and their remains. Foam cells form when macrophages or other cells uptake an excessive amount of LDL, and die. An oxidative hypothesis of atherosclerosis was proposed in 1989 and suggested modification of LDL as a primary reason of foam cell formation and development of atherosclerosis (Steinberget al, 1989; Parthasarathy et al., 2010). A massive amount of confirming data was collected since then. It is well accepted now that oxidative processes and oxidized lipids play pivotal role in initiation and progression of the disease.

LDL is a microparticle consisting of one ApoB protein molecule and a mixture of triacylglycerol, cholesterol and its esters, phospholidpids, and vitamin E. Oxidation of LDL is a gradual process starting with oxidation of vitamin E and polyunsaturated fatty acids. Peroxides, the primary oxidation products, undergo further transformations with generation of aldehydes among other products. Aldehydes modify amino acid residues of ApoB, primarily lysine, resulting in malondialdehyde modified ApoB (MDA-ApoB) and 4-hydroxy-2-nonenal modified ApoB (4-HNE-ApoB). Biological effect of oxidized LDL varies greatly depending on the grade of oxidation. There are several terms for oxidized LDL that indicate the level of oxidation, such as MM-LDL (minimally modified LDL), fully oxidized LDL, and MDA-LDL (malondialdehyde-modified LDL). It is difficult to determine the level of oxidation in many cases. The term OxLDL (oxidized LDL) is used for any oxidized LDL regardless of the extent of oxidation.

Development of atherosclerotic lesion starts with accumulation of OxLDL in intima, the innermost part of vessel, consisting of single layer of endothelial cells that rest on basement membrane. Intimal basement membrane separates endothelial cells and smooth muscle cells in arterial blood vessels. It consists of extracellular matrix, mostly collagen and proteoglycans, with sparse immune cells and smooth muscle cells (SMC) in it.

There is detectable level of OxLDL in circulating blood, and OxLDL is observed in vascular wall. Immunoglobulin M (IgM) is essential for noninflamatory clearance of OxLDL by macrophages. IgM co-localizes with CD68-positive macrophages in lesions. Double knockout Ldlr-/- and soluble IgM-/- mice develop lesions seven time bigger than Ldlr-/- control. C1qa is a complement participating in IgM-mediated clearance. There is a pronounced increase in the size of aortic root lesion in double knockout Ldlr-/-, C1qa-/- mouse as compared to Ldlr-/- mouse/- (Lewis et al., 2009).

Immunization of atherosclerosis-prone Ldlr-/- mice with MDA-LDL or native LDL before feeding with cholesterol-rich atherogenic diet resulted in smaller lesion areas without significant reduction of plasma cholesterol (Freigang et al., 1998). Both type of immunization generated antibodies that recognize a wide pattern of modified and oxidized LDL likely because of some oxidation of LDL during immunization. Binding of OxLDL with antibodies demonstrated antiatherogenic effect, whether it limits the influx of OxLDL into artery wall or helps to clear retained OxLDL. Similar results were obtained in rabbit (Ameli et al., 1996).

While immunization with MDA-LDL prior or at initial stages of atherosclerosis suppresses growth of lesions in mouse and rabbit, there is a controversy in whether higher titer of antibodies to OxLDL in blood correlates with higher or lower grade of atherosclerosis (Palinski et al., 1995; Tsimikas et al., 2007, reviewed in Shoenfeld et al., 2004).

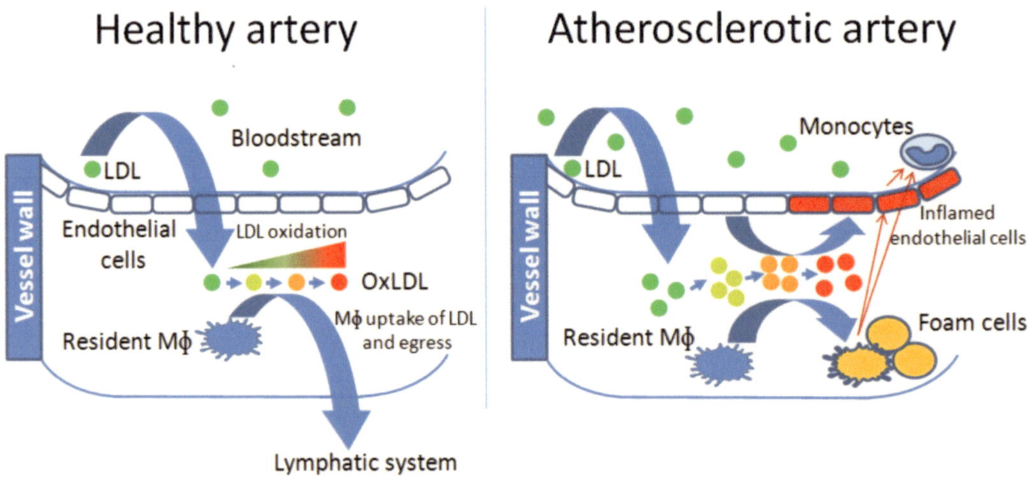

Fig. 1. **OxLDL effects and fate in healthy and atherosclerotic artery wall.** LDL (green circles) enter vessel wall and become gradually oxidized (depicted by changing circle color from green to red). In healthy artery tissue lymphocytes, primarily macrophages (Mϕ), uptake OxLDL, and egress the vessel to lymphatic system. The removal of OxLDL is impaired in atherosclerotic artery. Macrophages get overloaded with OxLDL and die generating foam cells. Overloaded macrophages release inflammatory signals that affect endothelial cells and patrolling leukocytes on the vessel surface (depicted with red arrows). Endothelial cells respond to accumulating OxLDL by inflammation as well.

Currently, the general consensus is that oxidation of LDL occurs mostly within vascular wall. Both native LDL and OxLDL are able to pass through endothelial layer passively through interendothelial junctions, or by endothelial transcytosis, an active transport process (von Eckardstein & Rohrer, 2009). LDL and OxLDL are retained in intima through interaction of the LDL protein ApoB-100 and proteoglycans. LDL undergoes oxidation in intima and becomes absorbed by macrophages through scavenger receptors. There are many scavenger receptors that vary in the substrate specificity, expression in different tissues, and biological roles. Some of them play essential role in atherosclerosis (Table 1). Excessive loading of macrophages by OxLDL convert them to dysfunctional "foam" cells. OxLDL itself or products of spontaneous or enzyme-assisted decomposition act as pro-inflammatory, chemotactic, growth-promoting factors (Fig 1).

2.1 Induction of oxidative stress by OxLDL

OxLDL are cytotoxic for all spectra of atherosclerosis-related cells: T-cells (Alcouffe et al., 1999), macrophages, endothelial cells, smooth muscle cells. OxLDL cytotoxicity in human fibroblasts is mediated through OxLDL-derived lipid peroxides and hydroperoxides, but not superoxide (Coffey et al., 1995).

High load of OxLDL induces two separate lethal processes in macrophages. The first process is activation of caspases-3 in Fas-independent manner. Other caspases, caspase-6, caspase-8, caspase-9, are likely involved as well. It ultimately leads to apoptosis with characteristic DNA fragmentation. The second process is OxLDL-induced plasma membrane lysis (necrosis) mediated by reactive oxygen species (ROS). Both processes occur concurrently, however lysis of plasma membrane is likely the actual reason for macrophages death.

Caspase activation might contribute to macrophage death, however some experiments demonstrate that the extent of the activation is not enough for OxLDL cytotoxicity, since a higher level of caspase-3 activity through activation of Fas is not lethal for macrophages. At the same time inhibitors of caspase-3 do not suppress macrophage lysis by OxLDL, while peroxyl radical scavengers Trolox, and N,N'-diphenyl-1,4-phenylene diamine (DPPD) inhibit cytotoxicity of OxLDL. Generation of peroxyl radical as primary reactive oxygen species (ROS) in OxLDL-activated macrophages was confirmed with several specific ROS-sensitive fluorescent dyes. So, OxLDL cytotoxicity is mediated by peroxyl radicals, but not superoxide. ROS-mediated lysis and caspase activation are independent processes since inhibitors of caspase-3 do not suppress macrophage lysis by OxLDL, and Trolox does not inhibit caspase activation when it inhibits OxLDL-induced macrophage lysis (Asmis & Begley, 2003).

In response to OxLDL, macrophages start to generate intracellularly an increased amount of ROS. Excessive load with OxLDL and ROS generation leads to necrosis of foam cells. There are several NADPH oxidases expressed in macrophages. Nox2 (Gp91phox), a heme-containing subunit of NADPH oxidase, is the major source of ROS during phagocytosis. Nox2 likely does not contribute to atherosclerosis, since Nox2 knockout mouse does not slow development of lesions (Kirk et al., 2000).

Nox4 is another NADPH oxidase. Protein expression of Nox4 and its binding partner p22phox in macrophages is increased by OxLDL but not by native LDL through MEK1/2 pathway. Inhibition of MEK1/2 or siRNA knockdown of Nox4 suppresses ROS production and macrophage death assessed by membrane integrity (Lee et al., 2010).

2.2 NF-κB response to OxLDL and atherosclerosis

NF-κB is a family of transcription factors and their precursors sharing Rel homology domain. They function as homo or heterodimers, such as RelA/p50. In resting cells, NF-κB dimer is associated with IκB, an inhibitory subunit of NF-κB. There are several members in IκB family. The canonical pathway of NF-κB activation is IκB phosphorylation by activated IκB kinase complex consisting of IKKα and IKKβ subunits and regulatory protein NEMO. Phosphorylated IκB becomes ubiquitinated and undergoes degradation. Degradation of inhibitory subunit releases NF-κB dimer, which translocates from cytoplasm to nucleus and initiates transcription of target genes. Various signals activate IKK complex including tumor necrosis factor (TNF) and interleukin-1 (IL-1). In an alternative pathway, activated NF-κB inducing kinase (NIK) phosphorylates precursor protein p100 that results in ubiquitination and proteasomal processing of a precursor protein p100 into mature p52 subunit. The subunit binds with RelB, and RelB/p52 dimer is an active transcription factor. B-cell–activating factor and other stimuli can activate NIK and thus initiate the alternative pathway. Factors such as lipopolysaccharide (LPS), CD40 ligand can activate both pathways, canonical and alternative. However, there is no data yet on regulation of NF-κB via alternative pathway in smooth muscle cells, macrophages, and endothelial cells (de Winther et al., 2005). OxLDL initiates inflammatory response in endothelial cells and leukocytes. Inflamed cells induce factors that attract leukocytes. Activation of NF-κB is one of the pathways that are involved in atherosclerosis. Activation of this pathway is observed in lesions in endothelial cells, macrophages and SMC (Brand et al., 1996).

OxLDL exerts dual effect on NF-κB activation in monocytes and macrophages. It activates NF-κB in short term, and suppresses it in long term (Brand et al., 1997; Eligini et al., 2002). Activation of NF-κB by OxLDL in atherosclerotic endothelial cells is more stable. An essential mechanism of NF-κB activation is mediated through scavenger receptor LOX-1 (lectin-like oxidized low-density lipoprotein receptor 1). Binding of OxLDL to LOX-1 induces superoxide and hydrogen peroxide generation, and NF-κB activation trough activation of p38 MAP kinase, PI3K, ERK1/2 pathway (Cominacini et al., 2000; Tanigawa et al., 2006). Knockdown of LOX-1 gene suppresses endothelial cell injury measured as LDH release, abates expression of MCP-1 and decreases monocyte adhesion to endothelial cells (Li & Mehta, 2000). Knockout of LOX-1 in Ldlr-/- mouse suppresses activation of p38 MAPK, decreases NF-κB p65 protein level, and inhibits development of atherosclerosis (Mehta et al., 2007).

The importance of NF-κB in endothelial cells in progression of atherosclerosis is demonstrated in ApoE-/- mouse. NF-κB pathway was disrupted by ablation of NEMO/IKKγ or expression of dominant-negative IκBα in endothelial cells. In both cases the lesions developed slower than in control ApoE-/- mouse (Gareus et al., 2008).

Inflammation is central process in development of atherosclerosis. Presentation of P-, E-, L-selectins by endothelial cells initiates vascular recruitment of circulating monocytes through selectin ligands that are expressed on surface of leukocytes, such as PSGL-1 (Yang et al., 1999; Sperandio et al., 2003). Inhibition of leukocyte recruitment slows development of atherosclerosis. Indeed, P-selectin knockout mice have smaller lesions than control animals (Dong et al., 2000). NF-κB regulates expression of P-selectin and other inflammation-related genes including E-selectin, ICAM-1, VCAM-1, and MCP-1 (Cominacini et al., 1997).

MCP-1 is another cytokine essential for development of atherosclerosis: Ldlr-/- Mcp1-/- mouse has smaller lesions compare to Ldlr-/- (Gu et al., 1998). VCAM-1 on endothelial cells participates in tight adhesion of monocytes. VCAM-1 knockout is lethal for mouse; however a study of a transgenic mouse with suppressed expression of VCAM-1(D4D) demonstrated reduced lesion development (Cybulsky et al., 2001).

While NF-κB pathway responds to OxLDL, activation of NF-κB stimulates expression of Lox-1 and OxLDL uptake. A study of transgenic ApoE-/-, SIRT1+/- mouse with decreased SIRT1 function revealed that NF-κB inhibition decreases expression of Lox-1 and Ox-LDL uptake. SIRT1, a NAD-dependent class III deacetylases, is known to inhibit NF-κB activity by deacetylating RelA/p65. Indeed transgenic ApoE-/-, SIRT1+/- mouse has decreased SIRT1 activity an increased level of Lox-1 in aorta, and develops atherosclerosis faster compared to ApoE-/-, SIRT1+/+ mouse. Experiments with bone marrow transplantation revealed that pro-atherogenic effect of decreased SIRT1 function is mostly associated with leukocytes. ApoE-/-, SIRT1+/- peritoneal thioglycolate-elicited macrophages uptake showed increased uptake of OxLDL (Stein et al., 2010).

3. Lipid peroxidation: NO Implication

It is believed that lipid peroxidation is involved in the oxidative modification of low density lipoprotein (LDL) and the formation of the potent oxidant peroxynitrite (ONOO−) (Roger et al., 1994). Despite intensive research into this key step, the identity of the radical is still a mystery, especially for the in vivo situation. It may result from preformed or lipoxygenase-derived lipid hydroperoxides or hydrogen peroxide, which decompose in the presence of metal ions to lipid alkoxyl radicals and lipid peroxyl radicals and to hydroxyl radical, respectively. Once formed, the carbon-centred PUFA radical reacts very quickly with molecular oxygen yielding a lipid peroxyl radical which in turn abstracts a hydrogen atom from an adjacent PUFA, yielding a lipid hydroperoxide and a new PUFA radical. It is the latter reaction that carries the lipid peroxidation chain. If no chain termination took place, a single initiating event could convert all LDL. The precise length of the chain, i.e., the number of PUFAs oxidized per one initiating radical depends on many factors especially on the antioxidants. The antioxidants of LDL compete with chain propagation by very efficiently scavenging lipid peroxyl radicals.

Lipid peroxidation can be measured in a laboratory setting by a variety of methods. Oxidized lipid extracts is measurable in spectrophotometer technique. Recent methods of analysis includes the free oxygen radicals monitor (FORM) system (Garelnabi et al, 2008), Electron Spin Resonance Spin Trapping Techniques (ESRT), and several other traditional techniques. Peroxidation of fatty acids containing three or more double bonds will produce malondialdehyde (MDA). Malondialdehyde produced by peroxidation can cause cross-linking and polymerization of membrane components (Nielsen, 1981). This can alter intrinsic membrane properties such as deformability, ion transport, enzyme activity, and the aggregation state of cell surface determinants. Because MDA is diffusible, it will also react with nitrogenous bases of DNA (Bruce & James 1982). Increased formation of MDA has been associated with arachidonic acid metabolism and platelet aggregation (Marie, 1979; Macfarlane et al., 1977; Garelnabi et al. 2008; Garelnabi et al. 2010). Experimental studies have shown that free radicals promote platelet aggregation and thrombosis and chain breaking antioxidants, such as vitamin E, inhibit or delay arterial thrombogenesis (Ikeda et al., 1994; Jourdan et al., 1995).

Scavenger receptor	Expression	LDL-related substrates	Other substrates	Effect of knockout in mouse
Class A: SR-AI, SR-AII	Tissue macrophages, arterial endothelial cells, smooth muscle cells	Acetylated LDL, lower affinity for OxLDL; recognize modified ApoB	Apoptotic cells, beta-amyloid peptide, anionic phospholipids, advanced glycation end-products, Gram-negative and Gram-positive pathogen-related molecules	Controversial results on atherosclerosis development in knockout of both SR-AI and SR-AII genes (Msr-/-) in Apo-/- or Ldlr-/- mice
Class B: SR-B1 (and another minor splice variant of the same gene SR-B2)	Liver, macrophages; adrenal glands, ovaries, and testes - reverse cholesterol transport	OxLDL	Native LDL, HDL, apoptotic cells, beta-amyloid, anionic phospholipids, advanced glycation end-products, amyloid	Srb1 knockout in Apoe-/- or Ldlr-/- mouse promotes atherosclerosis
Class B: CD36	Macrophages, dendritic cells, endothelial cells	Moderately oxidized LDL, POV-PC (1-palmytoyl-2-(5-oxovaleryl)-snglycero-3-phosphocholine) ; does not bind acetylated LDL or extensively oxidized LDL	Native LDL, HDL, apoptotic cells, beta-amyloid, anionic phospholipids, advanced glycation end-products, thrombospondin-1, collagen, fatty acids, protozoan and bacterial peptides and lipopeptides	Knockout of Cd36 in Apoe-/- mouse partly protects from atherosclerosis
Class E: LOX-1	Endothelial cells, macrophages, SMC	OxLDL		Lox1 knockout inhibits atherosclerosis in Ldlr-/- mouse (Mehta et al,. 2007)

Less studied scavenger receptors such as MARCO, SRCL (Class A), CD68 (Class D), SREC-1 (Class F), SR-PSOX/CXCL16 (Class G) are not included in the table. The table is based on review (Moore & Freeman, 2006)

Table 1. Scavenger receptors involved in atherosclerosis

The autoxidation of polyunsaturated lipids is an irreversible destructive process; and in tissues it may be associated with accelerated cell aging and premature cell death. Because such biological autoxidation is essentially slow process, the quantitative measurement of susceptibility to oxidation requires standard experimental stress conduction (Dildar et al., 1998).

4. Cellular defenses against ROS

The biochemical defenses that protect organism from the ROS include both small molecules (low molecular weight compounds such as antioxidants and free radical scavengers) and complex enzyme systems. These defenses serve to lower concentrations of free radical species such as superoxide ($O_2^{\bullet -}$), nitric oxide ($^{\bullet}NO$) hydroxyl radical ($^{\bullet}OH$), lipid peroxyl radicals (L-OO$^{\bullet}$), and strong oxidants and precursors of free radicals such as hydrogen peroxide (H_2O_2) and peroxynitrite ($ONOO^-$). If ROS generation exceeds defense capacity of the cell, ROS will cause excessive damage to cell components. ROS scavengers have also been used to characterize the production, nature, and toxicity of free radical species in *in vitro* and *in vivo* systems.

4.1 Lipid soluble scavengers

A variety of molecules that preferentially partition into membranes function by reducing lipophilic free radical species to less toxic forms. Vitamin E (a series of isomers of tocopherol) will reduce superoxide ($O_2^{\bullet -}$), hydroxyl radical ($^{\bullet}OH$), singlet oxygen ($^1O_2$), lipid peroxy radicals, and other radical species. Ascorbate is proposed to have similar properties and may serve to maintain tocopherols in the reduced active form. Ascorbate serves as a water-soluble reductant and radical scavenger (Bruce & James 1982). The ascorbate-glutathione pathway represent an avenue through which ascorbate consumed in H2O2 reduction get recycled at the expense of NADPH. In the first step of this pathway, H_2O_2 is reduced to water by ascorbate peroxidase (APX) using ascorbate as the electron donor. The oxidized ascorbate (monodehydroascorbate) is regenerated by monodehydroascorbate; a radical and if not rapidly reduced it disproportionates into ascorbate and dehydroascorbate. Dehydroascorbate is reduced to ascorbate by dehydroascorbate reductase at the expense of GSH, yielding oxidized glutathione GSSG which is reduced by glutathione reductase (GR) using NADPH as electron donor (Fig 2), (Blokhina and Fagerstedt KV, 2010; Palma et. al, 2009; Halliwell, 2009). Enzymatic ROS scavengers: Catalase and peroxidases lower the steady state concentration of H_2O_2 which is a precursor of potent radical species. Thus, the cytotoxic potential of H_2O_2 is in large part a function of intracellular catalase and peroxidase activities that scavenge H_2O_2, and concentration of free ions of transition metals that promote generation of $^{\bullet}OH$ from H_2O_2. Three glutathione peroxidase (GPx; EC1.11.1.9) isozymes are known, cellular GPx, extracellular GPx, and phospholipid hydroperoxide GPx, and each contains a selenocysteine in its catalytic center. Cellular GPx; the most characterized form, can react with hydrogen peroxide and organic peroxides but not lipid hydroperoxide (Michio et al., 1995). Platelet GPx has been shown to influence the platelet arachidonic acid metabolism by stimulating lipoxygenase and inhibiting cyclooxygenase, since oxidative stress enhances the arachidonic acid metabolism and thereby creates greater demands on the regulatory systems (Malmgren et al., 1990). Phospholipid hydroperoxide glutathione peroxidase (PHGPx) is an intracellular antioxidant selenoenzyme which interacts directly with peroxidized phospholipids and cholesterol and cholesteryl esters (Imai and Nakagawa 2003) . Selenium (Se) is an essential micronutrient for animals and humans that exerts its biological functions through selenoproteins. These proteins contain Se in the form of selenocysteine (Sec), Phospholipid hydroperoxide glutathione peroxidase (PHGPx or GPx4, E.C. 1.11.1.12) is characterized by the presence of selenocysteine at the active site, and belongs to the important family of glutathione peroxidases (GPx). Since the discovery of PHGPx, a number of studies have demonstrated that this seleno-enzyme is essential to organisms. However on the other hand glutaghione-S-transferase possessing glutathione peroxidase activity toward lipid peroxides, but not having selenocysteine in its active site (Ursini et al. 1982; Yagi et. al 1996)

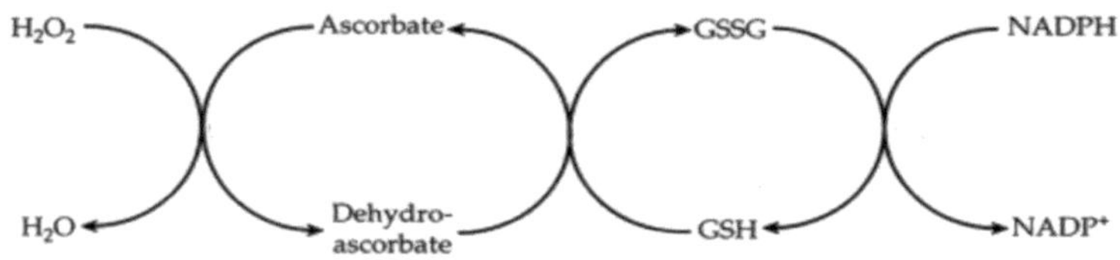

Fig. 2. The glutathione-ascorbate cycle.

Superoxide dismutases (SOD; EC 1.15.1.1) are metalloproteins that catalyze dismutation of superoxide anion radical to H_2O_2. Several types of SOD have been discovered. Mn-SOD (MW 85,000) has been found in mitochondria matrices and CuZn-SOD (MW 33,000) is contained in cellular cytosol. However, Mn-SOD and CuZn-SOD have been found also in extracellular fluids (Wesiger & Fridovich, 1973; Marklund et al., 1982). The superoxide radical has been reported as being produced from stimulated platelets (Levine et al., 1981) but its biological value in platelet function is not clearly understood (Violi et al., 1985). A decrease in cytosolic SOD the main defense against superoxide, could lead to increased cellular peroxides. Role of diet in the activity of Cu,Zn-SOD in platelets was studied and found to be influenced by the availability of Cu in diet (Catherine et al., 1993). Furthermore insufficiency in dietary copper was found to increase platelet thromboxane production, which in turn significantly correlated with endogenous lipid hydroperoxides. Evidence obtained from *in vitro* experiments indicates that superoxide dismutase may also inhibit platelet aggregation. That is, SOD given as adjuvant therapy with thrombolysis may both blunt free radicals mediated reperfusion injury and limit the incidence of spontaneous reocclusion after restoration of blood flow (Karin & Robert, 1993). Superoxide dismutase may protect endogenous $^{\bullet}NO$ from inactivation by scavenging superoxide anion. *In vitro* the inhibitory action of $^{\bullet}NO$ on platelet aggregation as well as their adhesion to endothelium induced by thrombin is potentiated by SOD consistent with its preventing inactivation of endothelium-derived $^{\bullet}NO$ (Meng et al., 1995).

Nitric oxide derived reactive nitrogen species (RNS) such as nitrogen dioxide ($^{\bullet}NO_2$) and peroxynitrite ($ONOO^-$) are indicated in the mediation of oxidative damage.Nitric oxide reacts very rapidly with oxygen radicals. Thus $^{\bullet}NO$ reacting with $O_2^{\bullet-}$ generates peroxynitrite (IUPAC–recommended name is oxoperoxonitrate $O{=}N{-}O{-}O^-$). The peroxynitrite anion ($ONOO^-$) is relatively stable but its acid form (ONOOH) decays to nitrite with a half life of at most 1 sec at physiological pH and temperature (Ducrocq et al., 1999). Peroxynitrite mediates several of the cytotoxic effects of $^{\bullet}NO$ such as the destruction of FeS centres in enzymes. Persistent blockade of cytochrome c oxidase by •NO may lead to the release of free calcium ions (Ca^{2+}) from the mitochondrial matrix into the cell cytosol. Nitric oxide also reacts with lipophilic peroxyl radicals, important propagating species in biological chain reaction of lipid peroxidation, to generate alkyl peroxynitrites (LOONO). These appear far more stable than $ONOO^-$. If LOONO derivatives can be metabolised without the release of toxic free radicals then the reaction of •NO with peroxyl radicals is potentially beneficial because it allows •NO to stop lipid peroxidation. •NO inhibits platelet and phagocyte adhesion to the endothelium. However, in atherosclerotic lesions excess production of $O_2^{\bullet -}$ may cause loss of the modulatory action of •NO and at the same time yield $ONOO^-$ which is pro-aggregatory and so could commit platelets in this environment to thrombus formation (Roger et al., 1994).

Protective mechanism: Several antioxidants can scavenge $ONOO^-$, a molecule responsible for irreversibly oxidation of thiols to higher oxidation states, but nitrosothiols can also form, and later may act as •NO donors. Indeed, when isolated vascular tissues are exposed to $ONOO^-$ vasorelaxation occurs by a mechanism characteristic of release of •NO from a carrier molecule such as nitrosothiol (Liu et al., 1994). Repeated exposure to $ONOO^-$ results in a progressive decrease in the efficiency of the vasorelaxing effect.

4.2 Benefits of antioxidants against lipid peroxidation

There are a vast number of studies on the role of anti-oxidants particularly in the area of atherosclerosis and CVD. These studies are controversial, and do not provide clear evidences on the benefits of antioxidants for prevention or treatment of the diseases. Supplementation of antioxidant vitamins such as α-tocopherol, ascorbic acid and β-carotene used alone or in combination had long been considered to be cardio protective. However, controlled clinical trials using antioxidant vitamin supplements to prevent CVD have yielded conflicting results (Raghavamenon et al., 2009). While some secondary prevention interventions have been shown with α-tocopherol supplementation alone or in combination with ascorbic acid is reported to reduce CVD risk, other studies have shown no effect of α-tocopherol supplementation in both primary and secondary prevention.

Vitamin E (α-tocopherol) is found in plant oils (Honarbakshsh & Schachter, 2009). This vitamin is extensively studied as a possible antioxidant agent against oxidation-induced cardiovascular diseases. Administration of 1000 IU/day α-tocopherol has been shown to reduce LDL oxidation (Princen et al., 1992). A human study shown that α-tocopherol supplementation of 150 IU/day to 1200 IU/day increases it level in plasma and in LDL in concentration-dependent manner. *In vitro* oxidation of LDL was partly inhibited in LDL with higher tocopherol content (Dieber-Rotheneder et al., 1991). α-Tocopherol is reported to reduce plasma OxLDL levels at 25 IU/day in both men and women, and the effect rises with increased supplementation until 800 IU/day (Princen et al., 1995). Tocopherol accumulation in monocytes decreases stress-induced adhesion of monocytes to endothelial cells (Islam et al., 1998; Devraj et al., 1996; Faruqi et al., 1994; Zapolska-Downar et al., 2000), which in turn inhibit the formation of atherosclerotic lesions. Overall, a number of *in vitro* studies demonstrate anti-atherogenic effect of vitamin E by decreasing the production of ROS, lipid oxidation, monocyte endothelial cell adhesion and cytokines secretion. However clinical studies have not revealed anti-atherogenic effect in human (Yusuf et al., 2000).

Vitamin C (ascorbic acid) is principally found in citrus fruits, broccoli, red pepper, and cauliflowers, etc. Ascorbate acts in combination with vitamin E and beta-carotene to protect them from excretion and recycle them for further use. It is also reported to inhibit OxLDL formation indirectly by protecting vitamin E and beta-carotene (Jialal & Grundy, 1991; Kagan et al., 1992). Apart from this vitamin C is reported to inhibit endothelial apoptosis initiated by inflammatory cytokines *in vitro*, and reduces circulating apoptotic microparticles in human (Rössig et al., 2001). Adhesion proteins such as ICAM-1 can be involved in atherosclerosis. Ascorbate supplementation of subjects with low baseline level of this vitamin suppresses mRNA and protein expression of ICAM-1 in monocytes (Rayment et al, 2003). While these and other studies suggest that vitamin C might have anti-atherogenic effect, there is no conclusive clinical evidence of such effect.

β-Carotene is indicated in preventing oxidation of lipids which might decrease atherosclerotic lesions formation. β-Carotene is proposed to be efficient scavenger of singlet oxygen and it attenuates oxidative stress, however it does not directly inhibit lipid peroxidation (Briviba et al., 2004).

Polyphenols are another group of antioxidants which are abundant in vegetables and fruits and are found to reduce the risk of CVD (Naderi et al., 2003). They contain both hydrophilic and hydrophobic moieties (Woodman & Chan, 2004). Polyphenols are suggested to inhibit lipid peroxidation (Madrau et al, 2009). It has also been reported that flavonoids chelates copper and iron ions, rendering them inactive to participate in free radical generating reactions (Fernandez et al., 2002). Polyphenols are also known to inhibit enzymes responsible for generation of ROS such as NADPH oxidase, lipoxygenase, phospholipase A2, and xanthine oxidase (Rice-Evans et al., 1997). Indirectly inhibiting the formation of OxLDL, the benefits of flavonoids goes beyond the protection against LDL oxidation to protect the HDL-associated paraoxonase activity (Patel et al., 2007). The antiatherogenic effect of mulberry leaf extracts (MLE) and the polyphenolic extracts (MLPE), which contain polyphenols including quercetin (11.70%), naringenin (9.01%) and gallocatechin gallate (10.02%) was studied by Yang et al. 2011. Both MLE and MLPE inhibited the oxidation and lipid peroxidation of LDL, while MLPE was shown to be more potent.

5. Clinical studies: OxLDL and antioxidants

A number of studies have demonstrated an association of circulating OxLDL with atherosclerosis disease (Itabe & Ueda, 2007; Hulthe & Fagerberg, 2002). The size of LDL particles might have an effect on LDL oxidation. Smaller LDL was associated with higher level of OxLDL. However the association was observed in diabetic subjects, but not in non-diabetic subjects (Scheffer et al., 2003).

OxLDL level normalized to LDL or ApoB protein levels was increased in diabetic subject with macrovascular diseases compared to diabetic subjects without such diseases. Increased OxLDL normalized level was associated with TT genotype of 108C/T polymorphism in PON1 promoter with lower level of expression of the gene (Tsuzura et al., 2004; Brinkley et al., 2009) have demonstrated for the first time that plasma OxLDL levels are related to arterial stiffness in elderly men and women; suggesting that the oxidative modification of LDL may be associated with changes in the elastic properties of blood vessels. Their findings suggest that while antioxidant supplementation trials have been found to be largely ineffective in preventing cardiovascular outcomes, other interventions including aerobic exercise training and pharmacological treatment with lipid and blood pressure-lowering medications may have significant antioxidant effects that are related to reductions in CVD risk. Another study have shown that oxidized lipoprotein(a) is significantly correlated with blood glucose level among healthy young women, suggesting that lipoprotein(a) may be oxidized with increased glucose concentration even within the normal glucose level (Kotani et al., 2010).

There is some controversy on the role of antioxidants on development of atherosclerosis. A number of clinical studies have demonstrated an anti-atherosclerotic effect of antioxidants while a group of other studies do not see any appreciable benefit of the use of antioxidants. The following are examples of these studies that have suggested an inhibiting effect of antioxidants on lesion development. Gey & Puska (1989) have reported that vitamin E and A concentrations in the plasma were inversely proportional to cardiovascular risks. A study of 667 cases of atherosclerosis-induced coronary disease developed in originally healthy (not diagnosed with coronary heart disease, diabetes, or hypercholesterolemia) 39,910 US men have shown a protective effect of vitamin E but not vitamin C. Carotene appeared to be protective in non-smoking men, however increased the risk of coronary disease among smokers (Rimm et al., 1993). A protective effect of vitamin E was observed in similar study of 87,245 women developed 552 cases of major coronary disease in eight years (Stampher et al., 1993).

However a large the Heart Outcomes Prevention Evaluation (HOPE) study did not show any anti-atherogenic effect of vitamin E (Yusuf et al., 2000). Subjects who were taking vitamin E and placebo developed atherosclerosis-related diseases such as myocardial infarction, stroke, unstable angina, congestive heart failure at the same rate. Potential explanation for the failure of antioxidants in clinical studies may include the type of dose, duration, time of introduction, i.e. stages of the disease at which the treatment/supplementation were introduced and the selection of an optimal doses of antioxidants. Also, most of the studies did not measure the oxidative stress markers in the plasma to take it into account (Parthasarathy et al., 2001).

Research has provided strong evidence that LDL oxidation plays an important role in the pathogenesis of atherosclerosis and cardiovascular diseases. The involvement of lipid peroxidation in the propagation of the disease is well supported by clinical and scientific research using cell culture and animal models; these studies clearly point that modification of the LDL and the accompanied oxidative damage trigger an inflammation response that mediate the development of the atherosclerosis. One may assume that antioxidants should inhibit the oxidative damage and slow the inflammation processes that lead to CVD and associated with metabolic disorders. However despite of some positive findings, antioxidant compounds did not consistently prove to be potent protective agents against atherosclerosis. In animal atherosclerosis, which is studied in the short term, the emphasis is on establishing the lesions. Thus, antioxidants, such as α-tocopherol, might affect predominantly the initial formation and progression of the lesion. In humans, particularly in those who already have clinically significant events, the early steps might have already occurred. In such cases, α-tocopherol and similar antioxidants could affect the conversion of aldehydes into carboxylic acids. The latter, are presumed to be nonatherogenic and are easily degraded *via* fatty-acid degradation pathways (Raghavamenon et al., 2009). Based on these arguments it may be necessary for the scientific community to revisit the topic and investigate in well structured studies the type, dose, duration of the anitoxidants on a well defined population of subjects with various stages of CVD and its associated metabolic disorders such as diabetes, obesity and hyperlipidemia.

Anti-oxidants	Mechanism	References
β-carotene	Scavenging ROS and excellent trapper of singlet oxygen, acts against LDL oxidation	Honarbakshsh & Schachter, 2009. Princen et al., 1992
Vitamin C	Scavenging ROS, reactivating other anti-oxidants such as Vitamin E; inhibit formation of OxLDL, Il-1β secretion or chemokines and monocyte - endothelial cell adhesion and β-carotene which are anti-atherogenic	Dunstan et al., 2007 Honarbakshsh & Schachter, 2009. Jialal & Grundy, 1991. Kagan et al, 1992. Rössig et al, 2001. Gokce et al., 1999, Rayment et al., 2003. Heller et al., 1999
Vitamin E	Scavenging ROS, reported to inhibit formation of OxLDL, Il-1β secretion or chemokines and monocyte -endothelial cell adhesion	Dunstan et al., 2007 Honarbakshsh & Schachter, 2009. Princen et al., 1992. Islam et al., 1998. Devraj et al., 1996. Faruqi et al, 1994. Zapolska-Downar et al., 2000
Selenium	Cofactor for glutathione peroxidase. Has antioxidant capacity.	Michiels et al., 1994
Zinc	Cofactor for superoxide dismutase. Protects cells from oxidative damage.	Michiels et.al., 1994
Curcumin	Chelating of iron and copper ions, scavenging of ROS, inhibiting lipid peroxidation Protects anti-oxidant enzymes.	Wongcharoen & Phrommintikul, 2009
Quercetin	Scavenging of metals ions, and inhibition ROS. Activation of NF-κB, which is involved in development of atherosclerosis.	Cho et al., 2003
Resevetrol	Inhibits ROS production and lipid peroxidation	Ramprasath & Jones, 2010
Ergothioneine	Protects endothelial cells from oxidative damage by reactive nitrogen species.	Martin, 2010

The table describes the currently investigated antioxidants and their relation to markers of CVD.

Table 2. Role of Antioxidants in Cardiovascular Disease

Clinical study	Findings	No of patients	References
Department of Internal Medicine, Kochi Medical School, Kochi, Japan.	OxLDL increased in subjects with PON1 genotype that lead to decreased expression of PON1 protein	155	Tsuzura et al., 2004
AIR study	OxLDL role in atherosclerosis and inflammation	391	Hulthe & Fagerberg, 2002
CARDIA study	OxLDL indication metabolic syndrome and in abdominal obesity, hyperglycemia and hypertriglyceridemia	1889	Holvoet et al., 2008
Metabolic Laboratory, Department of Clinical Chemistry study, Netherlands	Smaller LDL are associated with higher level of OxLDL	116	Scheffer et al., 2003
HOPE Study	No effect of vitamin E on development of CVD	9541	Yusuf et al., 2000

Table summarizes some clinical studies measured OxLDL in plasma

Table 3. Clinical studies on OxLDL

6. Conclusions and perspectives

The low density lipoprotein oxidation hypothesis is pivotal to the explanation of the formation of fatty streak lesions. A wide range of atherogenic processes has been reported to be influenced by OxLDL and its components. The presence of OxLDL in lesions and plasma of patients with various forms of coronary artery diseases and other related metabolic disorder confirms the role of oxidized lipids in atherosclerosis. This conclusion led to numerous studies on the role of antioxidants in the prevention or treatment of atherosclerosis. However they did not yield uniformed outcome on the role of antioxidants in suppressing of the atherosclerotic process. Possible reasons might include discrepancies in experimental models, study designs, and schemes of treatment. Results shown in cell culture or animal models do not necessarily translate to similar results in human due to the major difference between the atherosclerosis development and stages in the animal models and human. Another factor that has not been tested yet is a possible inhibition of oxidation of OxLDL-released aldehydes by antioxidants. If oxidation of aldehydes is inhibited, they modify proteins and cause wide spectra of biological effects that exaggerate atherosclerotic processes. The future studies on the role of antioxidants in atherosclerosis should take in consideration these factors.

7. References

Alcouffe J, Caspar-Bauguil S, Garcia V, Salvayre R, Thomsen M, Benoist H. (1999). Oxidized low density lipoproteins induce apoptosis in PHA-activated peripheral blood mononuclear cells and in the Jurkat T-cell line. *J Lipid Res.*;40(7):1200-10.

Ameli S, Hultgårdh-Nilsson A, Regnström J, Calara F, Yano J, Cercek B, Shah PK, Nilsson J. (1996). Effect of immunization with homologous LDL and oxidized LDL on early atherosclerosis in hypercholesterolemic rabbits. *Arterioscler Thromb Vasc Biol.*;16(8):1074-9.

Asmis R, Begley JG. (2003). Oxidized LDL promotes peroxide-mediated mitochondrial dysfunction and cell death in human macrophages: a caspase-3-independent pathway. *Circ Res.* 10;92(1):e20-9

Blokhina O, Fagerstedt KV (2010). Reactive oxygen species and nitric oxide in plant mitochondria: origin and redundant regulatory systems. Physiol Plant. Apr;138(4):447-62.

Brand K, Eisele T, Kreusel U, Page M, Page S, Haas M, Gerling A, Kaltschmidt C, Neumann FJ, Mackman N, Baeurele PA, Walli AK, Neumeier D. (1997). Dysregulation of monocytic nuclear factor-kappa B by oxidized low-density lipoprotein. *Arterioscler Thromb Vasc Biol.*; 17: 1901–1909.

Brand K, Page S, Rogler G, Bartsch A, Brandl R, Knuechel R, Page M, Kaltschmidt C, Baeuerle PA, Neumeier D. (1996). Activated transcription factor nuclear factor-kappa B is present in the atherosclerotic lesion. *J Clin Invest.*;97(7):1715-22.

Brinkley TE, Nicklas BJ, Kanaya AM, Satterfield S, Lakatta EG, Simonsick EM, Sutton-Tyrrell K, Kritchevsky SB. (2009).Plasma oxidized low-density lipoprotein levels and arterial stiffness in older adults: the health, aging, and body composition study. *Hypertension.*;53(5):846-52

Briviba K, Schnäbele K, Rechkemmer G, Bub A (2004). Supplementation of a diet low in carotenoids with tomato or carrot juice does not affect lipid peroxidation in plasma and feces of healthy men. *J Nutr.*; 134(5):1081-3.

Bruce, A.F., James D.C. (1982). Biology of disease. Free radicals and tissue injury. *J. Lab. Invest.*, 47: 412-426.

Catapano AL, Maggi FM, Tragni E. (2000). Low density lipoprotein oxidation, antioxidants, and atherosclerosis. *Curr Opin Cardiol.*;15(5):355-63

Catherine, M., Kenneth, D., Malvin, M. (1993). Thromboxane production in copper-deficient and marginal platelets: Influence of superoxide and lipid hydroperoxides. *P.S.E.BM.*, 202: 167-173.

Cho SY, Park SJ, Kwon MJ, Jeong TS, Bok SH, Choi WY, Jeong WI, Ryu SY, Do SH, Lee CS, Song JC, Jeong KS. (2003). Quercetin suppresses proinflammatory cytokines production through MAP kinases and NF-kappa B pathway in lipopolysaccharide-stimulated macrophage. *Mol Cell Biochem.* 243(1-2):153-60.

Coffey MD, Cole RA, Colles SM, Chisolm GM. (1995). In vitro cell injury by oxidized low density lipoprotein involves lipid hydroperoxide-induced formation of alkoxyl, lipid, and peroxyl radicals. *J Clin Invest.* 96: 1866–1873.

Cominacini L, Garbin U, Fratta Pasini A, Paulon T, Davoli A, Campagnola M, Marchi E, Pastorino AM, Gaviraghi G, Lo Cascio V. (1997). Lacidipine inhibits the activation of the transcription factor NF-kappaB and the expression of adhesion molecules induced by pro-oxidant signals on endothelial cells. J Hypertens.;15(12 Pt 2):1633-40.

Cominacini L, Pasini AF, Garbin U, Davoli A, Tosetti ML, Campagnola M, Rigoni A, Pastorino AM, Lo Cascio V, Sawamura T. (2000). Oxidized low density lipoprotein (OxLDL) binding to OxLDL receptor-1 in endothelial cells induces the activation of NF-kappaB through an increased production of intracellular reactive oxygen species. *J Biol Chem.*;275(17):12633-8.

Cybulsky MI, Iiyama K, Li H, Zhu S, Chen M, Iiyama M, Davis V, Gutierrez-Ramos JC, Connelly PW, Milstone DS. (2001). A major role for VCAM-1, but not ICAM-1, in early atherosclerosis. *J Clin Invest.* ;107(10):1255-62.

Daley, S., Klemp, K., Guyton, J., Rogers, K. (1994). Cholesterol-fed and Casein-fed rabbit models of atherosclerosis. Part 2 : Differing morphological severity of atherogenesis despite matched plasma cholesterol levels. *Arterioscler. Thromb.*, 14: 105-114.

Darley-Usmar V, Wiseman H, Halliwell B. (1995) Nitric oxide and oxygen radicals: a question of balance. *FEBS Lett.*; 369(2-3):131-5.

de Winther MP, Kanters E, Kraal G, Hofker MH. (2005). Nuclear factor kappaB signaling in atherogenesis. *Arterioscler Thromb Vasc Biol.*;25(5):904-14.

del Río LA, Corpas FJ, Sandalio LM, Palma JM, Barroso JB (2003). Plant peroxisomes reactive oxygen metabolism and nitric oxide. IUBMB Life. Feb;55(2):71-81.

DeMaio S, King SB, Lembo NJ, Roubin GS, Hearn JA, Bhagavan HN, Sgoutas DS. (1992). Vitamin E supplementation, plasma lipids and incidence of restenosis after percutaneous transluminal coronary angioplasty (PTCA). *J Am Coll Nutr*, 11:68–73.

Devraj S, Li D & Jialal I (1996). The effects of alpha tocopherol supplementation on monocyte function. Decreased lipid oxidation, interleukin 1 beta secretion, and monocyte adhesion to endothelium. *J Clin Invest.* 98(3): 756–763.

Dieber-Rotheneder M, Puhl H, Waeg G, Striegl G, Esterbauer H. (1991). Effect of oral supplementation with D-alpha-tocopherol on the vitamin E content of human low density lipoproteins and resistance to oxidation. *J Lipid Res.*;32(8):1325-32.

Dildar Konukglu, Tulay Akcay, Tijen Erdem (1998). Susceptibility of erythrocyte lipid to oxidation and erythrocyte antioxidant status in myocardial infarction. *Clini. Biochem.*, 31: 667-671.

Dong ZM, Brown AA, Wagner DD. (2000). Prominent role of P-selectin in the development of advanced atherosclerosis in ApoE-deficient mice. *Circulation.* ;101(19):2290-5.

Drüeke TB, Nguyen Khoa T, Massy ZA, Witko-Sarsat V, Lacour B, Descamps-Latscha B. (2001). Role of oxidized low-density lipoprotein in the atherosclerosis of uremia. *Kidney Int Suppl.*;78:S114-9.

Ducrocq, C., Blanchard, B., Pignatelli, B., Ohshima, H. (1999). Peroxynitrite: an endogenous oxidizing and nitrating agent. *CMLS*, 55: 1068-1077.

Dunstan JA, Breckler L, Hale J, Lehmann H, Franklin P, Lyons G, Ching SY, Mori TA, Barden A, Prescott SL. (2007). Supplementation with vitamins C, E, b-carotene and selenium has no effect on anti-oxidant status and immune responses in allergic adults: a randomized controlled trial. *Clin Exp Allergy*.37(2):180-7.

Eligini S, Brambilla M, Banfi C, Camera M, Sironi L, Barbieri SS, Auwerx J, Tremoli E. (2002). Colli S. Oxidized phospholipids inhibit cyclooxygenase-2 in human macrophages via nuclear factor-kappaB/IkappaB-and ERK2-dependent mechanisms. *Cardiovasc Res*; 55: 406–415.

Faruqi R, de la Motte C & DiCorleto PE (1994). Alpha-tocopherol inhibits agonist-induced monocytic cell adhesion to cultured human endothelial cells. *J Clin Invest* ;94,592-600.

Fernandez MT, Mira ML, Florêncio MH and Jennings KR.(2002). Iron and copper chelation by flavonoids: an electrospray mass spectrometry study. *J Inorg Biochem*.92(2):105-11.

Freigang S, Hörkkö S, Miller E, Witztum JL, Palinski W. (1998). Immunization of LDL receptor-deficient mice with homologous malondialdehyde-modified and native LDL reduces progression of atherosclerosis by mechanisms other than induction of high titers of antibodies to oxidative neoepitopes. *Arterioscler Thromb Vasc Biol.*;18(12):1972-82.

Friedman, J., Stemerman, B., Wenz, B., et al., (1977). The effect of thrombocytopenia on experimental arteriosclerotic lesion formation in rabbits: Smooth muscle cell proliferation and re-endothelization. *J. Clin. Invest.*, 60: 1191-1201.

Garelnabi M, Brown WV, Le NA. (2008). Evaluation of a novel colorimetric assay for free oxygen radicals as marker of oxidative stress. *Clin Biochem.*;41(14-15):1250-4.

Garelnabi M, Gupta V, Mallika V, Bhattacharjee J. (2010). Platelets oxidative stress in Indian patients with ischemic heart disease. *J Clin Lab Anal.* 24(1):49-54.

Garelnabi M. (2010). Emerging Evidences from the Contribution of the Traditional and New Risk Factors to the Atherosclerosis Pathogenesis. *J of Med Sci*, 10; 136-144.

Gareus R, Kotsaki E, Xanthoulea S, van der Made I, Gijbels MJ, Kardakaris R, Polykratis A, Kollias G, de Winther MP, Pasparakis M. (2008). Endothelial cell-specific NF-kappaB inhibition protects mice from atherosclerosis. *Cell Metab.*; 8(5):372-83.

Gey KF and Puska P. (1989). Plasma vitamins E and A inversely correlated to mortality from ischemic heart disease in cross-cultural epidemiology. *Ann N Y Acad Sci.* 570:268-82.

Gokce N, Keaney JF Jr, Frei B, Holbrook M, Olesiak M, Zachariah BJ, Leeuwenburgh C, Heinecke JW, Vita JA (1999). Long-term ascorbic acid administration reverses endothelial vasomotor dysfunction in patients with coronary artery disease. *Circulation.* 99(25):3234-40.

Gu L, Okada Y, Clinton SK, Gerard C, Sukhova GK, Libby P, Rollins BJ. (1998). Absence of monocyte chemoattractant protein-1 reduces atherosclerosis in low density lipoprotein receptor-deficient mice. *Mol Cell.*;2(2):275-81.

Haker, A., Harlan, M., Ross, R. (1983). Effect of sulfinpyrozone on homocysteine- induced endothelial injury and arteriosclerosis in baboons. *Circ. Res.*, 53: 731-739.

Halliwell B (2009). The wanderings of a free radical. Free Radic Biol Med, Mar 1;46(5):531-42.

Heller R, Münscher-Paulig F, Gräbner R, Till U (1999). L-Ascorbic acid potentiates nitric oxide synthesis in endothelial cells. *J Biol Chem.*274(12):8254-60.

Holvoet P, Lee DH, Steffes M, Gross M, Jacobs DR Jr.(2008). Association between circulating oxidized low-density lipoprotein and incidence of the metabolic syndrome. *JAMA.*299(19):2287-93.

Honarbakshsh S and Schachter M. (2009). Vitamins and cardiovascular disease. British *Journal of Nutrition.* 101,1113-1131.

Hulsmans M, De Keyzer D, Holvoet P. (2011). MicroRNAs regulating oxidative stress and inflammation in relation to obesity and atherosclerosis. *FASEB J.* ;25(8):2515-27.

Hulthe J and Fagerberg B. (2002). Circulating oxidized LDL is associated with subclinical atherosclerosis development and inflammatory cytokines (AIR Study). *Arterioscler Thromb Vasc Biol.*;22(7):1162-7.

Ikeda, H., Koga, Y., Oda, T. (1994). Free Oxygen radicals contribute to platelets aggregation and cyclic flow variations in stenosed and endothelium-injured canine coronary arteries. *J. Am. Coll. Cardiol.*, 24: 1749-1756.

Imai H.; Nakagawa Y. (2003) Biological significance of phospholipid hydroperoxide glutathione peroxidase (PHGPx, GPx4) inmammalian cells. Free Radic. Biol. Med. 34: 145–169.

Islam KN, Devraj S & Jialal I (1998). Alfa-tocopherol enrichment of monocytes decreases agonist-induced adhesion to human endothelial cells. *Circulation;* 98,2255-2261.

Itabe H, Ueda M. (2007). Measurement of plasma oxidized low-density lipoprotein and its clinical implications. *J Atheroscler Thromb.*;14(1):1-11.

Jialal I & Grundy SM (1991). Preservation of the endogenous anti-oxidants in low density lipoprotein by ascorbate but not probucol during oxidative modification. *J Clin Invest* 87,597-601.

Jourdan, A., Aguejouf, O., Imbault, P. (1995). Experimental thrombosis model induced by free radicals. Application to aspirin and other different substances. *Thromb. Res.*, 129: 109-112.

Kagan VE, Serbinova EA, Forte T, Scita G, Packer L (1992). Recycling of vitamin E in human low density lipoproteins. *J Lipid Res.*;33(3):385-97.

Karin, K., and Robert, K. (1993). Oxygen radical scavenging agents as adjuvant therapy with tissue plasminogen activator in a canine model of coronary thrombolysis. *Cardiov. Res.*, 27: 925-934.

Kirk EA, Dinauer MC, Rosen H, Chait A, Heinecke JW, LeBoeuf RC. (2000). Impaired superoxide production due to a deficiency in phagocyte NADPH oxidase fails to inhibit atherosclerosis in mice. *Arterioscler Thromb Vasc Biol.*;20:1529 –1535.

Kotani K, Yamada S, Uurtuya S, Yamada T, Taniguchi N, Sakurabayashi I. (2010).The association between blood glucose and oxidized lipoprotein(a) in healthy young women. *Lipids Health Dis.*;9:103.

Lee CF, Qiao M, Schröder K, Zhao Q, Asmis R. (2010). Nox4 is a novel inducible source of reactive oxygen species in monocytes and macrophages and mediatesoxidized low density lipoprotein-induced macrophage death. *Circ Res*;106(9):1489-97.

Levine, H., Sladdin, D., Krinsky, I. (1981). Superoxide Xanthine oxidase and platelet reactions further studies on mechanism by which oxidants influence platelets. *Thromb. Haemost.*, 45: 290-293.

Lewis MJ, Malik TH, Ehrenstein MR, Boyle JJ, Botto M, Haskard DO. (2009). Immunoglobulin M is required for protection against atherosclerosis in low-density lipoprotein receptor-deficient mice. *Circulation.*;120(5):417-26.

Li D, Mehta JL. (2000). Antisense to LOX-1 inhibits oxidized LDL-mediated upregulation of monocyte chemoattractant protein-1 and monocyte adhesion to human coronary artery endothelial cells. *Circulation.*;101(25):2889-95.

Liu S, Beckman JS, Ku DD. (1994). Peroxynitrite, a product of superoxide and nitric oxide, produces coronary vasorelaxation in dogs. *J Pharmacol Exp Ther.*;268(3):1114-21.

Mabile L, Bruckdorfer KR, Rice-Evans C. (1999). Moderate supplementation with natural alpha tocopherol decreases platelet aggregation and low density lipoprotein oxidation. *Atherosclerosis*, 147:177-185.

Macfarlane, D., Sheila, G., Carol, L. Mills, B. (1977). Malondialdehyde Production by Platelets during secondary aggregation. *Thrombos. Haemostas. (Stuttg.)*, 38: 1002-1009.

Madrau MA, Piscopo A, Sanguinetti AM, Del Caro A, Poiana M, Romeo FV and Piga A.(2009). Effect of drying temperature on polyphenolic content and antioxidant activity of apricots. *European food research and technology*. 228, 441-448

Malmgren, R., Unge, G., Zetterstrom, O. (1990). Lowered platelet glutathione peroxidase activity in patients with intrinsic asthma. *Allergy*, 45: 523-527.

Marie, J. (1979). Platelet malonyldialdehyde formation: An indicator of platelet hyperfunction. *Thrombos. Haemostas. (Stuttg.)*, 42: 549-654.

Marklund, L., Holme, E., Hellner, L. (1982). Superoxide dismutase in extracellular fluids. *Clin. Chim. Acta.*, 126: 41-51.

Martin KR (2010). The bioactive agent ergothioneine, a key component of dietary mushrooms, inhibits monocyte binding to endothelial cells characteristic of early cardiovascular disease. *J Med Food.*;13(6):1340-6.

Mehta JL, Sanada N, Hu CP, Chen J, Dandapat A. Sugawara F, Satoh H, Inoue K, Kawase Y, Jishage K, Suzuki H, Takeya M, Schnackenberg L, Beger R, Hermonat PL, Thomas

M, Sawamura T. (2007). Deletion of LOX-1 reduces atherogenesis in LDLR knockout mice fed high cholesterol diet. *Circ Res*;100(11):1634-42.

Meng, Y., Jeffrey, T., Una, S., Abendschein, R. (1995). Potentiation of endogenous nitric oxide with superoxide dismutase. Inhibits platelet-mediated thrombosis in injured and stenotic arteries. *J. Am. Coll. Cardiol.*, 25: 269-275

Michiels C, Raes M, Toussaint O, Remacle J(1994). Importance of Se-glutathione peroxidase, catalase, and Cu/Zn-SOD for cell survival against oxidative stress. *Free Radic Biol Med.*;17(3):235-48.

Michio A., Junichi, F., Keiichiro, S., et al. (1995). Inactivation of glutathione peroxidase by nitric oxide. *J. Biol. Chem.*, 270: 21035-21039.

Mitra S, Deshmukh A, Sachdeva R, Lu J, Mehta JL. (2011). Oxidized low-density lipoprotein and atherosclerosis implications in antioxidant therapy. *Am J Med Sci.*;342(2):135-42.

Moore KJ, Freeman MW. (2006). Scavenger receptors in atherosclerosis: beyond lipid uptake. *Arterioscler Thromb Vasc Biol.*;26(8):1702-11.

Naderi GA, Asgary S, Sarraf-Zadegan N and Shirvany H. (2003). Anti-oxidant effect of flavonoids on the susceptibility of LDL oxidation. *Mol Cell Biochem.* 246(1-2):193-6.

Nielsen, H. (1981). Covalent binding of peroxidized phospholipid to protein. III. Reaction of individual phospholipids with different proteins. *Lipids*, 16: 215.

Palinski W, Tangirala RK, Miller E, Young SG, Witztum JL. (1995). Increased autoantibody titers against epitopes of oxidized LDL in LDL receptor-deficient mice with increased atherosclerosis. *Arterioscler Thromb Vasc Biol.*;15(10):1569-76.

Palma JM, Corpas FJ, del Río LA (2009). Proteome of plant peroxisomes: new perspectives on the role of these organelles in cell biology. Proteomics. May;9(9):2301-12.

Parthasarathy S, Khan-Merchant N, Penumetcha M, Khan BV and Santanam N. (2001). Did the antioxidant trials fail to validate the oxidation hypothesis? *Curr Atheroscler Rep.*;3(5):392-8.

Parthasarathy S, Raghavamenon A, Garelnabi O, Santanam N. (2010). Oxidized low-density lipoprotein. *Methods Mol Biol.*;610:403-17.

Parthasarathy S., Litvinov D., Selvarajan K., Garelnabi M., (2008). Lipid peroxidation and decomposition — Conflicting roles in plaque vulnerability and stability. *Biochimica et Biophysica Acta* ;1781, 221–231

Patel R, Garg R, Erande S and B Maru G.(2007). Chemopreventive herbal anti-oxidants: current status and future perspectives. *J Clin Biochem Nutr.*;40(2):82-91.

Princen HM, van Duyvenvoorde W, Buytenhek R, van der Laarse A, van Poppel G, Gevers Leuven JA, van Hinsbergh VW.(1995). Supplementation with low doses of vitamin E protects LDL from lipid peroxidation in men and women. Arterioscler Thromb Vasc Biol.15(3):325-33.

Princen HM, van Poppel G, Vogelezang C, Buytenhek R, Kok FJ. (1992) Supplementation with vitamin E but not beta-carotene in vivo protects low density lipoprotein from lipid peroxidation in vitro. Effect of cigarette smoking. *Arterioscler Thromb.*;12(5):554-62.

Raghavamenon A, Garelnabi M, Babu S, Aldrich A, Litvinov D, Parthasarathy S. (2009). Alpha-tocopherol is ineffective in preventing the decomposition of preformed lipid peroxides and may promote the accumulation of toxic aldehydes: a potential explanation for the failure of antioxidants to affect human atherosclerosis. *Antioxid Redox Signal.*;11(6):1237-48.

Ramprasath VR, Jones PJ. (2010). Anti-atherogenic effects of resveratrol. *Eur J Clin Nutr.* 64(7):660-8.

Rao VS, Nagaraj RK, Hebbagodi S, Kadarinarasimhiah NB, Kakkar VV.(2010).Association of Inflammatory and Oxidative Stress Markers with Metabolic Syndrome in Asian Indians in India. *Cardiol Res Pract.* ;2011:295976.

Rayment SJ, Shaw J, Woollard KJ, Lunec J, Griffiths HR (2003). Vitamin C supplementation in normal subjects reduces constitutive ICAM-1 expression. *Biochem Biophys Res Commun.* 308(2):339-45.

Rayment SJ, Shaw J, Woollard KJ, Lunec J, Griffiths HR (2003). Vitamin C supplementation in normal subjects reduces constitutive ICAM-1 expression. *Biochem Biophys Res Commun.*;308(2):339-45.

Rice-Evans CV, Nicholas Miller and George Pagangal. (1997). Antioxidant properties of phenolic compounds. *Trends in Plant Science.* 2,152-159.

Rimm EB, Stampfer MJ, Ascherio A, Giovannucci E, Colditz GA, Willett WC.(1993). Vitamin E consumption and the risk coronary heart disease in men. *N Engl J Med;* 328:1450-1456.

Roger, C., Tomm, B., Ling-Yi C., James C., et al., (1994). Superoxide and peroxynitrite in atherosclerosis, *Proc. Natl. Acad. Sci. USA*, 91: 1044-1048.

Ross R (1986). The Pathogenesis of atherosclerosis –an update. *New Eng. J. Med.*, 314: 488-500.

Ross R (1993). The Pathogenesis of atherosclerosis : a perspective for the 1990s. *Nature*, 362: 801-809.

Rössig L, Hoffmann J, Hugel B, Mallat Z, Haase A, Freyssinet JM, Tedgui A, Aicher A, Zeiher AM, Dimmeler S (2001). Vitamin C inhibits endothelial cell apoptosis in congestive heart failure. *Circulation.* ;104(18):2182-7.

Scheffer PG, Bos G, Volwater HG, Dekker JM, Heine RJ, Teerlink T.(2003).Associations of LDL size with in vitro oxidizability and plasma levels of in vivo oxidized LDL in Type 2 diabetic patients. *Diabet Med.* 20(7):563-7.

Shargorodsky M, Debby O, Matas Z, Zimlichman R (2010). Effect of long-term treatment with antioxidants (vitamin C, vitamin E, coenzyme Q10 and selenium) on arterial compliance, humoral factors and inflammatory markers in patients with multiple cardiovascular risk factors. *Nutr Metab (Lond).* ;7:55.

Shoenfeld Y, Wu R, Dearing LD, Matsuura E. (2004). Are anti-oxidized low-density lipoprotein antibodies pathogenic or protective? *Circulation.*;110(17):2552-8.

Sperandio M, Smith ML, Forlow SB, Olson TS, Xia L, McEver RP, Ley K. (2003). P-selectin glycoprotein ligand-1 mediates L-selectin-dependent leukocyte rolling in venules. *J Exp Med.;* 197: 1355–1363.

Stampher MJ, Hennekens CH, Manson JE, Colditz GA, Rosner B, Willett WC.(1993). Vitamin E consumption and the risk coronary heart disease in women. *N Engl J Med;* 328:1444-1449.

Stein S, Lohmann C, Schäfer N, Hofmann J, Rohrer L, Besler C, Rothgiesser KM, Becher B, Hottiger MO, Borén J, McBurney MW, Landmesser U, Lüscher TF, Matter CM. (2010). SIRT1 decreases Lox-1-mediated foam cell formation in atherogenesis. *Eur Heart J.*;31(18):2301-9.

Steinberg D, Parthasarathy S, Carew TE, Khoo JC, Witztum JL. (1989). Beyond cholesterol. Modifications of low-density lipoprotein that increase its atherogenicity. *N Engl J Med.*;320(14):915-24.

Tanigawa H, Miura S, Matsuo Y, Fujino M, Sawamura T, Saku K. (2006). Dominant-negative lox-1 blocks homodimerization of wild-type lox-1-induced cell proliferation through extracellular signal regulated kinase 1/2 activation. *Hypertension.*;48(2):294-300.

Tanner, C., Noll, G., Boulanger, M., Luscher, F. (1990). Oxidized low density lipoproteins inhibit relaxations of porcine coronary arteries : role of scavenger receptor and endothelium-derived nitric oxide. *Circulation*, 83: 2012-2020.

Tsimikas S, Brilakis ES, Lennon RJ, Miller ER, Witztum JL, McConnell JP, Kornman KS, Berger PB. (2007). Relationship of IgG and IgM autoantibodies to oxidized low density lipoprotein with coronary artery disease and cardiovascular events. *J Lipid Res.*;48(2):425-33.

Tsuzura S, Ikeda Y, Suehiro T, Ota K, Osaki F, Arii K, Kumon Y and Hashimoto K. (2004).Correlation of plasma oxidized low-density lipoprotein levels to vascular complications and human serum paraoxonase in patients with type 2 diabetes. *Metabolism.* 53(3):297-302.

Ursini F, Maiorino M, Valente M, Ferri L, Gregolin C. (1982) Purification from pig liver of a protein which protects liposomes and biomembranes from peroxidative degradation and exhibits glutathione peroxidase activity on phosphatidylcholine hydroperoxides. Biochim Biophys Acta. 710:197-211

Violi, F., Iuliano, L. Alessandri, C., Ghiselli, A., Balsano, F. (1985). A simple method for evaluating platelet superoxide dismutase. *Scand. J. Clin. Lab. Invest.*, 45: 713-716.

von Eckardstein A, Rohrer L. (2009). Transendothelial lipoprotein transport and regulation of endothelial permeability and integrity by lipoproteins. *Curr Opin Lipidol.* 20(3):197-205.

Wesiger, R., Fridovich, I. (1973). Superoxide dismutase organelle specificity. *J. Biol. Chem.*, 248: 358-392.

Wongcharoen W and Phrommintikul A. (2009).The protective role of curcumin in cardiovascular diseases. *Int J Cardiol.* 133(2):145-51.

Woodman OL and Chan ECh. (2004). Vascular and anti-oxidant actions of flavonols and flavones. *Clin Exp Pharmacol Physiol.* 31(11):786-90.

World Health Organization WHO, Tech. Rep. Serv., (1985). 1453: 1-20.

Yagi K.; Komura S.; Kojima H.; Sun Q.; Nagata N.; Ohishi N.; Nishikimi M. (1996) Expression of human phospholipid hydroperoxide glutathione peroxidase gene for protection of host cells from lipid hydroperoxide-mediated injury. Biochem. Biophys. Res. Commun. 219: 486–491.

Yang J, Hirata T, Croce K, Merrill-Skoloff G, Tchernychev B, Williams E, Flaumenhaft R, Furie BC, Furie B. (1999).Targeted gene disruption demonstrates that P-selectin glycoprotein ligand 1 (PSGL-1) is required for P-selectin-mediated but not E-selectin-mediated neutrophil rolling and migration. *J Exp Med.*; 190: 1769–1782.

Yang MY, Huang CN, Chan KC, Yang YS, Peng CH, Wang CJ. (2011(Mulberry leaf polyphenols possess antiatherogenesis effect via inhibiting LDL oxidation and foam cell formation. J Agric Food Chem. 9;59(5):1985-95.

Yusuf S, Dagenais G, Pogue J, Bosch J and Sleight P. (2000). Vitamin E supplementation and cardiovascular events in high risk patients. The Heart Outomes prevention evaluation study Investigators. *N Engl J Med.* 342;154-160.

Zapolska-Downar D, Zapolski-Downar A, Markiewski M (2000). Slective inhibition by alpha-tocopherol of vascular cell adhesion molecule-1 expression in human endothelial cells. *Biochem Biophys Res Commun* 274, 609-615.

Zhang W, Salomon RG. (2005). Oxidized phospholipids, isolevuglandins, and atherosclerosis. *Mol Nutr Food Res.*;49(11):1050-62.

7

Oxidative Damage in Cardiac Tissue from Normotensive and Spontaneously Hypertensive Rats: Effect of Ageing

Juliana C. Fantinelli*, Claudia Caldiz*,
María Cecilia Álvarez, Carolina D. Garciarena,
Gladys E. Chiappe de Cingolani and Susana M. Mosca
Centro de Investigaciones Cardiovasculares,
Facultad de Ciencias Médicas,
Universidad Nacional de La Plata
Argentina

1. Introduction

The spontaneously hypertensive rat (SHR) is a laboratory model of naturally developing hypertension and heart failure that appears to be similar in many aspects to essential hypertension in humans (Trippodo & Frohlich, 1981). Systolic blood pressure in SHR rapidly increases during 5 to 10 weeks of age and develops cardiac hypertrophy between 9 and 12 weeks of age (Shimamoto et al., 1982). Increasing evidence from different experimental models supports the concept that oxidative stress contributes to the pathogenesis of myocardial hypertrophy and in the process of myocardial remodeling leading to heart failure (Yücel et al., 1998; Lasségue & Griendling, 2004).

The oxidative stress is the result of an increase of reactive oxygen species (ROS) and/or inadequate antioxidant defense mechanisms. It has been shown that an increase in the activity and expression of myocardial NAD(P)H oxidase (NOX) is the main source of ROS in cardiac hypertrophy (Bendall et al., 2002; Griendling et al., 2000; Xiao et al et al., 2002). However, existing data about the antioxidant status in hypertension are inconsistent. Some studies have shown that the activities of one or more antioxidant enzymes are lower (Ito et al, 1995; Newaz & Nawal, 1999), higher (Czonka et al., 2000) or without changes (Gómez-Amores et al., 2006; Girard et al, 2005) compared with normotensive controls. Although the underlying causes of these discrepancies are unknown, it may be possibly due to the use of different hypertension models, animals at different hypertensive stages and/or different experimental preparations.

On the other hand, ROS are thought to be a key mechanism in the aging process (Beckman & Ames, 1998; Colavitti & Finkel, 2004; Harman, 1988) and there are arguments that NOX-

* These authors contributed equally to the present work

derived ROS may lead to cellular senescence (Ago et al., 2010a; Ago et al., 2010b; Imanishi et al., 2005). Thus, lipid peroxidation and oxidative modification of proteins by ROS like peroxynitrite-the product of combination of superoxide ($O_2^{-\cdot}$) and nitric oxide (NO)- are implicated in the pathogenesis of hypertrophy (Nadruz et al., 2004) and in cardiac normal aging (Beal, 2002).

The aim of this study was to assess the oxidative stress in hearts from young and old SHR compared to age-matched Wistar rats.

2. Methods

Experiments were conducted with 40 days and 4-, 11- and 19-month-old male SHR and age-matched Wistar rats. All animals were identically housed under controlled lighting (12 hs) and temperature (20 °C) conditions with free access to standard rat chow and tap water. The experiments were conducted in accordance with the Guide for the Care and Use of Laboratory Animals published by the US National Institutes of Health (NIH Publication No. 85-23, revised in 1996). Systolic blood pressure (SBP) was recorded by the tail-cuff method (Camilión de Hurtado et al., 2002). Left ventricular hypertrophy (LVH) was evaluated by the ratio between heart weight (HW) and tibia length (TL) as previously described (Yin et al., 1982). Wistar strain was used as normotensive control rat. For the biochemical determinations SHR and Wistar rats of 4- and 19 months-old were used. The animals were decapitated and hearts were quickly removed and perfused with ice-cold saline solution (0.9% NaCl) to remove the blood. Left ventricle (LV) samples were taken to assay NOX activity, superoxide production and protein nitration. The rest of the heart was homogenized in 5 volume of 25 mM PO_4KH_2 - 140 mM ClK at pH = 7.4 containing protease inhibitors cocktail (Complete Mini Roche) with a Polytron homogenizer. An aliquot of heart homogenate was used to assess lipid peroxidation. The remaining homogenate was centrifuged at 12000 x g for 5 min at 4° C and the supernatant stored at -70 °C until superoxide dismutase (SOD), catalase (CAT) and glutathione peroxidase (GPx) activities were assayed. Protein concentration was evaluated by Bradford method (Bradford, 1976) using bovine serum albumin as a standard.

2.1 Assessment of lipid peroxidation

Lipid peroxidation was determined by measuring the level of thiobarbituric acid reactive substances (TBARS), expressed as nmol/mg protein. Heart homogenates were centrifuged at 2000 x g for 10 min. Supernatants (0.5 ml) were mixed with 1.5 ml trichloroacetic acid (30 % w/v), 1 ml thiobarbituric acid (0.7% w/v) and 0.5 ml water followed by boiling during 15 min. After cooling, absorbance was determined spectrophotometrically at 535 nm, using a ε value of 1.56×10^5 M^{-1} cm^{-1} (Buege & Aust, 1978).

2.2 Assessment of protein nitration

The interaction of peroxynitrite leads to nitrotyrosine formation actually considered as an indirect marker of oxidative /nitrosative stress (Halliwell, 1997). Thus, we assessed nitrotyrosine level by Western blot analysis. A sample of left ventricle was homogenized in lysis buffer (300 mM sucrose; 1 mM DTT; 4 mM EGTA, protease inhibitors cocktail: 1 tablet/15 ml of buffer; 20 mM Tris-HCl, pH 7.4). After a brief centrifugation proteins were denatured and equal amounts of protein subjected to PAGE and electrotransferred to PVDF membranes. Membranes were incubated with an anti-nitrotyrosine polyclonal antibody (Cayman Chemical). A peroxidase-conjugated, anti-rabbit IgG (Santa Cruz Biotechnology) was used as secondary antibody, and finally bands were visualized with ECL-Plus chemiluminescence detection system (Amersham). Autoradiograms were analyzed by densitometric analysis (Scion Image).

2.3 Determination of NAD(P)H oxidase (NOX) activity

Left ventricular slices (LVS, 1 x 5 mm, 3 – 3.5 mg dry weight) were incubated for 5 min at 37 °C in Krebs-Hepes buffer (in mmol/l: 99 ClNa, 4.69 ClK, 1.87 Cl_2Ca, 1.2 SO_4Mg, 1.03 K_2PO_4, 25 CO_3HNa, 20 Hepes, 11.1 glucose) bubbled with 95% O_2 - 5% CO_2 to maintain pH 7.4 and then transferred to glass scintillation vials containing the same buffer with 5 μM lucigenin. Chemiluminiscence was assessed at 37°C over 15 minutes in a Scintillation counter (Packard 1900 TR) at 1-minute intervals. Vials containing all components without tissue were previously counted and the values were substracted from the chemiluminiscence signals obtained in the presence of LVS. NOX activity was measured in the presence of 100 mM NAD(P)H and expressed as cpm/mg dry weight of LVS (Souza et al., 2002).

2.4 Measurement of superoxide ($O_2^{\cdot-}$) production

Superoxide production was measured in LVS with lucigenin-enhanced chemiluminiscence in Krebs-Hepes buffer with 5 μM lucigenin (Khan et al., 2004). The chemiluminiscence in arbitrary units (AU) was recorded with a luminometer (Chameleon, Hidex) during 30 seconds each with 4.5 min interval during 30 minutes. $O_2^{-\cdot}$ production was expressed as AU per mg dry weight per minute. To determine the involvement of NOX in $O_2^{-\cdot}$ production, the slices were pretreated during 30 min with 300 μM apocynin.

2.5 SOD, CAT and GPx activities assays

SOD activity was determined by inhibition of formazan production (produced by nitroblue tetrazolium (NBT) reduction by superoxide anion) at pH 10.2 and 25° C. The reaction mixture consists in: 100 μM xanthine, 100 μM EDTA, 25 μM NBT, 50 mM CO_3Na_2, pH 10.2. The reaction was started by the addition of xanthine oxidase, reading the absorbance at 560 nm each 30 sec for 5 min (Beauchamp & Fridovich, 1971). One unit of SOD assay was defined as the amount of enzymatic protein required to inhibit 50 % of NBT reduction.

CAT activity was determined by the procedure of Aebi (1984). Decrease in absorbance at 240 nm by the addition of 30 mM H_2O_2 was monitored each 15 sec and for 30 sec. One unit of CAT assay was defined as the amount of the enzyme that decomposed 1 μmol of H_2O_2.

The GPx activity was measured according to Lawrence and Burk method (1976). The assay reaction comprised 50 mM K_2HPO_4 buffer, 1 mM EDTA, 1 mM NaN_3, 1 mM reduced glutathione, 0.2 mM NADPH, 0.25 mM H_2O_2 and 1 U/ml glutathione reductase. Gpx activity was assayed by following NADPH oxidation at 340 nm, measuring the absorbance each 15 sec for 5 min. The activity was calculated using a molar extinction coefficient for NADPH of 6.22 10^3 M^{-1} x cm^{-1} at 340 nm. One unit of the enzyme was represented the decrease of 1 μmol of NADPH/min under assay conditions.

2.6 Statistical analysis

Data are presented as mean ± SE. Differences between Wistar and SHR, young and old groups were analyzed using two-way analysis of variance (ANOVA) with the Newman-Keul's post-hoc test used for multiple comparisons among groups, considering $P < 0.05$ as statistically significant.

3. Results

Comparing to age-matched W rats, SBP of SHR was higher at all ages examined. The analysis of the time course of SBP showed that as early as at 40-day-old the SHR exhibited higher SBP values compared to age-matched W rats. At 4-month-old SBP increased more in comparison to the youngest rats and it remained elevated throughout the last stage studied. LVH significantly increased in SHR at 4, 11 and 19-month-old compared to age-matched W rats. Higher values were obtained at 11 and 19-month-old SHR when compared to younger SHR. An increase in LVH was also observed in W rats with aging (11 and 19-month-old) compared to younger rats (Table 1).

	SHR		Wistar	
	SBP (mmHg)	**LVH**	**SBP (mmHg)**	**LVH**
40 days-old	154 ± 5 *	2.04 ± 0.11	115 ± 5	1.56 ± 0.15
4 months-old	187 ± 2 *#	2.72 ± 0.17 *	116 ± 3	2.05 ± 0.12
11 months-old	178 ± 1.5 *#	3.18 ± 0.23 *#	116 ± 3	2.56 ± 0.09 §
19 months-old	191 ± 5 *#	3.40 ± 0.26 *#	107 ± 6	2.46 ± 0.04 §

Table 1. Values of systolic blood pressure (SBP) and left ventricular hypertrophy (LVH) of SHR and Wistar rats of 40 days and 4, 11 and 19 months-old. * $P < 0.05$ in SHR vs. Wistar; # $P < 0.05$ in SHR vs. 40-day-old; § $P < 0.05$ in Wistar vs.to 40-day-old.

Fig. 1 shows TBARS content in hearts from 4-, and 19-month-old SHR and Wistar rats. In hearts from SHR there was a significantly higher TBARS level of approximately 87% at 19-month-old compared to age-matched Wistar rats. No differences in TBARS with aging were observed in Wistar rats.

Nitrotyrosine levels from hearts of 4 and 19-month-old Wistar and SHR are depicted in Fig. 2. Immunoblotting assays showed a statistically significant increase of approximately 40 % in nitrotyrosine levels at 19-month-old SHR compared to age-matched Wistar rats. The oldest SHR and Wistar rats exhibited an increase of 200 and 120 %, respectively, in nitrotyrosine levels compared to their respective younger group.

Although there were no significant differences in NOX between SHR and Wistar hearts from young animals, an increase in aged rats (approximately 30% for Wistar and 60% for SHR) was obtained showing SHR the highest values (Fig. 3).

Similar $O_2^{-\cdot}$ production was obtained in hearts from Wistar rats and SHR at 4 months of age, whereas in older animals SHR showed a significantly higher $O_2^{-\cdot}$ production (approximately 170%) in comparison with age matched Wistar rats (approximately 70%) (Fig. 4). Anyway, aged rats produced a higher $O_2^{-\cdot}$ amount that younger. The addition of the selective NOX inhibitor apocynin decreased $O_2^{-\cdot}$ production in hearts of aged SHR and Wistar rats. In 4-month-old SHR and Wistar rats $O_2^{-\cdot}$ production was lower in the presence of apocynin, but

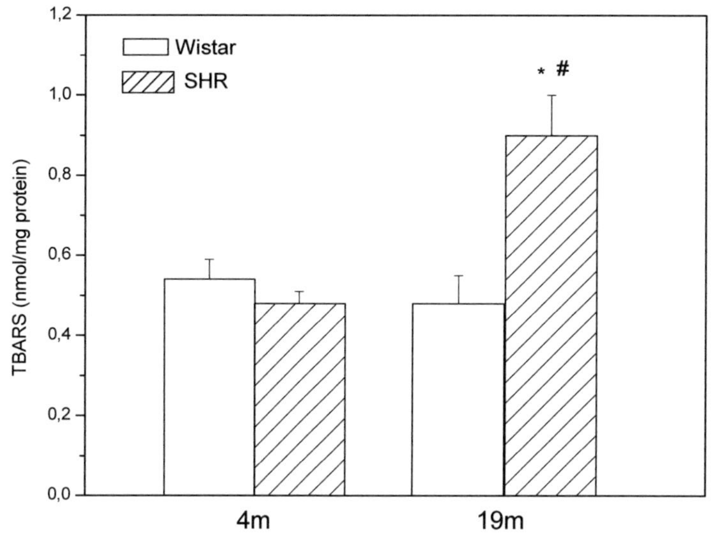

Fig. 1. TBARS content in nmol/mg protein, expressed in nmol/mg protein in hearts from SHR and Wistar rats at 4, and 19 months-old . * P < 0.05 in SHR vs Wistar ; # P < 0.05 vs 4 months-old SHR.

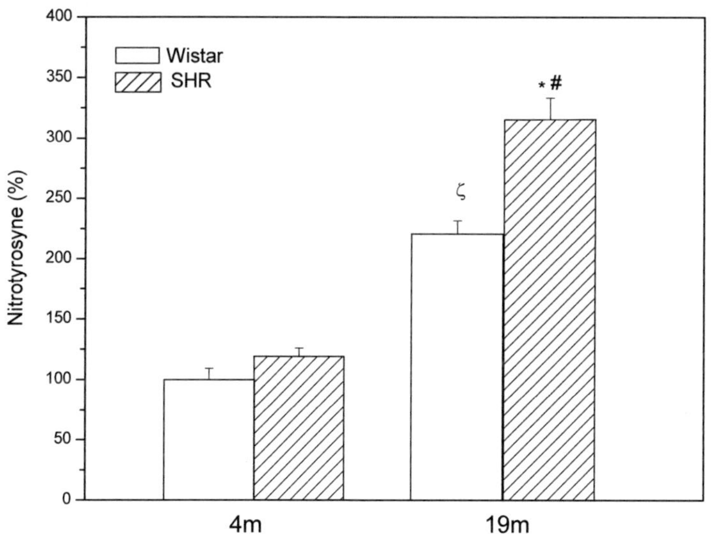

Fig. 2. Nitrotyrosine content, expressed as percentage with respect to 4-month-old Wistar rats in hearts from SHR and Wistar rats at 4 and 19 months-old. * P < 0.05 in SHR vs Wistar ; # P < 0.05 vs 4 months-old SHR; ς P < 0.05 vs 4-month-old Wistar rats.

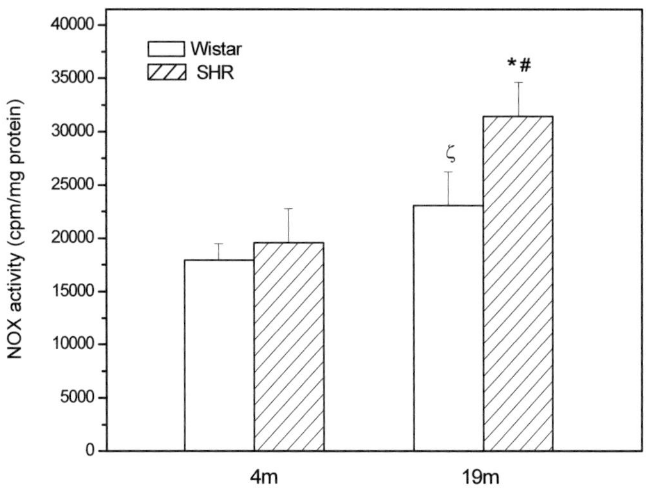

Fig. 3. NOX (NAD(P)H oxidase) activity, expressed as cpm/mg protein in hearts from SHR and Wistar rats at 4 and 19-month-old. * $P < 0.05$ in SHR vs Wistar; # $P < 0.05$ in 19- vs 4-month-old SHR; ς $P < 0.05$ in 19- vs 4-month-old Wistar.

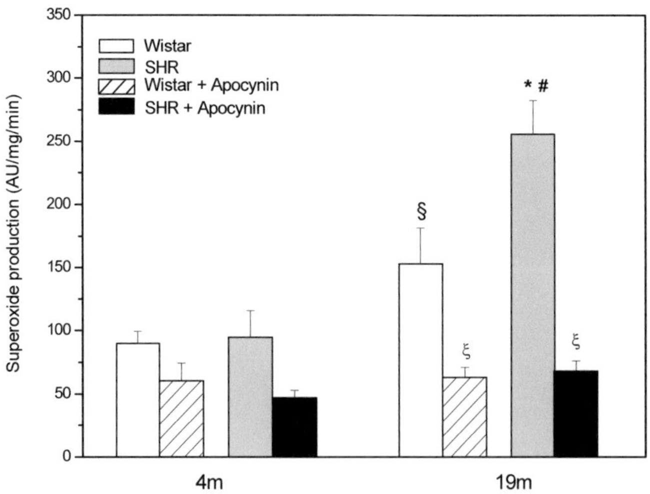

Fig. 4. Superoxide production, expressed as arbitrary units AU/mg/min, in hearts from SHR and Wistar rats at 4 and 19 months of age in the absence and presence of apocynin. *$P < 0.05$ in SHR vs. Wistar rats, # $P < 0.05$ in 19- vs. 4-month-old SHR, § $P< 0.05$ in 19- vs. 4-month-old Wistar rats, ξ $P < 0.05$ in 19-month-old SHR and Wistar rats in the presence vs. absence of apocynin.

the difference was not statistically significant. This may have been because the lucigenin method was unable to detect very small differences in $O_2^{-\cdot}$ levels that were only slightly above the background levels (Dikalov et al., 2007).

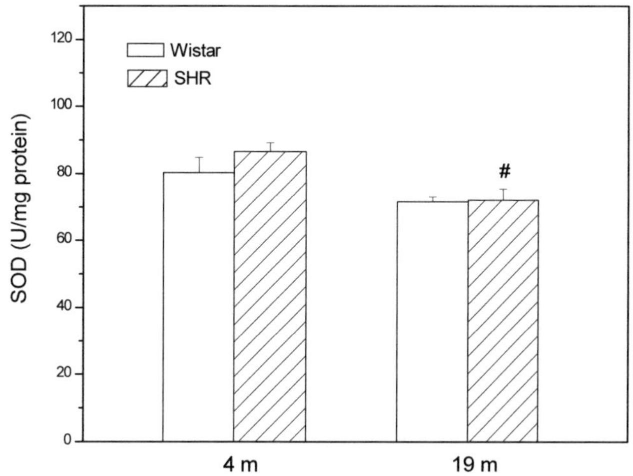

Fig. 5. Superoxide dismutase (SOD) activity, expressed as U/mg protein, in SHR and Wistar hearts of 4 and 19-month-old. # $P < 0.05$ in 19- vs 4-month-old SHR.

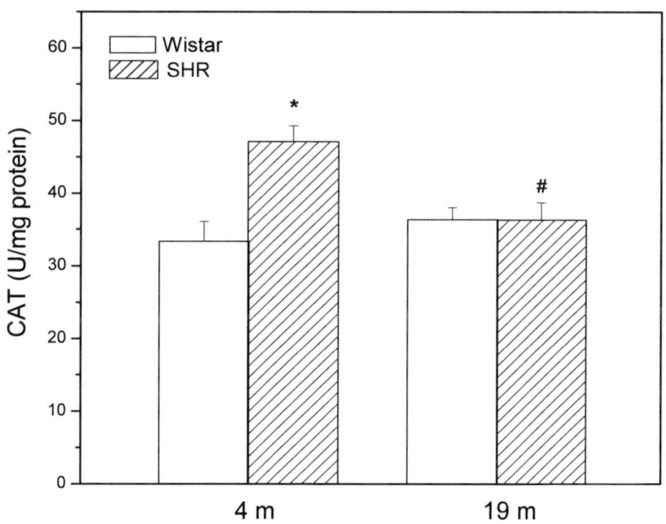

Fig. 6. Catalase (CAT) activity, expressed as U/mg protein, in SHR and Wistar hearts of 4 and 19-month-old. * $P < 0.05$ in SHR vs Wistar ; # $P < 0.05$ in 19- vs 4-month-old SHR.

The activities of antioxidant enzymes are shown in Fig. 5, 6 and 7. SOD activity significantly decreased in older hearts from SHR (approximately 17 %) while not significant differences were detected in Wistar rats with aging (Fig. 5).

Hearts from 4-month-old SHR exhibited a higher catalase activity (approximately 40%) in comparison to hearts from age-matched Wistar rats and it decreased in 19-month-old SHR. In Wistar rats CAT activity did not change with aging (Fig. 6).

Compared to younger animals, a significant decrease of GPx activity was detected in hearts from 19-month-old SHR and Wistar rats. No differences were detected between SHR and age-matched Wistar rats (Fig. 7).

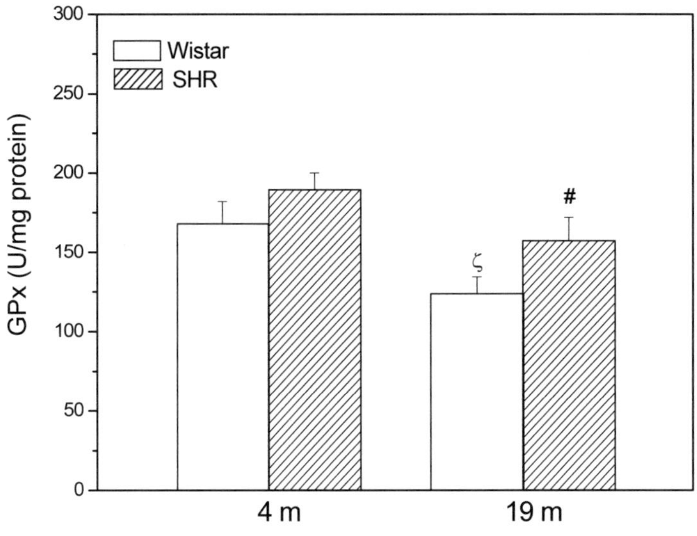

Fig. 7. Glutathione peroxidase (GPx) activity, expressed as U/mg protein, in SHR and Wistar hearts of 4 and 19-month-old. # $P < 0.05$ in 19- vs 4-month-old SHR; ς $P < 0.05$ in 19- vs 4-month-old Wistar.

4. Discussion

The present study shows an increase of oxidative stress associated to ageing in both rat strains, showing SHR the highest values. Oxidative stress is a major contributor to the aging process (Fukagawa, 1999) and appears to be a common feature of hypertensive disorders from diverse origins (Ito et al., 1995; Dobrian et al., 2003; Vaziri & Sica, 2004; Swei et al., 1997). The damage caused by oxidative stress during aging becomes more evident when analyzing the effect of ROS on organic macromolecules, like proteins and lipids. Lipid peroxidation is a major contributor to the age-related loss of membrane fluidity, especially related to increase in the levels of two aldehydic lipid peroxidation products, malonyldialdehyde (MDA) and 4-hydroxy-2-nonenal (HNE). Therefore, it is not surprising that lipid peroxidation is increased in the aged heart as demonstrated by higher levels of

MDA (Cocco et al., 2005) or HNE (Judge et al., 2005). However, in the present study, in accordance with previously reported data (Muscari et al., 1990; Navarro-Arévalo et al., 1999; Cand & verdetti, 1989), we did not find any increase of TBARS in hearts from normotensive rats with aging. These results can be explained considering that the normal hearts have a reduced amount of substrate for the lipoperoxidation (Cand & Verdetti, 1989) or /and the end products of lipoperoxidation are readily metabolized (Muscari et al., 1990) or possess efficient antioxidant defence system . However, we detected an increase in TBARS content with aging in hearts from SHR, compared to age-matched Wistar rats. Moreover, 19-month-old SHR exhibited the highest hypertrophy index and level of lipid peroxidation suggesting that an increase of oxidative damage can be the consequence or the reason for the persistent elevated systolic blood pressure and/or increased cardiac hypertrophy in addition to aging.

Nitric oxide (NO) plays pivotal roles in the maintenance of blood pressure and vascular tone (Loscalzo & Welch, 1995). Superoxide avidly reacts with NO and in the process produces highly reactive and cytotoxic products, like peroxynitrite (ONOO-). Peroxynitrite, in turn, reacts with and modifies various molecules, namely lipids, DNA, and proteins. For instance, peroxynitrite reacts with the tyrosine and cysteine residues in protein molecules to produce nitrotyrosine and nitrocysteine, leading to inactivation of important antioxidant enzymes, like SOD (Mac Millan-Crow & Cruthirds, 2001; Alvarez et al., 2004). In addition to these and other harmful biochemical reactions, the oxidation of NO by ROS inevitably results in functional NO deficiency, which can contribute to pathogenesis and maintenance of hypertension and its long-term consequences. In agreement with previous findings in the vasculature of hypertensive animals (Mc Intyre et al., 1999; Zalba et al., 2001), we detected a higher $O_2^{-\cdot}$ production in cardiac tissue of aged SHR compared to age-matched normotensive Wistar rats. The fact that blood pressure of SHR decreased with antioxidant therapy implies that oxidative stress is involved in the genesis and/or maintenance of hypertension (Vaziri et al., 2000). Recent investigations using hypertensive models other than SHR have shown that an increase of cellular tolerance to oxidative stress is one of the mechanisms responsible for the efficacy of anti hypertensive treatments such as calcium antagonists (Umemoto et al., 2004; Hirooka et al., 2006), angiotensin II type 1 receptor antagonists, or angiotensin-converting enzyme inhibitors (Takai et al., 2005; Tanaka et al., 2005). In our study, hearts from 4-month-old SHR and Wistar rats showed a similar nitrotyrosine content. In addition to lipid peroxidation data, this result is another demonstration that the higher LVH observed in young SHR relative to age-matched Wistar rats was not accompanied by higher nitrosative damage. Aged Wistar rats exhibited an increase in nitrotyrosilation compared with young animals. This increase was lower in Wistar in comparison to SHR, indicating that the addition of hypertrophy to aging process leads to a high degree of nitration due to an increased imbalance in myocardial production of either NO or $O_2^{-\cdot}$. Although we did not measure the expression or activity of NOS, it has been reported that aged hearts exhibited increased myocardial NOS-cGMP signaling associated with an up-regulation of NOS (Zieman et al., 2001; Llorens et al., 2005). Therefore, higher levels of nitrotyrosine in aged SHR hearts would be attributed to an increase of peroxynitrite derived from an excessive production of both reactive species, NO and $O_2^{-\cdot}$. Another possibility for explaining the higher oxidative and nitrosative stress of aged SHR compared to Wistar rats is a decrease in NO availability due to an increase in $O_2^{-\cdot}$ production.

Mitochondria occupy a central position in the metabolism of ROS, supporting the so-called "free radical theory of aging" (Beckman & Ames, 1998; Hardman, 1956; Hardman, 1988). Other cardiovascular sources of ROS include the enzymes xanthine oxidoreductase (Berry & Hare, 2004), NOX (multisubunit membrane complexes) (Griedling et al., 2000) and eNOS uncoupling (Kuzkaya et al., 2003; Landmesser et al., 2003). This eNOS transformation takes place when its essential cofactor (6R)-5,6,7,8-tetrahydro-L-biopterin (BH4) is oxidized by ONOO- then a functional NOS is converted into a dysfunctional $O_2^{-\cdot}$ generating enzyme that contributes to oxidative stress. Abnormal activation and expression of myocardial NOX have been suggested to be the mains sources of ROS in the hypertrophic and failing myocardium (Bendall et al., 2002; Li et al., 2002). A recent paper of Miyagawa et al. (2007) shows that the production of $O_2^{-\cdot}$ by NOX in femoral arteries of SHR in comparison to WKY is enhanced, resulting in the inactivation of NO and impairment of endothelial modulations of vascular contractions. In our study, whereas young SHR showed a similar NOX activity as age-matched Wistar, an increase in the activity of this enzyme was detected in aged SHR, suggesting that NOX-dependent ROS production would be mediating both the hypertrophic response and aging. Apocynin is a well characterized inhibitor of NOX (Meyer & Schmitt, 2000). It acts by impeding the assembly of the p47-phox and p67-phox subunits within the membrane NOX complex (Meyer & Schmitt, 2000; Hamilton et al., 2001). Some of the effects of apocynin treatment are protection of the endothelium from the initiating events of atherosclerosis (Hamilton et al., 2001), a reduction of p22-phox mRNA expression and cardiac hypertrophy in aldosterone-infused rats (Park et al., 2004), and a prevention of hyperglycemia-induced intracellular ROS elevation and myocyte dysfunction (Privratsky et al., 2003). Aponycin has also been shown to reduce oxidative stress in stroke-prone spontaneously hypertensive rats, leading to the suppression of cardiac hypertrophy, inflammation and fibrosis (Yamamoto et al., 2006). Under our experimental conditions, apocynin blunted the $O_2^{-\cdot}$ production in hearts from aged SHR and Wistar rats. Although a significant increase in NOX activity was only evident in aged SHR hearts, we suggest that NOX–dependent ROS production would mediate both the hypertrophic response and aging.

In the myocardium, as in other tissues, antioxidant enzymes protect cells by maintaining ROS at low levels, thus preventing oxidative damage to biological molecules. SOD rapidly converts $O_2^{-\cdot}$ to H_2O_2, which is further degraded by CAT and GPx. The levels of the antioxidant enzymes are sensitive to the oxidative stress and increased or decreased levels have been reported in different pathologies in which an enhancement of ROS is cause or consequence of the disease (Navarro-Arévalo et al., 1999; Ulker et al., 2003). Our data show that SOD activity in hearts from young SHR was slightly but not significantly higher than Wistar rats. The lack of significant difference between SOD activities of hearts from both rat strains is in accordance with previous findings (Gómez-Amores et al., 2006; Wilson & Johnson, 2000; Robin et al., 2004). GPx activity was slightly but no significantly higher in hearts from young SHR compared to age-matched Wistar rats whereas CAT activity showed a significant increase. An opposite result has been recently demonstrated in thoracic aorta of SHR in which a CAT activity decreased and a concomitant increase of H_2O_2 were detected (Ulker et al., 2003). Although we did not have experimental evidence, the increase in CAT activity without GPx one changes detected in young SHR would indicate that CAT is acting as compensatory mechanism. This action could lead to a diminution of H_2O_2 amount in our preparations and could explain the similar TBARS and nitrotyrosine content obtained in young hearts from both rat strains. Aged Wistar rats did not exhibit any change in SOD and GPx activities. However, a significant diminution of antioxidant enzymes was evident in aged compared to younger SHR.

These data are in concordance with those reported by Ito et al. (1995) and opposed to recent observations of Csonka et al. (2000). In addition, both rat strains of 19 months old showed similar antioxidant enzyme activity. Therefore, this fact could not explain the differences of oxidative damage detected between aged SHR and W rats. These differences could be attributed to a significantly higher NOX activity in aged than young SHR in accordance with the increased $O_2^{-\cdot}$ production with aging, indicating that the compensatory mechanism detected in young rats will be abnormal in cardiac tissue from aged SHR. In this regard, it is worth noting a previous report that an increase of SOD pharmacology potency by lecithinization is able to protect endothelial cells against alterations induced by ROS (Igarashi et al., 1992). Another explanation to the differences observed would be related to angiotensin II content, which appears involved in the genesis of oxidative stress in another tissue than heart in the SHR model (De Godoy & Rattan, 2006). This hypothesis was supported by the recent experiments performed in vascular tissue of stroke-prone SHR (Takai et al., 2005; Tanaka et al., 2005) in which the inhibition of angiotensin receptor or angiotensin-converting enzyme system produced a reduction of ROS production. Our results are also consistent with investigations showing that cardioprotective treatments are mediated by a restoration or up-regulation of antioxidant enzyme (Umemoto et al., 2004; Tanaka et al., 2005). Accumulating evidence has suggested that ROS are capable to activate directly intracellular cascades involved in the regulation of hypertrophic growth (Takano et al., 2003). It has been reported that Rho family proteins, specially Rac1, play critical roles in mechanical stress-induced hypertrophy responses and are involved in ROS-mediated activation of MAP kinases (such as p38, ERK1/2) and activation of nuclear factor-κB. Moreover, Rac 1 is essential for assembly of plasma membrane NOX (Griendling et al., 2000). Thus, in our experimental conditions, sustained hemodynamic load in SHR would modulate the action of extracellular stimuli (such as angiotensin II, norepinephrine, tumor necrosis factor-α, epidermal growth factor) on Rac1 activation leading to NOX activation. The increase in $O_2^{-\cdot}$ production by NOX would, in presence of a deficient endogenous antioxidant system, activate redox-sensitive kinase cascades and transcription factors. These actions would produce an induction of immediate early genes, reexpression of fetal genes, increased mRNA content and protein synthesis thus leading to the increase in myocyte cross-sectional area and fibrosis observed in aged SHR heart.

5. Conclusion

This study shows that an increase in $O_2^{-\cdot}$ production in NOX dependent way and consequently higher oxidative damage appears associated to the aging process and to the increase in cardiac hypertrophy detected in hearts of SHR compared to age-matched Wistar rats. Thus, oxidative stress would be the cause and/or consequence of hypertrophy development in the SHR model.

6. Acknowledgement

This work was supported in part by the grant PICT 1046 from Agencia Nacional de Promoción Científica y Técnica of Argentina to Dr Susana M Mosca.

7. References

Aebi, H. (1984). Catalase in Vitro. *Methods in Enzymology,* Vol. 105, pp. 121-126, ISSN 0076-6879.

Ago, T.; Kuroda, J.; Pain, J.; Fu, C.; Li, H. & Sadoshima, J. (2010a). Upregulation of Nox4 by hypertrophic stimuli promotes apoptosis and mitochondrial dysfunction in cardiac myocytes. *Circulation Research,* Vol. 106, No. 7 (April 2010), pp. 1253–64, ISSN 0009-7330.

Ago, T.; Matsushima, S.; Kuroda, J.; Zablocki, D.; Kitazono, T. & Sadoshima. J. (2010b). The NADPH oxidase Nox4 and aging in the heart. *Aging (Albany NY),* Vol. 2, No. 12, (December 2010), pp. 1012-6, ISSN 1945-4589.

Alvarez, B.; Demicheli, V.; Duran, R.; Trujillo, M.; Cervenansky, C.; Freeman, B.A. & Radi, R. (2004). Inactivation of human Cu,Zn superoxide dismutase by peroxynitrite and formation of histidinyl radical. *Free Radical Biology & Medicine,Vol.* 37, No. 6 (September 2004), pp. 813–822, ISSN 0891-5849.

Beal, M.F. (2002). Oxidatively modified proteins in aging and disease. *Free Radical Biology & Medicine,* Vol. 32, No. 9, (May 2002), pp. 797-803, ISSN 0891-5849.

Beauchamp, Ch. & Fridovich, I. (1971). Superoxide dismutase: improved assays and an assay applicable to acrylamide gels. *Analytical Biochemistry,* Vol. 44, No. 1, (November 1971), pp. 276-287, ISSN 0003-2697.

Beckman, K.B. & Ames, B.N. (1998). The free radical theory of aging matures. *Physiological Reviews,* Vol. 78, No. 2, (April 1998), pp. 547–581, ISSN 0031-9333.

Bendall, J.K.; Cave, A.C.; Heymes, C.; Gall, N. & Shah, A.M. (2002). Pivotal role of a gp91(phox)-containing NADPH oxidase in angiotensin II-induced cardiac hypertrophy in mice. *Circulation,* Vol. 105, No. 3 (January 2002), pp. 293-296, ISSN 0009-7322.

Berry, C.E. & Hare, J.M. (2004). Xanthine oxidoreductase in the cardiovascular system: molecular mechanisms and pathophysiologic implications. *Journal of Physiology,* Vol. 555, No. 3, (March 2004), pp. 589-606, ISSN 00219738.

Bradford, M.M. (1976). A rapid and sensitive for the quantitation of microgram quantitites of protein utilizing the principle of protein-dye binding. *Analytical Biochemistry,* Vol. 72 , (May 1976), pp. 248-254, ISSN 0003-2697.

Buege, J.A. & Aust, S.D.(1978). Microsomal lipid peroxidation. *Methods in Enzymology,* Vol. 52, pp. 302–310, ISSN 0076-6879.

Camilión de Hurtado, M.C., Portiansky, E.L., Pérez, N.G., Rebolledo, O.R., Cingolani, H.E. (2002). Regression of cardiomyocyte hypertrophy in SHR following chronic inhibition of the Na^+/H^+ exchanger. *Cardiovascular Research,* Vol. 53, No. 4, (March 2002), pp. 862–868, ISSN 0008-6363.

Cand, F. & Verdetti, J. (1989). Superoxide dismutase, glutathione peroxidase, catalase, and lipid peroxidation in the major organs of the aging rats. *Free Radical Biology & Medicine, Vol.* 7, No. 1, (January 1989), pp. 59-63, ISSN 0891-5849.

Cocco, T.; Sgobbo, P.; Clemente, M.; Lopriore, B.; Grattagliano, I.; Di Paola, M. & Villani, G. (2005). Tissue-specific changes of mitochondrial functions in aged rats: effect of a long-term dietary treatment with N-acetylcysteine. *Free Radical Biology & Medicine,* Vol. 38, No. 6, (March 2005), pp. 796-805, ISSN 0891-5849.

Colavitti, R. & Finkel, T. (2004). Reactive oxygen species as mediators of cellular senescence. *International Union of Biochemistry and Molecular Biology (IUBMB) Life,* Vol. 57, No. 4-5, (April-May 2004), pp. 277–281, ISSN 1521-6543.

Csonka, C.; Pataki, T.; Kovacs, P.; Müller, S.L.; Schroeter, M.L.; Tosaki, A. & Blasig, I.E. (2000). Effects of oxidative stress on the expression of antioxidative defense enzymes in spontaneously hypertensive rat hearts. *Free Radical Biology & Medicine,* Vol. 29, No. 7, (October 2000), pp. 612–619, ISSN 0891-5849.

De Godoy, M.A. & Rattan, S. (2006). Angiotensin-converting enzyme and angiotensin II receptor subtype 1 inhibitors restitute hypertensive internal anal sphincter in the spontaneously hypertensive rats. *Journal of Pharmacology and Experimental Therapeutics*, Vol. 318, No. 2, (August 2006), pp. 725-734, ISSN 0022-3565.

Dikalov, S.; Griendling, K.K. & Harrison, D.G. (2007). Measurement of reactive oxygen species in cardiovascular studies. *Hypertension*, Vol. 49, No. 4, (April 2007), pp. 717-727, ISSN 0194911X.

Dobrian, A.D.; Schriver, S.D.; Lynch, T. & Prewitt, R.L. (2003). Effect of salt on hypertension and oxidative stress in a rat model of diet-induced obesity. *American Journal of Renal Physiology*, Vol. 285, No.4, (October 2003), pp. F619-F628, ISSN 1931-857X.

Fukagawa, N.K. (1999). Aging: is oxidative stress a marker or is it causal? *Proceedings of Society Experimental Biology& Medicine*, Vol. 222, No. 3, (December 1999), pp. 293-298. ISSN 0025.7680.

Girard, A.; Madani, S.; El Boustani, E.S.; Belleville, J. & Prosa, J. (2005). Changes in lipid metabolism and antioxidant defense status in spontaneously hypertensive rats and Wistar rats fed a diet enriched with fructose and saturated fatty acids. *Nutrition*, Vol. 21, No. 5, (May 2005), pp. 240-248, ISSN 0899-9007.

Gómez-Amores, L.; Mate, A.; Revilla, E.; Santa-Maria, C. & Vázquez, C.M. (2006). Antioxidant activity of propionyl-L-carnitine in liver and heart of spontaneously hypertensive rats. *Life Sciences*, Vol. 78, No. 17, (March 2006), pp. 1945-1952, ISSN 0024-3205.

Griendling, K.K.; Sorescu, D. & Ushio-Fukai, M. (2000). NAD(P)H oxidase: role in cardiovascular biology and disease. *Circulation Research*, Vol. 86, No. 5, (March 2000), pp. 494-501, ISSN 0009-7330.

Halliwell, B. (1997). What nitrates tyrosine? Is nitrotyrosine specific as a biomarker of peroxynitrite formation in vivo? *FEBS Letter*, Vol. 411, No. 2-3 (July 1997), pp. 157–160, ISSN 0014-5793.

Hamilton, C.A.; Brosnan, M.J.; McIntyre, M.; Graham, D. & Dominiczak, A.F. (2001). Superoxide excess in hypertension and aging: a common cause of endothelial dysfunction. *Hypertension*, Vol. 37, No. 2 Part 2, (February 2001), pp. 529-534, ISSN 0194911X.

Harman, D. (1956). Aging: a theory based on free radical and radiation chemistry. The *Journals of Gerontology*, Vol. 11, No. 3, (July 1956), pp. 298–300, ISSN 1079-5006.

Harman, D. (1988). Free radicals in aging, *Molecular and Cellular Biochemistry*, Vol. 84, No. 2, (December 1988), pp. 155–161, ISSN 0300-8177.

Hirooka Y.; Kimura Y.; Nozoe M.; Sagara Y.; Ito K. & Sunagawa K. (2006). Amlodipine-induced reduction of oxidative stress in the brain is associated with sympatho-inhibitory effects in stroke-prone spontaneously hypertensive rats. *Hypertension Research, Vol. 29, No.1* (January 2006), pp. 49-56, ISSN 0916-9636.

Igarashi, R.; Hoshino, J.; Takenaga, M.; Kawai, S.; Morizawa, Y.; Yasuda, A.; Otani, M. & Mizushima, Y. (1992). Lecithinization of superoxide dismutase potentiates its protective effect against Forssman antiserum-induced elevation in guinea pig airway resistance. *Journal of Pharmacology and Experimental Therapeutics*, Vol. 262, No. 3, (September 1992), pp. 1214-1219, ISSN 0022-3565.

Imanishi, T.; Hano, T. & Nishio, I. (2005). Estrogen reduces angiotensin II-induced acceleration of senescence in endothelial progenitor cells. *Hypertension Research*, Vol. 28, No. 3, (March 2005), pp. 263–271, ISSN 0916-9636.

Ito, H.; Torii, M. & Suzuki, T. (1995). Decreased superoxide dismutase activity and increased superoxide anion production in cardiac hypertrophy of spontaneously hypertensive rats. *Clinical & Experimental Hypertension,* Vol. 17, No. 5, (July 1995), pp. 803-816, ISSN 1064-1963.

Judge, S.; Jang, Y.M.; Smith, A.; Hagen, T. & Leeuwenburgh, C. (2005). Age-associated increases in oxidative stress and antioxidant enzyme activities in cardiac interfibrillar mitochondria: implications for the mitochondrial theory of aging. *FASEB Journal, Vol.* 19, No. 3, (March 2005), pp. 419-421, ISSN 0892-6638.

Khan, S.A.; Lee, K.; Minhas, K.M.; Gonzalez, D.R.; Raju, S.V.; Tejani, A.D.; Li, D. Berkowitz, D.E. & Hare, JM. (2004). Neuronal nitric oxide synthase negatively regulates xanthine oxidoreductase inhibition of cardiac excitation-contraction coupling. *Proceedings of National Academy of Sciences USA*, Vol. 101, No. 45, (November 2004), pp. 15944-15948, ISSN 0027-8424.

Kuzkaya, N.; Weissmann, N.; Harrison, D.G. & Dikalov, S.(2003). Interactions of peroxynitrite, tetrahydrobiopterin, ascorbic acid, and thiols-implications for uncoupling endothelial nitric-oxide synthase. *Journal of Biological Chemistry,* Vol. 278, No. 25, (June 2003), pp. 22546-22554, ISSN 0021-9258.

Landmesser, U.; Dikalov, S.; Price, S.R.; McCann, L.; Fukai, T.; Holland, S.M.; Mitch, W.E. & Harrison D.G.(2003). Oxidation of tetrahydrobiopterin leads to uncoupling of endothelial cell nitric oxide synthase in hypertension. *Journal of Clinical Investigation,* Vol. 111, No. 8, (April 2003), pp. 1201-1209, ISSN 00219738.

Lassègue, B. & Griendling, K.K. (2004). Reactive oxygen species in hypertension: An update. *American Journal of Hypertension,* Vol. 17, No. 9, (September 2004), pp. 852-860, ISSN 0895-7061.

Lawrence, R.A. & Burk, R.F. (1976). Glutathione peroxidase activity in selenium-deficient rat liver. *Biochemical & Biophysic Research Communication,* Vol. 71, No. , (August 1976), pp. 952-958, ISSN 0006-291X.

Li, J.M.; Gall, N.P.; Grieve, D.J.; Chen, M. & Shah, A.M. (2002). Activation of NAD(P)H oxidase during progression of cardiac hypertrophy to failure. *Hypertension,* Vol. 40, No. 4, (October 2002), pp. 477-484, ISSN 0194911X.

Llorens, S.; Salazar, F.J. & Nava, E. (2005). Assessment of the nitric oxide system in the heart, aorta and kidney of aged Wistar-Kyoto and spontaneously hypertensive rats. *Journal of Hypertension*, Vol. 23, No. 8, (August 2005), pp. 1507-1514, ISSN 0263-6352.

Loscalzo, J. & Welch, G. (1995). Nitric oxide and its role in the cardiovascular system. *Progression Cardiovascular Disease,* Vol. 38, No. 2, (September 1995), pp. 87-104, ISSN 0033-0620.

Mac Millan-Crow, L.A. & Cruthirds, D.L. (2001). Invited review: manganese superoxide dismutase in disease. *Free Radical Research,* Vol. 34, No. 4, (April 2001), pp. 325-336, ISSN 1071-5762.

McIntyre, M.; Bohr, D.F. & Dominiczak, A.F. (1999). Endothelial function in hypertension: the role of superoxide anion. *Hypertension*, Vol. 34, No.4 Pt 1, (October 1999), pp. 539–545, ISSN 0194911X.

Meyer, J.W. & Schmitt, M.E. (2000).A central role for the endothelial NADPH oxidase in atherosclerosis. *FEBS Letter*, Vol. 472, No. 1, (April 2000), pp. 1-4, ISSN 0014-5793.

Miyagawa, K.; Ohashi, M.; Yamashita, S.; Kojima, M.; Sato, K.; Ueda, R. & Dohi, Y. (2007). Increased oxidative stress impairs endothelial modulation of contractions in arteries from spontaneously hypertensive rats. *Journal of Hypertension*, Vol. 25, No. 2, (February 2007), pp. 415-421, ISSN 0263-6352.

Muscari, C.; Caldarera, C.M. & Guarnieri, C. (1990). Age-dependent production of mitochondrial hydrogen peroxide, lipid peroxides and fluorescent pigments in the rat heart. *Basic Research of Cardiology, Vol.* 85, No. 2, (March-April 1990), pp. 172-178, ISSN 0300-8428.

Nadruz, W.Jr.; Lagosta, V.J.; Moreno, H.Jr.; Coelho, O.R. & Franchini, K.G. (2004). Simvastatin prevents load-induced protein tyrosine nitration in overloaded hearts. *Hypertension*, Vol. 43, No. 5, (May 2004), pp. 1060-1066, ISSN 0194-911X.

Navarro-Arévalo, A.; Canavate, C. & Sánchez-del-Pino, M.J. (1999). Myocardial and skeletal muscle aging and changes in oxidative stress in relationship to rigorous exercise training. *Mechanism of Ageing Development,* Vol. 108, No. 3, (May 1999), pp. 207-217, ISSN 0047-6374.

Newaz, M.A. & Nawal, N.N. (1999). Effect of gamma-tocotrienol on blood pressure, lipid peroxidation and total antioxidant status in spontaneously hypertensive rats (SHR). *Clinical & Experimental Hypertension,* Vol. 21, No. 8, (November 1999), pp. 1297-1313, ISSN 0148-3927.

Park, Y.M.; Park, M.Y.; Suh, Y.L. & Park, J.B. (2004). NAD(P)H oxidase inhibitor prevents blood pressure elevation and cardiovascular hypertrophy in aldosterone-infused rats. *Biochemical and Biophysical Research Communications,* Vol. 313, No. 3, (January 2004), pp. 812–817, ISSN 0006-291X.

Privratsky, J.R.; Wold, L.E.; Sowers, J.R.; Quinn, M.T. & Ren, J. (2003). AT1 blockade prevents glucose-induced cardiac dysfunction in ventricular myocytes: role of the AT1 receptor and NADPH oxidase. *Hypertension*, Vol. 42, No. 2, (August 2003), pp. 206–212, ISSN 0194911X.

Robin, S. ; Courderot-Masuyer, C. ; Nicod, L. ; Jacqueson, A. ; Richert, L. & Berthelot, A. (2004). Opposite effect of methionine-supplemented diet, a model of hyperhomocysteinemia, on plasma and liver antioxidant status in normotensive and spontaneously hypertensive rats. *Journal of Nutrition Biochemistry,* Vol. 15, No. 89, (February 2004), pp. 80-89, ISSN 0955-2863.

Shimamoto, N.; Goto, N.; Tanabe, M.; Imamoto, T.; Fujiwara, S. & Hirata, M. (1982). Myocardial energy metabolism in the hypertrophied hearts of spontaneously hypertensive rats. *Basic Research in Cardiology,* Vol. 77, No. 4, (July-August 1982), pp. 359-367, ISSN 0300-8428.

Souza, H.P.; Liu, X.; Samouilov, A.; Kuppusamy, P.; Laurindo, F.R. & Zweier, J.L. (2002). Quantitation of superoxide generation and substrate utilization by vascular NAD(P)H oxidase. Souza *American Journal of Physiology Heart and Circulatory Physiology,* Vol. 282, No. 2, (February 2002), pp. H466-H474, ISSN 0363-6135.

Swei, A.; Lacy, F.; DeLano, F.A. & Schmid-Schonbein, G.W. (1997). Oxidative stress in the Dahl hypertensive rat. *Hypertension*, Vol. 30, No. 6, (December 1997), pp. 1628-1633, ISSN 0194911X.

Takai, S.; Kirimura, K.; Jin, D.; Muramatsu, M.; Yoshikawa, K.; Mino, Y. & Miyazaki, M.T. (2005). Significance of angiotensin II receptor blocker lipophilicities and their protective effect against vascular remodeling. *Hypertension Research*, Vol. 28, No. 7, (July 2005), pp. 593-600, ISSN 0916-9636.

Takano, H.; Zou, Y.; Hasegawa, H.; Akazawa, H.; Nagai, T. & Komuro, I. (2003). Oxidative stress-induced signal transduction pathways in cardiac myocytes: involvement of ROS in heart diseases. *Antioxidant &Redox Signaling,* Vol. 5, No. 6, (December 2003), pp. 789-794, ISSN 1523-0864.

Tanaka, M.; Umemoto, S.; Kawahara, S.; Kubo, M.; Itoh, S.; Umeji, K. & Matsuzaki M. (2005). Angiotensin II type 1 receptor antagonist and angiotensin-converting enzyme inhibitor altered the activation of Cu/Zn-containing superoxide dismutase in the heart of stroke-prone spontaneously hypertensive rats. *Hypertension Research*, Vol. 28, No. 1, (January 2005), pp. 67-77, ISSN 0916-9636.

Trippodo, N.C. & Frohlich, E.D. (1981). Similarities of genetic (spontaneous) hypertension: man and rat. *Circulation Research*, Vol. 48, No 3. (March 1981), pp. 309-319, ISSN 0009-7330.

Ulker, S.; McMaster, D.; McKeown, P.P. & Bayraktutan, U. (2003). Impaired activities of antioxidant enzymes elicit endothelial dysfunction in spontaneous hypertensive rats despite enhanced vascular nitric oxide generation. *Cardiovascular Research, Vol.* 59, No. 2, (August 2003), pp. 488-500, ISSN 0008-6363.

Umemoto, S.; Tanaka, M.; Kawahara, S.; Kubo, M.; Umeji K.; Hashimoto, R. & Matsuzaki M. (2004). Calcium antagonist reduces oxidative stress by upregulating Cu/Zn superoxide dismutase in stroke-prone spontaneously hypertensive rats. *Hypertension Research*,Vol. 27, No. 11, (November 2004), pp. 877-885, ISSN 0916-9636.

Vaziri, N.D.; Ni, Z. & Tarnavsky-Hobbs, D.L. (2000). Effect of antioxidant therapy on blood pressure and nitric oxide synthase expression in hypertensive rats. *Hypertension*, Vol. 36, No. 6, (December 2000), pp. 957–964, ISSN 0194911X.

Vaziri, N.D. & Sica, D.A. 2004. Lead-induced hypertension: role of oxidative stress. *Current of Hypertension Reports* , Vol. 6, No. 4, (August 2004), pp. 314-320, ISSN 1522-6417.

Wilson, D.O. & Johnson, P. (2000). Exercise modulates antioxidant enzyme gene expression in rat myocardium and liver. *Journal of Applied Physiology*, Vol. 88, No. 5, (May 2000), pp. 1791-1796, ISSN 0021-8987.

Xiao, L.; Pimentel, D.R.; Wang, J.; Singh, K.; Colucci, W.S. & Sawyer, D.B. (2002). Role of reactive oxygen species and NAD(P)H oxidase in alpha(1)-adrenoceptor signaling in adult rat cardiac myocytes. *American Journal of Physiology-Cell Physiology, Vol.* 282, No. 4, (April 2002), pp. C926-C934, ISSN 0363-6143.

Yamamoto, E.; Lai, Z.F.; Yamashita, T.; Tanaka, T.; Kataoka, K.; Tokutomi, Y.; Ito, T.; Ogawa, H. & Kim-Mitsuyama., S. (2006). Enhancement of cardiac oxidative stress by tachycardia and its critical role in cardiac hypertrophy and fibrosis. *Journal of Hypertension,* Vol. 24, No. 10, (October 2006), pp. 2057-2069, ISSN 0263-6352.

Yin, F.C.; Spurgeon, H.A.; Rakusan, K.; Weisfeldt, M.L. & Lakatta, E.G. (1982). Use of tibial length to quantify cardiac hypertrophy: application in the aging rat. *American Journal of Physiology-Heart and Circulatory Physiology,* Vol. 243, No. 6, (December 1982), pp. H941-H947, ISSN 0363-6135.

Yücel, D.; Aydoğdu, S.; Cehreli, S.; Saydam, G.; Canatan, H.; Seneş, M.; Ciğdem Topkaya, B. & Nebioğlu, S. (1998). Increased oxidative stress in dilated cardiomyopathic heart failure. *Clinical Chemistry,* Vol. 44, No. 1, (January 1998), pp. 148–154, ISSN 0009-9147.

Zalba, G.; San José, G.; Moreno, M.U.; Fortuno, M.A.; Fortuno, A.; Beaumont, F.J. & Diez, J. (2001). Oxidative stress in arterial hypertension. Role of NAD(P)H oxidase. *Hypertension, Vol.* 38, No. 6, (December 2001), pp. 1395–1399, ISSN 0194911X.

Zieman, S.J.; Gerstenblith, G.; Lakatta, E.G.; Rosas, G.O.; Vandegaer, K.; Ricker, K.M. & Hare J.M.(2001). Upregulation of the nitric oxide-cGMP pathway in aged myocardium: physiological response to l-arginine. *Circulation Research,* Vol. 88, No. 1, (January 2001), pp. 97-102, ISSN 0009-7300.

8

Oxidative Stress and Mitochondrial Dysfunction in Cardiovascular Diseases

Sauri Hernández-Reséndiz, Mabel Buelna-Chontal,
Francisco Correa and Cecilia Zazueta
*Departamento de Bioquímica,
Instituto Nacional de Cardiología, Ignacio Chávez,
México*

1. Introduction

Reactive oxygen species (ROS) include a wide variety of molecules and free radicals derived from molecular oxygen. O_2 being highly electrophilic can be reduced by one electron at a time producing relatively stable intermediates, such as superoxide anion ($O_2\bullet^-$), precursor of most ROS and a relevant mediator in many biological reactions. Dismutation of $O_2\bullet^-$ produces hydrogen peroxide (H_2O_2), which, in turn, may be fully reduced to water or partially reduced to hydroxyl radical (•OH), one of the strongest oxidants in nature. The formation of •OH is catalyzed by reduced transition metals. On the other hand, superoxide anion is able to reduce transition metals and intensify in this way hydroxyl generation. In addition, $O_2\bullet^-$ may react with other radicals, in particular, with nitric oxide (•NO) in a reaction controlled by the rate of diffusion of both radicals. The product, peroxynitrite, is very powerful oxidant. The oxidants derived from •NO have been recently called reactive nitrogen species (RNS). Oxidative stress is an expression used to describe various deleterious processes resulting from an imbalance between the formation and elimination of ROS and/or RNS by antioxidant defenses. While small fluctuations in the steady-state concentration of these oxidants play an important role in intracellular signaling, uncontrolled increase in their concentration produces free radical-mediated chain reactions, which indiscriminately target proteins, lipids, polysaccharides, and DNA. Mitochondria are a major source of ROS, converting as much as 0.2-2% of molecular oxygen to superoxide as a by-product of the electron transfer activity (Wittenberg & Wittenberg, 1989; Alvárez et al., 2003). Other enzymatic sources of ROS include NADPH oxidases, located on the cell membrane of polymorphonuclear cells, macrophages, endothelial and other cells, and cytochrome P450-dependent oxygenases, along with the proteolytic conversion of xanthine dehydrogenase to xanthine oxidase, which produces both $O_2\bullet^-$ and H_2O_2.

Mitochondria's critical role in cardiomyocyte survival and death has become an exciting finding in the field of cardiac biology. Indeed, it is accepted that mitochondrial dysfunction plays a crucial role in the pathogenesis of multiple cardiac diseases, mainly due to the imbalance of the fine interplay between aerobic metabolism, calcium homeostasis, and ROS production. Reactive oxygen species generated in the mitochondria, unless adequately neutralized, cause mitochondrial oxidative stress and, through reactions with polyunsaturated fatty acids, form lipid hydroperoxides and unsaturated aldehydes that propagate among cellular compartments and react with proteins and nucleic acids. In the myocardium, the oxidative stress cascade impairs several functions, like mitochondrial biogenesis, fatty acid metabolism, ionic homeostasis, and antioxidant defense mechanisms, leading to diminished cardiac energetic efficiency, altered bioenergetics, apoptosis and degradation. Besides the obvious relevance of mitochondria in energy production, new processes like mitochondrial fusion and fission are reported to be linked to ROS generation and now are included in the cast of key players in cardiac disease. In this chapter, we explore the mechanisms of mitochondrial dysfunction driven by ROS generation associated with the pathophysiology of cardiovascular diseases.

2. Mitochondrial reactive oxygen species generation

The standard reduction potential for the conversion of molecular oxygen to $O_2{\bullet}^-$ is -0.160 V (Wood, 1987). Given the highly reducing intramitochondrial environment, various respiratory components, including complexes I and III of the mitochondrial respiratory chain (Paradies et al., 2001; Tompkins et al., 2006), flavoproteins (Prosser et al., 2011), iron-sulfur clusters (Napoli et al., 2006), and ubisemiquinone (Wen & Garg, 2008) are thermodynamically capable to donate one electron to oxygen. Moreover, most steps in the respiratory chain involve single-electron reactions, further favoring the monovalent reduction of oxygen. On the other hand, the mitochondrion possesses various antioxidant defenses designed to eliminate both $O_2{\bullet}^-$ and H_2O_2. As a result, the steady state concentrations of $O_2{\bullet}^-$ and H_2O_2 have been estimated to be around 1×10^{-10} M and 5×10^{-9} M, respectively (Cadenas & Davies, 2000). Mitochondrial sources of $O_2{\bullet}^-$ include several respiratory complexes and individual enzymes. Superoxide formation occurs on the outer mitochondrial membrane, in the matrix, and on both sides of the inner mitochondrial membrane (Table 1, Figure 1). While superoxide anion generated in the matrix is mainly eliminated in that compartment, part of the $O_2{\bullet}^-$ produced in the intermembrane space may be carried to the cytoplasm via voltage-dependent anion channels (Han et al., 2003). The relative contribution of every site to the overall $O_2{\bullet}^-$ production varies from organ to organ and also depends on whether mitochondria are actively respiring (State 3) or if the respiratory chain is highly reduced (State 4) (Barja, 1999). Complex III appears to be responsible for most of the $O_2{\bullet}^-$ produced in heart mitochondria (Turrens & Boveris, 1980; Turrens et al., 1982), although Complex I is thought to be the primary source of ROS in a variety of pathological scenarios ranging from ageing to Parkinson's disease (Betarbet et al., 2002; Sherer et al., 2003a). The rate of $O_2{\bullet}^-$ formation by the respiratory chain is controlled primarily by mass action law, increasing both when electron flow slows down (the concentration of electron donors, R• is higher) and when the concentration of oxygen increases[1] (Turrens et al., 1982).

$$d[O_2]/dt = k\,[O_2]\,[R\bullet] \qquad (1)$$

The electron flow through the respiratory chain establishes an H^+ gradient across the inner mitochondrial membrane, used to drive ATP synthesis through the ATP synthase complex (Complex V). In the absence of ADP, the movement of H^+ through ATP synthase is ceased and the H^+ gradient builds up causing slowdown of electron flow and reduction of the respiratory chain (State 4). As a result, the physiological steady state concentration of O_2•⁻ formation increases. The formation of O_2•⁻ may be further increased in the presence of certain inhibitors (for example rotenone, which inhibits Complex I, or antimycin an inhibitor of Complex III), which cause those carriers upstream from the site of inhibition to become fully reduced. In Complex I, the primary source of O_2•⁻ appears to be one of the iron-sulfur clusters, whereas in Complex III, most of O_2•⁻ results from ubisemiquinone auto-oxidation, both on the outer and inner sides of the inner mitochondrial membrane (Table 1).

Component	Localization	References
Complex I (NADH dehydrogenase)	Inner membrane/ inner side	(Turrens & Boveris, 1980; Turrens *et al.* 1982; Genova *et al.* 2001; Kushnareva *et al.* 2002)
Complex II (succinate dehydrogenase)	Inner membrane/ inner side	(Zhang *et al.* 1998; Lenaz, 2001)
Complex III (ubiquinol–cytochrome *c* reductase)	Inner membrane/ inner side	(Boveris *et al.* 1976; Cadenas *et al.* 1977; Turrens *et al.* 1985)
Complex III (ubiquinol–cytochrome *c* reductase)	Inner membrane/ outer side	(Han *et al.* 2001; Starkov & Fiskum, 2001)
External NADH dehydrogenase (yeast)	Inner membrane/ outer side	(Fang & Beattie, 2003)
Glycerolphosphate dehydrogenase	Inner membrane/ outer side	(Drahota *et al.* 2002)
Dehydroorotate dehydrogenase	Matrix	(Forman & Kennedy, 1976)
Mono amino oxidase	Outer membrane/ inner side	(Hauptmann *et al.* 1996; Cadenas & Davies, 2000)

Table 1. Compartmental localization of the main mitochondrial sources of superoxide anion. Modified from Turrens, 2003.

Although O_2•⁻ production increases as the respiratory chain becomes more reduced, not all mitochondrial inhibitors have this effect. Most of the production of O_2•⁻ by Complex III is actually inhibited if electron flow between the Rieske Fe–S protein and oxygen is blocked, for example by myxothiazol, cyanide or cytochrome *c* depletion (Turrens et al., 1985). This inhibitory effect indicates that O_2•⁻ must be produced as a result of the autoxidation of semiquinone (Q•), an intermediate produced in Complex III during the Q-cycle (Trumpower, 1990; Figure 2). Coenzyme Q is fully reduced and converted to ubiquinol (QH_2) in the inner side of the mitochondrial membrane and then migrates to the outer side of the inner membrane carrying two protons that become part of the pool needed to sustain ADP phosphorylation. Once on the outer side of the membrane, one electron is transferred to cytochrome *c*1 (via the Rieske Fe–S protein), resulting in the formation of Q•. In a second cycle, a new QH_2 transfers one of its electrons to the iron-sulphur protein (ISP) and then to cytochrome c1, whereas the second electron reduces cytochrome b_{566} and then cytochrome b_{540} (Turrens et al., 2003). This second electron reduces the Q• produced in the first cycle, yielding QH_2. Despite the high efficiency of redox reactions in the Q cycle, some electrons leak and react with oxygen producing O_2•⁻ (Figure 1).

Another modulator of mitochondrial ROS production is the membrane potential ($\Delta\psi_m$), thus it has been reported that both, uncouplers and uncoupling proteins (UCPs), minimize ROS production by enhancing proton leak and providing a negative feedback loop for mitochondrial ROS production. A direct impact of ROS on the glutathionylation status of UCPs has been invoked to explain the activation of such proteins (Mailloux & Harper, 2011).

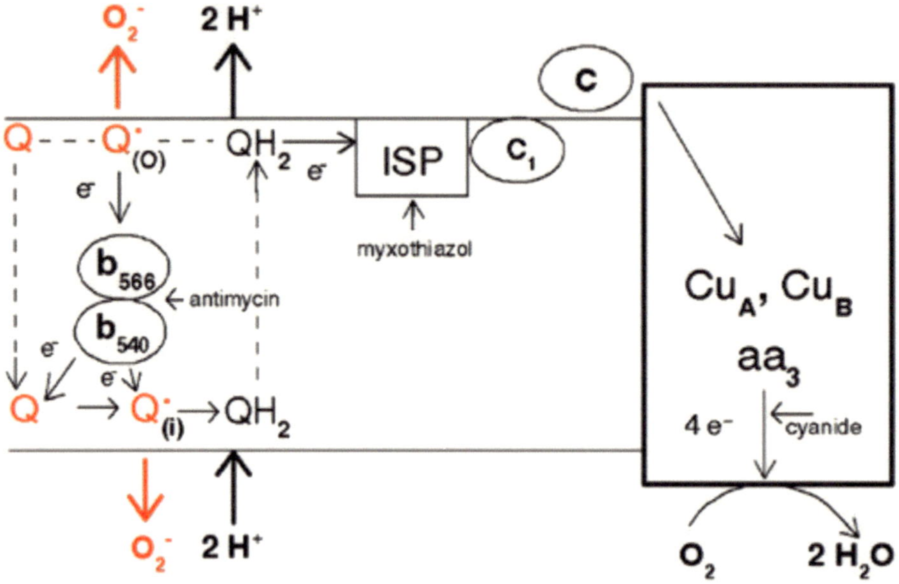

Fig. 1. Electron flow in the Q-cycle. Ubiquinone (Q) is reduced by electrons transferred from NADH or succinate producing ubiquinol (QH_2). The reduced form undergoes a two-cycle reoxidation in which the semiquinone (Q•) is a stable intermediate that transfers electrons to oxygen via the Rieske iron-sulfur protein (ISP), cytochrome *c*1 (c1) and cytochrome *c* (c). The terminal oxidase catalyzes the oxidation of reduced cytochrome c and the concomitant four-electron reduction of one O_2 molecule producing water. Superoxide may be produced on both sides of the inner membrane via the autoxidation of Q, but the contribution of each pool has not yet been determined.

Special mention is worth about how Ca^{2+} modulates mitochondrial ROS generation. The primary role of this cation in mitochondria is the stimulation of oxidative phosphorylation by allosteric activation of pyruvate dehydrogenase, isocitrate dehydrogenase, α-ketoglutarate dehydrogenase, as well as other proteins of the phosphorylating machinery (Brooks et al., 2004). Thus, the stimulation of oxidative phosphorylation would enhance ROS production, as mitochondria are being forced to work faster and to consume more O_2. Experimental observations are diverse, overall it appears that physiological $[Ca^{2+}]_m$ has no direct effect on respiratory chain function or oxidation/reduction process, however pathological mitochondrial Ca^{2+} overload can lead to ROS increase. Possible mechanisms include Ca^{2+} stimulated increase of metabolic rate; Ca^{2+} stimulated nitric oxide production, which inhibits complex IV; Ca^{2+} induced cytochrome c dissociation that would inhibit the distal respiratory chain; Ca^{2+} induced cardiolipin peroxidation and Ca^{2+} induced mitochondrial permeability transition pore opening (Peng & Jou, 2010).

On the other hand, simultaneous formation of $O_2^{\bullet-}$ and nitric oxide can produce peroxynitrite, a very strong oxidant and nitrating agent. Nitric oxide is a vasodilator resulting from the convertion of arginine to citrulline, in a reaction catalyzed by a family of NADPH-dependent enzymes called nitric oxide synthases. It has been reported that the mitochondrial matrix contains a unique form of nitric oxide synthase (Alvarez et al., 2003). Although its physiological role is still unclear, the formation of nitric oxide in mitochondria may have important pathological consequences, as it binds to the heme group of cytochrome oxidase, inhibiting respiration (Poderoso et al., 1996). ROS are also produced within mitochondria at sites other than the inner mitochondrial membrane (Dowrakowski et al., 2008), by proteins such as monoamine oxidase (MAO) and p66Shc (reviewed in Di Lisa et al., 2009).

3. Antioxidant systems in mitochondria

Mammalian mitochondria possess a multi-leveled ROS defense network of enzymes and non-enzymatic antioxidants. Thus, constantly generated ROS, essential for normal cellular physiology and signaling process, are maintained at specific levels by intrinsic antioxidant defenses, avoiding oxidative stress. In healthy mitochondria, ROS contention is driven by manganese-dependent superoxide dismutase (MnSOD), gluthatione peroxidase (GPx), thioredoxin ($TrxSH_2$) and thioredoxin reductase (TrxR), peroxiredoxin (Prx), and glutaredoxin (Grx), as well as water- and lipid-soluble antioxidants, i.e. vitamins C, α-tocopherol (α-toc), reduced glutathione (GSH), and melatonin. It has been proposed that under certain circumstances, the mitochondrial respiratory chain can also contribute to mitochondrial antioxidant defense.

3.1 Non-enzymatic antioxidants

The tripeptide GSH is the main non-protein molecule, containing reactive thiol (-SH) groups, with scavenging properties, that provides an abundant source of reducing equivalents (Stowe & Camara, 2009). GSH reacts with hydroxyl radical (•OH), hypochlorous acid (HOCl), peroxyl radical (RO_2•), carbon-centered radicals, and peroxynitrite anion ($ONOO^-$) producing thiyl radical (GS•), which potentially generates $O_2{•}^-$ among other ROS (Ježek & Hlavatá, 2005). Despite its exclusive synthesis in the cytosol, GSH is distributed in intracellular organelles, including the endoplasmic reticulum (RE), nucleus, and mitochondrion (Marí et al., 2009; Figure 2). GSH synthesis involves a two step reaction that requires ATP. Glutamate and cysteine are converted to γ-glutamyl-cysteine in a rate-limiting reaction driven by γ-glutamylcysteine synthetase. Then, γ-glutamylcysteine and glycine produce GSH by the action of the enzyme GSH synthetase (Figure 2). The first reaction is inhibited by GSH, a mechanism that regulates cellular GSH concentration (Marí et al., 2009). In the cytosol, GSH concentration is around 11 mM (Griffith & Meister, 1979; Mårtensson et al., 1990) and is transported into the mitochondrial matrix through a non-described high affinity carrier and a low affinity carrier, that could be the mitochondrial oxoglutarate carrier (Coll et al., 2003) or the dicarboxylate carrier (Lash et al., 2002). In mitochondria, GSH levels may fluctuate from 5 to 11 mM (Valko et al., 2007). Mitochondrial GSH plays a critical role in cell survival, as toxic cell death often correlates better with depletion of the mitochondrial GSH pool than with overall intracellular GSH depletion (Orrenius et al., 2007).

The importance of UCPs in the control of mitochondrial ROS generation remains unclear: it is known that UCPs are inner membrane carriers that transfer protons across the mitochondrial inner membrane (MIM), by-passing ATPase (Stuart et al., 2001). A putative

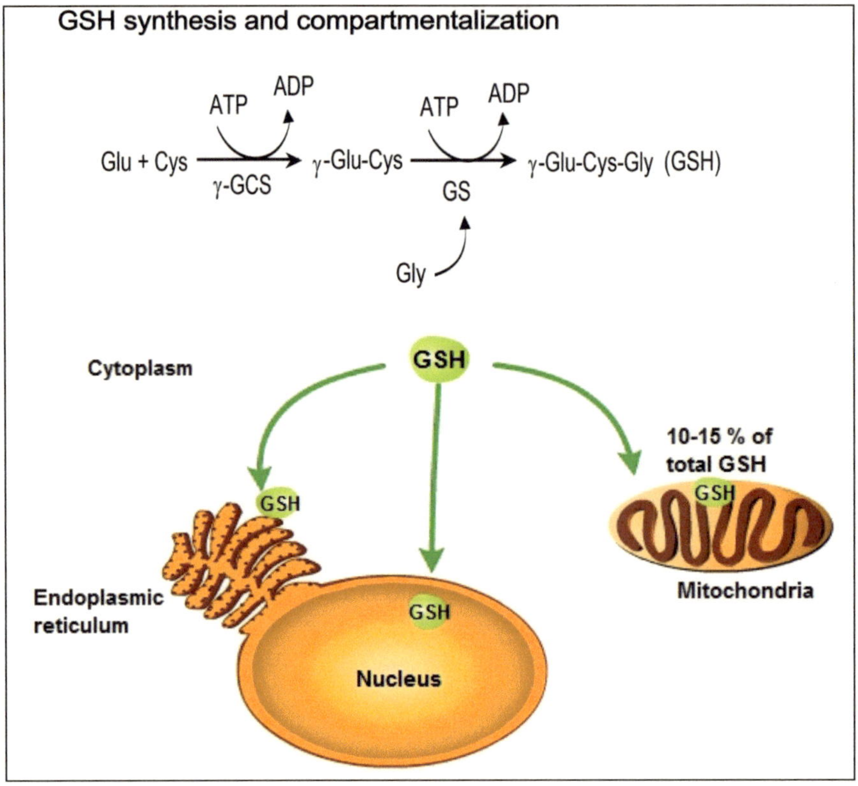

Fig. 2. GSH synthesis and compartmentalization. GSH is synthesized by γ-glutamylcysteine synthetase (γ-GCS) and glutathione synthetase (GS) in the cytoplasm and then redistributed to mitochondria, nucleus, and endoplasmic reticulum.

role in redox homeostasis control has been associated with their capacity to reduce mitochondrial ROS production by modulating $\Delta\psi_m$ (Haines et al., 2010). In fact, UCPs reduce the damaging effects of ROS during cardiac ischemia/reperfusion injury (Barreiro et al., 2009). UCP1 isoform is involved in thermogenesis and expressed specifically in brown adipose tissue mitochondria, in which it confers a regulated proton leak across the inner membrane, whereas the physiologic functions of the other isoforms remain unclear. UCP2 and UCP3 are present in the heart and provide cardioprotection. In rat neonatal cardiomyocytes, UCP overexpression confers tolerance against oxidative stress by a mechanism related with calcium uptake (Sack, 2006b).

α-Tocopherol and melatonin scavenge lipid peroxyl radicals much faster than these radicals can react with adjacent fatty acid side-chains, so they are probably the most important inhibitors of the free-radical chain reaction of lipid peroxidation in animals (Maroz et al., 2009; Gavazza & Catalá, 2009). Aside from its various physiological functions, melatonin could acts as a scavenger of the particularly toxic •OH and carbonate radical, which is important because of their presumed role in mitochondrial damage (Srinivasan et al., 2009, Hardeland & Coto-Montes, 2010). Besides, melatonin could act as an indirect antioxidant promoting *de novo* synthesis of GSH, stimulating the activity of *γ*-glutamylcysteine synthetase and also through its effects on GPx, Grx, SOD, and CAT gene expression

(Rodríguez et al., 2004), helping in GSH recycling and maintaining a high GSH/GSSG ratio. Melatonin is synthesized and released to the circulation by the pineal gland, and its amphiphilic properties lead to its free access to all compartments in the cell, being concentrated especially in the nucleus and mitochondria (Escames et al., 2010). A direct role of melatonin in regulation of Complex I and IV activity and in other mitochondrial functions has been suggested. This effect, not shared by other antioxidants, would reflect redox interactions with the electron transfer chain complexes, stimulating electron flow, limiting electron leakage, and ROS generation (Escames et al., 2010). Interestingly, it has also been reported that melatonin protects mitochondria from oxidative damage by preventing cardiolipin oxidation (Paradies et al., 2010).

3.2 Enzymatic antioxidants

MnSOD converts superoxide anion ($O_2 \bullet^-$) to hydrogen peroxide (H_2O_2) in the matrix side of the inner mitochondrial membrane (Liochev & Fridovich, 2010), while some $O_2 \bullet^-$ released into the intermembrane space is partially dismutated by copper-zinc containing superoxide dismutase (CuZnSOD) (Figure 3). Disruption of the MnSOD gene in mice has been

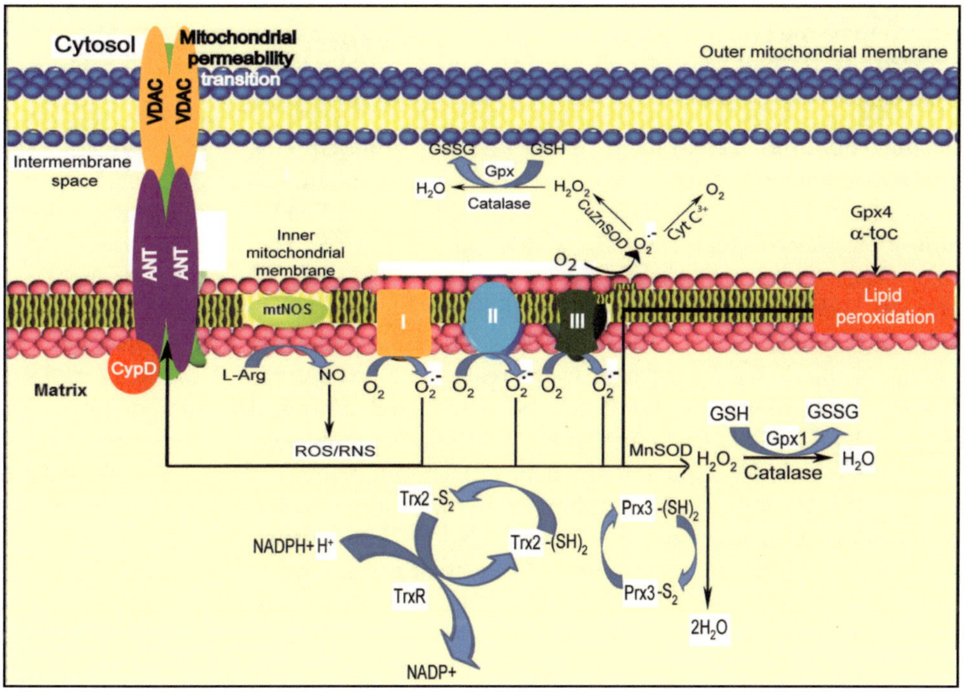

Fig. 3. Mitochondrial antioxidant network. Mitochondria are normally protected from oxidative damage by a network of mitochondrial antioxidant systems. See text for further details. α-toc: α-tocoferol; Cyt *c*3+ (reduced cytochrome *c*) ; CuZnSOD: copper-zinc superoxide dismutase; Gpx: glutathione peroxidase; GSH: reduced glutathione, GSSG: oxidized glutathione; L-Arg: L-arginine; mtNOS: mitochondrial nitric oxide synthase, NO: nitric oxide; Prx3-$(SH)_2$: peroxiredoxine 3 reduced, Prx3-S_2: peroxiredoxine 3 oxidized; ROS: reactive oxygen species, RNS: reactive nitrogen species; Trx2-$(SH)_2$: tioredoxine 2 reduced, Trx2-S_2: tioredoxine oxidized.

associated with early postnatal lethality (Li et al., 1995), while MnSOD overexpression was shown to protect mitochondrial function and block apoptosis (Holley et al., 2010). The activity of MnSOD should be coordinated with H_2O_2-removing enzymes. Thus, H_2O_2 produced by MnSOD could be metabolized by Gpx, Prx, or by catalase that has been found in extremely small amounts in the mitochondrial matrix.

Besides of the importance of GSH as a direct antioxidant, it participates in multiple GSH-linked enzymatic defense systems. Among others, GSH acts as electron donor in the reduction of H_2O_2 and different hydroperoxides by GPx1 and GPx4 (Camara et al., 2011). Five different isoforms of GPx have been identified GPx1, GPx2, GPx3, GPx 4, and GPx 6. GPx1 is the major isoform and is localized predominantly in the cytosol, but a small proportion is also present within the mitochondrial matrix (Orrenius et al., 2007). GPx4 is a unique intracellular antioxidant enzyme that directly reduces peroxidized lipids produced in cell membranes (Nomura et al., 2000). Because GPx4 is membrane-associated, with a fraction localized in the intermembrane space of the mitochondria, possibly at the contact sites of the two membranes, and due to its small size and large hydrophobic surface it can interact with, and detoxify, membrane lipid hydroperoxides much more efficiently than the alternative pathway, phospholipase A_2-GPx1 (PLA2) (Antunes et al., 1995). Hence, GPx4 is considered to be the primary enzymatic defense system against oxidative damage to cellular membranes. Accordingly, GPx4-null mice are embryonically lethal, while the heterozygotes are more sensitive to oxidants than wild type mice (Ran et al., 2003).

Other mitochondrial GSH-linked enzymes are glutaredoxins (Grx), which catalyze glutathione-dependent dithiol reaction, reducing protein disulfides, and monothiol reactions reducing mixed disulfides between proteins and GSH. An interesting member of this family is glutaredoxin 2 (Grx2), which was cloned and found to be present as both mitochondrial and nuclear isoforms (Lundberg et al., 2001). Modeling suggests that the GSH binding site and the hydrophobic surface of Grx2 are similar to those of Grx1 (Lundberg et al., 2001), although Grx2 lacks one of the conserved non-active site cysteine residues of Grx1 (Lundberg et al., 2001), hence it is more resistant to oxidants and oxidized glutathione (GSSG) action. Furthermore, Grx2 can be reactivated directly by thioredoxin reductase (TrxR) as well as by GSH (Johanson et al., 2004). GSSG is reduced by glutathione reductase (GR) with NADPH as a cofactor. In turn, mitochondrial NADPH can be regenerated by matrix dehydrogenases and by reaction of hydride ion transfer, which is proton motive force-dependent, utilizing intramitochondrial NADPH to reduce $NADP^+$. Besides NADPH *per se* can serve directly as a non-enzymatic antioxidant, according to some authors (Kirsch & De Groot, 2001). Another potential source of disulfide reductase activity in mitochondria is the thioredoxin system, which includes thioredoxin 2 (Trx2) and thioredoxin reductase (TrxR2). Trx2 catalyzes the reduction of protein disulfides at much higher rates than Grx (Arner & Holmgren, 2000). This enzyme is important for life, given that disruption of the Trx2 gene in the homozygous mouse causes massive apoptosis and, finally, results in embryonic lethality (Nonn et al., 2003). Specific glutathione S-transferase (GST) isoforms: GSTα1-1, GSTα4-4, and GSTμ1-1, which neutralize reactive molecules such as 4-hydroxy-2-noneal (4-HNE), incorporating GSH to the radical molecule, have been found in mitochondria (Raza et al., 2002).

The intermembrane space of mitochondria contains ~0.7 mM cytochrome *c* (Hackenbrock et al., 1986) capable of superoxide removal. Cytochrome *c* can be alternatively reduced by the respiratory chain or superoxide. A diminution in its concentration may inhibit the distal respiratory chain and increase ROS production. Indeed, it has been reported that upon cytochrome *c* release during apoptosis initiation, mitochondrial ROS production increases (Cai & Jones, 1998).

As mentioned before, ubiquinone (Q) acts as a pro-oxidant in its semiquinone form, however when fully reduced it acts as an antioxidant. Ubiquinol (UQH_2) contains phenolic hydrogen atoms that can be donated to a carbon- or oxygen centered radical, converting it to a non-radical molecule (Ježek & Hlavatá, 2005). Lipid peroxidation prevention by UQH_2 has been reported (James et al., 2004). Preferential succinate oxidation can provide a tool against excessive accumulation of ROS by increasing the proportion of fully reduced ubiquinone. The antioxidant activity of UQH_2 is independent from the effect of α-tocopherol (Ernster et al., 1992), which acts as a chain-breaking antioxidant, inhibiting the propagation of lipid peroxidation (Maroz et al., 2009). Even more, UQH_2 can efficiently sustain the effect of α-tocopherol by regenerating it from the tocopheroxyl radical, which otherwise must rely on water-soluble agents such as ascorbate (vitamin C) (Ernster & Forsmark-Andree, 1993).

4. Oxidative stress and cardiovascular diseases

The pathological role of increased mitochondrial ROS in heart disease has been established from studies in gene-modified mice with altered mitochondrial antioxidant levels. Deletion of mitochondrial thioredoxin reductase 2 is embryonically lethal in mice because of impaired hematopoiesis and impaired cardiac function (Conrad et al., 2004). Fatal dilated cardiomyopathy in mice is developed after complete deletion of mitochondrial Mn superoxide dismutase (Li et al., 1995). In contrast, attenuated left ventricular remodeling after myocardial infarct was observed in transgenic mice overexpressing mitochondrial peroxiredoxin III (Matsushima et al., 2006) or glutathione peroxidase (Shiomi et al., 2004). Also, mice with a mitochondrial-targeted overexpression of catalase have a prolonged life span and improved cardiac function (Schriner et al., 2005).

A critical role of intracellular Ca^{2+} overload and oxidative stress in the genesis of myocyte dysfunction is well established in cardiovascular diseases like atherosclerosis, hypertension, ischemia/reperfusion damage, cardiac hypertrophy, and heart failure (HF). In general, Ca^{2+} overload can be induced by direct effect of ROS on Ca^{2+} handling proteins or indirectly, by inducing membrane lipid peroxidation (Santos et al., 2011). Recent evidence suggests that redox modification of ryanodine receptor (RyR2) may contribute to abnormal Ca^{2+} handling in disease states. RyR2 dysfunction with an increase in diastolic Ca^{2+} leak from the sarcoplasmic reticulum (SR) may reduce calcium transients and contribute to a reduced contractile force in the failing heart, as well as an increased likelihood of arrhythmia (González et al., 2010). In humans, increased cytosolic calcium ($[Ca^{2+}]_c$) has been related with augmented oxidative stress in atherosclerosis. A growing body of evidence indicates that the production of ROS is tightly linked with Angiotensin II-induced action. In this respect, a causative link between superoxide production and hypertension has been established in experiments in which SOD reduced blood pressure by 50 mm Hg in vascular smooth muscle cells (VSCM) from Angiotensin II-infused rats (Laursen et al., 1997). Much less attention has been paid to other reactions catalyzed by ROS. However, it is known that ATPase activity and inhibition of ATP-independent Ca^{2+} binding are severely depressed in sarcolemmal membranes exposed to hydrogen peroxide and Fe^{2+} (Kukreja et al., 1992, Kaneko et al., 1989). In addition, augmented levels of iron pool in atherosclerotic lesions suggest that iron-catalyzed formation of free radicals may take place in the development of this pathology (Yuan & Li, 2003). High-fat diets stimulate stress response (heat shock protein 70) and signal transduction genes (Ras, MAPK1), inhibiting SOD and GPx gene expression. These effects could be prevented by scavengers of peroxides and antioxidant supplementation of the high-fat diet and caloric restriction (Rosier & Saes, 2006).

5. Mitochondrial dysfunction

Mitochondrial myopathies were described in the early 1960s, when systematic ultrastructural and histochemical studies revealed excessive proliferation of abnormally looking mitochondria in muscle of patients with weakness or exercise intolerance (Shy & Gonatas, 1964). Mitochondrial dysfunction, reflected in the structure, function and number of mitochondria within the cardiomyocyte, leads to diminished energy production, loss of myocyte contractility, altered electrical properties, and eventual cardiomyocyte cell death (Capetanaki, 2002). In addition, cardiotoxic stimuli often lead to excessive production of ROS and to Ca^{2+} overload in the mitochondrial matrix (Ragoni & Condolini, 2009). Evidences for a pathological role of mitochondrial ROS comes from studies in animal models of myocardial infarction, in which increased mitochondrial ROS production was observed, accompanied by decreases in mtDNA copy numbers, in mitochondrial-encoded gene transcripts, and in related enzymatic activities (complexes I, III, and IV), and from studies of genetically modified animals. Overexpression of Prx-3 (a mitochondrial antioxidant protein) improved post-myocardial infarction left ventricular function by restoring mitochondrial activity and DNA copy numbers (Matsushima et al., 2006). Other examples are studies in mice with complete deletion of mitochondrial MnSOD, which developed severe fatal dilated cardiomyopathy (Li et al., 1995). Decreased vascular SOD activities have also been associated with increased susceptibility to ischemia/reperfusion mediated damage; whereas overexpression of mitochondrial antioxidants increased cardiac tolerance to ischemia (Madamanchi, et al., 2005). Recently, the causal role of mitochondrial ROS in Angiotensin II-induced cardiomyopathy was shown by the observation that mice that overexpress catalase targeted to mitochondria, but not mice that overexpress wild-type peroxisomal catalase, are resistant to cardiac hypertrophy, fibrosis and mitochondrial damage induced by angiotensin II (Dai et al., 2011). Monoamine oxidase (MAO) has been shown to play a prominent role in myocardial injury caused by post-ischemic reperfusion (Bianchi et al., 2005a) and to contribute to the maladaptive evolution from myocardial hypertrophy to heart failure (Kaludercic et al., 2010). MAO-mediated ROS production has been related with serotonin-induced myocyte hypertrophy *in vitro* (Bianchi et al., 2005b) and in mitogenic signaling induction by a process that may involve the activation of the metalloproteinase MMP-2, in smooth muscle cells (Coatrieux et al., 2007).

Mitochondria isolated from hearts of rabbits exposed to hypercholesterolemic diet showed significantly reduced respiration rates (state 3 and state 4) (Kojik et al., 2011), whereas increased cholesterol is related with diminution of the mitochondrial membrane potential and mitochondrial pore opening (Chávez et al., 1998; Martínez Abundis et al., 2007) and activation of apoptosis (Martínez-Abundis et al., 2009).

5.1 Metabolic adaptation

Complex mechanisms have evolved to maintain the balance between myocardial O_2 supply and O_2 consumption under pathological stresses such as hypoxia, ischemia, pressure, and volume overload. These mechanisms induce changes in cardiomyocyte structure and/or function through coordinated changes in gene and protein expression and/or the activities of various proteins. Redox mechanisms are involved in the signaling pathways underlying many of these mechanisms, both via the direct effects of O_2 levels in the cardiomyocyte and through the effects of ROS (Santos et al., 2011). Metabolically, the adult mammalian heart normally uses lipids as the major fuel, and mitochondria supply over 90% of the total ATP through β-oxidation of plasma fatty acids (Opie & Sack, 2002). During hypoxia, under ischemia or settings of increased cardiac workload, there is a substantial increase in glycolytic ATP generation, which may be cardioprotective during ischemia/reperfusion by ensuring an adequate ATP supply for membrane and sarcoplasmic reticulum ion pumps (Opie & Sack, 2002; Correa et al., 2008a). Recent studies suggest that a metabolic shift to glycolysis is related with the redox status in the heart. NADPH has been recognized as a critical modulator of the antioxidant defense through the regeneration of reduced pools of glutathione, while G6PDH activity was shown to be of major importance for the maintenance of redox status, Ca^{2+} homeostasis, and contractile function in cardiomyocytes subjected to oxidative stress (Jain et al., 2003) .

5.2 Mitochondrial biogenesis

Mitochondrial biogenesis can be defined as a chain of events that promote growth and division of preexisting organelles. Mitochondrial biogenesis includes the synthesis, import and incorporation of proteins and lipids, as well as the replication of mitochondrial DNA (mtDNA). Replication and transcription of mtDNA are controlled by mtTFA (mitochondrial transcription factor A), and two specific transcription factors TFB1M and TFB2M (mitochondrial transcription factor B1/B2), an RNA polymerase (POLRMT), and a mitochondrial transcription termination factor (mTERF). The coordination between the expression of mitochondrial and nuclear genes is directed by nuclear respiratory factor (NRF-1 and/or NRF-2), the peroxisome proliferator-activated receptors (PPARs), estrogen receptor (ERR), and co-activators of peroxisome proliferator-activated receptor gamma (PGC-1α) (Scarpulla, 2008). PGC-1α is also involved in regulation of fatty acid oxidation (FAO) and in co-activation of ERRα (Figure 4).

Mitochondrial biogenesis decreases in aging, obesity, insulin resistance, dyslipidemia, and hypertension, co-morbidities associated with cardiovascular diseases. Impaired activation of the renin-angiotensin-aldosterone system (RAAS) has been associated with such pathologies (Cooper et al., 2007). In fact, elevated levels of angiotensin II (Ang II) and aldosterone promote alterations in insulin metabolism, endothelial dysfunction, and loss of myocardial function (Kim et al., 2008; Sowers et al., 2009). RAAS increases the activity of NADPH oxidase and stimulates ROS generation resulting in mitochondrial damage, decreased ATP production, diminished NO availability, and attenuated mitochondrial biogenesis. Clinical and experimental observations report the loss of expression of PGC-1α, and mtTFA NRFs in hypertension (Whaley-Connell et al., 2009). In addition, down-regulation of the mitochondrial biogenesis co-activator PGC-1α and its downstream nuclear factors have been associated with myocardial contractile dysfunction, intracellular Ca^{2+} mishandling, ROS accumulation, mitochondrial damage, and loss of mitochondrial density and mtDNA content in high-fat diet–induced obesity (Dong et al., 2007).

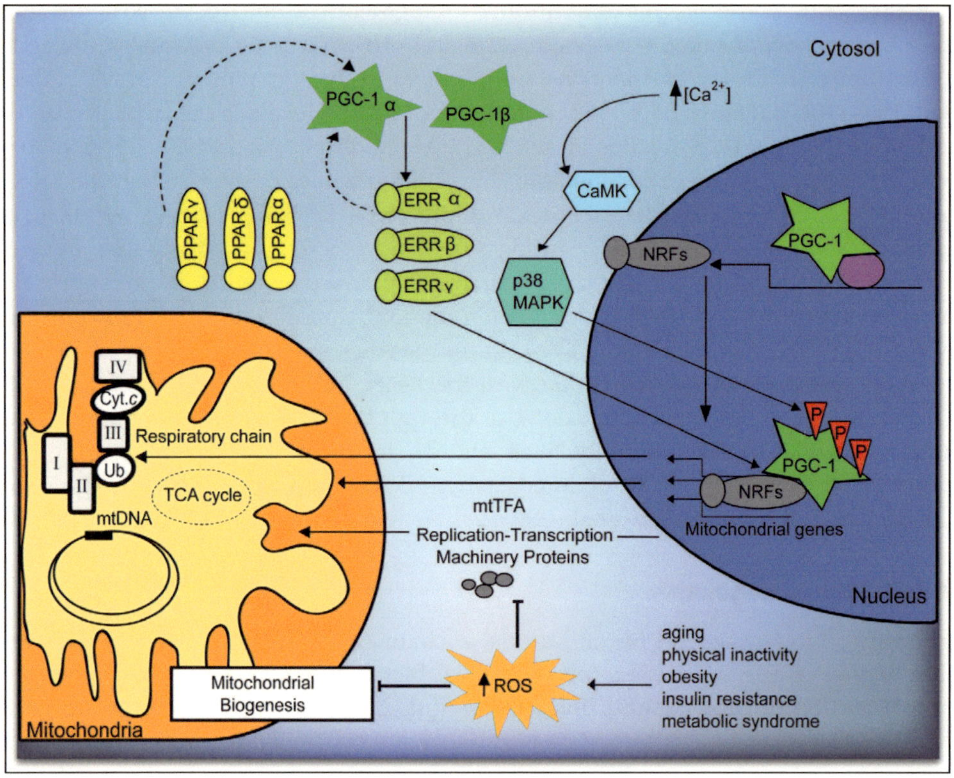

Fig. 4. The transcriptional network that controls mitochondrial biogenesis. See text for further details.

5.3 Mitochondrial ion channels

5.3.1 Permeability transition pore

General membrane damage secondary to ROS-mediated lipid peroxidation is one mechanism by which changes in mitochondrial permeability can occur; however, severe oxidative stress accompanied by calcium overload in the mitochondrial matrix favors the formation of the pathological and non-specific mitochondrial permeability transition pore (mPTP). Opening of the mPTP induces depolarization of the mitochondrial inner membrane (MIM) leading to ATP depletion and further ROS production. The increase in MIM permeability enhances colloidal osmotic pressure in the mitochondrial matrix ultimately leading to matrix swelling and rupture of the mitochondrial outer membrane (MOM). Rupture of the MOM results in release of pro-apoptotic proteins from the mitochondrial intermembrane space to the cytoplasm initiating both caspase-dependent and caspase-independent apoptosis. Permeabilization of the MOM may also occur due to formation of non-selective channels induced by translocation of pro-apoptotic Bcl-2 family proteins to mitochondria. Due to its central role in cell death triggering, the mPTP represents a potential therapeutic target in some cardiovascular diseases. Studies performed over 20 years have demonstrated that acute cardiac ischemia followed by reperfusion damage is associated with mPTP opening (Arteaga et al., 1992; Griffiths & Halestrap, 1993; Chipuk et al., 2006; Lucken-Ardjomande et al., 2008; Halestrap and Pasdois, 2009). Furthermore, pharmacological and conditional inhibition of mPTP formation significantly improved cardiac function reducing ischemic injury and myocardial infarction size in animal models (Argaud et a., 2005; Hausenloy & Yellon, 2003; Correa et al., 2008b) and in patients (Shanmuganathan et al., 2005; Piot et al., 2008). mPTP opening also causes cell death in isolated endothelial and vascular smooth muscle cells. Indeed, atherosclerosis is exacerbated when mitochondrial antioxidant defenses are hampered and a decrease in mitochondrial ROS formation reduces atherogenesis.

Regulation of the mPTP by a variety of signaling molecules and cellular metabolites and ions is a complex process, and mPTP formation ultimately depends on the balance between factors favoring and inhibiting pore opening (Figure 5). The precise metabolic role of mPTP formation

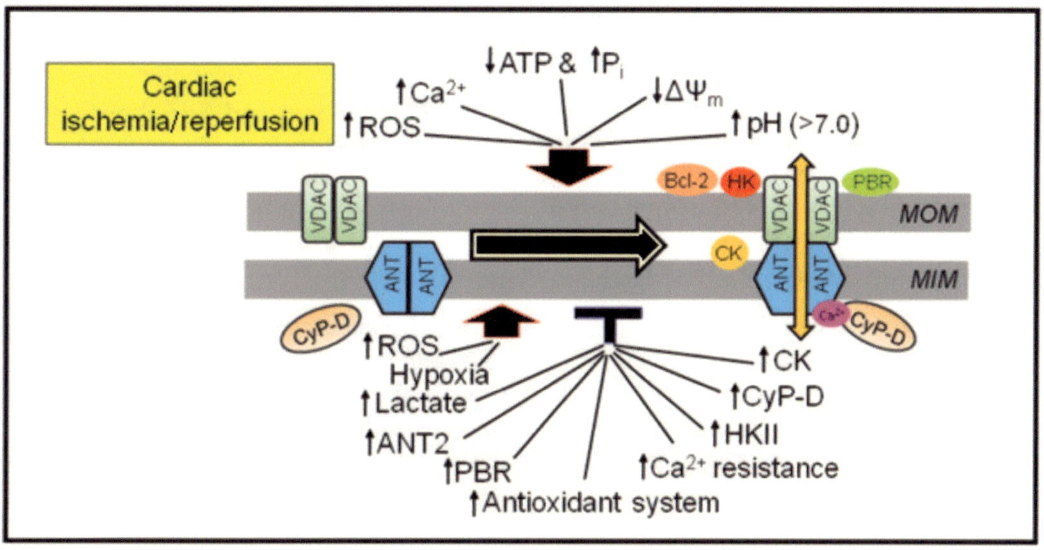

Fig. 5. Metabolic inducers and inhibitors of mPTP opening in cardiac ischemia/reperfusion and tumorigenesis. ANT, adenine nucleotide translocase; CK, creatine kinase; CyP-D, cyclophilin D; HK, hexokinase; MIM, mitochondrial inner membrane; MOM, mitochondrial outer membrane; Pi, inorganic phosphate; PBR, peripheral benzodiazepine receptor; SOD, superoxide dismutase; VDAC, voltage-dependent anion channel.

under physiological conditions is still being debated; reverse pore opening with a low conductance may be attributed to regulation of mitochondrial Ca^{2+}. Low conductive mPT-induced matrix swelling and increased mitochondrial Ca^{2+} can regulate ATP synthesis through the tricarboxylic acid cycle, electron transport chain, and oxidative phosphorylation. Induction of mitochondrial permeability transition (mPT) in response to pathological stresses can also be regulated with the signaling protein kinases: PKA, PKCε (protein kinase Cε) and GSK-3β (glycogen synthase kinase-3), which interact with the voltage-dependent anion channel (VDAC) (Bera et al., 1995; Baines et al, 2003; Javadov et al., 2009).

5.3.2 Structure of the mPTP complex

Although the crucial role of mPTPs in pathological conditions has been intensively studied in the heart, brain, and liver (Chipuk et al., 2006; Bernardi et al., 2006; Robertson et al., 2009), the actual molecular composition of the mPTP complex remains unclear. Until recently, three proteins had been accepted as key structural components of this megachannel: adenine nucleotide translocase (ANT), cyclophilin D (CyP-D), and the voltage-dependent anion channel (VDAC) located in the MIM, in the matrix and in the MOM, respectively. However, recent studies from different groups have questioned the molecular identity of the mPTP. A new model of the mPTP consisting of a phosphate carrier and ANT has been proposed where Ca^{2+} sensitivity of the pore is regulated by CyP-D binding to the phosphate carrier (Leung et al., 2008). Many studies have provided strong evidence that CyP-D plays a major regulatory role in mPTP formation (Baines et al., 2005; Nakagawa et al., 2005). Mitochondria isolated from CyP-D knockout mice were desensitized to the onset of the mPT, and required much higher concentrations of Ca^{2+} to induce pore opening compared to wild type animals, which is consistent with the role of CyP-D to regulate Ca^{2+}-mPTP interactions (Nakagawa et al., 2005). Recent studies on transgenic mice questioned the role of ANT and VDAC as essential components of the mPTP suggesting a regulatory, rather than structural role in pore formation.

5.3.3 mPTP formation in cardiac Ischemia/Reperfusion (I/R)

mPTP opening has been examined extensively in cardiac pathological conditions, mostly in I/R (Chipuk et al., 2006; Correa et al., 2007; Halestrap & Pasdois, 2009). Acute I/R does not affect the expression of mPTP compounds due to its short duration, although it induces conformational changes in essential mPTP proteins, modifying their interactions with the pore effectors in the cytoplasm and mitochondrial matrix. Although many factors that induce pore opening are present during ischemia, including ATP depletion, Ca^{2+} overload, increased phosphate and ROS levels, it has been demonstrated that pore opening occurs during reperfusion rather than during ischemia (Griffiths and Halestrap, 1995). This is explained, in part, by the acidic conditions resulting from lactate and other acidic intermediates accumulation in the mitochondrial matrix. We and others demonstrated that delayed pHi recovery during reperfusion exerts beneficial effects on post-ischemic cardiac function, associated with improved mitochondrial function and inhibition of mPTP opening (Javadov et al., 2008; Correa et al., 2008a). In this regard, inhibition of the Na^{+}/H^{+} exchanger 1(NHE-1) may be a promising therapeutic strategy against I/R damage (Linz & Busch, 2003; Karmazyn et al., 2001). mPTP opening causes mitochondrial uncoupling, thereby ATP is hydrolyzed rather than synthesized in the post-ischemic heart leading to myocardial death (Correa et al., 2005). mPTP opening also increases in Ca^{2+}-induced cardiomyopathy (Nakayama et al., 2007), in diabetic cardiomyopathy (Oliveira et al., 2003), in heart failure following myocardial infarction (Javadov et al., 2005), and in intracoronary microembolization (Sharov et al., 2007).

5.3.4 Mitochondrial K_{ATP} channels

Mitochondrial ATP-sensitive potassium channels (mK^+_{ATP}) were described about 20 years ago in mitoplasts obtained from rat liver mitochondria. First advances in mK^+_{ATP} research demonstrated that different drugs stimulate the opening of mK^+_{ATP} channels decreasing mitochondrial potential ($\Delta\psi_m$) and that mK^+_{ATP} channels are involved in mechanisms regulating cell volume (Garlid, 1988). Latter, it was observed that bradykinin (Yang et al., 2004), opioids (Jang et al., 2008), and adenosine (Kin H, 2005), activate signaling cascades that induce the opening of mK^+_{ATP} and provide cardioprotection against ischemia/reperfusion injury. Recently a causative link between the opening of mK^+_{ATP} and cardioprotection conferred by post-conditioning has been proposed. Garlid et al. (2008) suggested that post-conditioning induces protection via an early redox-sensitive mechanism, followed by persistent mK^+_{ATP} activation. A complex signaling system involving mitochondrial PKCε 1 and 2 may prevent the formation of the mPTP. The putative signaling cascade includes the activation of Gi protein-coupled receptors and cGMP-dependent protein kinase (PKG). At mitochondrial level, this kinase binds to a hypothetic receptor, called "R1" in the mitochondrial outer membrane. This receptor may phosphorylate PKCε 1 (Jaburek et al., 2006), which, in turn, phosphorylates the mK^+_{ATP} channel favoring its opening. Once activated, the entry of K^+ may produce alkalinization of the mitochondrial matrix and promote ROS production by Complex I. ROS could activate the mitochondrial matrix PKCε 2, and prevent the formation of mPTP, reducing cell death and infarction size (Costa et al., Garlid et al., 2009) (Figure 6).

Other proposals have been invoked to explain cardioprotection. One hypothesis is that K^+ flow into the matrix may depolarize the inner membrane and reduce the driving force that sustains Ca^{2+} overload (Holmuhamedov et al., 1991; Murata et al., 2001). However, although Ca^{2+} reduction in the mitochondrial matrix may reduce mPTP opening in the post-ischemic heart, it is difficult to explain how a small depolarizing effect generated by activation of mK^+_{ATP} channels could avoid Ca^{2+}-overload. Another assumption is that discrete mitochondrial swelling associated with K^+ flow would change the architecture and respiratory control of mitochondria, creating a state of mitochondrial "super-efficiency" (Garlid, 2000). Whatever the mechanism involved in mK^+_{ATP} opening, its association with myocardial protection is clear.

6. Programmed cell death and autophagy

ROS/RNS can cause cell death by non-physiological (necrotic) or regulated pathways (apoptotic) in many cardiovascular diseases such as atherosclerosis, ischemic heart disease, heart failure, stroke, hypertension, and diabetes. The mechanisms by which ROS/RNS cause or regulate apoptosis typically are caspase-dependent and include the activation of membrane receptors, Bcl-2 family proteins, and mitochondrial dysfunction. Autophagy, a caspase-independent mechanism of cell death that protects cells against oxidative damage and is involved in the degradation and recycling of oxidized proteins and damaged organelles in cells, yields amino acids for *de novo* protein synthesis or energy provision (Nishida et al., 2009). While programmed cell death participation in cardiovascular diseases is well established, insights into caspase-independent mechanisms of cell death have emerged recently.

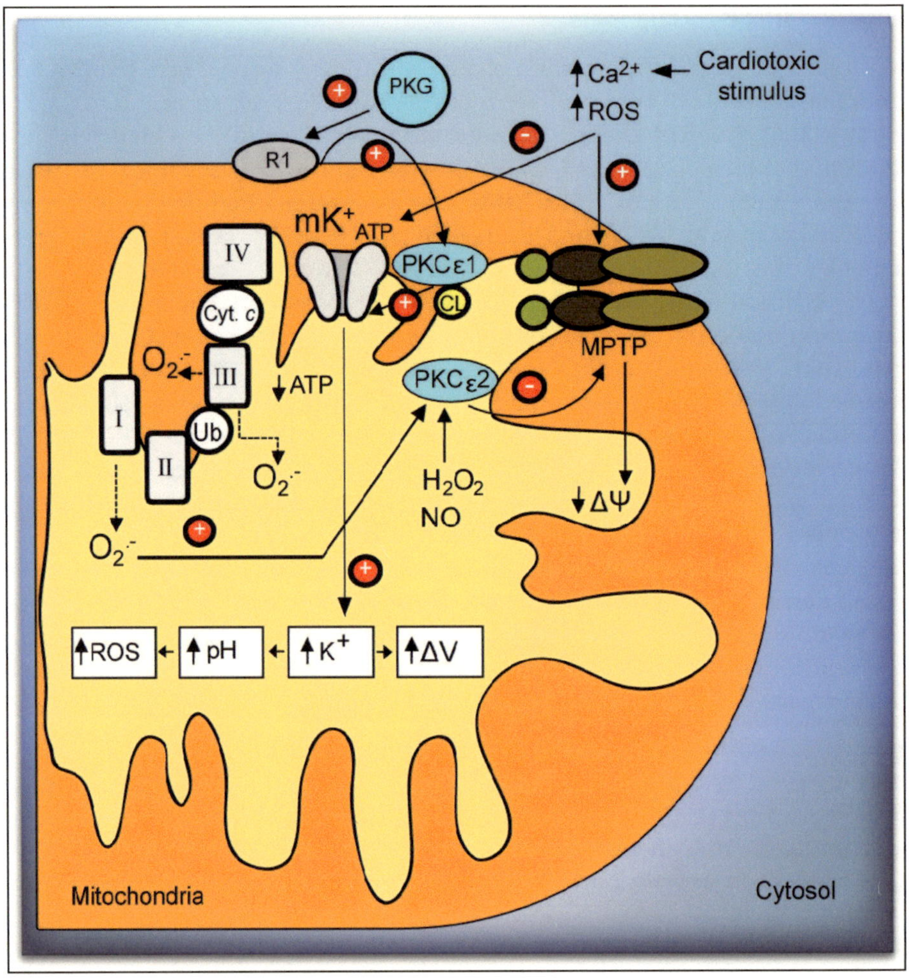

Fig. 6. Intramitochondrial signaling pathways. The pathways leading to mK^{+}_{ATP} opening, ROS production, and MPT inhibition are shown.

6.1 Apoptotic mitochondrial pathway

Mitochondria contain diverse pro-apoptotic factors within their intermembrane space, such as cytochrome *c*, apoptosis-inducer factor, and Smac / Diablo, which are released and propagate the death cascade. Two different pores have been described as pathways for cytochrome *c* release (reviewed in Kinally & Antonsson, 2007). The first one is the mitochondrial apoptosis-induced channel (MAC) formed by Bax and VDAC proteins (Shimizu et al., 2000). There are also reports indicating that only Bax-forming channels could account for cytochrome *c* release (Kuwana et al., 2002). In this sense, the contribution of Bax channels to cytochrome *c* release after reperfusion has been explored by Bombrun et al., 2003. A second possible pathway described for cytochrome *c* release is the mPTP. These proteins could be assembled into a continued unspecific channel, promoting mitochondrial swelling, MOM rupture, and pro-apoptotic proteins release (Figure 7).

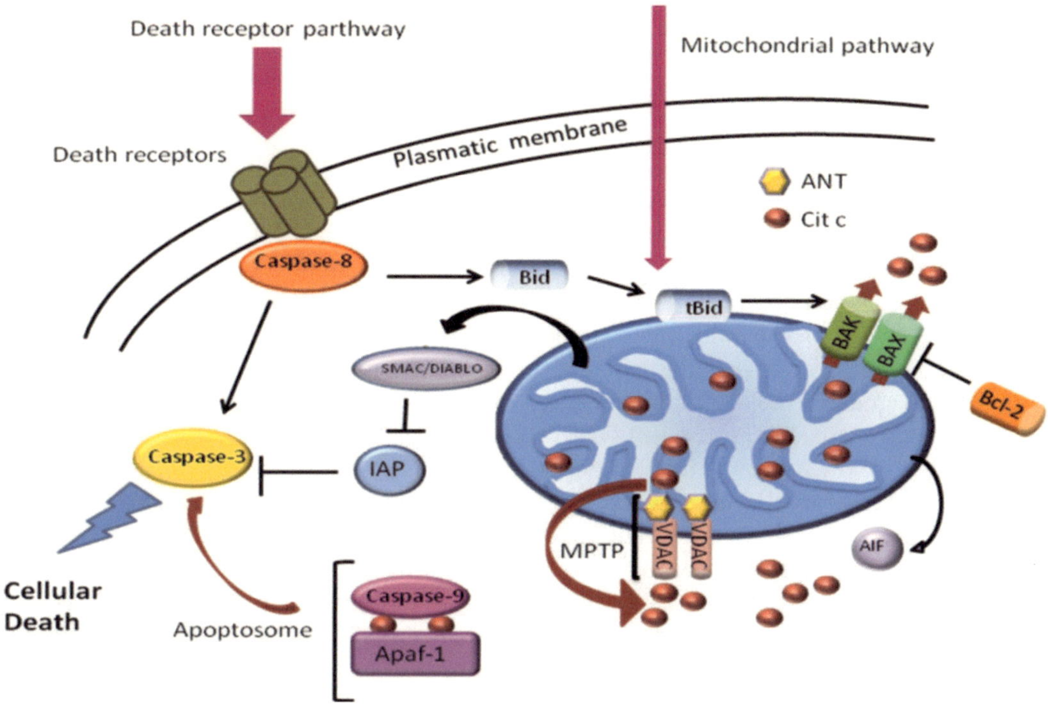

Fig. 7. Simplified model of cellular apoptotic pathways. Specific ligands bind to death receptors, activating initiator and executioner caspases. In the mitochondrial pathway, several stimuli are processed favoring membrane permeabilization and the release of pro-apoptogenic factors as cytochrome *c*, AIF, and Smac/DIABLO to the cytosol, through membrane pore forming proteins, such as BAK/BAX or as a consequence of the mPTP opening. Once in the cytosol, cytochrome c and APAF-1 bind to caspase-9, activating caspase-3. The extrinsic pathway could activate the mitochondrial pathway, through the Bcl-2 family member (Bid) that promotes BAX and BAK oligomerization.

Overexpression of antioxidant proteins in several models sustains the relevance of oxidative stress in cardiomyocyte apoptosis. Catalase, glutathione peroxidase 1, metalothionein, mitochondrial glutaredoxin-2, and peroxiredoxin 2 over- expression reduce apoptosis and improve contractile dysfunction after ischemia/reperfusion injury (Shiomi et al., 2004; Nagy et al., 2008; Zhao et al., 2009). As indicated, oxidative stress may activate the intrinsic apoptotic pathway in cardiomyocytes through multiple mechanisms, such as the induction of mPTP opening, DNA damage-induced, translocation of Bax and Bad to the mitochondria, and caspase activation. However, an alternative mode of oxidative stress-induced activation of the intrinsic apoptotic pathway may also involve induction of the ER stress response, leading to caspase-12 activation and/or Ca^{2+}-dependent opening of the mPTP (Foo et al., 2005). Catecholamines, angiotensin II, prostaglandin $F_{2\alpha}$, or endothelin-1, which interact with G-protein coupled receptors and induce cardiomyocyte hypertrophy, may also induce apoptosis. A well characterized mechanism is a $G_{\alpha q}$-mediated PKC-dependent transcriptional upregulation of the Bcl-2 family member Nix, which activates the mitochondrial death pathway (Yussman et al., 2002)

6.2 Autophagy

Autophagy is a physiological process that is necessary for cell survival and maintains stable levels of nutrients to sustain cellular homeostasis. It is also involved in various pathophysiological processes, and shows increased activity in response to extracellular and intracellular stimulation such as nutrient starvation and hypoxia. During autophagy, cytoplasmic constituents are sequestered into the autophagosome, a closed double membrane vacuole that eventually fuses with a lysosome. In the new structure, named autolysosome, the contents are degraded and recycled for protein synthesis (Cuervo, 2004). ROS act as signaling molecules in the early events of autophagy induction. If the pro-survival attempt fails, ROS cause cell death which, depending on the experimental context, involves either the autophagic or the apoptotic pathway. Mitochondria are both the major source of intracellular ROS and, at the same time, targets of ROS. An enhanced oxidative stress may activate a signaling cascade involving the PKCβ-dependent phosphorylation of p66 protein and its translocation to the mitochondrial matrix. Damaged mitochondria are degraded by a specialized form of autophagy, called mitophagy, in which mitochondrial calcium plays an active role. Normally calcium homeostasis is tightly regulated and occurs at ER-mitochondria contacts where microdomains of high calcium concentration are present. This event causes a variety of responses depending on the amount of Ca^{2+} increase, from stimulation of metabolism and ATP production to ROS production, mPTP opening, and apoptosis (Figure 8). In this respect, recent data have proposed a role of p66Shc in mediating the response of mitochondria to ROS-induced apoptosis or autophagy (Mammucari & Rizzuto, 2010).

Autophagy increases in response to acute myocardial ischemia (AMI), chronic myocardial ischemia, heart failure, and cardiomyopathy degeneration (Cuervo, 2004). The effect of autophagy upregulation is under debate, as some studies have demonstrated that it leads to myocyte death after ischemia/reperfusion (Valentim et al., 2006), but others indicate that autophagy has a cardioprotective effect during myocardial ischemia. Three mechanisms are invoked to explain protection: 1) generation of free amino acids and fatty acids that contributes to maintain the mitochondrial energy supply, improving cell survival (Matsui et al., 2007), 2) elimination of disordered structural proteins, harmful to cardiac myocytes, and 3) removal of damaged mitochondria. In human myocardial depression associated to endotoxemia, Hickson-Bick et al. (2008) described that mitochondrial biogenesis observed in cardiomyocytes may reflect an effort to replace the mitochondria eliminated by autophagy. In HL-1 cells subjected to oxidative stress, the induction of autophagy by rapamycin suppressed ROS production and protected cells against death (Yuan et al., 2009). These results are consistent with the notion that autophagy is a protective mechanism in this setting and limits the production of harmful ROS, either by removing damaged mitochondria or by supporting *de novo* glutathione biosynthesis through the delivery of amino acids.

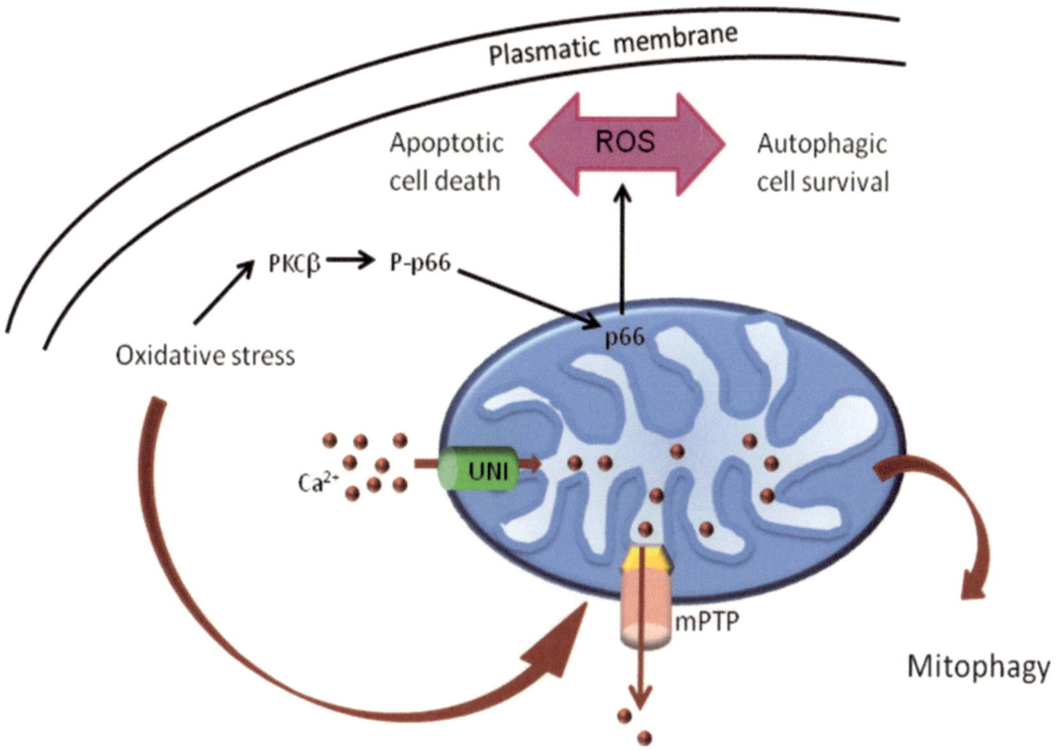

Fig. 8. Signaling pathways, regulating mitochondrial function. ROS production is induced by oxidative stress, which activates a signaling cascade involving the PKCβ-dependent phosphorylation of p66 its translocation to the mitochondrial matrix. Mitochondria are also targets of ROS damage. Damaged mitochondria are removed by mitophagy, a specialized form of autophagy, which is regulated by different pathways.

7. Mitochondrial fission and fusion

Mitochondria are highly dynamic organelles that undergo constantly fusion and fission as part of their normal function (Detmer & Chan, 2007). These two opposite processes are accurately coordinated and necessary for proper morphology and function and are thought to play critical roles during development, cell division, and apoptosis (Cerveny et al., 2007; Chan, 2006). Disruption of mitochondrial fission and fusion has been linked to the development and progression of some diseases.

Mitochondrial fusion facilitates the exchange of materials between mitochondria for the maintenance of functional mitochondria, whereas mitochondrial fission contributes to the elimination of damaged mitochondrial fragments through mitophagy and contributes to the proper distribution of mitochondria in response to the local demand for ATP. Multiple proteins have been identified to mediate mitochondrial fission and fusion processes (Chan, 2006). These two opposing processes are regulated by the mitochondrial fusion proteins, mitofusin 1 (Mfn1) and mitofusin 2 (Mfn2, Fzo1 in yeast) (Eura et al., 2003), and optic atrophy protein 1 (Opa1, Mgm1 in yeast) (Cipolat et al., 2004), and the mitochondrial fission proteins dynamin-related protein 1 (Drp1, Dnm1 in yeast) (Frank et al., 2001; Smirnova et al., 2001; Ingerman et al., 2005), and human mitochondrial fission protein 1 (hFis1) (Yoon et al., 2003). The balance between mitochondrial fusion and fission within a cell can be disrupted by a myriad of factors, including oxidative stress (Frank et al., 2001) and simulated ischemia (Brady et al., 2006), and has also been linked to aging (Kowald & Kirkwood, 2011) (Figure 9).

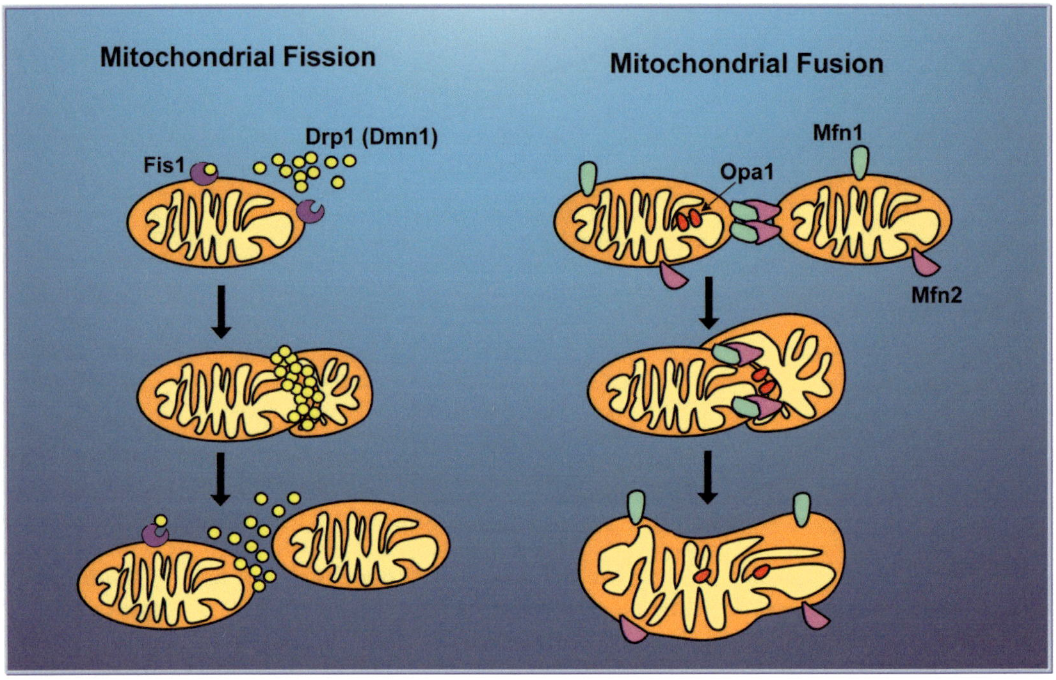

Fig. 9. Mitochondrial fission and fusion. Mitochondrial fission involves the action of Drp1, which can self-assemble into polymeric spirals and is recruited into the mitochondrial membrane by hFis1 and Mdv1/Caf4. Drp1 polymers wrap around the mitochondrion and constrict the membrane until fission occurs. Mitochondrial fusion involves the interaction of Mfn1 and Mfn2 proteins located in the outer mitochondrial membrane of two mitochondria until outer membranes fuse, consequently, inner mitochondrial membrane fusion occurs through interaction of Opa1 proteins. See text for further details.

7.1 Mitochondrial fusion

Data on fission and fusion proteins' role in heart diseases are scarce. Recently it has been reported that cardiac myocyte mitochondria, lacking the fusion protein Mfn2, are pleiomorphic and show enlarged morphopology. Consistent with an underlying mild mitochondrial dysfunction, Mfn2-deficient mice display modest cardiac hypertrophy accompanied by slight functional deterioration (Papanicolau et al., 2011). Expression of OPA1 is decreased in both human and rat failing hearts, which show small and fragmented mitochondria indicative of decreased fusion. OPA1 mRNA levels did not differ between failing and normal hearts, suggesting post-transcriptional control, possibly through degradation by proteases activated by ATP (Baricault et al., 2007).

7.2 Mitochondrial fission

It has been suggested that defects in mitochondrial fusion and fission processes are responsible for abnormal mitochondrial morphologies observed in many cardiac diseases. In cultured neonatal ventricular myocytes, inhibition of mitochondrial fission, by over-expressing a dominant-negative mutant form of Drp1, prevents ROS production, mitochondrial permeability transition pore opening, and subsequent cell death after ceramide treatment (Parra et al., 2008). An increase in the level of cytosolic Ca^{2+} induced by thapsigargin (Tg) causes cardiac mitochondrial fission associated to ROS generation in a Drp1-dependent pathway (Hom et al., 2010). Because calcium overload is a common feature in heart failure (HF), this may increase mitochondrial fission and dysfunction, thus further contributing to the decrease in the metabolic demand of the heart and increasing its injury.

8. Conclusion

Mitochondrial redox signaling is paramount to the maintenance of cardiomyocyte homeostasis. Therefore, oxidative deregulation of mitochondrial key players, like mK^{+}_{ATP}, mPTP, ionic transporters, metabolism enzymes, and apoptotic machinery, has enormous impact on cardiovascular function. Intense research is devoted to obtain a better understanding of the complex regulatory mechanisms ruling these systems and to enable the development of more specific therapeutic strategies for heart diseases. In addition, fascinating links are beginning to be discovered between mitochondrial function and cardiac physiology and diseases in the context of diverse signaling mechanisms. Besides, proteins with previously known function, like those driving mitochondrial fusion and fission, are now reported to have emergent functions in intracellular calcium homeostasis, apoptosis, and vascular smooth muscle cell proliferation, all, key issues in cardiac disease. These processes broaden the traditional role in energy production undertaken by mitochondria and provide new directions for research in cardiovascular diseases.

9. Acknowledgment

This work was partially supported by grant 80791-M to C. Zazueta

10. References

Alvarez, S.; Valdez, L.; Zaobornyj, T. & Boveris A (2003). Oxygen dependence of mitochondrial nitric oxide synthase activity. *Biochemical and Biophysical Research Community*. Vol. 305, 771–775.

Antunes, F.; Salvador, A. & Pinto, R. (1995). PHGPx and phospholipase A2/GPx: comparative importance on the reduction of hydroperoxides in rat liver mitochondria. *Free Radical Biology & Medicine*. Vol. 19, 669-77.

Argaud, L.; Gateau-Roesch, O.; Muntean, D.; Chalabreysse, L.; Loufouat, J.; Robert, D. & Ovize, M. (2005). Specific inhibition of the mitochondrial permeability transition prevents lethal reperfusion injury. *Journal of Molecular Cell Cardiology*. Vol. 38, 367-374.

Arteaga, D.; Odor, O.; Lopez, R.; Contreras, G.; Aranda, A. & Chávez, E. (1992) Impairment by cyclosporine A of reperfusion-induced arrhythmias. *Life Sciences*, 1127-1134.

Arnér, E. & Holmgren, A. (2000). Physiological functions of thioredoxin and thioredoxin reductase. *European Journal of Biochemistry. Vol.* 267, 6102-9.

Baines, C.; Kaiser, R.; Purcell, N.; Blair, N.; Osinska, H.; Hambleton, M.; Brunskill, E.; Sayen, M.; Gottlieb, R.; Dorn, G.; Robbins, J. & Molkentin, J. (2005). Loss of cyclophilin D reveals a critical role for mitochondrial permeability transition in cell death. *Nature.* Vol. 434, 658-662.

Baines, C.; Song, C.; Zheng, Y.; Wang, G.; Zhang, J.; Wang, O.; Guo, Y.; Bolli, R.; Cardwell, E. & Ping, P. (2003). Protein kinase Cepsilon interacts with and inhibits the permeability transition pore in cardiac mitochondria. *Circulation Research.* Vol. 92, 873- 880.

Baricault, L.; Ségui, B.; Guégand, L.; Olichon, A.; Valette, A.; Larminat, F. & Lenaers, G. (2007). OPA1 cleavage depends on decreased mitochondrial ATP level and bivalent metals. *Experimental Cell Research.* Vol. 313, 3800-8.

Barja, G. (1999). Mitochondrial oxygen radical generation and leak: sites of production in states 4 and 3, organ specificity and relation to aging and longevity. *Journal of Bioenergetics and Biomembranes.* Vol. 31, 347–366.

Barreiro, E.; Garcia-Martinez, C.; Mas, S.; Ametller, E.; Gea, J.; Argiles, J.; Busquets, S. & Lopez-Soriano, F. J. (2009). UCP3 overexpression neutralizes oxidative stress rather than nitrosative stress in mouse myotubes. *FEBS Letters.* Vol. 583, 350–356.

Bera, A.; Ghosh, S. & Das, S. (1995). Mitochondrial VDAC can be phosphorylated by cyclic AMP-dependent protein kinase. *Biochemical & Biophysical Research Community.* Vol. 209, 213-217.

Bernardi, P.; Krauskopf, A.; Basso, E.; Petronilli, V.; Blachly-Dyson, E.; Di Lisa, F. & Forte, M. (2006). The mitochondrial permeability transition from in vitro artifact to disease target. *FEBS Journal.* Vol. 273, 2077- 2099.

Betarbet R, Sherer TB & Greenamyre JT (2002). Animal models of Parkinson's disease. *Bioessays* 24, 308–318.

Bianchi, P.; Kunduzova, O.; Masini, E.; Cambon, C.; Bani, D.; Raimondi, L.; Seguelas, M.; Nistri, S.; Colucci, W.; Leducq, N. & Parini, A. (2005a). Oxidative stress by monoamine oxidase mediates receptor-independent cardiomyocyte apoptosis by serotonin and postischemic myocardial injury. *Circulation.* Vol. 112, 3297–3305.

Bianchi, P.; Pimentel, D.; Murphy, M.; Colucci, W. & Parini, A. (2005b). A new hypertrophic mechanism of serotonin in cardiac myocytes: receptor-independent ROS generation. *FASEB Journal.* Vol. 19, 641–643

Bombrun, A.; Gerber, P.; Casi, G.; Terradillos, O.; Antonsson, B. & Halazy, S. (2003). 3,6-Dibromocarbazole piperazine derivates of 2-propanol as first inhibitors of cytochrome c release *via* Bax channels modulation. *Journal of Medical Chemistry.* Vol. 46, 4365-68

Brady, N.; Hamacher-Brady, A.;Westerhoff, H. & Gottlieb, R. (2006). A wave of reactive oxygen species (ROS)-induced ROS release in a sea of excitable mitochondria. *Antioxidants & Redox Signal.* Vol. 8, 1651–1665.

Brigelius-Floé, R. (2006). Glutathione peroxidases and redox-regulated transcription factors. *Biological Chemistry.* Vol. 387, 1329-35.

Brookes, P.; Yoon, Y.; Robotham, J.; Anders, M. & Sheu, S. (2004). Calcium, ATP and ROS: a mitocondrial love-hate triangle. *American Journal of Physiology & Cell Physiology.* Vol. 287, C817-C833.

Cadenas, E. & Davies, K. (2000). Mitochondrial free radical generation oxidative stress and aging. *Free Radical Biological Medicine,* Vol. 29, 222–230.

Cai, J. & Jones, D. (1988). Superoxide in apoptosis. Mitochondrial generation triggered by cytochrome c loss. *Journal of Biological Chemistry Vol.* 273, 11401-4.

Camara, A.; Bienengraeber, M. & Stowe, D. (2011). Mitochondrial approaches to protect against cardiac ischemia and reperfusion injury. *Frontiers in Physiology.* Vol. 12, 2-13.

Capetanaki, Y. (2002). Desmin cytoskeleton: a potential regulator of muscle mitochondrial behavior and function. *Trends in Cardiovascular Medicine.* Vol. 12, 339-348.

Cerveny, K.; Tamura, Y.; Zhang, Z.; Jensen, R. & Sesaki, H. (2007). Regulation of mitochondrial fusion and division. *Trends in Cellular Biology.* Vol. 17, 563-9.

Chan, D. (2006). Mitochondrial fusion and fission in mammals. *Annual Reviews Cellular & Development Biology.* Vol. 22, 79–99.

Chipuk, J.; Bouchier-Hayes, L. & Green, D. (2006). Mitochondrial outer membrane permeabilization during apoptosis: the innocent bystander scenario. *Cell Death & Differentiation.* Vol. 13, 1396-1402.

Cipolat, S.; Martins de Brito, O.; Dal Zilio, B. & Scorrano, L. (2004). OPA1 requires mitofusin 1 to promote mitochondrial fusion. *Proceedings of the National Academic of Sciences U S A.* Vol. 101, 15927–15932.

Coatrieux, C.; Sanson, M.; Negre-Salvayre, A.; Parini, A.; Hannun, Y.; Itohara, S.; Salvayre, R. & Auge, N. (2007). MAO-A induced mitogenic signaling is mediated by reactive oxygen species, MMP-2, and the sphingolipid pathway. Free Radical Biology & Medicine. Vol. 43, 80–89

Coll, O.; Colell, A.; García-Ruiz, C.; Kaplowitz, N. & Fernández-Checa, J. (2003). Sensitivity of the 2-oxoglutarate carrier to alcohol intake contributes to mitochondrial glutathione depletion. *Hepatology.* Vol. 38, 692-702.

Conrad, M.; Jakupoglu, C.; Moreno, S.; Lippl, S.; Banjac, A.; Schneider, M.; Beck, H.; Hatzopoulos, A.; Just, U.; Sinowatz, F.; Schmahl, W.; Chien, K.; Wurst, W.; Bornkamm, G. & Brielmeier, M. (2004). Essential role for mitochondrial thioredoxin reductase in hematopoiesis, heart development and heart function. *Molecular & Cell Biology.* Vol. 21, 9414-23.

Cooper, S.; Whaley-Connell, A. & Habibi, J. (2007). Renin-angiotensin-aldosterone system and oxidative stress in cardiovascular insulin resistance. *American Journal of Physiology & Heart Circulation Physiology.* Vol. 293, H2009-H2023.

Correa F.; García, N.; Robles, C.; Martínez-Abundis, E. & Zazueta, C. (2008b). Relationship between oxidative stress and mitochondrial function in the post-conditioned heart. *Journal of Bioenergetics & Biomembranes.* Vol. 40, 599-606.

Correa, F.; García, N.; Gallardo, J.; Carreño, L.; Rodríguez-Enríquez, S.; Marín, A. & Zazueta, C. (2008a). Post-conditioning preserves glycolytic ATP during early reperfusion: A survival mechanism for the reperfused heart. *Cellular Physiology & Biochemistry.* Vol. 22, 635-644.

Correa, F.; Soto, V. & Zazueta , C. (2007). Mitochondrial permeability transition relevance for apoptotic triggering in the post-ischemic heart. *International Journal of Biochemistry & Cell Biology.* Vol. 39, 787-798.

Costa, A. & Garlid, K. (2008). Intramitochondrial signaling: interactions among mitoKATP, PKCε , ROS, and MPT. American Journal of Physiology. Vol. 295, H874–82.

Cuervo A. (2004). Autophagy in sickness and in health. *Trends in Cell Biology.* Vol. 14, 70-77.

Chávez, E.; Franco, M.; Reyes-Vivas, H.; Zazueta, C.;Ramírez, J. & Carrillo, R. (1998) Hypothyroidism renders liver mitochondria to the opening of membrane permeability transition pore. *Biochimica and Biophysica Acta*. Vol. 1407, 243-248.

Dai, D.F.; Johnson, S.C.; Villarin, J.J.; Chin, M.T.; Nieves-Cintrón, M.; Chen, T.; Marcinek, D.J.; Dorn, G.W. 2nd, Kang, Y.J.; Prolla, T.A.; Santana, L.F. & Rabinovitch, P.S. (2011). Mitochondrial oxidative stress mediates angiotensin II-induced cardiac hypertrophy and Galphaq overexpression-induced heart failure. *Circulation Research*. Vol. 108, 837-46.

Detmer, S. & Chan, D. (2007). Functions and dysfunctions of mitochondrial dynamics. *Nature Reviews Molecular Cell Biology*. Vol. 8, 870–879.

Di Lisa, F.; Kaludercic, N.; Carpi, A.; Menabò, R. & Giorgio, M. (2009). Mitochondria and vascular pathology. *Pharmacology Reports*. Vol. 61, 123-30.

Dong, F.; Li, Q.; Sreejayan, N.; Nunn, J. & Ren, J. (2007). Metallothionein prevents high-fat diet induced cardiac contractile dysfunction: role of peroxisome proliferator activated receptor gamma coactivator 1-alpha and mitochondrial biogenesis. *Diabetes*. Vol. 56, 2201-12.

Dworakowski, R.; Alom-Ruiz, S. & Shah, A. (2008). NADPH oxidase-derived reactive oxygen species in the regulation of endothelial phenotype. *Pharmacology Reports*. Vol. 60, 21–28

Ernster, L. & Forsmark-Andrée, P. (1993). Ubiquinol: an endogenous antioxidant in aerobic organisms. *Clinical Investigations*. Vol. 71, S60-5.

Escames, G.; López, A.; García, J.; García, L.; Acuña-Castroviejo, D.; García, J. & López, L. (2010). The role of mitochondria in brain aging and the effects of melatonin. *Current Neuropharmacology*, Vol. 8, 182–193.

Eura Y, et al. (2003). Two mitofusin proteins, mammalian homologues of FZO, with distinct functions are both required for mitochondrial fusion. *Journal of Biochemistry*. Vol. 134, 333–344.

Foo, R.; Mani, K. & Kitsis, R. (2005). Death begets failure in the heart . *Journal of Clinical Investigation*. Vol. 115, 565-71.

Frank, S.; Gaume, B.; Bergmann-Leitner, E.; Leitner, W.; Robert, E.; Catez, F.; Smith, C.; & Youle, R. (2001). The role of dynamin-related protein 1, a mediator of mitochondrial fission, in apoptosis. *Developmental Cell*. Vol. 1, 515-25.

Garlid, K. (1988). Mitochondrial volume control. In: *Integration of Mitochondrial Function*. New York: Plenum, p.p. 257–276.

Garlid, K. (2000). Opening mitochondrial K(ATP) in the heart—what happens, and what does not happen. *Basic Research in Cardiology*. Vol. 95, 275–79.

Gavazza, M. & Catalá, A. (2009) Relative efficacies of alpha-tocopherol, N-acetyl-serotonin, and melatonin in reducing non-enzymatic lipid peroxidation of rat testicular microsomes and mitochondria. *Molecular & Cellular Biochemistry*. Vol. 321, 37-43.

Gonzalez, D.; Treuer, A.; Castellanos, J.; Dulce, R. & Hare, J. (2010). Impaired S-nitrosylation of the ryanodine receptor caused by xanthine oxidase activity contributes to calcium leak in heart failure. *Journal of Biological Chemistry. Vol.* 285, 28938–28945.

Griffith, O. & Meister, A. (1979). Potent and specific inhibition of glutathione synthesis by buthionine sulfoximine (S-n-butyl homocysteine sulfoximine). *Journal of Biological Chemistry* 254, 7558-7560.

Griffiths, E. & Halestrap. A. (1993) Protection by Cyclosporin A of ischemia/reperfusion-induced damage in isolated rat hearts. *J Mol Cell Cardiol.* 25, 1461-9.

Griffiths, E. & Halestrap, A. (1995). Mitochondrial non-specific pores remain closed during cardiac ischaemia, but open upon reperfusion. *Biochemical Journal.* Vol. 307,93-98.

Hackenbrock, C.; Chazotte, B. & Gupte S. (1986). The random collision model and a critical assessment of diffusion and collision in mitochondrial electron transport. *Journal of Bioenergetics & Biomembranes.* Vol. 18, 331-68.

Haines, B.; Mehta, S.; Pratt, S.; Warden, C.; & Li, P. (2010). Deletion of mitochondrial uncoupling protein-2 increases ischemic brain damage after transient focal ischemia by altering gene expression patterns and enhancing inflammatory cytokines. *Journal of Cerebral Blood Flow Metabolism.* Vol. 30, 1825–1833.

Halestrap, A. & Pasdois, P. (2009). The role of the mitochondrial permeability transition pore in heart disease. *Biochimical & Biophysical Acta.* Vol. 1787,1402-1415.

Halestrap, A.P.; Connern, C.P.; Griffiths, E.J. & Kerr, P.M. (1997). Cyclosporin A binding to mitochondrial cyclophilin inhibits the permeability transition pore and protects heart from ischemia. *Molecular & Cellular Biochemistry.* Vol. 174, 167-72.

Han, D.; Antunes, F.; Canali, R.; Rettori, D. & Cadenas, E. (2003). Voltage-dependent anion channels control the release of the superoxide anion from mitochondria to cytosol. *Journal of Biological Chemistry.* Vol. 278, 5557-63.

Hardeland, R. & Coto-Montes, A. (2010). New vistas on oxidative damage and aging. *The Open Biology Journal.* Vol. 3, 39–52.

Hausenloy, D. & Yellon, D. (2003). The mitochondrial permeability transition pore: its fundamental role in mediating cell death during ischaemia and reperfusion. *Journal of Molecular Cell Cardiology.* Vol. 35, 339-341.

Hickson-Bick, D.; Jones, C. & Buja, L. (2008). Stimulation of mitochondrial biogenesis and autophagy by lipopolysaccharide in the neonatal rat cardiomyocyte protects against programmed cell death. *Journal of Molecular & Cell Cardiology.* Vol. 44, 411–418.

Holley, A.; Dhar, S.; Xu, Y. & St Clair, D. (2010). Manganese superoxide dismutase: beyond life and death. *Amino Acids.* Ë-pub ahead of print.

Holmuhamedov, E.; Wang, L. & Terzic, A. (1999). ATP-sensitive K^+ channel openers prevent Ca^{2+} overload in rat cardiac mitochondria. *Journal of Physiology.* Vol. 519, 347–60.

Hom, J.; Yu, T.; Yoon, Y.; Porter, G. & Sheu, S. (2010). Regulation of mitochondrial fission by intracellular Ca(2+) in rat ventricular myocytes. *Biochimical & Biophysical Acta.* Vol. 1797, 913-21.

Ingerman, E.; Perkins, E.; Marino, M.; Mears, J.; McCaffery, J.; Hinshaw, J.; & Nunnari, J. (2005). Dnm1 forms spirals that are structurally tailored to fit mitochondria. *Journal of Cell Biology.* Vol. 170, 1021-1027.

Jaburek, M.; Costa, A.; Burton, J.; Costa, C. & Garlid, K. (2006). Mitochondrial PKCepsilon and mitoKATP co-purify and co-reconstitute to form a functioning signaling module in proteoliposomes. *Circulation Research.* Vol. 99, 878–83.

Jain, M.; Brenner, D.; Cui, L.; Lim, C.; Wang, B.; Pimentel, D.; Koh, S.; Sawyer, D.; Leopold, J.; Handy, D.; Loscalzo, J.; Apstein, C.; & Liao, R. (2003). Glucose-6-phosphate dehydrogenase modulates cytosolic redox status and contractile phenotype in adult cardiomyocytes. *Circulation Research.* Vol. 93, e9–e16.

James, A.; Smith, R. & Murphy, M. (2004). Antioxidant and prooxidant properties of mitochondrial Coenzyme Q. *Archives of Biochemistry & Biophysics.* Vol. 423, 47-56.

Jang, Y.; Xi, J.; Wang, H.; Mueller, R.A.; Norfleet, E.A & Xu, Z. (2008). Postconditioning prevents reperfusion injury by activating delta-opioid receptors. *Anesthesiology.* Vol. 108, 243-250.

Javadov, S.; Choi, A.; Rajapurohitam, V.; Zeidan, A.; Basnakian, A. & Karmazyn, M. (2008). NHE-1 inhibition-induced cardioprotection against ischaemia/reperfusion is associated with attenuation of the mitochondrial permeability transition. *Cardiovascular Research.* Vol. 77, 416-424.

Javadov, S.; Huang, C.; Kirshenbaum, L. & Karmazyn, M. (2005). NHE-1 inhibition improves impaired mitochondrial permeability transition and respiratory function during postinfarction remodelling in the rat. *Journal of Molecular & Cell Cardiology.* Vol. 38,135-143.

Javadov, S.; Rajapurohitam, V.; Kilic, A.; Zeidan, A.; Choi, A. & Karmazyn, M. (2009) Antihypertrophic effect of NHE-1 inhibition involves GSK-3beta-dependent attenuation of mitochondrial dysfunction. *Journal of Molecular & Cell Cardiology.* Vol. 46, 998-1007.

Jezek, P. & Hlavatá, L. (2005) Mitochondria in homeostasis of reactive oxygen species in cell, tissues, and organism. *International Journal of Biochemistry and Cell Biology.* Vol. 37, 2478-503.

Johansson, C.; Lillig, C. & Holmgren, A. (2004). Human mitochondrial glutaredoxin reduces S-glutathionylated proteins with high affinity accepting electrons from either glutathione or thioredoxin reductase. *Journal of Biological Chemistry.* Vol. 279, 7537-43.

Kaludercic, N.; Takimoto, E.; Nagayama, T.; Feng, N.; Lai, E.; Bedja, D.; Chen, K.; Gabrielson, K.; Blakely, R.; Shih, J.; Pacak, K.; Kass, D.; Di Lisa, F. & Paolocci, N. (2010). Monoamine oxidase A-mediated enhanced catabolism of norepinephrine contributes to adverse remodeling and pump failure in hearts with pressure overload. *Circulation Research. Vol.* 106,193-202.

Kaneko, M.; Elimban, V. & Dhalla, N. (1989). Mechanism for depression of heart sercolemmal Ca2+ pump bye oxygen free radicals. *American Journal of Physiology.* Vol. 257, H804-H811.

Karmazyn, M.; Sostaric, J. & Gan, X. (2001). The myocardial Na+/H+ exchanger: a potential therapeutic target for the prevention of myocardial ischaemic and reperfusion injury and attenuation of postinfarction heart failure. *Drugs.* Vol. 61, 375-389.

Kim, J.; Wei, Y. & Sowers, J. (2008). Role of mitochondrial dysfunction in insulin resistance. *Circulation Research.* Vol. 102, 401-414.

Kin, H.; Zatta, A.J.; Lofye, M.T.; Amerson, B.S.; Halkos, M.E.; Kerendi, F.; Zhao, Z.Q.; Guyton, R.A.; Headrick, J.P. & Vinten-Johansen J. (2005). Postconditioning reduces infarct size via adenosine receptor activation by endogenous adenosine. *Cardiovascular Research.* Vol.67, 124-133.

Kinnally, K. & Antonsson, B. (2007). A tale of two mitochondrial channels, MAC and PTP, in apoptosis. *Apoptosis.* Vol. 12, 857-68.

Kirsch, M. & De Groot, H. (2001). NAD(P)H, a directly operating antioxidant? *FASEB Journal.* Vol. 15, 1569-74.

Kojic, Z.; Gopcevic, K.; Marinkovic, D. & Tasic, G. (2011). Effect of captopril on serum lipid levels and cardiac mitochondrial oxygen consumption in experimentally-induced hypercholesterolemia in rabbits. *Physiological Research.* In press.

Kowald, A. & Kirkwood, T. (2011). Evolution of the mitochondrial fusion-fission cycle and its role in aging. *Proceedings of the National Academy of Sciences U S A.* Vol. 108, 10237-42.

Kukreja, R. & Hess, M. (1992). The oxygen free-radical system- From equations through membrane-protein interactions to cardiovascular injury and protection. *Cardiovascular Research.* Vol. 26, 641-655.

Kuwana, T.; Mackey, M.R.; Perkins, G.; Ellisman, M.H.; Latterich, M.; Schneiter, R.; Green, D.R. & Newmeyer, D.D. (2002). Bid, Bax and lipids cooperate to form supramolecular openings in the outer mitochondrial membrane. *Cell.* Vol. 111, 331-42.

Laursen, J.; Rajagopalan, S.; Galis, Z.; Tarpey, M.; Freeman, B. & Harrison, D. (1997). Role of superoxide in angiotensin-II induced but not catecholamine-induced hypertension. *Circulation,* Vol. 95, 588–593.

Leung, A.; Varanyuwatana, P. & Halestrap, A. (2008). The mitochondrial phosphate carrier interacts with cyclophilin D and may play a key role in the permeability transition. *Journal of Biological Chemistry.* Vol. 283, 26312-26323.

Li, Y.; Huang, T.; Carlson, E.; Melov, S.; Ursell, P.; Olson. J.; Noble, L.; Yoshimura, M.; Berger, C.; Chan, P.; Wallace, D. & Epstein, C. (1995). Dilated cardiomyopathy and neonatal lethality in mutant mice lacking manganese superoxide dismutase. *Nature Genetics.* Vol. 11, 376-81.

Linz, W. & Busch, A. (2003). NHE-1 inhibition: from protection during acute ischaemia/ reperfusion to prevention/reversal of myocardial remodelling. *Naunyn Schmiedebergs Archives of Pharmacology.* Vol. 368, 239-246.

Liochev, S. & Fridovich, I. (2010). Mechanism of the peroxidase activity of Cu, Zn superoxide dismutase. *Free Radical Biology and Medicine.* Vol. 48, 1565–1569.

Lucken-Ardjomande, S.; Montessuit, S. & Martinou, J. (2008). Contributions to Bax insertion and oligomerization of lipids of the mitochondrial outer membrane. *Cell Death & Differentiation.* Vol. 15, 929-937.

Lundberg, M.; Johansson, C.; Chandra, J.; Enoksson, M.; Jacobsson, G.; Ljung, J.; Johansson, M. & Holmgren A. (2001). Cloning and expression of a novel human glutaredoxin (Grx2) with mitochondrial and nuclear isoforms. *Journal of Biological Chemistry.* Vol. 276, 26269-75.

Madamanchi, N.; Vendrov, A. & Runge, M. (2005). Oxidative stress and vascular disease. *Arteriosclerosis & Thrombosis Vascular Biology.* Vol. 25, 29–38.

Mailloux, R. & Harper, E. (2011). Uncoupling proteins and the control of mitochondrial reactive oxygen species production. *Free Radical Biological Medicine.* Jun 24. (Epub ahead of print).

Mammucari, C. & Rizzuto, R. (2010). Signaling pathways in mitochondrial dysfunction and aging. *Mechanisms of ageing and development. Vol.* 131, 536-43.

Marí, M.; Morales, A.; Colell, A.; García-Ruiz, C. & Fernández-Checa, J. (2009) Mitochondrial Glutathione, a Key Survival Antioxidant. *Antioxidants & Redox Signals.* Vol. 11, 2685-700.

Maroz, A.; Anderson, R.; Smith, R. & Murphy, M. (2009). Reactivity of ubiquinone and ubiquinol with superoxide and the hydroperoxyl radical: implications for in vivo antioxidant activity. *Free Radical Biology & Medicine.* Vol. 46, 105–109.

Mårtensson, J.; Lai, J. & Meister, A. (1990). High-affinity transport of glutathione is part of a multicomponent system essential for mitochondrial function. *Proccedings of the National Academic Science U S A.* Vol. 87, 7185-9.

Martínez-Abundis, E.; García, N.; Correa, F.; Franco, M. & Zazueta, C. (2007). Change in specific lipids regulates BAX-induced mitochondrial permeability transition. *FEBS Journal.* Vol. 274, 6500-6510.

Martínez-Abundis, E.; Correa, F.; Pavón, N. & Zazueta, C. (2009). Bax distribution into mitochondrial detergent-resistant microdomains is related to ceramide and cholesterol content in postischemic hearts. *FEBS Journal.* Vol. 276, 5579-5588.

Matsui, Y.; Takagi, H.; Qu, X.; Abdellatif, M.; Sakoda, H.; Asano, T.; & Sadoshima, J. (2007). Distinct roles of autophagy in the heart during ischemia and reperfusion: roles of AMP-activated protein kinase and Beclin 1 in mediating autophagy. *Circulation Research.* Vol. 100, 914-922.

Matsushima, S; Ide, T.; Yamato, M.; Matsusaka, H.; Hattori, F.; Ikeuchi, M.; Kubota, T.; Sunagawa, K.; Hasegawa, Y.; Kurihara, T.; Oikawa, S.; Kinugawa, S. & Tsutsui, H. (2006). Overexpression of mitochondrial peroxiredoxin-3 prevents left ventricular remodeling and failure after myocardial infarction in mice. *Circulation.* Vol. 113, 1779-86.

Murata, M.; Akao, M.; O'Rourke, B. & Marbán, E. (2001). Mitochondrial ATP-sensitive potassium channels attenuate matrix Ca^{2+} overload during simulated ischemia and reperfusion: possible mechanism of cardioprotection. *Circulation Research.* Res. Vol. 89, 891–98.

Nagy, N.; Malik, G.; Tosaki, A.; Ho, Y.; Maulik, N. & Das, D. (2008). Overexpression of glutaredoxin-2 reduces myocardial cell death by preventing both apoptosis and necrosis. *Journal of Molecular & Cell Cardiology.* Vol. 44, 252-60.

Nakagawa, T.; Shimizu, S.; Watanabe, T.; Yamaguchi, O.; Otsu, K.; Yamagata, H.; Inohara, H.; Kubo, T. & Tsujimoto, Y. (2005). Cyclophilin D-dependent mitochondrial permeability transition regulates some necrotic but not apoptotic cell death. *Nature* Vol. 434,652-658.

Nakayama, H.; Chen, X.; Baines, C.; Klevitsky, R.; Zhang, X.; Zhang, H.; Jalee, N.; Chua, B.; Hewett, T.; Robbins, J.; Houser, S. & Molkentin, J. (2007). Ca2+- and mitochondrial-dependent cardiomyocyte necrosis as a primary mediator of heart failure. *Journal of Clinical Investigation.* Vol. 117, 2431- 2444.

Napoli, E.; Taroni, F. & Cortopassi, G.A. (2006) Frataxin, iron sulfur clusters, heme, ROS and aging. *Antioxidant & Redox Signaling.* Vol. 8, 506-16.

Nishida, K.; Kyoi, S.; Yamaguchi, O.; Sadoshima, J. & Otsu, K. (2009). The role of autophagy in the heart. *Cell Death & Differentiation.* Vol. 16, 31–38.

Noma A. (1983). ATP-regulated K^+ channels in cardiac muscle. *Nature.* Vol. 305, 147-148.

Nomura, K.; Imai, H.; Koumura, T.; Kobayashi, T. & Nakagawa, Y. (2000) Mitochondrial phospholipid hydroperoxide glutathione peroxidase inhibits the release of cytochrome c from mitochondria by suppressing the peroxidation of cardiolipin in hypoglycaemia-induced apoptosis. *Biochemical Journal.* Vol. 351, 183-93.

Nonn, L.; Williams, R,; Erickson, R. & Powis, G. (2003). The absence of mitochondrial thioredoxin 2 causes massive apoptosis, exencephaly, and early embryonic lethality in homozygous mice. *Molecular & Cellular Biology.* Vol. 1, 682-9.

Oliveira, P.; Seica, R.; Coxito, P.; Rolo, A.; Palmeira, C.; Santos, M. & Moreno, A. (2005). Enhanced permeability transition explains the reduced calcium uptake in cardiac mitochondria from streptozotocin- induced diabetic rats. *FEBS Letters*. Vol. 554, 511-514.

Opie, L. & Sack, M. (2002). Metabolic plasticity and the promotion of cardiac protection in ischemia and ischemic preconditioning. *Journal of Molecular & Cellular Cardiology*. Vol. 34, 1077–1089.

Orrenius, S.; Gogvadze, V. & Zhivotovsky, B. (2007). Mitochondrial oxidative stress: implications for cell death. *Annual Review of Pharmacology & Toxicology*. Vol. 47,143-83.

Papanicolaou, K.; Khairallah, R.; Ngoh, G.; Chikando, A.; Luptak, I.; O'Shea, K.; Riley, D.; Lugus, J.; Colucci, W.; Lederer, W. & Walsh K. (2011). Mitofusin-2 maintains mitochondrial structure and contributes to stress-induced permeability transition in cardiac myocytes. *Molecular & Cell Biology*. Vol. 31, 1309-28.

Paradies, G.; Petrosillo, G.; Pistolese, M. & Ruggiero, F.M. (2001). Reactive oxygen species generated by the mitochondrial respiratory chain affect the complex III activity via cardiolipin peroxidation in beef-heart submitochondrial particles. *Mitochondrion*. Vol. 1, 151-9.

Paradies, G.; Petrosillo, G.; Paradies, V.; Reiter, R. & Ruggiero, F. Melatonin. (2010) Cardiolipin and mitochondrial bioenergetics in health and disease. *Journal of Pineal Research*. Vol. 48, 297-310.

Parra, V.; Eisner, V.; Chiong, M.; Criollo, A.; Moraga, F.; Garcia, A.; Härtel, S.; Jaimovich, E.; Zorzano, A.; Hidalgo, C. & Lavandero, S. (2008). Changes in mitochondrial dynamics during ceramide-induced cardiomyocyte early apoptosis. *Cardiovascular Research*. Vol. 77, 387-97.

Peng, T. & Jou, M. (2010). Oxidative stress caused by mitochondrial calcium overload. *Annals of the New York Academy of Science*. Vol. 1201,183-8.

Piot, C.; Croisille, P.; Staat, P.; Thibault, H.; Rioufol, G.; Mewton, N.; Elbelghiti, R.; Cung, T.; Bonnefoy, E.; Angoulvant, D.; Macia, C.; Raczka, F.; Sportouch, C.; Gahide, G.; Finet, G.; Andre-Fouet, X.; Revel, D.; Kirkorian, G.; Monassier, J.; Derumeaux, G. & Ovize, M. (2008). Effect of cyclosporine on reperfusion injury in acute myocardial infarction. *New England Journal of Medicine*. Vol. 359, 473-481.

Poderoso, J.; Carreras, M.; Lisdero, C.; Riobó, N.; Schöpfer, F. & Boveris, A (1996). Nitric oxide inhibits electron transfer and increases superoxide radical production in rat heart mitochondria and submitochondrial particles. *Archives of Biochemistry and Biophysics*. Vol. 328, 85–92.

Prosser, B.L.; Ward, C.W. & Lederer, W.J. (2011). X-ROS signaling: rapid mechano-chemo transduction in heart. *Science*. Vol. 333, 1440-5.

Ragone, M. & Consolini, A. (2009) Cardiac role of the mitochondrial Ca2+ transporters in the high-[K+](o) cardioprotection of rat hearts under ischemia and reperfusion: a mechano-energetic study. *Journal of Cardiovascular Pharmacology*. Vol..54, 213-22.

Ran, Q.; Van Remmen, H.; Gu, M.; Qi, W.; Roberts, L. 2nd; Prolla, T. & Richardson, A. (2003). Embryonic fibroblasts from Gpx4+/- mice: a novel model for studying the role of membrane peroxidation in biological processes. *Free Radical Biology & Medicine*. Vol. 35, 1101-9.

Raza, H.; Robin, M.; Fang, J. & Avadhani, N. (2002). Multiple isoforms of mitochondrial glutathione S-transferases and their differential induction under oxidative stress. *Biochemical Journal*. Vol. 366, 45-55.

Robertson, C.; Scafidi, S.; McKenna, M. & Fiskum, G. (2009). Mitochondrial mechanisms of cell death and neuroprotection in pediatric ischemic and traumatic brain injury. *Experimental Neurology*. Vol. 218, 371-380.

Rodríguez, C.; Mayo, J.; Sáinz, .R.; Antolín, I.; Herrera, F.; Martín, V. & Reiter, R. (2004). Regulation of antioxidant enzymes: a significant role for melatonin. *Journal of Pineal Research*, Vol. 36, 1–9.

Rosier, O. & Saes, P. (2006), Soy isoflavones reduce heat shock proteins in experimental atherosclerosis. *European Journal of Nutriology*. Vol. 45, 178-86.

Sack, M. N. (2006b). Mitochondrial depolarization and the role of uncoupling proteins in ischemia tolerance. *Cardiovascular Research*. Vol. 72, 210–219.

Santos, C.; Anilkumar, N.; Zhang, M.; Brewer, A . & Shah, A. (2011). Redox signaling in cardiac myocytes. *Free Radical Biology & Medicine*. Vol. 50, 777-93.

Scarpulla R. (2008). Transcriptional paradigms in mammalian mitochondrial biogenesis and function. *Physiological Revisions*. Vol. 88, 611-38.

Schriner, S.; Linford, N.; Martin, G.; Treuting, P.; Ogburn, C.; Emond, M.; Coskun, P.; Ladiges, W.; Wolf, N.; Van Remmen, H.; Wallace, D. & Rabinovitch, P. (2005). Extension of murine life span by overexpression of catalase targeted to mitochondria. *Science*. Vol.. 308, 5730.

Shanmuganathan, S.; Hausenloy, D.; Duchen, M. & Yellon, D. (2005). Mitochondrial permeability transition pore as a target for cardioprotection in the human heart. *American Journal of Physiology & Heart Circulation Physiology*. Vol. 289, H237-242.

Sharov, V.; Todor, A.; Khanal, S.; Imai, M. & Sabbah, H. (2007). Cyclosporine A attenuates mitochondrial permeability transition and improves mitochondrial respiratory function in cardiomyocytes isolated from dogs with heart failure. *Journal of Molecular & Cell Cardiology*. Vol. 42,150-158.

Sherer TB, Betarbet R, Kim JH & Greenamyre JT (2003*a*). Selective microglial activation in the rat rotenone model of Parkinson's disease. *Neuroscience Letters* 341, 87–90.

Shimizu, S.; Ide, T.; Yanagida, T. & Tsujimoto, Y. (2000). Electrophysiological study of a novel large pore formed by Bax and the Voltage-dependent Anion Channel that is permeable to cytocrome c. *Journal of Biological Chemistry*. Vol.275, 12321-25.

Shiomi T,; Tsutsui, H.; Matsusaka, H.; Murakami, K.; Hayashidani, S.; Ikeuchi, M.; Wen, J.; Kubota, T.; Utsumi, H. & Takeshita, A. (2004). Overexpression of glutathione peroxidase prevents left ventricular remodeling and failure after myocardial infarction in mice. *Circulation*. Vol. 109, 544-9.

Shy, G. & Gonatas, N. (1964). Human Myopathy with giant abnormal mitochondrila. *Science*. Vol. 145: 493-6.

Smirnova, E.; Griparic, L.; Shurland, D. & van der Bliek, A. (2001) Dynamin-related protein Drp1 is required for mitochondrial division in mammalian cells. *Molecular & Biology Cell*. Vol. 12, 2245-2256.

Sowers, J.; Whaley Connell, A. & Epstein, M. (2009). The emerging clinical implications of the role of aldosterone in the metabolic syndrome and resistant hypertension. *Annual International Medicine*. Vol. 150, 776-785.

Srinivasan, V.; Spence, W.; Pandi-Perumal, S.; Zakharia, R.; Bhatnagar, K. & Brzezinski, A. Melatonin and human reproduction: shedding light on the darkness hormone. *Gynecological Endocrinology.* Vol. 25, 779–785.

Stowe, D. & Camara, A. (2009). Mitochondrial reactive oxygen species production in excitable cells: modulators of mitochondrial and cell function. *Antioxidant Redox Signaling.* Vol. 6, 1373-414.

Stuart, J.; Cadenas, S.; Jekabsons, M.; Roussel, D. & Brand, M. D. (2001). Mitochondrial proton leak and the uncoupling protein 1 homologues. *Biochimical & Biophysical Acta.* Vol. 1504, 144–158.

Tompkins, A.J.; Burwell, L.S.; Digerness, S.B.; Zaragoza, C.; Holman, W.L. & Brookes, P.S. (2006). Mitochondrial dysfunction in cardiac ischemia-reperfusion injury: ROS from complex I, without inhibition. *Biochimica & Biophysica Acta.* Vol. 1762, 223-31.

Trumpower, B. (1990). The protonmotive Q cycle. *Journal of Biological Chemistry.* Vol. 265, 11409–11412.

Turrens, J. & Boveris, A. (1980). Generation of superoxide anion by the NADH dehydrogenase of bovine heart mitochondria. *Biochemistry Journal.* Vol. 191, 421–427.

Turrens, J.; Alexandre, A. & Lehninger, A. (1985). Ubisemiquinone is the electron donor for superoxide formation by complex III of heart mitochondria. *Archives of Biochemistry and Biophysics.* Vol. 237, 408–414.

Turrens, J.; Freeman, B.; Levitt, J. & Crapo, J. (1982). The effect of hyperoxia on superoxide production by lung submitochondrial particles. *Archives of Biochemistry and Biophysics.* Vol. 217, 401–410.

Turrens, J. (2003). Mitochondrial formation of reactive species. *Journal of Physiology.* Vol. 552, 335–344.

Valentim, L.; Laurence, K.; Townsend, P.; Carroll, C.; Soond, S.; Scarabelli, T.; Knight, R.; Latchman, D. & Stephanou, A. (2006). Urocortin inhibits Beclin1-mediated autophagic cell death in cardiac myocytes exposed to ischaemia/reperfusion injury. *Journal of Molecular & Cell Cardiology.* Vol. 40, 846-852.

Valko, M.; Leibfritz, D.; Moncol, J.; Cronin, M.; Mazur, M. & Telser, J. (2007). Free radicals and antioxidants in normal physiological functions and human disease. *International Journal of Biochemistry & Cell Biology.* Vol. 39, 44-84.

Wen, J.J. & Garg, N.J. (2008). Mitochondrial generation of reactive oxygen species is enhanced at the Q(o) site of the complex III in the myocardium of Trypanosoma cruzi-infected mice: beneficial effects of an antioxidant. *Journal of Bioenergetics and Biomembranes.* Vol. 40, 587-98.

Whaley- Connell, A. & Sowers, J. (2009). Hypertension and insulin resistance. *Hypertension.* Vol. 54, 462-464.

Wittenberg BA & Wittenberg JB (1989). Transport of oxygen in muscle. *Annu Rev Physiol* 51, 857–878.

Wood, P. (1987). The two redox potentials for oxygen reduction to superoxide.*Trends Biochemical Science.* Vol. 12, 250–251.

Yang, X.M.; Krieg, T.; Cui, L.; Downey, J.M. & Cohen, M.V. (2004). NECA and bradykinin at reperfusion reduce infarction in rabbit hearts by signaling through PI3K, ERK, and NO. *Journal of Molecular & Cellular Cardiology.* Vol. 36, 411-421.

Yoon, Y.; Krueger, W.; Oswald, B. & McNiven, M. (2003). The mitochondrial protein hFis1 regulates mitochondrial fission in mammalian cells through an interaction with the dynamin-like protein DLP1. *Molecular & Cellular Biology*. Vol. 23, 5409–5420.

Yuan, H.; Perry, C.; Huang, C.; Iwai-Kanai, E.; Carreira, R.; Glembotski, C. & Gottlieb, R. (2009). LPS-induced autophagy is mediated by oxidative signaling in cardiomyocytes and is associated with cytoprotection. *American Journal of Physiology & Heart Circulation Physiology*. Vol. 296, H470-9.

Yuan, X. M. & Li, W. (2003). The iron hypothesis of atherosclerosis and its clinical impact. *Annals of Medicine*.Vol. 35, 578–591.

Yussman, M.; Toyokawa, T.; Odley, A.; Lynch, R.; Wu, G.; Colbert, M.; Aronow, B.; Lorenz, J. & Dorn, G. 2nd. (2002). Mitochondrial death protein Nix is induced in cardiac hypertrophy and triggers apoptotic cardiomyopathy. *Nature Medicine*. Vol. 8, 725-30.

Zhao, W.; Fan, G.; Zhang, Z.; Bandyopadhyay, A.; Zhou, X. & Kranias, E.G. (2008). Protection of peroxiredoxin II on oxidative stress-induced cardiomyocyte death and apoptosis. *Basic Research Cardiology*. Vol. 104, 377-89.

9

Oxidatively Modified Biomolecules: An Early Biomarker for Acute Coronary Artery Disease

Sarawut Kumphune
Department of Medical Technology,
Faculty of Allied Health Sciences, Naresuan University,
Thailand

1. Introduction

Cardiovascular disease is the worldwide major cause of mortality and morbidity. The 2009 annual report from World Health Organization (WHO) highlighted the mortality rate prediction of the population worldwide that, in 2030, cardiovascular disease will become the major cause of deaths, and the mortality rate will higher than other infectious diseases such as HIV, Tuberculosis, malaria infection (World Heatlh Organization ,2009). Moreover, this report also mentioned that, among cardiovascular diseases, ischemic heart disease and cerebrovascular disease, which were reported as top 2 cause of mortality in 2004, are expected to still be the major cause of death in next 20 years (World Heatlh Organization ,2009). Coronary artery disease is a sequence of pathophysiologic processes in coronary arteries, myocardial ischemia and infarction (Wudkowska et al.2010). Therefore, the early diagnostic of myocardial ischemia and infarction, will lead to the rapid and more effective of medical intervention, and safe the patients' life. The standard diagnosis of coronary artery disease focuses on clinical assessment such as history of chest pain associated with electrocardiogram (ECG) changes, and elevation of cardiac specific-biochemical markers (Maneewong K. et al.2011).

Determination of serum or plasma level of cardiac specific-biochemical markers is one of the most essential and effective way for diagnosing myocardial ischemia/infarction. The ideal cardiac markers should have high specificity, high sensitivity, rapidly released after the onset of the symptoms, abundant in cardiac tissue but less in other tissues, long half life in blood circulation, and capable of representing the prognosis and estimating the infarct size.

It has been known that coronary artery disease, especially myocardial ischemia and ischemia-reperfusion injury is the phenomenon that related to an oxidative stress (Buja2005), which is an imbalance and inadequate production of reactive oxygen species (ROS), subsequently resulted in biochemical modifications of major principle biomolecules such as proteins, lipids, and nucleic acids (Valko et al.2007;Sbarouni et al.2008a;Sbarouni et al.2008b;Sbarouni et al.2008c;le-Donne et al.2003a;le-Donne et al.2003c). Some oxidatively modified biomolecules such as Ischemia Modified Albumin or IMA, has been approved by US Food and drug Administration (FDA) and used as a rule-out marker for acute myocardial ischemia (Apple et al.2005;Bar-Or et al.2000;Sbarouni et al.2008c;Sbarouni et al.2008a;Sbarouni et al.2008b;Van et al.2010). In addition, many of oxidatively modified biomolecules have been reported to correlate with the severity of coronary artery disease and possibly used as a marker for myocardial ischemia (Apple et al.2005;Bar-Or et al.2001c; Bar-Or et al.2000;le-Donne et al.2003b;Berlett & Stadtman1997;Kiyici et al.2010;Turedi et al.2010; Melanson & Tanasijevic2005;Van et al.2010;Shen et al.2010;Pantazopoulos et al.2009; Bhagavan et al.2003;Santalo et al.2003;Sinha et al.2003;Mutlu-Turkoglu et al.2005;Mocatta et al.2007; Beal2002;Docherty2010;Wudkowska et al.2010;Charpentier et al.2010;Maneewong K. et al.2011; Sbarouni et al.2008a; Sbarouni et al.2008b;Sbarouni et al.2008c;le-Donne et al.2003a; le-Donne et al.2003d).

In this chapter, studies of oxidatively modified biomolecules such as proteins, lipids, and nucleic acids, related to coronary artery diseases will be discussed. Moreover, clinical usefulness of determining these oxidatively modified biomolecules as a biomarker for coronary artery disease will also be addressed.

2. Oxidative stress

The term oxidative stress has been commonly mentioned or explained the underline pathophysiological mechanism of some diseases during the last thirty years (Hensley et al.2000). Oxidative stress is referred to an inadequate of free radicals generation and/or insufficient removal of the radicals by antioxidants, radical scavengers. Free radicals can also be defined as atoms or molecules containing one or more unpaired electrons on an open shell configuration (Lushchak2011), which generate the highly reactivity properties of the molecules. There are 2 major types of free radicals such as reactive oxygen species (ROS) and reactive nitrogen species (RNS).

2.1 Reactive Oxygen Species

Reactive oxygen species (ROS) are generated from oxygen metabolism include superoxide anion ($O_2^{\bullet -}$), peroxyl ($RO^{\bullet}_2$), hydroperoxyl ($HRO_2^{\bullet -}$), and hydroxyl radical ($^{\bullet}OH$). In addition, ROS can also be non-radical species such as hydrogen peroxide (H_2O_2) and hydrochlorous acid (HOCl). ROS can be generated from regular metabolic processes or from external sources such as X-ray exposure, air pollutants, cigarette smoking, and etc. The primary source of intracellular free radicals generated by the addition of one oxygen electron, which is resulted in superoxide ($O_2^{\bullet -}$) (equation 1).

$$O2 + e- \longrightarrow O_2^{\bullet -} \quad (1)$$

Intracellular mechanism to balance the generation of superoxide is achieved by specific enzyme called superoxide dismutase (SOD), which catalyze the changing of superoxide to oxygen and hydrogen peroxide (H_2O_2) (equation 2).

$$2\,O_2^{\bullet -} + 2H^+ \xrightarrow{\text{SOD}} O_2 + H_2O_2 \quad (2)$$

This hydrogen peroxide (H_2O_2) that is generated from equation 2 has a property of being an oxidizing agent and serve as a major source of $^{\bullet}OH$, which is one of the very harmful reactive oxygen species to the cell. According to hydrogen peroxide is non-radical and weak polar, it can penetrate through the lipid bilayer of cell membrane or mitochondrial membrane, and destroy some biological molecules such as proteins, lipids, and nucleic acids. Cellular balancing mechanism for H_2O_2 is the enzyme catalase, which convert two molecules of H_2O_2 to oxygen and water (equation 3)

$$2\,H_2O_2 \xrightarrow{\text{(Catalase)}} 2H_2O + O_2 \qquad (3)$$

Another alternative mechanism generating ROS in the cell is the Haber-Weiss reaction, which is a chemical catalysis of superoxide and hydrogen peroxide by ferric ion (Fe^{3+}) to generate hydroxyl radical ($^{\bullet}OH$) (equation 4)

$$O_2^{\bullet -} + H_2O_2 + O_2 \xrightarrow{Fe^{3+}/CU^{2+}} OH^- + {}^{\bullet}OH \qquad (4)$$

In addition, superoxide can reduce ferric ion to form ferrous ion (equation 5), the reaction called "Fenton reaction". The production of ferrous ion in first Fenton reaction can react with H_2O_2 in the second reaction and result in OH^- and $^{\bullet}OH$ generation (equation 6).

$$Fe^{3+} + O_2^{\bullet -} \longrightarrow Fe^{2+} + O_2 \qquad (5)$$

$$Fe^{2+} + H_2O_2 \longrightarrow Fe^{3+} + OH^- + {}^{\bullet}OH \qquad (6)$$

2.2 Reactive Nitrogen Species

Reactive nitrogen species (RNS) are generated from the reaction of nitric oxide (NO), which is enzymatically generated by nitric oxide synthetase (NOS). The NOS oxidized the amino acid L-arginine or L-citrulline. The member of RNS include nitric oxide (NO) and nitrogen dioxide ($NO^{\bullet}_2$), as well as non radicals nitrogen species e.g. peroxynitrite ($ONOO^-$), nitrousoxide (HNO_2), and alkyl peroxynitrates (RONOO). Among these RNS molecules, $^{\bullet}NO$, and $ONOO^-$ are the most investigated species, which have significant impact in cardiovascular complication (Kumar et al.2010).

2.3 Antioxidants

Antioxidants are either endogenous or exogenous compounds that prevent the generation of harmful free radicals, reduce the generated radicals, inactivate their harmful reactivity, and thereby block the chain reactions of these oxidants. The primary or chain breaking antioxidants so called "scavenger" which is neutralize the free radicals by donating one of their own electrons (Kumar et al.2010). The secondary or preventative antioxidants work by sequestration of transition metal ions or removal the peroxides by catalase and glutathione peroxidase. The tertiary antioxidants defense is the repairing of damaged molecules, in attempt to avoid the accumulative damages (Kumar et al.2010).

3. The oxidative modification of biomolecules

Reactive oxygen species readily attack a variety of important biomolecules, including carbohydrates, proteins, lipids, and nucleic acids. Interaction between ROS and these biomolecules resulted in biochemical modifications, which alter the functions as well as the properties of these biomolecules (Figure 1).

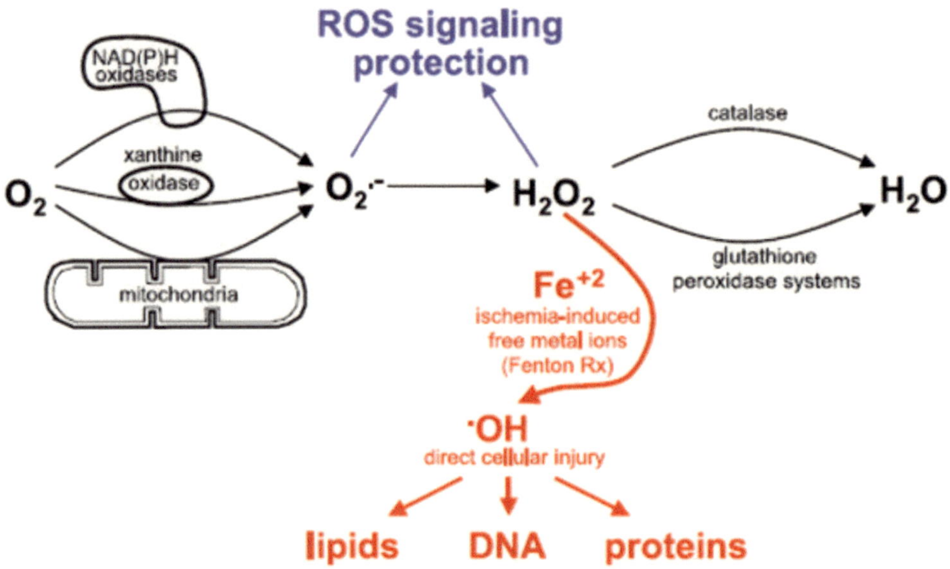

Fig. 1. Oxidative modification of biomolecules (Becker2004). In normal physiological conditions, superoxide and hydrogen peroxide are generated. Generation of intracellular ROS may activate the intracellular signaling pathways for cardiac protection, for example in ischemic preconditioning. The generated hydrogen peroxide, especially in myocardial ischemia, reacts with ferrous ion in Fenton reaction, which results in hydroxyl radicals. Over production of the hydroxyl radical causes oxidative modification of biomolecules, such as lipids, proteins, and nucleic acids.

3.1 Proteins

It has become manifested that proteins are also concerned as a target of free radical destruction. The mechanism involved in the oxidation modification of proteins is thought to occur at the monomeric level of amino acids, especially cysteine, tyrosine, phenylalanine, tryptophan, histidine, and methionine. The process of proteins oxidation creates new functional groups such as hydroxyl groups and carbonyl groups. These added up new functional groups can be generated by different mechanisms and can also indicate the degree of oxidative modification. The outcomes of the oxidative modification of proteins cause proteins fragmentation, cross-linking and unfolding, which may activate or hinder proteolytic and proteasome-mediated turnover. The biomarkers of oxidatively modified proteins include protein carbonyl, ischemia-modified albumin, and etc. Ischemia modified albumin (IMA) and protein carbonyl (PC) are oxidatively modified proteins found in many oxidative related disorders such as myocardial ischemia, renal ischemia, (Apple et al.2005;Pantke et al.1999;Bar-Or et al.2000;Kiyici et al.2010;Turedi et al.2010;Melanson & Tanasijevic2005). According to this, many studies suggested the ability of these two oxidatively modified proteins as the early biomarkers for diagnosis of coronary artery disease.

3.2 Lipids

Lipids are the basic biomolecules found throughout the cells, such as phospholipids component of the cell membrane. Therefore, lipids can be one of an oxidative modification targets, similar to proteins. Oxidative modification of lipids are the chain reactions, lead to the degradation of lipids or so-called "lipid peroxidation", which mediated by free radicals abstract electrons from lipid molecules such as aldehyde group e.g. Malonaldehyde (MDA). Polyunsaturated fatty acids are more sensitive to the lipid peroxidation according to these lipids contain multiple double bonds in between methylene- CH_2- groups that easily react with reactive hydrogen atoms (Lu et al.2010). The reactions of oxidative modified lipids consist of three major steps including; the initiation step, where is a fatty acid radicals are produced. The propagation is the direct reaction with oxygen molecules produced peroxyl fatty acid radials that react with another free fatty acid producing a different fatty acid radical and lipid peroxide or a cyclic peroxide and termination. The destruction of lipid molecules by lipid peroxidation can cause membrane permeability alteration, loss in fluidity, decreasing in electrical resistance, change in phospholipids bilayer membrane disruption, membrane-bound enzyme malfunction and loose of integrity ionic gradient, disruption or activation of enzyme function, and cellular injury (Ayres1984). Biomarkers of lipid peroxidation include malonaldehyde, F2-Isoprostanes, and etc.

3.3 Nucleic acid

Nucleic acid is one of the basic biomolecules that play many essential roles in the cell. The nucleic acids-DNA and RNA- are the principal informational molecules of the living cells. During aging processes, free radicals such as $^{\bullet}OH$ can be generated and can bind to DNA molecules. Association and reaction of free radical to DNA can lead to DNA bases damaging, both purines and pyrimidines, and result in DNA strand break (Valavanidis et al.2009). Alteration of purines and pyrimidines play a significant role in large variety of pathological stages such as cancer (Kasai1997). Biomarkers of oxidative modified nucleic acid include 8-hydroxy-2'-deoxyguanosine, 8-nitroguanin, and etc.

4. Oxidatively modified biomolecules as cardiac markers for coronary artery disease

4.1 Ischemia modified albumin

Generation of reactive oxygen species resulted in the modification of proteins, which introduce new functional groups such as hydroxyl groups and carbonyl groups (le-Donne et al.2003b;Berlett & Stadtman1997). Among these proteins, ischemia-modified albumin (IMA) was reported as an early biomarker in many pathological disorders (Kiyici et al.2010;Montagnana et al.2006;Abboud et al.2007;Gunduz et al.2009;Sharma et al.2007).

Ischemia Modified Albumin (IMA) is serum albumin that modified at the N-terminal portion, especially at aspartate-alanine-histidine-lysine sequences, by oxidative stress generated during ischemia (Bar-Or et al.2001b). This modification reduced the ability of albumin to bind with metal ions such as cobalt, copper, and nickel (Bar-Or et al.2001a) (Figure 2). The ischemic mechanism initiated with the insufficiency of oxygen supply during ischemia, which caused cardiomyocytes cellular anaerobic metabolism. Within a few seconds after occlusion of a major coronary artery tissue oxygen content decreases and mitochondrial oxidative metabolism becomes inhibited. At this point, a compensatory increase in anaerobic glycolysis for ATP production leads to accumulation of hydrogen ions and lactate, resulting in intracellular acidosis and inhibition of glycolysis (Reimer & Ideker1987). An aerobic glycolysis cannot provide sufficient ATP to meet the demand of myocardium. The depletion of ATP also causes the interruption of cellular ion-pumps and calcium influx to the cells. The excess intracellular calcium activates calcium-dependent proteases such as calpain, calmodulin, generates $O_2^{\bullet -}$ and converts to H_2O_2. Blood consist of transition metals such as copper and iron, which can interact with $O_2^{\bullet -}$ and H_2O_2 and form the strong oxidant $^{\bullet}OH$, which lead to cellular destruction. Proteins, predominantly albumin, are damaged by free radicals especially at amino terminus (N-terminus), resulting in the albumin N-terminal derivatives. Human serum albumin, a major protein in circulation, consists of 585 amino acid residues with half life in circulation approximately 19 days. The metal binding properties of albumin depend on the three dimensional structure binding sites, which are distributed over the molecule (Bar-Or et al.2001b;Takahashi et al.1987). The modification of albumin during ischemia is independent on cell death, and can be an early biomarker for such an early stage of ischemia.

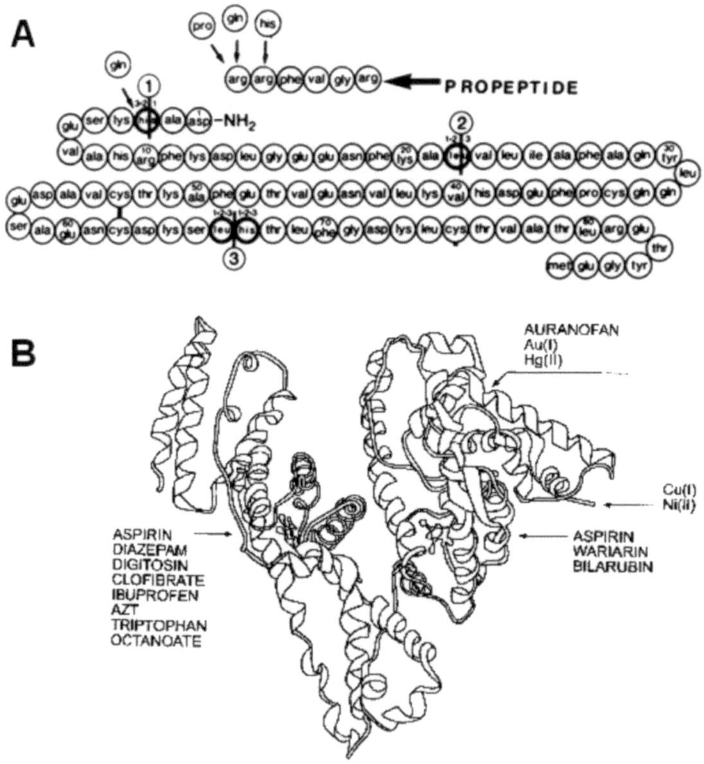

Fig. 2. The amino acid sequences (A) and molecular structure of albumin (B). This figure is modified from figure3 of Takahashi et al. (Takahashi et al.1987). Proteins albumin is oxidatively modified at NH_2 terminal of albumin.

Determination of serum or plasma IMA can be performed by Albumin Cobalt Binding (ACB) method. In 2003, US Food and drug Administration (FDA) approved that ACB method is the diagnostic test for acute myocardial infarction (Van et al.2010). The principle of ACB method is based on the principle of free radicals, which is generated during ischemia, alters the metal ions binding capacity of serum albumin (Sbarouni et al.2008a) (Figure 3). The test is currently called IMA test instead of the ACB test. It has been reported that IMA test could be used for screening the patients with chest pain, who suspected AMI, at the emergency department, excluded patients from the other causes of chest pain (Bar-Or et al.2000). Many studies show that IMA levels increased in patients with acute coronary syndrome and also elevated in myocardial ischemia (Sbarouni et al.2008a). The analytical sensitivity of the test is 13 u/ml, with 98% recovery (Sbarouni et al.2008a). Moreover, there were reports mentioned of non-interfering effect from bilirubin, hemoglobin, cholesterol, total proteins, and number of cardiac drugs (Govender et al.2008). It was also reported that no biological variation of IMA regarding race and gender (Govender et al.2008).

According to the ability to detect IMA as a result of ischemia, the event of reduce oxygen supply prior to cardiomyocytes necrosis, make IMA test good enough to be an earlier cardiac marker (Sbarouni et al.2008a). It was reported that the serum IMA level increased and can be detected within 6-10 minutes after ischemia and returned back to baseline within 6 hours (Bhagavan et al.2003). This could be an advantage of IMA, in comparison to the other conventional cardiac markers such as cardiac troponin and CK-MB, which are necrotic marker and could not be detected until 4-6 hours after onset of chest pain/ischemia (Wu et al.1999). Determination of IMA has been used triage patient who suspected from cardiac ischemia. Low level of serum IMA, would estimate low risk for a cardiac ischemic event and make a rapid consideration to exclude or discharge patient. Low level of serum IMA perhaps indirectly predicts the low level of cardiac troponin (Sbarouni et al.2008a). So, it can make a clear distinct when the negative results from IMA, troponin, and ECG can exclude the patients from ACS (Bhagavan et al.2003). The assay method can be easily and rapidly performed by spectrophotometric method. It has been shown that IMA test has high method sensitivity more than troponin as it gave positive results in 84% of patient who suspect ACS while cardiac troponin could detect only 42% (Takhshid et al.2010). Combination with triple tests including ECG, IMA, and cardiac troponin could increase the negative predictive value for ACS to 96% (Takhshid et al.2010). Furthermore, IMA test might reduce in the number of diagnostic tests such as determination of serum high sensitivity C-reactive proteins (hsCRP), NT-proBNP elevation, and cTnT release (Kazanis et al.2009), invasive imaging, which have high cost (Keating et al.2006).

However, it seems like IMA test lack of specificity. High serum IMA level can also be detected in other diseases such as cancer, acute infections, end renal disease, and liver cirrhosis, (Kazanis et al.2009). Therefore, the negative results from cTnT test and IMA allow more confident to exclude the patients, who suspected AMI. However, a positive IMA alone still need further investigation. Moreover, it has been reported that serum IMA level can also be elevated in plasma from healthy subjects, 24-48 hours after exercise (Kim et al.2008). Therefore, utilization of IMA test as cardiac marker for coronary artery disease need to be further investigated to ensure the value of the test.

4.2 Proteins carbonyl

The carbonyl (CO) groups in proteins compose of aldehyde and ketone groups. Proteins Carbonyl groups (PC) is a product of oxidative modification on amino acid residues, especially proline, arginine, lysine, and threonine from free radicals reactions, forming protein carbonyl groups [53]. In addition, protein carbonyl groups can be generated from an indirect mechanism of the hydroxyl radical-mediated oxidation of lipids (Figure 4). The product of lipid peroxidation, which will be described latter in this chapter, can diffuse across cell membrane, allowing the reactive aldehyde-containing lipids, which will covalently modified proteins in the cell (Grimsrud et al.2008). Proteins oxidation changes proteins functions by changing in pattern of proteins folding, which is important for their activity, decrease catalytic activity of enzyme, and finally breakdown of proteins by proteases (Almroth et al.2009). The cleavage of proteins may occur by either the amidation pathway or by oxidation of glutamyl side chain. Redox cycling cation such as Fe^{2+} or Cu^{2+} can bind to cation binding location on proteins. Free radical attack by H_2O_2 or $O_2^{\bullet -}$ can transform side chain of amine groups into carbonyls.

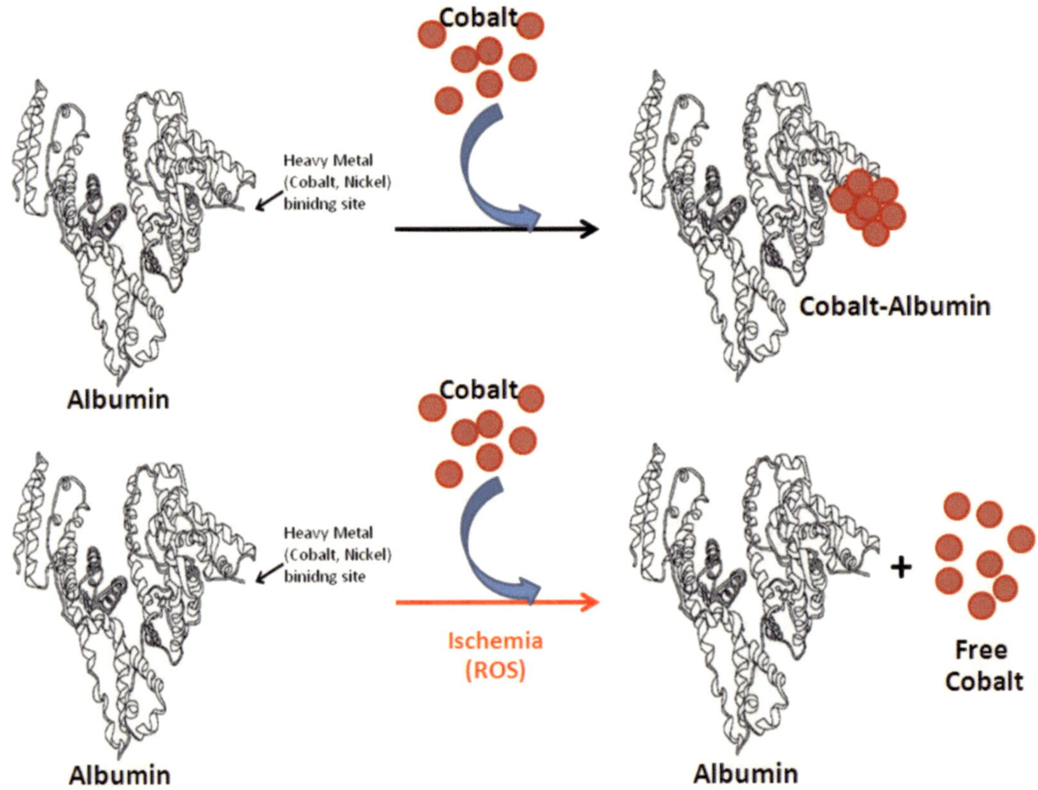

Fig. 3. Principle of Albumin cobalt binding (ACB) assay. In physiological conditions, albumin capable of binding with metal ions such as cobalt, copper, and nickel, at amino terminal end of the protein. During ischemia, N-terminal portion of albumin, especially at aspartate-alanine-histidine-lysine sequences, is modified and result in the reduction in albumin-metal ions binding ability.

Laboratory measurement of PC can be performed by variety of methods, for example, spectrophotometric assay, HPLC, ELISA, and immnunoblotting (le-Donne et al.2003a;le-

Donne et al.2003b;le-Donne et al.2006). Spectrophotometric assay for PC can be perform by 2,4-dinitrophenylhydrazine (DNPH spectrophotometric method), which based on the formation of a stable dinitrophenyl (DNP) hydrazone reacts in acidic pH solution. Spectrophotometric DNPH assay showed high sensitivity detection of carbonyl content level in purified proteins (le-Donne et al.2003b;Levine et al.1994). This method does not require any expensive or specialized equipments. It has been shown that the serum level of PC increased rapidly in blood stream and still remained at least 24 hours (Mutlu-Turkoglu et al.2005). Mutlu-Turkoglu *et al.* demonstrated that serum PC level increased in coronary artery disease, atherosclerotic lesion in human, and during ischemia-reperfusion (Mutlu-Turkoglu et al.2005). As it has also been reported that PC can be generated following the onset of myocardial infarction (Paton et al.2010) suggested the diagnostic value of PC and may be used as biomarker for coronary artery disease. The stability of this assay remained in hours and days, whereas lipid oxidation products can be removed within minutes (Mutlu-Turkoglu et al.2005). In AMI, serum PC level was significantly increased when compared with normal control (Paton et al.2010). Diagnosed value of PC in human can also be used in environmental studies, monitoring in subjects who exposed to the bunker oil (Almroth et al.2009). Although PC has been proven as a sensitive marker, but it was shown to has less specificity, similar to IMA. The increasing in serum level of PC can be detected in other human diseases such as Alzheimer' disease, cataract genesis, chronic hepatitis, diabetics, cigarette smoker, and after doing exercise (Mutlu-Turkoglu et al.2005). According to the time consuming and proteins precipitation is required in spectrophotometric method, this technique is inappropriate to determine the PC level in large number of clinical samples. Therefore, other techniques, for example ELISA, were developed. Recently, the findings from our study demonstrated that PC could be an early marker for myocardial ischemia. Serum PC level in non-ST elevation myocardial infarction (NSTEMI) was significantly higher than that in ST elevation myocardial infarction (STEMI) and healthy controls, suggesting that PC is an early marker. Moreover, combinatorial determination of PC with IMA helps to improve the diagnostic power of these two markers (Maneewong et al.2011).

4.3 8-hydroxy-2'-deoxyguanosine

As mentioned in the previous section, free radicals can attack DNA and cause molecular structural alterations of DNA and result in DNA strand break. The interaction of $^{\bullet}OH$ with the nucleobases of DNA, such as guanine, form the C8-hydroxyguanine (8-OHGua) or its nucleoside form deoxyguanosine (8-hydroxy-2′-deoxyguanine) or so called 8-OH-dG. The 8-OH-dG can be further oxidized and produced 8-oxo-7,8-dihydro-2′-deoxyguanine or 8-oxodG (Valavanidis et al.2009) (Figure 4). Although the other nucleic acids in DNA molecules can react with $^{\bullet}OH$ in the same manner, the 8-oxodG is the major form of oxidative modified nucleic acids in DNA, and known as a potential biomarker of carcinogenesis (Kasai1997). These days, the 8-OHdG can be a biomarker of oxidative stress, aging and cancer. This molecule can be measured and analyzed using high sensitivity by high performance liquid chromatography (HPLC), gas-chromatography-mass spectrometry (GC-MS), and liquid chromatography-mass spectrometry- mass spectrometry (LC-MS-MS), immunohistochemical methods, and single cell electrophoresis (Griffiths et al.2002;Halliwell & Whiteman2004;Collins et al.2004). There are many reports that the elevation of 8-OHdG related to some pathological disorders, for example, urinary 8-OHdG has been established as a marker to evaluate oxidative stress in carcinogenic exposure, environment pollutants and cigarette smoking (Kiyosawa et al.1990;Asami et al.1996). Elevation of 8-OHdG has been found in the plasma and myocardium of the patients with heart failure (Kono et al.2006). Recently, Himmetoglu *et al*. reported that the plasma level of 8-OHdG increased in patients with myocardial infarction and the level of this molecule decreased after reperfusion therapy in patients with MI, suggested that 8-OHdG could possibly be biomarker for monitoring or determining the prognosis of the patients (Himmetoglu et al.2009). In addition, Nagayoshi *et al* demonstrated that the urinary levels of 8-OHdG were significantly higher in cardiac patients when assessed the serial alteration of oxidative stress of patients with AMI (Nagayoshi et al.2005).

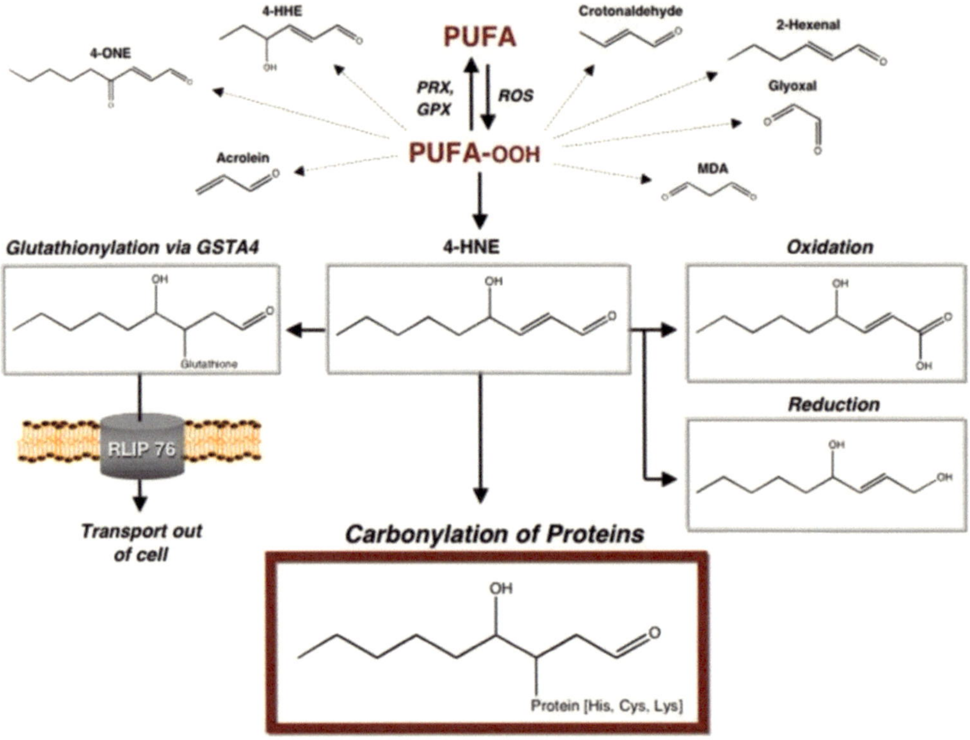

Fig. 4. Mechanism of ROS stimulates lipids peroxidation induced proteins carbonylation (Grimsrud et al.2008). Proteins carbonylation can be induced by the oxidative modification of polyunsaturated fatty acids (PUFA), which then undergo to lipid peroxidation reaction generating products such as α,β-unsaturated aldehyde 4-HNE. These molecules act as electrophiles in the covalently modification of proteins via non-enzymatic addition reactions.

It is known that reactive nitrogen species or RNS such as nitric oxide (NO) and peroxynitrite ($ONOO^-$) can modify the molecular structure of DNA (Ohshima et al.2006). The 8-nitroguanine is the example of nucleic acid in DNA, which can be oxidatively modified by RNS. There is overwhelm data showed that 8-nitroguanine is undetectable in normal tissues, which indicating that this molecule may be a candidate as a biomarker for DNA damage induced by RNS (Akaike et al.2003;Ma et al.2004;Horiike et al.2005;Pinlaor et al.2004). Several techniques have been developed for determining 8-nitroguanine in clinical samples, for example, HPLC with electrochemical detection, HPLC with a UV detector, GC-MS, and immunohistochemistry (Halliwell & Whiteman2004;Ohshima et al.2006;Sawa et al.2006). Many studies showed that 8-nitroguanine increased in inflammation, carcinogenesis, and cigarette smoke (Hiraku2010). However, there are no any evidence of the increasing in 8-nitoguanine in coronary heart diseases. Therefore, further investigation of 8-nitoguanine in coronary heart diseases is still need to be further investigated.

4.4 MDA

One of the most frequently used biomarkers indicating lipid peroxidation is plasma concentration of malondialdehyde (MDA). This molecule is one of the end products of lipid peroxidation in the cell membrane or in low-density lipoproteins (LDL) (Ogino & Wang2007). Quantification of plasma MDA level can be performed by thiobarbituric acid (TBA) test (Nielsen et al.1997). TBA-reactive substances (TBARS) formed in plasma, urine, or tissue samples that need to be calibrated by sample pretreatment procedure, which forms a red adduct with 2 molecules of TBA (MDA-TBA2). The adducted compounds are separated by an HPLC method, which originally described by Wong *et. al.*(Wong et al.1987) and Carbonneau *et. al.* (Carbonneau et al.1991). The GC-MS method has been used to analyze the plasma MDA as well (Yeo et al.1994). It has been reported that the plasma from patients with coronary artery disease also had higher level of MDA than the healthy subjects, suggested that MDA could be one of the candidate biomarkers for coronary artery disease (Rajesh et al.2011;Rao & Kiran2011;Mogadam et al.2008;Pasupathi et al.2009). A recent report also suggested that serum levels of TBARS, which was determined by reverse-phase HPLC and spectrophotometric method, were a good predictive marker in patients with stable coronary artery disease (Walter et al.2004).

4.5 F_2-Isoprostanes

Isoprostanes are a complex family of compounds generated from arachidonic acid via a free radical's catalyzed mechanism. This compound was firstly discovered in 1990 by Morrow *et. al.* who discovered prostaglandin-F_2-like compounds, and termed this newly discovered compound as ***F_2-isoprostanes*** (Morrow et al.1990). The F_2 -isoprostanes can be generated by the oxidative induced peroxidation of arachidonic acid (Figure 5).

Determination of F_2-isoprostanes is similar to other techniques measuring the products from lipid peroxidation including GC-MS, which might be associated with an immunoaffinity extraction, GC-tandem MS, and LC-tandem MS (Halliwell2000). Although these techniques have high specificity, the budget cost of these techniques is the impediment of their routine use (Milne et al.2005). Determination of 15- F_{2t}-IsoP in urine samples, by radioimmunoassay, has been validated and easier alternative to GC-MS. In addition, the new technique is developed, for example enzyme-immunoassay for detecting F_2-isoprostanes (Milne et al.2005).

F_2-isoprostanes can be measured in varieties of clinical samples, for example urine, plasma, bronchoalveolar lavage fluid, bile, cerebrospinal, seminal and pericardial fluids (Iuliano et al.2001;Lindsay et al.1999;Delanty et al.1997;Cipollone et al.2000;Reilly et al.1997). In addition, F_2-isoprostanes can be detected in normal tissues, including umbilical cords (Chu et al.2003). The level of F_2-isoprostanes increased in cigarette smoking, similar to other oxidative modified molecules, which is known that the increasing in smoking can cause the oxidative stress (Reilly et al.1996;Morrow et al.1995). The measurement of isoprostanes in biological fluids has prompted clinical investigations on the pathophysiological role of lipid peroxidation in cardiovascular diseases. In coronary artery disease, the quantified isoprostanes was mostly in 15- F_{2t}-IsoP and 5- F_{2t}-IsoP, which can be measured in urine samples (Haschke et al.2007). The urinary level of 15- F_{2t}-IsoP and 5- F_{2t}-IsoP was found to increase in, unstable angina, reperfusion following myocardial infarction and cardiopulmonary bypass, coronary angioplasty (Sakamoto et al.2002). These findings suggested that isoprostane could be biomarker for coronary artery disease.

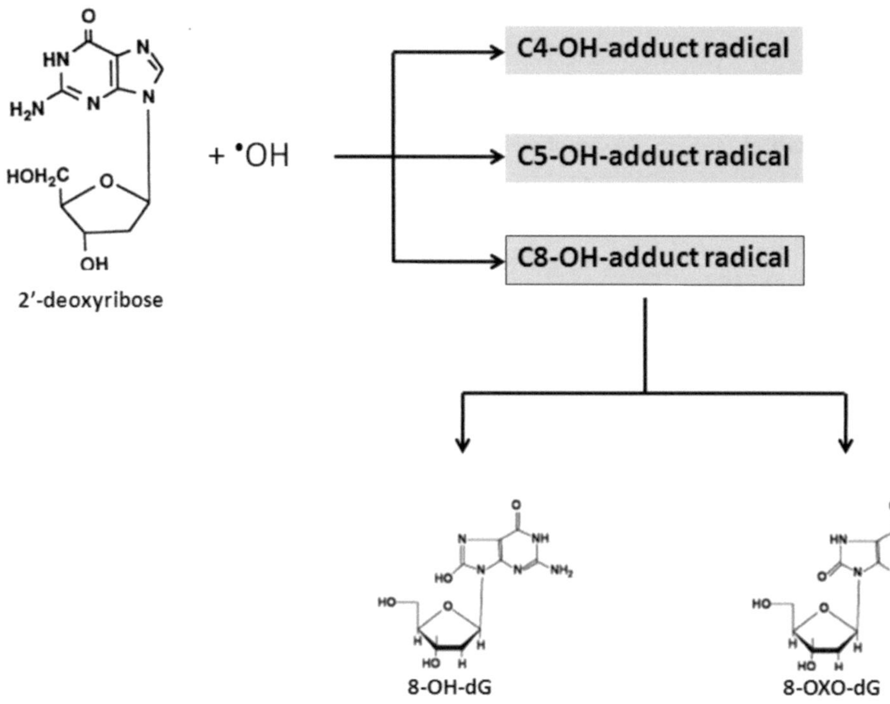

Fig. 5. The Chemical reaction of 2′-deoxyguanosine with hydroxyl radicals. The Oxidative modification reactions of 2′-doxyguanosine cause by hydroxyl radicals. This radical adducts are oxidized to 8-hydroxy-2′-deoxyguanosine (8-OHdG), or it tautomer 8-oxo-7-hydro-2′-deoxyguanosine (8-oxodG).

4.6 Advanced Glycation End-Produces (AGEs)

Advanced glycation end-produces (AGEs) are products of non-enzymatic glycation of proteins by reducing sugars (Zieman & Kass2004). AGEs was firstly discovered in early of 1900s by Louis Camille Mailard by the non-enzymatic chemical reaction between reducing sugars and amino groups on proteins to form protein-protein crosslink and complex yellow-brown pigments (Zieman & Kass2004). The Maillard reaction occurs when the reducing sugars, such as glucose, react with an amine groups, result in the formation of an unstable Shift bases (Figure 6). The produced unstable Shift bases that transform to an Amadori product, which can further rearrange to form advanced glycation endproducts (AGEs) capable of crosslinking proteins (Figure 7, 8).

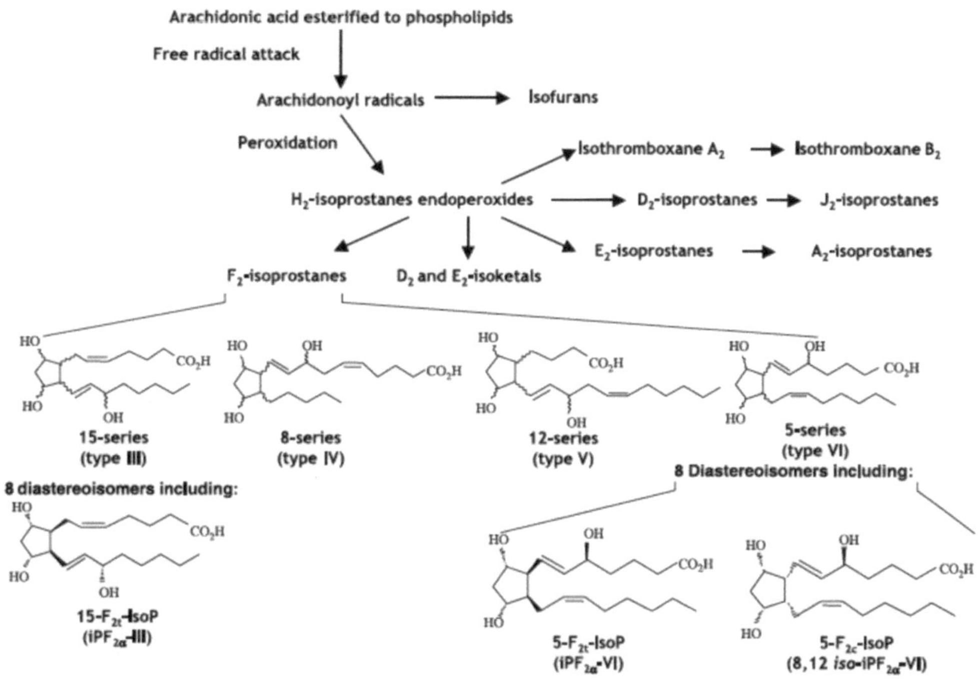

Fig. 6. Metabolic pathways of isoprostane (Cracowski & Durand2006). Free radicals interact with arachidonic acid produce arachidonyl radicals; these molecules were continue to the lipids peroxidation reaction and generated four types of prostaglandin-H_2-like compounds, which subsequently reduced to be 4 prostaglandin F2α.

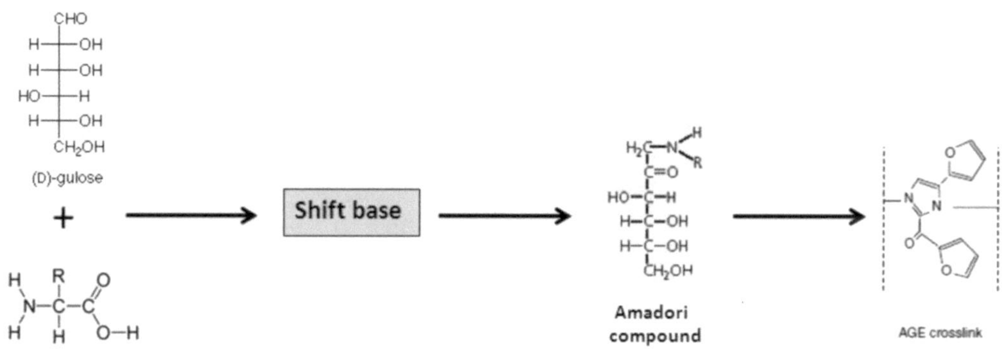

Fig. 7. The Maillard reaction is chemical reaction between a reducing sugar, such as glucose, and amino acid groups. The outcome from this reaction is the formation of unstable Schiff bases that can transform to an Amadori products, which can rearrange to form advanced glycation endproducts (AGEs) (Zieman & Kass2004).

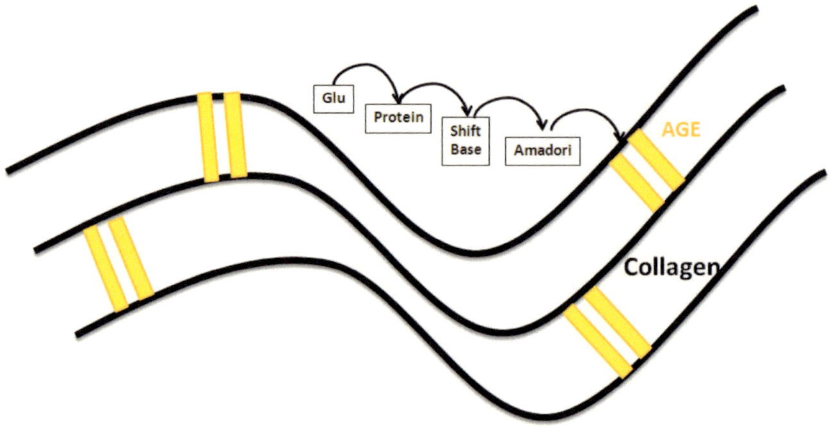

Fig. 8. The formation of collagen-collagen-AGEs crosslinking, this figure was modified from Zieman et. al. AGEs from the Maillard reaction can accelerate enzymatically crosslinking reaction of collagens strands (Zieman & Kass2004).

It has been known that AGEs play important role in the pathogenesis of diabetic vascular complications, as they lead to an abnormal leakage of proteins from the circulation and a progressive constriction of the luminal area of vessel (Brownlee et al.1988;Makita et al.1991;Ono et al.1998). Moreover, AGEs have been recognized as factors in the pathogenesis of other diabetic complications, such as nephropathy and retinopathy (Makita et al.1991;Ono et al.1998). In addition, the level of serum concentration of AGEs was associated with severity of coronary arthrosclerosis and development of this pathology in type 2 diabetic patients (Kiuchi et al.2001). Interestingly, it has been reported that the serum level of AGEs were elevated and correlated significantly with oxidized LDL, especially in diabetic patients (Lopes-Virella et al.2011). A recent evidence of 18-year study showed that the serum level of AGEs could predict the mortality from cardiovascular disease and coronary heart disease in non-diabetic women (Kilhovd et al.2005).

Determination of AGEs is similar to other techniques, used in determining other oxidative modified biomarkers, such as HPLC, GC-MS, ELISA, and immunochemistry (Ogino & Wang2007). The accuracy and reproducibility of these techniques have not been well examined according to lack of universally established unit of measurement, for comparing study findings from different laboratories (Ogino & Wang2007). Furthermore, AGEs has been reported to increase in cigarette smoking, similar to the findings found in other biomarkers (Nicholl & Bucala1998).

5. Early cardiac biomarkers for diagnostic acute coronary syndrome

The biochemical markers have been routinely used to assess myocardial damage, especially in patients suspected with ACS. World health organization criteria, formulated in 1979, have classically diagnosed in ACS patients if the patient present two (probable) or three (definite) diagnostic criteria of acute coronary syndrome. The criteria including clinical history of ischemic type chest pain lasting for more than 20 minutes, changes in serial ECG tracings, and elevation of serum cardiac biomarkers. Patients with ACS are subdivided into the following 2 major categories based on the results from electrocardiogram (ECG) including those whose ECG show ST-elevation that is diagnostic of acute ST-elevation myocardial infarction (STEMI) and those who present other patterns of ECG change, but not categorized in STEMI, called non- ST elevation ACS (NSTEACS). The latter include unstable angina (UA) and non-ST-elevation myocardial infarction (NSTEMI) (Morrow et al.2007;Wiviott & Braunwald2004). The ECG in NSTEMI can be interpreted in the way that the artery is only partially blocked, or only transiently occlusive, and results in coronary ischemia without the appearance of ST-segment elevation. The ECG is the most readily available tool for diagnosing STEMI. However, the limitation of ECG is usually occur in acute chest pain, according to the low sensitivity of the baseline ECG, which is only 60% (Panteghini2002). Undetectable of ST-elevation of ECG lead to delay in final diagnosis and affect treatment and clinical outcome. Therefore, determination of high sensitivity, specificity and early ischemic biomarker is useful for diagnosis of acute myocardial ischemia, particularly in NSTEMI patients. There are many types of conventional cardiac biomarkers such as creatine kinase- MB isoenzyme (CK-MB), cardiac troponin I or T (cTnI, cTnT). These conventional cardiac markers are known to release in blood circulation as a result of cellular necrosis, not early enough to detect the early phase of myocardial ischemia that may not excess the reference range of biochemical markers of myocardial necrosis. Determination of plasma/serum cardiac biomarkers in patients, who has arrived hospital after the onset of symptoms, may not be detected. Therefore, screening method, for measuring the early cardiac biomarkers that actually reflect the early phase of cellular injury, is extremely useful. The more rapid diagnosis, the more effective intervention and treatment, the less cost for hospital stay, secondary prevention and reduce effective budget for screening test to exclude myocardial infarction patients (Figure 9)

Creatine kinase (CK) is an enzyme responsible for transferring a phosphate group from ATP to creatine. The molecular weight of this enzyme is approximately 80,000 dalton. It is composed of M and/or B subunits build up at least 3 isoenzymes including CK-BB, CK-MB, and CK-MM or CK-1, CK-2 and CK-3, respectively. Moreover, there are one more isoenzymes that have been reported e.g. mitochondrial isoenzyme. CK-2 or CK-MB is sometime called the cardiac isoenzyme as it is predominant isoenzyme in myocardium, whereas there is only 2-5% in skeletal muscle. CK-MB can be found in large amount of infarcted myocardium and can rise up in the circulation within 3-6 hours after ischemia, peaks in 10-48 hours, and returns to normal within 72 hours (Wu et al.1999). However, an elevated serum CK-MB may occur in people with severe skeletal muscle damage (such as in muscular dystrophy, accident) and renal disease (Green et al.1986). In such cases, the ratio of CK-MB per total CK, or CK index, is very helpful. If the index is under 4%, a non-myocardial source of high CK-MB should be concerned. One of the limitations of determining serum CK-MB is undetectable of minimal myocardial injury, late rise in the setting of AMI.

Cardiac Troponin is a useful cardiac marker, localized in myofibrils. Troponin consists of 3 subunits including inhibitory subunit (cTnI), calcium binding subunit (cTnC), and tropomyosin binding subunit (cTnT). The troponin complex is located on the thin filaments of the contractile muscles and regulates the calcium mediated interaction of myocardial myosin and actin filaments. The specificity, sensitivity, and reliability of troponin assay for diagnosed myocardial necrosis make cardiac troponin be an ideal cardiac marker. In addition, the minimal concentration in serum cardiac troponin, from healthy people without cardiac disease, cannot be detected (Adams, III et al.1993). Among those 3 forms of cardiac troponin, troponin C cannot be used as cardiac marker according to non-specific expression in various tissues, not only the heart (Adams, III et al.1993). Cardiac troponin I (cTnI) and cardiac troponin T (cTnT) are 2 forms that normally used as cardiac marker. It has been known that, after myocardial ischemia, elevated cTnT last for 10 days to 2 weeks. The advantages of cTnT include highly sensitive for detecting MI, cTnT level may also help to risk stratify afterward, qualitative test run in 10 minutes. In contrast, the disadvantage of using cTnT assays as cardiac markers due to non specificity of cTnT, which can be found in unstable angina, chronic renal failure (Wood et al.2003). The cTnI is also being an ideal marker for ACS, according to high sensitivity and specificity of this marker in AMI. However, these two markers could not counted as the early marker, as it need increase around 6 hours after ischemia, until the level of cTnT is significantly higher than normal level.

The oxidatively modified markers such as PC and IMA have been proven as potential cardiac marker for diagnosis of ACS. However, determining of oxidative modified markers is not specific for myocardial ischemia. For example, it has been reported that the plasma level of IMA can be increased in cerebral, gastrointestinal intestinal and skeletal muscular ischemia as well as myocardial ischemia (Matthews et al.1990;Siegel et al.1995). Therefore, it is recommended that the interpretation of a positive IMA finding should be combined with other clinical indices (Shen et al.2010). Recently, our study showed the usefulness of determining serum IMA and PC content level to identify acute myocardial infarction, particularly in STEMI. The level of both serum IMA and PC content were significantly higher in STEMI compared to healthy control and determination of serum IMA level in combination of serum PC content level improved test performance (Kumphune et al.2010). However, the results from our recent study reported that diagnosis of NSTEMI was not improved by combination of serum IMA and PC level, in contrast, individual determination of serum PC content showed a good area under ROC curve and high PPV for NSTEMI diagnosis (Maneewong et al.2011). Charpentier *et. al.* also demonstrated in a large cohort study of patients admitted to an emergency department for chest pain that IMA did not provide valuable information for ACS diagnosis (Charpentier et al.2010). The possible explanation is NSTEMI patients did not have major myocardial necrosis, unlike in patients with STEMI. Therefore, the minor myocardial damage possibly has less degree of ROS mediated proteins oxidation.

Another limitation of using oxidative modified biomarkers is the interpretation in elder patients. It has been reported that oxidative modified forms of proteins were accumulated during aging (Berlett & Stadtman1997). For example, increases in proteins carbonyls occur in rat hepatocytes, drosophila, brain, and kidney of mice and in brain tissue of gerbils (Beal2002). In humans proteins carbonyls increase with age in brain, muscle, and human eye lens (Beal2002). The carbonyl content of human fibroblasts also increases as a function of age of the donor (Beal2002).

There are some reports determining other oxidative modified molecules, such as 8-OH-dG, isoprostane, and AGEs, in ACS. However, those reports were indicated only the incidences of elevated markers in ACS, but not the efficiency of the test. Therefore, determination of analytical method efficiency of those markers is challenge and need to be further investigated.

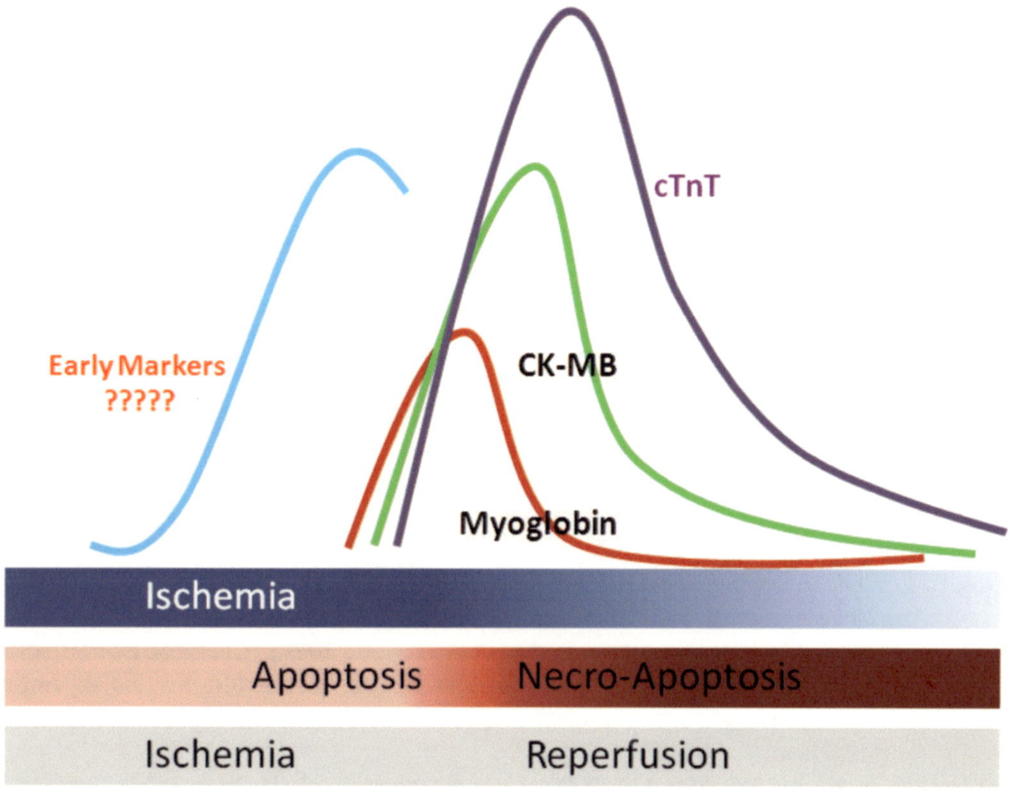

Fig. 9. The kinetics curve of conventional biomarkers. The rise and fall pattern of conventional cardiac biomarkers such as myoglobin, CK-MB, and cTnT. These markers release to circulation many hours after the onset of chest pain, post ischemia. Novel early markers, probably oxidatively modified markers, which release into blood stream, right after the onset of ischemia, will helpful.

6. Conclusion

Early cardiac biomarkers are essential for diagnosis of acute coronary syndrome. Conventional markers might not early enough to detect the early phase of cellular injury according to ischemia. Many oxidatively modified biomolecules were studied and known to have potential as cardiac markers. Further intensive investigation of these cardiac markers, especially the diagnostic power, is very helpful and can be used in real clinical investigation of coronary artery disease.

7. Acknowledgement

This study was supported by Naresuan University research endowment fund, and Faculty of Allied Health Sciences, Naresuan University.

8. References

Abboud, H., Labreuche, J., Meseguer, E., Lavallee, P.C., Simon, O., Olivot, J.M., Mazighi, M., Dehoux, M., Benessiano, J., Steg, P.G., and Amarenco, P., 2007. Ischemia-modified albumin in acute stroke. Cerebrovasc.Dis. 23, 216-220.

Adams, J.E., III, Abendschein, D.R., and Jaffe, A.S., 1993. Biochemical markers of myocardial injury. Is MB creatine kinase the choice for the 1990s? Circulation 88, 750-763.

Akaike, T., Okamoto, S., Sawa, T., Yoshitake, J., Tamura, F., Ichimori, K., Miyazaki, K., Sasamoto, K., and Maeda, H., 2003. 8-nitroguanosine formation in viral pneumonia and its implication for pathogenesis. Proc.Natl.Acad.Sci.U.S.A 100, 685-690.

Almroth, B.C., Sturve, J., Berglund, A., and Forlin, L., 2009. Oxidative damge in eelpout (Zoarces viviparus), measured as protein carbonyls and TBARS, as biomarkers. Aquatic Toxicology 73, 171-180.

Apple, F.S., Wu, A.H., Mair, J., Ravkilde, J., Panteghini, M., Tate, J., Pagani, F., Christenson, R.H., Mockel, M., Danne, O., and Jaffe, A.S., 2005. Future biomarkers for detection of ischemia and risk stratification in acute coronary syndrome. Clin.Chem. 51, 810-824.

Asami, S., Hirano, T., Yamaguchi, R., Tomioka, Y., Itoh, H., and Kasai, H., 1996. Increase of a type of oxidative DNA damage, 8-hydroxyguanine, and its repair activity in human leukocytes by cigarette smoking. Cancer Res. 56, 2546-2549.

Ayres, P.G., 1984. The interation between environmental stress injury and biotic disease physiology. Ann.Rev.Phytopathol 22, 53-75.

Bar-Or, D., Curtis, G., Rao, N., Bampos, N., and Lau, E., 2001a. Characterization of the Co(2+) and Ni(2+) binding amino-acid residues of the N-terminus of human albumin. An insight into the mechanism of a new assay for myocardial ischemia. Eur.J.Biochem. 268, 42-47.

Bar-Or, D., Lau, E., and Winkler, J.V., 2000. A novel assay for cobalt-albumin binding and its potential as a marker for myocardial ischemia-a preliminary report. J.Emerg.Med. 19, 311-315.

Bar-Or, D., Rael, L.T., Lau, E.P., Rao, N.K., Thomas, G.W., Winkler, J.V., Yukl, R.L., Kingston, R.G., and Curtis, C.G., 2001b. An analog of the human albumin N-terminus (Asp-Ala-His-Lys) prevents formation of copper-induced reactive oxygen species. Biochem.Biophys.Res.Commun. 284, 856-862.

Bar-Or, D., Winkler, J.V., Vanbenthuysen, K., Harris, L., Lau, E., and Hetzel, F.W., 2001c. Reduced albumin-cobalt binding with transient myocardial ischemia after elective percutaneous transluminal coronary angioplasty: a preliminary comparison to creatine kinase-MB, myoglobin, and troponin I. Am.Heart J. 141, 985-991.

Beal, M.F., 2002. Oxidatively modified proteins in aging and disease. Free Radic.Biol.Med. 32, 797-803.

Becker, L.B., 2004. New concepts in reactive oxygen species and cardiovascular reperfusion physiology. Cardiovasc.Res. 61, 461-470.

Berlett, B.S. and Stadtman, E.R., 1997. Protein oxidation in aging, disease, and oxidative stress. J.Biol.Chem. 272, 20313-20316.

Bhagavan, N.V., Lai, E.M., Rios, P.A., Yang, J., Ortega-Lopez, A.M., Shinoda, H., Honda, S.A., Rios, C.N., Sugiyama, C.E., and Ha, C.E., 2003. Evaluation of human serum albumin cobalt binding assay for the assessment of myocardial ischemia and myocardial infarction. Clin.Chem. 49, 581-585.

Brownlee, M., Cerami, A., and Vlassara, H., 1988. Advanced glycosylation end products in tissue and the biochemical basis of diabetic complications. N.Engl.J Med 318, 1315-1321.

Buja, L.M., 2005. Myocardial ischemia and reperfusion injury. Cardiovasc.Pathol. 14, 170-175.

Carbonneau, M.A., Peuchant, E., Sess, D., Canioni, P., and Clerc, M., 1991. Free and bound malondialdehyde measured as thiobarbituric acid adduct by HPLC in serum and plasma. Clin Chem. 37, 1423-1429.

Charpentier, S., Ducasse, J.L., Cournot, M., Maupas-Schwalm, F., Elbaz, M., Baixas, C., Juchet, H., Lang, T., and Lauque, D., 2010. Clinical assessment of ischemia-modified albumin and heart fatty acid-binding protein in the early diagnosis of non-ST-elevation acute coronary syndrome in the emergency department. Acad.Emerg.Med. 17, 27-35.

Chu, K.O., Wang, C.C., Rogers, M.S., and Pang, C.P., 2003. Quantifying F2-isoprostanes in umbilical cord blood of newborn by gas chromatography-mass spectrometry. Anal.Biochem 316, 111-117.

Cipollone, F., Ciabattoni, G., Patrignani, P., Pasquale, M., Di, G.D., Bucciarelli, T., Davi, G., Cuccurullo, F., and Patrono, C., 2000. Oxidant stress and aspirin-insensitive thromboxane biosynthesis in severe unstable angina. Circulation 102, 1007-1013.

Collins, A.R., Cadet, J., Moller, L., Poulsen, H.E., and Vina, J., 2004. Are we sure we know how to measure 8-oxo-7,8-dihydroguanine in DNA from human cells? Arch.Biochem Biophys. 423, 57-65.

Cracowski, J.L. and Durand, T., 2006. Cardiovascular pharmacology and physiology of the isoprostanes. Fundam.Clin Pharmacol. 20, 417-427.

Delanty, N., Reilly, M.P., Pratico, D., Lawson, J.A., McCarthy, J.F., Wood, A.E., Ohnishi, S.T., Fitzgerald, D.J., and FitzGerald, G.A., 1997. 8-epi PGF2 alpha generation during coronary reperfusion. A potential quantitative marker of oxidant stress in vivo. Circulation 95, 2492-2499.

Docherty, A., 2010. Acute medical management of the non-ST-segment elevation acute coronary syndromes (NSTE-ACS) in older patients. Arch.Gerontol.Geriatr. 51, 129-134.

Govender, R., De, G.J., Delport, R., Becker, P.J., and Vermaak, W.J., 2008. Biological variation of ischaemia-modified albumin in healthy subjects. Cardiovasc.J.Afr. 19, 141-144.

Green, T.R., Golper, T.A., Swenson, R.D., Pulliam, J.P., and Morris, C.D., 1986. Diagnostic value of creatine kinase and creatine kinase MB isoenzyme in chronic hemodialysis patients: a longitudinal study. Clin Nephrol. 25, 22-27.

Griffiths, H.R., Moller, L., Bartosz, G., Bast, A., Bertoni-Freddari, C., Collins, A., Cooke, M., Coolen, S., Haenen, G., Hoberg, A.M., Loft, S., Lunec, J., Olinski, R., Parry, J., Pompella, A., Poulsen, H., Verhagen, H., and Astley, S.B., 2002. Biomarkers. Mol.Aspects Med. 23, 101-208.

Grimsrud, P.A., Xie, H., Griffin, T.J., and Bernlohr, D.A., 2008. Oxidative stress and covalent modification of protein with bioactive aldehydes. J Biol.Chem. 283, 21837-21841.

Gunduz, A., Turkmen, S., Turedi, S., Mentese, A., Yulug, E., Ulusoy, H., Karahan, S.C., and Topbas, M., 2009. Time-dependent variations in ischemia-modified albumin levels in mesenteric ischemia. Acad.Emerg.Med. 16, 539-543.

Halliwell, B., 2000. Lipid peroxidation, antioxidants and cardiovascular disease: how should we move forward? Cardiovasc.Res. 47, 410-418.

Halliwell, B. and Whiteman, M., 2004. Measuring reactive species and oxidative damage in vivo and in cell culture: how should you do it and what do the results mean? Br.J Pharmacol. 142, 231-255.

Haschke, M., Zhang, Y.L., Kahle, C., Klawitter, J., Korecka, M., Shaw, L.M., and Christians, U., 2007. HPLC-atmospheric pressure chemical ionization MS/MS for quantification of 15-F2t-isoprostane in human urine and plasma. Clin Chem. 53, 489-497.

Hensley, K., Robinson, K.A., Gabbita, S.P., Salsman, S., and Floyd, R.A., 2000. Reactive oxygen species, cell signaling, and cell injury. Free Radic.Biol.Med. 28, 1456-1462.

Himmetoglu, S., Dincer, Y., Bozcali, E., Ali, V., V, and Akcay, T., 2009. Oxidative DNA damage and antioxidant defense after reperfusion in acute myocardial infarction. J Investig.Med. 57, 595-599.

Hiraku, Y., 2010. Formation of 8-nitroguanine, a nitrative DNA lesion, in inflammation-related carcinogenesis and its significance. Environ Health Prev Med 15, 63-72.

Horiike, S., Kawanishi, S., Kaito, M., Ma, N., Tanaka, H., Fujita, N., Iwasa, M., Kobayashi, Y., Hiraku, Y., Oikawa, S., Murata, M., Wang, J., Semba, R., Watanabe, S., and Adachi, Y., 2005. Accumulation of 8-nitroguanine in the liver of patients with chronic hepatitis C. J Hepatol. 43, 403-410.

Iuliano, L., Pratico, D., Greco, C., Mangieri, E., Scibilia, G., FitzGerald, G.A., and Violi, F., 2001. Angioplasty increases coronary sinus F2-isoprostane formation: evidence for in vivo oxidative stress during PTCA. J Am.Coll.Cardiol. 37, 76-80.

Kasai, H., 1997. Analysis of a form of oxidative DNA damage, 8-hydroxy-2'-deoxyguanosine, as a marker of cellular oxidative stress during carcinogenesis. Mutat.Res. 387, 147-163.

Kazanis, K., Dalamaga, M., Nounopoulos, C., Manolis, A.S., Sakellaris, N., Jullien, G., and onyssiou-Asteriou, A., 2009. Ischemia modified albumin, high-sensitivity c-reactive protein and natriuretic peptide in patients with coronary atherosclerosis. Clin Chim.Acta 408, 65-69.

Keating, L., Benger, J.R., Beetham, R., Bateman, S., Veysey, S., Kendall, J., and Pullinger, R., 2006. The PRIMA Study: presentation ischaemia-modified albumin in the emergency department. Emergency Medicine Journal 23, 764-768.

Kilhovd, B.K., Juutilainen, A., Lehto, S., Ronnemaa, T., Torjesen, P.A., Birkeland, K.I., Berg, T.J., Hanssen, K.F., and Laakso, M., 2005. High serum levels of advanced glycation end products predict increased coronary heart disease mortality in nondiabetic women but not in nondiabetic men: a population-based 18-year follow-up study. Arterioscler.Thromb.Vasc.Biol. 25, 815-820.

Kim, J.H., Choi, J.H., Lee, H.K., Bae, W.H., Chun, K.J., Kim, Y.S., Lee, S.K., Kim, H.H., Hong, T.J., and Shin, Y.W., 2008. Ischemia-modified albumin (IMA) is not useful for detecting myocardial ischemia during symptom-limited exercise stress tests. Korean J Intern.Med. 23, 121-126.

Kiuchi, K., Nejima, J., Takano, T., Ohta, M., and Hashimoto, H., 2001. Increased serum concentrations of advanced glycation end products: a marker of coronary artery disease activity in type 2 diabetic patients. Heart 85, 87-91.

Kiyici, A., Mehmetoglu, I., Karaoglan, H., Atalay, H., Solak, Y., and Turk, S., 2010. Ischemia-modified albumin levels in patients with end-stage renal disease patients on hemodialysis: does albumin analysis method affect albumin-adjusted ischemia-modified albumin levels? J.Clin.Lab Anal. 24, 273-277.

Kiyosawa, H., Suko, M., Okudaira, H., Murata, K., Miyamoto, T., Chung, M.H., Kasai, H., and Nishimura, S., 1990. Cigarette smoking induces formation of 8-hydroxydeoxyguanosine, one of the oxidative DNA damages in human peripheral leukocytes. Free Radic.Res.Commun. 11, 23-27.

Kono, Y., Nakamura, K., Kimura, H., Nishii, N., Watanabe, A., Banba, K., Miura, A., Nagase, S., Sakuragi, S., Kusano, K.F., Matsubara, H., and Ohe, T., 2006. Elevated levels of oxidative DNA damage in serum and myocardium of patients with heart failure. Circ.J 70, 1001-1005.

Kumar, S.V., Saritha, G., and Fareedullah, Md., 2010. Role of antioxidants and oxidative stress in cardiovascular disease. Annals of Biological Research 1, 158-173.

Kumphune, S., Mekrungruangwong, T., Luangaram, S., Putaloon, A., Yathingchai, A., Intuyot, K., Opanun, M., Srihawong, P., Samranphat, S., and Thongsri, T., 2010. Diagnostic performance of combinatorial determination of ischemia modified albumin and protein carbobyl in ST elevation myocardial infarction. Journal of medical technology association of Thailand 38, 3418-3431.

le-Donne, I., Aldini, G., Carini, M., Colombo, R., Rossi, R., and Milzani, A., 2006. Protein carbonylation, cellular dysfunction, and disease progression. J Cell Mol.Med. 10, 389-406.

le-Donne, I., Giustarini, D., Colombo, R., Rossi, R., and Milzani, A., 2003a. Protein carbonylation in human diseases. Trends Mol.Med. 9, 169-176.

le-Donne, I., Rossi, R., Giustarini, D., Milzani, A., and Colombo, R., 2003c. Protein carbonyl groups as biomarkers of oxidative stress. Clin Chim.Acta 329, 23-38., 2003d. Protein carbonyl groups as biomarkers of oxidative stress. Clin Chim.Acta 329, 23-38., 2003b. Protein carbonyl groups as biomarkers of oxidative stress. Clin.Chim.Acta 329, 23-38.

Levine, R.L., Williams, J.A., Stadtman, E.R., and Shacter, E., 1994. Carbonyl assays for determination of oxidatively modified proteins. Methods Enzymol. 233, 346-357.

Lindsay, T.F., Luo, X.P., Lehotay, D.C., Rubin, B.B., Anderson, M., Walker, P.M., and Romaschin, A.D., 1999. Ruptured abdominal aortic aneurysm, a "two-hit" ischemia/reperfusion injury: evidence from an analysis of oxidative products. J Vasc.Surg. 30, 219-228.

Lopes-Virella, M.F., Hunt, K.J., Baker, N.L., Lachin, J., Nathan, D.M., and Virella, G., 2011. Levels of oxidized LDL and advanced glycation end products-modified LDL in circulating immune complexes are strongly associated with increased levels of carotid intima-media thickness and its progression in type 1 diabetes. Diabetes 60, 582-589.

Lu, J.M., Lin, P.H., Yao, Q., and Chen, C., 2010. Chemical and molecular mechanisms of antioxidants: experimental approaches and model systems. J Cell Mol.Med. 14, 840-860.

Lushchak, V.I., 2011. Environmentally induced oxidative stress in aquatic animals. Aquat.Toxicol. 101, 13-30.

Ma, N., Adachi, Y., Hiraku, Y., Horiki, N., Horiike, S., Imoto, I., Pinlaor, S., Murata, M., Semba, R., and Kawanishi, S., 2004. Accumulation of 8-nitroguanine in human gastric epithelium induced by Helicobacter pylori infection. Biochem Biophys.Res.Commun. 319, 506-510.

Makita, Z., Radoff, S., Rayfield, E.J., Yang, Z., Skolnik, E., Delaney, V., Friedman, E.A., Cerami, A., and Vlassara, H., 1991. Advanced glycosylation end products in patients with diabetic nephropathy. N.Engl.J Med 325, 836-842.

Maneewong K., Mekrungruangwong T., Luangaram S., Thongsri T., and Kumphune S., 2011. Combinatorial Determination of Ischemia Modified Albumin and Protein Carbonyl in the Diagnosis of Non ST-Elevation Myocardial Infarction. Ind J Clin Biochem.

Matthews, J.N., Altman, D.G., Campbell, M.J., and Royston, P., 1990. Analysis of serial measurements in medical research. BMJ 300, 230-235.

Melanson, S.F. and Tanasijevic, M.J., 2005. Laboratory diagnosis of acute myocardial injury. Cardiovasc.Pathol. 14, 156-161.

Milne, G.L., Musiek, E.S., and Morrow, J.D., 2005. F2-isoprostanes as markers of oxidative stress in vivo: an overview. Biomarkers 10 Suppl 1, S10-S23.

Mocatta, T.J., Pilbrow, A.P., Cameron, V.A., Senthilmohan, R., Frampton, C.M., Richards, A.M., and Winterbourn, C.C., 2007. Plasma concentrations of myeloperoxidase predict mortality after myocardial infarction. J.Am.Coll.Cardiol. 49, 1993-2000.

Mogadam, R.A., Nemati, A., and Baghi A.N., 2008. Serum MDA as a Diagnostic's Biomarker in Stable Coronary Heart Disease. Research Journal of Bological Sciences 3, 206-210.

Montagnana, M., Lippi, G., Volpe, A., Salvagno, G.L., Biasi, D., Caramaschi, P., and Cesare, G.G., 2006. Evaluation of cardiac laboratory markers in patients with systemic sclerosis. Clin Biochem 39, 913-917.

Morrow, D.A., Cannon, C.P., Jesse, R.L., Newby, L.K., Ravkilde, J., Storrow, A.B., Wu, A.H., Christenson, R.H., Apple, F.S., Francis, G., and Tang, W., 2007. National Academy of Clinical Biochemistry Laboratory Medicine Practice Guidelines: clinical characteristics and utilization of biochemical markers in acute coronary syndromes. Clin Chem. 53, 552-574.

Morrow, J.D., Frei, B., Longmire, A.W., Gaziano, J.M., Lynch, S.M., Shyr, Y., Strauss, W.E., Oates, J.A., and Roberts, L.J., 1995. Increase in circulating products of lipid peroxidation (F2-isoprostanes) in smokers. Smoking as a cause of oxidative damage. N.Engl.J Med 332, 1198-1203.

Morrow, J.D., Hill, K.E., Burk, R.F., Nammour, T.M., Badr, K.F., and Roberts, L.J., 1990. A series of prostaglandin F2-like compounds are produced in vivo in humans by a non-cyclooxygenase, free radical-catalyzed mechanism. Proc.Natl.Acad.Sci.U.S.A 87, 9383-9387.

Mutlu-Turkoglu, U., Akalin, Z., Ilhan, E., Yilmaz, E., Bilge, A., Nisanci, Y., and Uysal, M., 2005. Increased plasma malondialdehyde and protein carbonyl levels and lymphocyte DNA damage in patients with angiographically defined coronary artery disease. Clin.Biochem. 38, 1059-1065.

Nagayoshi, Y., Kawano, H., Hokamaki, J., Miyamoto, S., Kojima, S., Shimomura, H., Tsujita, K., Sakamoto, T., Yoshimura, M., and Ogawa, H., 2005. Urinary 8-hydroxy-2'-deoxyguanosine levels increase after reperfusion in acute myocardial infarction and may predict subsequent cardiac events. Am.J Cardiol. 95, 514-517.

Nicholl, I.D. and Bucala, R., 1998. Advanced glycation endproducts and cigarette smoking. Cell Mol.Biol.(Noisy.-le-grand) 44, 1025-1033.

Nielsen, F., Mikkelsen, B.B., Nielsen, J.B., Andersen, H.R., and Grandjean, P., 1997. Plasma malondialdehyde as biomarker for oxidative stress: reference interval and effects of life-style factors. Clin Chem. 43, 1209-1214.

Ogino, K. and Wang, D.H., 2007. Biomarkers of oxidative/nitrosative stress: an approach to disease prevention. Acta Med.Okayama 61, 181-189.

Ohshima, H., Sawa, T., and Akaike, T., 2006. 8-nitroguanine, a product of nitrative DNA damage caused by reactive nitrogen species: formation, occurrence, and implications in inflammation and carcinogenesis. Antioxid.Redox.Signal. 8, 1033-1045.

Ono, Y., Aoki, S., Ohnishi, K., Yasuda, T., Kawano, K., and Tsukada, Y., 1998. Increased serum levels of advanced glycation end products in NIDDM patients with diabetic complications. Diabetes Care 21, 1027.

Pantazopoulos, I., Papadimitriou, L., Dontas, I., Demestiha, T., Iakovidou, N., and Xanthos, T., 2009. Ischaemia modified albumin in the diagnosis of acute coronary syndromes. Resuscitation 80, 306-310.

Panteghini, M., 2002. Acute coronary syndrome: biochemical strategies in the troponin era. Chest 122, 1428-1435.

Pantke, U., Volk, T., Schmutzler, M., Kox, W.J., Sitte, N., and Grune, T., 1999. Oxidized proteins as a marker of oxidative stress during coronary heart surgery. Free Radic.Biol.Med. 27, 1080-1086.

Pasupathi, P., Rao, Y.Y., Farook, J., Saravanan, G., and Bakthavathsalam, G., 2009. Oxidative stress and cardiac biomakrers in patients with acute myocardial infarction. European Journal of Scientific Research 27, 275-285.

Paton, L.N., Mocatta, T.J., Richards, A.M., and Winterbourn, C.C., 2010. Increased thrombin-induced polymerization of fibrinogen associated with high protein carbonyl levels in plasma from patients post myocardial infarction. Free Radic.Biol.Med. 48, 223-229.

Pinlaor, S., Ma, N., Hiraku, Y., Yongvanit, P., Semba, R., Oikawa, S., Murata, M., Sripa, B., Sithithaworn, P., and Kawanishi, S., 2004. Repeated infection with Opisthorchis viverrini induces accumulation of 8-nitroguanine and 8-oxo-7,8-dihydro-2'-deoxyguanine in the bile duct of hamsters via inducible nitric oxide synthase. Carcinogenesis 25, 1535-1542.

Rajesh, K.G., Surekha, R.H., Mrudula, S.K., Prasad, Y., Sanjib, K.S., and Prathiba, N., 2011. Oxidative and nitrosative stress in association with DNA damage in coronary heart disease. Singapore Med J 52, 283-288.

Rao, V. and Kiran, R., 2011. Evaluation of correlation between oxidative stress and abnormal lipid profile in coronary artery disease. J Cardiovasc.Dis.Res. 2, 57-60.

Reilly, M., Delanty, N., Lawson, J.A., and FitzGerald, G.A., 1996. Modulation of oxidant stress in vivo in chronic cigarette smokers. Circulation 94, 19-25.

Reilly, M.P., Delanty, N., Roy, L., Rokach, J., Callaghan, P.O., Crean, P., Lawson, J.A., and FitzGerald, G.A., 1997. Increased formation of the isoprostanes IPF2alpha-I and 8-epi-prostaglandin F2alpha in acute coronary angioplasty: evidence for oxidant stress during coronary reperfusion in humans. Circulation 96, 3314-3320.

Reimer, K.A. and Ideker, R.E., 1987. Myocardial ischemia and infarction: anatomic and biochemical substrates for ischemic cell death and ventricular arrhythmias. Hum.Pathol. 18, 462-475.

Sakamoto, H., Corcoran, T.B., Laffey, J.G., and Shorten, G.D., 2002. Isoprostanes--markers of ischaemia reperfusion injury. Eur.J Anaesthesiol. 19, 550-559.

Santalo, B.M., Guindo, S.J., and Ordonez, L.J., 2003. [Biological markers of myocardial necrosis]. Rev.Esp.Cardiol. 56, 703-720.

Sawa, T., Tatemichi, M., Akaike, T., Barbin, A., and Ohshima, H., 2006. Analysis of urinary 8-nitroguanine, a marker of nitrative nucleic acid damage, by high-performance liquid chromatography-electrochemical detection coupled with immunoaffinity purification: association with cigarette smoking. Free Radic.Biol.Med. 40, 711-720.

Sbarouni, E., Georgiadou, P., Kremastinos, D.T., and Voudris, V., 2008a. Ischemia modified albumin: is this marker of ischemia ready for prime time use? Hellenic.J Cardiol. 49, 260-266.

Sbarouni, E., Georgiadou, P., Panagiotakos, D., Kyrzopoulos, S., Tsiapras, D., Voudris, V., and Kremastinos, D.T., 2008b. Ischemia modified albumin in relation to pharmacologic stress testing in coronary artery disease. Clin Chim.Acta 396, 58-61.

Sbarouni, E., Georgiadou, P., Panagiotakos, D., Livanis, E., Theodorakis, G.N., and Kremastinos, D.T., 2008c. The ischemia-modified albumin in relation to pacemaker and defibrillator implantation. Pacing Clin Electrophysiol. 31, 83-87.

Sharma, R., Gaze, D.C., Pellerin, D., Mehta, R.L., Gregson, H., Streather, C.P., Collinson, P.O., and Brecker, S.J., 2007. Evaluation of ischaemia-modified albumin as a marker of myocardial ischaemia in end-stage renal disease. Clin Sci.(Lond) 113, 25-32.

Shen, X.L., Lin, C.J., Han, L.L., Lin, L., Pan, L., and Pu, X.D., 2010. Assessment of ischemia-modified albumin levels for emergency room diagnosis of acute coronary syndrome. Int J.Cardiol.

Siegel, A.J., Lewandrowski, K.B., Strauss, H.W., Fischman, A.J., and Yasuda, T., 1995. Normal post-race antimyosin myocardial scintigraphy in asymptomatic marathon runners with elevated serum creatine kinase MB isoenzyme and troponin T levels. Evidence against silent myocardial cell necrosis. Cardiology 86, 451-456.

Sinha, M.K., Gaze, D.C., Tippins, J.R., Collinson, P.O., and Kaski, J.C., 2003. Ischemia modified albumin is a sensitive marker of myocardial ischemia after percutaneous coronary intervention. Circulation 107, 2403-2405.

Takahashi, N., Takahashi, Y., and Putnam, F.W., 1987. Structural changes and metal binding by proalbumins and other amino-terminal genetic variants of human serum albumin. Proc.Natl.Acad.Sci.U.S.A 84, 7403-7407.

Takhshid, M.A., Kojuri, J., Kojuri, S., Tavasouli, A.R., Heidary, S., and Tabandeh, M., 2010. Early Diagnosis of Acute Coronary Syndrome with Sensitive Troponin I and Ischemia Modified Albumin. Iranian Cardiovascular Research Journal 4, 144-151.

Turedi, S., Cinar, O., Yavuz, I., Mentese, A., Gunduz, A., Karahan, S.C., Topbas, M., Cevik, E., Yildirim, A.O., Uzun, A., and Kaldirim, U., 2010. Differences in ischemia-modified albumin levels between end stage renal disease patients and the normal population. J.Nephrol. 23, 335-340.

Valavanidis, A., Vlachogianni, T., and Fiotakis, C., 2009. 8-hydroxy-2' -deoxyguanosine (8-OHdG): A critical biomarker of oxidative stress and carcinogenesis. J Environ.Sci.Health C.Environ.Carcinog.Ecotoxicol.Rev. 27, 120-139.

Valko, M., Leibfritz, D., Moncol, J., Cronin, M.T., Mazur, M., and Telser, J., 2007. Free radicals and antioxidants in normal physiological functions and human disease. Int J.Biochem.Cell Biol. 39, 44-84.

Van, B.E., Dallongeville, J., Vicaut, E., Degrandsart, A., Baulac, C., and Montalescot, G., 2010. Ischemia-modified albumin levels predict long-term outcome in patients with acute myocardial infarction. The French Nationwide OPERA study. Am.Heart J. 159, 570-576.

Walter, M.F., Jacob, R.F., Jeffers, B., Ghadanfar, M.M., Preston, G.M., Buch, J., and Mason, R.P., 2004. Serum levels of thiobarbituric acid reactive substances predict cardiovascular events in patients with stable coronary artery disease: a longitudinal analysis of the PREVENT study. J Am.Coll.Cardiol. 44, 1996-2002.

Wiviott, S.D. and Braunwald, E., 2004. Unstable angina and non-ST-segment elevation myocardial infarction: part I. Initial evaluation and management, and hospital care. Am.Fam.Physician 70, 525-532.

Wong, S.H., Knight, J.A., Hopfer, S.M., Zaharia, O., Leach, C.N., Jr., and Sunderman, F.W., Jr., 1987. Lipoperoxides in plasma as measured by liquid-chromatographic separation of malondialdehyde-thiobarbituric acid adduct. Clin Chem. 33, 214-220.

Wood, G.N., Keevil, B., Gupta, J., Foley, R., Bubtana, A., McDowell, G., and Ackrill, P., 2003. Serum troponin T measurement in patients with chronic renal impairment predicts survival and vascular disease: a 2 year prospective study. Nephrol.Dial.Transplant. 18, 1610-1615.

World Heatlh Organization, 2009 World Heath Statistics 2008.

Wu, A.H., Apple, F.S., Gibler, W.B., Jesse, R.L., Warshaw, M.M., and Valdes, R., Jr., 1999. National Academy of Clinical Biochemistry Standards of Laboratory Practice: recommendations for the use of cardiac markers in coronary artery diseases. Clin Chem. 45, 1104-1121.

Wudkowska, A., Goch, J., and Goch, A., 2010. Ischemia-modified albumin in differential diagnosis of acute coronary syndrome without ST elevation and unstable angina pectoris. Kardiol.Pol. 68, 431-437.

Yeo, H.C., Helbock, H.J., Chyu, D.W., and Ames, B.N., 1994. Assay of malondialdehyde in biological fluids by gas chromatography-mass spectrometry. Anal.Biochem 220, 391-396.

Zieman, S.J. and Kass, D.A., 2004. Advanced glycation endproduct crosslinking in the cardiovascular system: potential therapeutic target for cardiovascular disease. Drugs 64, 459-470.

Section 4

Diabetes Mellitus

10

Oxidative Stress in Diabetes Mellitus: Is There a Role for Hypoglycemic Drugs and/or Antioxidants?

Omotayo O. Erejuwa
Department of Pharmacology,
School of Medical Sciences,
Universiti Sains Malaysia,
Malaysia

1. Introduction

The most recent statistics indicate that the global prevalence of diabetes mellitus, estimated as 366 million in 2011, will increase to 522 million by 2030 (Whiting et al., 2011). Diabetes mellitus is a metabolic disorder of multiple etiology characterized by chronic hyperglycemia with disturbances of carbohydrate, fat and protein metabolism resulting from defects in insulin secretion and/or insulin action (ADA, 2011). There are basically two types of diabetes mellitus: type 1 and type 2 diabetes mellitus. Type 1 diabetes mellitus, an autoimmune disease, is characterized by the loss of pancreatic β-cells resulting in absolute insulin deficiency. It accounts for about 5-10 % of all newly diagnosed diabetes mellitus (ADA, 2011). On the other hand, type 2 diabetes mellitus is characterized by insulin resistance and β cell dysfunction. It remains the most common form of diabetes mellitus and constitutes about 90-95 % of all diabetes cases (ADA, 2011). In spite of the availability of different classes of oral hypoglycemic drugs, the incidence of microvascular complications (nephropathy, retinopathy and neuropathy) and macrovascular complications atherosclerosis, coronary artery disease, peripheral arterial disease and stroke continues to rise unabated in diabetic patients, even with treatment (Roglic and Unwin, 2010).

Pharmacological agents with different mechanisms of action are often combined to achieve optimal glycemic control (Turner et al., 1999). However, despite the use of multiple drugs, a lot of diabetic patients do not achieve the optimal glycemic goal (Turner et al., 1999). The Diabetes Control and Complications Trial (DCCT) and the United Kingdom Prospective Diabetes Study (UKPDS) have demonstrated that intensive treatment of hyperglycemia reduces risk of developing microvascular and macrovascular complications (DCCT, 1993, UKPDS, 1998). However, recent findings indicate that intensive treatment of hyperglycemia is associated with higher incidence of weight gain, hypoglycemia and mortality than conventional therapy (Ismail-Beigi et al., 2010). These findings suggest that intensive therapy is not only detrimental, but limited and may not be the best. Besides, these findings may suggest that it is high time "hyperglycemia alone" was made the "culprit" in the management of diabetes mellitus. Generally, hypoglycemic drugs are incapable to prevent pancreas degeneration, worsening of glycemic control and diabetic complications (DCCT, 1993, UKPDS, 1998, Turner et al., 1999, Ball et al., 2000). All these have been linked to increased oxidative stress in diabetes mellitus (Figueroa-Romero et al., 2008, Giacco and Brownlee, 2010). The aim of this chapter is to shed more light on the prospective of managing diabetes mellitus more effectively by targeting both "hyperglycemia and oxidative stress simultaneously". The data presented in this chapter convincingly suggest that the current management of diabetes mellitus may be improved upon by targeting hyperglycemia and oxidative stress as two potential therapeutic targets in diabetes mellitus.

2. General overview of oxidative stress

Considering the aim of this chapter, the general concept of oxidative stress will be discussed only in brief. Oxidative stress can defined as an "imbalance between oxidants and antioxidants in favor of the oxidants, potentially leading to damage" (Sies, 1991). According to Halliwell, "oxidative stress refers to a serious imbalance between reactive species production and antioxidant defenses" (Halliwell and Gutteridge, 2007). It occurs due to an increased generation and/or reduced elimination of reactive species (RS) by the antioxidant defense system. Oxidative stress is usually associated with oxidative damage, which is defined as "the biomolecular damage caused by attack of RS upon the constituents of living organisms" (Halliwell and Gutteridge, 2007). Most of the biologically relevant RS are either reactive oxygen species (ROS) or reactive nitrogen species (RNS). ROS include free radicals such as superoxide ($O_2^{\bullet-}$) and hydroxyl ($^{\bullet}OH$), and non-free radicals such as hydrogen peroxide (H_2O_2). Reactive nitrogen species include free radicals such as nitric oxide ($^{\bullet}NO$) and nitrogen dioxide ($NO_2^{\bullet-}$), and non-free radicals such as peroxynitrite ($OONO^-$) (Sies, 1991, Halliwell and Gutteridge, 2007). The generation of RS by aerobic organisms may occur as by products of metabolism (e.g. during operation of electron transfer chains), intentionally (e.g. during inflammation), or as a result of accidents of chemistry (such as the autoxidation of unstable biomolecules, e.g. dopamine) (Halliwell, 2011). Of all the RS, significant roles of $O_2^{\bullet-}$, $^{\bullet}NO$, and $OONO^-$ have been implicated in diabetic cardiovascular complications (Johansen et al., 2005). In order to prevent oxidative damage, it is important that excess RS is eliminated from the cells. Oxidative damage to cellular components impairs cellular functions. Besides their toxicities, ROS are also required in certain conditions and for physiological functions. For instance, during inflammation, the phagocytes release ROS which kill invading bacteria. ROS generated during mild or moderate exercise constitute part of the mechanism of exercise- or training-induced adaptation (Sachdev and Davies, 2008).

The ability of cells or tissues to withstand oxidative stress is largely dependent on the efficiency of the overall antioxidant defense system to scavenge excess RS, without compromising the physiological roles of ROS (Halliwell, 2011). The antioxidant defense system consists of endogenously-synthesized antioxidants which include antioxidant enzymes, glutathione, vitamins, small molecules and micronutrients (Sies, 1991, Halliwell and Gutteridge, 2007). An antioxidant is defined as "any substance that delays, prevents or removes oxidative damage to a target molecule" (Halliwell and Gutteridge, 2007). Antioxidant enzymes are enzymes which scavenge or eliminate a variety of RS including those generated during biological processes (Sies, 1991, Halliwell and Gutteridge, 2007). The main antioxidant enzymes are superoxide dismutase (SOD), catalase (CAT) and glutathione peroxidase (GPx) (Halliwell, 2011). SOD maintains the cellular levels of $O_2^{\bullet -}$ within the physiological concentrations by converting $O_2^{\bullet -}$ to H_2O_2, a more stable ROS (Halliwell and Gutteridge, 2007, Fukai and Ushio-Fukai, 2011). CAT metabolizes H_2O_2 to O_2 and H_2O (Halliwell and Gutteridge, 2007). CAT exerts two enzymatic activities, depending on the concentrations of its substrate (H_2O_2) (Scibior and Czeczot, 2006). It elicits a catalytic function at high concentrations of H_2O_2, whereas it produces a peroxidatic effect at lower concentrations of H_2O_2 (Scibior and Czeczot, 2006). GPx enzymatically reduces H_2O_2 to O_2 and H_2O using a hydrogen donor, glutathione (GSH) which is oxidized to glutathione disulfide (GSSG) (Lubos et al., 2011). Unlike CAT, GPx has a broader spectrum of substrates, detoxifying organic hydroperoxides and lipid peroxides (Lubos et al., 2011). However, CAT compared to GPx has a higher K_M for H_2O_2 and thus can protect against a higher concentration of H_2O_2 (Halliwell and Gutteridge, 2007).

The other antioxidant enzymes include glutathione reductase (GR), glutathione S-transferase (GST), peroxiredoxin, thioredoxin and thioredoxinreductase (Andreyev et al., 2005). GR scavenges $O_2^{\bullet -}$ and $^{\bullet}OH$ non-enzymatically or by serving as an electron donor to certain enzymes involved in the metabolism of ROS (Andreyev et al., 2005, Slonchak and Obolens'ka, 2009). GR helps to regenerate GSH via reduction of oxidized glutathione (GSSG) (Slonchak and Obolens'ka, 2009). GST comprises a family of multifunctional phase II biotransformation enzymes with a broad spectrum for a variety of substrates including epoxides, carcinogens, mutagens, 4-hydroxy-2-nonenal and malondialdehyde (MDA) (Andreyev et al., 2005, Slonchak and Obolens'ka, 2009). It catalyzes the conjugation of many electrophilic compounds with GSH (Andreyev et al., 2005). These enzymes work co-operatively together in order to scavenge RS and xenobiotics and thereby protect cells against oxidative damage (Halliwell, 2011). Generally, antioxidant enzymes differ from one another in terms of structure, tissue distribution, co-factor requirement, function, substrate specificity and affinity. The uniqueness of the antioxidant defense system lies in its capability to maintain the RS at certain steady-state levels thereby create and maintain a balance between the beneficial and injurious effects of RS (Lushchak, 2010). More detailed information on oxidative stress including free radicals, ROS, RNS, antioxidant enzymes, antioxidants, antioxidant defense system, and markers of oxidative stress can be obtained from following references (Sies, 1991, Johansen et al., 2005, Halliwell and Gutteridge, 2007, Halliwell, 2011).

3. Oxidative stress and its sources in diabetes mellitus

Under normal conditions and in most diseases including diabetes mellitus, mitochondria are the main source of RS and oxidative stress. Under physiological conditions, e.g. during mitochondrial oxidative metabolism, the bulk of oxygen (O_2) utilized is reduced to H_2O, while less than 2% of O_2 consumed is converted to $O_2^{\bullet -}$ (Brand, 2010). $O_2^{\bullet -}$ is an important ROS because it may be converted to other RS including H_2O_2, OH and $ONOO^-$ (Andreyev et al., 2005). Within physiological conditions, the body is protected from the detrimental effects of these free radicals by a network of antioxidant defense system. However, this defense system becomes impaired in diabetes mellitus and is further exacerbated by chronic hyperglycemia which generates ROS, resulting in oxidative stress. Some of the various sources of ROS and oxidative stress in diabetes mellitus include:

3.1 Hyperglycemia

Chronic hyperglycemia is the hallmark of diabetes mellitus. Evidence implicates mitochondrial generation of $O_2^{\bullet-}$ as a significant source of ROS (Andreyev et al., 2005). With persistent hyperglycemia, disproportionate amounts of glucose are delivered to the cells. This results in enhanced glucose flux through glycolysis and the tricarboxylic acid (TCA) cycle (Drews et al., 2010). This leads to an overdrive of the mitochondrial electron transport chain, which generates greater amounts of $O_2^{\bullet-}$ more than mitochondrial SOD can dismutase (Wiernsperger, 2003, Brand, 2010). This tilts the normal delicate balance between mitochondrial ROS production and mitochondrial ROS degradation in favor of mitochondrial ROS generation, and oxidative stress ensues (Brand, 2010). Evidence indicates that hyperglycemia-induced excessive mitochondrial $O_2^{\bullet-}$ production plays an important role in generating other RS in diabetes mellitus (Nishikawa et al., 2000b). Furthermore, glucose autooxidation produces ROS in the presence of transition metal ions (Johansen et al., 2005). Elevated glucose in diabetes may also react with lipids, resulting in the generation of RS (Johansen et al., 2005). Through non-enzymatic glycation reaction, glucose can react with proteins to produce several intermediate products such as Amadori and Sciff base products before generating advanced glycosylation endproducts (AGEs) (Johansen et al., 2005). Evidence indicates ROS are generated at each step of these reactions. Moreover, with excessive glucose in diabetes, it has been shown that glucose is diverted to other pathways such as sorbitol and hexosamine pathways where glucose is metabolized and ROS are generated (Johansen et al., 2005, Figueroa-Romero et al., 2008, Giacco and Brownlee, 2010).

3.2 Impaired antioxidant defense system

Impaired antioxidant defense system, such as reduced levels of endogenous antioxidants, reduced/enhanced antioxidant enzyme activities and increased levels of oxidative stress markers such as MDA, is very common in diabetes mellitus (Maritim et al., 2003, Johansen et al., 2005, Rahimi et al., 2005, Erejuwa et al., 2010a). The insufficient scavenging of RS as a result of impaired antioxidant defense system in diabetes may contribute to increased oxidative damage. The mechanisms for the impaired antioxidant defenses in diabetes mellitus remain poorly understood. It may be due to non-enzymatic glycation of these enzymes by hyperglycemia and thereby impairs their individual functions. Furthermore, evidence indicates that the antioxidant enzymes produce optimal protection when they function together (Michiels et al., 1994). Thus, glycation of any of these antioxidant enzymes may impair the efficiency of the entire antioxidant defense system or network. For instance, if SOD activity is impaired, this may result in $O_2^{\bullet-}$ build-up. On the other hand, if SOD activity is up-regulated, this may result in increased levels of H_2O_2. In either case, this may affect the activity of CAT or GPx. Similarly, if GR activity is impaired, there may be increased steady-state GSSG levels which will prevent regeneration of GSH, an endogenous antioxidant.

3.3 Increased activity of ROS-generating enzymes

The activities of many ROS-generating enzymes such as cyclooxygenase, xanthine oxidase, lipoxygenases, myeloperoxidase, NADPH oxidases and eNOS are augmented in diabetes (Wiernsperger, 2003). Besides, evidence implicates a role of endothelial NO synthase (eNOS). The eNOS produces NO which scavenges $O_2^{\bullet-}$ in non-diabetic subjects. However, the eNOS has been found to be uncoupled in diabetic blood vessels where it produces O_2•− instead of •NO (Wiernsperger, 2003). Hyperglycemia might play an important role in the upregulation and uncoupling of ROS-generating enzymes.

3.4 Hyperinsulinemia

Insulin resistance characterized by hyperinsulinemia is frequent in the majority of the individuals with type 2 diabetic mellitus. Insulin induces the release of H_2O_2 when activating its receptors (Wiernsperger, 2003). Even though H_2O_2 is a non-free radical, it is membrane permeable and can diffuse to other sites, different from its site of production (Sies, 1991, Halliwell and Gutteridge, 2007). Chronic hyperinsulinemia together with the impaired antioxidant defenses in diabetes will lead to inefficient scavenging of H_2O_2. In the presence of transition metals such as copper and iron, H_2O_2 undergoes Fenton reaction to generate •OH which is implicated in the initiation and propagation of lipid peroxidation. Thus, hyperinsulinemia via H_2O_2 formation may increase RS and contribute to oxidative stress and damage in diabetes mellitus. Besides, insulin stimulates the release of many neurotransmitters, via activation of sympathetic nervous system. Many of these neurotransmitters are known to generate ROS and induce oxidative stress (Wiernsperger, 2003).

3.5 Insulin deficiency

Insulin deficiency is frequently observed in the diabetic patients. In some type 2 diabetic patients, insulin deficiency may be so severe such that the injection of exogenous insulin is required to control hyperglycemia (Turner et al., 1999, Cook et al., 2005). Insulin deficiency augments the activity of fatty acyl coenzyme A oxidase. Fatty acyl coenzyme A oxidase is an enzyme which is responsible for the oxidation of fatty acids, resulting in the increased generation of H_2O_2 (Schonfeld et al., 2009). H_2O_2 is well recognized for its role in exerting deleterious effects on cellular components such as proteins, nucleic acid and lipids including polyunsaturated fatty acids (PUFAs) (Sies, 1991, Halliwell and Gutteridge, 2007). These injurious effects of H_2O_2 can be mediated directly or indirectly through •OH formation or reaction with transition metals (such as copper or iron) to form toxic aldehydes, which are highly susceptible to free radical attack (Sies, 1991, Halliwell and Gutteridge, 2007). This sets up a chain reaction which further propagates the formation of more free radicals or RS and thereby contributes to or exacerbate oxidative stress.

3.6 Other sources of ROS and oxidative stress in diabetes mellitus

Diabetes mellitus is characterized by lipid abnormalities such as elevated LDL and cholesterol (ADA, 2011). These abnormalities are further exacerbated by the increased oxidizing environment which enhances the formation of oxidized LDLs (oxLDLs), glycated LDL and oxysterols (formed from the oxidation of cholesterol) (Johansen et al., 2005). These oxidized lipid products bind to specific receptor proteins or activate inflammatory proteins which generate ROS (Johansen et al., 2005). The import of oxLDLs in the vascular wall is the main mechanism by which ROS and oxidative stress induce atherosclerosis (Sies, 1991, Wiernsperger, 2003, Halliwell and Gutteridge, 2007). Evidence indicates that the levels of certain pro-oxidants such as ferritin and homocysteine are elevated in diabetes (Penckofer et al., 2002). Free iron can increase ROS generation and the oxidation of LDL cholesterol. Similarly, homocysteine can generate ROS in the presence of transition metals which may enhance the oxidation of LDL cholesterol (Penckofer et al., 2002). Another source of ROS in diabetes mellitus is leptin. Elevated levels of leptin are associated with insulin resistance and diabetes mellitus. Evidence implicates a role of leptin in inducing ROS and oxidative stress in aortic endothelial cells in a dose-dependent manner while it produces additive effects with those of glucose (Wiernsperger, 2003). Other potential sources of ROS include aging, menopause, diet and physical activity (Penckofer et al., 2002). Increased ROS is reported in older people. Menopause may also enhance ROS production in older women. The levels of oestrogen, an antioxidant which decreases the oxidation of LDL cholesterol, usually decline during menopause (Penckofer et al., 2002). Aging and menopause may exacerbate oxidative stress since a large number of type 2 diabetics are older men and women. Consumption of foods rich in carbohydrates and fats, as opposed to antioxidant-enriched diets, may also enhance ROS formation. Sedentary lifestyle may predispose to increased ROS generation. This is corroborated by evidence which indicates mild or moderate, but not strenuous, exercise induces antioxidant defenses (Sachdev and Davies, 2008).

4. Role of oxidative stress in the pathogenesis of diabetes mellitus

Evidence implicates the role of oxidative stress in the different stages of the development of diabetes mellitus, starting from the pre-diabetes state, impaired glucose tolerance, postprandial hyperglycemia, mild diabetes and finally to overt diabetes mellitus (Ceriello et al., 1998). Loss of β-cell function, resulting from impaired secretory capacity and increased apoptosis, is a main occurrence in the pathogenesis of both types of diabetes (Drews et al., 2010). Besides β-cell dysfunction, insulin resistance is also a major characteristic feature of type 2 diabetes mellitus (Evans et al., 2003). Oxidative stress plays an important role in the pathogenesis of both β-cell dysfunction and insulin resistance (Evans et al., 2003, Drews et al., 2010).

4.1 Role of oxidative stress in β-cell dysfunction

The β-cells express low level of antioxidant enzymes such as SOD, CAT and GPx and thereby increase their susceptibility to oxidative stress (Tiedge et al., 1997). Increased mitochondrial ROS production in the β-cells results from enhanced glucose or fatty acid flux through glycolysis and the TCA cycle (Drews et al., 2010). This generates excess $O_2^{\bullet -}$ which gives rise to other ROS and RNS. The insufficiency of antioxidant enzymes to scavenge these ROS leads to oxidative stress. Besides mitochondria, NADPH oxidases, nitric oxide synthases, and phagocytes are other key sources of ROS in the β-cells (Drews et al., 2010). In type 1 diabetes mellitus, evidence implicates the role of ROS in impaired β-cell function caused by autoimmune reactions, cytokines and inflammatory proteins (Drews et al., 2010). Similarly, in type 2 diabetes mellitus, the role of ROS is implicated in the β-cell dysfunction as well as insulin resistance (Drews et al., 2010). The pancreas is highly susceptible to oxidative stress as evidenced by studies which show that H_2O_2 impairs insulin secretion in pancreatic β-cells (Maechler et al., 1999) and products of oxidative stress inhibit glucose-stimulated insulin secretion (Miwa et al., 2000). Other evidence shows that overexpression of antioxidant enzymes in islets or transgenic mice and antioxidants such as N-acetyl-L-cysteine (NAC) protect against ROS-induced β-cell toxicity (Tiedge et al., 1998, Drews et al.,

2010). Research within the last decade has recognized the role of glucotoxicity as the main causal determinant of β-cell dysfunction (Drews et al., 2010). The role of glucotoxicity in β-cell dysfunction is demonstrated by studies which indicate increased glucose concentrations impair insulin release in non-diabetic subjects (Marchetti et al., 2008). In contrast, improved glycemic control results in improved insulin secretion in patients with type 2 diabetes (Marchetti et al., 2008). The fact that antioxidants reduce or prevent the toxicities of elevated glucose on the expression of insulin mRNA, insulin content and secretion lends support to the role of oxidative stress in mediating the toxic effects of glucotoxicity (Tanaka et al., 1999). Besides glucotoxicity, lipotoxicity may also play a role in impaired β-cell function. Free fatty acids have been shown to uncouple mitochondrial oxidative phosphorylation and increase ROS formation in rat pancreatic islets (Carlsson et al., 1999), deplete pancreatic β-cell insulin content (Bollheimer et al., 1998) and inhibit glucose-induced insulin secretion and biosynthesis (Zhou and Grill, 1994). Both glucotoxicity and lipotoxicity may be involved in β-cell dysfunction in diabetes mellitus (Marchetti et al., 2008). The role of oxidative stress is also implicated in β-cell deficit, as well as increased apoptosis observed in humans with type 2 diabetes (Drews et al., 2010).

4.2 Role of oxidative stress in insulin resistance

Insulin resistance precedes the onset of diabetes mellitus and is influenced by factors such as genetic make-up and environmental factors including increased calorie intake, sedentary lifestyle, obesity, pregnancy and abnormally elevated levels of certain hormones (Evans et al., 2003). The role of oxidative stress is implicated in the pathogenesis of insulin resistance (Kim et al., 2006). Both pyruvate and fatty acids can serve as energy substrate in muscle and adipose tissue. Pyruvate is derived from glucose and other sugars, while fatty acids originate from fats. Once transported across the inner mitochondrial membrane, these fuel substrates are converted to acetyl CoA by mitochondrial enzymes. During citric acid cycle, oxidation of the carbon atoms of the acetyl groups in acetyl CoA generates CO_2. Besides CO_2 formation, the citric acid cycle generates high-energy electrons which are carried by NADH and $FADH_2$. The increased uptake of energy substrate in the muscle and adipose tissue enhances citric acid cycle activity. This in turn generates mitochondrial NADH more than required. This leads to an overdrive of the oxidative phosphorylation which increases the mitochondrial transmembrane proton gradient. These high-energy electrons are then transferred to O_2 leading to production of $O_2^{\bullet-}$ which is further converted to other ROS. This sets the stage for oxidative stress (Talior et al., 2003). A recent study showed that the skeletal muscle of high-fat diet-induced insulin-resistant rats liberated more mitochondrial H_2O_2 and had impaired ability to maintain normal redox balance compared to the data obtained in the skeletal muscle of the insulin-sensitive control rats (Anderson et al., 2009). Similar findings were observed in insulin-resistant, morbidly obese human subjects (Anderson et al., 2009). This study provides strong evidence in support of a role of mitochondrial ROS production and oxidative stress in the pathogenesis of insulin resistance.

Various mechanisms by which oxidative stress contributes to insulin resistance have been identified. These include oxidative stress-impaired insulin-induced GLUT4 translocation in adipocytes (Rudich et al., 1998), oxidative stress-induced impairment in insulin stimulation of protein kinase B and glucose transport in adipocytes (Rudich et al., 1999), oxidative stress-induced interactions between the PI3-kinase-dependent signaling pathway and activation of p38 MAPK (Kim et al., 2006), and interruption of insulin-induced cellular redistribution of insulin receptor substrate-1 and phosphatidylinositol 3-kinase in adipocytes (Tirosh et al., 1999). Other studies indicate that oxidative stress can directly induce considerable insulin resistance in skeletal muscle by interfering with insulin signaling, glucose uptake and glycogen synthesis (Dokken et al., 2008). This oxidative stress-induced insulin resistance is mediated in part through reduced insulin-modulated suppression of glycogen synthase kinase-3 (GSK-3beta) (Dokken *et al.*, 2008; Henriksen, 2010). Evidence has also implicated a role of inducible nitric oxide synthase and •NO donor in the degradation of insulin receptor substrate-1. Increased S-nitrosylation of certain molecules or pathways involved in insulin signaling such as insulin receptor, insulin receptor substrate-1, and protein kinase B/Akt in skeletal muscle have also been reported to play an important role in insulin resistance (Carvalho-Filho et al., 2009).

In order to protect against increased glucose-induced oxidative stress (Talior et al., 2003), cells tend to respond by limiting more energy fuel or substrates from gaining access into the cells. Cells may utilize various mechanisms, including inhibition of α-ketoglutarate dehydrogenase, to limit the amount of NADH available for the oxidative phosphorylation. Therefore, to limit insulin-dependent nutrient uptake into the cells, the insulin receptors become less sensitive to the action of insulin. This marks the onset of insulin resistance - a phenomenon whereby normal amounts of insulin can no longer activate the glucose transport system in insulin-sensitive tissues such as skeletal muscle and adipose tissue. This results in enhanced steady-state glucose levels in the blood. It is suggested that, in this setting, insulin resistance may be a compensatory mechanism employed by the cells to prevent further uptake of insulin-stimulated glucose and fatty acids (Hoehn et al., 2009). This compensatory mechanism may result in reduced formation and accumulation of RS leading to reduced oxidative stress and damage. With persistently increased blood glucose levels, hyperglycemia ensues leading to overt type 2 diabetes mellitus.

4.3 Could antioxidants play a role in preventing diabetes mellitus and/or its progression?

In view of evidence which implicates a role of oxidative stress in β-cell dysfunction and insulin resistance, the question that arises is: could antioxidants play a role in preventing diabetes mellitus and/or its progression? As discussed earlier, there is a possibility for such a role of antioxidants. Antioxidants such as vitamin C, vitamin E, β-carotene, α-lipoic acids and honey have been shown to ameliorate hyperglycemia through increased β-cell mass and insulin secretion. However, at the moment, the evidence to recommend or prescribe antioxidants for the prevention of diabetes mellitus is very weak. Instead, efforts should be made to create and increase the awareness on (1) the role of ROS and oxidative stress in the pathogenesis and/or progression of diabetes mellitus and (2) the importance of increased consumption of antioxidant-enriched diets including fruits and vegetables, as opposed to increased calorie intake. The recommendation for increased consumption of fruits and vegetables is very important because even in the developed countries, majority of the population do not meet these requirements. The importance of exercise should also not be left out. These could be achieved by incorporating into educational curricula - at all levels of education. In addition, those who are already diabetic should be enlightened on the importance of maintaining good glycemic control in order to prevent or delay the progression or complications of diabetes mellitus. Diabetic patients also need to be informed on the need for adherence to dietary regimens and compliance to prescribed medications. These recommendations could also be an important component of training received by healthcare providers.

5. Role of oxidative stress in the complications of diabetes mellitus

There is strong evidence implicating a role of oxidative stress in diabetic nephropathy, retinopathy and neuropathy which constitute the microvascular complications (Figueroa-Romero et al., 2008, Giacco and Brownlee, 2010, Brownlee, 2005). Similarly, a role of oxidative stress is implicated in the macrovascular complications (coronary artery disease, peripheral arterial disease and cerebrovascular disease) (Giacco and Brownlee, 2010, Brownlee, 2005). This section highlights the different mechanisms by which hyperglycemia causes diabetic complications.

5.1 Hyperglycemia-enhanced polyol pathway

The polyol pathway comprises two enzymes: aldose reductase (AR) and sorbitol dehydrogenase (SDH) (Brownlee, 2005). AR reduces a broad spectrum of substrates such as glucose, galactose, methylglyoxal, glucosone, deoxyglucosone and lipid-derived aldehydes (Petrash, 2004). Under euglycemic conditions, glucose is not reduced by AR. The bulk of glucose is normally phosphorylated by hexokinase to produce glucose-6-phosphate, a substrate for glycolysis and pentose phosphate pathway. However, under hyperglycemic conditions, AR reduces glucose to sorbitol (Brownlee, 2005). Sorbitol is oxidized to fructose by SDH (Giacco and Brownlee, 2010). With chronic hyperglycemia, the AR pathway becomes enhanced leading to increased formation of sorbitol. As a result of activated AR pathway, there is increased consumption of NADPH (as an obligate co-factor) by AR (Figueroa-Romero et al., 2008). The GR also requires NADPH, as co-factor, for the regeneration of GSH, an endogenous scavenger of ROS. Therefore, increased utilization of NADPH caused by enhanced activity of AR reduces intracellular concentration of GSH. Reduced levels of GSH will impair the activity of GPx which utilizes GSH as a hydrogen donor (Halliwell and Gutteridge, 2007). Taken together, decreased NADPH impairs GR activity, reduces GSH level and impairs GPx activity. This impairs the antioxidant defense network and increases cellular susceptibility to oxidative stress. NO• has been shown to inhibit AR activity in diabetes (Chandra et al., 2002). In view of evidence which indicates ROS can decrease NO• bioavailability, therefore, increased oxidative stress in diabetes will further augment AR activity. Thus, hyperglycemia-enhanced polyol pathway will exacerbate oxidative stress in diabetes mellitus.

Besides, the increased levels of sorbitol caused by enhanced AR activity increase the osmolality of intracellular milieu. Sorbitol, myoinositol, glycerophosphorylcholine, betaine and taurine are physiological osmolytes which help to maintain homeostasis in cells such as renal medullary cells (Yancey and Burg, 1989). Thus, as a compensatory mechanism, this leads to efflux of intracellular osmolytes (Figueroa-Romero et al., 2008). Some of these osmolytes e.g. myoinositol play a vital role in signaling transduction, while others such as taurine are endogenous antioxidants (Figueroa-Romero et al., 2008). Hence, increased sorbitol formation reduces endogenous antioxidants and other important osmolytes. This further impairs cellular function and increases intracellular susceptibility to oxidative stress. In contrast, the SDH pathway generates fructose from sorbitol. Similar to AR pathway, chronic hyperglycemia increases the activity of SDH which results in the formation of high amounts of fructose (Figueroa-Romero et al., 2008). Increased SDH activity result in an increased NADH:NAD^+ ratio, which may inhibit oxidation of triose phosphates (Nishikawa et al., 2000a). Accumulation of triose phosphates increases *de novo* synthesis of diacylglycerols (DAG) which activate protein kinase C. Increased levels of triose phosphate may also increase generation of methylglyoxal, a potent AGE-precursor. Besides, increased fructose levels may enhance glycation and further contribute to reduced levels of NADPH, impaired antioxidant defenses and formation of AGEs.

5.2 Hyperglycemia-enhanced formation of advanced glycation end products

Advanced glycation end products (AGEs) are adducts formed non-enzymatically by the reaction between reducing carbohydrates and proteins, DNA, or lipids (Ahmed, 2005). AGEs also include products that are formed non-enzymatically from the reaction between AGE precursors, glycated sugars or oxidized products of fatty acid (in arterial endothelial cells) and protein (Giacco and Brownlee, 2010). They are produced through three major pathways: (1) convertion of glucose to glyoxal; (2) degradation of Amadori products to 3-deoxyglucosone; and (3) conversion of glyceraldehyde-3-phosphate to methylglyoxal (Nishikawa et al., 2000a, Ahmed, 2005, Figueroa-Romero et al., 2008). In diabetes mellitus, the levels of AGEs become elevated as a result of chronic hyperglycemia (Duran-Jimenez et al., 2009). The formation of AGEs occurs in different stages. During these stages of AGE formation, a number of highly reactive intermediates and cross-linkers, which enhance the binding affinity of AGEs to proteins, are also formed (Ahmed, 2005). AGEs can inhibit the antiproliferative effects of nitric oxide (Maritim et al., 2003). AGEs bind to and modify intracellular proteins thereby altering their functions (Giacco and Brownlee, 2010). In the vasculature, AGEs interact with cell surface protein or extracellular matrix components resulting in the formation of cross-linked proteins which enhance stiffening within the arterial vessel (Ahmed, 2005). AGEs can also modify plasma proteins which in turn activate receptor for advanced glycation end products (RAGE) on cells such as macrophages, vascular endothelial and smooth muscle cells (Giacco and Brownlee, 2010). AGEs can bind directly to and activate the receptors for AGEs.(Griesmacher *et al.*, 1995, Ahmed, 2005).

The binding of AGEs or AGE-modified plasma proteins to RAGE induces the release of ROS (Nishikawa et al., 2000a; Ahmed, 2005; Giacco and Brownlee, 2010). The ROS activate the expression of several genes and proteins that are involved in inflammatory cascade and implicated in the pathogenesis of diabetic cardiovascular disease. These genes and proteins include nuclear factor kappa β, tumor necrosis factor α, interleukin-1 and granulocyte-macrophage colony-stimulating factor (Nishikawa et al., 2000a, Ahmed, 2005, Giacco and Brownlee, 2010).

5.3 Hyperglycemia-activated protein kinase C pathway

Protein kinase C (PKC) is an enzyme that modulates the functions of other proteins through their phosphorylation. PKC is activated by the elevated level of DAG, derived from enhanced formation of triose phosphate via hyperglycemia (Giacco and Brownlee, 2010). Hyperglycemia may also increase DAG content through phosphatidylcholine hydrolysis (Nishikawa et al., 2000a). In diabetes, elevated levels of triose phosphate occur through increased *de novo* synthesis due to inhibition of glycolytic enzyme glyceraldehyde phosphate dehydrogenase (GAPDH) by increased ROS (Giacco and Brownlee, 2010). Besides DAG, evidence indicates that AGEs can also activate PKC pathway to increase the expression of vascular endothelial growth factor (VEGF) (Ahmed, 2005). Similarly, increased ROS levels in vascular endothelial cells may also enhance PKC pathway (Nishikawa et al., 2000a). Enhanced PKC activity induces several cytokines and protein signals including plasminogen activator inhibitor (PAI-1), NF-κB, NAD(P)H oxidases, endothelin-1, transforming growth factor β (TGF-β) and extracellular matrix (ECM) (Nishikawa et al., 2000a). These pathological alterations have been implicated in basement membrane thickening, vasoconstriction, altered capillary permeability, hypoxia and activation of angiogenesis (Nishikawa et al., 2000a, Figueroa-Romero et al., 2008).

5.4 Hyperglycemia-enhanced hexosamine pathway

Evidence has implicated the role of hexosamine pathway in the toxic or adverse effects of hyperglycemia in diabetes mellitus (Schleicher and Weigert, 2000). Under physiological conditions, a small quantity of fructose-6 phosphate derived from glycolysis is diverted to the hexosamine pathway. Glutamine: fructose-6 phosphate amidotransferase (GFAT) then converts fructose-6 phosphate to glucosamine-6 phosphate, which is converted to uridine diphosphate-N-acetylglucosamine (UDP-GlcNAc) (Schleicher and Weigert, 2000). The enzyme O-GlcNAc transferase then utilizes UDP-GlcNAc as a substrate, fixing O-GlcNAC to protein residues of transcription factors such as Sp1 and thus modify their expression (Figueroa-Romero et al., 2008). Similar to the other pathways, with chronic hyperglycemia, the hexosamine pathway becomes enhanced (Figueroa-Romero et al., 2008, Schleicher and Weigert, 2000). This leads to increased formation of UDP-GlcNAc and increased activity of O-GlcNAc transferase, with consequent alterations in gene expression (Figueroa-Romero et al., 2008). This pathway is implicated in the hyperglycemia-mediated increases in the transcription of TGF-α and TGF-β_1. Over-expression of these transcription factors such as TGF-β_1 is known to activate the proliferation of collagen matrix, basement membrane thickening and inhibition of mesangial cell mitogenesis, thus contributing to microvascular complications such as nephropathy (Schleicher and Weigert, 2000).

5.5 Hyperglycemia-activated Poly-ADP Ribose Polymerase (PARP) pathway

Poly(ADP-ribose) polymerase (PARP) is a family of enzymes that detect single- and double-stranded DNA and repair damaged DNA (Virag and Szabo, 2002). Activation of PARP is a direct cellular response to metabolic- or chemical-induced DNA damage. Once PARP senses and identifies a damaged DNA, it binds to the DNA and forms homodimers and catalyzes the cleavage of nicotinamide adenine dinucleotide (NAD^+) into nicotinamide and ADP-ribose (Virag and Szabo, 2002). It then uses ADP-ribose to synthesize a poly(ADP-ribose) chain (PAR) which serves as a signal for several DNA repairing enzymes such as DNA ligase III and DNA polymerase beta (polβ). In hyperglycemic environment, there is increased ROS formation leading to oxidative damage which activates PARP. As a result of NAD^+ utilization, this depletes cellular NAD^+ stores and induces a progressive ATP depletion. This further increases the vulnerability of cells to oxidative stress and damage as well as cell death (Figueroa-Romero et al., 2008). Available evidence suggests that PARP's catalytic activity may cause altered gene expression, increased oxidative stress and diversion of glycolytic intermediates to other pathogenic pathways (Figueroa-Romero et al.,

2008). A recent study demonstrated the beneficial effects of PARP inhibition in diabetic complications (Lupachyk et al., 2011).

5.6 Hyperglycemia-induced mitochondrial O2•⁻ overproduction

Recent data indicates that hyperglycemia-induced mitochondrial $O_2^{\bullet-}$ overproduction is the sole underlying mechanism (directly or indirectly) by which hyperglycemia induces cellular damage (Giacco and Brownlee, 2010). During mitochondrial oxidative phosphorylation, $O_2^{\bullet-}$ is generated due to leakage of electrons from electron transport chain (ETC) on molecular oxygen. In euglycemic environment, about 0.2–2% of O_2 utilized by the mitochondria is reduced to $O_2^{\bullet-}$ (Bashan et al., 2009, Brand, 2010). The antioxidant defense network maintains the mitochondrial level of ROS within physiological concentrations (Andreyev et al., 2005, Brand, 2010). However, in hyperglycemic environment, enhanced glucose flux through glycolysis and TCA causes an overdrive of the mitochondrial ETC resulting in mitochondrial dysfunction and increased ROS formation (Bashan *et al.*, 2009; Brand, 2010). Elevated levels of ROS lead to oxidative stress and damage. Oxidative damage to DNA can activate Poly(ADP-ribose) polymerase (PARP) pathway (Wei, 1998).

Besides this pathway, evidence suggests that hyperglycemia, via $O_2^{\bullet-}$ overproduction , inhibits G6PDH. G6PDH is the rate-limiting enzyme of the pentose phosphate pathway necessary for generating reducing equivalents to the antioxidant defense system (Brand, 2010). Inhibition of G6PDH leads to increased levels of glycolytic intermediates resulting in increased flux into these pathways. For instance, glyceraldehyde 3-phosphate can non-enzymatically be converted to methylglyoxal which activates AGEs pathway (Giacco and Brownlee, 2010). Similarly, glyceraldehyde 3-phosphate is a precursor of DAG which can activate PKC pathway. Increased levels of fructose 6-phosphate will increase flux through the hexosamine pathway (Giacco and Brownlee, 2010). Furthermore, reduced levels of G6PDH result in increased glucose concentrations which further enhances flux through the polyol pathway. The aldose reductase pathway becomes intensified leading to increased formation of sorbitol. This sets up a chain reaction that continuously activates one pathway or the other generating ROS which may cause DNA damage. This causes activation of PARP pathway. Thus, virtually all these pathways, namely polyol pathway, formation of AGEs pathway, PKC pathway, hexosamine pathway, and poly-ADP ribose polymerase (PARP) pathway, can be activated by hyperglycemia-induced mitochondrial $O_2^{\bullet-}$ overproduction.

6. Interrelation among glycemic control, oxidative stress and diabetic complications

So far, this chapter has identified the various sources of oxidative stress in diabetes mellitus. It has also presented evidence that indicates hyperglycemia enhances formation of ROS in diabetes mellitus. It has also shown that hyperglycemia-induced oxidative stress plays an important role in the activation of several pathogenic pathways implicated in the pathogenesis of diabetic complications. Generally, the mechanisms by which hyperglycemia causes cellular damage can be classified into two groups (Nishikawa et al., 2000a). The first group of mechanisms entails constant acute fluctuations in cellular metabolism which are reversible following restoration of euglycemia. The second group of mechanisms involves cumulative changes in long-lived macromolecules which are irreversible even after euglycemia is restored (Nishikawa et al., 2000a). Studies have demonstrated the beneficial effects of reduced hyperglycemia or glycemic control on the risk of developing diabetic complications (DCCT, 1993, UKPDS, 1998). Nevertheless, recent findings suggest that treatment of chronic hyperglycemia to achieve optimal glycemic goal in diabetic patients is limited and detrimental (Ismail-Beigi et al., 2010). It is recommended that the consequences (higher mortality rate, hypoglycemia and weight gain) should be weighed against the benefits of intensive therapy (Ismail-Beigi et al., 2010). Besides, available evidence indicates that achieving and/or maintaining optimal glycemic control in diabetic patients is difficult (Turner et al., 1999, Cook et al., 2005). The difficulty in maintaining optimal glycemic control is attributed to deterioration of pancreatic β-cell function, which is linked to hyperglycemia-induced oxidative stress (Drews et al., 2010). Interestingly, even in diabetic patients given pancreatic transplants, diabetic complications such as nephropathy continued to deteriorate at least five years after their diabetes had been cured (Fioretto et al., 1998). This contradicts evidence that links hyperglycemia to diabetic complications. Therefore, this section attempts to explain the interrelation among glycemic control, oxidative stress and diabetic complications and possible role of hypoglycemic drugs (and/or insulin) and antioxidants in the management of diabetic complications by answering the following questions:

1. Does reduced or intensive therapy of hyperglycemia prevent induction or development of oxidative stress?
2. Does reduced or intensive therapy of hyperglycemia prevent diabetic complications?
3. Why does reduced or intensive therapy of hyperglycemia not prevent diabetic complications?
4. Could there be a role of antioxidants in the management of diabetic complications?
5. Could there be a role of hypoglycemic drugs (and/or insulin) and antioxidants in the management of diabetic complications?

6.1 Does reduced or intensive therapy of hyperglycemia completely restore or ameliorate oxidative stress?

Hyperglycemia induces oxidative stress in diabetes mellitus. However, does evidence indicate that reduced or intensive treatment of hyperglycemia completely prevent development of oxidative stress? This section aims to answer this important question by presenting both experimental and clinical data. In diabetic rats, after two months of poor glycemic control, re-institution of good glycemic control for seven additional months partially reduced the elevated caspase-3 activity, levels of NF-kβ, lipid peroxides and nitric oxides with no beneficial effect on nitrotyrosine formation. In contrast, after six months of poor glycemic control, re-institution of good glycemic control for seven additional months demonstrated no significant effects on the elevated caspase-3 activity, NF-kβ, and oxidative stress parameters (Kowluru, 2003, Kowluru *et al.*, 2004). In another follow up study, after six months of poor glycemic control, normalization of hyperglycemia for another 6 months also had no significant effect on retinal nitrotyrosine levels, neither did oxidative stress parameters improve (Kowluru et al., 2007). Other studies have also shown that reduced hyperglycemia does not completely restore redox status (Rahimi et al., 2005, Erejuwa et al., 2010a, Erejuwa et al., 2011b).

Evidence suggests that proteins (collagen) are likely to be glycated irrespective of blood glucose levels (Monnier et al., 1999). In patients with type 2 diabetes mellitus, insulin treatment only partially improved oxidative stress parameters (Seghrouchni et al., 2002). This is evidenced by the elevated levels of thiobarbituric acid reactive substances and reduced erythrocyte GSH (Seghrouchni et al., 2002). In type 2 diabetic patients, treatment with gliclazide for 12 weeks ameliorated oxidative stress better than did glibenclamide (Fava et al., 2002). Available data from DCCT and Epidemiology of Diabetic Complications and Interventions (EDIC) Trial indicated that type 1 diabetic patients in the intensive therapy group still had increased levels of protein glycation products and AGEs despite intensive treatment (Genuth et al., 2005). However, protein glycation and AGE formation were less compared with those in the conventional treatment group (Genuth et al., 2005).

The data highlighted in this section reveal that reduced or intensive therapy of hyperglycemia does not completely prevent induction of oxidative stress. In other words, once hyperglycemia (either via mitochondrial $O_2^{\bullet -}$ overproduction or other mechanisms) activates any of these mechanistic pathways (especially the polyol pathway), intensive therapy or even normalization of hyperglycemia (which is even difficult with the current hypoglycemic drugs) would have limited effects on oxidative stress. Once oxidative stress is induced in diabetes mellitus, it can enhance the generation of ROS and initiate redox-chain reactions which may activate various inflammatory proteins and signaling pathways including all the abovementioned mechanistic pathways. Even if normal glucose level is restored, these inflammatory proteins and signaling pathways on their own could cause oxidative stress and/or sustain the oxidative stress originally or previously induced by hyperglycemia. Thus, with or without hyperglycemia, the resulting ROS and oxidative stress secondary to hyperglycemia would suffice to activate some of these pathways and set the stage for oxidative stress or exacerbate the already developed or existing oxidative stress. Besides, evidence implicates a role of oxidative stress in many neurodegenerative disorders such as hypertension, cancer and Alzheimer's disease. All of these disorders are characterized by euglycemia. Therefore, it means or suggests that oxidative stress can be an entirely independent phenomenon which can exist even with normalization of hyperglycemia.

6.2 Does reduced or intensive therapy of hyperglycemia prevent diabetic complications?

Data from animal and human studies indicate that intensive therapy may delay the progression of diabetic complications, but does not prevent diabetic complications. A study that investigated the effect of improved glycemic control on the progression of retinopathy in diabetic dogs found that diabetic dogs with 5-year poor glycemic control developed diabetic retinopathy while those with 5-year good glycemic control had no diabetic retinopathy (Engerman and Kern, 1987). The third group comprised diabetic dogs with 2.5-year poor glycemic control. It was observed that these diabetic dogs did not develop diabetic retinopathy. However, the dogs later developed diabetic retinopathy despite 2.5-year good glycemic control (Engerman and Kern, 1987). The study further revealed that the extent of pathology of diabetic retinopathy in the third group (with 2.5-year poor glycemic control + 2.5-year good glycemic control) was similar to that of the dogs with 5-year poor glycemic control (Engerman and Kern, 1987). Similarly, in sucrose-fed diabetic rats, cure of diabetes via islet transplantation at 12 weeks (but only at 6 weeks after the confirmation of diabetes) did not prevent lesions or progression of diabetic retinopathy (Hammes et al., 1993). Kowluru and colleagues (2007) also reported that after 6 months of poor glycemic control in rats, normalization of hyperglycemia for 6 months had no effect on the lesions or pathology of diabetic retinopathy.

In type I diabetic patients whose diabetes had been cured (through pancreas transplantation) but still had diabetic nephropathy, the thickness of glomerular and tubular basement membranes was still similar at 5 years versus baseline values. In contrast, it was significantly reduced only by the 10th year versus baseline values. The study further showed that while mesangial fractional volume had increased by the 5th year, it significantly decreased by the 10th year (Fioretto et al., 1998). In the DCCT, due to the considerable benefits of intensive therapy, patients in the conventional therapy group were transitioned to intensive therapy group (DCCT, 1993). A long-term follow-up study under the EDIC Trial (DCCT/EDIC, 2002, DCCT/EDIC, 2003, Pop-Busui et al., 2009) showed that patients who were formerly in the intensive therapy group had lower incidence of diabetic microvascular complications than the patients who were originally in the conventional treatment group, despite 8 years of similar and normalized glycemic control in the EDIC trial (DCCT/EDIC, 2002). It was further reported that the conventionally treated-DCCT patients who were transitioned to intensive therapy group in the EDIC trial still had greater incidence of macrovascular pathology or complications (Nathan et al., 2003, Nathan et al., 2005, Cleary et al., 2006, Patel et al., 2008). Evidence from clinical trials also suggests that the incidence or development of diabetic complications is more likely to depend on the intensity of oxidative stress than on the level of glycemic control (Monnier et al., 1999, Genuth et al., 2005). Besides, evidence indicates that the degree of insulin resistance correlates with the onset of diabetic complications, independently of glycemic levels (Chillaron et al., 2009). In type 2 diabetic patients, it was reported that gliclazide treatment delayed the progression of diabetic nephropathy only, whereas it produced no significant effect on the development or progression of retinopathy or macrovascular complications (Patel et al., 2008). These findings are very important because gliclazide is one of the few hypoglycemic agents with an antioxidant effect (Fava et al., 2002).

It is evident from the different aforementioned hyperglycemia-induced mechanistic pathways and the data (both experimental and clinical) presented in this section that the pathogenesis of diabetic complications is a complex process. It involves oxidative stress and ROS-activated pathways including several inflammatory proteins, cytokines and growth factors. It is clear that hyperglycemia exerts long-term injurious effects in patients with type 1 and type 2 diabetes mellitus. Similar long-lasting detrimental effects of hyperglycemia also occur in animals (dogs). In both animals and humans with diabetes, glycemic control only delays the development or progression of diabetic complications. It does not prevent or completely restore diabetic complications. This is understandable in view of the fact that these diabetic complications are not primary effects of hyperglycemia but are its sequelae (secondary effects). In fact, in few cases in which normalization of hyperglycemia or cure of diabetes mellitus do prevent diabetic complications, it has to be initiated at a very early stage of the disease and maintained for several years. Overall, these findings clearly show that intensive therapy or normalization of hyperglycemia does not prevent diabetic complications.

6.3 Why does reduced or intensive therapy of hyperglycemia not prevent diabetic complications?

Investigators have introduced different phrases to describe this concept or observation in which reduced or intensive therapy of hyperglycemia does not prevent diabetic complications. Some of these phrases include ''glycemic memory", "hyperglycemic memory", "metabolic memory'' or "lasting memory". Glycemic memory is a term that refers to the development of diabetic complications during post-hyperglycemic normoglycemia

(Nishikawa et al., 2000a). It is a phenomenon whereby early glycemic milieu or environment is remembered in many target organs such as heart, eye, nerve and kidney. Evidence suggests that oxidative stress may contribute to the inability of reduced or intensive treatment of hyperglycemia to prevent diabetic complications (Ceriello et al., 2009). It is proposed that glycemic memory could involve two stages: induction and perpetuation (Nishikawa et al., 2000a). During induction, hyperglycemia generates increased ROS levels. This may result from increased production of reducing equivalents formed from overdrive of the mitochondrial ETC. As a result of increased ROS, cellular dysfunction and mutations in mitochondrial DNA may occur (Wei, 1998). On the other hand, perpetuation, which is glycemic memory itself, could occur because ROS-induced mutated mitochondrial DNA would encode defective ETC subunits (Nishikawa et al., 2000a). This hypothesis of defective mitochondrial DNA subunits seems valid. Two years after this hypothesis, a study demonstrated that methylglyoxal modified mitochondrial proteins causing disturbances in mitochondria in kidney of rats (Rosca *et al.*, 2002). The study further showed that methylglyoxal produced an inhibitory effect on the tricarboxylic acid (TCA) cycle and the electron respiratory chain in kidney of rats. In another related study, it was shown that methylglyoxal-modified mitochondria considerably augmented $O_2^{\bullet-}$ production,, independently of the level of hyperglycemia, and were characterized by oxidative damage (Rosca *et al.*, 2005).

Furthermore, Ihnat and colleagues (2007) also provided evidence in support of the role of oxidative stress in mediating the hyperglycemic memory (Ihnat et al., 2007). The authors showed that in human endothelial and ARPE-19 retinal cells, the levels of protein kinase C-beta, NAD(P)H oxidase subunit p47phox, BCL-2-associated X protein, 3-nitrotyrosine, ffibronectin and poly (ADP-ribose) remained elevated for 1 week after the levels of glucose had normalized. The study showed that inhibition of ROS production using antioxidant alpha-lipoic acid prevented the induction of these glucose-induced oxidative stress markers (Ihnat et al., 2007). Similar findings were also reported in aortic endothelial cells both *in vitro* and in non-diabetic mice (El-Osta et al., 2008). The study showed that short-term hyperglycemic spikes produced long-lasting effects on vascular cells (El-Osta et al., 2008). This suggests that transient spikes of hyperglycemia may be an HbA1c-independent risk factor for diabetic complications (El-Osta et al., 2008). A recent study also indicated that elevated glucose levels caused continual changes in cell viability and apoptosis-related gene expressions even after recovery of normoglycemia (Wei et al., 2011). The changes were associated with increased ROS production (Wei et al., 2011). Besides, evidence implicates the role of protein glycation and formation of AGEs in metabolic memory (Genuth et al., 2005, Ceriello et al., 2009). AGEs may reduce NADPH and impair antioxidant system which in turn can generate more ROS (Ahmed, 2005). Data from the DCCT suggest that the tendency of collagen to be glycated is less dependent on the level of blood glucose (Monnier et al., 1999). It was also demonstrated that both conventional and intensive therapies did not prevent protein glycation and formation of AGEs (Genuth et al., 2005). The data further revealed that the incidences of retinopathy and nephropathy were significantly associated with the levels of protein glycation and AGEs (Genuth et al., 2005). This phenomenon termed "glycemic memory" has also been corroborated in several other studies (Nathan et al., 2005, Holman et al., 2008).

Recent findings indicate that elevated oscillating glucose concentrations may contribute to increased risk for cardiovascular diabetic complications (Ceriello et al., 2008). As demonstrated by Ceriello and colleagues (2008), using a euinsulinemic hyperglycemic clamp, glucose at 5, 10, and 15 mmol/l was given in rising steps as a single "spike", and oscillating between basal and high levels over 24-hour in non-diabetic subjects and type 2 diabetic patients. The authors reported that glucose at 10 and 15 mmol/l led to a concentration-dependent fasting blood glucose-independent impaired endothelial function and increased intensity of oxidative stress in both non-diabetic subjects and type 2 diabetic patients (Ceriello et al., 2008). The study also revealed that oscillating glucose concentrations between 5 and 15 mmol/l every 6 hour for 24 hours caused further significant impairments in endothelial function and induced oxidative stress compared with continuous 10 or 15 mmol/l glucose (Ceriello et al., 2008). These findings are very relevant because the current management of diabetes mellitus (including intensive therapy) does not control postprandial hyperglycemia. Besides, both endothelial function and oxidative stress are implicated in the pathogenesis of diabetic micro- and macrovascular complications. Oxidative stress also plays an important role in endothelial dysfunction (Sies, 1991, Halliwell and Gutteridge, 2007). This study is also remarkable because it shows that oscillating levels of glucose result in endothelial dysfunction and induced oxidative stress even in non-diabetic subjects (euglycemia). These postprandial hyperglycemia fluctuations may contribute to the continuous deterioration of diabetic complications, despite restoration of euglycemia. Therefore, postprandial hyperglycemia-induced endothelial dysfunction and oxidative stress may explain the mechanism of glycemic or hyperglycemic memory.

The findings indicate that ROS-induced mutated DNA mitochondria may continuously generate RS (Nishikawa et al., 2000a). The data also reveal that AGEs can modify or glycate protein content of mitochondrial TCA cycle and the electron respiratory chain (Ceriello, 2009, Ceriello et al., 2009). Irrespective of the level of glycemic control, all these will generate RS and trigger cellular injury. Hence, it does suggest that oxidative stress in diabetes mellitus can exist as an independent entity. As explained previously, oxidative stress is also implicated in other disorders characterized by euglycemia. Since hyperglycemia enhances the pathogenic pathways of diabetic complications via oxidative stress, therefore, whether hyperglycemia is normalized or the recommended optimal glycemic goal ≤ 6.5% HbA1c is achieved and/or maintained, the already existing oxidative stress can activate these same mechanistic pathways and thus propagate glycemic memory (induce diabetic complications).

6.4 Could there be a role of antioxidants in the management of diabetic complications?

Since oxidative stress is implicated in the pathogenesis of diabetes and its complications, there ought to be a place for antioxidants in the treatment of diabetes mellitus. However, previous clinical trials using antioxidants have yielded both promise and inconsistent results. Even though the data from the large scale clinical trials are inconclusive, it is noteworthy that many of those clinical trials were characterized by inappropriate study designs or several limitations (Johansen et al., 2005, Penckofer et al., 2002, Wierzba, 2005, Robinson et al., 2006, Willcox et al., 2008). These include: trials did not address specific diabetic populations; some studies included both healthy and unhealthy subjects; no data establishing the occurrence of oxidative stress in the patients before treatment and comparing such data with those obtained after treatment; the short duration of treatment; most of the trials were performed with vitamins A, C and E without consideration for other antioxidants; the use of vitamin E supplementation without the concurrent use of vitamin C (Johansen et al., 2005, Penckofer et al., 2002, Wierzba, 2005, Robinson et al., 2006, Willcox et al., 2008). Other limitations include: some trials are gender-specific (comprising either men or women); lack of pharmacokinetic data of these antioxidants, before and after treatment, so as to ascertain if these antioxidants reached the target cells/tissues in adequate concentrations; no data to show that effects of different doses of each antioxidant were investigated so as to obtain and select optimal dose; the suppression of gamma-tocopherol by alpha-tocopherol; vitamins inappropriately administered relative to meal ingestion; and poor patient compliance are some of the issues that may contribute to the failure of antioxidants in clinical studies (Johansen et al., 2005, Penckofer et al., 2002, Wierzba, 2005, Robinson et al., 2006, Willcox et al., 2008). Some endpoints that were not directly related to oxidative stress such as mortality were used in some trials (Johansen et al., 2005). Hence, limited research and findings are available on the effects of antioxidants in diabetic patients. However, available evidences in small or medium sample-sized diabetic studies, both experimental and clinical, suggest antioxidants might play a role in the management of diabetes mellitus.

In diabetic rats with neuropathy, α-lipoic acid supplementation ameliorated oxidative stress parameters and improved lesions of diabetic neuropathy such as conduction velocity of the digital nerve, deficits in nerve conduction and nerve blood flow (Coppey et al., 2001). Evidence suggests that antioxidants can inhibit some of the pathways of diabetic complications such as protein kinase C-signaled increases in TGF-β in mesangial cells (Scott and King, 2004). Similarly, antioxidant treatment prevented the elevation in the levels of protein kinase C-beta, NAD(P)H oxidase subunit p47phox, BCL-2-associated X protein, 3-nitrotyrosine, fibronectin and poly (ADP) ribose in the retina of diabetic rats (Ihnat et al., 2007). In the kidney of diabetic rats, honey supplementation considerably reduced hyperglycemia, attenuated antioxidant enzymes, ameliorated oxidative stress markers and reduced mesangial matrix expansion and glomerular basement membrane thickness (Erejuwa et al., 2010a, Erejuwa et al., 2010c).

In patients with type 1 diabetes, supplementation with vitamins E and/or C combination ameliorated oxidative stress and improved endothelium-dependent vasorelaxation (Johansen et al., 2005, Rahimi et al., 2005). A study found that supplementation with combined chromium (Cr) and vitamins C and E ameliorated oxidative stress, reduced fasting blood glucose, HbA1c and insulin resistance in type 2 diabetes (Lai, 2008). Similarly, a recent study reported that vitamin E supplementation significantly reduced malondialdehyde (MDA) levels and increased the concentrations of GSH and vitamin E in type 1 diabetic patients (Gupta et al., 2011). The study also found a negative correlation between oxidative stress marker (MDA) and antioxidants (vitamin E and GSH) and a positive correlation between exogenously administered antioxidant (vitamin E) and endogenous antioxidant (GSH) (Gupta et al., 2011). However, the study showed that vitamin E supplementation in type 1 diabetic patients did not produce significant effects in metabolic parameters (Gupta et al., 2011). In patients with type 1 diabetes mellitus, vitamins C and E supplementation ameliorated oxidative stress markers, improved vascular dysfunction, retinal blood flow and creatinine clearance (Scott and King, 2004). These studies indicate that antioxidants could play a role in the management of diabetes mellitus. However, considering that diabetes mellitus is a disorder with multiple etiology and metabolic derangements, antioxidant supplementation alone is likely to be less effective.

This is corroborated by findings of Gupta and co-workers (2011). That could also explain the failure of antioxidants in clinical trials.

6.5 Could there be a role of hypoglycemic drugs (and/or insulin) and antioxidants in the management of diabetic complications?

A closer look at the various mechanistic pathways implicated in the pathogenesis of diabetic complications indicates that hyperglycemia-enhanced polyol pathway (via depletion of intracellular NADPH) and $O_2^{\bullet-}$ inhibition of G6PDH (via hyperglycemia-enhanced $O_2^{\bullet-}$ overproduction) would play a major role in impairing antioxidant defenses. This will increase intracellular susceptibility to oxidative stress during diabetes. As regards evidence, very few studies have investigated the effects of combined hypoglycemic agents and antioxidants in diabetic rodents or patients. Interestingly, all these studies found beneficial effects of combination of these two agents in both animals and human with diabetes mellitus. A study that investigated the effects of 4-week insulin and/or antioxidant (vitamin E and C) supplementation in diabetic rats found that the antioxidant treatment improved some of the oxidative stress parameters whereas insulin treatment prevented weight loss and ameliorated the activities and expression of antioxidant enzymes. In contrast, the combination of insulin and antioxidants resulted in normalization of all measurements including oxidative stress parameters (Sindhu et al., 2004).

Similarly, comparison of the effects of glibenclamide alone or combined with honey in pancreas of diabetic rats indicated that, even though glibenclamide reduced hyperglycemia, it only partially ameliorated oxidative stress parameters (most of the data were insignificant) (Erejuwa et al., 2011b). However, the combination of glibenclamide and honey significantly reduced hyperglycemia and ameliorated oxidative stress parameters in pancreas of diabetic rats (Erejuwa et al., 2011b). A similar study also showed that a combination of glibenclamide and metformin produced a limited antioxidant effect compared to when they were combined with honey in pancreas of diabetic rats (Erejuwa et al., 2010b). In the kidney of diabetic rats treated with metformin and/or glibenclamide, impaired antioxidant defenses were reported. In contrast, metformin and/or glibenclamide combined with honey significantly ameliorated oxidative stress parameters and restored the activities of antioxidant enzymes in the kidney of diabetic rats (Erejuwa et al., 2011a).

In type 1 and type 2 diabetic patients, a study found that while optimal glycemic control reduced the levels of MDA and increased the levels of GSH and vitamin E, it did not normalize the oxidative stress parameters (Chugh et al., 1999). However, after 4 weeks of vitamin E supplementation, the levels of oxidative stress markers were further reduced while those of endogenous antioxidants were increased compared to the optimal control values (without antioxidant treatment) (Chugh et al., 1999). A similar beneficial effect of vitamin E supplementation and optimal glycemic control was also reported in type 2 diabetic patients (Sharma et al., 2000). A number of other studies have also shown that antioxidants reduce glucose levels, improve insulin secretion and insulin resistance during diabetes (Penckofer et al., 2002). Moreover, a study found that in type 1 diabetic patients, normalization of glucose levels did not ameliorate hyperglycemia-induced endothelial dysfunction (Ceriello et al., 2007). The authors reported that, neither insulin nor vitamin C was able to ameliorate oxidative stress or normalize endothelial dysfunction (Ceriello et al., 2007). On the contrary, combination of insulin and vitamin C significantly decrease the intensity of oxidative stress and normalized endothelial dysfunction in type 1 diabetic patients (Ceriello et al., 2007).

A critical analysis of the mechanistic pathways of hyperglycemia-induced diabetic complications indicates that they are all characterized by increased formation of ROS and impaired antioxidant defense network, which would further exacerbate oxidative stress and damage. In other words, these pathways begin and end with oxidative stress. Besides, evidence indicates that postprandial hyperglycemic fluctuations can cause endothelial dysfunction and induce oxidative stress in diabetic subjects and even in euglycemic subjects. Hence, findings from these studies clearly indicate that it is oxidative stress all over in diabetes mellitus and its complications. Moreover, the data from experimental and clinical studies indicate that there is a role for co-administration of hypoglycemic drugs or insulin and antioxidants in diabetes mellitus. It is possible that normalization of hyperglycemia may be achieved with hypoglycemic drugs, insulin, their combinations or even via pancreatic transplant. However, in patients with diabetic complications, whether euglycemia is achieved and/or maintained, oxidative stress (and oxidative stress-induced sequelae) becomes an independent entity. Thus, oxidative stress, as a possible independent entity, in diabetes mellitus necessitates antioxidant therapy. On account of these observations, findings and data, there seems little doubt that antioxidant therapy or other therapeutic intervention of oxidative stress in combination with hypoglycemic drugs or insulin should result in better management of diabetes mellitus. This should also prevent or reduce ROS-linked diabetic complications.

6.6 Other potential beneficial effects of hypoglycemic drugs (and/or insulin) and antioxidants in diabetes mellitus

Diabetes mellitus is characterized by impairments in renal and hepatic function as well as impaired metabolism of glucose, lipid and protein. Lipid abnormalities and induction of oxidative stress enhance the oxidation and glycation of low-density lipoproteins (LDLs), thereby exacerbate endothelial dysfunction (Penckofer et al., 2002). Studies have shown that antioxidants and some hypoglycemic drugs can prevent oxidation of LDL (Fava et al., 2002, Maritim et al., 2003, Rahimi et al., 2005). Besides, evidence indicates that antioxidants can ameliorate lipid abnormalities (Rahimi et al., 2005, Erejuwa et al., 2011d). The beneficial effects of antioxidants on glycemic control (blood glucose, fructosamine and glycosylated hemoglobin) in diabetes have also been documented (Rahimi et al., 2005, Lai, 2008, Erejuwa et al., 2010a; 2011d). Furthermore, antioxidants improve C-peptide and insulin levels as well as insulin resistance in diabetes mellitus (Rahimi et al., 2005, Lai, 2008, Erejuwa et al., 2011d). Co-administration of hypoglycemic drugs (glibenclamide or metformin) and antioxidant (honey) considerably improved glycemic control and lipid parameters in diabetic rats more than the effects produced by individual hypoglycemic drug (Erejuwa et al., 2011d). It is worth mentioning that other non-antioxidant constituents of honey, such as fructose and oligosaccharides, might contribute to this improved glycemic control and lipid parameters. In addition, antioxidants ameliorated and improved impaired renal function which has been documented in diabetes mellitus (Slyvka et al., 2009, Erejuwa et al., 2011d) or in combination with hypoglycemic drugs may produce synergism (Erejuwa et al., 2011d).

In the duodenum and jejunum of diabetic rats, a number of alterations in the brush border membrane (BBM) fluidity, non-enzymatic glycation, oxidative stress and damage have been reported (Bhor and Sivakami, 2003). Similarly, increased protein glycation and lipid peroxidation might exacerbate diabetes-related alterations in BBM fluidity (Watala and Winocour, 1992). Therefore, antioxidants may ameliorate intestinal oxidative stress and improve BBM fluidity, thereby promote healing and enhance gastrointestinal tract health in diabetes mellitus. This might impact positively on glycemic control. Antioxidants may also augment bioavailability of essential macronutrients or co-administered hypoglycemic drugs (Faria et al., 2009). Furthermore, antioxidants may help to ameliorate liver damage and hepatic oxidative stress which are common in diabetes mellitus (Dias et al., 2005, Erejuwa et al., 2012b). Considering the role of liver in glucose homeostasis and the fact that some hypoglycemic agents (e.g. glibenclamide) mediate their effects via liver, these hepatic effects of antioxidants combined with those of hypoglycemic drugs may enhance liver functions and contribute to improved glycemic control. Moreover, evidence suggests that the use of antioxidants is associated with reduced weight gain (Razquin et al., 2009, Erejuwa et al., 2012a), therefore, co-administration of antioxidants and hypoglycemic agents, especially glibenclamide, may be beneficial in type 2 diabetic patients, majority of whom are obese. Majority of diabetic patients end up developing hypertension which further increases the risk of developing diabetic complications including cardiovascular events. Interestingly, oxidative stress is also implicated in the pathogenesis and/or complications of hypertension. Therefore, a combination of hypoglycemic drugs and antioxidants, via improved glycemic control and amelioration of oxidative stress, may help to prevent or delay the development of hypertension and diabetic complications (Erejuwa et al., 2011c, 2012a). Besides, the combination of both agents may help to minimize the adverse effects or toxicities of hypoglycemic agents. The use of antioxidants may necessitate lower doses of hypoglycemic agents to achieve the same therapeutic effect, thereby limiting the side or adverse effects of these drugs.

7. Conclusions

These studies indicate that hyperglycemia exerts long-term injurious effects in patients with type 1 and type 2 diabetes mellitus. Similar long-lasting detrimental effects of hyperglycemia also occur in diabetic animals. In both animals and humans with diabetes, glycemic control only delays the development or progression of diabetic complications. It does not prevent or completely restore diabetic complications. In few cases in which good glycemic control or cure of diabetes does prevent diabetic complications, it has to be initiated at a very early stage of the disease and maintained for several years. This is probably impracticable in the larger diabetic population. Evidence indicates it is not easy to achieve and/or maintain glycemic control in many diabetic patients close to the physiological range commonly observed in their healthy counterparts. Together with recent findings which demonstrate the deleterious effect of intensive therapy of hyperglycemia, it can be inferred that any therapeutic option that target hyperglycemia alone is not only limited and ineffective but may also be detrimental in diabetic patients. In view of the alarming rate of global prevalence of diabetes mellitus and the associated complications, morbidity and mortality, there is an urgent need for a better or new therapeutic management. While efforts are being made by researchers and scientists to unravel the main cause(s) of diabetes mellitus, it is high time clinicians, physicians and diabetologists began to look for an alternative and/or a complementary therapy to the current management of diabetes mellitus.

At the moment, one of such options or alternatives is the prospective of managing diabetes mellitus by targeting both hyperglycemia and oxidative stress simultaneously. As the data presented in this chapter have revealed, co-administration of oral hypoglycemic drugs (and/or insulin) and antioxidants might prove to be a better therapy in the management of diabetes mellitus. This is because, with the combination, hypoglycemic drugs (and/or insulin) will target hyperglycemia to improve glycemic control and reduce hyperglycemia-enhanced ROS production. In addition, administration of antioxidants will help to scavenge or eliminate RS including those generated in the various pathways highlighted in this chapter. Besides, many antioxidants have hypoglycemic effect which may also contribute to improved glycemic control. The co-administration of these two agents will help to minimize the level of oxidative stress in the vasculature and other targets of diabetic complications such as kidney (reducing diabetic nephropathy), retina (reducing diabetic retinopathy), nerves (reducing diabetic neuropathy) and heart (reducing diabetic cardiomyopathy). Moreover, evidence has shown that the pancreas and the liver are also target of oxidative stress in diabetes mellitus. Hence, co-administration of antioxidants will help to ameliorate oxidative stress in these tissues and organs (pancreas and liver) which play key roles in glucose homeostasis in diabetes mellitus.

In addition to improved glycemic control and amelioration of oxidative stress, evidence suggests that co-administration of hypoglycemic drugs and antioxidants may exert other beneficial effects on gastrointestinal tract, lipid profile, renal function and others which will contribute to better management of diabetic patients. Considering the limitations with antioxidants, coupled with the latest advances in our understanding of the various mechanisms involved in ROS formation, other interventions such as inhibition of the mitochondrial ROS overproduction, developing mitochondria-targeted antioxidants, blockage of hyperglycemia-induced mechanistic pathways are viable therapeutic options. This chapter has shown that the prospective of managing diabetes mellitus more effectively by targeting both hyperglycemia and oxidative stress simultaneously holds much promise. This new therapeutic option is worth investigating in patients with diabetes mellitus. Hence, both small and large, well designed, randomized clinical trials that examine the effect of combination of hypoglycemic drugs (and/or insulin) and specific antioxidants in patients with type 1 or type 2 diabetes mellitus are recommended. This may revolutionize the management of diabetes mellitus, at least in the interim, while attempts are being made to discover its main cause(s) and develop more potent and effective antidiabetic drugs.

8. Dedication

This chapter is dedicated to the memory of my dad, Educator Sephaniah Adeyemi Erejuwa, who battled diabetes mellitus and later succumbed to its complications. It is also dedicated to millions of people globally who are suffering from this disorder and its complications

9. References

ADA (2011). American Diabetes Association. Diagnosis and classification of diabetes mellitus. *Diabetes Care,* Vol. 34 Suppl 1, No. pp. S62-69.

Ahmed, N. (2005). Advanced glycation endproducts--role in pathology of diabetic complications. *Diabetes Res Clin Pract,* Vol. 67, No. 1, pp. 3-21.

Anderson, E. J., Lustig, M. E., Boyle, K. E., Woodlief, T. L., Kane, D. A., Lin, C. T., Price, J. W., 3rd, Kang, L., Rabinovitch, P. S., Szeto, H. H., Houmard, J. A., Cortright, R. N., Wasserman, D. H. & Neufer, P. D. (2009). Mitochondrial H2O2 emission and cellular redox state link excess fat intake to insulin resistance in both rodents and humans. *J Clin Invest,* Vol. 119, No. 3, pp. 573-581.

Andreyev, A. Y., Kushnareva, Y. E. & Starkov, A. A. (2005). Mitochondrial metabolism of reactive oxygen species. *Biochemistry (Mosc),* Vol. 70, No. 2, pp. 200-214.

Ball, A. J., Flatt, P. R. & McClenaghan, N. H. (2000). Desensitization of sulphonylurea- and nutrient-induced insulin secretion following prolonged treatment with glibenclamide. *Eur J Pharmacol,* Vol. 408, No. 3, pp. 327-333.

Bashan, N., Kovsan, J., Kachko, I., Ovadia, H. & Rudich, A. (2009). Positive and negative regulation of insulin signaling by reactive oxygen and nitrogen species. *Physiol Rev,* Vol 89, No. 1, pp. 27-71.Bhor, V. M. & Sivakami, S. (2003). Regional variations in intestinal brush border membrane fluidity and function during diabetes and the role of oxidative stress and non-enzymatic glycation. *Mol Cell Biochem,* Vol. 252, No. 1-2, pp. 125-132.

Bollheimer, L. C., Skelly, R. H., Chester, M. W., McGarry, J. D. & Rhodes, C. J. (1998). Chronic exposure to free fatty acid reduces pancreatic beta cell insulin content by increasing basal insulin secretion that is not compensated for by a corresponding increase in proinsulin biosynthesis translation. *J Clin Invest,* Vol. 101, No. 5, pp. 1094-1101.

Brand, M. D. (2010). The sites and topology of mitochondrial superoxide production. *Exp Gerontol,* Vol. 45, No. 7-8, pp. 466-472.

Brownlee, M. (2001). Biochemistry and molecular cell biology of diabetic complications. *Nature,* Vol. 414, No. 6865, pp. 813-820.

Brownlee, M. (2005). The pathobiology of diabetic complications: a unifying mechanism. *Diabetes,* Vol. 54, No. 6, pp. 1615-1625.

Carlsson, C., Borg, L. A. & Welsh, N. (1999). Sodium palmitate induces partial mitochondrial uncoupling and reactive oxygen species in rat pancreatic islets in vitro. *Endocrinology,* Vol. 140, No. 8, pp. 3422-3428.

Carvalho-Filho, M. A., Ropelle, E. R., Pauli, R. J., Cintra, D. E., Tsukumo, D. M., Silveira, L. R., Curi, R., Carvalheira, J. B., Velloso, L. A. & Saad, M. J. (2009). Aspirin attenuates insulin resistance in muscle of diet-induced obese rats by inhibiting inducible nitric oxide synthase production and S-nitrosylation of IRbeta/IRS-1 and Akt. *Diabetologia,* Vol. 52, No. 11, pp. 2425-2434.

Ceriello, A., Bortolotti, N., Motz, E., Crescentini, A., Lizzio, S., Russo, A., Tonutti, L. & Taboga, C. (1998). Meal-generated oxidative stress in type 2 diabetic patients. *Diabetes Care,* Vol. 21, No. 9, pp. 1529-1533.

Ceriello, A., Esposito, K., Piconi, L., Ihnat, M. A., Thorpe, J. E., Testa, R., Boemi, M. & Giugliano, D. (2008). Oscillating glucose is more deleterious to endothelial function and oxidative stress than mean glucose in normal and type 2 diabetic patients. *Diabetes,* Vol. 57, No. 5, pp. 1349-1354.

Ceriello, A., Ihnat, M. A. & Thorpe, J. E. (2009). Clinical review 2: The "metabolic memory": is more than just tight glucose control necessary to prevent diabetic complications? *J Clin Endocrinol Metab,* Vol. 94, No. 2, pp. 410-415.

Ceriello, A., Kumar, S., Piconi, L., Esposito, K. & Giugliano, D. (2007). Simultaneous control of hyperglycemia and oxidative stress normalizes endothelial function in type 1 diabetes. *Diabetes Care,* Vol. 30, No. 3, pp. 649-654.

Chandra, D., Jackson, E. B., Ramana, K. V., Kelley, R., Srivastava, S. K. & Bhatnagar, A. (2002). Nitric oxide prevents aldose reductase activation and sorbitol accumulation during diabetes. *Diabetes,* Vol. 51, No. 10, pp. 3095-3101.

Chillaron, J. J., Goday, A., Flores-Le-Roux, J. A., Benaiges, D., Carrera, M. J., Puig, J., Cano-Perez, J. F. & Pedro-Botet, J. (2009). Estimated glucose disposal rate in assessment of the metabolic syndrome and microvascular complications in patients with type 1 diabetes. *J Clin Endocrinol Metab,* Vol. 94, No. 9, pp. 3530-3534.

Chugh, S. N., Kakkar, R., Kalra, S. & Sharma, A. (1999). An evaluation of oxidative stress in diabetes mellitus during uncontrolled and controlled state and after vitamin E supplementation. *J Assoc Physicians India,* Vol. 47, No. 4, pp. 380-383.

Cleary, P. A., Orchard, T. J., Genuth, S., Wong, N. D., Detrano, R., Backlund, J. Y., Zinman, B., Jacobson, A., Sun, W., Lachin, J. M. & Nathan, D. M. (2006). The effect of intensive glycemic treatment on coronary artery calcification in type 1 diabetic participants of the Diabetes Control and Complications Trial/Epidemiology of Diabetes Interventions and Complications (DCCT/EDIC) Study. *Diabetes,* Vol. 55, No. 12, pp. 3556-3565.

Cook, M. N., Girman, C. J., Stein, P. P., Alexander, C. M. & Holman, R. R. (2005). Glycemic control continues to deteriorate after sulfonylureas are added to metformin among patients with type 2 diabetes. *Diabetes Care,* Vol. 28, No. 5, pp. 995-1000.

Coppey, L. J., Gellett, J. S., Davidson, E. P., Dunlap, J. A., Lund, D. D. & Yorek, M. A. (2001). Effect of antioxidant treatment of streptozotocin-induced diabetic rats on endoneurial blood flow, motor nerve conduction velocity, and vascular reactivity of epineurial arterioles of the sciatic nerve. *Diabetes,* Vol. 50, No. 8, pp. 1927-1937.

DCCT (1993). Diabetes Control and Complications Trial Research Group. The effect of intensive treatment of diabetes on the development and progression of long-term complications in insulin-dependent diabetes mellitus. . *N Engl J Med,* Vol. 329, No. 14, pp. 977-986.

DCCT/EDIC (2002). Writing Team for the Diabetes Control and Complications Trial/Epidemiology of Diabetes Interventions and Complications Research Group. Effect of intensive therapy on the microvascular complications of type 1 diabetes mellitus. *JAMA,* Vol. 287, No. 19, pp. 2563-2569.

DCCT/EDIC (2003). Sustained effect of intensive treatment of type 1 diabetes mellitus on development and progression of diabetic nephropathy: the Epidemiology of Diabetes Interventions and Complications (EDIC) study. *JAMA,* Vol. 290, No. 16, pp. 2159-2167.

Dias, A. S., Porawski, M., Alonso, M., Marroni, N., Collado, P. S. & Gonzalez-Gallego, J. (2005). Quercetin decreases oxidative stress, NF-kappaB activation, and iNOS overexpression in liver of streptozotocin-induced diabetic rats. *J Nutr,* Vol. 135, No. 10, pp. 2299-2304.

Dokken, B. B., Saengsirisuwan, V., Kim, J. S., Teachey, M. K. & Henriksen, E. J. (2008). Oxidative stress-induced insulin resistance in rat skeletal muscle: role of glycogen synthase kinase-3. *Am J Physiol Endocrinol Metab,* Vol. 294, No. 3, pp. E615-621.

Drews, G., Krippeit-Drews, P. & Dufer, M. (2010). Oxidative stress and beta-cell dysfunction. *Pflugers Arch,* Vol. 460, No. 4, pp. 703-718.

Duran-Jimenez, B., Dobler, D., Moffatt, S., Rabbani, N., Streuli, C. H., Thornalley, P. J., Tomlinson, D. R. & Gardiner, N. J. (2009). Advanced glycation end products in extracellular matrix proteins contribute to the failure of sensory nerve regeneration in diabetes. *Diabetes,* Vol. 58, No. 12, pp. 2893-2903.

El-Osta, A., Brasacchio, D., Yao, D., Pocai, A., Jones, P. L., Roeder, R. G., Cooper, M. E. & Brownlee, M. (2008). Transient high glucose causes persistent epigenetic changes and altered gene expression during subsequent normoglycemia. *J Exp Med,* Vol. 205, No. 10, pp. 2409-2417.

Engerman, R. L. & Kern, T. S. (1987). Progression of incipient diabetic retinopathy during good glycemic control. *Diabetes,* Vol. 36, No. 7, pp. 808-812.

Erejuwa, O. O., Gurtu, S., Sulaiman, S. A., Ab Wahab, M. S., Sirajudeen, K. N. & Salleh, M. S. (2010a). Hypoglycemic and antioxidant effects of honey supplementation in streptozotocin-induced diabetic rats. *Int J Vitam Nutr Res,* Vol. 80, No. 1, pp. 74-82.

Erejuwa, O. O., Sulaiman, S. A., Wahab, M. S., Sirajudeen, K. N., Salleh, M. S. & Gurtu, S. (2010b). Antioxidant protective effect of glibenclamide and metformin in combination with honey in pancreas of streptozotocin-induced diabetic rats. *Int J Mol Sci,* Vol. 11, No. 5, pp. 2056-2066.

Erejuwa, O. O., Sulaiman, S. A., Wahab, M. S., Sirajudeen, K. N., Salleh, M. S. & Gurtu, S. (2010c). Antioxidant protection of Malaysian tualang honey in pancreas of normal and streptozotocin-induced diabetic rats. *Ann Endocrinol* (Paris), Vol. 71, No. 4, pp. 291-296.

Erejuwa, O. O., Sulaiman, S. A., Wahab, M. S., Sirajudeen, K. N., Salleh, M. S. & Gurtu, S. (2011a). Comparison of antioxidant effects of honey, glibenclamide, metformin, and their combinations in the kidneys of streptozotocin-induced diabetic rats. *Int J Mol Sci,* Vol. 12, No. 1, pp. 829-843.

Erejuwa, O. O., Sulaiman, S. A., Wahab, M. S., Sirajudeen, K. N., Salleh, M. S. & Gurtu, S. (2011b). Effect of Glibenclamide alone versus Glibenclamide and Honey on Oxidative Stress in Pancreas of Streptozotocin-Induced Diabetic Rats. *Int J Appl Res Nat Prod,* Vol. 4, No. 2, pp. 1-10.

Erejuwa, O. O., Sulaiman, S. A., Wahab, M. S., Sirajudeen, K. N., Salleh, M. S. & Gurtu, S. (2011c). Differential responses to blood pressure and oxidative stress in streptozotocin-induced diabetic wistar-kyoto rats and spontaneously hypertensive rats: effects of antioxidant (honey) treatment. *Int J Mol Sci,* Vol. 12, No. 3, pp. 1888-1907.

Erejuwa, O. O., Sulaiman, S. A., Wahab, M. S., Sirajudeen, K. N., Salleh, M. S. & Gurtu, S. (2011d). Glibenclamide or metformin combined with honey improves glycemic control in streptozotocin-induced diabetic rats. *Int J Biol Sci,* Vol. 7, No. 2, pp. 244-252.

Erejuwa, O. O., Sulaiman, S. A., Ab Wahab, M. S., Sirajudeen, K. N., Salleh, M. S. & Gurtu, S. (2012a). Honey supplementation elicits antihypertensive effect in spontaneously hypertensive rats via amelioration of renal oxidative stress. *Oxid Med Cell Longev,* Vol. 2012, No. 374037, pp. 1-14.

Erejuwa, O. O., Sulaiman, S. A., Wahab, M. S., Sirajudeen, K. N., Salleh, M. S. & Gurtu, S. (2012b). Hepatoprotective effect of tualang honey supplementation in streptozotocin-induced diabetic rats. *Int J Appl Res Nat Prod,* Vol. 4, No. 4, pp. 37-41.

Evans, J. L., Goldfine, I. D., Maddux, B. A. & Grodsky, G. M. (2003). Are oxidative stress-activated signaling pathways mediators of insulin resistance and beta-cell dysfunction? *Diabetes,* Vol. 52, No. 1, pp. 1-8.

Faria, A., Monteiro, R., Pestana, D., Freitas, V., Mateus, N., Azevedo, I. & Calhau, C. (2009). Intestinal oxidative state can alter nutrient and drug bioavailability. *Oxid Med Cell Longev,* Vol. 2, No. 5, pp. 322-327.

Fava, D., Cassone-Faldetta, M., Laurenti, O., De Luca, O., Ghiselli, A. & De Mattia, G. (2002). Gliclazide improves anti-oxidant status and nitric oxide-mediated vasodilation in Type 2 diabetes. *Diabet Med,* Vol. 19, No. 9, pp. 752-757.

Figueroa-Romero, C., Sadidi, M. & Feldman, E. L. (2008). Mechanisms of disease: the oxidative stress theory of diabetic neuropathy. *Rev Endocr Metab Disord,* Vol. 9, No. 4, pp. 301-314.

Fioretto, P., Steffes, M. W., Sutherland, D. E., Goetz, F. C. & Mauer, M. (1998). Reversal of lesions of diabetic nephropathy after pancreas transplantation. *N Engl J Med,* Vol. 339, No. 2, pp. 69-75.

Fukai, T. & Ushio-Fukai, M. (2011). Superoxide dismutases: role in redox signaling, vascular function, and diseases. *Antioxid Redox Signal,* Vol. 15, No. 6, pp. 1583-1606.

Genuth, S., Sun, W., Cleary, P., Sell, D. R., Dahms, W., Malone, J., Sivitz, W. & Monnier, V. M. (2005). Glycation and carboxymethyllysine levels in skin collagen predict the risk of future 10-year progression of diabetic retinopathy and nephropathy in the diabetes control and complications trial and epidemiology of diabetes interventions and complications participants with type 1 diabetes. *Diabetes,* Vol. 54, No. 11, pp. 3103-3111.

Giacco, F. & Brownlee, M. (2010). Oxidative stress and diabetic complications. *Circ Res,* Vol. 107, No. 9, pp. 1058-1070.

Griesmacher, A., Kindhauser, M., Andert, S. E., Schreiner, W., Toma, C., Knoebl, P., Pietschmann, P., Prager, R., Schnack, C., Schernthaner, G. & et al. (1995). Enhanced serum levels of thiobarbituric-acid-reactive substances in diabetes mellitus. *The American journal of medicine,* Vol. 98, No. 5, pp. 469-475.

Gupta, S., Sharma, T. K., Kaushik, G. G. & Shekhawat, V. P. (2011). Vitamin E supplementation may ameliorate oxidative stress in type 1 diabetes mellitus patients. *Clin Lab,* Vol. 57, No. 5-6, pp. 379-386.

Halliwell, B. (2011). Free radicals and antioxidants - quo vadis? *Trends Pharmacol Sci,* Vol. 32, No. 3, pp. 125-130.

Halliwell, B. & Gutteridge, J. M. C. (2007) Free Radicals in Biology and Medicine 4th. Edn, Clarendon Press, Oxford.

Hammes, H. P., Klinzing, I., Wiegand, S., Bretzel, R. G., Cohen, A. M. & Federlin, K. (1993). Islet transplantation inhibits diabetic retinopathy in the sucrose-fed diabetic Cohen rat. *Invest Ophthalmol Vis Sci,* Vol. 34, No. 6, pp. 2092-2096.

Henriksen, E. J. (2010). Dysregulation of glycogen synthase kinase-3 in skeletal muscle and the etiology of insulin resistance and type 2 diabetes. *Curr Diabetes Rev,* Vol. 6, No. 5, pp. 285-293.

Hoehn, K. L., Salmon, A. B., Hohnen-Behrens, C., Turner, N., Hoy, A. J., Maghzal, G. J., Stocker, R., Van Remmen, H., Kraegen, E. W., Cooney, G. J., Richardson, A. R. & James, D. E. (2009). Insulin resistance is a cellular antioxidant defense mechanism. *Proc Natl Acad Sci U S A,* Vol. 106, No. 42, pp. 17787-17792.

Holman, R. R., Paul, S. K., Bethel, M. A., Matthews, D. R. & Neil, H. A. (2008). 10-year follow-up of intensive glucose control in type 2 diabetes. *N Engl J Med,* Vol. 359, No. 15, pp. 1577-1589.

Ihnat, M. A., Thorpe, J. E., Kamat, C. D., Szabo, C., Green, D. E., Warnke, L. A., Lacza, Z., Cselenyak, A., Ross, K., Shakir, S., Piconi, L., Kaltreider, R. C. & Ceriello, A. (2007). Reactive oxygen species mediate a cellular 'memory' of high glucose stress signalling. *Diabetologia,* Vol. 50, No. 7, pp. 1523-1531.

Ismail-Beigi, F., Craven, T., Banerji, M. A., Basile, J., Calles, J., Cohen, R. M., Cuddihy, R., Cushman, W. C., Genuth, S., Grimm, R. H., Jr., Hamilton, B. P., Hoogwerf, B., Karl, D., Katz, L., Krikorian, A., O'Connor, P., Pop-Busui, R., Schubart, U., Simmons, D., Taylor, H., Thomas, A., Weiss, D. & Hramiak, I. (2010). Effect of intensive treatment of hyperglycaemia on microvascular outcomes in type 2 diabetes: an analysis of the ACCORD randomised trial. *Lancet,* Vol. 376, No. 9739, pp. 419-430.

Johansen, J. S., Harris, A. K., Rychly, D. J. & Ergul, A. (2005). Oxidative stress and the use of antioxidants in diabetes: linking basic science to clinical practice. *Cardiovasc Diabetol,* Vol. 4, No. 1, pp. 5.

Kim, J. S., Saengsirisuwan, V., Sloniger, J. A., Teachey, M. K. & Henriksen, E. J. (2006). Oxidant stress and skeletal muscle glucose transport: roles of insulin signaling and p38 MAPK. *Free Radic Biol Med,* Vol. 41, No. 5, pp. 818-824.

Kowluru, R. A. (2003). Effect of reinstitution of good glycemic control on retinal oxidative stress and nitrative stress in diabetic rats. *Diabetes,* Vol. 52, No. 3, pp. 818-823.

Kowluru, R. A., Chakrabarti, S. & Chen, S. (2004). Re-institution of good metabolic control in diabetic rats and activation of caspase-3 and nuclear transcriptional factor (NF-kappaB) in the retina. *Acta Diabetol,* Vol. 41, No. 4, pp. 194-199.

Kowluru, R. A., Kanwar, M. & Kennedy, A. (2007). Metabolic memory phenomenon and accumulation of peroxynitrite in retinal capillaries. *Exp Diabetes Res,* Vol. 2007, No. pp. 21976.

Lai, M. H. (2008). Antioxidant effects and insulin resistance improvement of chromium combined with vitamin C and e supplementation for type 2 diabetes mellitus. *J Clin Biochem Nutr,* Vol. 43, No. 3, pp. 191-198.

Lubos, E., Loscalzo, J. & Handy, D. E. (2011). Glutathione peroxidase-1 in health and disease: from molecular mechanisms to therapeutic opportunities. *Antioxid Redox Signal,* Vol. 15, No. pp. 1957-1997.

Lupachyk, S., Shevalye, H., Maksimchyk, Y., Drel, V. R. & Obrosova, I. G. (2011). PARP inhibition alleviates diabetes-induced systemic oxidative stress and neural tissue 4-hydroxynonenal adduct accumulation: correlation with peripheral nerve function. *Free Radic Biol Med,* Vol. 50, No. 10, pp. 1400-1409.

Lushchak, V. (2010). Oxidative stress in yeast. *Biochemistry* (Moscow), Vol.75, pp. 281-296.

Maechler, P., Jornot, L. & Wollheim, C. B. (1999). Hydrogen peroxide alters mitochondrial activation and insulin secretion in pancreatic beta cells. *J Biol Chem,* Vol. 274, No. 39, pp. 27905-27913.

Marchetti, P., Dotta, F., Lauro, D. & Purrello, F. (2008). An overview of pancreatic beta-cell defects in human type 2 diabetes: implications for treatment. *Regul Pept,* Vol. 146, No. 1-3, pp. 4-11.

Maritim, A. C., Sanders, R. A. & Watkins, J. B., 3rd (2003). Diabetes, oxidative stress, and antioxidants: a review. *J Biochem Mol Toxicol,* Vol. 17, No. 1, pp. 24-38.

Michiels, C., Raes, M., Toussaint, O. & Remacle, J. (1994). Importance of Se-glutathione peroxidase, catalase, and Cu/Zn-SOD for cell survival against oxidative stress. *Free Radic Biol Med,* Vol. 17, No. 3, pp. 235-248.

Miwa, I., Ichimura, N., Sugiura, M., Hamada, Y. & Taniguchi, S. (2000). Inhibition of glucose-induced insulin secretion by 4-hydroxy-2-nonenal and other lipid peroxidation products. *Endocrinology,* Vol. 141, No. 8, pp. 2767-2772.

Monnier, V. M., Bautista, O., Kenny, D., Sell, D. R., Fogarty, J., Dahms, W., Cleary, P. A., Lachin, J. & Genuth, S. (1999). Skin collagen glycation, glycoxidation, and crosslinking are lower in subjects with long-term intensive versus conventional therapy of type 1 diabetes: relevance of glycated collagen products versus HbA1c as markers of diabetic complications. DCCT Skin Collagen Ancillary Study Group. Diabetes Control and Complications Trial. *Diabetes,* Vol. 48, No. 4, pp. 870-880.

Nathan, D. M., Cleary, P. A., Backlund, J. Y., Genuth, S. M., Lachin, J. M., Orchard, T. J., Raskin, P. & Zinman, B. (2005). Intensive diabetes treatment and cardiovascular disease in patients with type 1 diabetes. *N Engl J Med,* Vol. 353, No. 25, pp. 2643-2653.

Nathan, D. M., Lachin, J., Cleary, P., Orchard, T., Brillon, D. J., Backlund, J. Y., O'Leary, D. H. & Genuth, S. (2003). Intensive diabetes therapy and carotid intima-media thickness in type 1 diabetes mellitus. *N Engl J Med,* Vol. 348, No. 23, pp. 2294-2303.

Nishikawa, T., Edelstein, D. & Brownlee, M. (2000a). The missing link: a single unifying mechanism for diabetic complications. *Kidney Int Suppl,* Vol. 77, No. pp. S26-30.

Nishikawa, T., Edelstein, D., Du, X. L., Yamagishi, S., Matsumura, T., Kaneda, Y., Yorek, M. A., Beebe, D., Oates, P. J., Hammes, H. P., Giardino, I. & Brownlee, M. (2000b). Normalizing mitochondrial superoxide production blocks three pathways of hyperglycaemic damage. *Nature,* Vol. 404, No. 6779, pp. 787-790.

Patel, A., MacMahon, S., Chalmers, J., Neal, B., Billot, L., Woodward, M., Marre, M., Cooper, M., Glasziou, P., Grobbee, D., Hamet, P., Harrap, S., Heller, S., Liu, L., Mancia, G., Mogensen, C. E., Pan, C., Poulter, N., Rodgers, A., Williams, B., Bompoint, S., de Galan, B. E., Joshi, R. & Travert, F. (2008). Intensive blood glucose control and vascular outcomes in patients with type 2 diabetes. *N Engl J Med,* Vol. 358, No. 24, pp. 2560-2572.

Penckofer, S., Schwertz, D. & Florczak, K. (2002). Oxidative stress and cardiovascular disease in type 2 diabetes: the role of antioxidants and pro-oxidants. *J Cardiovasc Nurs,* Vol. 16, No. 2, pp. 68-85.

Petrash, J. M. (2004). All in the family: aldose reductase and closely related aldo-keto reductases. *Cell Mol Life Sci,* Vol. 61, No. 7-8, pp. 737-749.

Pop-Busui, R., Low, P. A., Waberski, B. H., Martin, C. L., Albers, J. W., Feldman, E. L., Sommer, C., Cleary, P. A., Lachin, J. M. & Herman, W. H. (2009). Effects of prior intensive insulin therapy on cardiac autonomic nervous system function in type 1 diabetes mellitus: the Diabetes Control and Complications Trial/Epidemiology of Diabetes Interventions and Complications study (DCCT/EDIC). *Circulation,* Vol. 119, No. 22, pp. 2886-2893.

Rahimi, R., Nikfar, S., Larijani, B. & Abdollahi, M. (2005). A review on the role of antioxidants in the management of diabetes and its complications. *Biomed Pharmacother,* Vol. 59, No. 7, pp. 365-373.

Razquin, C., Martinez, J. A., Martinez-Gonzalez, M. A., Mitjavila, M. T., Estruch, R. & Marti, A. (2009). A 3 years follow-up of a Mediterranean diet rich in virgin olive oil is associated with high plasma antioxidant capacity and reduced body weight gain. *Eur J Clin Nutr,* Vol. 63, No. 12, pp. 1387-1393.

Robinson, I., de Serna, D. G., Gutierrez, A. & Schade, D. S. (2006). Vitamin E in humans: an explanation of clinical trial failure. *Endocr Pract,* Vol. 12, No. 5, pp. 576-582.

Roglic, G. & Unwin, N. (2010). Mortality attributable to diabetes: estimates for the year 2010. *Diabetes Res Clin Pract.,* Vol. 87, No. 1, pp. 15-19.

Rosca, M. G., Monnier, V. M., Szweda, L. I. & Weiss, M. F. (2002). Alterations in renal mitochondrial respiration in response to the reactive oxoaldehyde methylglyoxal. *Am J Physiol Renal Physiol,* Vol. 283, No. 1, pp. F52-9.

Rosca, M. G., Mustata, T. G., Kinter, M. T., Ozdemir, A. M., Kern, T. S., Szweda, L. I., Brownlee, M., Monnier, V. M. & Weiss, M. F. (2005). Glycation of mitochondrial proteins from diabetic rat kidney is associated with excess superoxide formation. *Am J Physiol Renal Physiol,* Vol. 289, No. 2, pp. F420-30.

Rudich, A., Tirosh, A., Potashnik, R., Hemi, R., Kanety, H. & Bashan, N. (1998). Prolonged oxidative stress impairs insulin-induced GLUT4 translocation in 3T3-L1 adipocytes. *Diabetes,* Vol. 47, No. 10, pp. 1562-1569.

Rudich, A., Tirosh, A., Potashnik, R., Khamaisi, M. & Bashan, N. (1999). Lipoic acid protects against oxidative stress induced impairment in insulin stimulation of protein kinase B and glucose transport in 3T3-L1 adipocytes. *Diabetologia,* Vol. 42, No. 8, pp. 949-957.

Sachdev, S. & Davies, K. J. (2008). Production, detection, and adaptive responses to free radicals in exercise. *Free Radic Biol Med,* Vol. 44, No. 2, pp. 215-223.

Schleicher, E. D. & Weigert, C. (2000). Role of the hexosamine biosynthetic pathway in diabetic nephropathy. *Kidney Int Suppl,* Vol. 77, No. pp. S13-18.

Schonfeld, P., Dymkowska, D. & Wojtczak, L. (2009). Acyl-CoA-induced generation of reactive oxygen species in mitochondrial preparations is due to the presence of peroxisomes. *Free Radic Biol Med,* Vol. 47, No. 5, pp. 503-509.

Scibior, D. & Czeczot, H. (2006). [Catalase: structure, properties, functions]. *Postepy Hig Med Dosw (Online),* Vol. 60, No. pp. 170-180.

Scott, J. A. & King, G. L. (2004). Oxidative stress and antioxidant treatment in diabetes. *Ann N Y Acad Sci,* Vol. 1031, No. pp. 204-213.

Seghrouchni, I., Drai, J., Bannier, E., Riviere, J., Calmard, P., Garcia, I., Orgiazzi, J. & Revol, A. (2002). Oxidative stress parameters in type I, type II and insulin-treated type 2 diabetes mellitus; insulin treatment efficiency. *Clin Chim Acta,* Vol. 321, No. 1-2, pp. 89-96.

Sharma, A., Kharb, S., Chugh, S. N., Kakkar, R. & Singh, G. P. (2000). Effect of glycemic control and vitamin E supplementation on total glutathione content in non-insulin-dependent diabetes mellitus. *Ann Nutr Metab,* Vol. 44, No. 1, pp. 11-13.

Sies, H. (1991) Oxidative stress: introduction. In Oxidative Stress: Oxidants and Antioxidants, Academic Press London.

Sindhu, R. K., Koo, J. R., Roberts, C. K. & Vaziri, N. D. (2004). Dysregulation of hepatic superoxide dismutase, catalase and glutathione peroxidase in diabetes: response to insulin and antioxidant therapies. *Clin Exp Hypertens,* Vol. 26, No. 1, pp. 43-53.

Slonchak, A. M. & Obolens'ka, M. (2009). [Structure and functions of glutathione S-transferase P1-1]. *Ukr Biokhim Zh,* Vol. 81, No. 1, pp. 5-13.

Slyvka, Y., Inman, S. R., Malgor, R., Jackson, E. J., Yee, J., Oshogwemoh, O., Adame, J. & Nowak, F. V. (2009). Protective effects of antioxidant-fortified diet on renal function and metabolic profile in obese Zucker rat. *Endocrine,* Vol. 35, No. 1, pp. 89-100.

Talior, I., Yarkoni, M., Bashan, N. & Eldar-Finkelman, H. (2003). Increased glucose uptake promotes oxidative stress and PKC-delta activation in adipocytes of obese, insulin-resistant mice. *Am J Physiol Endocrinol Metab,* Vol. 285, No. 2, pp. E295-302.

Tanaka, Y., Gleason, C. E., Tran, P. O., Harmon, J. S. & Robertson, R. P. (1999). Prevention of glucose toxicity in HIT-T15 cells and Zucker diabetic fatty rats by antioxidants. *Proc Natl Acad Sci U S A,* Vol. 96, No. 19, pp. 10857-10862.

Tiedge, M., Lortz, S., Drinkgern, J. & Lenzen, S. (1997). Relation between antioxidant enzyme gene expression and antioxidative defense status of insulin-producing cells. *Diabetes,* Vol. 46, No. 11, pp. 1733-1742.

Tiedge, M., Lortz, S., Munday, R. & Lenzen, S. (1998). Complementary action of antioxidant enzymes in the protection of bioengineered insulin-producing RINm5F cells against the toxicity of reactive oxygen species. *Diabetes,* Vol. 47, No. 10, pp. 1578-1585.

Tirosh, A., Potashnik, R., Bashan, N. & Rudich, A. (1999). Oxidative stress disrupts insulin-induced cellular redistribution of insulin receptor substrate-1 and phosphatidylinositol 3-kinase in 3T3-L1 adipocytes. A putative cellular mechanism for impaired protein kinase B activation and GLUT4 translocation. *J Biol Chem,* Vol. 274, No. 15, pp. 10595-10602.

Turner, R. C., Cull, C. A., Frighi, V. & Holman, R. R. (1999). Glycemic control with diet, sulfonylurea, metformin, or insulin in patients with type 2 diabetes mellitus: progressive requirement for multiple therapies (UKPDS 49). UK Prospective Diabetes Study (UKPDS) Group. *JAMA,* Vol. 281, No. 21, pp. 2005-2012.

UKPDS (1998). UK Prospective Diabetes Study (UKPDS) Group. Intensive blood-glucose control with sulphonylureas or insulin compared with conventional treatment and risk of complications in patients with type 2 diabetes (UKPDS 33). *Lancet,* Vol. 352, No. 9131, pp. 837-853.

Virag, L. & Szabo, C. (2002). The therapeutic potential of poly(ADP-ribose) polymerase inhibitors. *Pharmacol Rev,* Vol. 54, No. 3, pp. 375-429.

Watala, C. & Winocour, P. D. (1992). The relationship of chemical modification of membrane proteins and plasma lipoproteins to reduced membrane fluidity of erythrocytes from diabetic subjects. *Eur J Clin Chem Clin Biochem,* Vol. 30, No. 9, pp. 513-519.

Wei, W. P., Xue, Y. M., Gao, F., Zhu, B. & Li, C. Z. (2011). [Cellular memory of high glucose exposure in normoglycemia is probably mediated by reactive oxygen species in INS-1 cells]. *Nan Fang Yi Ke Da Xue Xue Bao,* Vol. 31, No. 4, pp. 682-685.

Wei, Y. H. (1998). Oxidative stress and mitochondrial DNA mutations in human aging. *Proc Soc Exp Biol Med,* Vol. 217, No. 1, pp. 53-63.

Wiernsperger, N. F. (2003). Oxidative stress as a therapeutic target in diabetes: revisiting the controversy. *Diabetes Metab,* Vol. 29, No. 6, pp. 579-585.

Whiting, D.R., Guariguata, L., Weil, C., Shaw, J. (2011). IDF Diabetes Atlas: Global estimates of the prevalence of diabetes for 2011 and 2030. *Diabetes Res Clin Pract,* Vol. 94, pp. 311–321.

Whiting, D.R., Guariguata, L., Weil, C., Shaw, J. (2011). IDF Diabetes Atlas: Global estimates of the prevalence of diabetes for 2011 and 2030. Diabetes Res Clin Pract, Vol. 94, pp. 311–321.

Wiernsperger, N.F. (2003). Oxidative stress as a therapeutic target in diabetes: revisiting the controversy. Diabetes Metab, Vol. 29, pp. 579–585.

Wierzba, T. H. (2005). [Unexpected failure of antioxidant clinical trials]. *Kardiol Pol,* Vol. 63, No. 4 Suppl 2, pp. S472-482.

Willcox, B. J., Curb, J. D. & Rodriguez, B. L. (2008). Antioxidants in cardiovascular health and disease: key lessons from epidemiologic studies. *Am J Cardiol,* Vol. 101, No. 10A, pp. 75D-86D.

Yancey, P. H. & Burg, M. B. (1989). Distribution of major organic osmolytes in rabbit kidneys in diuresis and antidiuresis. *Am J Physiol,* Vol. 257, No. 4 Pt 2, pp. F602-607.

Zhou, Y. P. & Grill, V. E. (1994). Long-term exposure of rat pancreatic islets to fatty acids inhibits glucose-induced insulin secretion and biosynthesis through a glucose fatty acid cycle. *J Clin Invest,* Vol. 93, No. 2, pp. 870-876.

11

Oxidative Stress and Novel Antioxidant Approaches to Reduce Diabetic Complications

Sih Min Tan, Arpeeta Sharma and Judy B. de Haan
Oxidative Stress Laboratory, Diabetic Complications Division, Baker IDI Heart and Diabetes Institute, Melbourne, Australia

1. Introduction

In 1995, the International Diabetes Federation estimated the prevalence of diabetes to be approximately 135 million patients worldwide. More recently in 2010, it was estimated that around 285 million people were diabetic and this number is predicted to reach 438 million by 2030, accounting for 7.7% of the population aged 20-79 (Shaw et al 2010). However, despite greater knowledge of the disease, approximately one-third of people with diabetes remain undiagnosed. Although intensive blood glucose and blood pressure control have reduced the risk of diabetes-associated microvascular (nephropathy, retinopathy, neuropathy) and macrovascular complications (atherosclerosis), diabetes remains a major risk factor for cardiovascular complications, cardiomyopathy, end-stage renal disease (ESRD), blindness and neuropathy. There is therefore an urgent need to develop more effective therapeutic strategies to prevent and/or halt the progression of diabetic complications.

Accumulating evidence suggests that oxidative stress plays a pivotal role in the aetiology of diabetic complications. Many biochemical pathways associated with hyperglycaemia increase the production of free radicals leading to oxidative stress, including glucose auto-oxidation, the polyol pathway, prostanoids synthesis, protein glycation and the protein kinase C (PKC) pathway (Giugliano et al 1996). Hyperglycaemia alters reactive oxygen species (ROS) production, particularly in the mitochondria, leading to increased intracellular ROS and activated stress-sensitive pathways such as nuclear factor κB (NFκB), p38 mitogen-activated protein kinase (MAPK), and the c-Jun NH2-terminal kinase/stress-activated protein kinase (JNK/SAPK) pathways (Johansen et al 2005). Subsequently, PKC activity, advanced glycation end-products (AGE) and sorbitol levels increase and this can lead to more ROS generation in a positive regulatory feedback loop to chronically stimulate stress-sensitive pathways. ROS can also inflict direct damage upon cellular macromolecules which, in turn, result in further oxidative stress (Evans et al 2002).

Under physiological conditions, reactive oxygen and reactive nitrogen species (RNS) are produced and maintained at steady-state levels within a cell (Lushchak 2011). On the other hand, oxidative stress arises when an imbalance occurs between the production of ROS/RNS and the antioxidant defences that neutralise them, shifting the balance in favour of enhanced ROS levels. The consequence of this shift is cellular damage to biologically important molecules and organelles (Sies 1997). Elevations in ROS/RNS levels are mainly caused by an imbalance between the activity of endogenous pro-oxidant enzymes, such as nicotinamide adenine dinucleotide phosphate (NADPH) oxidase, xanthine oxidase or the mitochondrial respiratory chain, and the antioxidant enzymes, such as superoxide dismutase (SOD), glutathione peroxidase (GPx), heme oxygenase (HO), thioredoxin (Trx) peroxidase/peroxiredoxin, catalase and paraoxonase (Forstermann 2008). ROS include the superoxide anion ($^{\bullet}O_2^-$) and the hydroxyl radical ($^{\bullet}OH$), as well as non-radical species such as hydrogen peroxide (H_2O_2). RNS include the free radicals nitric oxide ($^{\bullet}NO$) and non-radical species such as peroxynitrite ($ONOO^-$) and nitrogen dioxide (NO_2)(Johansen et al 2005). In a hyperglycaemic milieu, $^{\bullet}O_2^-$ increases through the enhanced activity of enzymatic sources, including NADPH oxidase and xanthine oxidase, and non-enzymatic sources such as the mitochondrial respiratory chain, glucose autoxidation, AGE formation and activation of the polyol pathway. In addition, antioxidant defences are known to decrease in a hyperglycaemic milieu, shifting the balance away from steady-state levels of ROS towards an environment of oxidative stress.

2. Oxidative stress and diabetic complications

2.1 Diabetes-associated atherosclerosis

Atherosclerosis is a major cause of mortality and morbidity in patients with diabetes (Beckman et al 2002). The buildup of fat and cholesterol along the walls of arteries is progressive; it thickens and hardens, forming calcium deposits, and may eventually block the arteries. Blockage of the arteries and/or rupture of vulnerable plaques is a common cause of heart attack and stroke. Diabetes has been shown to accelerate the clinical course of atherosclerosis in the coronary arteries (coronary artery disease, including myocardial infarction), lower extremities (peripheral arterial disease) and extracranial carotid arteries (cerebrovascular disease, including stroke) (Beckman et al 2002).

An understanding of the underlying mechanisms that accelerate diabetes-associated atherosclerosis is important in the search for treatments to protect against or retard the progression of this disease. The abnormal metabolic state associated with diabetes, which includes chronic hyperglycaemia, dyslipidemia and insulin resistance can alter the function of multiple cell types including endothelial cells, smooth muscle cells and platelets. The single layer of endothelial cells that line the vessels of the circulatory system, provide a metabolically active interface between the blood and the underlying tissue to facilitate blood flow and nutrient delivery. Disruption of the integrity of the endothelium leads to inflammation, activation of platelets, coagulation, and thrombosis (Cines et al 1998). To protect against this, the endothelium synthesises important bioactive substances such as endothelial-derived NO (EDNO), prostaglandins, endothelin (ET) and angiotensin II (Ang II) that regulate blood vessel function and structure (Beckman et al 2002). It is now known that hyperglycaemia-mediated dysregulation of these vasoprotective agents either enhances the intensity of oxidative stress directly or is affected by oxidative stress. The consequences of hyperglycaemia-driven enhanced ROS/RNS on the vasculature will be discussed below.

2.1.1 The role of ROS in diabetes-associated atherosclerosis

Due to its vasorelaxation, anti-inflammatory and anti-proliferative properties, EDNO is often viewed as vasculoprotective. Diabetes is associated with an attenuation of EDNO bioavailability, which is lowered by either decreased formation or enhanced removal of $^{\bullet}NO$. One way in which hyperglycaemia attenuates the level of EDNO is by blocking the function of endothelial NOS (eNOS) synthase in endothelial and vascular smooth muscle cells (De Vriese et al 2000). However, evidence now points most strongly at the prevention of EDNO reaching its molecular target, rather than its attenuated production as being critical for the loss of EDNO bioavailability in diabetes. An increase in ROS, such as $^{\bullet}O_2^-$ within the endothelium is one of the most significant factors known to decrease EDNO (de Haan & Cooper 2011). Increased $^{\bullet}O_2^-$ can reduce EDNO bioavailability due to its propensity to react with $^{\bullet}NO$, producing the highly reactive oxidant, $ONOO^-$ (Beckman 1996). Loss of functional EDNO causes impaired relaxation of the vessel wall and inhibition of the proliferative effects of EDNO (Maritim et al 2003a). In addition, $ONOO^-$ can induce cell damage via lipid peroxidation, and the inactivation of enzymes and structural proteins by oxidation and nitration. Furthermore, $ONOO^-$ can activate matrix metalloproteinases (MMPs), trigger the release of pro-apoptic factors such as cytochrome c and induce DNA damage (Pacher & Szabo 2006). $ONOO^-$ is also involved in oxidising tetrahydrobiopterin (BH_4), an important cofactor of eNOS, thereby uncoupling eNOS which then produces $^{\bullet}O_2^-$ instead of EDNO (Maritim et al 2003a).

It is also known that a reduction in $^{\bullet}NO$, as evident in diabetes, stimulates endothelial angiotensin-converting enzyme (ACE) activity and the generation of Ang II and $^{\bullet}O_2^-$ (Schulman et al 2006). While EDNO inhibits the production of endothelin-1 (ET-1) which is a vasoconstricting peptide (Boulanger & Luscher 1990), increased Ang II can stimulate the endothelial cell to synthesise and release ET-1, thereby contributing to vascular smooth muscle dysfunction (Sasser et al 2002). A disruption in vascular smooth muscle function may lead to plaque destabilisation and rupture, with often fatal consequences (Beckman et al 2002). Since EDNO also limits inflammation by reducing leukocyte adhesion and migration (Chen et al 1998), lowering EDNO will also promote atherogenesis via accelerated pro-inflammatory pathways. Additionally, EDNO is also involved in the inhibition of platelet activation (Loscalzo 2001). A reduction in the bioavailability of EDNO in diabetes therefore potentiates platelet activation, adhesion and aggregate formation, leading to thrombosis. Hence, the increased presence of $^{\bullet}O_2^-$, as seen in diabetes, limits the protective effects of EDNO in the vasculature leading to increased inflammation, thrombosis, plaque destabilisation and plaque rupture (Fig.1).

The effects of hyperglycaemia-mediated increases in $^{\bullet}O_2^-$ levels in the mitochondria are numerous and mostly detrimental to the cells of the vasculature. For example, $^{\bullet}O_2^-$ has been shown to activate the nuclear enzyme poly(ADP-ribose) polymerase (PARP) which in turn leads to metabolic alterations that activate NFκB, AGE/receptor for AGE (RAGE) and the polyol pathways (Pacher & Szabo 2006). Upregulation of these pathways results in more $^{\bullet}O_2^-$ production, while NFκB activation increases the expression of many proinflammatory mediators, leading to endothelial dysfunction. Furthermore, it is well accepted that ROS such as $^{\bullet}O_2^-$ are involved in the oxidation of low-density lipoprotein (ox-LDL), which is not recognised by the LDL receptor and is preferentially taken up by scavenger receptors on macrophages, leading to foam cell formation and atherosclerotic plaques (Boullier et al 2001).

Finally, it is important to highlight that increased $^{\bullet}O_2^-$ via enzymatic antioxidant conversion (see Fig.2) gives rise to increased levels of H_2O_2, an important ROS implicated in pro-inflammatory processes that are further amplified as diabetes develops (Nicolls et al 2007). H_2O_2 has also been shown to upregulate vascular cell adhesion molecule-1 (VCAM-1), an important adhesion molecule that aids in the migration of leukocytes from the blood into the tissue (Cook-Mills 2006). It is therefore clear that elevations in hyperglycaemia-mediated ROS lead to cellular, molecular and functional vascular alterations that initiate, mediate and ultimately hasten cardiovascular complications associated with diabetes.

2.2 Diabetic cardiomyopathy

Diabetic cardiomyopathy is considered a distinct clinical entity first recognised by Rubler et al. (1972) in 4 diabetic patients with congestive heart failure without evidence of hypertension, coronary artery disease or congenital heart disease. The Framingham study showed that diabetic men and women had a 2- and 5-fold greater incidence of heart failure respectively, even after taking into account other common risk factors such as coronary artery disease, age, blood pressure, weight and cholesterol (Kannel et al 1974). Diabetic cardiomyopathy is characterised by early diastolic dysfunction and late systolic impairment, and is accompanied by a wide range of structural abnormalities and pathophysiological impairments (Hayat et al 2004). Despite intensive investigations, the aetiology of diabetic cardiomyopathy remains elusive.

2.2.1 The role of ROS in diabetic cardiomyopathy

Hyperglycaemia is known to upregulate the production of Ang II, which is the overt hormone of the renin-angiotensin system (RAS). This has a profound effect on the myocardium given that most of the cellular components of the RAS including angiotensinogen, renin and the angiotensin II type I (AT_1) receptor are found in myocytes (Fiordaliso et al 2000). Although Ang II is known to contribute to the development of diabetic cardiomyopathy through its hemodynamic vasoconstrictor effects and its ability to act as a proinflammatory mediator, it is now becoming increasingly clear that Ang II mediates its effects on the myocardium via its ability to enhance production of $^{\bullet}O_2^-$ (Cooper 2004). Indeed, Privratsky et al. (2003) found that hyperglycaemia induces cardiac myopathies via the AT_1 receptor, with activation of NADPH oxidase and increased ROS generation. Furthermore, $^{\bullet}O_2^-$ levels were attenuated with an ACE inhibitor (Fiordaliso et al 2006). However, other sources of ROS generation are known to contribute to the oxidative stress that accompanies diabetic cardiomyopathy. For example, treatment of diabetic mice with allopurinol, the xanthine oxidase inhibitor, improved type 2 diabetes-induced cardiac dysfunction by decreasing oxidative/nitrosative stress and fibrosis (Rajesh et al 2009).

The biochemical pathways described earlier for diabetes-associated atherosclerosis, including those leading to endothelial dysfunction and inflammation due to the overproduction of ROS, appear to play a causal role in the pathogenesis of diabetic cardiomyopathy (Fig.1). Several lines of evidence suggest that nitrosative stress and peroxynitrite-induced damage contribute to the pathogenesis of diabetic cardiomyopathies. In particular, Szabo et al. (2002) showed that a metalloporphyrin peroxynitrite decomposition catalyst, FP15, which neutralises $ONOO^-$, ameliorates cardiovascular dysfunction in STZ-induced murine models of diabetes. Treatment with FP15 prevented loss of endothelium-dependent relaxant ability of blood vessels and improved both diastolic and systolic dysfunction of the diabetic heart, supporting the concept that neutralisation of $ONOO^-$ can be of significant therapeutic benefit. Furthermore, hyperglycaemia-mediated oxidative stress has been shown to cause abnormal gene expression, altered signal transduction, and the activation of pathways leading to myocyte apoptosis (Cai & Kang 2001). Myocyte death causes a loss of contractile units, compensatory hypertrophy of myocytes and reparative fibrosis, all characteristics of diabetic cardiomyopathy (Kang 2001). In a study by Frustaci et al. (2000), increased levels of nitrotyrosine were associated with apoptosis and necrosis of cardiac cells including myocytes, endothelial cells and fibroblasts in patients with diabetes, as well as in STZ-induced diabetic mice (Cai et al 2005). However, the mechanisms underlying hyperglycaemia-induced myocyte loss are still poorly understood.

Recently, it was shown that hyperglycaemia-induced oxidative stress results in the activation of the hexosamine biosynthetic pathway (HBP), leading to increased *O*-GlcNAcylation (endproduct of HBP) of the pro-apoptotic peptide, BAD. In this manner oxidative stress is linked to increased cardiac myocyte death (Rajamani & Essop 2010). Other known mediators of hyperglycaemia-induced cardiac cell death include AGEs (Li et al 2007), apoptosis signal-regulating kinase 1 (ASK1) (Thandavarayan et al 2008) and mitochondrial dysfunction (Duncan 2011). All of these pathways appear to induce myocyte apoptosis via an increase in oxidative stress in the diabetic heart. Myocyte loss and myocyte injury are believed to contribute to systolic dysfunction due to the impairment in the ability of the myocardium to develop force, resulting in reduced contractility, decreased pump function, and decreased ejection fraction (Fang et al 2004).

For destructive $ONOO^-$ to form within the diabetic myocardium, as detailed above, $^{\bullet}O_2^-$ must interact with and reduce the bioavailability of $^{\bullet}NO$. Since $^{\bullet}NO$ is one of the most important regulators of myocardial function, it is not surprising that hemodynamic studies have indicated that endothelium-dependent vasodilatory responses are impaired in the diabetic milieu (Farhangkhoee et al 2006). Indeed, the bioavailability of vasodilatory $^{\bullet}NO$ was found to be reduced with the progression of diabetic cardiomyopathy (Joffe et al 1999). In the heart, both eNOS and inducible NOS (iNOS) are the principal producers of $^{\bullet}NO$. Under physiological conditions, low levels of $^{\bullet}NO$ produced by eNOS increase diastolic relaxation and decrease oxygen consumption in cardiac myocytes, whereas high levels of $^{\bullet}NO$ produced by iNOS decrease the contraction of cardiac myocytes and induce apoptosis (Khullar et al 2010). Under pathological conditions, such as diabetes, both enzymes can produce highly reactive $^{\bullet}O_2^-$ and increase oxidative stress and inflammation (Razavi et al 2005). Additionally, loss of $^{\bullet}NO$ bioavailability in diabetes causes endothelial cell dysfunction, resulting in increased permeability of the vessel wall and reduced blood flow through the myocardium causing tissue ischemia. In response, endothelial cells release growth factors, such as transforming growth factor-β (TGF-β), resulting in increased basement membrane thickening, extracellular matrix (ECM) deposition and interstitial fibrosis (Farhangkhoee et al 2006).

Diabetes-mediated increases in ROS are also known to affect structural proteins pertinent to the integrity of the myocardium, as well as proteins that affect its function. ROS have been shown to cause alterations in the function of regulatory and contractile proteins such as the sarcoplasmic reticulum Ca^{2+}-ATPase and Na^{+}-Ca^{2+} exchanger in the heart (Fang et al., 2004). This leads to diminished calcium sensitivity of proteins involved in the regulation of the cardiac actomyosin system, a reduction in the sarcoplasmic reticulum Ca^{2+}-ATPase and a decrease in the sarcoplasmic reticulum calcium (SERCA2a) pump protein (Abe et al., 2002). These deficits may all contribute to impaired LV function. Indeed, abnormal diastolic and systolic function was normalised in streptozotocin-induced diabetic rat hearts when SERCA2a was overexpressed (Trost et al., 2002).

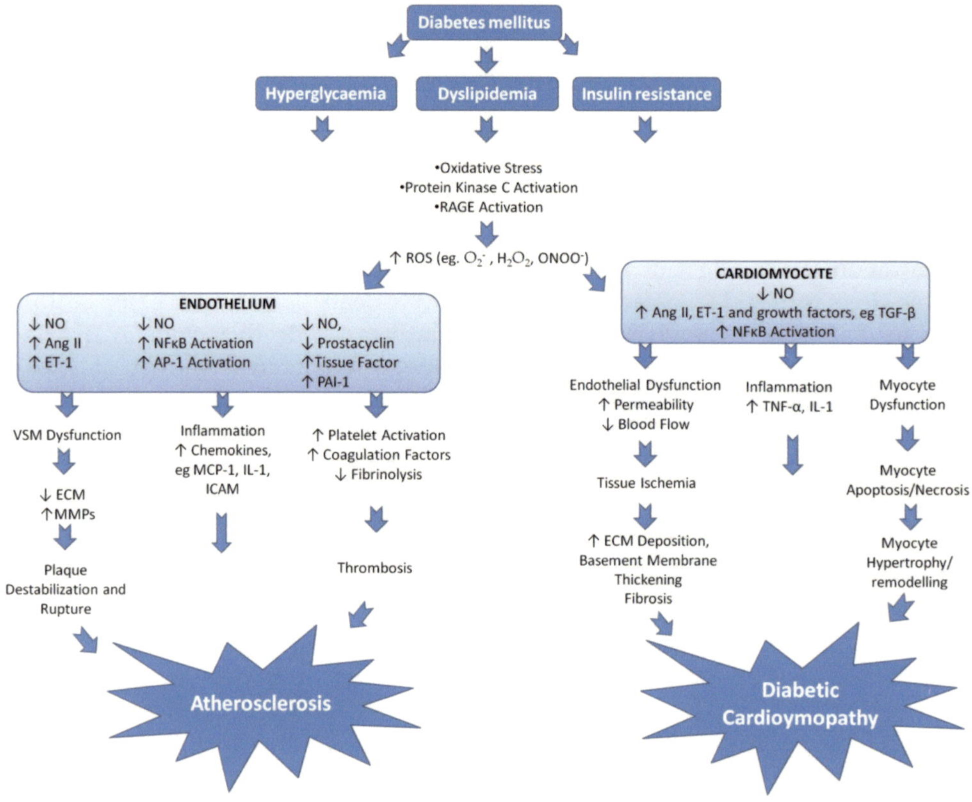

Fig. 1. Roles of reactive oxygen species (ROS) in the pathophysiology of diabetic macrovascular complications, namely atherosclerosis and diabetic cardiomyopathy.

2.3 Diabetic nephropathy

Diabetic nephropathy (DN) has become a worldwide epidemic, accounting for approximately one third of all cases of ESRD (Rossing 2006). DN is classically defined as the increase in protein excretion in the urine. The early stage of DN is characterised by a small increase in urinary albumin excretion (microalbuminuria), while overt diabetic nephropathy is defined as the presence of macroalbuminuria or proteinuria (Zelmanovitz et al 2009).

The earliest structural changes associated with diabetic nephropathy are the expansion of glomerular mesangial area, mesangial cell hypertrophy and thickening of the glomerular basement membrane (Gilbert & Cooper 1999), leading to a progressive reduction in the filtration surface of the glomerulus, a process known as glomerulosclerosis (Kalant 1978). Furthermore, there is now compelling evidence to suggest that disruption of the tubulointerstitial architecture is as important, if not more important in contributing to kidney injury as glomerular damage (Nangaku 2004).

Despite intensive glucose control and blockade of the RAS (Barit & Cooper 2008; Keane et al 2006), DN continues to progress in a significant proportion of patients and often leads to organ failure and the need for dialysis and/or kidney transplantation. Therefore, the development of novel targeted therapeutics is warranted to reduce or eliminate kidney disease in diabetic patients.

2.3.1 The role of ROS in diabetic nephropathy

An upregulation of ROS in diabetes has been implicated in the pathogenesis of kidney injury (Forbes et al 2008). ROS activate a number of signalling pathways including PKC, p38 MAPK, p42/p44 MAPK and the transcription factor NF-κB, which leads to the increased activation of growth factors such as TGF-β that contribute to the pathogenesis of DN. In the diabetic kidney, enhanced glucose uptake occurs in many of the cell populations including glomerular epithelial cells, mesangial cells and proximal tubular epithelial cells, leading to the excessive production of intracellular ROS, making these cells particularly susceptible to the diabetic milieu (Forbes et al 2008).

Sufficient evidence exists, from both clinical and pre-clinical studies, to suggest that oxidative stress accompanies the progression of diabetic nephropathy. Hyperglycaemia has been shown to increase 8-hydroxy-2′-deoxyguanosine (8-OHdG), a marker of oxidative mitochondrial DNA damage in diabetic rat kidneys (Kakimoto et al 2002). In this study, intervention by insulin treatment normalised renal 8-OHdG level in diabetic rats, clearly linking the diabetic milieu and increased oxidative stress in this pre-clinical model (Kakimoto et al 2002). In type 2 diabetic patients, it was found that urinary 8-OHdG excretion was significantly higher than in healthy controls and furthermore, that this increase was proportional to the severity of the tubulointerstitial lesion observed in the kidneys of these patients (Kanauchi et al 2002). In addition, it was reported that the 24-hour urinary content of 8-oxo-7,8-dihydro-2'-deoxyguanosine (8-oxodG), a product of oxidative DNA damage, strongly predicted the progression of DN in type 2 diabetic patients in a 5-year follow up study (Hinokio et al 2002).

Several studies have examined the pathways through which increased ROS may mediate its damaging effects on glomerular and tubular injury in the diabetic kidney. One study showed that ROS mediates high glucose-induced activation of PKC in mesangial cells, leading to an increase in TGF-β expression (Studer et al 1997). Ha et al. (2002) have demonstrated that by inhibiting ROS with a series of antioxidants, high glucose-induced activation of NFκB and NFκB-dependent monocyte chemoattractant protein-1 (MCP-1) expression was inhibited in mesangial cells. Furthermore, increased ROS led to accelerated glomerulosclerosis through TGF-β-mediated plasminogen activator inhibitor-1 (PAI-1) upregulation in mesangial cells (Jiang et al 2003b). Similarly, it was proposed that ROS mediate kidney fibrosis in renal cells through the upregulation of the transcription factors NFκB and activator protein-1 (AP-1), that in turn increase MCP-1, TGF-β and PAI-1, resulting in the increased accumulation of ECM (Lee et al 2003). Using several disparate antioxidants, another study found that the TGF-β-induced cellular ROS, the phosphorylation of Smad2, p38 MAPK and extracellular signal-regulated kinase (ERK), as well as endothelial-mesenchymal transition (EMT) were inhibited, further suggesting an important role for ROS in TGF-β-dependent pathways in renal tubular epithelial cells (Rhyu et al 2005).

3. A role for antioxidant defence in diabetic complications

Evidence suggests that glucose alters antioxidant defences in endothelial cells (Ceriello et al 1996) and in patients with diabetic complications such as DN (Ceriello et al 2000; Hodgkinson et al 2003). Fibroblasts derived from type 1 diabetic patients susceptible to microvascular complications were unable to upregulate their protective antioxidative defences after exposure to high glucose compared with skin fibroblasts from normal subjects, suggesting a failure of antioxidant defences in diabetic patients with nephropathy (Ceriello et al 1996). In addition, the concentration of the antioxidant glutathione (GSH) is found to decrease in a range of organs including the liver, kidney, pancreas, plasma, and red blood cells of chemically induced diabetic animals (Maritim et al 2003b). Given that reduced GSH functions as a direct free-radical scavenger and a cosubstrate for GPx activity, as well as a cofactor for many enzymes, reductions in this antioxidant induced by the hyperglycaemic environment is likely to impact on the progression of diabetic complications. Thus, these findings suggest that increased ROS in diabetes is not only the result of their increased production, as detailed in section 2, but also a consequence of impaired antioxidant defences.

3.1 Glutathione peroxidase

Pre-clinical and clinical evidence are now mounting in support of an important role for GPx in the protection against diseases such as atherosclerosis, both in a non-diabetic and a diabetic setting. The selenocysteine-containing GPx family of antioxidant enzymes attenuates oxidative stress by utilising GSH to reduce hydrogen and lipid peroxides to water and their corresponding alcohol (Fig.2). Additionally, GPx also functions to remove harmful $ONOO^-$. Thus the major role for GPx in the protection against pathogenesis may reside in the fact that it is the only antioxidant enzyme that metabolises three major ROS, H_2O_2, lipid peroxide (LOOH) and $ONOO^-$ (Fig.2). Several isoforms of GPx have been identified and they are each encoded by separate genes, which vary in cellular location, substrate specificity and tissue-specific functions (Brigelius-Flohé 1999).

3.1.1 Different isoforms of GPx

GPx1, also known as cellular GPx, was first identified as an erythrocyte enzyme that protects haemoglobin from oxidative injury (Mills 1957). Its ubiquitous expression in almost all tissues, together with its abundant expression in organs such as the kidney and liver have meant that this isoform is one of the most well-characterised of the GPx family (Lei 2001). GPx2 is most prominent in the gastrointestinal tract and its role is mainly to protect intestinal epithelium from oxidative stress (Chu et al 1997; Esworthy et al 1998). GPx3 is secreted by the kidney and is the main source of plasma GPx; however GPx3 is also expressed in other tissues, for example in the heart (Reeves & Hoffmann 2009). GPx4 reduces phospholipid hydroperoxides (Conrad et al 2007; Thomas et al 1990) and is thought to play a protective role in oxidative stress-induced apoptosis, possibly through the mitochondrial death pathway (Nomura et al 1999; Seiler et al 2008).

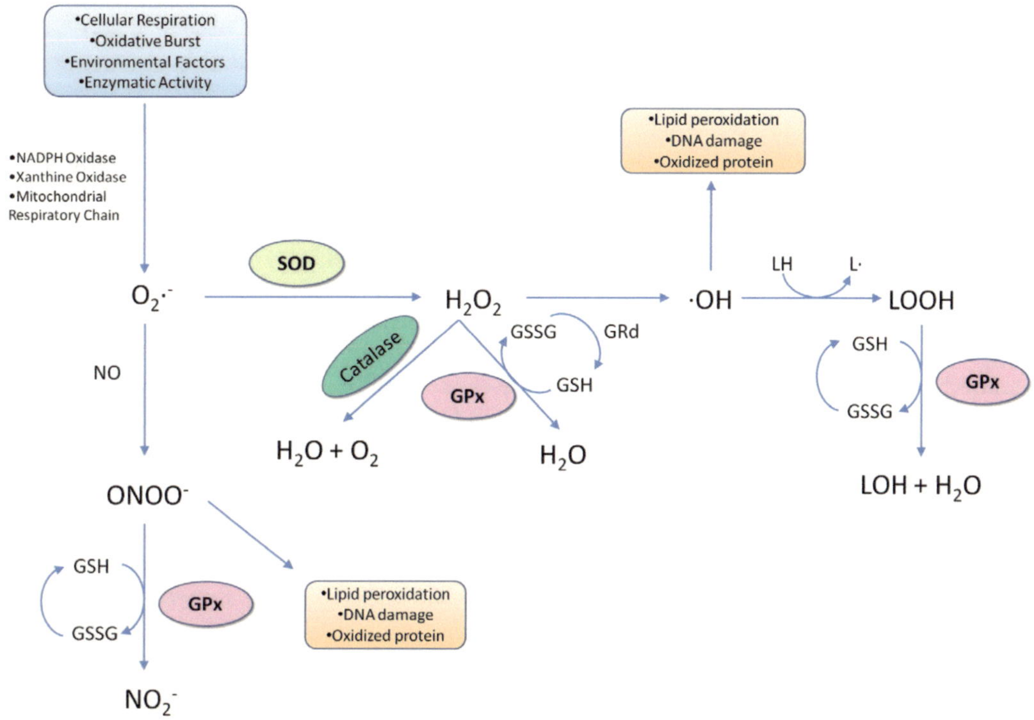

Fig. 2. Removal of reactive oxygen species (ROS) by antioxidant defence systems. Superoxide radical ($^{\bullet}O_2^-$) is generated in low levels under physiological states but its production is greatly enhanced under pathological situations via enzymes such as NADPH oxidase, xanthine oxidase and a dysfunctional mitochondrial respiratory chain. $^{\bullet}O_2^-$ is neutralised to water via a two-step process involving superoxide dismutase (SOD) in the first step, and glutathione peroxidase (GPx) or catalase in a second step. Increased production of $^{\bullet}O_2^-$ and/or impairment of antioxidant defence systems lead to a build-up of the intermediate hydrogen peroxide (H_2O_2). H_2O_2 forms the toxic oxygen species hydroxyl anion ($^{\bullet}OH$) via Fenton biochemistry, which is highly reactive and causes lipid peroxidation forming lipid hydroperoxides (LOOH). The functional importance of GPx resides in its ability to remove H_2O_2 and LOOH and neutralise these to water and lipid alcohol, respectively. Additionally, the increase in $^{\bullet}O_2^-$ also favours the formation of peroxynitrite ($ONOO^-$) which reduces the bioavailability of nitric oxide ($^{\bullet}NO$). GPx also functions to neutralise $ONOO^-$.

3.1.2 GPx in diabetes-associated complications

GPx activity is decreased in patients with type 1 diabetes, as well as in experimentally-induced diabetic rats (Chiu et al 2005; Dominguez et al 1998), although some studies have shown opposite results (Maritim et al 2003b). The decrease in GPx activity may contribute to the progression of diabetic complications due to the build-up of ROS such as H_2O_2 and $ONOO^-$, leading to lipid peroxidation and oxidative injury.

Clinical evidence has shown that diabetic patients with cardiovascular complications have significantly lower enzymatic antioxidant defences, including an impairment in GPx activity, with this defect being more pronounced in younger patients (Čolak et al 2005). GPx activity is also found to decrease in diabetic rats in the heart, kidney and brain, leading to enhanced oxidative stress and secondary organ damage (Aliciguzel et al 2003). In particular, glomerular expression of GPx is significantly reduced in both human and rats with diabetes (Chiu et al 2005). Furthermore, diabetic rats with reduced glomerular GPx expression were found to have more severe glomerulosclerosis and mesangial expansion (Chiu et al 2005). Moreover, patients with type 1 diabetes together with DN displayed a defective GPx defence mechanism, in contrast to patients with type 1 diabetes but without DN (Ceriello et al 2000). Several studies have linked selenium deficiency to a reduction in GPx mRNA expression and activity in the kidney together with elevated plasma glucose, albuminuria and glomerulosclerosis (Fujieda et al 2007; Reddi & Bollineni 2001). These changes may be mediated by the profibrotic growth factor, TGF-β, since inhibition of TGF-β with a TGF-β neutralising antibody, abrogated the reduction in GPx activity, as well as the increase in lipid peroxidation, albuminuria and glomerular injury in rats fed with a selenium-deficient diet (Reddi & Bollineni 2001).

Several clinical studies have linked reduced GPx1 levels with diabetes-associated atherogenesis (Čolak et al 2005; Hamanishi et al 2004). Polymorphisms identified within the GPx1 gene resulting in reduced GPx1 activity have been linked with increased intima-media thickness of carotid arteries and an increased risk of cardiovascular and peripheral vascular disease in type 2 diabetic patients (Hamanishi et al 2004). Moreover, a reduction in red blood cell GPx1 activity has been associated with an increased risk of cardiovascular events in a prospective cohort study assessing the extent of atherosclerosis (Espinola-Klein et al 2007; Winter et al 2003), while atherosclerotic plaques of patients with carotid artery disease have reduced GPx1 activity (Lapenna et al 1998). These evidence, although correlative, suggest that GPx1 is a key enzyme for the protection of vessels against oxidative stress and atherogenesis, particularly in the highly pro-oxidant diabetic environment (de Haan & Cooper 2011).

The roles of GPx in mediating diabetes-associated heart injury are less well understood. Current evidence suggest that the compensatory upregulation of antioxidant enzymes, including GPx1 is impaired in the heart of severely hyperglycaemic mice (Fujita et al 2005). More recently, GPx3 is reported to be upregulated in the heart of STZ-diabetic mice, suggesting that GPx3 is the major antioxidative enzyme of the heart in the cellular defence against oxidative stress under hyperglycaemia (Iwata et al 2006). However, these were short term studies of only 4 to 10 weeks of diabetes, therefore further studies are required to investigate whether diabetes has long term effects on the expression and/or activity of GPx3 in the heart.

3.1.3 The GPx1 knockout mouse: a model of enhanced intensity of oxidative stress

GPx1 knockout (-/-) mice, generated in our laboratory (de Haan et al 1998) and by others (Cheng et al 1997; Esposito et al 2000; Yoshida et al 1997) have become an important research tool to specifically study the protective role of GPx1 in the ROS-mediated progression and promotion of oxidative stress-mediated injury. Most studies investigating the role of GPx do so by limiting selenium intake which results in non-specific reductions of all selenium-dependent enzymes (Reddi & Bollineni 2001; Rosenblat & Aviram 1998). Furthermore, studying GPx1 knockout mice allows us to draw meaningful conclusions about the protective role of this isoform of the GPx family, since standard assays do not discriminate between different isoforms (Lewis et al 2007). This specific knockout model also facilitates the distinction between the contribution of GPx1, catalase (a peroxisomal H_2O_2 metabolising enzyme) and thioredoxin reductase in the peroxidation of H_2O_2 to water (de Haan & Cooper 2011).

Forgione et al. first reported vascular functional changes in mice associated with both a heterozygous (Forgione et al 2002a) and homozygous deficiency of GPx1 compared to wildtype (WT) mice (Forgione et al 2002b). Mesenteric arterioles of GPx+/- and GPx-/- mice demonstrated paradoxical vasoconstriction to endothelium-dependent vasodilatory compounds such as acetylcholine and bradykinin, whereas WT arterioles showed dose-dependent vasodilation. Superfusion of GPx-/- vessels with an endothelium-independent vasodilator, sodium nitroprusside (SNP) resulted in dose-dependent arteriolar vasodilation that was similar in GPx-/- and WT vessels. These results suggest that GPx-/- mice may have a depletion of bioavailable EDNO. Furthermore, the observed endothelial dysfunction was accompanied by increased nitrotyrosine levels in the endothelial layer of the vessel wall, as well as elevated plasma isoprostanes, indicative that lack of GPx1 leads to oxidative stress in this tissue. By increasing intracellular thiol pools (GSH, cysteine) in the vascular tissue of GPx-/- mice using (L)-2-Oxothiazolidine carboxylic acid (OTC), endothelial dysfunction and oxidant stress was attenuated, further indicating the importance of GPx1 in maintaining normal endothelial function, as well as protecting the blood vessels from oxidative injury (Forgione et al 2002b).

Several isoforms of GPx are present in kidney, however GPx1 is the major isoform expressed in normal kidney, and accounts for >96% of the renal GPx activity (de Haan et al 1998). Protection against oxidative stress is therefore most likely due to lipid and H_2O_2 quenching effects of the GPx1 isoform in the kidney. Until recently, no study has directly linked GPx1 to the protection against DN (Chew et al 2010). Our initial studies using diabetic C57Bl/6J GPx-/- mice, surprisingly failed to show accelerated kidney injury compared with diabetic WT mice (de Haan et al 2005). Furthermore, an assessment of atherosclerosis, which is only possible in the aortic sinus after feeding mice diets rich in fats, cholesterol and choline, failed to reveal a protective role for GPx1 in G57Bl/J6 GPx-/- mice (de Haan et al 2006). As detailed below, the importance of GPx1 in limiting diabetes-associated atherosclerosis and diabetic nephropathy became evident in ApoE/GPx1 double knockout (dKO) mice, a murine model that encompasses three important risk factors, namely hyperglycaemia, hyperlipidemia and enhanced intensity of oxidative stress, seen in diabetic patients.

3.1.4 Diabetic ApoE/GPx1 double knockout mouse: a model of accelerated diabetes-associated atherosclerosis and diabetic nephropathy

Since the lack of GPx1 plays a major role in endothelial dysfunction (Forgione et al 2002b), which is known to be an important mediator of hyperglycaemia-induced atherosclerosis (Nakagami et al 2005), we hypothesised that a lack of GPx1 would accelerate atherosclerosis in a diabetic setting. Because rodents are more resilient than humans to the development of diabetic atherosclerosis, in order to generate a mouse model with similar disease progression and aetiology, we crossed our GPx1-/- mice with ApoE-deficient mice that were also on a C57/BL6 background (Lewis et al 2007). We then compared aortic lesion formation and atherogenic pathways in ApoE-deficient and ApoE/GPx1 dKO mice after these mice were rendered diabetic using the diabetogenic agent, streptozotocin (STZ). STZ destroys the pancreatic β-islet cells, thus providing a robust model of insulin deficient diabetes (Wilson & Leiter 1990).

In our study, we demonstrated that atherosclerotic lesions within the aortic sinus region, as well as lesions within the arch, thoracic and abdominal region were significantly increased in diabetic ApoE/GPx1 dKO aortas compared with diabetic ApoE-/- aortas (Lewis et al 2007). This increase in aortic lesions was accompanied by an increase in macrophages, α-smooth muscle actin (α-SMA), RAGE and various proinflammatory (VCAM-1, MCP-1) and profibrotic mediators (vascular endothelial growth factor (VEGF), connective tissue growth factor (CTGF)). Gene expression analyses also revealed a concomitant increase in RAGE, VCAM-1, VEGF and CTGF in diabetic dKO aortas compared with diabetic controls. Furthermore, the oxidative stress marker nitrotyrosine was also significantly increased in the diabetic dKO aortas. These findings were observed despite upregulation of other antioxidants, suggesting that a lack of functional GPx1 accelerates diabetes-associated atherosclerosis via upregulation of proinflammatory and profibrotic pathways in ApoE-/- mice. Similar results were reported in a separate study using ApoE/GPx1-/- dKO mice, but in this instance atherosclerosis was induced by high fat diet (Torzewski et al 2007). In particular, these authors demonstrated increased atherosclerosis in their dKO mice, which was accompanied by increased cellularity in atherosclerotic lesions, as well as increased nitrotyrosine levels in the aortic wall and a lower level of bioactive $^{\bullet}NO$ (Torzewski et al 2007).

As previously discussed, diabetic GPx1-deficient mice on a C57Bl/J6 background did not show accelerated kidney injury. However, on examination of the kidneys of diabetic dKO mice, we observed increased albuminuria and renal pathological changes which included mesangial expansion of the glomeruli and upregulation of profibrotic (collagen I and III, fibronectin, TGF-β) and proinflammatory mediators (VCAM-1, MCP-1) (Chew et al 2010). Thus, we believe that in the diabetic C57Bl/J6 GPx1-/- mice, the significance of a lack of GPx1 may not have been properly revealed since lipid levels were unaffected in this model (de Haan et al 2005). Elevated lipid levels have been shown to be critical in accelerating DN since clinical observation suggests that hyperlipidemia is an important contributory factor to the progression of diabetic renal disease (Jenkins et al 2003; Tolonen et al 2009). Importantly, we show enhanced staining for nitrotyrosine, which is a marker of $ONOO^-$ damage in diabetic ApoE/Gpx1 dKO glomeruli and tubules of the kidney compared to diabetic ApoE-/- controls. We have therefore established a role for GPx1 in limiting and/or preventing DN in the pathophysiologically relevant milieu of increased lipids known to accompany diabetes (Chew et al 2010).

3.2 Other antioxidant defence systems

3.2.1 Superoxide Dismutase (SOD)

The SOD family of enzymes catalyse the conversion of $^{\bullet}O_2^-$ into H_2O_2 and oxygen in the first step of the antioxidant pathway (Fig.2), thereby performing an important role in the removal of $^{\bullet}O_2^-$. Three isoforms exists in humans, Cu/Zn-SOD (also known as SOD1), Mn-SOD (also known as SOD2) and SOD3 with distinct cellular localisation, namely cytosolic, mitochondrial and extracellular, respectively.

Diabetes is associated with a decrease in SOD activity in most animal studies (Brocca et al 2008; Fujita et al 2009; Fukuda et al 2010). Lowered SOD levels are reported in serum and urine of STZ-treated Sprague-Dawley rats (Luo et al 2010), and decreased SOD1 and SOD3 levels are suggested to play a key role in the pathogenesis of diabetic nephropathy (Fujita et al 2009). Manipulations of SOD, through the use of SOD knockout mice or SOD overexpressing mice, have shown the importance of these enzymes in the protection against diabetic complications. Indeed, SOD1 knockout mice have clearly shown the importance of protection by SOD1 against superoxide-mediated DN. These mice demonstrated significant mesangial matrix expansion, renal cortical malondialdehyde content and severe tubulointerstitial injury compared with diabetic controls (DeRubertis et al 2007). Importantly, these pathological changes were attenuated in the presence of the SOD-mimetic, tempol (discussed in more detail in section 4.3.2). The significance of SOD2 was revealed in eMnSOD-Tg mice where the overexpression of mitochondrial-specific SOD targeted to the endothelium prevented diabetic retinopathy (Goto et al 2008). Furthermore, the targeted overexpression of Mn-SOD significantly attenuated morphological changes in diabetic hearts and improved contractility in diabetic cardiomyocytes (Shen et al 2006). Collectively, these studies show that targeted removal of $^{\bullet}O_2^-$, leads to improved outcomes in diabetic nephropathy and retinopathy.

3.2.2 Catalase

Catalase is present mainly in the peroxisomes of mammalian cells as a tetrameric enzyme of four identically arranged subunits; each containing a heme group and NADPH at its active centre (MatÉs et al 1999). Similar to GPx1, the enzyme neutralise H_2O_2 to water and oxygen (Fig.2). A role for catalase in the protection against atherosclerosis comes from the analysis of mice overexpressing catalase. In these experiments, overexpression of catalase significantly reduced the severity of lesions in ApoE-deficient mice (Yang et al 2004). However, the role of catalase in diabetes is debatable; studies have shown that onset and progression of diabetes is accompanied by reductions in catalase activity (Ali & Agha 2009; Kamboj et al 2010; Pari et al 2010; Patel et al 2009), while others report an increase in the activity of catalase (Kakkar et al 1996; Kesavulu et al 2000).

More recently, mutations within the catalase gene have been suggested to contribute to the increased risk of diabetes (Góth & Eaton 2000). However, other studies report no such association with catalase gene polymorphisms and the development of diabetic complications (Letonja et al 2011; Panduru et al 2010). For example, one study reported that blood catalase activity was lowered due to the downregulation of catalase synthesis, rather than specific catalase gene mutations in type 2 diabetic patients. This was also associated with increased H_2O_2 levels and dysfunctional insulin receptor signalling (Góth 2008).

3.2.3 Thioredoxin system

The mammalian Trx system is ubiquitously expressed and consists of Trx, Trx reductase and NADPH. The antioxidant properties of Trx is exerted mostly through the antioxidant enzymes, Trx peroxidase (also known as peroxiredoxin), which uses sulfhydryl (SH) groups as reducing equivalents (Chae et al., 1994). Trx reduces oxidised peroxiredoxin, which then scavenges H_2O_2 to produce water (Kang et al., 1998), thus attenuating oxidative stress in cells. The role of the Trx system in diabetic complications has gained considerable interest since thioredoxin-interacting protein (Txnip), which is an inhibitor of Trx activity, was discovered to be a highly upregulated hyperglycaemia-induced gene in both human and animal studies (Kobayashi et al 2003; Qi et al 2007; Shalev et al 2002). Txnip directly binds to the catalytic active site of Trx, thus inhibiting the reducing activity of Trx (Nishiyama et al 1999).

In vitro studies have shown Txnip expression to be significantly upregulated by glucose in mesangial cells (Kobayashi et al 2003), proximal tubule cells (Qi et al 2007) and distal tubule/collecting duct cells (Advani et al 2009; Kobayashi et al 2003). Overexpression of Txnip in STZ-treated diabetic rats was associated with an increase in ROS, as well as ECM accumulation in the kidney (Kobayashi et al 2003; Tan et al 2011). By reducing Txnip gene transcription with siRNA in kidney cells, high glucose-mediated increases in ROS production and ECM accumulation were attenuated, together with a restoration of Trx activity (Advani et al 2009). These results clearly delineate a role for Trx in maintaining redox homeostasis and highlight the importance of Txnip dysregulation in diabetic complications.

Txnip also plays an important role as a biomechanical effector of atherosclerosis (World et al 2006). In the endothelium of intact rabbit aorta, exposure to physiological fluid shear stress decreased Txnip expression and increased Trx activity, leading to a reduction in pro-inflammatory events mediated by the tumour necrosis factor (TNF)-ASK-1-JNK/p38 pathway, in association with a decrease in TNF-mediated VCAM1 expression (Yamawaki et al 2005). Furthermore, a calcium channel blocker promoted cardiac myocyte survival and improved cardiac function by reducing cardiac Txnip expression, suggesting a role for Txnip in mediating cardiac myocyte apoptosis in diabetic cardiomyopathy (Chen et al 2009).

4. Novel antioxidants to limit diabetic micro- and macrovascular disease

4.1 GPx1-mimetic ebselen

Ebselen (2-phenyl-1,2-benzisoselenazol-3[2H]-one) is a synthetic, lipid soluble, non-toxic seleno-organic compound (Sies & Masumoto 1997) with anti-inflammatory and antioxidant activities (Muller et al 1984). Ebselen eliminates hydroperoxides, including H_2O_2 and lipid peroxides due to its GPx mimetic activity (Maiorino et al 1988; Parnham et al 1987; Safayhi et al 1985). Additionally, ebselen also scavenges other ROS such as peroxyl radicals and $ONOO^-$ (Sies & Masumoto 1997). Several enzymes involved in inflammatory processes, including 5-lipoxygenases, NOS, NADPH oxidase, PKC and ATPase are also inhibited by ebselen (Sies & Masumoto 1997). Importantly, ebselen has shown tremendous potential in reducing injury in various experimental models. Ebselen conferred protection against endothelial dysfunction in stroke-prone hypertensive rats (Sui et al 2005) and improved cardiac function in a model of chronic iron overload (Davis & Bartfay 2004). Furthermore, ebselen partially restored endothelial dysfunction in Zucker diabetic rats (Brodsky et al 2004). Additionally, arterial lesions were reduced by ebselen in a superoxide-driven non-inflammatory transgenic murine model, suggesting a role for ebselen in reducing atherosclerosis (Khatri et al 2004). Importantly, in a clinical trial, ebselen has shown improved neurological outcomes in patients after cerebral infarction (Yamaguchi et al 1998) and a safety and pharmacokinetic profile of ebselen has been established in normal volunteers in a Phase I trial to determine whether ebselen is protective against noise-induced hearing loss (Lynch & Kil 2009).

4.1.1 Ebselen in experimental models of diabetes associated atherosclerosis and nephropathy

We hypothesised that ebselen, in its capacity to act as a mimetic of GPx, would attenuate oxidative stress and lessen diabetes-associated atherosclerosis (Chew et al 2009). Eight week-old male C57Bl/J6 ApoE-/- mice were rendered diabetic with STZ and assigned to ebselen-gavaged and non-gavaged groups. Ebselen was administered twice daily at 10mg/kg/day body weight starting at 10 weeks of age and continued for 20 weeks. Our analysis showed that ebselen reduced lesion formation in most regions of the aorta including the arch, thoracic and abdominal regions of diabetic ApoE-/- mice. In addition, ebselen attenuated aortic nitrotyrosine levels and the expression of the Nox2 subunit of NADPH oxidase. The cellularity of the aorta associated with a pro-atherosclerotic phenotype (increased α-SMA-positive cells and increased macrophage infiltration) was also decreased by ebselen, together with a reduction in the aortic expression of the pro-atherosclerotic mediators, RAGE and VEGF (Chew et al 2009). These data support the notion of Blankenberg et al. (2003) that bolstering GPx-like activity reduces atherosclerosis.

Furthermore, similar results were observed in our diabetic ApoE/GPx1 dKO mice where ebselen significantly reduced total aortic plaque, as well as regional plaque (arch, thoracic and abdominal) (Chew et al 2010). These reductions in plaque were also accompanied by a decrease in vascular oxidative stress (aortic 4-hydroxynonenal (HNE), nitrotyrosine, the Nox2 subunit of NADPH oxidase), as well as reductions in plasma hydroperoxides and urinary 8-isoprostanes. Additionally, the pro-inflammatory and pro-atherogenic mediators VCAM-1, MCP-1, CTGF and VEGF were attenuated by ebselen in diabetic ApoE/GPx1-deficient aortas. These data suggest that ebselen is able to replenish GPx1 activity in this model, thereby reducing atherosclerosis.

As mentioned in section 3.1.4, diabetic ApoE/GPx1 dKO mice demonstrated significant renal injury with an increase in albuminuria, hyperfiltration, mesangial expansion, oxidative stress (nitrotyrosine), pro-fibrotic (TGF-β, CTGF, collagen I, III and IV, fibronectin) and pro-inflammatory mediators (MCP-1, VCAM-1 and TNF-α) (Chew et al 2010). Ebselen significantly attenuated all of these parameters in diabetic dKO kidneys (Chew et al 2010). Our results are in agreement with Chander et al. (2004) where ebselen improved renal function and attenuated structural defects such as glomerulosclerosis, tubulointerstitial fibrosis and vasculopathy in the Zucker diabetic fat rat. Moreover, ebselen prevented the accumulation of lipid peroxidation products and 3-nitrotyrosine-modified proteins, and restored renal tissue levels of GSH (Chander et al 2004).

4.1.2 Mechanistic understanding of the actions of ebselen

Ebselen is well-characterised for its ability to act as a GPx mimic and can be catalytically maintained at the expense of GSH (Muller et al 1984; Sies & Masumoto 1997). Ebselen has been shown to reduce oxidative stress in several *in vivo* models; however this protective effect is unlikely to be solely due to the direct pro-oxidant interception by ebselen. Recently, ebselen has been reported to be an inducer of NF-E2-Related Factor 2- (Nrf-2)-dependent gene activation (Tamasi et al 2004). Nrf-2 is a member of the Cap'n'Collar family of basic region-leucine zipper (bZIP) transcription factors (Chui et al 1995). Genes upregulated by

Nrf-2 can be broadly classified into three separate classes; those that are involved in GSH synthesis (cystine membrane transporters), detoxication enzymes (rat glutathione S-transferase A2, a non-selenium-dependent glutathione peroxidase, and NAD(P)H:quinine oxidoreductase), and those directly involved in the amelioration of oxidative stress (heme oxygenase-1 (HO-1), peroxiredoxin MSP23, and Trx reductase) (Tamasi et al 2004). Tamasi et al. (2004) showed that ebselen can directly induce Nrf-2-dependent gene transcription, including the increase of intracellular GSH production, which acts as a substrate for GPx activity. These data showed that the activation of Nrf-2-dependent signalling by ebselen could indirectly augment cellular defences, independent of the direct interception of ROS by ebselen.

To further elucidate the mechanistic actions of ebselen observed in our diabetic experimental models, we examined the effect of ebselen on various signalling pathways implicated in atherosclerosis and nephropathy in human aortic endothelial cells (HAEC) (Chew et al 2009) and normal rat kidney (NRK) cells (Chew et al 2010). Pre-treatment of HAEC with 0.03 μM ebselen prior to exposure to 100 μM H_2O_2 reduced the H_2O_2-mediated increase in IkB-kinase (IKK) phosphorylation on critical activatory residues. Since IKK is a key regulator of NK-κB activation (Schmid & Birbach 2008), it is anticipated that by reducing IKK phosphorylation, ebselen anchors NF-κB in the cytoplasm thereby preventing the activation of pro-inflammatory genes. We further showed that ebselen reduced the H_2O_2-mediated increase in Nox2 expression; Nox2 is known to be regulated by NK-κB (Anrather et al 2006), further confirming the view that ebselen affects downstream targets of NF-κB.

The cytokine TNF-α is an important diabetes-associated pro-inflammatory mediator and is involved in the activation of NF-κB (Hacker & Karin 2006). Our *in vitro* data showed that H_2O_2-induced upregulation of TNF-α was reduced by ebselen. Our results support previous findings that ebselen inhibits TNF-α-induced pro-inflammatory responses in endothelial cells (Yoshizumi et al 2004) and other cell types (Sharma et al 2008; Tewari et al 2009). We also investigated the effects of ebselen on H_2O_2-mediated phosphorylation of JNK, a kinase involved in the activation of the transcription factor, AP-1. Our *in vitro* analysis showed that ebselen effectively attenuated H_2O_2-mediated phosphorylation of JNK, an important finding since phosphorylated JNK has been implicated in TNF-α-mediated endothelial activation (Min & Pober 1997) in particular through the interaction of AP-1 and NF-κB (Read et al 1997). Collectively, our results with ebselen have implications not only for inflammatory genes known to be regulated by these pathways, but also on the proatherosclerotic pathway itself, since inflammatory events are integrally linked with the development and progression of atherosclerosis.

Our *in vitro* studies in NRK cells further strengthen the notion that ebselen downregulates proinflammatory pathways in renal cells (Chew et al 2010). Similar to what we observed in HAEC, ebselen attenuated the phosphorylation of the pro-inflammatory mediator, IKK. Furthermore, stress-response kinases such as JNK and p38 MAPK phosphorylation were also attenuated by ebselen in NRK cells (Chew et al 2010).

4.2 Novel GPx1-mimetics

Novel GPx-mimetics, synthesised for their greater solubility and efficacy than ebselen are now available. Several laboratories have reported the synthesis and characterisation of novel small selenium compounds as functional mimics of GPx, either by modifying the basic structure of ebselen or by incorporating some structural features of the native enzyme (Alberto et al 2010; Back 2009; Bhabak & Mugesh 2010). These synthetic mimics can be classified into three major categories: (i) cyclic selenenyl amides having a Se-N bond, (ii) diaryl diselenides, and (iii) aromatic or aliphatic monoselenides (Bhabak & Mugesh 2010). The most widely studied among the novel GPx-mimetics is diphenyl selenide.

In addition to their GPx-like activity, the antioxidant activity of diphenyl diselenides may also be attributed to their capacity to be a substrate for mammalian Trx reductase (De Freitas et al 2010). In a study where acidosis was used to mediate oxidative stress in rat kidney homogenates, diphenyl diselenide significantly protected against lipid peroxidation, whilst the protection afforded by ebselen was only minor (Hassan et al 2009). Furthermore, diphenyl diselenide was also effective in protecting against acute renal failure induced by glycerol in rats (Brandão et al 2009). In cholesterol-fed rabbits, where animals exhibited hypercholesterolaemia and oxidative stress, diphenyl diselenide significantly reduced both of these risk factors of coronary artery disease in these animals (De Bem et al 2009). More recently, diphenyl diselenide has also been reported to attenuate atherosclerotic lesions in LDLr-/- mice by lowering oxidative stress and inflammation (Hort et al 2011).

The clinical benefits of ebselen and/or these novel GPx-mimetics in attenuating diabetes-associated complications are yet to be reported. Our pre-clinical assessments, as well as those of others, have highlighted the attractiveness of this class of therapeutic for their clinical use to prevent or attenuate both diabetes-associated atherosclerosis and DN, two co-morbidities often present in diabetic patients.

4.3 Other novel antioxidants

4.3.1 NOX inhibitors

Increased NADPH oxidase (NOX) activity, which catalyses the production of ROS, has been implicated in the pathogenesis of diabetic complications (Kakehi & Yabe-Nishimura 2008). NOX4 has been shown to not only mediate the increase in ROS, but also activate profibrotic pathways in type 2 DN (Sedeek et al 2010). Additionally, inhibition of NOX1 suppresses neointimal formation in the prevention of vascular complications associated with diabetes (Lee et al 2009).

Several small molecule and peptide inhibitors of the NOX enzymes have been developed and are showing promise in experimental studies, but issues of specificity, potency and toxicity militate against any of the existing compounds as candidates for drug development (Kim et al 2011; Williams & Griendling 2007). In a recent study, apocynin, a proven NADPH oxidase inhibitor, attenuated albuminuria, improved kidney structure (glomerular and mesangial expansion) and reduced oxidative stress (urinary 8-OHdG and malondialdehyde) in aged Otsuka Long Evans Tokushima Fatty (OLETF) rats (Nam et al 2009). However, apocynin is considered to be non-selective in its mode of action as it also targets other enzymes such as Rho-kinase (Heumüller et al 2008).

One of the most specific NOX inhibitors developed so far is gp91 (ds-tat), an 18-amino acid peptide which interferes with NOX assembly and activation (Rey et al 2001). This peptide functions by mimicking the binding region of NOX2, and possibly NOX1, which interacts with p47^{phox}. In doing so, it inhibits subunit assembly, resulting in the specific inhibition of $^{\bullet}O_2^-$ production from NOX and not from other oxidases such as xanthine oxidase. Gp91 (ds-tat) has shown promise in reducing vascular ROS associated with Ang II-mediated hypertension in mice (Rey et al 2001), as well as reducing endothelial dysfunction and vascular ROS in the Dahl salt-sensitive rat model (Zhou et al 2006). However, limited bioavailability of this peptide has hampered its usefulness as a therapeutic agent; at present, it can only be administered via intravenous injection (Williams & Griendling 2007). VAS2870 is a fairly new NOX inhibitor discovered via high-throughput screening and is specific for NADPH oxidase activity (ten Freyhaus et al 2006). It has been shown to attenuate platelet-derived growth factor (PDGF)-dependent smooth muscle cell chemotaxis *in vitro* via a mechanism that includes the complete abolition of NOX activation and ROS production (ten Freyhaus et al 2006).

Only limited *in vitro* and *in vivo* data are available for these novel compounds. Further testing in pre-clinical models is necessary to determine if these approaches represent feasible therapeutic strategies for diabetic complications.

4.3.2 SOD mimetics

As discussed in section 3.2.1, SOD is the first line of defence against both physiological and pathological ROS, by catalysing the dismutation of $^{\bullet}O_2^-$ to H_2O_2 (Fig.2). Protective and beneficial effects of SOD enzymes have been demonstrated in a broad range of superoxide-driven diseases, both pre-clinically and clinically (Muscoli et al 2003). When tested in humans, Orgotein (a bovine CuZn-SOD mimetic) showed promising results in acute and chronic conditions associated with inflammation; however, because of its non-human origin, the use of bovine native enzyme in the human context caused a variety of immunological disorders (Muscoli et al 2003). Since then, several synthetic, low-molecular weight mimetics of SOD have been produced with promising results in pre-clinical models.

The most well-characterised of the SOD-mimetics is tempol (4-hydroxy-2,2,6,6,-tetramethylpiperidine-*N*-oxyl). Tempol has been reported to protect animals and mammalian cells from cytotoxicity induced by oxygen radicals such as H_2O_2 and $^{\bullet}O_2^-$ (Mitchell et al 1990). One attractive attribute of tempol is its ability to penetrate cell membranes and hence react with ROS both intracellularly and extracellularly, as well as within important organelles such as the mitochondria (Simonsen et al 2009). Tempol has been shown to improve acetylcholine- and arachidonic acid-induced relaxation in skeletal muscle arteries and in coronary arteries from diabetic animals (Gao et al 2007; Xiang et al 2008). Furthermore, in an *in vivo* one-kidney one-clip hypertensive rat model, tempol improved endothelial function in small arteries exposed to high blood pressure (Christensen et al 2007). However, the use of tempol may be limited in some instances by its propensity to increase H_2O_2, thereby exacerbating the progression of disease. For instance, in an experimental model of glomerulonephritis, tempol increased proteinuria and crescentric glomerulonephritis with leukocyte infiltration, as well as accelerating mortality in the treated group (Lu et al 2010). Moreover, tempol upregulated p65-NFκB and osteopontin in the kidney and increased H_2O_2 levels in the urine. In another study, tempol could not prevent the development of hypertension in a hypertensive rat model induced by inhibiting renal medullary SOD with diethyldithiocarbamic acid (Chen et al 2003). These results may be due to the increased formation of H_2O_2, as a result of the dismutation of $^{\bullet}O_2^-$ by tempol, causing constriction of the medullary vessels, and counteracting the vasodilatory actions of tempol.

Manganese(II) complex with a bis(cyclohexylpyridine)-substituted macrocyclic ligand (M40403) is another SOD-mimetic which has high catalytic SOD activity and is chemically and biologically stable *in vivo*. Injection of M40403 into rat models of inflammation and ischemia-reperfusion injury protected the animals against tissue damage, possibly by preventing the formation of $ONOO^-$, as well as assisting in the direct removal of $^{\bullet}O_2^-$ (Salvemini et al 1999). M40403 also reversed endothelial dysfunction in ApoE-/- aortas *ex vivo* by decreasing NADPH oxidase-dependent $^{\bullet}O_2^-$ levels (Jiang et al 2003a).

4.3.3 Mitochondrially-targeted antioxidants

The targeted delivery of antioxidants to the mitochondria is an attractive approach to effectively remove or attenuate pathogenic ROS produced by the mitochondria. Animal studies using transgenic mice over-expressing mitochondrially-targeted SOD and catalase have already shown the potential of this strategy, since these transgenic mice were associated with significant reductions in cardiac mitochondrial oxidative stress and improvements in left ventricular function after antiretroviral-induced cardiomyopathy (Kohler et al 2009). Indeed, the development of antioxidants that specifically target the matrix-facing inner surface of the mitochondrial membrane is hypothesised to protect against mitochondrial oxidative damage (Ross et al 2005). Because of the high negative membrane potential of the inner mitochondrial membrane, antioxidants conjugated with a lipophilic triphenylphosphonium (TPP) cation such as mitoquinone, mitovitamin E and mitophenyltertbutyline accumulate in the mitochondrial matrix at concentrations several-fold greater than cytosolic non-mitochondrially targeted antioxidants (Subramanian et al 2010; Victor et al 2009). In particular, MitoQ, which has a TPP modification added to coenzyme Q is 100 times more potent than idebenone, a coenzymes Q derivative. Furthermore, MitoVitE (vitamin E attached to a TPP cation) is 350 times more potent than Trolox, a water soluble version of vitamin E, in fibroblasts from patients (Victor et al 2009). *In vitro* experiments using both mitoquinone and mitovitamin E have shown promising reductions in peroxide-mediated oxidant stress and apoptosis whilst maintaining proteasomal function in bovine aortic endothelial cells (BAEC) (Dhanasekaran et al 2004). Moreover, Mito-carboxy proxyl (Mito-CP), a mitochondrial-targeted SOD, significantly diminished glucose/glucose oxidase-induced formation of intracellular ROS and apoptosis in BAEC, while the "untargeted" carboxy proxyl (CP) nitroxide probe did not (Dhanasekaran et al 2005). Furthermore, a mitochondrial-targeted form of the Gpx1-mimetic, MitoPeroxidase, which contains an ebselen moiety covalently linked to a TPP cation, decreases glucose and H_2O_2-mediated apoptosis in a rat basophilic leukemia cell line (RBL-2H3) (Filipovska et al 2005). Several studies have shown the accumulation of these compounds in the mitochondria of various tissues including brain, heart, liver and kidney, in mice fed mitrochondrially-targeted antioxidant compounds for several weeks (Smith et al 1999). However, to date, their therapeutic potential in militating against diabetic complications has not been explored.

4.3.4 Bolstering antioxidant defences via the transcription factor Nrf2

Nrf2 is a redox sensitive transcription factor which regulates the expression of important cytoprotective enzymes (Kensler et al 2007). Nrf2 plays an important role in endogenous defence against sustained oxidative stress by upregulating important detoxifying phase II enzymes, such as NAD(P)H:quinine oxidoreductase (NQO1) and antioxidant proteins, such as HO-1, through an antioxidant response element (ARE)-dependent pathway. The protective role of Nrf2 in diabetes-mediated kidney injury has gained considerable attention recently. Diabetic Nrf2 knockout mice demonstrated increased glomerular ROS production and greater oxidative DNA damage and renal injury compared to control mice (Jiang et al 2010). In addition, in human renal mesangial (Jiang et al 2010) and coronary arterial endothelial cells (Ungvari et al 2011), high glucose induced ROS production and the enhanced expression of Nrf2 and its downstream genes, such as NQO1, glutathione S-transferase (GST), glutamate-cysteine ligase catalytic (GCLC) and HO-1. These effects of high glucose were significantly attenuated by silencing Nrf2 expression using siRNA or overexpression of kelch-like ECH-associated protein (Keap-1), which is an inhibitor of Nrf2 (Ungvari et al 2011). Furthermore, overexpression of Nrf2 inhibited the promoter activity of TGF-β1 in a dose-dependent manner, whereas knockdown of Nrf2 by siRNA enhanced TGF-β1 transcription and fibronectin production, suggesting that Nrf2 plays a protective role in attenuating diabetic nephropathy (Jiang et al 2010).

Hyperglycaemia is associated with the increased formation of AGE and enhanced oxidative stress, leading to the progression of diabetic cardiovascular disease (Thomas et al 2005). It was recently reported that Nrf2 is activated by AGE in BAEC, resulting in the induction of the antioxidant genes HO-1 and NQO1, thus confirming a protective role of Nrf2 against oxidative stress in diabetes (He et al 2011). Furthermore, to test the protective effects of Nrf2 under metabolic stress, which often occurs concurrently with diabetes, Nrf2-/- mice were subjected to high fat diet (Ungvari et al 2011). These mice failed to show significant increases in the gene expression of the Nrf2 downstream targets GCLC and HO-1. In addition, increased ROS and endothelial dysfunction was attenuated in Nrf2-/- aortas, in contrast to Nrf2+/+ controls, further confirming that an adaptive activation of the Nrf2/ARE pathway confers endothelial protection under diabetic conditions (Ungvari et al 2011).

Nonetheless, very few studies have directly demonstrated the therapeutic potential of increasing Nrf2 in pre-clinical models. Oltipraz, an Nrf2 activator, significantly prevented the development of insulin resistance and obesity in high fat diet (HFD)-induced C57BL/6J mice (Yu et al 2011). Control mice fed with HFD demonstrated reduced nuclear content of Nrf2 in adipose tissue, which was associated with increased Keap-1 mRNA expression and reduced HO-1 and NQO1; all of which were attenuated with oltipraz. Moreover, resveratrol, which is a polyphenolic phytoalexin that occurs naturally in many plant species, including grapevines and berries, was shown to attenuate STZ-induced diabetic nephropathy in rats, through the preservation of Nrf2 mRNA and protein expression, with an inhibitory effect on diabetes-induced upregulation of Keap-1 in diabetic kidneys (Palsamy & Subramanian 2011). As mentioned earlier, ebselen can directly upregulate the expression of Nrf2-dependent genes, in addition to its ability to quench H2O2 (Tamasi et al 2004). Furthermore, ebselen has been shown to modify Keap-1, thereby relieving the inhibitory effect of Keap-1 on Nrf2 (Sakurai et al 2006).

A recent clinical trial using the Nrf2 activator, bardoxolone methyl, (Pergola et al 2011) has generated particular interest in this type of drug to lessen the burden of DN. In this double-blind, randomized, placebo-controlled trial, bardoxolone significantly improved the estimated glomerular filtration rate (eGFR) in patients with type 2 diabetes and impaired renal function. Current interventions appear to slow the decline in renal function by less than 1 ml/min/1.73 m[2] per year, therefore (Brenner et al 2001), improvements with bardoxolone methyl of between 5-10 ml/min/1.73 m[2] are seen as a major advance over standard therapies. These results may lead to further pre-clinical and clinical activity to identify additional Nrf2 activators with possibly even greater efficacy. Indeed, the strategy of bolstering antioxidant defences by manipulating Nrf2 may represent a new class of therapy with potentially major advances over conventional therapy in the treatment of diabetic complications such as diabetic nephropathy.

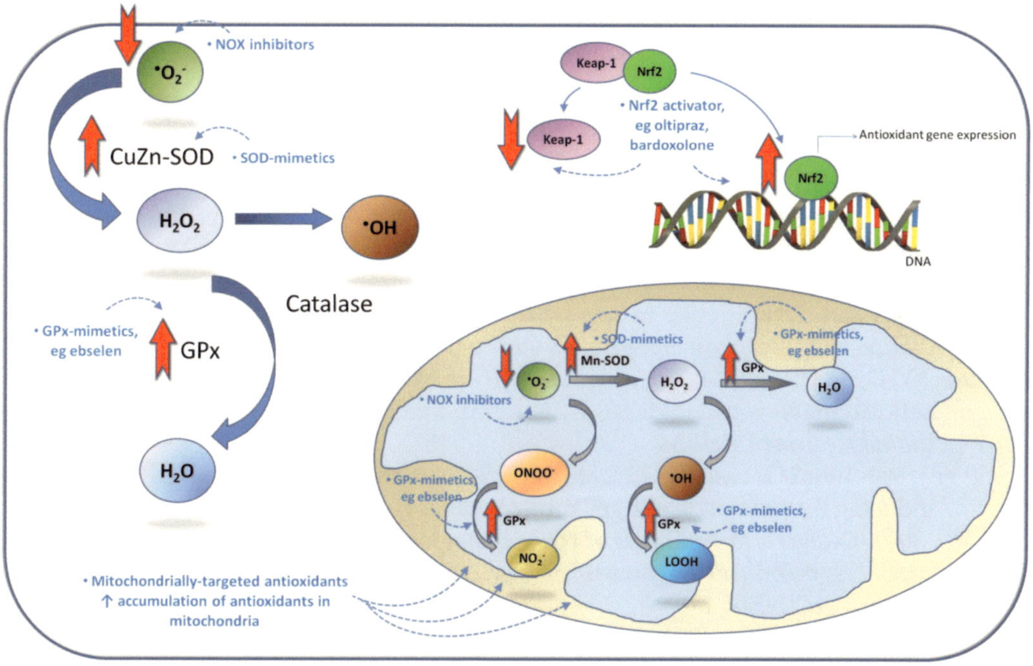

Fig. 3. Novel antioxidant strategies to attenuate increased cellular ROS production and/or increase the activity of endogenous antioxidant defence systems in diabetes-associated complications.

5. Conclusion

Increasing evidence has implicated a role for oxidative stress in mediating diabetes-associated complications. Despite this, very few therapies are currently available in clinical practice to effectively target oxidative stress and lessen the burden of diabetic complications. The use of vitamins in clinical trials have been mostly disappointing, showing no overall benefit for major cardiovascular events and in some instances, even increasing cardiovascular mortality (McQueen et al 2005). Failure of vitamins in the clinic may be due to their lack of specificity in not correctly targeting the ROS responsible for pathogenesis; conversely, total ablation of ROS could be detrimental as ROS are essential for basic cell signalling and homeostasis. Thus, the challenge for developing an effective antioxidant therapy for diabetes-associated complications would be to target either the production of specific ROS involved in diabetes-mediated injury or to eliminate ROS now appreciated to contribute to diabetes-associated-atherosclerosis such as hydrogen peroxide. A further challenge would be the maintenance of steady-state levels of ROS important for cellular processes including cell signalling. This is by no means an easy task; however, as highlighted in this review (Fig.3), several approaches are currently being investigated in pre-clinical models to lower the levels of those ROS involved in pathogenesis, or to activate specific antioxidant defences to lessen the diabetes-driven enhanced intensity of oxidative stress. The ultimate aim of these investigations is the clinical translation of novel targeted antioxidant therapies to lessen the burden of diabetic complications.

6. References

Advani A, Gilbert RE, Thai K, Gow RM, Langham RG, et al. 2009. Expression, Localization, and Function of the Thioredoxin System in Diabetic Nephropathy. *J Am Soc Nephrol* 20:730-41

Alberto EE, Nascimento VD, Braga AL. 2010. Catalytic application of selenium and tellurium compounds as glutathione peroxidase enzyme mimetics. *Journal of the Brazilian Chemical Society* 21:2032-41

Ali MM, Agha FG. 2009. Amelioration of streptozotocin-induced diabetes mellitus, oxidative stress and dyslipidemia in rats by tomato extract lycopene. *Scandinavian Journal of Clinical and Laboratory Investigation* 69:371-9

Aliciguzel Y, Ozen I, Aslan M, Karayalcin U. 2003. Activities of xanthine oxidoreductase and antioxidant enzymes in different tissues of diabetic rats. *The Journal of laboratory and clinical medicine* 142:172-7

Anrather J, Racchumi G, Iadecola C. 2006. NF-κB Regulates Phagocytic NADPH Oxidase by Inducing the Expression of gp91phox. *Journal of Biological Chemistry* 281:5657-67

Back TG. 2009. Design and synthesis of some biologically interesting natural and unnatural products based on organosulfur and selenium chemistry. *Canadian Journal of Chemistry* 87:1657-74

Barit D, Cooper ME. 2008. Diabetic patients and kidney protection: an attainable target. *Journal of hypertension. Supplement : official journal of the International Society of Hypertension* 26:S3-7

Beckman JA, Creager MA, Libby P. 2002. Diabetes and Atherosclerosis. *JAMA: The Journal of the American Medical Association* 287:2570-81

Beckman JS. 1996. Oxidative Damage and Tyrosine Nitration from Peroxynitrite. *Chemical Research in Toxicology* 9:836-44

Bhabak KP, Mugesh G. 2010. Functional Mimics of Glutathione Peroxidase: Bioinspired Synthetic Antioxidants. *Accounts of Chemical Research* 43:1408-19

Blankenberg S, Rupprecht HJ, Bickel C, Torzewski M, Hafner G, et al. 2003. Glutathione Peroxidase 1 Activity and Cardiovascular Events in Patients with Coronary Artery Disease. *New England Journal of Medicine* 349:1605-13

Boulanger C, Luscher TF. 1990. Release of endothelin from the porcine aorta. Inhibition of endothelium-derived nitric oxide. *Journal of Clinical Investigation* 85:587-90

Boullier A, Bird DA, Chang M-K, Dennis EA, Friedman P, et al. 2001. Scavenger Receptors, Oxidized LDL, and Atherosclerosis. *Ann NY Acad Sci* 947:214-23

Brandão R, Acker CI, Leite MR, Barbosa NBV, Nogueira CW. 2009. Diphenyl diselenide protects against glycerol-induced renal damage in rats. *Journal of Applied Toxicology* 29:612-8

Brenner BM, Cooper ME, de Zeeuw D, Keane WF, Mitch WE, et al. 2001. Effects of losartan on renal and cardiovascular outcomes in patients with type 2 diabetes and nephropathy. *N Engl J Med* 345:861-9

Brigelius-Flohé R. 1999. Tissue-specific functions of individual glutathione peroxidases. *Free Radical Biology and Medicine* 27:951-65

Brocca L, D'Antona G, Bachi A, Pellegrino MA. 2008. Amino Acid Supplements Improve Native Antioxidant Enzyme Expression in the Skeletal Muscle of Diabetic Mice. *The American journal of cardiology* 101:S57-S62

Brodsky SV, Gealekman O, Chen J, Zhang F, Togashi N, et al. 2004. Prevention and Reversal of Premature Endothelial Cell Senescence and Vasculopathy in Obesity-Induced Diabetes by Ebselen. *Circulation Research* 94:377-84

Cai L, Kang Y. 2001. Oxidative stress and diabetic cardiomyopathy: a brief review. *Cardiovasc Toxicol* 1:181-93

Cai L, Wang J, Li Y, Sun X, Wang L, et al. 2005. Inhibition of superoxide generation and associated nitrosative damage is involved in metallothionein prevention of diabetic cardiomyopathy. *Diabetes* 54:1829-37

Ceriello A, Dello Russo P, Amstad P, Cerutti P. 1996. High glucose induces antioxidant enzymes in human endothelial cells in culture; Evidence linking hyperglycemia and oxidative stress. *Diabetes* 45:471-7

Ceriello A, Morocutti A, Mercuri F, Quagliaro L, Moro M, et al. 2000. Defective intracellular antioxidant enzyme production in type 1 diabetic patients with nephropathy. *Diabetes* 49:2170-7

Chander PN, Gealekman O, Brodsky SV, Elitok S, Tojo A, et al. 2004. Nephropathy in Zucker Diabetic Fat Rat Is Associated with Oxidative and Nitrosative Stress: Prevention by Chronic Therapy with a Peroxynitrite Scavenger Ebselen. *Journal of the American Society of Nephrology* 15:2391-403

Chen J, Cha-Molstad H, Szabo A, Shalev A. 2009. Diabetes induces and calcium channel blockers prevent cardiac expression of proapoptotic thioredoxin-interacting protein. *Am J Physiol Endocrinol Metab* 296:E1133-9

Chen X-L, Tummala PE, Olbrych MT, Alexander RW, Medford RM. 1998. Angiotensin II Induces Monocyte Chemoattractant Protein-1 Gene Expression in Rat Vascular Smooth Muscle Cells. *Circ Res* 83:952-9

Chen Y-F, Cowley AW, Zou A-P. 2003. Increased H2O2 counteracts the vasodilator and natriuretic effects of superoxide dismutation by tempol in renal medulla. *American Journal of Physiology - Regulatory, Integrative and Comparative Physiology* 285:R827-R33

Cheng WH, Ho YS, Ross DA, Valentine BA, Combs Jr GF, Lei XG. 1997. Cellular glutathione peroxidase knockout mice express normal levels of selenium-dependent plasma and phospholipid hydroperoxide glutathione peroxidases in various tissues. *Journal of Nutrition* 127:1445-50

Chew P, Yuen DYC, Koh P, Stefanovic N, Febbraio MA, et al. 2009. Site-Specific Antiatherogenic Effect of the Antioxidant Ebselen in the Diabetic Apolipoprotein E–Deficient Mouse. *Arteriosclerosis, Thrombosis, and Vascular Biology* 29:823-30

Chew P, Yuen DYC, Stefanovic N, Pete J, Coughlan MT, et al. 2010. Antiatherosclerotic and renoprotective effects of ebselen in the diabetic apolipoprotein E/GPx1-double knockout mouse. *Diabetes* 59:3198-207

Chiu YIW, Kuo M-C, Kuo H-T, Chang J-M, Guh J-Y, et al. 2005. Alterations of glomerular and extracellular levels of glutathione peroxidase in patients and experimental rats with diabetic nephropathy. *Journal of Laboratory and Clinical Medicine* 145:181-6

Christensen FH, Stankevicius E, Hansen T, Jørgensen MM, Valverde VL, et al. 2007. Flow- and acetylcholine-induced dilatation in small arteries from rats with renovascular hypertension -- effect of tempol treatment. *European Journal of Pharmacology* 566:160-6

Chu FF, Esworthy RS, Ho YS, Bermeister M, Swiderek K, Elliott RW. 1997. Expression and Chromosomal Mapping of Mouse Gpx2 Gene Encoding the Gastrointestinal Form of Glutathione Peroxidase, GPX-GI. *Biomedical and Environmental Sciences* 10:156-62

Chui DHK, Tang WZ, Orkin SH. 1995. cDNA Cloning of Murine Nrf 2 Gene, Coding for a p45 NF-E2-Related Transcription Factor. *Biochemical and Biophysical Research Communications* 209:40-6

Cines DB, Pollak ES, Buck CA, Loscalzo J, Zimmerman GA, et al. 1998. Endothelial Cells in Physiology and in the Pathophysiology of Vascular Disorders. *Blood* 91:3527-61

Čolak E, Majkić-Singh N, Stanković S, Srecković-Dimitrijević V, Djordjević PB, et al. 2005. Parameters of antioxidative defense in type 2 diabetic patients with cardiovascular complications. *Annals of Medicine* 37:613-20

Conrad M, Schneider M, Seiler A, Bornkamm GW. 2007. Physiological role of phospholipid hydroperoxide glutathione peroxidase in mammals. *Biological Chemistry* 388:1019-25

Cook-Mills JM. 2006. Hydrogen peroxide activation of endothelial cell-associated MMPS during VCAM-1-dependent leukocyte migration. *Cellular and Molecular Biology* 52:8-16

Cooper ME. 2004. The role of the renin-angiotensin-aldosterone system in diabetes and its vascular complications. *American Journal of Hypertension* 17:S16-S20

Davis MT, Bartfay WJ. 2004. Ebselen Decreases Oxygen Free Radical Production and Iron Concentrations in the Hearts of Chronically Iron-Overloaded Mice. *Biological Research For Nursing* 6:37-45

De Bem AF, De Lima Portella R, Colpo E, Duarte MMMF, Frediane A, et al. 2009. Diphenyl diselenide decreases serum levels of total cholesterol and tissue oxidative stress in cholesterol-fed rabbits. *Basic and Clinical Pharmacology and Toxicology* 105:17-23

De Freitas AS, De Souza Prestes A, Wagner C, Sudati JH, Alves D, et al. 2010. Reduction of diphenyl diselenide and analogs by mammalian thioredoxin reductase is independent of their gluthathione peroxidase-like activity: A possible novel pathway for their antioxidant activity. *Molecules* 15:7699-714

de Haan JB, Bladier C, Griffiths P, Kelner M, O'Shea RD, et al. 1998. Mice with a Homozygous Null Mutation for the Most Abundant Glutathione Peroxidase, Gpx1, Show Increased Susceptibility to the Oxidative Stress-inducing Agents Paraquat and Hydrogen Peroxide. *Journal of Biological Chemistry* 273:22528-36

de Haan JB, Cooper ME. 2011. Targeted antioxidant therapies in hyperglycemia-mediated endothelial dysfunction. *Frontiers in bioscience (Scholar edition)* 3:709-29

de Haan JB, Stefanovic N, Nikolic-Paterson D, Scurr LL, Croft KD, et al. 2005. Kidney expression of glutathione peroxidase-1 is not protective against streptozotocin-induced diabetic nephropathy. *American Journal of Physiology - Renal Physiology* 289:F544-F51 de Haan JB, Witting PK, Stefanovic N, Pete J, Daskalakis M, et al. 2006. Lack of the antioxidant glutathione peroxidase-1 does not increase atherosclerosis in C57BL/J6 mice fed a high-fat diet. *Journal of Lipid Research* 47:1157-67

De Vriese AS, Verbeuren TJ, Van de Voorde J, Lameire NH, Vanhoutte PM. 2000. Endothelial dysfunction in diabetes. *Br J Pharmacol* 130:963-74

DeRubertis FR, Craven PA, Melhem MF. 2007. Acceleration of diabetic renal injury in the superoxide dismutase knockout mouse: effects of tempol. *Metabolism: clinical and experimental* 56:1256-64

Dhanasekaran A, Kotamraju S, Kalivendi SV, Matsunaga T, Shang T, et al. 2004. Supplementation of endothelial cells with mitochondria-targeted antioxidants inhibit peroxide-induced mitochondrial iron uptake, oxidative damage, and apoptosis. *Journal of Biological Chemistry* 279:37575-87

Dhanasekaran A, Kotamraju S, Karunakaran C, Kalivendi SV, Thomas S, et al. 2005. Mitochondria superoxide dismutase mimetic inhibits peroxide-induced oxidative damage and apoptosis: Role of mitochondrial superoxide. *Free Radical Biology and Medicine* 39:567-83

Dominguez C, Ruiz E, Gussinye M, Carrascosa A. 1998. Oxidative stress at onset and in early stages of type 1 diabetes in children and adolescents. *Diabetes Care* 21:1736-42

Duncan JG. 2011. Mitochondrial dysfunction in diabetic cardiomyopathy. *Biochimica et Biophysica Acta (BBA) - Molecular Cell Research* 1813:1351-9

Espinola-Klein C, Rupprecht HJ, Bickel C, Schnabel R, Genth-Zotz S, et al. 2007. Glutathione Peroxidase-1 Activity, Atherosclerotic Burden, and Cardiovascular Prognosis. *The American journal of cardiology* 99:808-12

Esposito LA, Kokoszka JE, Waymire KG, Cottrell B, MacGregor GR, Wallace DC. 2000. Mitochondrial oxidative stress in mice lacking the glutathione peroxidase-1 gene. *Free Radical Biology and Medicine* 28:754-66

Esworthy RS, Swiderek KM, Ho YS, Chu FF. 1998. Selenium-dependent glutathione peroxidase-GI is a major glutathione peroxidase activity in the mucosal epithelium of rodent intestine. *Biochimica et Biophysica Acta - General Subjects* 1381:213-26

Evans JL, Goldfine ID, Maddux BA, Grodsky GM. 2002. Oxidative Stress and Stress-Activated Signaling Pathways: A Unifying Hypothesis of Type 2 Diabetes. *Endocr Rev* 23:599-622

Fang ZY, Prins JB, Marwick TH. 2004. Diabetic Cardiomyopathy: Evidence, Mechanisms, and Therapeutic Implications. *Endocr Rev* 25:543-67

Farhangkhoee H, Khan ZA, Kaur H, Xin X, Chen S, Chakrabarti S. 2006. Vascular endothelial dysfunction in diabetic cardiomyopathy: Pathogenesis and potential treatment targets. *Pharmacology & Therapeutics* 111:384-99

Filipovska A, Kelso GF, Brown SE, Beer SM, Smith RAJ, Murphy MP. 2005. Synthesis and Characterization of a Triphenylphosphonium-conjugated Peroxidase Mimetic. *Journal of Biological Chemistry* 280:24113-26

Fiordaliso F, Cuccovillo I, Bianchi R, Bai A, Doni M, et al. 2006. Cardiovascular oxidative stress is reduced by an ACE inhibitor in a rat model of streptozotocin-induced diabetes. *Life Sciences* 79:121-9

Fiordaliso F, Li B, Latini R, Sonnenblick EH, Anversa P, et al. 2000. Myocyte Death in Streptozotocin-Induced Diabetes in Rats Is Angiotensin II- Dependent. *Lab Invest* 80:513-27

Forbes JM, Coughlan MT, Cooper ME. 2008. Oxidative Stress as a Major Culprit in Kidney Disease in Diabetes. *Diabetes* 57:1446-54

Forgione MA, Cap A, Liao R, Moldovan NI, Eberhardt RT, et al. 2002a. Heterozygous Cellular Glutathione Peroxidase Deficiency in the Mouse. *Circulation* 106:1154-8

Forgione MA, Weiss N, Heydrick S, Cap A, Klings ES, et al. 2002b. Cellular glutathione peroxidase deficiency and endothelial dysfunction. *American Journal of Physiology - Heart and Circulatory Physiology* 282:H1255-H61

Forstermann U. 2008. Oxidative stress in vascular disease: causes, defense mechanisms and potential therapies. *Nat Clin Pract Cardiovasc Med* 5:338-49

Frustaci A, Kajstura J, Chimenti C, Jakoniuk I, Leri A, et al. 2000. Myocardial Cell Death in Human Diabetes. *Circ Res* 87:1123-32

Fujieda M, Naruse K, Hamauzu T, Miyazaki E, Hayashi Y, et al. 2007. Effect of selenium-deficient diet on tubular epithelium in normal rats. *Pediatric Nephrology (Berlin, Germany)* 22:192-201

Fujita A, Sasaki H, Ogawa K, Okamoto K, Matsuno S, et al. 2005. Increased gene expression of antioxidant enzymes in KKAy diabetic mice but not in STZ diabetic mice. *Diabetes research and clinical practice* 69:113-9

Fujita H, Fujishima H, Chida S, Takahashi K, Qi Z, et al. 2009. Reduction of Renal Superoxide Dismutase in Progressive Diabetic Nephropathy. *Journal of the American Society of Nephrology* 20:1303-13

Fukuda M, Nakamura T, Kataoka K, Nako H, Tokutomi Y, et al. 2010. Ezetimibe Ameliorates Cardiovascular Complications and Hepatic Steatosis in Obese and Type 2 Diabetic db/db Mice. *Journal of Pharmacology and Experimental Therapeutics* 335:70-5

Gao X, Belmadani S, Picchi A, Xu X, Potter BJ, et al. 2007. Tumor Necrosis Factor-α Induces Endothelial Dysfunction in Leprdb Mice. *Circulation* 115:245-54

Gilbert RE, Cooper ME. 1999. The tubulointerstitium in progressive diabetic kidney disease: More than an aftermath of glomerular injury? *Kidney Int* 56:1627-37

Giugliano D, Ceriello A, Paolisso G. 1996. Oxidative stress and diabetic vascular complications. *Diabetes Care* 19:257-67

Góth L. 2008. Catalase deficiency and type 2 diabetes. *Diabetes Care* 31

Góth L, Eaton JW. 2000. Hereditary catalase deficiencies and increased risk of diabetes. *Lancet* 356:1820-1

Goto H, Nishikawa T, Sonoda K, Kondo T, Kukidome D, et al. 2008. Endothelial MnSOD overexpression prevents retinal VEGF expression in diabetic mice. *Biochemical and Biophysical Research Communications* 366:814-20

Ha H, Mi RY, Yoon JC, Kitamura M, Hi BL. 2002. Role of high glucose-induced nuclear factor-κB activation in monocyte chemoattractant protein-1 expression by mesangial cells. *Journal of the American Society of Nephrology* 13:894-902

Hacker H, Karin M. 2006. Regulation and Function of IKK and IKK-Related Kinases. *Sci. STKE* 2006:re13-

Hamanishi T, Furuta H, Kato H, Doi A, Tamai M, et al. 2004. Functional Variants in the Glutathione Peroxidase-1 (GPx-1) Gene Are Associated With Increased Intima-Media Thickness of Carotid Arteries and Risk of Macrovascular Diseases in Japanese Type 2 Diabetic Patients. *Diabetes* 53:2455-60

Hassan W, Ibrahim M, Rocha JBT. 2009. Towards the mechanism and comparative effect of diphenyl diselenide, diphenyl ditelluride and ebselen under various pathophysiological conditions in rat's kidney preparation. *Chemico-Biological Interactions* 182:52-8

Hayat SA, Patel B, Khattar RS, Malik RA. 2004. Diabetic cardiomyopathy: mechanisms, diagnosis and treatment. *Clin Sci* 107:539-57

He M, Siow RCM, Sugden D, Gao L, Cheng X, Mann GE. 2011. Induction of HO-1 and redox signaling in endothelial cells by advanced glycation end products: A role for Nrf2 in vascular protection in diabetes. *Nutrition, Metabolism and Cardiovascular Diseases* 21:277-85

Heumüller S, Wind S, Barbosa-Sicard E, Schmidt HHHW, Busse R, et al. 2008. Apocynin Is Not an Inhibitor of Vascular NADPH Oxidases but an Antioxidant. *Hypertension* 51:211-7

Hinokio Y, Suzuki S, Hirai M, Suzuki C, Suzuki M, Toyota T. 2002. Urinary excretion of 8-oxo-7, 8-dihydro-2'-deoxyguanosine as a predictor of the development of diabetic nephropathy. *Diabetologia* 45:877-82

Hodgkinson AD, Bartlett T, Oates PJ, Millward BA, Demaine AG. 2003. The Response of Antioxidant Genes to Hyperglycemia Is Abnormal in Patients With Type 1 Diabetes and Diabetic Nephropathy. *Diabetes* 52:846-51

Hort MA, Straliotto MR, Netto PM, Da Rocha JBT, De Bem AF, Ribeiro-Do-Valle RM. 2011. Diphenyl diselenide effectively reduces atherosclerotic lesions in LDLr -/- Mice by attenuation of oxidative stress and inflammation. *Journal of Cardiovascular Pharmacology* 58:91-101

Iwata K, Nishinaka T, Matsuno K, Yabe-Nishimura C. 2006. Increased Gene Expression of Glutathione Peroxidase-3 in Diabetic Mouse Heart. *Biological & Pharmaceutical Bulletin* 29:1042-5

Jenkins AJ, Lyons TJ, Zheng D, Otvos JD, Lackland DT, et al. 2003. Lipoproteins in the DCCT/EDIC cohort: Associations with diabetic nephropathy. *Kidney International* 64:817-28

Jiang F, Guo Y, Salvemini D, Dusting GJ. 2003a. Superoxide dismutase mimetic M40403 improves endothelial function in apolipoprotein(E)-deficient mice. *British Journal Of Pharmacology* 139:1127-34

Jiang T, Huang Z, Lin Y, Zhang Z, Fang D, Zhang DD. 2010. The Protective Role of Nrf2 in Streptozotocin-Induced Diabetic Nephropathy. *Diabetes* 59:850-60

Jiang Z, Seo JY, Ha H, Lee EA, Kim YS, et al. 2003b. Reactive oxygen species mediate TGF-β-induced plasminogen activator inhibitor-1 upregulation in mesangial cells. *Biochemical and Biophysical Research Communications* 309:961-6

Joffe II, Travers KE, Perreault-Micale CL, Hampton T, Katz SE, et al. 1999. Abnormal cardiac function in the streptozotocin-induced, non-insulin-dependent diabetic rat : Noninvasive assessment with Doppler echocardiography and contribution of the nitric oxide pathway. *Journal of the American College of Cardiology* 34:2111-9

Johansen J, Harris A, Rychly D, Ergul A. 2005. Oxidative stress and the use of antioxidants in diabetes: Linking basic science to clinical practice. *Cardiovascular Diabetology* 4:5

Kakehi T, Yabe-Nishimura C. 2008. NOX enzymes and diabetic complications. *Seminars in Immunopathology* 30:301-14

Kakimoto M, Inoguchi T, Sonta T, Yu HY, Imamura M, et al. 2002. Accumulation of 8-hydroxy-2'-deoxyguanosine and mitochondrial DNA deletion in kidney of diabetic rats. *Diabetes* 51:1588-95

Kakkar R, Mantha SV, Kalra J, Prasad K. 1996. Time course study of oxidative stress in aorta and heart of diabetic rat. *Clinical Science* 91:441-8

Kalant N. 1978. Diabetic glomerulosclerosis: Current status. *Canadian Medical Association Journal* 119:146-53

Kamboj SS, Vasishta RK, Sandhir R. 2010. N-acetylcysteine inhibits hyperglycemia-induced oxidative stress and apoptosis markers in diabetic neuropathy. *Journal of Neurochemistry* 112:77-91

Kanauchi M, Nishioka H, Hashimoto T. 2002. Oxidative DNA damage and tubulointerstitial injury in diabetic nephropathy. *Nephron* 91:327-9

Kang Y. 2001. Molecular and cellular mechanisms of cardiotoxicity. *Environ Health Perspect* 109:27-34

Kannel W, Hjortland M, Castelli W. 1974. Role of diabetes in congestive heart failure: the Framingham study. *Am J Cardiol* 34:29-34

Keane WF, Zhang Z, Lyle PA, Cooper ME, de Zeeuw D, et al. 2006. Risk Scores for Predicting Outcomes in Patients with Type 2 Diabetes and Nephropathy: The RENAAL Study. *Clinical Journal of the American Society of Nephrology* 1:761-7

Kensler TW, Wakabayashi N, Biswal S. 2007. Cell survival responses to environmental stresses via the Keap1-Nrf2-ARE pathway. pp. 89-116

Kesavulu MM, Girl R, Kameswara Rao B, Apparao CH. 2000. Lipid peroxidation and antioxidant enzyme levels in type 2 diabetics with microvascular complications. *Diabetes and Metabolism* 26:387-92

Khatri JJ, Johnson C, Magid R, Lessner SM, Laude KM, et al. 2004. Vascular Oxidant Stress Enhances Progression and Angiogenesis of Experimental Atheroma. *Circulation* 109:520-5

Khullar M, Al-Shudiefat AA-RS, Ludke A, Binepal G, Singal PK. 2010. Oxidative stress: a key contributor to diabetic cardiomyopathyThis review is one of a selection of papers published in a Special Issue on Oxidative Stress in Health and Disease. *Canadian Journal of Physiology and Pharmacology* 88:233-40

Kim JA, Neupane GP, Lee ES, Jeong BS, Park BC, Thapa P. 2011. NADPH oxidase inhibitors: A patent review. *Expert Opinion on Therapeutic Patents* 21:1147-58

Kobayashi T, Uehara S, Ikeda T, Itadani H, Kotani H. 2003. Vitamin D3 up-regulated protein-1 regulates collagen expression in mesangial cells. *Kidney Int* 64:1632-42

Kohler JJ, Cucoranu I, Fields E, Green E, He S, et al. 2009. Transgenic mitochondrial superoxide dismutase and mitochondrially targeted catalase prevent antiretroviral-induced oxidative stress and cardiomyopathy. *Lab Invest* 89:782-90

Lapenna D, de Gioia S, Ciofani G, Mezzetti A, Ucchino S, et al. 1998. Glutathione-Related Antioxidant Defenses in Human Atherosclerotic Plaques. *Circulation* 97:1930-4

Lee HB, Yu M-R, Yang Y, Jiang Z, Ha H. 2003. Reactive Oxygen Species-Regulated Signaling Pathways in Diabetic Nephropathy. *J Am Soc Nephrol* 14:S241-5

Lee MY, Martin AS, Mehta PK, Dikalova AE, Garrido AM, et al. 2009. Mechanisms of Vascular Smooth Muscle NADPH Oxidase 1 (Nox1) Contribution to Injury-Induced Neointimal Formation. *Arteriosclerosis, Thrombosis, and Vascular Biology* 29:480-7

Lei XG. 2001. Glutathione peroxidase-1 gene knockout on body antioxidant defense in mice. *Biofactors (Oxford, England)* 14:93-9

Letonja M, Nikolajević-Starčević J, Letonja MS, Petrovič D. 2011. Association of the-262C/T polymorphism in the catalase gene promoter with carotid atherosclerosis in Slovenian patients with type 2 diabetes. *Central European Journal of Medicine* 6:463-9

Lewis P, Stefanovic N, Pete J, Calkin AC, Giunti S, et al. 2007. Lack of the Antioxidant Enzyme Glutathione Peroxidase-1 Accelerates Atherosclerosis in Diabetic Apolipoprotein E–Deficient Mice. *Circulation* 115:2178-87

Li S-Y, Sigmon VK, Babcock SA, Ren J. 2007. Advanced glycation endproduct induces ROS accumulation, apoptosis, MAP kinase activation and nuclear O-GlcNAcylation in human cardiac myocytes. *Life Sciences* 80:1051-6

Loscalzo J. 2001. Nitric Oxide Insufficiency, Platelet Activation, and Arterial Thrombosis. *Circulation Research* 88:756-62

Lu H, Zhen J, Wu T, Peng A, Ye T, et al. 2010. Superoxide dismutase mimetic drug tempol aggravates anti-GBM antibody-induced glomerulonephritis in mice. *American Journal of Physiology - Renal Physiology* 299:F445-F52

Luo ZF, Feng B, Mu J, Qi W, Zeng W, et al. 2010. Effects of 4-phenylbutyric acid on the process and development of diabetic nephropathy induced in rats by streptozotocin: Regulation of endoplasmic reticulum stress-oxidative activation. *Toxicology and Applied Pharmacology* 246:49-57

Lushchak VI. 2011. Adaptive response to oxidative stress: Bacteria, fungi, plants and animals. *Comparative Biochemistry and Physiology Part C: Toxicology & Pharmacology* 153:175-90

Lynch E, Kil J. 2009. Development of ebselen, a glutathione peroxidase mimic, for the prevention and treatment of noise-induced hearing loss. *Seminars in Hearing* 30:47-55

Maiorino M, Roveri A, Coassin M, Ursini F. 1988. Kinetic mechanism and substrate specificity of glutathione peroxidase activity of ebselen (PZ51). *Biochemical Pharmacology* 37:2267-71

Maritim A, Sanders R, Watkins Jr. 2003a. Diabetes, oxidative stress, and antioxidants: A review. *Journal of Biochemical and Molecular Toxicology* 17:24-38

Maritim AC, Sanders RA, Watkins JB. 2003b. Diabetes, oxidative stress, and antioxidants: A review. *Journal of Biochemical and Molecular Toxicology* 17:24-38

MatÉs JM, Pérez-Gómez C, De Castro IN. 1999. Antioxidant enzymes and human diseases. *Clinical Biochemistry* 32:595-603

McQueen MJ, Lonn E, Gerstein HC, Bosch J, Yusuf S. 2005. The HOPE (heart outcomes prevention evaluation) study and its consequences. *Scandinavian Journal of Clinical and Laboratory Investigation, Supplement* 65:143-56

Mills GC. 1957. Hemoglobin catabolism. I. Glutathione peroxidase, an erythrocyte enzyme which protects hemoglobin from oxidative breakdown. *The Journal of biological chemistry* 229:189-97

Min W, Pober J. 1997. TNF initiates E-selectin transcription in human endothelial cells through parallel TRAF-NF-kappa B and TRAF-RAC/CDC42-JNK-c-Jun/ATF2 pathways. *The Journal of Immunology* 159:3508-18

Mitchell JB, Samuni A, Krishna MC, DeGraff WG, Ahn MS, et al. 1990. Biologically active metal-independent superoxide dismutase mimics. *Biochemistry®* 29:2802-7

Muller A, Cadenas E, Graf P, Sies H. 1984. A novel biologically active seleno-organic compound-I. Glutathione peroxidase-like activity in vitro and antioxidant capacity of PZ 51 (Ebselen). *Biochemical Pharmacology* 33:3235-9

Muscoli C, Cuzzocrea S, Riley DP, Zweier JL, Thiemermann C, et al. 2003. On the selectivity of superoxide dismutase mimetics and its importance in pharmacological studies. *British Journal Of Pharmacology* 140:445-60

Nakagami H, Kaneda Y, Ogihara T, Morishita R. 2005. Endothelial dysfunction in hyperglycemia as a trigger of atherosclerosis. *Current diabetes reviews* 1:59-63

Nam SM, Lee MY, Koh JH, Park JH, Shin JY, et al. 2009. Effects of NADPH oxidase inhibitor on diabetic nephropathy in OLETF rats: The role of reducing oxidative stress in its protective property. *Diabetes research and clinical practice* 83:176-82

Nangaku M. 2004. Mechanisms of Tubulointerstitial Injury in the Kidney: Final Common Pathways to End-stage Renal Failure. *Internal Medicine* 43:9-17

Nicolls MR, Haskins K, Flores SC. 2007. Oxidant Stress, Immune Dysregulation, and Vascular Function in Type I Diabetes. *Antioxidants & Redox Signaling* 9:879-89

Nishiyama A, Matsui M, Iwata S, Hirota K, Masutani H, et al. 1999. Identification of Thioredoxin-binding Protein-2/Vitamin D3 Up-regulated Protein 1 as a Negative Regulator of Thioredoxin Function and Expression. *J Biol Chem* 274:21645-50

Nomura K, Imai H, Koumura T, Arai M, Nakagawa Y. 1999. Mitochondrial Phospholipid Hydroperoxide Glutathione Peroxidase Suppresses Apoptosis Mediated by a Mitochondrial Death Pathway. *Journal of Biological Chemistry* 274:29294-302

Pacher P, Szabo C. 2006. Role of peroxynitrite in the pathogenesis of cardiovascular complications of diabetes. *Current Opinion in Pharmacology* 6:136-41

Palsamy P, Subramanian S. 2011. Resveratrol protects diabetic kidney by attenuating hyperglycemia-mediated oxidative stress and renal inflammatory cytokines via Nrf2-Keap1 signaling. *Biochimica et Biophysica Acta (BBA) - Molecular Basis of Disease* 1812:719-31

Panduru NM, Moța E, Moța M, Cimponeriu D, Serafinceanu C, Cheța DM. 2010. Polymorphism of catalase gene promoter in Romanian patients with diabetic kidney disease and type 1 diabetes. *Romanian journal of internal medicine = Revue roumaine de médecine interne* 48:81-8

Pari L, Karthikesan K, Menon VP. 2010. Comparative and combined effect of chlorogenic acid and tetrahydrocurcumin on antioxidant disparities in chemical induced experimental diabetes. *Molecular and Cellular Biochemistry* 341:109-17

Parnham MJ, Leyck S, Kuhl P. 1987. Ebselen: A new approach to the inhibition of peroxide-dependent inflammation. *International Journal of Tissue Reactions* 9:45-50

Patel SS, Shah RS, Goyal RK. 2009. Antihyperglycemic, antihyperlipidemic and antioxidant effects of Dihar, a polyherbal ayurvedic formulation in streptozotocin induced diabetic rats. *Indian Journal of Experimental Biology* 47:564-70

Pergola PE, Raskin P, Toto RD, Meyer CJ, Huff JW, et al. 2011. Bardoxolone methyl and kidney function in CKD with type 2 diabetes. *N Engl J Med* 365:327-36

Privratsky JR, Wold LE, Sowers JR, Quinn MT, Ren J. 2003. AT1 Blockade Prevents Glucose-Induced Cardiac Dysfunction in Ventricular Myocytes: Role of the AT1 Receptor and NADPH Oxidase. *Hypertension* 42:206-12

Qi W, Chen X, Gilbert RE, Zhang Y, Waltham M, et al. 2007. High Glucose-Induced Thioredoxin-Interacting Protein in Renal Proximal Tubule Cells Is Independent of Transforming Growth Factor-β1. *Am J Pathol* 171:744-54

Rajamani U, Essop MF. 2010. Hyperglycemia-mediated activation of the hexosamine biosynthetic pathway results in myocardial apoptosis. *American Journal of Physiology - Cell Physiology* 299:C139-C47

Rajesh M, Mukhopadhyay P, Bátkai S, Mukhopadhyay B, Patel V, et al. 2009. Xanthine oxidase inhibitor allopurinol attenuates the development of diabetic cardiomyopathy. *Journal of Cellular and Molecular Medicine* 13:2330-41

Razavi HM, Hamilton JA, Feng Q. 2005. Modulation of apoptosis by nitric oxide: implications in myocardial ischemia and heart failure. *Pharmacology & Therapeutics* 106:147-62

Read MA, Whitley MZ, Gupta S, Pierce JW, Best J, et al. 1997. Tumor Necrosis Factor α-Induced E-selectin Expression Is Activated by the Nuclear Factor-κB and c-JUN N-terminal Kinase/p38 Mitogen-activated Protein Kinase Pathways. *Journal of Biological Chemistry* 272:2753-61

Reddi AS, Bollineni JS. 2001. Selenium-deficient diet induces renal oxidative stress and injury via TGF-[bgr]1 in normal and diabetic rats. *Kidney Int* 59:1342-53

Reeves M, Hoffmann P. 2009. The human selenoproteome: recent insights into functions and regulation. *Cellular and Molecular Life Sciences* 66:2457-78

Rey FE, Cifuentes ME, Kiarash A, Quinn MT, Pagano PJ. 2001. Novel Competitive Inhibitor of NAD(P)H Oxidase Assembly Attenuates Vascular O2− and Systolic Blood Pressure in Mice. *Circulation Research* 89:408-14

Rhyu DY, Yang Y, Ha H, Lee GT, Song JS, et al. 2005. Role of reactive oxygen species in TGF-β1-induced mitogen-activated protein kinase activation and epithelial-mesenchymal transition in renal tubular epithelial cells. *Journal of the American Society of Nephrology* 16:667-75

Rosenblat M, Aviram M. 1998. Macrophage Glutathione Content and Glutathione Peroxidase Activity Are Inversely Related to Cell-Mediated Oxidation of LDL: In Vitro and In Vivo Studies. *Free Radical Biology and Medicine* 24:305-17

Ross MF, Kelso GF, Blaikie FH, James AM, Cochemé HM, et al. 2005. Lipophilic triphenylphosphonium cations as tools in mitochondrial bioenergetics and free radical biology. *Biochemistry (Moscow)* 70:222-30

Rossing P. 2006. Diabetic nephropathy: Worldwide epidemic and effects of current treatment on natural history. *Current Diabetes Reports* 6:479-83

Rubler S, Dlugash J, Yuceoglu Y, Kumral T, Branwood A, Grishman A. 1972. New type of cardiomyopathy associated with diabetic glomerulosclerosis. *Am J Cardiol* 30:595-602

Safayhi H, Tiegs G, Wendel A. 1985. A novel biologically active seleno-organic compound. V. Inhibition by ebselen (PZ 51) of rat peritoneal neutrophil lipoxygenase. *Biochemical Pharmacology* 34:2691-4

Sakurai T, Kanayama M, Shibata T, Itoh K, Kobayashi A, et al. 2006. Ebselen, a Seleno-organic Antioxidant, as an Electrophile. *Chemical Research in Toxicology* 19:1196-204

Salvemini D, Wang ZQ, Zweier JL, Samouilov A, Macarthur H, et al. 1999. A nonpeptidyl mimic of superoxide dismutase with therapeutic activity in rats. *Science (New York, N.Y.)* 286:304-6

Sasser JM, Pollock JS, Pollock DM. 2002. Renal endothelin in chronic angiotensin II hypertension. *American Journal of Physiology - Regulatory Integrative and Comparative Physiology* 283:R243-R8

Schmid JA, Birbach A. 2008. IκB kinase β (IKKβ/IKK2/IKBKB)—A key molecule in signaling to the transcription factor NF-κB. *Cytokine & growth factor reviews* 19:157-65

Schulman IH, Zhou MS, Raij L. 2006. Interaction between nitric oxide and angiotensin II in the endothelium: Role in atherosclerosis and hypertension. *Journal of Hypertension* 24:S45-S50

Sedeek M, Callera G, Montezano A, Gutsol A, Heitz F, et al. 2010. Critical role of Nox4-based NADPH oxidase in glucose-induced oxidative stress in the kidney: Implications in type 2 diabetic nephropathy. *American Journal of Physiology - Renal Physiology* 299:F1348-F58

Seiler A, Schneider M, Förster H, Roth S, Wirth EK, et al. 2008. Glutathione Peroxidase 4 Senses and Translates Oxidative Stress into 12/15-Lipoxygenase Dependent- and AIF-Mediated Cell Death. *Cell Metabolism* 8:237-48

Shalev A, Pise-Masison CA, Radonovich M, Hoffmann SC, Hirshberg B, et al. 2002. Oligonucleotide Microarray Analysis of Intact Human Pancreatic Islets: Identification of Glucose-Responsive Genes and a Highly Regulated TGF-β Signaling Pathway. *Endocrinology* 143:3695-

Sharma V, Tewari R, Sk UH, Joseph C, Sen E. 2008. Ebselen sensitizes glioblastoma cells to Tumor Necrosis Factor (TNFα)-induced apoptosis through two distinct pathways involving NF-κB downregulation and Fas-mediated formation of death inducing signaling complex. *International Journal of Cancer* 123:2204-12

Shaw JE, Sicree RA, Zimmet PZ. 2010. Global estimates of the prevalence of diabetes for 2010 and 2030. *Diabetes research and clinical practice* 87:4-14

Shen X, Zheng S, Metreveli NS, Epstein PN. 2006. Protection of Cardiac Mitochondria by Overexpression of MnSOD Reduces Diabetic Cardiomyopathy. *Diabetes* 55:798-805

Sies H. 1997. Oxidative stress: oxidants and antioxidants. *Experimental Physiology* 82:291-5

Sies H, Masumoto H. 1997. Ebselen as a glutathione peroxidase mimic and as a scavenger of peroxynitrite. *Advances in pharmacology (San Diego, Calif.)* 38:229-46

Simonsen U, Rodriguez-Rodriguez R, Dalsgaard T, Buus NH, Stankevicius E. 2009. Novel approaches to improving endothelium-dependent nitric oxide-mediated vasodilatation. *Pharmacological Reports* 61:105-15

Smith RAJ, Porteous CM, Coulter CV, Murphy MP. 1999. Selective targeting of an antioxidant to mitochondria. *European Journal of Biochemistry* 263:709-16

Studer RK, Craven PA, DeRubertis FR. 1997. Antioxidant inhibition of protein kinase C-signaled increases in transforming growth factor-beta in mesangial cells. *Metabolism: Clinical and Experimental* 46:918-25

Subramanian S, Kalyanaraman B, Migrino RQ. 2010. Mitochondrially targeted antioxidants for the treatment of cardiovascular diseases. *Recent Patents on Cardiovascular Drug Discovery* 5:54-65

Sui H, Wang W, Wang PH, Liu LS. 2005. Effect of glutathione peroxidase mimic ebselen (PZ51) on endothelium and vascular structure of stroke-prone spontaneously hypertensive rats. *Blood Pressure* 14:366-72

Szabó C, Mabley JG, Moeller SM, Shimanovich R, Pacher P, et al. 2002. Part I: Pathogenetic role of peroxynitrite in the development of diabetes and diabetic vascular complications: Studies with FP15, a novel potent peroxynitrite decomposition catalyst. *Molecular Medicine* 8:571-80

Tamasi V, Jeffries JM, Arteel GE, Falkner KC. 2004. Ebselen augments its peroxidase activity by inducing nrf-2-dependent transcription. *Archives of Biochemistry and Biophysics* 431:161-8

Tan SM, Zhang Y, Cox AJ, Kelly DJ, Qi W. 2011. Tranilast attenuates the up-regulation of thioredoxin-interacting protein and oxidative stress in an experimental model of diabetic nephropathy. *Nephrol. Dial. Transplant.* 26:100-10

ten Freyhaus H, Huntgeburth M, Wingler K, Schnitker J, Bäumer AT, et al. 2006. Novel Nox inhibitor VAS2870 attenuates PDGF-dependent smooth muscle cell chemotaxis, but not proliferation. *Cardiovascular Research* 71:331-41

Tewari R, Sharma V, Koul N, Ghosh A, Joseph C, et al. 2009. Ebselen abrogates TNFα induced pro-inflammatory response in glioblastoma. *Molecular oncology* 3:77-83

Thandavarayan RA, Watanabe K, Ma M, Veeraveedu PT, Gurusamy N, et al. 2008. 14-3-3 protein regulates Ask1 signaling and protects against diabetic cardiomyopathy. *Biochemical Pharmacology* 75:1797-806

Thomas JP, Maiorino M, Ursini F, Girotti AW. 1990. Protective action of phospholipid hydroperoxide glutathione peroxidase against membrane-damaging lipid peroxidation. In situ reduction of phospholipid and cholesterol hydroperoxides. *Journal of Biological Chemistry* 265:454-61

Thomas MC, Baynes JW, Thorpe SR, Cooper ME. 2005. The role of AGEs and AGE inhibitors in diabetic cardiovascular disease. *Current Drug Targets* 6:453-74

Tolonen N, Forsblom C, Thorn L, Wadén J, Rosengård-Bärlund M, et al. 2009. Lipid abnormalities predict progression of renal disease in patients with type 1 diabetes. *Diabetologia* 52:2522-30

Torzewski M, Ochsenhirt V, Kleschyov AL, Oelze M, Daiber A, et al. 2007. Deficiency of Glutathione Peroxidase-1 Accelerates the Progression of Atherosclerosis in Apolipoprotein E-Deficient Mice. *Arteriosclerosis, Thrombosis, and Vascular Biology* 27:850-7

Ungvari Z, Bailey-Downs L, Gautam T, Jimenez R, Losonczy G, et al. 2011. Adaptive induction of NF-E2-related factor-2-driven antioxidant genes in endothelial cells in response to hyperglycemia. *American Journal of Physiology - Heart and Circulatory Physiology* 300:H1133-H40

Victor VM, Apostolova N, Herance R, Hernandez-Mijares A, Rocha M. 2009. Oxidative stress and mitochondrial dysfunction in atherosclerosis: mitochondria-targeted antioxidants as potential therapy. *Current Medicinal Chemistry* 16:4654-67

Williams HC, Griendling KK. 2007. NADPH Oxidase Inhibitors: New Antihypertensive Agents? *Journal of Cardiovascular Pharmacology* 50:9-16 0.1097/FJC.0b013e318063e820

Wilson GL, Leiter EH. 1990. Streptozotocin interactions with pancreatic β cells and the induction of insulin-dependent diabetes. *Current Topics in Microbiology and Immunology* 156:27-54

Winter JP, Gong Y, Grant PJ, Wild CP. 2003. Glutathione peroxidase 1 genotype is associated with an increased risk of coronary artery disease. *Coronary Artery Disease* 14:149-53

World CJ, Yamawaki H, Berk BC. 2006. Thioredoxin in the cardiovascular system. *Journal of Molecular Medicine* V84:997-1003

Xiang L, Dearman J, Abram SR, Carter C, Hester RL. 2008. Insulin resistance and impaired functional vasodilation in obese Zucker rats. *American Journal of Physiology - Heart and Circulatory Physiology* 294:H1658-H66

Yamaguchi T, Sano K, Takakura K, Saito I, Shinohara Y, et al. 1998. Ebselen in Acute Ischemic Stroke : A Placebo-Controlled, Double-blind Clinical Trial. *Stroke* 29:12-7

Yamawaki H, Pan S, Lee RT, Berk BC. 2005. Fluid shear stress inhibits vascular inflammation by decreasing thioredoxin-interacting protein in endothelial cells. *J Clin Invest* 115:733-8

Yang H, Roberts LJ, Ming JS, Li CZ, Ballard BR, et al. 2004. Retardation of atherosclerosis by overexpression of catalase or both Cu/Zn-superoxide dismutase and catalase in mice lacking apolipoprotein E. *Circulation Research* 95:1075-81

Yoshida T, Maulik N, Engelman RM, Ho YS, Magnenat JL, et al. 1997. Glutathione peroxidase knockout mice are susceptible to myocardial ischemia reperfusion injury. *Circulation* 96:II216-II20

Yoshizumi M, Fujita Y, Izawa Y, Suzaki Y, Kyaw M, et al. 2004. Ebselen inhibits tumor necrosis factor-[alpha]-induced c-Jun N-terminal kinase activation and adhesion molecule expression in endothelial cells. *Experimental Cell Research* 292:1-10

Yu Z, Shao W, Chiang Y, Foltz W, Zhang Z, et al. 2011. Oltipraz upregulates the nuclear respiratory factor 2 alpha subunit (NRF2) antioxidant system and prevents insulin resistance and obesity induced by a high-fat diet in C57BL/6J mice. *Diabetologia* 54:922-34

Zelmanovitz T, Gerchman F, Balthazar A, Thomazelli F, Matos J, Canani L. 2009. Diabetic nephropathy. *Diabetology & Metabolic Syndrome* 1:10-26

Zhou M-S, Schulman IH, Pagano PJ, Jaimes EA, Raij L. 2006. Reduced NAD(P)H Oxidase in Low Renin Hypertension. *Hypertension* 47:81-6

12

Evaluation of Oxidative Stress and the Efficacy of Antioxidant Treatment in Diabetes Mellitus

Nemes-Nagy Enikő et al.*
University of Medicine and Pharmacy, Tîrgu-Mureş, Medical Biochemistry Department, Romania

1. Introduction

Studies on the efficacy of antioxidant treatment in type 1 diabetes mellitus is an interesting, actual research subject. Reactive oxygen species (ROS) are continuously produced and eliminated by living organisms normally maintaining ROS at certain steady-state levels. Under some circumstances, the balance between ROS generation and elimination is disturbed leading to enhanced ROS level causing oxidative stress [Lushchak, 2011]. Oxidative stress is involved in the development of several important diseases (cancer, ulcer, atherosclerosis, autoimmune diseases, ischaemia-reperfusion injury, emphysema, inflammation, etc.).

Oxidative stress due to increased production of reactive oxygen species and/or impaired antioxidant capacity of the body plays a special, important role in the development of type 1 diabetes mellitus and its complications [Baynes, 1991], [Giugliano et al., 1995], [Krippeit-Drews et al., 1994], [Nakazaki et al., 1995], [Nomikos et al., 1989], [Raes et al, 1995], [Shinn, 1998].

Under normal conditions, oxidative tissue damage is prevented by enzymatic and non-enzymatic antioxidants. Superoxide dismutase (SOD), glutathione peroxidase (GPx) and catalase (CAT) are three enzymes involved in detoxification of reactive oxygen species (superoxide radical, hydroxyl radical, and hydrogen peroxide). Pancreatic cells have a poor antioxidant defence system, so they are very vulnerable to oxidative stress, especially to superoxide mediated radical damage [Dejica, 2000].

Evaluation of oxidative status can be made by various methods, most of them very sophisticated, requiring laboratories with modern equipment, and are used almost exclusively for research purposes.

---

* V. Balogh-Sămărghiţan[1], Elena Cristina Crăciun[2], R. Morar[3], Dana Liana Pusta[3], Fazakas Zita[1], Szőcs-Molnár Terézia[4], Dunca Iulia[4], Sánta Dóra[5] and Minodora Dobreanu[6]

[1] *University of Medicine and Pharmacy, Tîrgu-Mureş, Medical Biochemistry Department, Romania*

[2] *University of Medicine and Pharmacy "Iuliu Haţieganu", Cluj-Napoca, Pharmaceutical Biochemistry and Clinical Laboratory Department, Romania*

[3] *Faculty of Veterinary Medicine, University of Agricultural Sciences and Veterinary Medicine, Cluj-Napoca, Romania*

[4] *II. Clinical Hospital of Pediatrics, Tîrgu-Mureş, Romania*

[5] *Santa Medical Unit, Tîrgu-Mureş, Romania,*

[6] *University of Medicine and Pharmacy, Tîrgu-Mureş, Clinical Biochemistry Department, Romania*

Exploring the body oxidative status can be made through the following ways:

1. Free radical measurement by absorption spectroscopy with electronic spin resonance (ESR) and electronic paramagnetic resonance (EPR) [Olinescu, 1994].
2. Measurement of chemical uptake (chemical trapping) by quantitative determination of the elimination of specific derivatives of salicylic acid, hydroxylated or nitrosylated compounds.
3. Measuring the antioxidant capacity of each antioxidant in part or total plasma antioxidant capacity.
4. Determination of antioxidant enzyme activites (SOD, CAT, GPX) and non-enzymatic antioxidants (tocopherols and tocotrienols, vitamin C, ubiquinone, glutathione, carotenoids and vitamin A, bilirubin, melatonin, uric acid, ceruloplasmin, vitamin K, lipoic acid) [Dejica, 2000, 2001].
5. The measurement of biological compounds resulting from oxidative processes:
   - lipid compounds - conjugated dienes, hydroperoxides, aldehydes (malondialdehyde, hydroxynonenal)
   - ethane and pentane measurements in expired gases
   - DNA beta-hydroxydeoxyguanosine
   - protein derivatives (carbonyl or thiol groups)
   - amino acids - methionine sulfoxide, ortho-tyrosine, dityrosine, nitrotyrosine, chlorotyrosine.
6. Measurement of the antioxidants / oxidizing substances ratio (eg. ascorbic acid / dehydroascorbic acid and reduced glutathione / oxidized glutathione) [Prior & Cao, 1999].

2. Antioxidants

Determination of trace elements is also of interest because some are in the active center of antioxidant enzymes: for example Cu, Zn and Mn are found in the structure of SOD, and Se is present in the active center of GPX, but also possesses antioxidant effect independent of this enzyme [Olinescu, 1994].

The variety of antioxidant substances in the body, the difficulty of measuring their individual level and the interactions between them require methods for measuring total antioxidant capacity (TAOC) in different biological samples [Cadenas & Packer, 2002].

By measuring TAOC one can assess not only the interaction effects of antioxidants known, but also the antioxidant action of unidentified components present in human plasma. In most methods uric acid is the major contributor to the TAOC of plasma, so increasing plasma levels of uric acid can mask the depletion of ascorbate or other antioxidants in some pathological conditions if only TAOC measurement is carried out.

TAOC are methods used to measure indirect inhibition involving a prooxidant (typically a free radical) and an oxidizable substrate. The prooxidant induces oxidative deterioration of the substrate, which is inhibited in the presence of the antioxidant.

Antioxidant capacity can be defined as the ability of a compound to reduce prooxidants. In biological systems, prooxidants are usually defined as toxic substances causing oxidative damage to lipids, proteins, nucleic acids, leading to a variety of pathological events, but not every prooxidant is necessary a toxic compound. Antioxidants are substances that, in low concentrations compared to an oxidizable substrate, prevent or delay oxidation initiated by a prooxidant [Dejica, 2001].

Several vitamins are well known for their antioxidant properties: vitamin C exhibits its effect in hydrophilic environment, while vitamin A and E protect especially the cell membranes, and act in hydrophobic phase. Many other, more complex antioxidant substances are found in plants.

3. Implication of oxidative stress and glycation process in diabetes mellitus

In type 2 diabetic patients, besides the relative insulin deficiency, there is a certain grade of insulin resistance. The relationship between reactive oxygen species and the effect of insulin has been studied, and the results showed that in elderly people, presenting intense exposure to oxidative stress, the ratio between GSH/GSSG is reduced, leading to intensified lipoperoxidation. This phenomenon might exhibit a negative influence on the integrity of plasma membranes, leading to their disfunction, regarding for instance the transmembrane glucose transport. There is a high probability that the periferal action of insulin is disturbed by the negative effect of reactive oxygen species on membrane ATP-ase activity [Dejica, 2000].

Peroxidation of lipids (especially LDL) plays an important role in inducing macrovascular lesions found in both diabetes and in atherosclerotic disease. Susceptibility to oxidation of lipoproteins seems to be a key element in the initiation and propagation of the atherogenic process [Dobreanu M., Módy, 1998]. In diabetic patients, lipid oxidation affects circulating lipids, and also those present in cell membranes or myelin layers. Hyperglycemia, excessive autooxidation and decreased antioxidant capacity registered in diabetic patients are responsible for intensified oxidative processes.

The speed of non-enzymatic glycation is proportional to the blood sugar level. Glucose (and fructose and galactose) are attached to the extreme N-terminal peptide chain, initially forming a Schiff base (aldimine), which is unstable, then by Amadori rearrangement a stable cetoimine is formed, and advanced glycation end products, leading to alterations in configuration, of the electronegative charge and molecular recognition of proteins.

Amadori-products can also be oxidized, by reactions catalyzed by transition metals, releasing eritronic acid and forming carboxymethylated lysine. Its level is double in the collagen of the skin of diabetic patients compared to non-diabetic subjects, and it is positively correlated with the presence of retino- and nephropathy in diabetic patients [Wolff, 1993].

All structural proteins and those circulating in the body can suffer non-enzymatic glycation processes. They can alter protein structure and function of vessels, nerves, liver, skin and other organs. Glycosylation of LDL lipoprotein particles decreases their catabolism and accelerates HDL catabolism, disorders that may explain in part the modifications present in macroangiopathy. Glycosylated proteins are more susceptible to attack by reactive oxygen species.

Enzymatic glycosylation of proteins is also important in development of chronic diabetic complications. The collagen molecules are thus glycosylated, glycoproteins and proteoglycans suffer similar processes. At the level of nerves, lens, livers or other organs, glycosylation of proteins is involved in the occurrence of diabetic neuropathy, cataracts, dysmetabolic hepatopathy [Gherasim, 1998], [Kovács, 2001].

Based on these evidences, antioxidant treatment is a promising approach for complementary therapy in diabetes mellitus. Several phytotherapeutical products contain a complexity of free radical scavengers and exhibit no side effects on long term treatment.

4. Evaluation of oxidative stress and the efficacy of antioxidant treatment in diabetes mellitus

4.1. Studies on animals

Some of the plants known for their high antioxidant power are: Allium sativa, Ricinus communis, Securinega virosa, Viscum album, pomegranates, berries (including strawberries, blueberries, and raspberries), walnuts, sunflower seeds, ginger and several plants of Indian traditional medicine: Emblica officinalis L., Curcuma longa L., Mangifera indica L., Momordica charantia L., Santalum album L, Swertia chirata Buch-Ham, Withania somnifera and Cassia auriculata [Capasso et al, 2003], [Dejica, 2001], [Moshi & Mbwambo, 2003], [Pari & Latha, 2003], [Pietta, 1998], [Scartezzini & Speroni, 2000], [Varga et al., 2001].

Our studies carried out in streptozotocin diabetic rats demonstrated that treatment with the blueberry (Eridiarom®) or blueberry and sea buckthorn concentrate (Diavit®) for two months had regenerative effect on pancreatic beta cells [Crăciun et al., 2007], [Morar et al., 2004].

The therapeutic properties of blueberry are attributed to its anthocyanosides which belong to a class of substances known as plant bioflavonoids. Pharmacologically, anthocyanosides are thought to decrease vascular permeability and improve microcirculation. They are also thought to have antioxidant activity.

Diavit® is a dietary supplement with a more complex composition compared to Eridiarom®, it contains quinolizidine alkaloids, anthocyanosides, sugars, carotenoids, vitamins (C, E, PP, B_1, B_2, folic acid), minerals (K, Ca, P, S, Mg, Cl, Mn, Fe), organic acids, flavonoids, etc..

Carotenoids are best recognized for their antioxidant capacity, they are considered the most potent biological quenchers of singlet oxygen [Morar, 2003], [Paiva & Russell, 1999], [Pizzorno & Murray, 2003], [Rombi, 1998], [Slosse & Hootele, 1981], [Timberlake & Henry, 1988], [Verette, 1984], [Zeb, 2004].

The experiment was carried out on 5 groups of male Wistar rats, the first five group received Streptozotocin i.v. 4 mg/100 g body weight to induce diabetes.

The toxicity of Streptozotocin can be counteracted by desferioxamine, suggesting that oxidative reactions catalyzed by transition metals could be responsible for the toxicity of this substance. Streptozotocin, being one of the glico-nitrosureas, could exhibit its diabetes-inducing effect also by inadequate NO release [Giugliano et al., 1995].

The first group served as a diabetic witness, the second group was treated with Siofor® ½ tablet/day/group (equivalent to 12 mg/kg), the third group received Meguan® (2 tablets of

0.5 g/group/day), the 4th group was treated with Eridiarom® (1.2 g/group/day), and the fifth group was given Diavit® (1.2 g/group/day). Healthy, normally fed rats formed the 6th, non streptozotocin-treated witness group.

After 5 days, and than each month glycaemia was measured, and after 100 days histopathologic examination (pancreas, liver, kidney, heart, muscles, eyes) were performed on 2 animals of each group, and the rest of the rats were kept under observation.

During the experiment one animal in each treated group died, and in the group treated with Siofor two animals died.

The dynamics of glycaemia increases at 7 days after the induction of subclinical diabetes (176.8 - 185.5 mg/dl +/- 3.0 - 5.6 SD) in each of the streptozotocin-treated groups compared to the initial values (103.2 - 105.3 mg/dl +/- 1.6 - 2.2 SD).

After 30 days the glycaemia is close to normal (120.1 - 127.8 mg/dl +/- 2.0 - 2.1 SD) in groups 4 and treated with the phytotherapeutic products Eridiarom® and Diavit®5 (14.6-22.6% higher than the initial values), and it is high (151.6 mg/dl +/- 4.0 - 4.1 SD) in groups 2 and 3 treated with the antidiabetic sulphamides Siofor® and Meguan® (45.46% higher than the initial values), but lower compared to the first, witness group (164.6 mg/dl +/- 4.2 SD). After 90 days the glycaemia is practically normalized in groups 4 and 5 (102.8 - 114.3 mg/dl +/- 1.5 -2.3 SD) (the final value 1.37% lower, and 9.6% higher than the initial values) and it is slightly increased in the first 3 groups (135.0 - 133.3 mg/dl +/- 3.3 - 4.0 mg/dl) (29,1-27.9% higher than the initial values).

The histopathologic examination of the pancreas (Trichromic stain) revealed a strong destructive action of streptozotocin against the endocrine and exocrine pancreas.

In the first witness group we can observe pancreatic cytonecrosis, atrophy with hypofunction and disturbing of the ratio between α and β secretory cells after administering streptozotocin. 100 days later the Langerhans islets of the rats in the first, witness group present partial regeneration and recovery of pseudolobules with β cells, general interstitial oedema, atrophy of the acini's level with the significant reducing of the cellular secretory pole.

In group 2, treated with Siofor®, 100 days after the beginning of the experiment partial recovery can be observed in the Langerhans islets, with β cells during the pseudolobules' reconstruction, and partial recovery of the exocrine secretor function by acinary and lobular hyperfunction.

In group 3 treated with Meguan®, 100 days after the initiation of the experiment regenerated Langerhans islets can be seen with α and β cells' reorganisation and the formation of sinusoidal capillary, and acinus-lobulary hyperfunction with the hypertrophy of the secretor pole in pancreatic acini.

In group 4, treated with Eridiarom®, 100 days after the beginning of the experiment, Langerhans islets with regenerated α and β cells can be observed, with increased mitotic index and complete recovery, and generalised acinus-lobulary functional hypertrophy.

In group 5, treated with Diavit®, 100 days after the initiation of the experiment, Langerhans islets with complete recovery of the cell-architectonics can be observed, specific for normal functioning Langerhans cells, and hyperthrophy with general acinus-lobulary moderate secretion.

Based on these experimental data we can conclude that the two phytotherapeutic products exhibited a powerful regenerative effect on the pancreatic cells, presenting a better efficacy compared to the widely used antidiabetic sulphamides [Crăciun et al., 2007], [Morar et al., 2004].

4.2 Studies on human subjects

In our research in humans we evaluated oxidative stress using several methods, measuring lipid peroxidation products in type 1 diabetic patients compared to non-diabetic subjects of the same age-group. We used the LPO 586 (R&D Systems) kit and two methods based on the reaction between malondialdehyde and thiobarbituric acid [Nemes-Nagy et al., 2004a], [Satoh, 1978].

After the incubation period, malondialdehyde concentration was determined by photometric dosage, in case of some methods comparing the results obtained for the samples with those for the reference series with known concentrations, previously prepared.

We revealed that oxidative stress was more intense in diabetic children (78 patients, aged 12.8 years +/- 4.2 SD) compared to healthy subjects of their age group (P=0.0022).

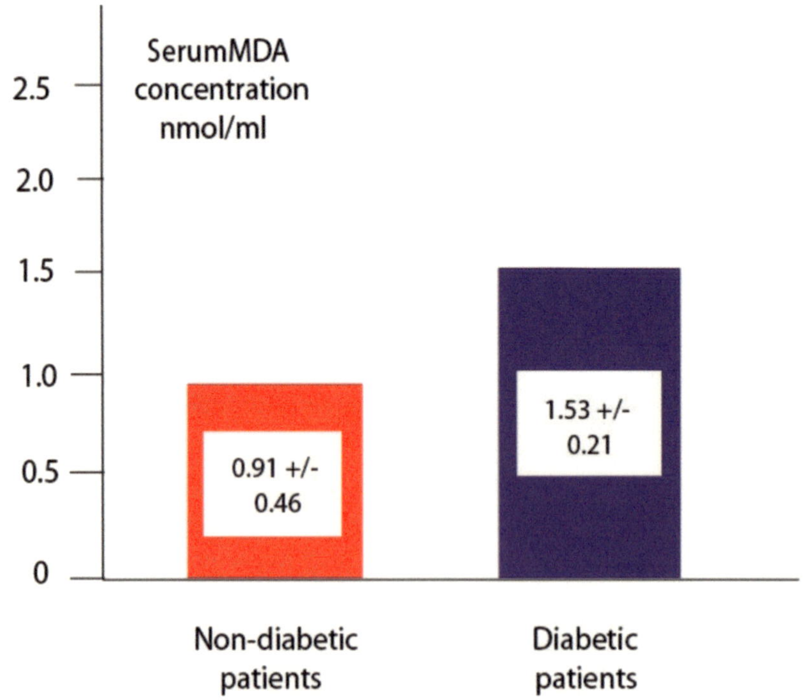

Fig. 1. Malondialdehyde concentration in diabetic and non-diabetic patients by Kei Satoh method

We obtained good correlation of the results provided by the three methods: r = 0.8087, P = 0.0151 comparing LPO-586 method with Fogelman procedure, r = 0.6580, P = 0.0007 comparing Fogelman method with the procedure described by Kei Satoh, and r = 0.9085, p = 0.0007 comparing the LPO-586 method with Kei Satoh procedure [Nemes-Nagy, 2004a].

In the diabetic children's group the average value of HbA1c was 10.0% +/- 1.9 (SD) (range 6.7 - 15.4 %), and the average malondialdehyde concentration was 3.7 nmol/ml +/- 1.04 (SD) (range 1.7 - 8.1 nmol/ml), and the MDA concentration was significantly higher ($P<0.001$) compared to the average value of children presenting glucose intolerance (2.6 nmol/ml +/- 1.1 SD).

HbA1c level highly correlated with malondialdehyde concentration ($r = 0.814$, $P<0.05$) in the diabetic children's group (60 patients).

HbA1c was determined by chromatographic method using venous blood samples collected on EDTA-K_2 as anticoagulant.

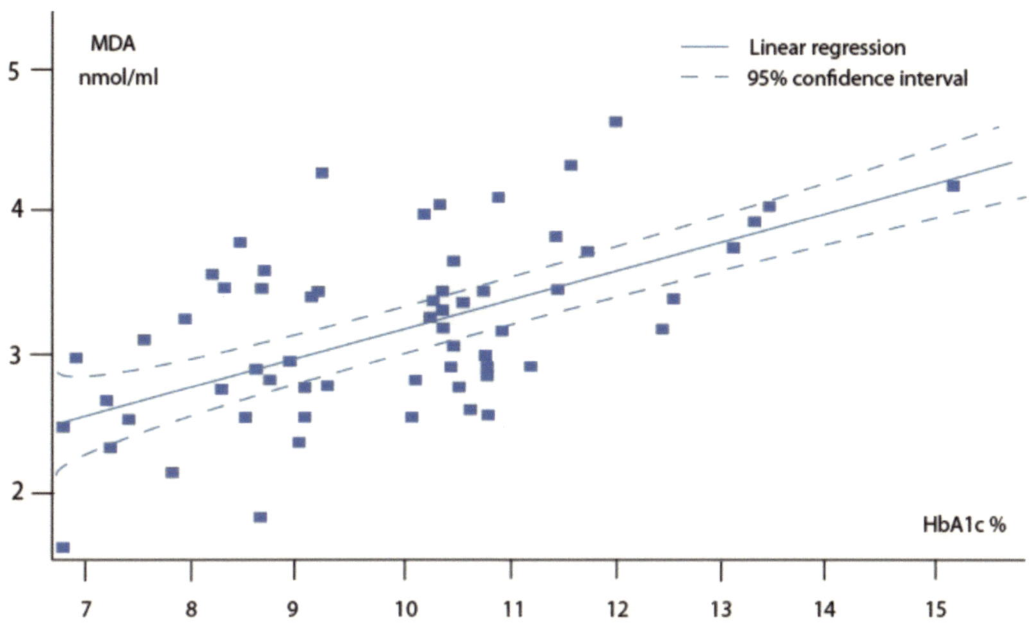

Fig. 2. Correlation between glycated hemoglobin level and serum malondialdehyde concentration in type 1 diabetic children

We also determined serum malondialdehyde concentration in three different groups of type 2 diabetic patients: subjects presenting cardiovascular (CV) diseases, patients having a high risk to develop such diseases, and those who had no other cardiovascular risk factor besides suffering from diabetes mellitus.

We obtained significant differences between the first and third (P = 0.0015), and the second and the third group (P = 0.0018) concerning malondialdehyde concentration, the patients in the third group having lower levels [Moldován, 2003] compared to those from the first two groups.

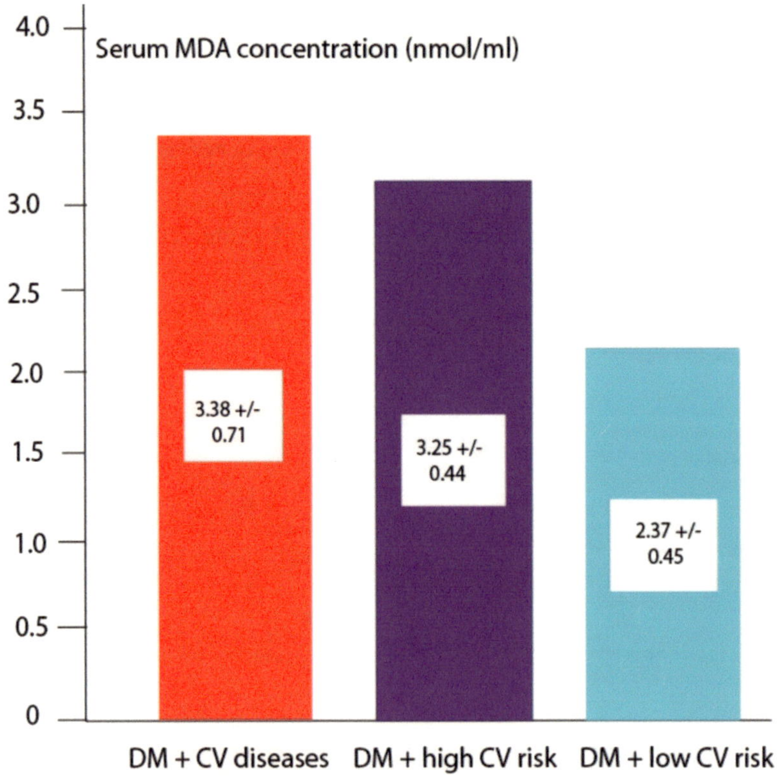

Fig. 3. Average values of serum malondialdehyde concentration in different cardiovascular risk groups of type 2 diabetic patients

We compared Cu/Zn SOD and GPX activities in diabetic children and a non-diabetic infant group of similar age. In diabetic infants we found significantly lower SOD activities (1200.8 U/gHb ± 101.4 SD) compared to the control group (1404.9 U/gHb +/- 125.4 SD), the difference is significant ($P<0.005$). No notable differences could be observed regarding GPX activity in the 2 studied groups of patients ($P>0.05$).

According to the literature normal values of erythrocyte SOD are considered between 1102-1601 U/gHb. In our diabetic group only 16,7% of the patients presented values lower than normal, the minimum SOD activity value was 1014.2 U/gHb and the maximum was 1386 U/gHb.

Physiological values of GPX activity are between 27.5-73.6 U/gHb, only one of the studied diabetic children exhibited a value slightly lower than normal [Jákó et al, 2009].

Our research team demonstrated the powerful antioxidant and hypoglycemic effect of a blueberry (*Vaccinium myrtillus*) concentrate (Eridiarom®) in diabetic children (initially this product was used for treatment of diarrhoea in humans). We selected 29 infants presenting poor carbohydrate metabolic balance to participate to the study.

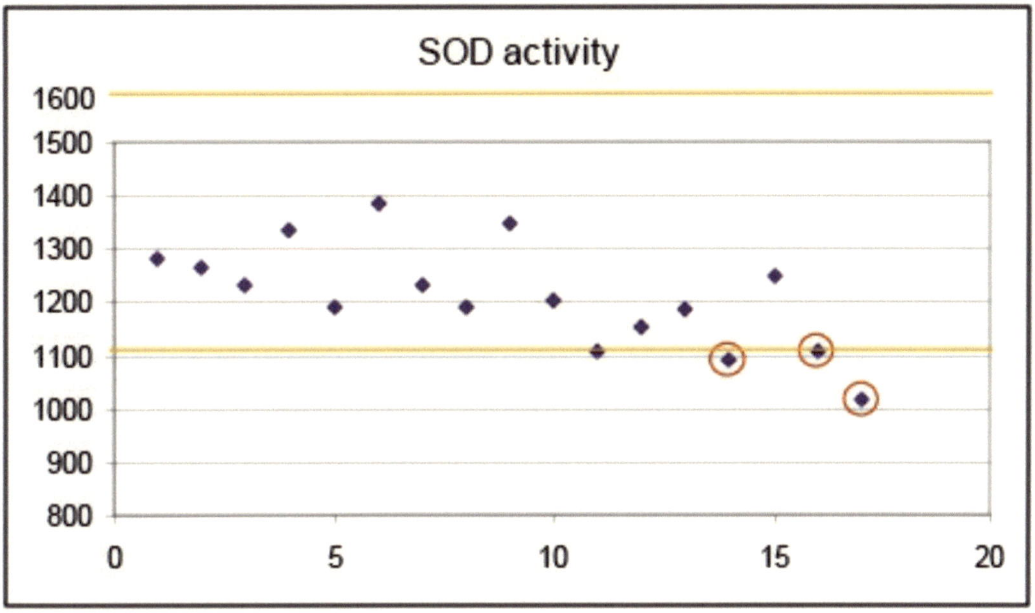

Fig. 4. Erythrocyte Cu-Zn superoxide dismutase activity in type 1 diabetic children

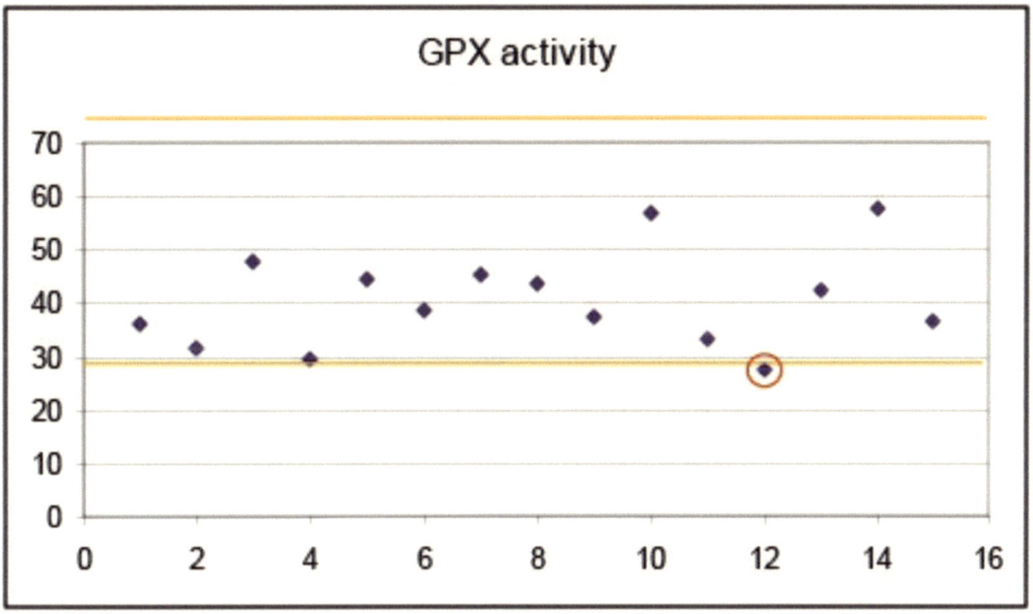

Fig. 5. Whole blood glutathione peroxidase dismutase activity in type 1 diabetic children

The average glycemic level at the beginning of the study was 179.4 mg/dl ± 39.2 (SD), after 3 months of Eridiarom® treatment the value decreased to 159.1 mg/dl +/- 40.7 (SD), the difference is significant ($P<0.005$).

Insulin doses (UI/kg) could be lowered in 78.6% of the patients. Initially the average dose was 0.98 UI/kg ± 0.2 (SD) and after 3 months of treatment 0.91 UI/kg ± 0.2 (SD), the difference is significant ($P<0.05$). This result can be explained by the regenerative effect of this phytotherapeutic product on the pancreatic beta cells, improving their insulin secretion.

We observed that the longer the treatment with this dietary supplement, better the results are.

After 3 months of Eridiarom® treatment HbA1c values presented decrease in 71.43% of the patients. Using the Student paired t test, we obtained significant differences ($P<0.05$) regarding the HbA1c values at the beginning of the study (9.6% ± 1.6 SD) and 8.5% ± 1.5 (SD) after 3 months of Eridiarom® treatment.

After 3 months of Eridiarom® treatment MDA concentration decreased in 92.9% of the patients, 7.1% showed practically no modification of the MDA level.

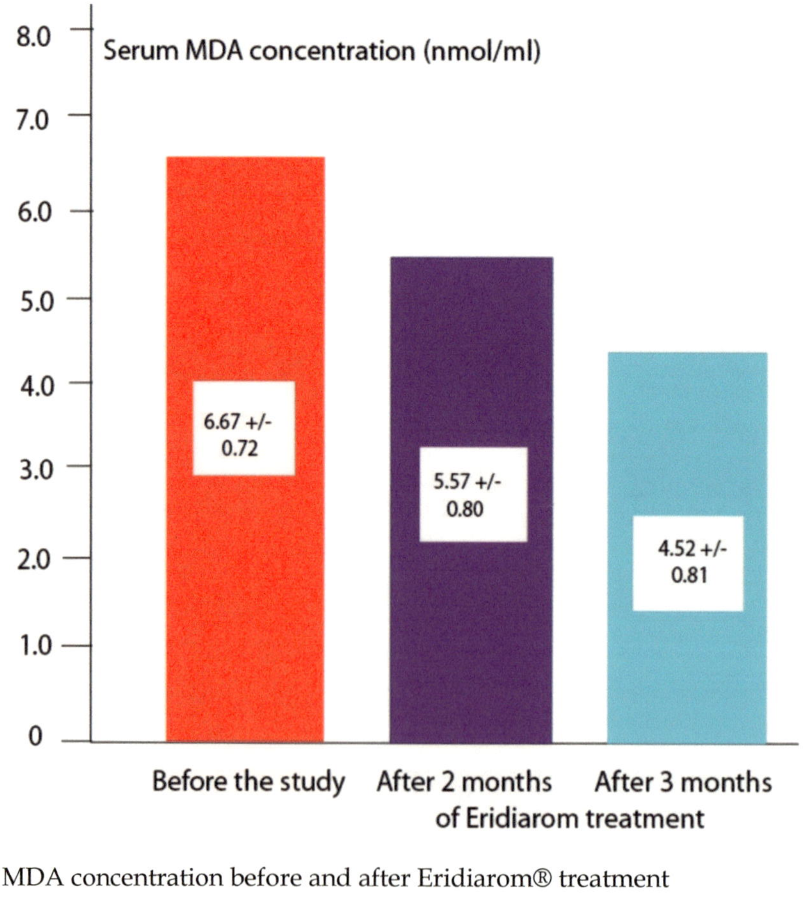

Fig. 6. Serum MDA concentration before and after Eridiarom® treatment

The average MDA concentration before the study was 6.7 nmol/ml ± 0.7 (SD), after 3 months of treatment the average value was 4.5 nmol/ml ± 0.8 (SD), the difference is significant (P<0.0001).

Prior to the study the serum magnesium and calcium concentrations were under the normal range in 43% of the patients. The average magnesium level at the beginning of the study was 1.7 mg/dl, while after 3 months of Eridiarom® treatment in case of all these patients the magnesium level turned to normal, the average value being 2.2 mg/dl; the difference is significant (P<0.0001) [Balogh-Sămărghiţan et al., 2004], [Nemes-Nagy et al., 2006].

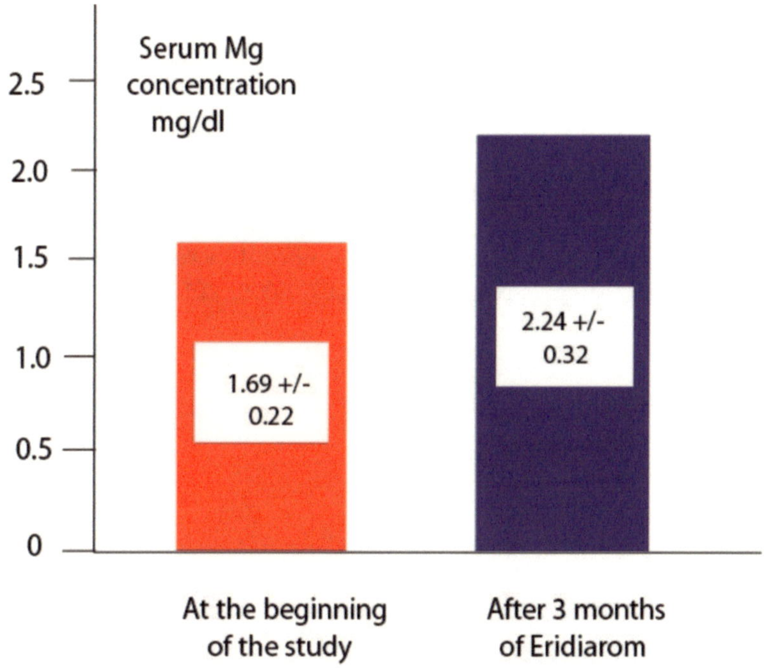

Fig. 7. Dynamics of serum magnesium concentration under blueberry containing Eridiarom® treatment

Several studies were made on the implications of magnesium in diabetes mellitus. Certain key enzymes of carbohydrate metabolism (glucokinase, hexokinase, glucose-6-phosphate dehydrogenase) and lipid metabolism (mevalonate kinase, lecithin-cholesterol acyl-transferase) are magnesium-dependent.

Insulin, along with catecholamines, has major effects on intracellular homeostasis of magnesium, being, besides vitamin D and taurine, an important magnesium-linking substance. Insulin receptors exhibit a magnesium-dependent kinase activity [Vereşiu, 2000].

Studies evaluating magnesium levels in diabetic patients compared to healthy controls showed decreases in case of diabetic subjects, and other studies have shown an increased risk for this disease in patients with magnesium deficiency. Possible correlation of Mg with chronic diabetes complications have been the subject of other studies, that have found lower values in patients with retinopathy [De Valk, 1999] and neuropathy [DeLourdes, 1998].

Effects of magnesium administration in patients with diabetes to improve glycemic control and prevention of chronic complications are conflicting and awaiting further confirmation.

A few years later we studied the effect of another dietary supplement (Diavit®), containing blueberry (*Vaccinum myrtillus*) and sea buckthorn (*Hippophae rhamnoides*) concentrate with a complex composition previously presented.

We compared glycaemic profile, glycated hemoglobin ($HbA1_C$) after 2 and 3 months of treatment, C peptide level and changes in antioxidant enzyme activity (Cu/Zn superoxide dismutase and glutation peroxidase) after two months of treatment with the Diavit® dietary supplement versus after placebo treatment.

Values for activity of erythrocyte Cu/Zn SOD, a scavenger of superoxide radicals, were significantly higher ($P<0.05$) in diabetic patients after two months of treatment with the concentrate (1260.9 ± 66.9 U/g Hb) compared to those obtained before treatment (1201.6 ± 105.6 U/g Hb).

There was no significant difference in GPX activity before (40.8 ± 9.2 U/g Hb) and after the study (43.9 ± 13.9 U/g Hb), only a slight, not significant increase could be observed ($P>0.05$) [Capasso et al, 2003], [Nemes-Nagy et al., 2007, 2008, 2010], [Paglia & Valentine, 1967], [Szőcs-Molnár et al., 2006].

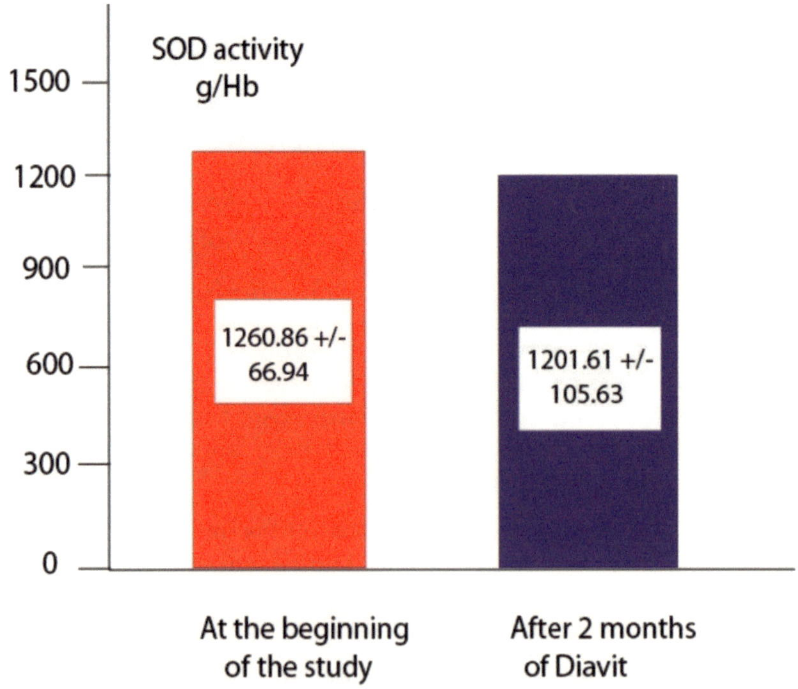

Fig. 8. Dynamics of blood SOD activity under blueberry and sea buckthorn containing Diavit® treatment

Hydrogen peroxide, formed by the reaction catalyzed by SOD, is decomposed by two enzymes: GPX and CAT. Dosage of blood catalase activity could have helped to have a better picture on the enzymatic antioxidant equipment of these diabetic patients under the treatment with this dietary supplement.

$HbA1_C$ levels were significantly lower after treatment with the dietary supplement (9.2 ±1.6 % versus 4the initial 10.2 ± 2.3 %; P<0.05) and C-peptide average value increased significantly (P<0.05) after 2 month of treatment with this dietary supplement (0.2 ng/ml ± 0.1 SD) compared to the initial average value (0.04 ng/ml ± 0.02 SD). Insulin requirement reduced significantly from the average of 0.96 ± 0.27 IU/kg bodyweight to 0.89 ± 0.28 IU/kg after 2 months of treatment with the product (P<0.05), insulin doses were reduced in 66.7% of the patients.

Lower blood glucose and HbA1c values may be due to a regenerative effect that the product has on pancreatic beta cells. Significantly higher C-peptide levels after 2 months of treatment with the extract support this hypothesis [Nemes-Nagy et al., 2008].

A scientific team in Harvard University, Howard Hughes Medical Institute, under the leadership of Prof. Douglas Melton, published their findings about the capacity of pancreatic beta cells to regenerate by self-duplication due to some latent embrional cell remains or adult stem cells [Zhou et al., 2008], and this regenerative process might explain our results with the product studied. We suppose that better results could be obtained if the treatment with the concentrate begins soon after the diabetic disease is diagnosed, maybe because long term insulin treatment causes the atrophy of pancreatic beta-cells, similar to corticosteroid-caused hypofunction of corticosuprarenals. This hypothesis should be verified in latter studies. Based on our experimental data it seems that the longer the treatment with these dietary supplements, the better the results are.

Hyperglycemia in diabetes mellitus produces increased oxidative stress via non-enzymatic glycation, glucose autooxidation, and alteration in polyol pathway activity. This is characterized by increased lipid peroxide production and decreased antioxidative defence (e.g. inactivation of SOD by glycation) which affects the entire body. Two months using Diavit® lead to a significant increase in SOD which may have occurred as a result of its antioxidant and hypoglycemic effects. The antioxidant effect of this product might be partially due to anthocyanosides, known as scavengers of superoxide anions, inhibitors of lipid peroxidation. Lower glycaemic levels during the study might cause lower superoxide radical production and decrease the inactivation rate of this antioxidant enzyme, leading to higher SOD levels than before.

Protection of free radical scavengers might help to maintain higher levels of antioxidants under treatment with this concentrate, and several components of the product (carotenoids, vitamin E, C) show important protective role against oxidative stress. According to recent studies, it might be a link between GPX and ascorbate: intracellular vitamin C cooperates in enhancing glutathione recovery after oxidative challenge thus providing cells with enhanced survival potential, while extracellular vitamin C is recycled through a mechanism involving the simultaneous neutralization of oxidant species [Montecinos et al., 2007].

Several data suggest that oxygen metabolits are involved in the pathogenesis of autoimmune destruction of pancreatic beta cells, involving inflammatory process, and especially superoxide radical is required for the expression of the disease. Pancreatic beta cells are particularly sensitive to superoxide mediated radical damage, having a poor antioxidant defence system. Superoxide itself or derivative radicals may be the direct cause of cell damage. Radical generation leads to breakage of cell DNA, which initiates the repair process resulting in depletion of cellular NADH + H^+ levels, leading to an inhibition of pro-insulin synthesis and renders the cell more sensitive to radical damage because NAD is involved in the electron-transport process required for radical scavenging by the cell. Oxygen radicals are also involved in the production of the cytokines (IL-1, TNF) by the cells of the inflammatory focus that could be involved in the cell damage [Nemes-Nagy et al., 2008].

Another important component of Diavit® is the phytoestrogen called resveratrol, which is a natural polyphenolic compound found largely in the skin of red grapes, but also in blueberries.

Growing evidence suggests that resveratrol may play an important role in the prevention of many human diseases. Many of the biological actions of this polyphenol have been attributed to its antioxidant properties, it exhibits anticoagulant, vasodilator, antiinflammatory effects, inhibits oxidation of LDL-cholesterol particles, thus preventing atherosclerosis, and also increases sensitivity to insulin.

Certain studies evaluated the effect of resveratrol on intracellular reduced glutathione (GSH) and membrane sulphydryl groups in erythrocytes subjected to oxidative stress in vitro to test the efficacy of the antioxidant effect of resveratrol on human erythrocytes. In one of these studies subjecting erythrocytes to oxidative stress (in vitro) by incubating them with t-BHP (10 micromolar) caused a significant decrease in the intracellular GSH level and membrane -SH content compared with basal values.

Incubation of erythrocytes/membranes with resveratrol (1-100 micromolar final concentration) resulted in significant protection against the t-BHP-induced oxidative stress as evidenced by the increase in GSH level and membrane -SH content. It was observed that the effect of resveratrol is dose/concentration and time-dependent, it protects erythrocytes experimentally exposed to oxidative stress. Since resveratrol is naturally present in many fruits and vegetables, a diet rich in resveratrol, or dietary supplements containing this substance may provide protection against degenerative diseases and prevent diabetes complications [Pandey & Rizvi, 2010].

A new promising study on humans demonstrated the effect of regular consumption of a resveratrol supplement and the health of patients with impaired glucose tolerance. Resveratrol has been tested in relation to diabetes before, but only in animal subjects or on cell lines. Those studies have repeatedly shown promising effects on insulin secretion, insulin sensitivity and glucose tolerance, leading to the initiation of this first-of-its-kind pilot clinical study on humans [Crandall, 2010].

5. Studies on antioxidant components of medicinal teas, fruit and vegetable juices

We also determined the flavonoid content and the antioxidant capacity of several medicinal teas used by diabetic patients. We found the highest amount of flavonoids in Juglandis folium, and the smallest amount of flavonoids was found in Phaseoli tegumen. The results were calculated in hyperoside units.

The highest concentration of malondialdehyde was found in Centauri herba (149 mmol/100g), smaller amounts were found in Myrtilli folium (146 mmol/100g), Mori folium (115 mmol/100g), Crataegi summitas (100 mmol/100g), Urticae herba (97 mmol/100g), Menthae piperitae (97 mmol/100g), Visci albae stipes (94 mmol/100g), Juglandis folium (89 mmol/100g), Millefolii flos (79 mmol/100g) and Phaseoli tegumen (73 mmol/100g). The antioxidant capacity of these plants is inversely proportional to their MDA contents, a measure of ROS-induced damage to lipids [Nemes-Nagy et al., 2004], [Lushchak Vl., 2011].

Medicinal teas	**Flavonoid content (g% hyperoside)**
Juglandis folium	1.79
Crataegi summitas	0.75
Menthae piperitae	0.70
Urticae herba	0.68
Mori folium	0.59
Myrtilli folium	0.31
Millefolii flos	0.24
Centauri herba	0.24
Visci albae stipes	0.18
Phaseoli tegumen	0.03

Table 1. Flavonoid content of medicinal teas

We measured, by photometric diclorphenol-indophenol method the vitamin C concentration in freshly squeezed juices and in those preserved, available in stores. As a result we found that lemon, orange and grapefruit contain the biggest ascorbate quantity, especially freshly squeezed (22.0 – 22.2 mg/dl) the same volume of juice contains higher ascorbate concentration compared to those sold in boxes (15.0 mg/dl – 21.9 mg/dl).

In case of orange juices, we compared the vitamin C content of 3 samples from juices sold in boxes from different firms (the results obtained were 20.5 mg/dl, 18.2 mg/dl and 15.0 mg/dl), so we concluded that the concentration of ascorbic acid was 7.7%, 18.0% and 32.0% lower compared to the result obtained from the freshly squeezed juices.

Freshly squeezed juices	**Vitamin C content (mg/dl)**
Orange	22.2
Lemon	22.2
Grapefruit	22.0
Grapes	17.2
Tomato	17.0

Table 2. Vitamin C contents of freshly squeezed juices

6. Vitamin C dynamics in human milk

We also followed the dynamics of ascorbate in human milk after juice and vitamin C tablet ingestion. The highest ascorbate level in milk was 1 hour after juice ingestion and half an hour after taking 1000 mg vitamin C containing tablets, the assimilation from natural sources being better. It is a close relationship between mothers' diet and the quality of their milk. We can recommend to consume juices one hour before brestfeeding, to offer the infant the highest amount of ascorbate [Jákó et al., 2008].

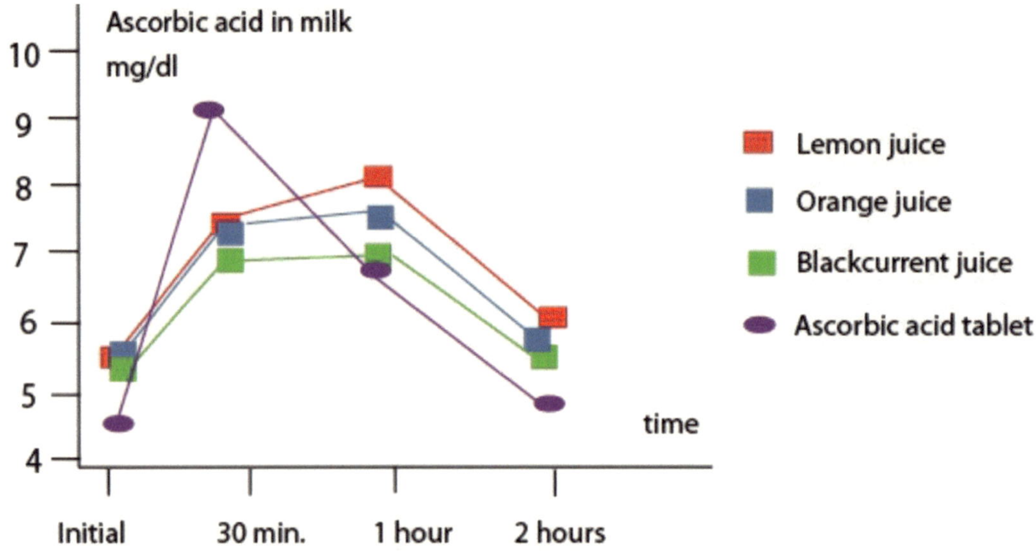

Fig. 9. The dynamics of ascorbic acid in human milk after ingestion of freshly squeezed juices and C vitamin tablets

7. Determination of carotenoid score in diabetic patients

Another study was made on adult subjects, we used Raman spectroscopy (a method that can identify carotene molecules in the skin) to determine the carotenoide score, which gives information on the antioxidant capacity of the body. Significantly lower average value was obtained in adult diabetic compared to the control non-diabetic group of similar age; the difference is significant ($P<0.05$) [Jákó et al, 2009].

Food carotenoids are transported into the skin, protecting the tegument against ultraviolet radiation. The skin carotenoid concentration undergoes smaller variation compared to that in the blood depending on the dietary intake. Skin carotenoid determination by HPLC method using bioptic material is an invasive procedure and cannot be introduced in the every day practice. A very good correlation can be found between the serum carotenoid concentration and that in the palm skin ($r = 0.78$, $P<0.001$) determined by Raman spectroscopy, and the biophotonic scanner operates based on this observation [Jákó et al, 2009], [Peng et al., 1995], [Smidt & Shieh, 2003]. Thus, skin carotenoid measurement appears to be a valuable biomarker of carotenoid nutritional status.

Raman scattering spectroscopy is a highly specific method for skin carotenoid determination. This method is able to discern carotenoids from other potentially interfering compounds present in the skin due to its ability to identify molecules with long conjugated double-bond structures. Raman spectroscopy involves a blue, low-energy laser light source of 470 - 490 nm, directed onto the surface of the skin, where Raman resonance light scattering events cause the carotenoids to emit a green signal at 510 – 530 nm, which is detected and quantified.

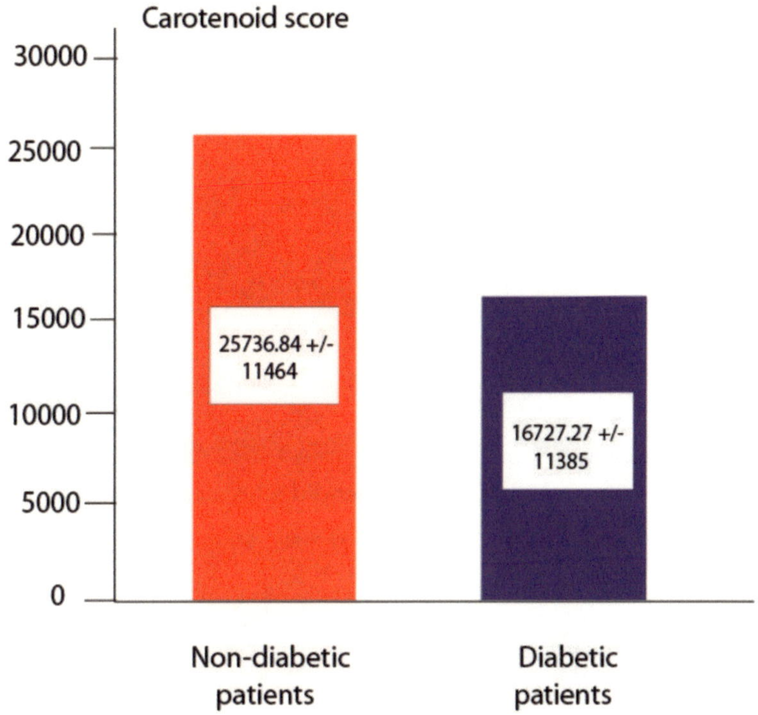

Fig. 10. Comparision of skin carotenoid score in diabetic and non-diabetic patients

Studies showed that the Raman spectroscopic method accurately reflects the presence of carotenoids in the human skin with high reproducibility. Significant differences in carotenoid concentrations were found between five different skin sites, the highest concentration being found in the palm.

An epidemiological study performed on a large number of healthy volunteers determined that the Raman spectroscopic method of measuring skin carotenoids is not really affected by gender, age or skin pigmentation.

Raman intensity measurements were positively related to the amount of fruit and vegetable intake and use of carotenoid-containing dietary supplements, and inversely related to body fat content and smoking. This study confirmed that skin carotenoids follow similar dietary and demographic patterns as in case of serum or plasma carotenoid measurements.

Before the measurement, every patient has to fill in a special questionnaire containing questions regarding its lifestyle, dietary habits and other aspects that could influence the result.

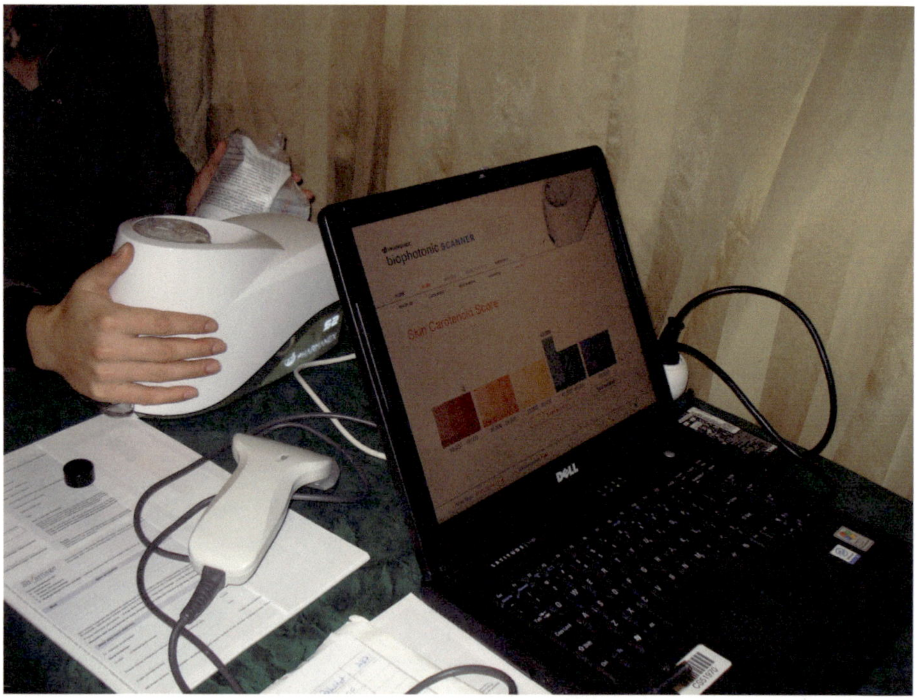

Fig. 11. Biophotonic scanner showing the carotenoid score of a non-diabetic patient

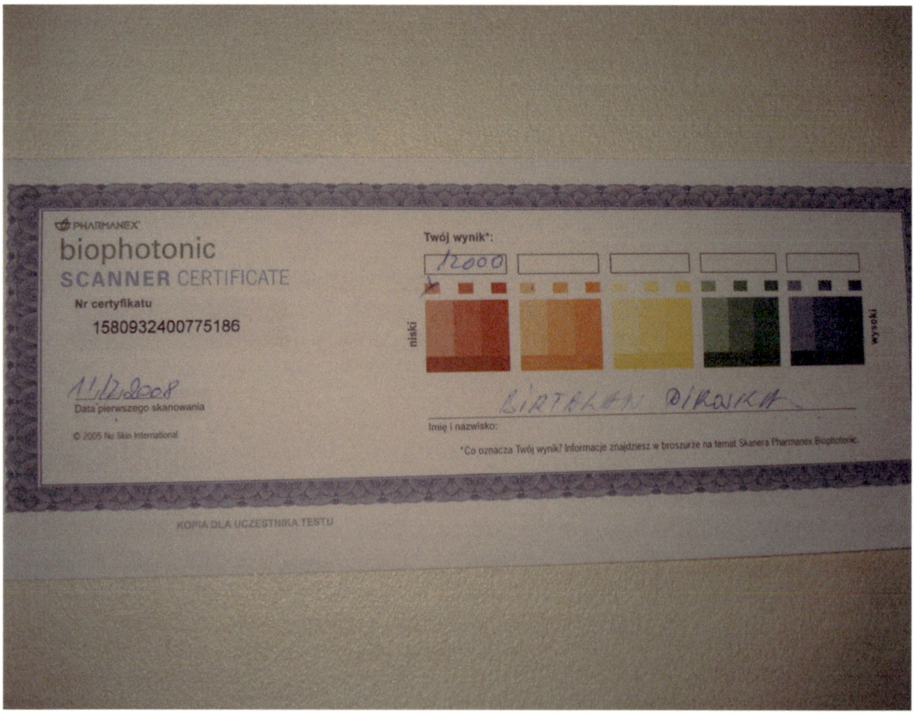

Fig. 12. Low carotenoid score of an old diabetic patient

8. Conclusion, perspectives

Regarding proper evaluation of antioxidant status in the human body, measuring lipoperoxidation products is a valuable tool because its high value positively correlates with the intensified oxidative stress. Interpretation of antioxidant enzyme activities could be sometimes difficult because it can decrease in case of intense consumption when free radical production is intensified, and in other situations even higher values can be observed due to compensatory mechanisms, being a way of adaptation to intensified oxidative stress.

We can conclude that proper nutrition including adequate fresh fruit and vegetable intake are important sources of natural antioxidants. Patients suffering from diseases like diabetes mellitus which involves high oxidative stress should take dietary supplements containing antioxidant vitamins, phytoterapeutical products and oligoelements, these could help diabetic patients to achieve a better metabolic balance and to prevent several complications of this disease.

It would be interesting to perform a placebo-controlled double-blind study on the effect of the dietary supplement Diavit®, containing blueberry and sea buckthorn concentrate, on a large group of type 2 diabetic patients followed for several years, to observe the long term effect of this phytotherapeutic product, or other, more complex dietary supplements could be used in similar studies. This could be a possibility to reduce the incidence of complications in diabetic patients, and to help them to achieve a proper metabolic balance without taking antidiabetic drugs, or at least lower the doses of their usual medication, decreasing the risk of developing side effects.

9. References

Balogh-Sămărghițan V., Nemes-Nagy E., I. Dunca, Szőcs T., Pap Z., Máthé J. & Şt. Hobai: Modificări ionice la copii cu diabet zaharat de tip 1 sub tratament cu Eridiarom® (Ionic modifications in type 1 diabetic children under Eridiarom treatment), in Diabetul - alternative fitoterapeutice, sub redacția Roman Morar, Dana Liana Pusta, Ed. Todesco, Cluj-Napoca, 2004, p. 105-115

Baynes J.W.: Role of oxidative stress in development of complications in diabetes, Diabetes, 1991, 40, 405-412

Capasso F., Gaginella TS., Grandolini G. & Izzo AA.: Phytotherapy A Quick Reference to Herbal Medicine, Ed. Springer, 2003

Cadenas E., Packer L. (eds): *Handbook of Antioxidants*, Ed. Marcel Dekker Inc., New York, 2002, p. 47-55

Crăciun E. C., Szőcs-Molnár T., Nemes-Nagy E., Dunca I., Balogh-Sămărghițan V., Hobai Şt., Pusta D. & Morar R.: Effect of dietary supplement Diavit® on antioxidant capacity in diabetes mellitus disease (poster), 2nd Symposium International - Nutrition, Oxygen Biology and Medicine, Paris, 11-13 April (2007), (abstract p. 31)

Crandall J.: Promising Results of First-Ever Human Clinical Trial of a Resveratrol Supplement's Impact on Pre-diabetes, ADA's 70th Annual Meeting, 2010

Dejica D.: Antioxidanți şi terapie antioxidantă (Antioxidants and antioxidant therapy), Ed. Casa Cărții de Ştiință, Cluj-Napoca, 2001

Dejica D.: Stresul oxidativ (Oxidative stress), Ed. Casa Cărții de Ştiință, Cluj-Napoca, 2000

DeLourdes M., Cruz T., Pousada J., et al: *The effect of Magnezium Supplementation in Increasing Doses on the Control of Type 2 Diabetes*, Diabetes Care, 1998, 21(5), p. 682-686

De Valk H., Hardus L.L.J., Van Rijn J.M. & Erkelens W.D.: *Plasma Magnesium Concentration and Progression of Rethinopathy*, Diabetes Care, 1999, 22(5), p. 864-865

Dobreanu M., Módy E.: Studiul influenței vitaminelor antioxidante asupra oxidării in vitro a lipoproteinelor cu densitate scăzută, Revista de Medicină şi Farmacie, Târgu-Mureş, 1998, 44, p. 3-4

Gherasim L.: Medicină internă, vol. III - Bolile cardiovasculare şi metabolice, Ed. Medicală, Bucureşti, 1998, p. 1167-1297

Giugliano, D., Ceriello, A., et. al.- Diabetes mellitus, hypertension and cardiovascular disease, which role for oxidative stress ? *Metabolism*, 1995, 44, 363-368

Jákó Zs., Nemes-Nagy E., Balogh-Sămărghițan V., Crăciun E.C., Baki L.B., Kósa B., Zöld G., Czédula A., Szőcs K., Szilveszter M., Sánta D. & Dobreanu M.: Az oxidatív stressz felmérésének módozatai cukorbetegeknél (Evaluation of oxidative stress in diabetic patients), Orvostudományi Értesítő, vol 82, nr, 4/2009 (ISSN 1453-0953, CNCSIS B/2008, cod 274), p. 261-264

Jákó Zs., Nemes-Nagy E., Szabó K.D., Szabó A., Balogh A., Baki L.B., Al-Aissa Z., Kósa B., Balogh-Sămărghițan V. & Fazakas Z.: Aszkorbinsav meghatározása gyümölcs-és zöldséglevekből, valamint a C-vitamin koncentráció dinamikája az anyatejben (Determination of ascorbic acid concentration in fruit and vegetable juices, and following the dynamics of vitamin C in the human milk), EME Orvostudományi Értesítő, (ISSN 1453-0953), Cluj Napoca, 2008, 81(2), p. 52-53

Kovács L.G.: Modern Aspects of Laboratory Diagnosis and Monitoring of Diabetes Mellitus, Klin. Kísérl. Lab. Med., 2001, 28, p. 98-107

Krippeit-Drews P., Lang F., Haussinger D. & Drews G.: H_2O_2 induced hyperpolarisation of pancreatic beta-cells, Pflugers Arch., 1994, 426, p. 552-554

Lushchak Vl.: Adaptive response to oxidative stress: Bacteria, fungi, plants and animals, Comp Biochem Physiol C Toxicol Pharmacol, 2011, 153(2), p. 175-190

Moldován M., Nemes-Nagy E., V. Balogh-Sămărghițan, Máthé J. & Pap Z.: A szérum malondialdehid koncentráció és érelmeszesedés összefüggése 2 típusú cukorbetegeknél (Correlation of serum malondialdehyde concentration and atherosclerosis in type 2 diabetic patients), EME Orvostudományi Értesítő, Cluj Napoca, vol. 76(3), 2003, p. 479-481

Montecinos V., Guzmán P. & Barra V.: Vitamin C Is an Essential Antioxidant That Enhances Survival of Oxidatively Stressed Human Vascular Endothelial Cells in the Presence of a Vast Molar Excess of Glutathione, J. Biol. Chem., 2007, Vol. 282, Issue 21, 15506-15515

Morar R.: Eridiarom, Erisol, Polivitarom sau alternative fitoterapeutice (Eridiarom, Erisol, Polivitarom or phytotheraperutical alternatives), Ed. Todesco, Cluj-Napoca, 2003.

Morar R., Pusta D, Toader S, Orboi A., Miclăuş V., Pasca I. & Cîmpean A.: Rezultate histologice şi biochimice obținute în tratamentul cu unele sulfamide hipoglicemiante şi produse fitoterapeutice originale în diabetul provocat (The histological and biochemical results obtained in the treatment with some hypoglycemiant sulphamides and original phytoterapeutic products of induced diabetes), In: Diabetul - alternative fitoterapeutice, eds: Roman Morar, Dana Liana Pusta, Ed. Todesco, Cluj-Napoca, 2004, p. 91-104.

Moshi M.J., Mbwambo Z.H.: Experience of Tanzanian traditional healers in the management of non-insulin dependent diabetes mellitus, Pharmaceutical Biology, 2003, 40(7), 552-560.

Nakazaki M., Kakei M., Koriyama N. & Tanaka H.: Involvement of ATP-sensitive K^+ channels in free radical-mediated inhibition of insulin secretion in rat pancreatic beta-cells, Diabetes, 1995, 44, 878-883.

Nemes-Nagy E., Balogh-Sămărghiţan V., Dunca I., Szőcs T., Pap Z., Máthé J. & Hobai Şt.: Áfonyakivonattal (Eridiarom®) történő kezelés hatékonysága 1. típusú cukorbetegeknél (Efficacy of treatment with a blueberry concentrate (Eridiarom®) in type 1 diabetic patients), EME Orvostudományi Értesítő, Cluj-Napoca, 2006, 79(1), 49-53

Nemes-Nagy E., E.C. Crăciun, R. Morar, D.L. Pusta, Szőcs-Molnár T., Dunca I., M. Dobreanu & V. Balogh-Sămărghiţan: Efficacy of phytotherapeutical products (Eridiarom, Diavit) in treatment of type 1 diabetes mellitus, p. 491-501, in: Handbook of Type I Diabetes Mellitus: Etiology, Diagnosis and Treatment, Leon Aucoin, Tristan Prideux (eds), Ed. Nova Science Publishers, Inc, New York, SUA, 2010, ISBN 978-1-60741-311-0

Nemes-Nagy E., Dobreanu M., Balogh-Sămărghiţan V., Simionescu A., Pap Z. & Hobai Şt.: Trei metode de determinare a produşilor de lipoperoxidare la copiii diabetici (Three methods for determination of lipid peroxidation products in diabetic children), Infomedica, Bucureşti, 2004, 2(120), p. 28-31

Nemes-Nagy E., Máthé J., V. Balogh-Sămărghiţan, Moldován M. & Hobai Şt.: Cukorbetegek által használt gyógyteák antioxidáns összetevőinek vizsgálata (Study on antioxidant components in medicinal teas used by diabetic patients), EME Orvostudományi Értesítő, Cluj-Napoca, 77(3), 2004, p. 348-351.

Nemes-Nagy E., Szőcs-Molnár T., Dunca I., V. Balogh-Sămărghiţan, Morar R., Kósa B., Ferenczi Attila, Gyenge O. & Şt. Hobai: A Diavit® táplálékkiegészítővel történő hosszú távú kezelés hatékonysága cukorbeteg gyermekeknél (The efficacy of long-term therapy with the dietary supplement Diavit® in diabetic children), EME Orvostudományi Értesítő, Cluj-Napoca, 80(2), 2007, p. 124-126

Nemes-Nagy E., Szőcs-Molnár T., Dunca I., V. Balogh-Sămărghiţan, Şt. Hobai, R. Morar, D.L. Pusta & E.C. Crăciun: Effect of a dietary supplement containing blueberry and sea buckthorn concentrate on antioxidant capacity in type 1 diabetic children, Acta Physiologica Hungarica, Akadémiai Kiadó, Budapest, vol. 95(4), 2008, p. 383-393, DOI-number: 10.1556/APhysiol.95.2008.4.5.

Nomikos I.N., Wang Y. & Lafferty K.J.: Involvement of O_2 radicals in "autoimmune" diabetes. Immunol Cell Biol., 1989, 67, 85-87.

Olinescu R: Radicali liberi în fiziopatologia umană (Free radicals in human physiopathology), Ed. Tehnică, 1994, Bucureşti

Paglia D.E., Valentine W.N.: Studies on the quantitative and qualitative characterisation of erythrocyte glutathione peroxidase, J. Lab. Clin. Med., 1967, 70, 158-169.

Paiva S., Russell R.: Beta-carotene and other carotenoids as antioxidans, J Am Coll Nutr., 1999, 18, 426-433

Pandey K.B., Rizvi S.I.: Protective effect of resveratrol on markers of oxidative stress in human erythrocytes subjected to in vitro oxidative insult, Phytother Res, 2010, 24 Suppl. 1, p. 11-14

Pari L., Latha M.: Antidiabetic activity of Cassia auriculata flowers: effect on lipid peroxidation in streptozotocin diabetes rats. Pharmaceutical Biology., 2003, 40(7), 512-517

Peng Y.M., Peng Y.S., Lin Y. et al: Concentrations and plasma-tissue-diet relationships of carotenoids, retinoids and tocopherols in humans, Nutrition and Cancer, 1995, 23:233-246

Pietta P., Simonetti P. & Mauri P. - Antioxidant activity of selected medicinal plants, J. Agricultural Food Chem., 1998, 46, p. 4487-4490

Pizzorno J. Jr, Murray M., eds: A textbook of natural medicine. Vol 1. WA: Bastyr University Publication, Seattle, 1993

Prior R.L., Cao G.: In vivo total antioxidant capacity: comparison of different analytical methods, Free Radic. Biol. Med., 1999, 27, p. 1173-1181

Raes M., Renard P., Remacle J.: Free radicals as second messengers. C R Seances Soc Biol Fil., 1995, 189, 355-366.

Rombi M.: 100 plantes médicinales. Composition, mode d'action et intérêt thérapeutique. Deuxième édition. Édition Romart, 1998, pp. 199-201

Satoh K.: Serum lipid peroxide in cerebrovascular disorders determined by a new colorimetric method, Clinica Chimica Acta, 1978, 90:37-43

Scartezzini P., Speroni E.: Review on some plants of Indian traditional medicine with antioxidant activity, J Ethnopharmacol, 2000, 71(1-2):23-24

Shinn S.H.: Oxidative stress and diabetic vascular complications. In: Recent advances on pathogenesis and management of diabetes mellitus, 1st ed, Elsevier Science Co., Singapore, 1998, pp 3-8.

Slosse P., Hootele C.: Myrtine and epimyrtine quinolizidine alkaloids from Vaccinium myrtillus. Tetrahedron, 1981, 37, 4287-4292.

Smidt C.R., Shieh D.: Non-invasive biophotonic assessment of skin carotenoids as a biomarker of human antioxidant status, FASEB Journal, 2003, 17:11-15

Szőcs-Molnár T., Nemes-Nagy E., Dunca I., Truţa I., Ferenczi A., Morar R., Balogh-Sămărghiţan V. & Sin A.: Influenţa suplimentului alimentar Diavit® asupra echilibrului metabolic la copii cu diabet zaharat de tip 1 (Influence of dietary supplement Diavit® on metabolic balance in type 1 diabetic children), Revista Română de Medicină de Laborator, 2006, 4(3), p. 36-39

Timberlake C., Henry B.: Anthocyanins as natural food colorants. In: Plant flavonoids in biology and medicine II: biochemical, cellular, and medicinal properties, eds. Cody V, Middleton E Jr, Harborne JB, Beretz A, New York, NY: Alan R. Liss, Inc; 1988, pp. 107-121.

Varga E., Kovács M., Dernovics M., Csedő K. & Pais I.: Szelénnel kezelt fokhagyma (Allium sativa L.) vizsgálata (Study on garlic (Allium sativa L.) treated with selenium). EME Orvostudományi Értesítő, Cluj-Napoca, 2001, 74, 347-351.

Vereşiu I.A.: Implicaţiile magneziului în diabetul zaharat (Implications of magnesium in diabetes mellitus), Infomedica, 2000, 3(73), p. 10-12

Verette E.: Fractionnement des composés polyphénoliques de la myrtille (Vaccinium myrtillus). Étude de leur activité antiradicalaire, determination des anthocyanes monomères. Thèse de Doctorat de Troisième cycle. Montpellier I (Pharmacie), 1984.

Wolff S.R.: Free radicals, transition metals and oxidative stress in the aethiology of diabetes mellitus and complications, Br Med Bull, 1993, 49, p. 642-652

Zeb A.: Chemical and nutritional constituents of sea buckthorn juice. Pakistan Journal of Nutrition, 2004, 3(2), 99-106

Zhou Q., Brown J., Kanarek A., Rajagopal J. & Melton D.A.: In vivo reprogramming of adult pancreatic exocrine cells to beta cells, Nature, 2008, 455, p. 627-632

13

Diabetes, Oxidative Stress, Antioxidants and Saliva: A Review

Natheer H. Al-Rawi
Dept. Oral & Craniofacial Health Science, College of Dentistry, University of Sharjah, UAE

1. Introduction

Diabetes mellitus is a devastating disease throughout the world. It has been estimated that the number of peoples affected with diabetes in the world will increase to 300 million by 2025 (1). Diabetes is associated with several mechanisms, one of which is oxidative stress. Increased oxidative stress is a widely accepted participant in the development and progression of diabetes and its complications (2,3). Oxidative stress is a general term used to describe the imbalance between the production and manifestation of reactive oxygen species and a biological system's ability to ready detoxify the reactive intermediates or to repair the resulting damage (4). Oxidative stress occurs when free radical production exceeds the body's ability to neutralize them. The imbalance may be due to either: decrease production of antioxidants; or excessive production of free radicals. In diabetes, free radicals are formed disproportionately by glucose oxidation, non-enzymatic glycation of proteins and the subsequent oxidative degradation of glycated proteins (5). Abnormally high levels of free radicals and the simultaneous decline of antioxidant defense mechanisms can lead to damage of cellular organelles and enzymes, increased lipid peroxidation and development of insulin resistance (6). These consequences of oxidative stress can promote the development of complications of diabetes mellitus.

2. Sources of oxidative stress in diabetes

There are multiple sources of oxidative stress in diabetes including non enzymatic, enzymatic and mitochondrial pathway.

Non enzymatic sources of oxidative stress originate from the oxidative biochemistry of glucose. Hyperglycemia can directly cause increased Reactive Oxygen Species (ROS) generation. Glucose can undergo autooxidation and generate hydroxyl $^*OH^-$ radicals (7). In addition, glucose reacts with proteins in a non enzymatic manner leading to the formation of advanced glycation end products (AGEs). ROS is generated at multiple steps during this process. In hyperglycemia, there is enhanced metabolism of glucose through the polyol (sorbitol) pathway, which also results in enhanced production of superoxides (*O2-) .

Enzymatic sources of augmented generation of reactive species in diabetes include Nitrous Oxide Species (NOS), NAD(P)H oxidase and xanthine oxidase (8-10). The mitochondrial respiratory chain is another source of non enzymatic generation of reactive species. Hyperglycemia-induced generation of $*O_2^-$ at the mitochondrial level is the initial trigger of vicious cycle of oxidative stress in diabetes (11,12).

3. Saliva as diagnostic fluid

Saliva in humans is a mouth fluid possessing several functions involved in oral health and homeostasis, with an active protective role in maintaining oral health. It plays a role in the preliminary digestion of food, fascilitates taste perception, maintains teeth enamel mineralization, buffers the acid components of food, and antimicrobial functions. The assay of saliva is an increasing area of research with implications of basic and clinical purposes. Recently, the use of saliva has provided a substantial addition to the diagnostic armamentarium as an investigative tool for disease processes and disorders. In addition to its oral indications, the analysis of saliva provides important information about the functioning of various organs within the body. Saliva analyses have been used mainly in dentistry and for studies in oral disease to help assess the risk of caries, by measuring buffering capacity and bacterial contents (13). Oral fluid is mainly utilized for research and diagnostic purposes concerning systemic diseases such as diabetes.

The determination of the oxidative stress and antioxidants require sometimes invasive techniques such as venepuncture. Whole saliva is an important physiologic fluid that contains a highly complex mixture of substances. Variable amounts of blood, serum markers that accurately reflect the redox status of the body can be determined in saliva and may have great clinical interest. The assay of salivary oxidative stress parameters has brought substantial insight into the pathogenesis and evolution of many systemic diseases including diabetes.

4. Mechanisms for increased oxidative stress in diabetes

1. Advanced glycation end products (AGEs):

AGEs are products of glycation and oxidation (glycol-oxidation), which are increased with age, and at accelerated rate in diabetes (14,15). The formation of AGEs is an important biochemical abnormality that accompanies diabetes mellitus. AGEs initiate oxidative reactions that promote the formation of oxidized LDL. Interaction of AGEs with endothelial cells as well as other cells accumulating within the atherosclerotic plaque, such as mononuclear phagocytes and smooth muscle cells provides a mechanism to augment vascular dysfunction (16)

Nuclear magnetic resonance spectra of AGEs were determined in saliva of 52 consecutive patients with diabetes mellitus and 47 age-matched healthy control subjects. Resonance spectra showed specific peaks at 2.3, 7.3, and 8.4 ppm in saliva from patients with diabetes mellitus, indicating the presence of advanced glycation endproducts which was associated with approximal plaque index. (17).

In a study of Garay-Sevilla et al (18) who measured AGEs in skin, serum and saliva of diabetic patients with complications they concluded that the AGEs measurement in saliva is useful to evaluate diabetes complications.

2. Alteration in glutathione metabolism:

Reduced glutathione detoxify reactive oxygen species such as hydrogen peroxide and lipid peroxide directly or in a glutathione peroxidase (GPX) catalyzed mechanism. Glutathione reductase (GRD) catalyzes the NAD(P)H dependent reduction of oxidized glutathione, serving to maintain intercellular glutathione stores and a favorable redox status (19).

Blood GSH was significantly decreased in different phases of type 2 diabetes mellitus such as: glucose intolerance and early hyperglycemia (20) and poor glycemic control (21)

Measurement of salivary GPX and GRD activities and GSSG/GSH ratio, provide a non-invasive method to assess the degree of oxidative stress in pathophysiologic status, such as diabetes (22).

The decrease in salivary reduced-glutathione levels in patients with type 1 DM may have a role in periodontal tissue destruction by predisposing tissues to oxidative stress.(23). Our previous study (24) identified GSH activity in serum and saliva of patients with type 2 diabetes which was significantly low when compared with control group. This finding was explained on the basis that oxidative stress may consumes some naturally occurring local antioxidants such as reduced glutathione and this reflects the overwhelming adaptive response to the challenge of oxidative stress in the diabetic state with or without complications

3. Impairment of SOD and catalase activity:

SOD and catalase are also major antioxidant enzymes, SOD exists in 3 different isoforms; Cu,Zn-SOD is mostly in the cytosol and dismutate superoxide to hydrogen peroxide, Extracellular SOD is found in the plasma and extracellular space and Mn-SOD is located in mitochondria. Catalase is H_2O_2 decomposing enzyme mainly localized to peroxicomes or microperoxicomes. Superoxide may react with other reactive oxygen species such as Nitric Oxide to form highly toxic species such as peroxynitrite (25).

The major reason for the decreased SOD activity is the glycosylation of Cu,Zn-SOD which has been shown to lead to enzyme inactivation both in vivo and in vitro (26). Salivary SOD was measured in saliva (27) .Belce et al suggested that the main reason for the decrease of salivary SOD activity may be increased glycation of the enzyme and/or deleterious effect of increased free oxygen radicals by glycated proteins on SOD activity in diabetes which could lead to oral complications in diabetic patients.However; Al-Rawi study (24) demonstrated an increase in the level of SOD in serum and saliva of diabetic patients, this increase could be due to the existance or increased free radicals production which could enhance the antioxidant defense system that couter-balance the pro-oxidant environment.

4. Polyol Pathway:

The polyol pathway consists of two enzymes. The first enzyme, aldose reductase (AR), reduces glucose to sorbitol with the aid of its co-factor NADPH, and the second enzyme, sorbitol dehydrogenase (SDH), with its co-factor NAD^+, converts sorbitol to fructose. In animal models, treatment with AR inhibitors (ARI) was shown to be effective in preventing the development of various diabetic complications, including cataract, neuropathy, and nephropathy (28). The possibility of determination of sorbitol and fructosamine in saliva has been studied in healthy volunteers and patients with diabetes. It was concluded that saliva sorbitol and fructosamine levels measurements may be used as diagnostic tests in diabetes and serve as indicators of efficacy of therapy in diabetes (29).

5. Lipid peroxidation and protein oxidation in diabetes

Lipid peroxidation: Lipid peroxidation end-products very commonly detected by the measurement of thiobarbituric acid reactive substance (TBARS). The use of TBARS as an index of lipid peroxidation has been increased in plasma of diabetic patients (30-35). Thiobarbituric acid reacting substances (TBARS) are produced during lipoperoxidation-oxidative stress-induced damage of lipids and are, thus, a widely used marker of oxidative stress (36,37). However, they represent a heterogeneous group of compounds - best known is malondialdehyde (MDA). TBARS is associated with parodontopathies when measured directly in the injured gingival tissue (38). In previous studies we have shown that TBARS can be found in measurable concentrations in saliva and that these levels are higher in patients with parodontopathies and their origin is unlikely to be plasma (39,40). Whether the difference in patients is caused by a rise of MDA or instead of and which other factors influence salivary TBARS levels is unknown.(40) thus, assume, that salivary TBARS may reflect the local oral oxidative stress, although the producer is still hidden (41). Salivary MDA levels are directly affected by sytemic oxidative stress, since MDA levels were also elevated in saliva of diabtetic patients without parodontopathies (24). Astaneie et al (42) have reported no difference in salivary versus serum MDA levels and presence of high Antioxidant activity (AOA) in type 1 diabetics. Studies conducted on diabetic rats have reported an increase in salivary and serum MDA with variable antioxidant activity (43). Celec et al (44) have found an increase in MDA levels in non diabetics which was attributed to age, altered periodontal status and smoking. Hodosy et al (45) suggest that MDA levels depend on the time of sampling and also are affected by factors like tooth brushing and antioxidative therapy received by the patients. Studies by Reznick et al (46)and Astaneie et al (42) have shown both salivary and serum antioxidants to increase depending on HbA1C levels and severity of diabetes. The AOA levels of both the groups did not show notable correlation with Fasting Plasma Glucosa (FPG) but a significant correlation existed between salivary MDA and FPG levels in the diabetic group.

6. Diabetes and antioxidants

Antioxidants are substances that inhibit the destructive eefects of oxidation. Some of the general antioxidants that are known are glutathione effects, glutathione peroxidase, vitamins A,C,E, catalase and SOD. The decreased efficiency of antioxidant defenses (both enzymatic and non-enzymatic) seems to correlate with the severity of pathological tissue changes in type 1 diabetes (47).

Administration of the antioxidants, for example, the vitamin C and free amino acids, get a better reaction to insulin and can supply extra benefit to the proposed reduction of oxidative stress in tissues (48,49). Experimental study on diabetic rats suggested that nutritional vitamin E supplementation helps fatty acids metabolism and lower lipid peroxidation in rat tissues (50). Oral vitamin C and vitamin E has the ability to lower the oxidative stress in eye (51) and the vascular endothelia function get better in type1 and not type 2 diabetes (52). Vitamin C and Vitamin E, probably have an important role in reducing the oxidative damage produced by nitric oxide and other free radicals. The estimation of vitamin levels and other antioxidants in saliva could provide a good insight about the body function against oxidative stress and it can be used to monitor therapy.

7. Conclusion

The saliva matrix is an upcoming area of research for basic and clinical application purposes, with considerable potential for growth and progress. Nevertheless, to date salivary assays are still little used compared with plasma assays, even it is possible to have a quantitative estimate of oxidative stress markers and antioxidants in saliva.

8. References

[1] Current Diabetes scenario in India. Br. J Diabetes Vasc Dis 2007; 7(1): 12-16

[2] Cerielo A. Oxidative stress and glycemic regulation. Metabolism 2000;49 (2)suppl 1:27-29

[3] Baynes JW, Thorpe SR. Role of oxidative stress in diabetic complications: a new perspective on the old paradigm. Diabetes 1999;48:1-9.

[4] Maritim AC, Sanders RA, Watkins JB 3rd . Diabetes, oxidative stress, and antioxidants: A review. J Biochem Mol Toxicol 2003;17(1):24-38.

[5] Atalay M, Laaksonen. Diabetes, Oxidative stress and physical exercise. J Sports Science & Med 2002;1:1-14.

[6] Johansen JS, Harris AK, Rychly DJ, Ergul A. Oxidative stress and the use of antioxidants in diabetes: Linking basic science to clinical practice. Cardiovascular Diabetology 2005;4:5.

[7] Turko IV, Marcondes S, Murad F. Diabetes-associated nitration of tyrosine and inactivation of succinyl-CoA:3-oxoacid CoA- transferase. Am J Physiol Heart Circul Physiol 2001;281(6):H2289-94.

[8] Cuzik TJ, West NE, Black E, McDonald D, Ratnatunga C, Pillai R, Channon KM. Vascular superoxide production by NAD(P)H oxidase:association with endothelial dysfunction and clinical risk factors. Circ Res 2000;86(9):E85-90.

[9] Cuzik TJ, Mussa S, Gastaldi D, Sadowski J, Ratnatunga C, Pillai R, Channon KM. Mechanisms of increased vascular superoxide production in human diabetes mellitus: role of NAD(P)H oxidase and endothelial nitric oxide synthase. Circulation 2002;105(14):1656-62.

[10] Aliciguzel Y, Ozen I, Aslan M, Karayalcin U. Activities of xanthine oxireductase and antioxidant enzymes in different tissues of diabetic rats. J Lab Clin Med 2003;142(3):172-77.

[11] Nishikawa T, Edelstein D, Du XL, Yamagishi S, Matsumura T, Kaneda Y, Yorek MA, Beebe D, Oates PJ, Hammes HP, et al. Normalizing mitochondrial superoxide production block three pathways of hyperglycemic damage. Nature 2000;404(6779):787-790.

[12] Brownlee M. Biochemistry and molecular cell biology of diabetic complications. Nature 2001;414(6865):813-20.

[13] Van Nieuw Amerongen AV, Bolscher JG, Veerman ECI. Salivary proteins: protective and diagnostic value in cariology: Caries Res 2004;38:247-53.

[14] Sell DR, Lapolla A, Odetti P, Fogarty J , Monnier VM. Pentosidine formation in skin correlates with severity of complications in individuals with long-standing IDDM. Diabetes 1992:41:1286-92.

[15] Dyer DG, Dunn JA, Thorpe SR, Bailie KE, Lyons TJ, McCance DR, Baynes JW. Accumulation of Maillard reaction products in skin collagen in diabetes and aging. J Clin Invest 1993;91:2463-69.

[16] Basta G, Schmidt AM, De Caterina R. Advanced glycation end products and vascular inflammation: implications for accelerated atherosclerosis in diabetes. Cardiovasc Res 2004;63:582-92.

[17] Yoon MS, Jankowski V, Montag S, Zidek W, Henning L, Schluter H, Tepel M,Jankowski A. Characterisation of advanced glycation endproducts in saliva from patients with diabetes mellitus. Biochem Biophys Res Commun. 2004 15;323(2):377-81.

[18] Garay-Sevilla ME, Regalado JC, Malacara JM, Nava LE, Wróbel-Zasada K, Castro-Rivas A, Wróbel K. Advanced glycosylation end products in skin, serum, saliva and urine and its association with complications of patients with type 2 diabetes mellitus. J Endocrinol Invest. 2005 Mar;28(3):223-30.

[19] Mannervik B, Danielson UH. Glutathione transferases-structure and catalytic activity. CRC. Critical Reviews in Biochemistry 1988;23:283-337.

[20] Vijayalingam S, Parthiban A, Shanmugasundaram KR, Mohan V. Abnormal antioxidant status in impaire glucose tolerance and non-insulin dependent diabetes mellitus. Diabetic Med 1996;13:715-19.

[21] Peuchant E, Delmas Beauvieux MC, Couchouron A, Dubourg L, Thomas MJ, Perromat A, Clerc M, Gin H. Short-term insulin therapy and normoglycemia. Effects on erythrocyte lipid peroxidation in NIDDM patients. Diabetes Care 1997;20:202-207.

[22] Arana C, Cutando A, Ferrera MJ, Gomez-Moreno G, Vander Worf C, Bolanos MJ, Escames G, Acuna-Castroviejo. Parameters of oxidative stress in saliva from diabetic and parenteral drug addict patients. J Oral Pathol Med 2006;35:554-9.

[23] Gümüş P, Buduneli N, Cetinkalp S, Hawkins SI, Renaud D, Kinane DF, Scott DA. Salivary antioxidants in patients with type 1 or 2 diabetes and inflammatory periodontal disease: a case-control study. J Periodontol. 2009;80(9):1440-6.

[24] Al-Rawi N. Oxidative stress, antioxidant status and lipid profile in the saliva of type 2 diabetics. Diabetes & Vas Dis Res 2011;8(1):22-28.

[25] Tesfamariam B. Free radicals in diabetic Endothelial cell dysfunction. Free rad Biol & Med 1994;16:383-91.

[26] Arai K, Iizuka S , Tada Y, Oikawa K, taniguchi N. Increase in the glycosylated form of erythrocyte CU-Zn_superoxide dismutase in diabetes and close association of the non enzymatic glycosylation with the enzyme activity. Biochemica et Biophysica Acta 1987;924:292-96.

[27] Belce A, Uslu E, Kucur M, Umut M, Ipbüker A, Seymen HO. Evaluation of salivary sialic acid level and Cu-Zn superoxide dismutase activity in type 1 diabetes mellitus. Tohoku J Exp Med. 2000;192(3):219-25.

[28] Oates PJ, Mylari BL: Aldose reductase inhibitors: Therapeutic implications for diabetic complications. Expert Opin Investig Drugs 1999; 8: 2095–2119.

[29] Morenkova SA. Comparative analysis of dependence of saliva sorbitol and fructosamine levels on blood glucose level in patients with diabetes. Biomed Khim. 2004;50(6):612-4

[30] Noberasco G, Odetti P, Boeri D, Maiello M, Adezati L. Malondialdehyde (MDA) level in diabetic subjects. Relationship with blood glucose and glycosylated hemoglobin. Biomedicine & Pharmacotherapy 1991;45:193-96.

[31] Altomare E, vendemiale G, Chicco D, Procacci V, Cirelli F. Increased lipid peroxidation in type 2 poorly controlled diabetic patients. Diabetes & Metabolism 1992;18:264-71.

[32] Jain SK, McVie R. Effect of glycemic control, race (white versus black), and duration of diabetes on reduced glutathione content in erythrocytes of diabetic patients. Metabolism 1994;43:306-9.

[33] Nourooz-Zadeh J, Tajaddini-Sarmadi J, McCarthy S, Betteridge DJ, Wolff SP. Elevated levels of authentic plasma hydroperoxides in NIDDM. Diabetes 1995;44:1054-58.

[34] Ozben T, Nacitarhan S, Tuncer N. Plasma and urine malondialdehyde levels in non-insulin-dependent diabetic patients with and without microalbuminemia. Int J Clin Lab Res. 1995;25:162-64.

[35] Freitas JP, Filipe PM, Rodrigo FG. Lipid peroxidation in type 2 normolipidemic diabetic patients. Diabetic res & Clin Practice.1997;36:71-75.

[36] Chapple Il. Reactive oxygen species and antioxidants in inflammatory diseases, *J Clin Periodontol* 1997;24 : 287–296.

[37] Moore S, Calder KA,. Miller NJ Rice-Evans CA. Antioxidant activity of saliva and periodontal disease, *Free RadicRes1994;* 21 :417–425.

[38] Tuter G, Kurtis B, Serdar M. Interleukin-1beta and thiobarbituric acid reactive substance (TBARS) levels after phase I periodontal therapy in patients with chronic periodontitis, *J Periodontol 2001;* 72 : 883–888.

[39] Celec P, Cervenka T, Hodosy J, Boor B, Vesela S, Halcak L, Ostatnikova D, Tomandlova A, Rendekova V, Podhradsky J. Thiobarbituric acid reacting substances and their relation to the gingival inflammation, *Timisoara Medical Journal* 54 (2004), 81–85.

[40] Makinen KK , Isotupa KP, Kivilompolo T, Makinen PL, Murtomaa S, Petaja J, Toivanen J , Soderling E. The effect of polyol-combinant saliva stimulants on S. mutans levels in plaque and saliva of patients with mental retardation, *SpecCare Dentist2002;* 22 : 187–193.

[41] Marton IJ , Balla G, Hegedus C, Redi P, Szilagyi Z, Karmazsin L, Kiss C. The role of reactive oxygen intermediates in the pathogenesis of chronic apical periodontitis, *Oral Microbiol Immunol 1993;8* : 254–257.

[42] Astaneie F, Afshari M, Mojtahedi A, Mostafalou S, Zamani MJ, Larijani B, Abdollahi M. Total antioxidant capacity and levels of epidermal growth factor and nitric oxide in blood and saliva of insulin dpendent diabetic patients. Arch Med Res 2005; 36(4): 376-81.

[43] Nogueira FN, Carvalho AM, Yamaguti PM, Nicolau J. Antioxidant parameters and lipid peroxidation in salivary glands of streptozotocin-induced diabetic rats. Clin Chim Acta 2005; 353 (1-2): 133-139.

[44] Celec P, Hodosy J, Celecová V, Vodrázka J, Cervenka T, Halcák L, Bozek P, Kopáni M, Kúdela M. Salivary thiobarbituric acid reacting substances and malondial-dehyde-their relationship to reported smoking and to parodontal status described by the papillary bleeding index. Dis Markers 2005; 21(3): 133-137.

[45] Hodosy J, Celec P. Daytime of sampling, tooth-brushing and ascorbic acid influence salivary thiobarbituric acid reacting substances—a potential clinical marker of gingival status. Dis Markers 2005; 21(4): 203-207.
[46] Reznick AZ, Shehadeh N, Shafir Y, Nagler RM. Freeradicals related effects and antioxidants in saliva and serum of adolescents free radicals Type 1 diabetes mellitus. Arch Oral Biol 2006; 51(8): 640-648.
[47] Santini SA, Marra G, Giardina B, Cotroneo P, Mordente A, Martorana GE, Manto A, Chirlanda G. Defective plasma antioxidant defenses and enhanced susceptibility to lipid peroxidation in uncomplicated IDDM. Diabetes 1997;46:1853-58.
[48] Paolisso G, D'Amore A, Balbi V, Volpe C, Galzerano D, Giugliano D, Sgambato S, Verricchio M, D'Onofrio F. Plasma vitamin C affects glucose homeostasis in healthy subjects and in non-insulin-dependent diabetics. Am J Physiol 1994;266:E261-8.
[49] Natarajan Sulochana K, Lakshmi S, Punitham R, Arokiasamy T, Sukumar B, Ramakrishnan S. Effects of oral supplementation of free aminoacids in type 2 diabetic patients. A pilot clinical trial. Med Sci Monit 2002; 8:CR131-137.
[50] Celik S, Baydas G, Yilmaz O. Influence of vitamin E on the levels of fatty acids and MDA in some tissues of diabetic rats. Cell biochem Funct 2002;20:67-71.
[51] Peponis V, Papathanasiou M, Kapranou A, Magkou C, Tyligada A, Melidonis A, Droses T, Sitaras NM. Protective role of oral antioxidant supplementation in ocular surface of diabetic patients. Br J Ophthalmol. 2002;86:1369-73.
[52] Beckman JA, Goldfine AB, Gordon MB, Garrett LA, Keaney JF, Creager MA. Oral antioxidant therapy improves endothelial function in type 1 and not type 2 diabetes mellitus. Am J Heart Circ Physiol 2003;285:H2392-98.

Section 5

Systemic, Neuronal and Hormonal Pathologies

14

The Role of Oxidative Stress in Female Reproduction and Pregnancy

Levente Lázár
1st Departmet of Obstetrics and Gynecology,
Semmelweis University Budapest,
Hungary

1. Introduction

In a healthy body, reactive oxygen species (ROS) and antioxidants remain in balance. Oxidative stress occurs when the generation of reactive oxygen species and other radical species exceeds the scavenging capacity by antioxidants of antioxidative agents in organism, due to excessive production of reactive oxidagen species and/or inadequate intake or increased utilization of antioxidants. Most ROS are formed at operation of electrone transport chains in mitochondria, endoplasmatic reticulum, plasmatic and nuclear membranes. Minor ROS amounts are generated by some enzymes through autooxidation of different molecules. Reactive oxygen specieses can also be formed by exogenous exposures such as alcohol, tobacco smoke, and environmental pollutants. Elimination of reactive oxygen species is catalysed by certain enzymes such as superoxide dismutses (SOD), catalases and peroxidases. Antioxidants (including vitamins C and E) and antioxidant cofactors (such as selenium, zinc, and copper) are capable to dispose, scavenge, or suppress ROS formation. „Oxidative stress" rises when due to some reasons the steady-state ROS concentration is increased, leading to oxidative modification of cellular constituents, resulting disturbance of cellular metabolism and regulatory pathways (Lushchak. 2011). Cellular ROS and their control by antioxidants are involved in the physiology of the female reproductive system. Physiological ROS levels play an important regulatory role through various signalling and transduction pathways in folliculogenesis, oocyte maturation, corpus luteum, uterine function, embryogenesis, embryonic implantation and fetoplacental development. Imbalances between antioxidants and ROS production are considered to be responsible for the initiation or development of pathological processes affecting female reproductive processes.

The establishment of pregnancy requires a receptive uterus able to respond to a variety of biochemical and molecular signals produced by the developing conceptus, as well as specific interactions between the uterine endometrium and the extra-embryonic membranes. Therefore, placental development and function are prerequisites for an adequate supply of nutrients and oxygen to the fetus and successful establishment of pregnancy. Oxidative stress has been proposed as the causative agent of female sterility, recurrent pregnancy loss and several pregnancy-related disorders as preeclampsia, intra-uterine growth restriction (IUGR) and gestational diabetes.

2. Effect of oxidative stress on female reproductive system

The female reproductive system is a complex multiorgan system which require an optimal biological environment. Aerobic metabolism utilizing oxygen is essential for reproductive homeostazis. Aerobic metabolism is associated with the generation of prooxidant molecules called ROS including hydroxyl radical, superoxide anion, hydrogen peroxide, and nitric oxide. The balance between the prooxidants and antioxidants maintain the cellular homeostasis, whenever there is an imbalance in this equilibrum leading to enhanced steady-state level a state of oxidative stress is initiated. Free radicals are key signal molecules modulating reproductive functions by the influence of the endometrial and fallopian tube function, maturation of oocytes, sperm, implantation of the preembryo and early embryo development (Figure 1.)

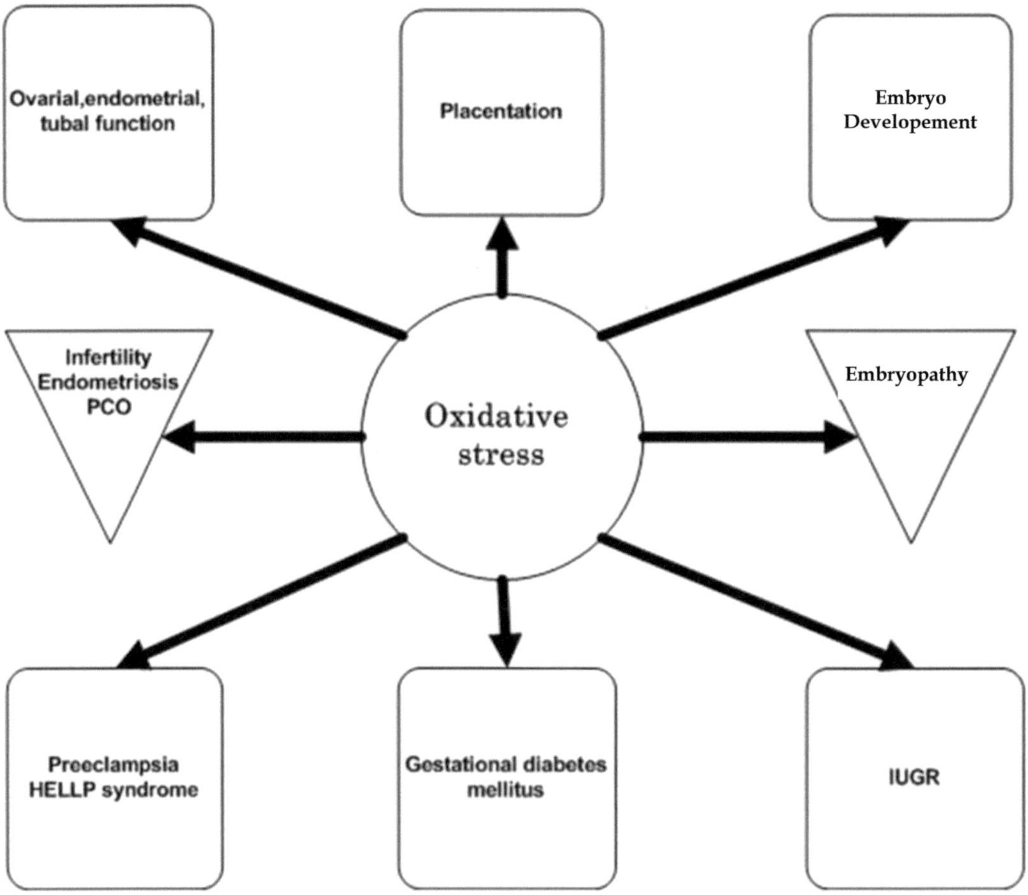

Fig. 1. Oxidative stress in female reproduction

2.1 Ovarian function

Aerobic metabolism utilizing oxygen is essential for developement of the gametes, also free radicals play a significant role in physiological processes within the ovary. The expression of various biomarkers of oxidative stress has been investigated in normal cycling human ovaries (Maruyama et al. 1997, Matsui et al., 1996), justifiing the regulatory role of ROS and antioxidants in oocyte maturation, folliculogenesis, ovarian steroidogenesis and luteolysis (Shiotani et al., 1991; Behrman et al., 2001; Sugino et al., 2004). Studies demonstrate intensified lipid peroxidation in the preovulatory Graafian follicle (Paszkovski et al., 1995). The significance of reactive oxygen specieses and antioxidant enzymes as copper zinc superoxide dismutase (Cu, Zn-SOD), manganese superoxide dismutase (Mn-SOD), and glutathione peroxidase, in oocyte maturation was provided by Riley et al. (1991) using immmunohistochemical localization and mRNA expression (Tamate et al., 1995). The antioxidant enzymes neutralize reactive oxygen specieses and protect the oocyte. In corpora lutea collected from pregnant and nonpregnant patients, it was observed that during normal situations Cu–Zn SOD expression rise from early luteal to midluteal phase and decrease during regression of the corpus luteum. Studies investigating the correlation between adrenal-4 binding protein (Ad4BP) and superoxide dismutase expression also suggest an association between oxidative stress and ovarian steroidogeneis (Matsui et al.,1996). Antibody to adrenal 4-binding protein (Ad4BP) was utilized to localize Ad4BP in the nuclei of theca and granulosa cells. Ad4BP is a steroidogenic transcription factor that induces transcription of the steroidogenic P450 enzyme. Both human granulosa and luteal cells respond to hydrogen peroxide with an extirpation of gonadotropin action and inhibition of progesterone secretion (Sabuncu et al., 2001). The production of both progesterone and estradiol hormones is reduced when hydrogen peroxide is added to a culture of human chorionic gonadotropin-stimulated luteal cells (Agrawal et al., 2006).

Levels of three oxidative stress biomarkers, conjugated dienes, lipid hydroperoxide and thiobarabituric acid reactive substances were found significantly lower in the follicular fluid compared with serum levels (Jozwik et al., 1999). The preovulatory follicle has a potent antioxidant defense, which is depleted by the intense peroxidation (Jozwik et al., 1999). Also the antioxidant enzymes glutathione peroxidase and Mn-SOD are considered to be markers for cytoplasmic maturation in metaphase II oocytes (El Mouattasim et al., 1999).

2.2 Changes in endometrium

Cyclical changes in the endometrium are accompanied by changes in the expression of antioxidants. Enzymes, such as thioredoxin, have a higher expression in the early secretory phase (Murayama et al, 1997). There is also a cyclical variation in the expression of superoxide dismutase in the endometrium. Superoxide dismutase activity decreased in the late secretory phase while ROS levels increased and ROS triggered the release of prostaglandin F2 α (Sugino et al., 1996). Estrogen or progesterone withdrawal led to increased expression of cyclooxygenase-2 (COX-2). Stimulation of the cyclooxygenase enzyme is brought about by ROS via activation of the transcription factor NF-κB, suggesting a mechanism for menstruation (Sugino et al., 2004).

Nitrogen monoxide (.NO) has also important role in decidualisation and preparation of the endometrium for implantation by regulatation of the endometrial, myometrial and microvascular functions. Expression of endothelial and inducible NO synthase (NOS) have been demonstrated in the human endometrium (Tseng et al., 1996), and the endometrial vessels (Taguchi et al,. 2000). Highest levels of transcripts of endothelial NOS mRNA have been reported in the late secretory phase of the endometrium (Tseng et al., 1996). These changes have been hypothesized to be important in the genesis of menstruation and endometrial shedding.

2.3 Fallopian tube function

Several studies demonstrated the presence of cytokines, prostaglandins, metabolites of lipid peroxidation and ROS in fluid samples of fallopain tube (Tamate et al., 1985). The eqilibrum of these components serves as an optimal milieu for fertilization and the transport of the preembryo. An endogenous nitrogen monoxide system exists in the fallopian tubes. Nitric oxide has a relaxing effect on smooth muscle and it has similar effects on tubular contractility. Deficiency of NO may lead to tubal motility dysfunction, resulting in retention of the ovum, delayed sperm transport and infertility. Increased NO levels in the fallopian tubes are cytotoxic to the invading microbes and also may be toxic to spermatozoa (Rosselli et al., 1995), leading to infetility.

2.4 Embryo implantation and placenta

The human embryo undergoes interstitial implantation by invading the maternal decidua at the blastocyst stage (Riley& Behrman, 1991). Although placental villi are bathed in maternal blood in the hemochorial placenta (Tamate et al., 1995), prior to 10 weeks of gestation maternal blood flow to the placenta is blocked by extravillous trophoblasts. Placentation is initiated when the blastocyst makes contact with the epithelial lining of the uterus shortly after implantation. Placental villi which consist of a mesenchymal core surrounded by a monolayer of mononuclear villous cytotrophoblast stem cells which either fuse to form the overlying multinucleated syncytiotrophoblast or, in anchoring villi, differentiate into extravillous trophoblasts which grow out from the villous and spread laterally around the placenta (Irving et al., 1995).

Invasive extravillous trophoblasts play an important role in adapting the decidua to sustain pregnancy. Extravillous trophoblasts invade the walls of the uterine spiral arteries and adapt these vessels into large bore conduits capable of delivering the increased blood supply required in the second and third trimesters (Robertson et al., 1967; Zhou et al., 1997). As the extravillous trophoblasts invade the spiral arteries early in pregnancy they form plugs which occlude the spiral arteries and prevent maternal blood from entering the intervillous space, creating a physiologic hypoxic environment (Hustin &nd Schaaps,1987; Jaffe et al., 1997; Burton et al., 1999).

Early placental and embryonic development occurs in a state of low oxygen in histiotroph manner (Evans et al., 2004). The early gestation placenta is poorly protected against oxidative damage, as the antioxidant enzymes Cu,Zn-SOD and Mn-SOD are not expressed by the syncytiotrophoblast until approximately 8–9 weeks of gestation (Watson et al., 1997). Premature perfusion of this space during this first 10 weeks of development increases the risk of pregnancy loss (Jauniaux et al., 2000). The low oxygen environment during early placental development is essential for normal placental angiogenesis, and this angiogenesis is promoted by hypoxia-induced transcriptional and post-transcriptional regulation of angiogenic factors, as vascular endothelial growth factor and placental growth factor (Charnock-Jones&Burton, 2000).

The partial oxygen tension in the intervillous space declines from the second to the third trimester, reaching about 40 mm Hg in the third trimester (Soothill et al., 1986). The exact mechanism by which trophoblasts sense oxygen tension is currently unclear; however, several potential pathways have been identified. Many of these pathways utilize the ROS formation, but it is currently unclear whether hypoxia results an increase or decrease in their cellular levels (DeMarco & Caniggia, 2002). In hypoxic conditions, trophoblast oxygen sensing mechanisms utilize several different pathways to control gene expression. These pathways often utilize redox-sensitive transcription factors, of which the hypoxia inducible factor (HIF) family are the best characterized. HIF-1α is a transcription factor and master regulator of the cellular response to low oxygen levels (Majmundar et al., 2010), showing prominent expression in first trimester villi (Wang&Semenza, 1993). HIF-1α regulates the expression of genes such as p53, p21, and Bcl-2 required for cells to adapt to a low oxygen environment and apoptosis. HIF-1α is able to be stabilized under normoxic conditions by a variety of growth factors and cytokines including epidermal growth factor (EGF), insulin, heregulin, insulin-like growth factors 1 and 2, transforming growth factor, and interleukin-1 (Zelzer et al., 1998; Feldser et al., 1999; Hellwig-Burgel et al., 1999; Laughner et al., 2001; Fukuda et al., 2002; Stiehl et al., 2002).

Several other transcription factors involved in trophoblast differentiation are responsive to hypoxia. The transcription factors Id1 stream stimulatory factor-1 and -2 (USF1 and USF2) mediate the effects of Mash2 are all up-regulated in 2% oxygen in comparison to 20% oxygen (Jiang et al., 2000; Jiang & Mendelson, 2003). The up-regulation of Mash2, USF1 and USF2 may inhibit cytotrophoblast fusion into syncytiotrophoblast (Jiang et al., 2000; Jiang& Mendelson, 2003). The elevation of intracellular Ca^{2+} is believed to activate an HIF-1-independent signalling pathway that involves the transcription factor activator protein-1 (AP-1), with cooperation between the HIF-1 and AP-1 pathways allowing fine regulation of gene expression under hypoxia (Laderoute et al., 2002; Salnikow et al., 2002). AP-1 is a dimeric transcription factor composed from the products of the Jun and Fos proto-oncogenes (c-Jun, JunB, JunD, c-Fos, FosB, Fra-1 and Fra-2) (Dakour et al., 1999). AP-1 transcription factors are believed to play an important role in trophoblast differentiation. In the villus, AP-1 transcription factor expression is limited; however, extravillous trophoblasts express c-Jun, JunB, c-Fos, FosB and Fra-2 both in the first trimester and later in gestation (Bamberger et al., 2004.)

The other protective system is formed by antioxidant enzymes, playing a key role in the response of trophoblast to the burst of perfusion by maternal blood. With the increase of oxygen saturation and oxidative stress the activity in intervillous space the placenta employs a number of physiologic adaptations (Burton, 2009). Levels and activity of antioxidant enzymes: catalase, glutathione peroxidase, manganese and cooper, zinc superoxide dismutase are increased within placental tissues. This response is evolved as a defense mechanism to reduce harm to placental tissues exposed to this burst of oxidative stress (Jauniaux et al., 2000).

We can summarize that the trophoblast differentiation is essential for the success of human pregnancy, and despite some conflicting experimental evidence, hypoxia appears to play a vital role in regulating trophoblast differentiation in the first trimester. The regulation of trophoblast differentiation by hypoxia is a result of complex interactions between factors associated with oxidative stress, oxygen sensing mechanisms and the release of inflammatory cytokines. Therefore, aberrations in any one of these factors, along with the temporal and spatial regulation of blood flow in the intervillous space has the potential to result in altered gene expression and trophoblast phenotype leading to fail of implantation.

3. The role of oxidative stress in embryo and fetal malformation

Basic principles of teratogenesis state that a teratogen must cause a specific malformation through a specific mechanism during a period in which the conceptus is susceptible to said mechanism (Karnofsky, 1965). Different mechanisms are responsible for malformations that are in agreement with these basic scientific principles.

A mechanism that has not been well described in teratology is oxidant induced or redox misregulation of developmental signals en route to dysmorphogenesis. The paucity of teratogenic study of redox misregulation is partially due to oxidative stress (Sies, 1985). Oxidizing and reducing equivalent imbalance in turn, leads to macromolecule damage, namely protein modification, lipid peroxidation, and DNA oxidation, and can lead to cell death. Unspecific oxidation of cellular components does not apply to basic principles of teratology or adequately explain the manifestation of teratogenic effects. If oxidative stress is the random, unspecific oxidation of cellular molecules, it does not adequately exemplify why or how specific teratogens that induce oxidative stress could cause a specific malformation. While untimely cell death during differentiation can have serious repercussions on the developing embryo, generalized cellular oxidation and subsequent apoptosis do not sufficiently describe specificity of malformations seen with most teratogens. To qualify as a plausible teratogenic mechanism, oxidative stress must be a controlled, specific event that alters cell function and/ or signal transduction pathways that would in turn cause specific dysmorphogenesis.

During particular periods in development, the embryo is more or less susceptible to oxidative stress. In early development, one-cell embryo relies on the Krebs cycle, whereas the blastocyst relies on glycolysis and anaerobic pathways as does the embryo during early organogenesis. Once the circulatory system is established, there is a higher reliance on oxidative and aerobic metabolism and more ROS are produced by mitochondria. Conversely, more antioxidants are available at this period to counteract and detoxify these reactive oxygen specieses (Hansen, 2006). Over the course of development, the delicate balance between oxidants and antioxidants can be disrupted by exogenous agents that simulate ROS production leading to oxidative stress.

Thalidomide is associated with multiple birth defects, including phocomelia (Lecutier, 1962; Taussig, 1962). The most sensitive organ to thalidomide toxicity is the limb. Although the mechanism of teratogenesis and determinants of risk remain unclear, related teratogenic xenobiotics are bioactivated by embryonic prostaglandin H synthase (PHS) producing reactive oxygen species, which cause oxidative damage to DNA and other cellular macromolecules. Similarly, thalidomide is bioactivated by horseradish peroxidase, and oxidizes DNA and glutathione, indicating free radical-mediated oxidative stress. Furthermore, thalidomide teratogenicity is reduced by the PHS inhibitor acetylsalicylic acid, indicating PHS-catalyzed bioactivation. This appears to be regulated through redox shift resulting from depletion of GSH and increased GSSG in the nucleus, and this may imply that various transcription factors are affected by thalidomide through redox regulation (Hansen et al., 2001, 2002).

Exposure to the anticonvulsant valproic acid during the first trimester of pregnancy is associated with an increased risk of congenital malformations including heart defects, craniofacial abnormalities, skeletal and limb defects, and most frequently, neural tube defects (NTDs). The mechanisms by which valproic acid induces teratogenic effects are not fully understood, although previous studies support a role for oxidative stress. Valproic acid can alter cell signaling through gene expression changes mediated through histone deacetylase inhibition (Phiel et al., 2001), and is a direct inhibitor of class I and II histone deacetylases. Several laboratories have shown that embryonic histone acetylation levels are increased following exposure to valproic acid (Menegola et al., 2005; Tung and Winn, 2010). Furthermore, studies have supported a role for histone deacetylase inhibition as a mechanism of teratogenesis as analogs of valproic acid that lack histone deacetylase inhibitory activity are less teratogenic (Gurvich et al., 2005). Gene microarray studies have also demonstrated that valproic acid targets genes regulated by histone deacetylase, including *Mt1* and *Mt2*, both of which are ROS-sensitive (Jergil et al., 2009). In addition, histone deacetylase inhibitors have also been shown to increase ROS production and induce apoptosis in several cancer cell lines (Carew et al., 2008). Therefore, alterations in gene expression and/or increases in ROS formation mediated by histone deacetylase inhibition during development may induce teratogenesis.

The widely used anticonvulsant, phenytoin, can double the incidence of structural and functional birth defects when used in pregnancy (Kaneko et al., 1991). It can induce vascular disruption, which leads to hypoxia and hypoperfusion (Danielsson et al.,1995). In addition, phenytoin results in oxidative DNA damage and dysmorphogenesis, which can be eliminated by antioxidants (Winn and Wells, 1995). Phenytoin also selectively increased NF-kB activity in targeted tissues. Blocking of these signaling events with p65 antisense oligonucleotides eliminated the associated embryopathies (Kennedy et al., 2004). Further evidence that oxidative stress is important in phenytoin mediated toxicity is exemplified by the fact that treatment with polyethylene-modified superoxide dismutase enhances embryo toxicity whereas antioxidant levels were modulated with phenytoin (Winn and Wells, 1999).

Chronic ethanol consumption can lead to the generation of ROS and, as a consequence, teratogenicity. Prolonged ethanol exposure lead to increased production of lipid peroxides and decreased expression of antioxidant enzymes. Ascorbic acid can prevent against ethanol toxicity through inhibition of ROS formation and NF-kB activation (Peng et al.,2005). Zebrafish embryos exposed to ethanol with lipoic acid and/or only partially attenuated ethanol embryo toxicity, suggesting that other mechanisms are also involved (Reimers et al., 2006).

4. Oxidative stress in pathological pregnancies

4.1 Preeclampsia

Preeclampsia is a complex multisystem disorder that occurs during the pregnancy. The disease affects 5-8% of all pregnancies and is one of the leading couses of maternal and fetal morbidity and mortality. It is characterized with hypertension and proteinuria. The systolic blood pressure ≥140 mmHg, diastolic blood pressure ≥ 90 mmHg and the proteinuria at least 300 mg in 24 h urine collection. Women with mild proteinuria generally have no symptoms. However, women with severe preeclampsia (blood presure ≥160/110 mmHg, proteinuria >2-5g/24h) may have simptoms such as renal insufficiency, liver disease, haematological and neurological disturbances. Preeclampsia is charactized by vasospasm, reduced placental perfusion and abnormal placentation. The main couse of fetal compromise is the disturbance in uteroplacental perfusion. The only cure is the delivery of the baby. With antihypertensive treatment may prolong the pregnancy, increasing the chances of the baby to survive. If the blood presure cannot be controlled, or the laboratory parameters entry in a critical value the baby must be delivered. Preeclampsia has been proposed as a two-stage disorder. In first stage the placenta produces cytotoxic factors, in the second stage the maternal response to the placental factors occurs. There are several theories regarding to the main couse of disorder: abnormal placentation, immunological background, abnormal inflamatory response, etc. Assuming preeclampsia literature we can conclude that all the theories are part of disorders etiology.

4.1.1 Oxidative agents

Some reserches suggest that the placental oxidative stress may be involved in the ethiopathogenesis of preeclampisa. As there was mentioned above, the oxidatives stress is described as an imbalance in the production of reactive oxygen specieses and the ability of atioxidant defense to scavenge them. Pregnancy is a state of oxidative stress arrising from the increased metabolic activity in the placenta and reduced scavenging power of antioxidants (Wisdom et al. 1991). During the gestation the oxygenation of the uteroplacental unit is changing. The placenta and fetus exist in a hypoxic enviromet during early pregnancy as the uterine oxygen tension is extremly low till 8-10. weeks of gestation (pO_2<20 mmHg, 5%O_2), prior to estabilishment of the blood flow into intervillous space. The onset of blood flow is processig from the periphery to the center of placental disc, with villous regression in the placental periphery envolving into the chorion leave (Jauniaux et al., 2003). The developing chorioallantoic villous trees are exposed to a marked increase of pO_2 in a range of 40-80 mm Hg (Sjostedt et al., 1960; Shaaps et al., 2005; Rooth et al., 1961). This reoxygenation of the uteroplacental unit results an oxidative burst, controlled by antioxidant mechanisms.

Proposed effect of oxidative stress on placental fatty acid metabolism.

As a consequence of abnormal trophoblast invasion, and maternofetal barrier preeclampsia is characterized by induced oxidative stress and decreased antioxidants (Patil et al., 2009). In preeclamptic women, maternal circulating levels, placental tissue levels and production rate of lipid peroxides are increased and several antioxidants are markedly decreased (Serdar et al., 2003; Orhan et al., 2003). Normal pregnancy is associated with physiological hyperlipidemia (Belo et al., 2004). Physiological alterations are manifested by increased levels of triglycerides and cholesterol in pregnancy, which decreases rapidly after delivery. Preeclampsia is characterized by further elevation of serum triglycerides and serum free fatty acids (Hubel et al., 1996). (Figure 2.) Increased lipid peroxidation has been reported in preeclampsia, IUGR (Liu et al., 2005; Gupta et al., 2004, Bretelle et al., 2004).

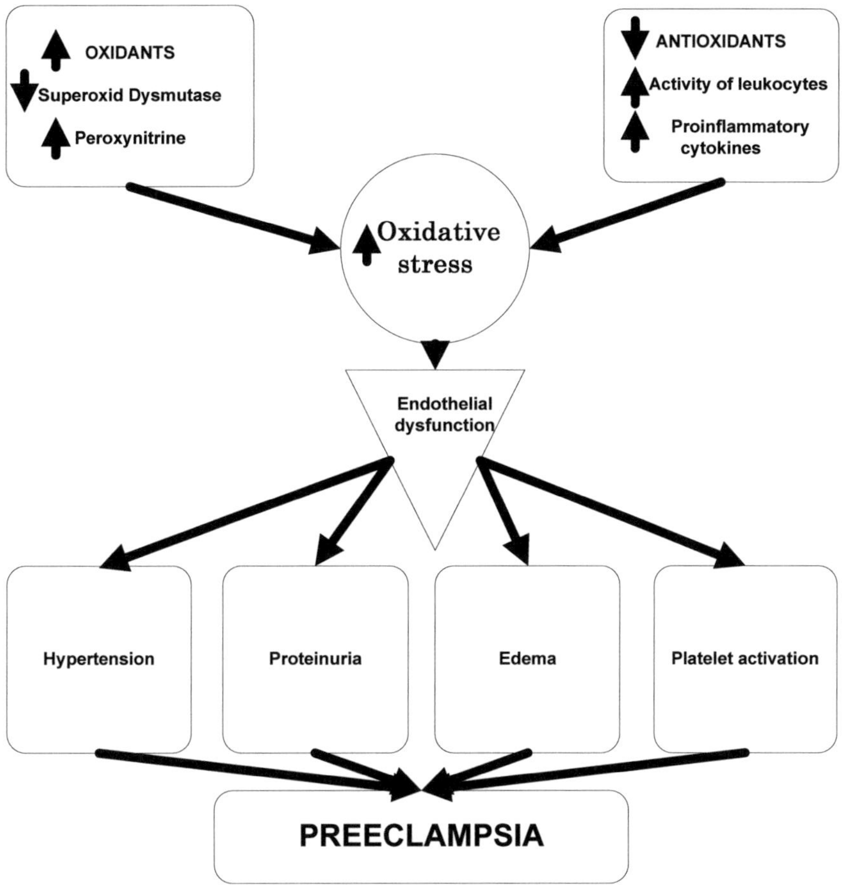

Fig. 2. Supposed oxidative stress pathway in preeclampsia

Nicotinamide adenine dinucleotide phosphate (NADPH) oxidase is an important enzyme that generates superoxide anion radical localized in the placenta syncytial microvillous membrane (Matsubara & Sato, 2001; Raijmakers et al., 2004). NADPH oxidase may play a role in placental lipid peroxidation by generating increased amounts of the superoxide anion radical. Poor antioxidant reserves can also tilt the balance in favor of prooxidation. Lipid peroxidation results in formation of primary lipid peroxidation products such as lipid hydroperoxides and secondary products such as malondialdehyde (MDA) and lipid peroxides. Lipid hydroperoxides are formed and bind to lipoproteins. They are then carried to distant sites where the hydroperoxides can cause ongoing lipid peroxidation and result in systemic oxidative stress. Increased placental production of lipid peroxides and thromboxane was demonstrated from both the trophoblast and the villous core components of placentas in patients with preeclampsia (Walsh & Wang, 1995).

Studies of women undergoing cesarean section showed significantly higher contents of lipid hydroperoxides, phospholipids, cholesterol and free 8-iso-prostaglandin F2α (8-iso-PGF2α), but not the total (free plus esterified) 8-iso-PGF2α in decidual tissues from women with preeclampsia as compared with tissues from normal pregnancies (Staff et al., 1999).

Moreover, tissue levels of free and total 8-iso-PGF2α are significantly higher in preeclamptic placenta than in normal placenta (Walsh et al., 2000). Isoprostanes like 8-iso-PGF2α are produced specifically by free radical-catalyzed peroxidation of arachidonic acid (Morrow et al., 1990). Free 8-iso-PGF2α has activities of relevance to preeclampsia, being a potent vasoconstrictor in kidney (Morrow et al., 1990) and placenta (Kwek et al., 1990), platelet activator (Minzu et al., 2002), and inducer of the release of endothelin from endothelial cells (Yura et al. 1999).

An increase in diastolic pressure correlates significantly with an increase in lipid peroxide levels, indicating that the severity of hypertension is correlated with the extent of lipid peroxidation (Aydin et al., 2004; Jain & Wise, 1995; Gupta et al., 2006). Women with preeclampsia have significantly higher mean plasma levels of malonaldehyde and significantly lower superoxide dismutase levels compared with normotensive pregnant women, (Aydin et al., 2004). The decrease in nitric oxide (NO) and superoxide dismutase (SOD) levels followed by a concomitant increase in levels of malonaledehyde, fibronectin, endothelin-1 (ET-1), and soluble-E selectin (sE-selectin) correlate with an increase in diastolic blood pressure (Aydin et al., 2004). In further studies, malonaldehyde levels in maternal erythrocytes were significantly elevated in women with developed preeclampsia. The risk of developing preeclampsia was 24-fold higher when malonaldehyde levels were above the cutoff value of 36 nmol/g (Basbug et al., 2003).

The cord plasma malonaldehyde and vitamin E levels were higher in patients with eclampsia than in patients with preeclampsia and in normotensive pregnant patients (Bowen et al. 2001).

Hyperhomocystinemia and altered eicosanoid synthesis has also been implicated in the pathophysiology of preeclampsia. Eicosanoids have vasoactive properties and enhance lipid peroxidation and decrease prostacyclin synthesis. The generation of the eicosanoid, 15-hydroxyeicosateranoic acid by the placenta was higher in women with preeclampsia than in normotensive control subjects. In preeclampsia, there is increased synthesis of thromboxane and reduced synthesis of prostacyclin. Lipid peroxides may also stimulate the cyclooxygenase enzyme to produce more thromboxane, resulting in a hypercoagulable state (Walsh, 2004).

4.1.2 Antioxidant agents

Antioxidants can be enzymatic or nonenzymatic. The enzymatic antioxidants are superoxide dismutase, thioredoxin, thioredoxin reductase, and glutathione peroxidase. The nonenzymatic antioxidants can be lipid-soluble such as vitamin E or water-soluble such as vitamin C. Serum levels of vitamin E and beta carotene (Serdar et al., 2003; Akyol et al., 2000), serum coenzyme Q10 and tocopherol levels (Palan et al., 2004), ascorbic acid were significantly reduced in pregnancies complicated by mild or severe preeclampsia, and the total antioxidant capacity was significantly reduced in pregnant women with mild and severe preeclampsia (Sagol et al., 1999). The balance between lipid peroxides and antioxidant vitamin E is tipped in favor of lipid peroxides in patients with mild and severe preeclampsia. A two-fold increase in the ratio between lipid peroxidation and antioxidant capacity was reported in the antepartum period in women with preeclampsia (Davidge et al., 1992). Significantly lower levels of vitamin C, E, and total thiol were seen in women with preeclampsia (Kharb et al., 2000). In patients with preeclampsia, antioxidants scavenge the increased free radicals, resulting in lowered antioxidant levels. Water-soluble antioxidants may function as a first line of antioxidants to scavenge excess of reactive oxygen species in plasma, whereas lipid soluble antioxidants such as tocopherol and carotene scavenge reactive oxygen species affecting the membrane lipids (Mikhail et al., 1994).

The activities of placental superoxide dismutase and glucose-6-phosphate dehydrogenase are decreased in preeclampsia compared to normal pregnancy (Poranen et al., 1996). Moreover, the activity and mRNA expression of Cu,Zn-SOD, glutathione peroxidase, and tissue levels of vitamin E are significantly lower in placental tissues from preeclampsia than from normal pregnancy (Wnag & Walsh, 1996). Glutathione and its related enzymes are antioxidants that help detoxify the increased generation of free radicals. Significantly reduced whole blood glutathione levels have been reported in women with preeclampsia and HELPP syndrome (Madazil et al., 2002; Knapen et al., 1998).

4.1.3 Leukocyte activation

The other main caracteristics of preeclampsia is the exacerbated inflamatory state (Bretelle et al., 2004; Holthe et al., 2005; Redman et al., 1999). Activated leukocytes, both monocytes and granulocytes, generate excess reactive oxygen specieses resulting in oxidative stress (Holthe et al., 2004). Compared with normotensive pregnant women, women with preeclampsia have higher levels of calprotectin, a protein involved in various physiological inflammatory processes, which is indicative of leukocyte activation (Holthe et al., 2005). The expression of surface adhesion molecules on cord blood neutrophils was significantly higher in infants born to women with preeclampsia than in infants born to the control subjects. Increased TNF secretion by leukocytes was detected in blood from patients with preeclampsia, providing further evidence of leukocyte activation (Beckman et al., 2004). TNF-α can activate the endothelial cells and upregulate the gene expression of numerous molecules such as platelet-derived growth factor, cell adhesion molecules, endothelin-1 and PAI-1. These molecules have been reported to have detrimental effects on the vasculature and also characterize preeclamptic pregnancy (Hajjar et al., 1987; van Hinsbrgh et al., 1988). Furthermore, chronic infusion of TNF-α into rats during late pregnancy results in a significant increase in renal vascular resistance and arterial pressure (Alexander et al., 2002; Giardina et al., 2002).

4.1.4 Endothelial cell dysfunction

Endothelial dysfunction is also one of the main pathogenic features of preeclampsia. The markers of endothelial dysfunction such as tissue plasminogen activator, von Willebrand factor, sE-selectin, and fibronectin are elevated in patients with preeclampsia (Aydin et al., 2004; Stubbs et al., 1984; Halligan et al., 1994). Although the exact mechanisms of vascular endothelial damage in preeclampsia are unclear, increased lipid peroxidation may lead to endothelial cell dysfunction (Davidge et al., 1996). Tumor necrosis factor (TNF), tissue factor (TF) of placental origin, endothelial nitric oxide synthase (NOS), and excessive activity of the enzyme polymerase may contribute to endothelial dysfunction. Compared with normotensive pregnant women, women with preeclampsia have reduced expression of constitutive nitrite oxidative stress -mRNA, and this lead to reduced production of NO.

NOS inhibition consequence is the increased endothelial permeability and an abnormal response of the endothelial cells to the stress (Wang et al., 2004). In preeclampsia greater nitrotyrosine immunostaining were found in placental villous vascular endothelium and its surrounding smooth muscle cells, and also in villous stromal cells compared to normal pregnant controls (Myatt et al., 2006). Moreover particularly intense immunoreactivity of nitrotyrosine was measured within the invasive cytotrophoblasts in placental biopsies and vascular endothelium in the floating villi obtained from women with preeclampsia (Many et al., 2000).

4.1.5 Vascular developement

Aberrant placental vasculature development and abnormal placental blood flow are characterized by increased impedance in Doppler velocimetry (Farag et al., 2004). These abnormalities significantly correlated with expression of tissue factor in the placenta of women with severe preeclampsia (Di Paolo et al., 2003). The expression of tissue factor was found to be markedly increased in the endothelial cells within the basal deciduus. Doppler impedance modifications were significantly correlated to the endothelial cell activation. Tumor necrosis factor, a circulating cytokine, has also been implicated as causing endothelial dysfunction in preeclampsia (Hung et al., 2004). Significantly higher tissue levels of tumor necrosis factor were demonstrated in the placenta from women with preeclampsia (Wang et al., 1996). Higher levels of tumor necrosis factor lead to increased generation of E-selectin, a marker of endothelial activation of umbilical endothelial cells.

4.2 Oxidative stress in gestational diabetes (GDM)

Gestational diabetes is defined as a carbohydrate intolerance of variable severity, which begins, or is identified during the pregnancy (Lopez et al. 2011). The prevalence of gestational diabetes mellitus is around 5% of all pregnancies (Ben Haroush et al., 2004). The presence of this disease increases the risk of macrosomia, perinatal morbido-mortality (Ostlund et al., 2003) and subsequent developement of type 2 diabetes mellitus. The pathophysiology of gestational diabetes remain unclear. Pregnant women with gestational diabetes have a reduction in insulin sensitivity (Catalano et al., 1999), hypergicemia, and hyperlipidemia. Oxidative stress implication in developement of the disease is a result of imbalance between the increase in the formation of reactive oxidative substances (Brownlee, 2001; Maddux et al., 2001) and the insufficience of antioxidative defence mechanisms (Chen et al., 2003).

4.2.1 Induction of oxidative stress in gestational diaetes pathways

Hyperglycemia induces oxidative stress and cell and tissue damage through several metabolic mechanisms.

These include the formation of advanced glycation endproducts (AGE), activation of protein kinase C (PKC), the hexosamine pathway, and increased reactive oxygen specieses production in the mitochondria. An important source of free radicals in diabetes is the interaction of glucose with proteins. Maillard reaction that form by nonenzymatic glycation through covalent attachment of highly reactive aldehyde or ketone groups of reducing

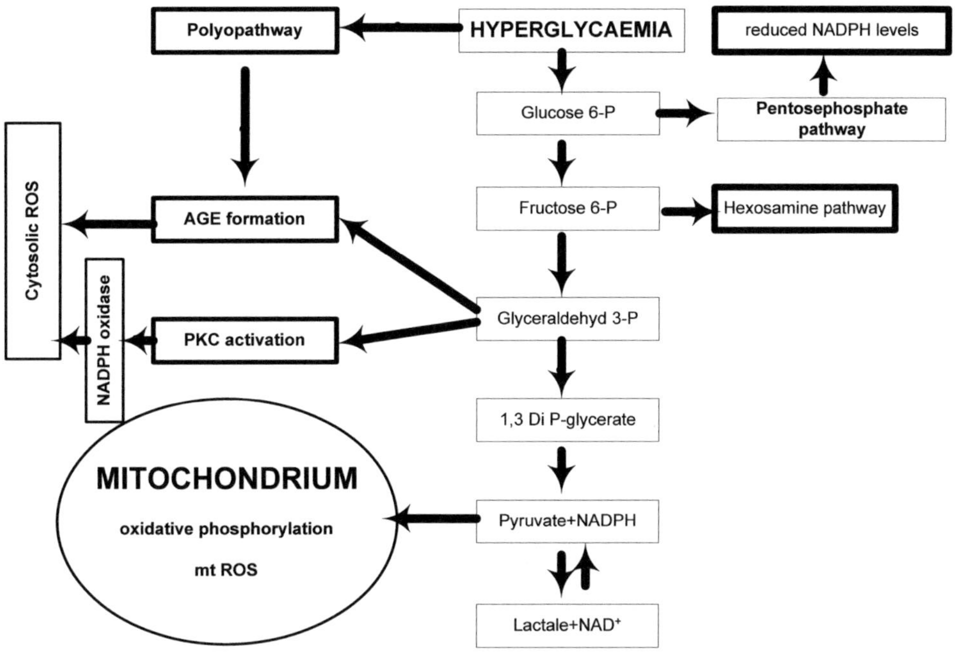

Fig. 3. Mechanisms by which hyperglycemia induces cellular dysfunction and damage.

carbohydtrates and the free amino groups on proteins, lipids, and nucleic acids. Elevated concentration of glucose leads to enhanced formation glycolytic products which together with the tricarboxylic acid (TCA) cycle intermediates provide glycation of intracellular proteins. The interaction of aldehyde groups of glucose with free amino groups on proteins generates a Schiff's base. Extracellular AGE can bind to the AGE receptor (RAGE), a multi-ligand member of the immunoglobulin superfamily. Engagement of RAGE by AGE results in activation of intracellular signaling molecules resulting in oxidative stress and inflammation. Since oxidative stress induction and inflammation are closely associated with gestational diabetes (Coughlan et al., 2001; Lappas et al., 2004), it is plausible that the AGE-RAGE system could play a role in the pathogenesis of this metabolic disease. During pregnancy, the AGE-RAGE axis may be involved in oxidative and inflammatory responses. Specifically, AGE-BSA stimulated the release of the pro-inflammatory cytokines IL-1β, IL-6, IL-8, and tumor necrosis factor (TNF)-α and prostaglandins PGE_2 and $PGF_{2\alpha}$. NF-κB and MAPK activate expression of several pro-inflammatory genes, including pro-inflammatory cytokines, the adhesion molecules vascular cell adhesion molecule (VCAM)-1, and intercellular cell adhesion molecule (ICAM)-1, and RAGE causing cellular inflammation. This is consistent with gestational diabetes being closely associated with low-grade inflammation (Kirwan et al., 2002) and atherosclerosis (Anastasiou et al., 1998; Hannemann et al., 2002). Additionally, the activation of cytokines by AGE in human placenta may also be involved in insulin resistance associated with gestational diabetes (Colomiere et al., 2009).

Hyperglycemia also activats hexosamine biosynthetic pathway (Rajapakse et al., 2009). This pathway of glucose metabolism uses fructose-6-phosphate derived from glycolysis to metabolize glucosamine-6-phosphate by glucosamine-6-phosphate amidotransferase.

Glucosamine-6-phosphate is a competitive inhibitor of glucose-6-phosphate dehydrogenase (G6PDH). Glucosamine-6 phosphate produced in the hexosamine pathway, leads to decreased NAPDH concentrations, diminished cellular GSH levels, and elevated oxidative stress. The activity of G6PDH also rapidly increases in response to intracellular reactive oxygen specieses production (Jian et al., 2003).

NADPH oxidase is a membrane enzyme complex accounting for ROS generation by electron transport chain and the enzyme is especially important in redox signaling. Under diabetic conditions it can be stimulated by AGE, insulin, and angiotensin II. Hypoxia possibly induces all these stimuli, which can activate NADPH oxidase. Once activated in response to high glucose levels, NADPH oxidase catalyzes the transfer of electrons from NADPH to molecular oxygen to produce $O_2^{\cdot-}$ convetred to H_2O_2. High glucose levels lead to generation of reactive oxygen specieses by stimulation of NADPH oxidase (Gao et al., 2009; Gupte et al., 2010).

Under physiological conditions reactive oxygen specieses are eliminated by cellular defense mechanisms, including diverse enzymes and vitamins. Imbalance of reactive oxygen specieses production and antioxidant systems of a cell can lead to an upregulation of expression of antioxidant enzyme encoding genes. Hyperglycemia causes excessive reactive oxygen specieses formation, thus activating the Nrf2/ARE pathway (Xue et al., 2008). NADPH oxidase was shown to be higher expressed and activated in endothelial cells of pregnant women with GDM (Sankaralingam et al., 2009). Protein kinase C (PKC) promotes the activation of mitochondrial NADPH oxidase, thereby leading to oxidative stress events. Once stimulated, NADPH oxidase reduces glutathione levels and impairs the cellular antioxidant defense systems (King et al., 2004).

4.2.2 Oxidant species

Maternal MDA levels in serum and plasma are increased in gestational diabete mellitus women compared to normal glucose tolerant (NGT) pregnant women (Chaudhari et al., 2003; Surapanieni et al., 2008). Higher levels of lipid peroxidation are evident in patients with poor glycemic control. Proteins undergo oxidative damage, they become increasingly susceptible to proteolytic degradation. Erythrocytes contain proteolytic enzymes that can degrade oxidatively damaged proteins such as hemoglobin, thus preventing the accumulation of nonfunctional proteins and protein fragments. GDM is associated with higher levels of maternal erythrocyte proteolytic activity than NGT controls (Kamath et al., 1998).

4.2.3 Antioxidants

The level of total superoxide dismutase in placental tissues of gestational diabetes mellitus (both diet- and insulin-controlled) patients is lower (Kinalski et al., 2001) or did not significantly change (Biri et al., 2006; Lappas et al., 2010). Relative ratio of Cu,Zn-SOD to 8-isoprostane or protein carbonyl was lower in gestational diabetes mellitus placentas, suggesting that the increase in superoxide deismutase is not sufficient to compensate for the developed oxidative stress (Coughlan et al., 2004).

Oxidative stress plays a significant role in both NO overproduction and loss of NO bioavailability (Gloire et al., 2006; Xia et al., 2007). Oxidative stress leads to NOS-dependent increases in NO production in different tissues. Reduction in NO-induced stress is related to diabetes-induced endothelial dysfunction, NOS activation can also be induced by diabetes. NO induces the expression of antioxidant enzymes Mn- and Cu,Zn-SODs, and heme oxygenase-1 and increases intracellular glutathione concentration (Moellering et al., 1999). Although NO stimulates O_2^--induced lipoperoxidation in membranes, it can also mediate protective reactions to inhibit O_2^- and $ONOO^-$ induced lipoperoxidation (Rubbo et al., 1994). NO production has been found increased in the placenta, placental veins and arteries, and in umbilical vein endothelial cells from estational diabetes mellitus patients (Figueroa et al., 2000; vonMadach et al., 2003). NOS expression is also altered, as NOS has been found overexpressed in the placenta and eNoxidative stress increased in umbilical vein endothelial cells from estational diabetes mellitus patients (SanMartin et al., 2006). In estational diabetes mellitus, increases in reactive oxygen specieses and NO production, evident in the placenta and umbilical vessels, lead to peroxynitrite formation. In platelets from estational diabetes mellitus patients, elevated NOS activity and peroxynitrite production have been reported, possibly associated with platelet dysfunction and membrane damage due to increased lipid peroxidation (Mazzanti et al. , 2004). Strong protein nitration is found in term placentas from diabetic rats. Collectively, these data provide evidence of reactive nitrogen species (RNS)-induced damage in estational diabetes mellitus in the placenta and the vasculature of the mother, the placenta, and the umbilical cord, produced as a resulting consequence of exacerbated NO and ROS production.

4.2.4 Role of oxidative stress in gestational diabetes-induced teratogenesis

Diabetes in pregnancy is associated with suboptimal decidualization (Garris et al., 1988). NO plays a key role in decidualization and embryo implantation (Norwitz et al., 2001). It increases vascular permeability, vasodilation, and blood flow in the uterus, and is a component of the decidual cell reaction (Valdes et al., 2009). Diabetes during pregnancy is associated with embryonic dysmorphogenesis. Due to its capacity to regulate cell survival, apoptosis, differentiation, oxidative and nitrosative stresses play a significant role in embryo organogenesis. Low and high levels of NO can lead to embryonic maldevelopment, possibly due to an improper regulation of apoptotic events. During embryo and fetal development, NO has been found to be relevant in regulating differentiation of lung branching morphogenesis, cephalic morphogenesis, heart development, and nephrogenesis (Bloch et al., 1999; Tain et al., 2010).

Transcription factors, as paired box (PAX)-3 and peroxisome proliferator-activated receptor (PPAR) δ, has been found to be involved in the induction of both neural tube and heart malformations, the most common malformations in gestational diabetes pregnants (Higa et al., 2007; Loeken et al., 2006). Different antioxidants such as α-tocopherol and gluthatione ethyl ester increase expression of *PAX-3* and prevent apoptosis and the induction of hyperglycemia-induced neural tube and heart defects (Chang et al., 2003; Morgan et al. 2008). The higher 8-isoprostane levels observed in the offspring of diabetic animals (Wentzel & Erikkson, 2002; Wentzel et al., 1999) have its own teratogenic potency. Diabetic embryopathy is also associated with inhibition of GAPDH activity resulting from an excess of reactive oxygen speciesesin the embryo (Wentzel et al., 2002). Oxidative glucose metabolism is low and about 80% of the glucose used by the placenta. The effect of oxidative stress on placental glucose metabolism is not known. However, in nongestational tissues, there is certainly evidence demonstrating oxidative stress regulates GLUT-1 and/or GLUT-3 dependent glucose uptake and transport. On the other hand estational diabetes mellitus placenta is less sensitive to oxidative stress due to the heightened level of antioxidants. Under normal conditions, physiological levels of reactive oxygen speciesespromote and stimulate adequate insulin signaling. The insulin signaling pathway leads to low levels of reactive oxygen species production itself and ROS act as second messengers of which disposal impairs insulin signaling. Insulin-induced reactive oxygen specieses production is accounted for by activation of the NADPH oxidase NOX4 through PI3K. The reactive oxygen speciespathway subsequently activates kinases or induces gene expression by redox-sensitive transcription (Omroy, 2007).

4.3 Intrauterine Growth Restriction (IUGR)

Fetal growth depends on the interactions of genetic and epigenetic determinants functioning against an environment of maternal, fetal, and placental influences (Gardosi *et al.,* 1992). Intrauterine growth restriction (IUGR) manifests as a variable syndrome of suboptimal growth and body disproportions rather than a well-defined etiologic entity. Causes for IUGR are diverse and include aneuploidies, non-aneuploid syndromes, infections, metabolic factors and placental disorders. IUGR places the fetus and neonate at risk of death or disability in the perinatal period (Baschat *et al.* 2000; Bernstein *et al.* 2000) and predisposes the child to a lifelong increased risk for hypertension, cardiovascular disorders and renal disease, among others (Murphy *et al.,* 2006). A common definition is an estimated fetal weight less than the 10th percent for gestational age. Diminished fetal arterial and venous Doppler flows in key vascular beds predict worsening fetal acid base status (Rizzo et al., 2001; Baschat *et al.* 2004) and such findings frequently lead to delivery of a markedly premature baby to avoid *in utero* demise.

A diverse number of stimuli and mediators contribute to the observed injury to the chorioallantoic villi but oxidative stress is high on the list as an injurious agent (Hung *et al.,* 2002). The production of reactive oxygen species during oxidative stress is linked with tissue injury in many diseases (Ryter *et al.,* 2007). Paper shows that the placentas of pregnancies with IUGR exhibit overt signs of oxidative stress, with reduced protein translation and particular reductions in key signalling proteins pathways (Yung *et al.,* 2008). Moreover, the syncytiotrophoblast shows signs of endoplasmatic reticulum (ER) stress by activating the unfolded protein response, which leads to an ER signal for enhanced apoptosis. The identified dysregulation of protein translation, signalling pathways and trophoblast turnover in placentas of pregnancies with IUGR (Burton *et al.,* 2009). Hypoxia, ischaemia/reperfusion, or both may contribute to placental injury through mechanisms other than reactive oxygen species generation, as variable blood flow to organs also activates the complement cascade (Levy *et al.,* 2000; Hung *et al.,* 2002; Heazell *et al,.* 2008). Activation of the complement cascade injure the feto-placental unit (Girardi *et al,.* 2003).

Clarifying the role of complement activation in pregnancies complicated by IUGR, and in placental dysfunction generally, may lead to new approaches to treatment for IUGR, as therapeutic options to modulate complement receptors and complement activity are on the horizon.

5. Role of antioxidant supplementation in pregnancy

Clinical and research centers are investigating the usefulness of antioxidant supplementation and their role in prevention of pathological pregnancies. Antioxidant supplementation, for example vitamin C and vitamin E, has been shown to have beneficial effects in preventing luteal phase deficiency and resultant increased pregnancy rate (Hemi et al., 2003; Crha et al., 2003). Meta-analysis investigating the intervention of vitamin-C supplementation in pregnancy was inconclusive (Rumbold et al, 2005). Another meta-analysis of women taking any of the vitamin supplements started prior to 20 weeks' gestation revealed no reduction in total fetal losses, or in early and late miscarriage, having used the fixed-effects model. Improved pregnancy rates were also reported with combination therapy with the antioxidants pentoxifylline and vitamin-E supplementation for 6 months in patients with thin endometria who were undergoing in vitro fertilization with oocyte donation (Ledee-Bataille et al., 2002). Supplementation with vitamin E has also been reported to prevent the deleterious effects of ethanol toxicity on cerebral development in the animal model (Peng et al., 2005). There are essential differences among the population groups and the dosage and duration of supplementation for prevention of preeclampsia. Although many advances are being made in the field of antioxidants therapy, the data are still debatable and need further controlled evaluations in larger populations (Ashok et al., 2006).

6. Conclusions

The establishment of pregnancy requires a harmonic hormonal, ovarial and fallopian tube function, a receptive uterus able to respond to a variety of biochemical and molecular signals produced by the developing conceptus, as well as specific interactions between the uterine endometrium and the extra-embryonic membranes. Therefore, the fetal, placental development and function are prerequisites for an adequate supply of nutrients and oxygen to the fetus and successful establishment of pregnancy. Oxidative stress is a complex system, affecting in a complex way the female fertility, and pregnancy outcome. The inbalance of the oxidative agents and antioxidants has been proposed as the causative agents of female sterility, recurrent pregnancy loss and several pregnancy-related disorders, most notably preeclampsia, intra-uterine growth restriction (IUGR) and gestational diabetes.

Preeclampsia is characterized by increased oxidative stress due to the imbalance between lipid peroxidation and antioxidant defense mechanisms, leading to endothelial dysfunction and free radical mediated cell injury. Other maternal factors including activated neutrophils and imbalance between anticoagulants and procoagulants aggravate the oxidative stress and endothelial dysfunction this plays crucial role in developement of the disease. There is no doubt that both hypoxia and hypoxia-reperfusion lead to reactive oxygen species production, but both may also arise from the same underlying problem of impaired conversion of the spiral arteries. The effects of the reduced trophoblast invasion associated with complicated pregnancies can easily be superimposed on this basic model. Reduced invasion will leave the spiral arteries vasoreactive, and thus more likely to undergo spontaneous transient vasoconstriction. They will be more responsive to endogenous and exogenous vasoactive stimuli. Partial obliteration of their lumens by atherotic changes will also impair flow. Excessive production of inflammatory cytokines, deportation of apoptotic microvillous placental fragments, activation of maternal leukocytes and platelets, or depletion of NO production may then cause or contribute to the maternal endothelial response. The degree of the oxidative stress will likely reflect the extent of the maternal vascular pathology.

There are a number of pathways that may contribute to oxidative stress observed in the gestational diabetes mellitus placenta. In the placenta, reactive oxygen species and reactive nitrite spesies are an important source of growth and signaling factors, and are susceptible to ROS-mediated apoptosis. The placenta is endowed with many antioxidants, some of which are increased in gestational diabetes mellitus. However, there is much data to indicate that maternal diabetes during pregnancy may induce oxidative stress in the newborn that may entail biochemical disturbances of the fetus (Hung et al., 2006). Given that The placenta provides the interface of the maternal and fetal circulations, it may play a crucial role in protecting the fetus from adverse effects of the maternal diabetic milieu (Lappas et al., 2011).

The investigation of oxidtive stress is inevitabile for better understanding of aerobe organism function. Evaluation of environmental factors effect on oxidative stress molecular pathways can sereve possible solutions for female reproductive malfunctions. The are several fertility and pregnancy related disease, as unexplained infertility, preeclampsia, HELLP syndrome where the reactive oxidative species and antioxidant mechanism play key role in pathogenesis of the disease. The antioxidant supplementation, avoidance of different enviromental factors, as polluted comestibles may lead to decrease of infertility rate and incidence of pregnancy related disorders.

7. References

Agarwal A, Allamaneni SS. (2004). Role of free radicals in female reproductive diseases and assisted reproduction. *Reprod Biomed Online*, 9, 338-47.

Allen RG. (1991). Oxygen-reactive species and antioxidant response during development. The metabolic paradox of cellular differentiation. *Soc Exp Biol Med*, 196, 117–129.

Anastasiou E, Lekakis JP, Alevizaki M, Papamichael CM, Megas J, Souvatzoglou A, Stamatelopoulos SF. (1998). Impaired endothelium-dependent vasodilatation in women with previous gestational diabetes. *Diabetes Care*, 21, 2111–2115.

Behrman HR, Kodaman PH, Preston SL, Gao S. (2001). Oxidative stress and the ovary. *J Soc Gynecol Investig*, 8, S40–S42.

Biri A, Onan A, Devrim E, Babacan F, Kavutcu M, Durak I. (2006). Oxidant status in maternal and cord plasma and placental tissue in gestational diabetes. *Placenta* 27, 327-332.

Bloch W, Fleischmann BK, Lorke DE, Andressen C, Hops B, Hescheler J, Addicks K. (1999). Nitric oxide synthase expression and role during cardiomyogenesis. *Cardiovasc Res*, 43: 675–684.

Carew JS, Giles FJ and Nawrocki ST (2008) Histone deacetylase inhibitors: mechanisms of cell death and promise in combination cancer therapy. *Cancer Lett* 269:7-17.

Chang TI, Horal M, Jain SK, Wang F, Patel R, Loeken MR. (2003). Oxidant regulation of gene expression and neural tube development: insights gained from diabetic pregnancy on molecular causes of neural tube defects. *Diabetologia,* 46, 538–545.

Chaudhari L, Tandon OP, Vaney N, Agarwal N. (2003). Lipid peroxidation and antioxidant enzymes in gestational diabetics. *Indian J Physiol Pharmacol* 47, 441–446.

Colomiere M, Permezel M, Riley C, Desoye G, Lappas M. (2009). Defective insulin signaling in placenta from pregnancies complicated by gestational diabetes mellitus. *Eur J Endocrinol* 160, 567–578.

Coughlan MT, Oliva K, Georgiou HM, Permezel JM, Rice GE. (2001). Glucose-induced release of tumour necrosis factor-alpha from human placental and adipose tissues in gestational diabetes mellitus. *Diabet Med,* 18, 921–927.

Coughlan MT, Vervaart PP, Permezel M, Georgiou HM, Rice GE. (2004). Altered placental oxidative stress status in gestational diabetes mellitus. *Placenta,* 25, 78–84.

Crha I, Hrubá D, Ventruba P, Fiala J, Totusek J, Visnová H. (2003). Ascorbic acid and infertility treatment. *Cent Eur J Public Health,* 11,63–67.

El Hage S, Singh SM. (1990). Temporal expression of genes encoding free radical-metabolizing enzymes is associated with higher mRNA levels during in vitro development in mice. *Dev Genet,* 11, 149–159.

El Mouatassim S, Guerin P, Menezo Y. (1999). Expression of genes encoding antioxidant enzymes in human and mouse oocytes during the final stages of maturation. *Mol Hum Reprod,* 5, 720–725.

Evans MD, Dizdaroglu M, Cooke MS. (2004). Oxidative DNA damage and disease: induction, repair and significance. *Mutat Res,* 567, 1-61.

Figueroa R, Martinez E, Fayngersh RP, Tejani N, Mohazzab HK, Wolin MS. (2000). Alterations in relaxation to lactate and H(2)O(2) in human placental vessels from gestational diabetic pregnancies. *Am J Physiol Heart Circ Physiol,* 278, 706–713.

Gao L, Mann GE. (2009). Vascular NAD(P)H oxidase activation in diabetes: a double-edged sword in redox signalling. *Cardiovasc Res,* 82, 9–20.

Garris DR. (1988). Effects of diabetes on uterine condition, decidualization, vascularization, and corpus luteum function in the pseudopregnant rat. *Endocrinology,* 122, 665–672.

Gloire G, Legrand-Poels S, Piette J. (2006). NF-kappaB activation by reactive oxygen species: fifteen years later. *Biochem Pharmacol,* 72, 1493–1505.

Gupta S, Agarwal A, Sharma RK. (2005). The role of placental oxidative stress and lipid peroxidation in preeclampsia. *Obstet Gynecol Surv,* 12, 807-816.

Gupta S, Labinskyy N, Gupte R, Csiszar A, Ungvari Z, Edwards JG. (2010). Role of NAD(P)H oxidase in superoxide generation and endothelial dysfunction in Goto-Kakizaki (GK) rats as a model of nonobese NIDDM. *PLoS One,* 5, 11800.

Gurvich N, Berman MG, Wittner BS, Gentleman RC, Klein PS and Green JBA (2005) Association of valproate-induced teratogenesis with histone deacetylase inhibition in vivo. *FASEB J* 19,1166-1180.

Halliwell B, Gutteridge JMC, Cross C. (1992). Free radicals, antioxidants and human diseases: where are we now? *Lab Clin Med,* 119, 598–613.

Halliwell B, Gutteridge JMC. (1995). Free radicals in biology and medicine, *Clarendon Press,* Oxford.

Halliwell B. (1990). How to characterize a biological antioxidant. *Free Radic Res Commun,* 9, 1–32.

Hannemann MM, Liddell WG, Shore AC, Clark PM, Tooke JE. (2002). Vascular function in women with previous gestational diabetes mellitus. *J Vasc Res*, 39, 311–319.

Hass M, Iqbal J, Clearch LB, Brank L, Massaro D.(1989). Cu, Zn superoxide dismutase, isolation and sequence of full-length cDNA and studies of enzyme induction. *J Clin Invest*, 83, 1241–1245.

Henmi H, Endo T, Kitajima Y, Manase K, Hata H, Kudo R. (2003). Effects of ascorbic acid supplementation on serum progesterone levels in patients with a luteal phase defect. *Fertil Steril*, 80, 459–461.

Higa R, Gonzalez E, Pustovrh MC, White V, Capobianco E, Martinez N, Jawerbaum A. (2007). PPARdelta and its activator PGI2 are reduced in diabetic embryopathy: involvement of PPARdelta activation in lipid metabolic and signalling pathways in rat embryo early organogenesis. *Mol Hum Reprod*, 13, 103–110.

Hung TH, Burton GJ. (2006). Hypoxia and reoxygenation: a possible mechanism for placental oxidative stress in preeclampsia. *Taiwan J Obstet Gynecol*, 3,189-200.

Jain M, Brenner DA, Cui L, Lim CC, Wang B, Pimentel DR, Koh S, Sawyer DB, Leopold JA, Handy DE, Loscalzo J, Apstein CS, Liao R. (2003). Glucose-6-phosphate dehydrogenase modulates cytosolic redox status and contractile phenotype in adult cardiomyocytes. *Circ Res*, 93, 9–16.

Jauniaux E, Watson AL, Hempstock J, Bao YP, Skepper JN, Burton GJ. (2000). Onset of maternal arterial blood flow and placental oxidative stress. A possible factor in human early pregnancy failure. *Am J Pathol*, 157, 2111–2122.

Jergil M, Kultima K, Gustafson A, Dencker L and Stigson M (2009) Valproic acid–induced deregulation in vitro of genes associated in vivo with neural tube defects. *Toxicol Sci* 108,132-148.

Jiang B, Mendelson R. (2003). USF1 and USF2 mediate inhibition of human trophoblast differentiation and CYP19 gene expression by Mash-2 and hypoxia. *Mol Cell Biol*, 23, 6117-6128.

Jozwik M, Wolczynski S, Szamatowicz M. (1999). Oxidative stress markers in preovulatory follicular fluid in humans. *Mol Hum Reprod*, 5, 409-413.

Kamath U, Rao G, Raghothama C, Rai L, Rao P. (1998). Erythrocyte indicators of oxidative stress in gestational diabetes. *Acta Paediatr*, 87, 676–679.

Karowicz-Bilinska A, Suzin J, Sieroszewsk P. (2002). Evaluation of oxidative stress indices during treatment in pregnant women with intrauterine growth retardation. *Med Sci Monit*, 3, 211-6.

Kinalski M, Sledziewski A, Telejko B, Kowalska I, Kretowski A, Zarzycki W, Kinalska I. (2001). Lipid peroxidation, antioxidant defence and acid-base status in cord blood at birth: the influence of diabetes. *Horm Metab Res*, 33, 227–231.

King GL, Loeken MR. (2004). Hyperglycemia-induced oxidative stress in diabetic complications. *Histochem Cell Biol*, 122, 333–338.

Kirwan JP, Hauguel-De Mouzon S, Lepercq J, Challier JC, Huston-Presley L, Friedman JE, Kalhan SC, Catalano PM. TNF-alpha is a predictor of insulin resistance in human pregnancy. *Diabetes*, 51, 2207–2213.

Kohen R, Nyska A. (2002). Oxidation of biological systems: oxidative stress phenomena, antioxidants, redox reaction and methods for their quantitation. *Toxicol Pathol*, 30, 620–650.

Lappas M, Hiden U, Desoye G, Froehlich J, Mouzon SH, Jawerbaum A. (2011). The Role of Oxidative Stress in the Pathophysiology of Gestational Diabetes Mellitus. *Antioxid Redox Signal.* (epubl).

Lappas M, Mitton A, Permezel M. (2010). In response to oxidative stress, the expression of inflammatory cytokines and antioxidant enzymes are impaired in placenta, but not adipose tissue, of women with gestational diabetes. *J Endocrinol,* 204, 75–84.

Lappas M, Permezel M, Ho PW, Moseley JM, Wlodek ME, Rice GE. (2004). Effect of nuclear factor-kappa B inhibitors and peroxisome proliferator-activated receptor-gamma ligands on PTHrP release from human fetal membranes. *Placenta,* 25, 699–704.

Lédée-Bataille N, Olivennes F, Lefaix JL, Chaouat G, Frydman R, Delanian S. (2002). Combined treatment by pentoxifylline and tocopherol for recipient women with a thin endometrium enrolled in an oocyte donation programme. *Hum Reprod,* 17, 1249–1253.

Loeken MR. (2006). Advances in understanding the molecular causes of diabetes-induced birth defects. *J Soc Gynecol Investig* 13, 2–10.

López-Tinoco C, Roca M, García-Valero A, Murri M, Tinahones FJ, Segundo C, Bartha JL, Aguilar-Diosdado M. (2011). Oxidative stress and antioxidant status in patients with late-onset gestational diabetes mellitus. *Acta Diabetol,* (epubl)

Lushchak VI. (2011). Adaptive response to oxidative stress: Bacteria, fungi, plants and animals. Comp Biochem Physiol C *Toxicol Pharmacol* 153,175-90.

Lushchak VI. (2011). Environmentally induced oxidative stress in aquatic animals. *Aquat Toxicol* 101,13-30.

Maruyama T, Kitaoka Y, Sachi Y, Nakanoin K, Hirota K, Shiozawa T, Yoshimura Y, Fujii S, Yodoi J. (1997). Thioredoxin expression in the human endometrium during the menstrual cycle. *Mol Hum Reprod,* 3, 989–993.

Matsui M, Oshima M, Oshima H, Takaku K, Maruyama T, Yodoi J, Taketo MM. (1996). Early embryonic lethality caused by targeted disruption of the mouse thioredoxin gene. *Dev Biol,* 178, 179–185.

Mazzanti L, Nanetti L, Vignini A, Rabini RA, Grechi G, Cester N, Curzi CM, and Tranquilli AL. (2004). Gestational diabetes affects platelet behaviour through modified oxidative radical metabolism. *Diabet Med,* 21, 68–72.

Menegola E, Di Renzo F, Broccia ML, Prudenziati M, Minucci S, Massa V and Giavini E (2005) Inhibition of histone deacetylase activity on specific embryonic tissues as a new mechanism for teratogenicity. *Birth Defects Res B Dev Reprod Toxicol* 74, 392-398.

Moellering D, Mc Andrew J, Patel RP, Forman HJ, Mulcahy RT, Jo H, and Darley-Usmar VM. (1999). The induction of GSH synthesis by nanomolar concentrations of NO in endothelial cells: a role for gamma-glutamylcysteine synthetase and gamma-glutamyl transpeptidase. *FEBS Lett,* 448, 292–296.

Morgan SC, Relaix F, Sandell LL, Loeken MR. (2008). Oxidative stress during diabetic pregnancy disrupts cardiac neural crest migration and causes outflow tract defects. *Birth Defects Res A Clin Mol Teratol,* 82, 453–463.

Myatt L, Cui X. (2004). Oxidative stress in the placenta. *Histochem Cell Biol,* 122, 369-382.

Norwitz ER, Schust DJ, Fisher SJ. (2001). Implantation and the survival of early pregnancy. *N Engl J Med,* 345, 1400–1408.

Ornoy A, Zaken V, Kohen R. (1999). Role of reactive oxygen species (ROS) in the diabetes-induced anomalies in rat embryos in vitro: reduction in antioxidant enzymes and LMWA may be the causative factor for increased anomalies. *Teratology*, 60, 376–386.

Ornoy A. (2007). Embryonic oxidative stress as a mechanism of teratogenesis with special emphasis on diabetic embryopathy. *Reprod Toxicol*. 24, 31-41.

Papaccio G, Pisanti FA, Frascatore S. (1986). Acetyl homocysteine thiolactone induced increase: superoxide dismutase counteracts the effect of sub diabetogenic doses of streptozocin. *Diabetes*, 35, 470–474

Paszkowski T, Traub AI, Robinson SY, McMaster D.(1995). Selenium dependent glutathione peroxidase activity in human follicular fluid. *Clin Chim Acta*, 236, 173–180.

Peng Y, Kwok KH, Yang PH, Ng SS, Liu J, Wong OG, He ML, Kung HF, Lin MC. (2005). Ascorbic acid inhibits reactive oxygen speciesesproduction, NF-kappa B activation and prevents ethanol-induced growth retardation and microencephaly. *Neuropharmacology*, 48, 426–434.

Phiel CJ, Zhang F, Huang EY, Guenther MG, Lazar MA and Klein PS (2001) Histone Deacetylase Is a Direct Target of Valproic Acid, a Potent Anticonvulsant, Mood Stabilizer, and Teratogen. *J Biol Chem* 276, 36734-36741.

Rajapakse AG, Ming XF, Carvas JM, Yang Z. (2009). The hexosamine biosynthesis inhibitor azaserine prevents endothelial inflammation and dysfunction under hyperglycemic condition through antioxidant effects. *Am J Physiol Heart Circ Physiol*, 296, 815–822.

Riley JC, Behrman HR. (1991). Oxygen radicals and reactive oxygen species in reproduction. *Proc Soc Exp Biol Med*, 198, 781–791.

Rosselli M, Dubey RK, Imthurn B, Macas E, Keller PJ. (1995). Effects of nitric oxide on human spermatozoa: evidence that nitric oxide decreases sperm motility and induces sperm toxicity. *Hum Reprod*, 10, 1786-1790.

Rubbo H, Radi R, Trujillo M, Telleri R, Kalyanaraman B, Barnes S, Kirk M, Freeman BA. (1994). Nitric oxide regulation of superoxide and peroxynitrite-dependent lipid peroxidation. Formation of novel nitrogen-containing oxidized lipid derivatives. *J Biol Chem*, 269, 26066–26075.

Rumbold A, Crowther CA. (2005). Vitamin C supplementation in pregnancy. *Cochrane Database Syst Rev*, (CD004072).

Sabuncu T, Vural H, Harma M. (2001). Oxidative stress in polycystic ovary syndrome and its contribution to the risk of cardiovascular disease. *Clin Biochem*, 34, 407–413.

San Martin R, Sobrevia L. (2006). Gestational diabetes and the adenosine/L-arginine/nitric oxide (ALANO) pathway in human umbilical vein endothelium. *Placenta*, 27, 1–10.

Sankaralingam S, Xu Y, Sawamura T, Davidge ST. (2009). Increased lectin-like oxidized low-density lipoprotein receptor-1 expression in the maternal vasculature of women with preeclampsia: role for peroxynitrite. *Hypertension*, 53, 270–277.

Shiotani M, Noda Y, Narimoto K, Imai K, Mori T, Fujimoto K, Ogawa K. (1991). Immunohistochemical localization of superoxide dismutase in the human ovary. *Hum Reprod*, 6, 1349–1353.

Siddiqui IA, Jaleel A, Tamimi W, Al Kadri HM. (2010). Role of oxidative stress in the pathogenesis of preeclampsia. *Arch Gynecol Obstet*, 282, 469-474.

Sugino N, Karube-Harada A, Sakata A, Takiguchi S, Kato H. (2002). Nuclear factor-kappa B is required for tumor necrosis factor-alpha-induced manganese superoxide dismutase expression in human endometrial stromal cells. *J Clin Endocrinol Metab*, 87, 3845–3850.

Sugino N, Karube-Harada A, Taketani T, Sakata A, Nakamura Y. (2004). Withdrawal of ovarian steroids stimulates prostaglandin F2alpha production through nuclear factor-kappaB activation via oxygen radicals in human endometrial stromal cells: potential relevance to menstruation. *J Reprod Dev*, 50, 215–225.

Sugino N, Shimamura K, Takiguchi S, Tamura H, Ono M, Nakata M, Nakamura Y, Ogino K, Uda T, Kato H. (1996). Changes in activity of superoxide dismutase in the human endometrium throughout the menstrual cycle and in early pregnancy. *Hum Reprod*, 11, 1073-1078.

Surapaneni KM, Vishnu Priya V. (2008). Antioxidant enzymes and vitamins in gestational diabetes. *J Clin Diagn Res*, 2, 1081–1085.

Taguchi M, Alfer J, Chwalisz K, Beier HM, Classen-Linke I. (2000). Endothelial nitric oxide synthase is differently expressed in human endometrial vessels during the menstrual cycle. *Mol Hum Reprod* , 6, 185-190.

Tain YL, Hsieh CS, Lin IC, Chen CC, Sheen JM, and Huang LT. (2010). Effects of maternal L-citrulline supplementation on renal function and blood pressure in offspring exposed to maternal caloric restriction: the impact of nitric oxide pathway. *Nitric Oxid*, 23, 34–41.

Tamate K, Sengoku K, Ishikawa M. (1995). The role of superoxide dismutase in the human ovary and fallopian tube. *J Obstet Gynaecol*, 21, 401–409.

Telfer JF, Lyall F, Norman JE, Cameron IT. (1995). Identification of nitric oxide synthase in human uterus. *Hum Reprod*, 10, 19-23.

Tseng L, Zhang J, Peresleni T, Goligorsky MS. (1996). Cyclic expression of endothelial nitric oxide synthase mRNA in the epithelial glands of human endometrium. *J Soc Gynecol Investig*, 3, 33-38.

Tung EWY and Winn LM (2010) Epigenetic modifications in valproic acid-induced teratogenesis.*Toxicol Appl Pharmacol* 248, 201-209.

Valdes G, Kaufmann P, Corthorn J, Erices R, Brosnihan KB, Joyner-Grantham J. (2009). Vasodilator factors in the systemic and local adaptations to pregnancy. *Reprod Biol Endocrinol*, 7, 79.

von Mandach U, Lauth D, and Huch R. (2003). Maternal and fetal nitric oxide production in normal and abnormal pregnancy. *J Matern Fetal Neonatal Med*, 13, 22–27.

Wentzel P and Eriksson UJ. (2002). 8-Iso-PGF(2alpha) administration generates dysmorphogenesis and increased lipid peroxidation in rat embryos in vitro. *Teratology*, 66, 164–168.

Wentzel P, Ejdesjö A, Eriksson UJ. (2003). Maternal diabetes in vivo and high glucose in vitro diminish GAPDH activity in rat embryos. *Diabetes*, 52, 1222–1226.

Wentzel P, Welsh N, Eriksson UJ. (1999). Developmental damage, increased lipid peroxidation, diminished cyclooxygenase-2 gene expression, and lowered prostaglandin E2 levels in rat embryos exposed to a diabetic environment. *Diabetes* 48, 813–820.

Xia Y. (2007). Superoxide generation from nitric oxide synthases. *Antioxid Redox Signal* 9, 1773–1778.

Xue M, Qian Q, Adaikalakoteswari A, Rabbani N, Babaei-Jadidi R, Thornalley PJ. (2008). Activation of NF-E2-related factor-2 reverses biochemical dysfunction of endothelial cells induced by hyperglycemia linked to vascular disease. *Diabetes* 57, 2809–2817.

Zimmerman EF, Potturi RB, Resnick E, Fisher JE. (1994). Role of oxygen free radicals in cocaine-induced vascular disruption in mice. *Teratology*, 49, 192–201.

15

Effects of Oxidative Stress on the Electrophysiological Function of Neuronal Membranes

Zorica Jovanović
Department of Pathological Physiology, Faculty of Medicine, Kragujevac, Serbia

1. Introduction

Numerous experimental and clinical observations suggest that reactive oxygen species (ROS) play a significant role in several pathological conditions of the central nervous system where they directly injure tissue and where their formation may also be a consequence of tissue injury. Reactive oxygen metabolites are particularly active in the brain and neuronal tissue, and they are involved in numerous cellular functions, including cell death and survival. In comparison with other organs of the body, the brain may, for a number of biochemical, physiological and anatomical reasons, be especially vulnerable to oxidative stress and ROS mediated injury. A high metabolic rate (the brain consumes approximately 20% of total-body oxygen) and an abundant supply of transition metals, make the brain an ideal target for free radical attack (Facchinetti et al., 1998; Gutowicz, 2011). In addition, the brain has high susceptibility to oxidative stress due to high polyunsaturated fatty acid content and relatively lower regenerative capacity in comparison with other tissues. On the other hand, the brain is poor in catalytic activity and has moderate amounts of glutathion peroxidase and superoxyde dismutase. Of all the cell types in the body, neuronal cells may be among the most vulnerable to oxidative stress. These cells are continuously exposed to ROS. Accumulating evidence demonstrating that the defense of nerve cells against ROS-mediated oxidative damage is essential for maintaining functionality of nerve cells. Because hydrogen peroxide (H_2O_2) is the peroxide generated in the highest quantity in the brain, the defense against the oxidative stress appears to be particularly important. When production exceeds antioxidant protection, oxidative stress leads to molecular damage. An important component of the cellular detoxification of ROS is the antioxidant glutathione (GSH) (Dringen & Gutterer, 2002; Dringen & Hirrlinger, 2003). Because neurons have limited antioxidant capacity, they rely heavily on their metabolic coupling with astrocytes to combat oxidative stress. Evidence is growing that glutathione plays an important role in the detoxification of H_2O_2 and organic hydroperoxides in the brain and that glutathione is the main antioxidant molecule in neurons (Aoyama et al., 2008; Haskew-Layton et al., 2010; Limon-Pacheco & Gonsebat, 2010). Ongoing studies have shown that neuron-glial compartmentalization of antioxidants is critical for neuronal signaling by H_2O_2, as well as neuronal protection. The neurons are more vulnerable to oxidative stress than astrocytes, due to an insufficient detoxification of ROS via their glutathione system (Dringen et al., 1999; Martin & Teismann, 2009). But, the concentration of glutathione is in relatively lesser quantities in the brain in comparison to the other organs of the body (Skaper et al., 1999). In contrast to other ROS, H_2O_2 is neither a free radical nor an ion, which limits its reactivity (Cohen, 1994). However, in the presence of transition metals such as iron or copper, H_2O_2 can give rise to the indiscriminately reactive and toxic hydroxyl radical ($HO^{\bullet}$) by Fenton chemistry. H_2O_2 is able to diffuse across biological membranes, and therefore can diffuse freely from a site of generation (Bienert et al., 2007; Makino et al., 2004) so that it is well-suited as a diffusible messenger. Increasing evidence indicates that H_2O_2 is a particularly intriguing candidate as an intracellular and intercellular signaling molecule because it is neutral and membrane-permeable (Nistico et al., 2008; Forman et al., *2010)*. Recent research into mechanisms of ROS-induced modifications in ion transport pathways involves: oxidation of sulfhydryl (SH) groups on the ion transport proteins, lipid peroxidation, and alterations of calcium (Ca^{2+}) homeostasis, a major second messenger system (Kourie, 1998). Increases in Ca^{2+} initiate inappropriate activation of several enzyme systems e.g., nitric oxide synthase and phospholipase A_2. Overactivation of these enzymes results in the breakdown of proteins and phospholipids and initiates several cascades that damage cells (Lee et al., 1999). It has been described that elevation in cytoplasmic Ca^{2+} levels activates the mitogen-activated protein kinase (MAPK) cascade (Liu & Templeton, 2008; Son et al., 2011) and the phosphatidylinositol 3′-kinase (PI3K)-Akt pathway (Cheng et al., 2003). ROS produce cell damage through multiple mechanisms, including excitotoxicity, metabolic dysfunction and disturbance of intracellular homeostasis of Ca^{2+} (Halliwell & Gutteridge, 1984; Del Maestro et al., 1980; Bracci, 1992). Activation of glutamate ionotropic receptors promptly triggers membrane depolarization and Ca^{2+} influx, resulting in the activation of several different protein kinases (Ca^{2+}-calmodulin-dependent kinase, protein kinase C and MAPK) and transcription factors, such as cyclic AMP response element binding protein (CREB). Neurons efficiently repair glutamate-induced oxidative DNA damage by a process involving CREB-mediated up-regulation of apurinic endonuclease 1 (APE1) (Yang et al., 2011).

Studies have demonstrated that ROS can induce or mediate the activation of the MAPK pathways (McCubrey et al., 2006). The mechanisms by which ROS can activate MAPK pathways are unclear. Because ROS can alter protein structure and function by modifying critical amino acid residues of proteins (Thannickal & Fanburg, 2000), the oxidative modification of signaling proteins by ROS may be one of the plausible mechanisms for the activation of MAPK pathways. However, the precise molecular target(s) of ROS is unknown. The prevention of oxidative stress by antioxidants blocks MAPK activation after cell stimulation with cellular stimuli indicating the involvement of ROS in activation of MAPK pathways. The recent observations provide a strong argument for activation of MAPK pathways by direct exposure of cells to exogenous H_2O_2 (Ruffels et al., 2004; Son et al., 2011).

The cell membrane would seem of special interest because of its large surface area and because of the susceptibility of membrane unsaturated fatty acids and proteins containing oxidizable amino acids (such as cysteine and methionine) to oxidant attack. Oxidative stress affects cellular membrane lipids and proteins. Cell membranes are either a source of neurotoxic lipid oxidation products or the target of pathogenic processes that cause permeability changes or ion channel formation (Axelsen, 2011). Reactive oxygen metabolites modify ion transport mechanisms either directly via ion transport pathway proteins and regulatory proteins or indirectly via peroxidation of membrane lipids. The nature and sequence of events that lead to the disruptions of these ion transport pathways are not fully understood. Early studies revealed that the effects of ROS on membrane properties could be deduced from electrophysiological parameters of the membrane. These include changes in membrane potential and current, ionic gradients, action potential duration and amplitude, spontaneous activity and excitability (Tarr et al., 1995; Tarr & Valenzeno, 1989; Beleslin et al., 1998). Oxygen-derived free radicals are thought to induce alterations in nervous electrical activity, however, the underlying membrane ionic currents affected by ROS and the mechanisms by which ROS induce their effects on ion channels in the nerve cells are not well defined. Considering neuronal function, ROS can attack ion channels and transporters directly, or indirectly by causing lipid peroxidation (Kourie, 1998; Carmeliet, 1999) and affecting associated signaling molecules (Hool, 2006). The mechanism of initiation of ROS peroxidation is not understood completely. The hydroxyl radical ($HO^•$), a highly reactive oxidant, has been proposed as the initiating species. The ability of the $HO^•$ to initiate lipid peroxidation has been questioned by some investigators. In addition to initiating lipid peroxidation, the $HO^•$ has been implicated in direct cellular damage. Peroxidation of membrane phospholipids has been demonstrated to affect various transmembrane processes, such as receptor activation and formation of intracellular second messengers and Ca^{2+} homeostasis. Ca^{2+} ions also play a central role in the control of neuronal excitability. ROS oxidatively modify numerous membrane-bound proteins including ion channels. ROS can also react with proteins directly and in this case seem to have a prevalence for SH groups or disulfide bridges on the ion transport proteins (Van der Vliet & Bast, 1992). Oxidative sensitivity of ion channels is often conferred by amino acids containing sulfur atoms (Su et al., 2007). The mechanism of ROS-induced modifications in ion transport pathways involves the inhibition of membrane-bound regulatory enzymes and modification of the oxidative phosphorylation and ATP levels.

Studies have demonstrated that oxidative stress, perturbations in the cellular thiol level and redox balance, affects many cellular functions, including signaling pathways. In the CNS, cells respond to oxidative stress by initiating endogenous protective cascades often regulated at the transcriptional level. The transcription factor, nuclear factor erythroid 2-related factor 2 (Nrf2) plays an integral role in astrocyte-mediated protection of neurons from oxidative stress. Previous studies have reported that MAPKs may play a role in the induction and regulation of the Nrf2 system in the brain (Clark & Simon, 2009). When cells are exposed to oxidative stress, the Nrf2 binds to the antioxidant responsive element (ARE). The Nrf2–ARE pathway elicits transcriptional activation of antioxidant genes and detoxifying genes that protect cells and organisms from oxidative stress. Activation of this pathway protects cells from oxidative stress-induced cell death (Hur and Gray, 2011). The NRF2/KEAP1 signaling pathway is the main pathway responsible for cell defense against oxidative stress and maintaining the cellular redox state (Stepkowski & Kruszewski, 2011). The Nrf2-mediated GSH biosynthesis and release from astrocytes protects neurons from oxidative stress (Shih et al., 2003). Increased levels of GSH may be a major component of the protection observed by Nrf2 activation. In the CNS, Nrf2 plays an integral role in astrocyte-mediated protection of neurons from oxidative stress. Neuronal viability is enhanced significantly by an increased supply of GSH precursors from Nrf2-overexpressing glia. Thus Nrf2-dependent enhancement of glial GSH release appears to be necessary and sufficient for neuronal protection. The observations of Correa et al. (2011) suggest that activated microglia can stimulate or reduce the GSH-related anti-oxidant defense in cultured astrocytes. Recently, Zou et al. (2011) reported that overexpression of Nrf2 increased GSH content and efficiently protected t-BHP-induced mitochondrial membrane potential loss and apoptosis in cultured human retinal pigment epithelial cells.

Ion channels and transporters are susceptible to oxidative stress. For example, voltage-dependent Na^+, K^+ and Ca^{2+} channels, Ca^{2+}-activated K^+ channels, and K_{ATP} channels have all been identified as targets for ROS (Hool, 2006). Several previous studies indicate that H_2O_2 alters energy metabolism, ATP- sensitive K^+currents, L-type Ca^{2+}currents (Goldhaber & Liu, 1994; Racay et al., 1997), as well as delayed rectifier K^+ currents (Goldhaber et al., 1989). However in literature the data concerning the effect of ROS on potassium current are controversal. For example, Cerbai et al. (1991) and Ward & Giles (1997) did not observe any effect, in contrast to Tarr & Valenzeno (1989) who obtained a decrease in the outward, delayed rectifier potassium current. The results of Hasan et al. (2007) suggest that oxidative stress, which inhibits the delayed-rectifier current, can alter neural activity. Ward and Giles (1997) studied the effects of H_2O_2 on action potentials and underlying ionic currents in isolated rat ventricular myocytes. They showed that H_2O_2 caused no significant changes in either the Ca^{2+}-independent transient outward K^+ current (Ito) or the inwardly rectifying K^+ current (I_{K1}). The most prominent effect of H_2O_2 on the ionic currents which underlie the action potential is a slowing of inactivation of the I_{Na}. Potassium channels constitute a highly diverse class of ion channel and thus participate in multiple modulatory functions. Although altered potassium dynamics play a major role in this type of neuronal activity (Dudek et al., 1998) the role of K^+ channels is still incompletely understood. The voltage-activated K^+ channels are responsible for the establishment of the resting membrane potential, repolarization during action potentials and regulation of action potential frequency (Vacher et al., 2008). Three principal K^+ currents were identified in LRNC (Stewart et al., 1989). These differed in their time courses of activation and inactivation and in their responses to Ca^{2+} channel blockers. K^+ currents of the A-type (I_A) with rapid activation and inactivation kinetics, were not affected by Ca^{2+} channel blockers. The A-type K^+ currents were a minor component of the outward current in LRNC. A Ca^{2+} activated K^+ current (I_{Ca}), that inactivated more slowly and was reduced by Ca^{2+} channel blockers, constituted the major outward current in LRNC. The third K^+ current resembled the delayed rectifier currents (I_{K1} and I_{K2}) of squid axons, activated and inactivated slowly. Modifications of K^+ channel activity by ROS in the brain would lead to drastic changes in the electrical excitability of neuronal cells and could easily explain a tendency to brain hyperexcitability, or even neuronal death.

2. Materials and methods

All experiments were carried out at room temperature (22-25°C) on the Retzius nerve cells of isolated abdominal segmental ganglia of the ventral nerve cord of the horse leech *Haemopis saguisuga.* The dissection procedure, the recording method and point voltage clamp technique were employed as described previously (Beleslin et al., 1988). Dissected segments of 4 ganglia were immediately transferred to a 2.5 ml plastic chamber with a leech Ringer and fixed by means of fine steel clips. The plastic chamber was then placed in a grounded Faraday's cage mounted on a fixed table in a manner that prevents vibrations. Identification and penetration of the cells was performed in the cage under a stereomicroscope. Retzius neurons were identified based on the position within the ganglion, the size and the bioelectrical properties of the cells. The Retzius cells, are the largest neurons (40-60 μm in diameter) situated on the ventral side of the ganglia. It is well known that the resting potential of Retzius nerve cells of medical and horse leeches are lower than in other neurons (Hagiwara & Morita, 1962; Beleslin, 1985). Theoretically, this can be due to the low resting potassium permeability or the high membrane permeability to sodium. The Retzius cell is spontaneously active and responds to depolarization with an increased firing rate proportional to the depolarization (Lent, 1977). In leech Retzius nerve cells three classes of K^+ channels (fast, slow calcium-activated and late voltage-regulated) have been identified (Beleslin et al., 1982; Beleslin, 1985). To change the solution, the chamber was flushed continuously with a volume of fluid at least five times that of the chamber volume. The perfusion rate was kept low so that implanted microelectrodes remained inside the cells during the perfusion. The bath volume was 2 ml and the solution changes were completed within 30 sec.

2.1 Electrical methods

In this study, we investigated the time-dependent changes in action potential configuration and changes in steady-state membrane currents in leech Retzius nerve cells. The spontaneous spike activity was recorded with a conventional 3 M KCl microelectrode. Membrane voltage and current were recorded using voltage-clamp techniques. This was shown in voltage-clamped neurons by long depolarizing steps (to 500 ms) from the holding potential which was more negative than –40 mV in a sodium free leech Ringer, in order to induce fast and slow K^+ outward currents. The recording electrodes were prepared from 1.5 mm borosilicate capillaries (Clark Electromedical Instruments, UK) and filled with a 3 M KCl-containing solution. The pipette resistance ranged from 5 to 10 MΩ (when filled with 3M KCl solution). Microelectrodes with a tip potential less than 5 mV in an artificial solution, were selected for use. Usually the microelectrode was connected through a Ringer bridge and Ag-AgCl electrode via a negative capacitance high input resistant amplifier "Bioelectric Instrument DS2C" to a computer. Command pulses were derived from a "Tektronix 161" pulse generator. The signals were digitized by the use of an analog-to-digital converter (Digidata 1200; Axon Instruments) and saved in a computer for off-line analysis.

2.2 Solutions

Pharmacological agents were prepared and dissolved immediately before application in the physiological salt solution at the concentrations stated. H_2O_2, cumene hydroperoxide (CHP) and reduced glutathione (GSH), were added to the leech or Tris-Ringer. All drugs were administered sufficient to reach a steady-state response (up to 30 min). The bath volume was 2 ml and the solution changes were completed within 30 sec. The ganglia were bathed in a leech Ringer containing (mM): 115 NaCl, 4 KCl, 2 $CaCl_2$, 1.2 Na_2HPO_4, 0.3 NaH_2PO_4 (pH 7.2). In the Na^+-free Ringer, 115 mM NaCl was completely replaced with an equal amount of Tris (hydroxy-methyl)aminomethane-Cl (Tris Ringer) and Na_2HPO_4 and NaH_2PO_4 were omitted.

Solutions containing H_2O_2 were prepared freshly before their use from 30% H_2O_2 solution (Zorka Pharma, Sabac) and added to the Ringer solution (or Tris-Ringer) at final concentrations of 1, 5 and 10 mM. CHP and GSH were added to the normal or Tris-Ringer solution. The CHP was obtained from Sigma (St. Louis, U.S.A.), dissolved in 0.01% dimethyl sulfoxide (Sigma, St. Louis, U.S.A.) and added to the Ringer solution (or Tris-Ringer) in a concentrations of 0.25, 1 and 1.5 mM. A GSH (Sigma, St. Louis, U.S.A.) was added to the Ringer solution to produce a final concentration of 0.2 mM.

2.3 Data analysis

Data are expressed as mean ± SEM. Comparisons between the mean values were made with a Student's t-analysis. P values <0.05 were considered significant.

3. Results

3.1 Effects of cumene hydroperoxide on the spontaneous spike potential of leech Retzius nerve cells

In our work we used CHP to stimulate lipid peroxidation as the mechanism of free radical-induced cell membrane damage. We investigated the time-dependent changes in action potential configuration and changes in steady-state membrane currents in LRNC. Superfusion of leech abdominal ganglia with CHP (0.25, 1 and 1.5 mM) caused an extreme change to the shape and action potential duration (APD) in LRNC. Exposure of LRNC to CHP prolonged the duration of the action potentials of the LRNC in a concentration-dependent manner. Figure 1 illustrates the representative record obtained 15, 20, 25 and 30 min after the exposure of an isolated ganglia to 1 mM of CHP. A cardiac-like action potential with a rapid depolarization, followed by a sustained depolarization or plateau and fast repolarization was recorded. During the 20 min of exposure with leech Ringer containing 1 mM CHP, early after depolarization was recorded. Higher concentration of CHP led to appearance of repetitive firing only a few minutes after application of CHP, which was followed by loss of excitability of leech Retzius nerve cells.

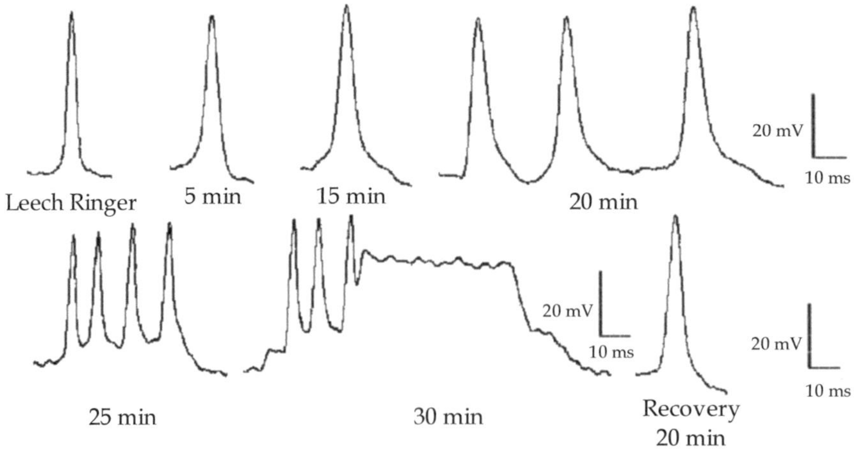

Fig. 1. Early after depolarization and repetitive firing recorded in LRNC after exposure of isolated ganglion to 1 mM CHP

Table 1 summarizes the values of the APD in a leech Ringer and after adding CHP (0.25, 1 and 1.5 mM). Table 1 shows that CHP caused a concentration-dependent increase in APD.

	Leech Ringer	5 min	15 min	20 min	30 min	Recovery 20 min
0.25 mM CHP n= 6	10.45±0.98	12.33±1.74	13.50±2.13	13.50±1.39	14.4±0.80 $P>0.05$	15.66±1.05
1 mM CHP n= 6	9.66±0.52	13.17±4.02	25.17±2.91	31.05±5.96	35.33±13.60 $P\leq0.01$	26.50±8.38
1.5 mM CHP n= 11	9.66±2.18	16.09±3.15	41.64±8.27*	68.72±13.4*	127.80±15.95* $P\leq0.01$	23.43±4.61

Table 1. Values of the APD (in ms) of LRNC before, 5, 15, 20 and 30 minutes after the adding of CHP (0.25, 1 and 1.5 mM) and during the recovery. Data are expressed as mean ± SEM; n=number of cells. * *repetitive firing*

3.2 Effects of hydrogen peroxide on the spontaneous spike potential of leech Retzius nerve cells

Previous investigations have shown that H_2O_2 is involved in cascades of pathological events affecting neural cells. The background of this study were the findings that 1 mM CHP treatment caused an extreme change in the duration of the action potential and suppression of Ca^{2+} activated outward K^+ currents of LRNC. The aim of the present experiments was to examine the effect of the higher concentrations of H_2O_2 on LRNC. H_2O_2 in concentrations up to 10 mM in the reaction mixture had no effect on spontaneous spike potential. Extracellular application of H_2O_2 (1, 5 and 10 mM) did not significantly change ($P > 0.05$) the duration of the action potential of the LRNC. H_2O_2 is ineffective in generating either cardiac-like action potential or early after depolarization in LRNC.

3.3 Effects of glutathione on the cumene hydroperoxide-induced change of the spontaneous spike potential of leech Retzius nerve cells

The background of this study were the findings that the hydroxyl radical scavenger, mannitol (5 mM) significantly reduced neurotoxic effect of CHP on the spontaneous spike electrogenesis of LRNC (Jovanović, 2010).

Taking in to consideration that it has been proved that CHP affects the lasting action potentials of Retzius nerve cells, the possibility of recovering the changes by the effect of antioxidant, GSH was also examined. Firstly, Retzius cells were exposed to the effect of CHP (1 mM) then GSH was added in a concentration of 0.2 mM to the Leech Ringer solution. The application of GSH, a free radical scavenger, to a bathing solution reverses the CHP effects. The GSH, largely inhibited the effects of CHP on the APD. In the presence of the GSH the APD has been extended by 9.22±1.14 ms (in controlled conditions, before the application of

CHP and GSH) to 12.45±1.56 ms (30 min after adding CHP and GSH to the Leech Ringer solution), which did not have any significant statistical result (Table 2). In the presence of GSH repetitive firings has not been registered in any examined cells.

	Leech Ringer	5 min	15 min	20 min	30 min	Recovery 20 min
CHP+GSH n=10	9.22±1.14	8.87±2.34	9.67±1.44	10.76±2.32	12.45±1.56 P>0.05	10.34±1.21

Table 2. Effects of GSH on CHP-induced prolongation of the APD in LRNC.

The APD of LRNC before and after the adding of CHP (1 mM) and GSH (0.2 mM). Data are expressed as mean ± SEM; n=number of cells

The application of 0.2 mM GSH solution significantly decreased the bursting frequency, duration and amplitude of depolarization plateaus, and the number of spikes per plateau. These observations point out the significance of GSH in the protection of SH groups of membrane proteins as well as lipids in oxidative stress caused by CHP.

3.4 Modulation of Ca^{2+} activated K^{+} current in leech Retzius nerve cells by cumene hydroperoxide

The elongation of action potentials by CHP suggested that CHP decreased the magnitude of ion currents needed for the repolarization phase of action potentials. The action potentials of **leech** Retzius nerve cells elongated after the exposure to 1mM of CHP, suggested that CHP modified the outward K^{+} currents that form action potentials together with the Na^{+} current. In order to explore the ionic mechanism by which CHP prolongs spike potential, we examined its effects on membrane K^{+}currents. Several studies have reported the possibility that ROS alter ionic channel function. The K^{+} channels, key regulators of neuronal excitability, are targets of ROS. It is well known that outward K^{+} current are essential for maintaining normal APD. The K^{+} currents contributing to the resting membrane potential and repolarization of the action potential were studied in voltage-clamped Retzius neurones. Modifications of voltage-sensitive K^{+} channel activity by ROS would lead to changes in APD and the electrical excitability of neuronal cells. To test this hypothesis, the effect of CHP on Ca^{2+} activated K^{+} current was studied.

This was shown in voltage-clamped neurons by long depolarizing steps (to 500 ms) from the holding potential which was more negative than –40 mV in the sodium free leech Ringer in order to induce fast and slow K^{+} outward currents. Figure 2 illustrates the typical outward currents elicited in a CHP responsive neuron, depolarized in steps from a holding potential of -56 mV to +4 mV. Both components of the delayed outward K^{+} current, Ikr and Iks were inhibited by external CHP.

Application of CHP (in a concentration of 1 mM) caused suppression of fast and slow Ca^{2+} activated outward K^{+} currents. The fast and slow steady part of the K^{+} outward current was reduced by 40% and 31%, respectively. Figure 2 shows K^{+} current amplitudes measured before and during exposure to CHP.

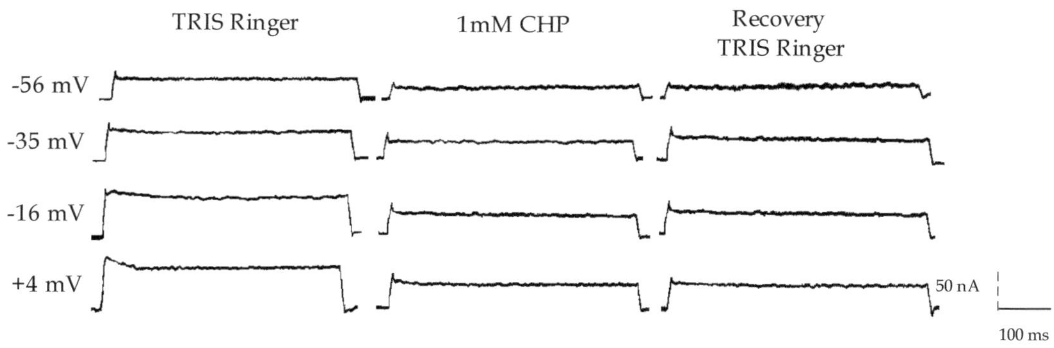

Fig. 2. Patterns of voltage clamp current record obtained from Retzius nerve cell in Tris-Ringer, after adding 1 mM CHP and again in an Na-free fluid (recovery) during displacement of holding potential from -56 mV to +4 mV.

Figure 3 shows the current-voltage relationship, separately, for the peak and established a steady level of depolarizing K^+ outward current. At the test potential of +4 mV the fast and late steady part of the K^+ outward current dropped from 60 to 36 nA (40%) and from 33 to 23 nA (31%). These results demonstrate the marked electrophysiological effects of CHP in leech Retzius nerve cells. Upon washout of the CHP, the fast and slow steady part of the K^+ outward current recovered by approximately 30% and 40% within 15 min.

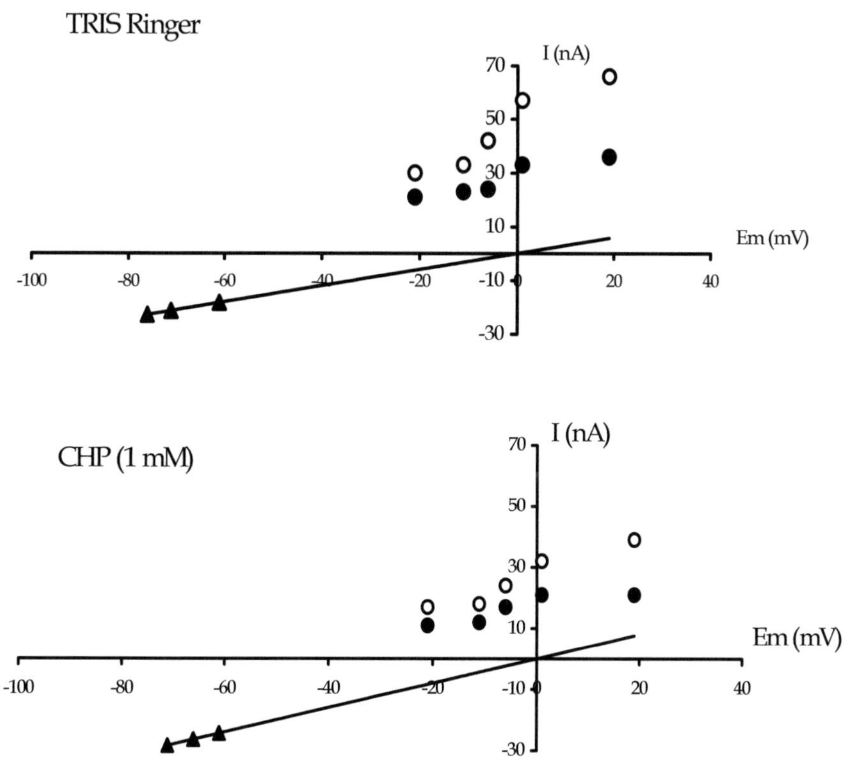

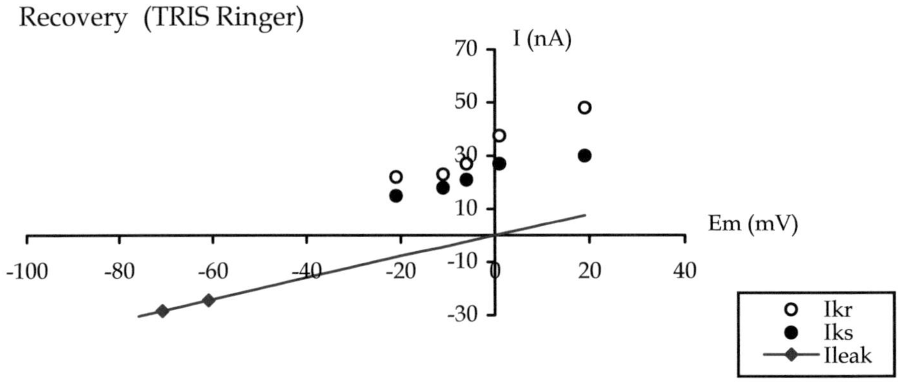

Fig. 3. The current-voltage relationship for the same cell, measured at the peak of the K^+ outward current (open circles) and at the end of stimulation (solid circles) in the Tris-Ringer, 25 min after adding 1 mM CHP and during the recovery.

3.5 Effects of hydrogen peroxide on the Ca^{2+} activated K^+ current of leech Retzius nerve cells

Modification of on membrane potassium currents by H_2O_2, a membrane-permeable form of ROS, in LRNC was examined using the voltage clamp technique. Using a two-electrode voltage clamp, we examined the H_2O_2 effect on the K^+ outward current. In contrast to the effect of CHP, application of the H_2O_2 failed to inhibit fast and slow outward K^+ currents in leech Ringer. At the test potential of -14 mV from holding potential of -77 mV, the fast and late steady part of K^+ outward current dropped by 7.48% and 6.07%, respectively. In the current-voltage relationship (Fig. 4) there were no significant changes on the early or late part of the K^+ outward current in the presence of H_2O_2. Voltage clamp experiments using double microelectrode methods revealed that H_2O_2 reduced a fast and slow K^+ outward current by 7.48% and 6.07% respectively at the test potential of -14 mV, after 25 min.

Ikr- rapid Ca^{2+} activated K^+ current; Iks- slow Ca^{2+} activated K^+ current; Ileak - passive leak current

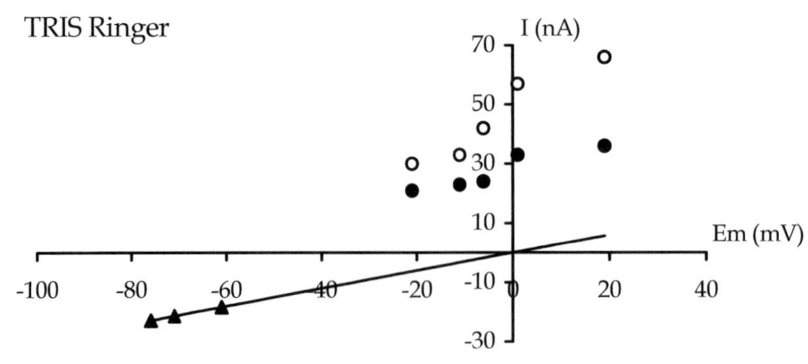

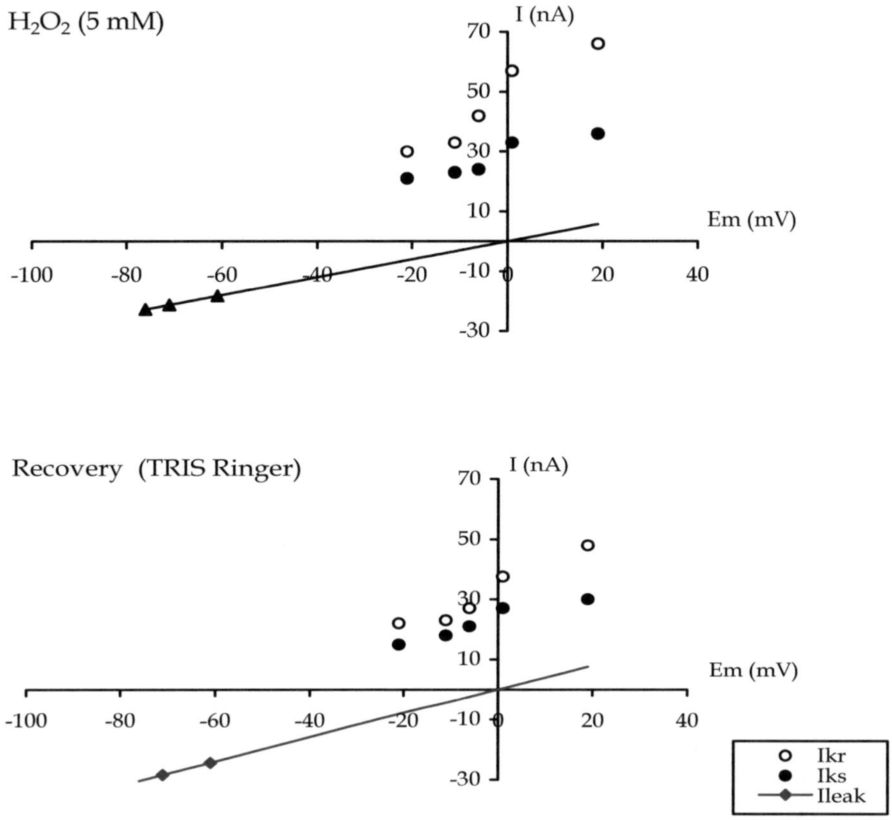

Fig. 4. Current-voltage relationship for the same cell measured at the peak of the K^+ outward current (open circles) and at the end of stimulation (solid circles) in Tris-Ringer, 25 min after adding 5 mM H_2O_2 and during the recovery.

Ikr- rapid Ca^{2+} activated K^+ current; Iks- slow Ca^{2+} activated K^+ current; Ileak - passive leak current

3.6 Effects of glutathione on cumene hydroperoxide-induced suppression of the Ca^{2+} activated K^+ current of leech Retzius nerve cells

Reduced glutathione applied in a concentration of 0.2 mM partially blocked the effect of CHP on Ca^{2+} activated outward K^+ currents. Figure 5 illustrates the effect of GSH on Ca^{2+} activated K^+ currents. The application of the GSH reduced fast and slow K^+ outward currents in the leech Ringer. At the test potential of -17 mV from the holding potential of -57 mV, the fast and late steady part of the K^+ outward current dropped by 21% and 12%, respectively.

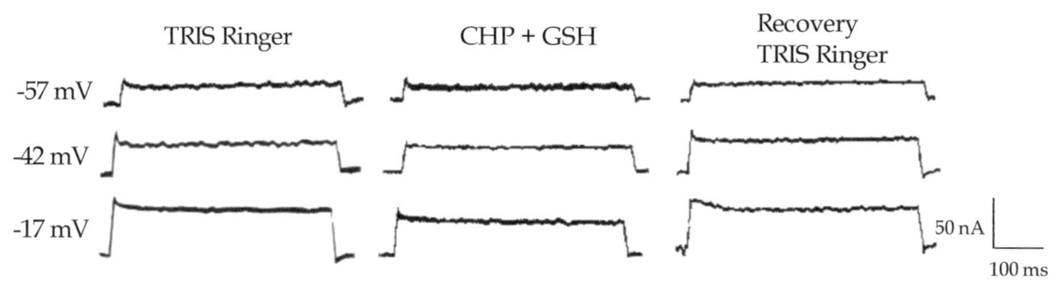

Fig. 5. Patterns of the voltage clamp current record obtained from Retzius nerve cell in the Tris-Ringer, after adding 1 mM CHP and 0.2 mM GSH, and in Na-free fluid (recovery) during displacement of the holding potential from -57 mV to -17 mV.

In the corresponding current-voltage relationship (Fig. 6) there were no significant changes on the early or late part of the K^+ outward current in the presence of 1 mM CHP and 0.2 mM GSH. At the test potential of -17 mV the fast and late steady part of the K^+ outward current dropped from 65 to 51 nA (21%) and from 46 to 38 nA (12%).

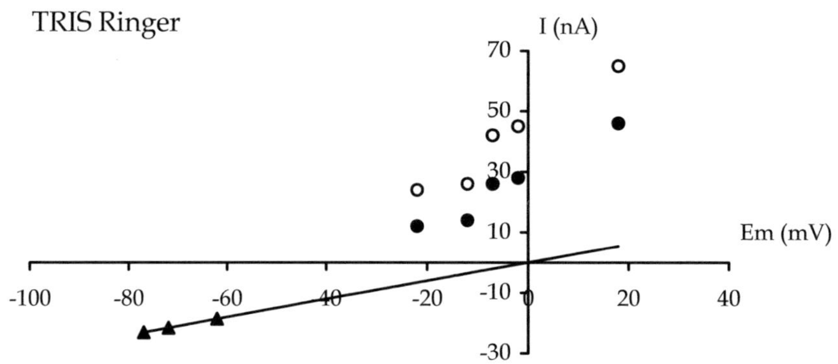

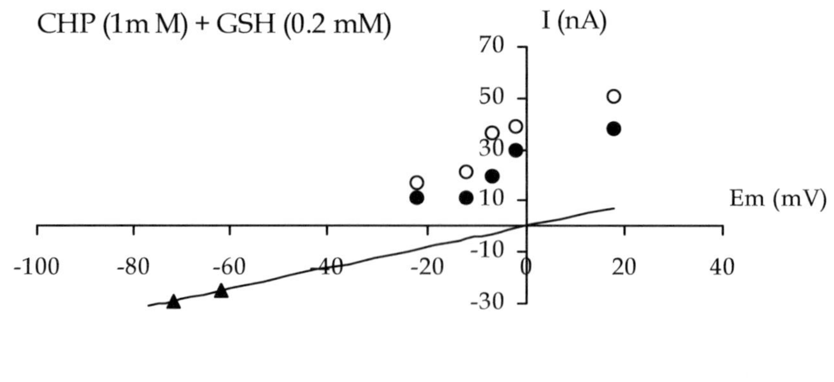

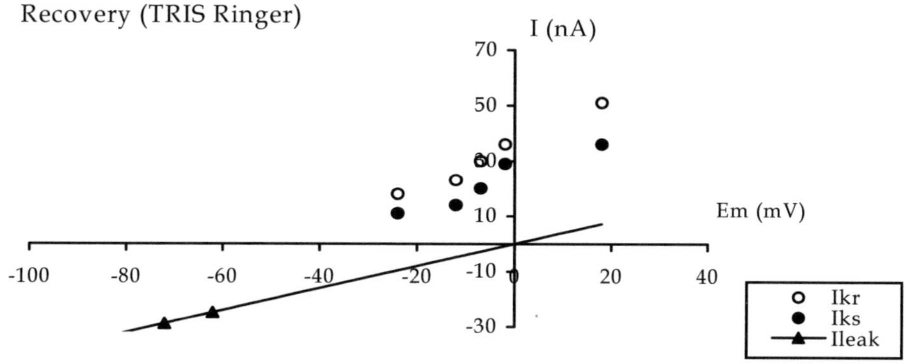

Fig. 6. Current-voltage relationship for the same cell measured at the peak of the potassium outward current (open circles) and at the end of stimulation (solid circles) in the Tris-Ringer, 25 min after adding 1 mM CHP and 0.2 mM GSH, and during the recovery.

Ikr- rapid Ca^{2+} activated K^+ current; Iks- slow Ca^{2+} activated K^+ current; Ileak - passive leak current

4. Discussion

The interest in H_2O_2 as a biologically active oxygen-derived intermediate is evident, because it is associated to a series of alterations and effects in different types of cells. The present data show that H_2O_2 did not significantly change, within 30 min, the shape of the amplitude of spontaneous spike potentials of LRNC. In the voltage clamp experiments, H_2O_2 was ineffective in the supression of fast and slow Ca^{2+} activated K^+ currents. The background of this study were the findings that a 1 mM H_2O_2 treatment with or without $FeCl_2$ did not significantly change the resting membrane potential of LRNC (Jovanović & Beleslin, 1996; Jovanović & Beleslin, 1997; Jovanović & Beleslin, 2004).

The present results suggest that leech ganglia have an efficient system against oxidative stress. There are several explanations why leech Retzius nerve cells should be resistant to H_2O_2. The simplest could be that leech Retzius nerve cells have a low concentration of polyunsaturated fatty acids, which are very sensitive to radical injury. This possibility is unlikely since neuronal membrane are rich in lipids (Whittemore et al., 1995; Wilson, 1997). Another explanation could be that they have an efficient scavenging enzyme system which reacts rapidly with H_2O_2. Peroxidation of lipids that inactivates membrane-associated enzymatic protein, increases membrane permeability. However, since we have insignificant changes in action potential with H_2O_2, it is reasonable to suppose that lipid membrane peroxidation did not occur. On the other hand, since changes in the action potential were not significant, it could further be expected that H_2O_2 was decomposed by a number of enzymatic and nonenzymatic antioxidant systems. A possible explanation for weak responses of LRNC to H_2O_2 is that the extracellular H_2O_2 application, results in an intracellular concentration some 7–10-fold below that of extracellular (Stone, 2004). It is well known that concentration as well as time of exposure plays an important role in the response generated by ROS. The range of [H_2O_2] used by different authors varies from 0.1 to 50 mM (Kourie, 1998).

When cells are exposed to external H_2O_2, the intracellular consumption of H_2O_2 catalyzed by anti-oxidants and enzymes is able to generate a gradient of H_2O_2 across membranes, which makes the intracellular H_2O_2 concentration lower than the extracellular one. Previous studies have reported that H_2O_2 did not affect channel activity when added to the extracellular side (Soto, 2002). In particular, oxidation of free SH groups of cysteines, present in a greater proportion at the intracellular side, could explain the observed difference. These results provide evidence for an intracellular site(s) of H_2O_2 action. It has been recently demonstrated that H_2O_2 activates TRPC6 channels via modification of thiol groups of intracellular proteins (Graham et al., 2010). H_2O_2 is a weaker oxidizing agent than other ROS. H_2O_2 is not by itself reactive enough to oxidize organic molecules in an aqueous environment. Nevertheless, the biological importance of H_2O_2 stems from its participation in the production of more reactive chemical species such as $HO^•$ and its role as a source of free radicals has been emphasized rather than its chemical reactivity. However, because of its extremely short half-life, $HO^•$ is effective only near the locus of its production.

The results reported in this paper show that an alkyl-hydroperoxide, CHP is a more efficient oxidant than H_2O_2. In contrast to H_2O_2, CHP, induced dose and time dependent membrane depolarization with a marked prolongation of spontaneous repetitive activity. These actions appear to underlie the prolongation of the action potential, and contribute to repetitive firing. Several mechanisms have been proposed for the plateau of the prolonged action potential, such as sustained inward Na^+ current, block of Ca^{2+} activated K^+ channels, modification of Ca^{2+} channels or its transformation in Na^+ channels. Our findings support the second proposal. A possible explanation is that CHP form free radicals that are more stable than the $HO^•$. H_2O_2 and organic hydroperoxides, generate distinct ROS. $HO^•$ generated by one-electron reduction of the H_2O_2, damages adjacent molecules at diffusion controlled rates. By contrast, the organic hydroperoxide triggers the generation of the free radical intermediates peroxyl and alkoxyl radicals, which can cross cellular membranes and evoke the production of the $HO^•$ (Hwang et al., 2009). It was well known that $HO^•$ generated from H_2O_2 could cause peroxidation of lipids that inactivates membrane-associated protein, increasing membrane permeability. This metabolic and physico-chemical alteration of a cell membrane would produce intracellular Ca^{2+} overload. CHP is more hydrophobic than H_2O_2. The most important finding of the present study is that CHP modulates Ca^{2+} activated K^+ channels in leech Retzius nerve cells. In the voltage clamp experiments, fast and slow Ca^{2+} activated outward K^+ currents were suppressed with CHP. The present results support the view that CHP stimulates lipid peroxidation, as the mechanism of ROS-induced cell membrane injury.

Although several previous investigations have described electrophysiological effects of H_2O_2 and CHP, the literature describing these effects is sometimes contradictory. For example, Cerbai et al. (1991) and Ward and Giles (1997) did not observe any effect, in contrast to Tarr and Valenzeno (1989) who obtained a decrease in the rectifying current. Vega-Saenz de Miera and Rudy (1992) reported that H_2O_2 inhibited three cloned voltage-gated K^+ channels expressed in Xenopus oocytes. A recent paper reported that ROS donors (H_2O_2 and t-BHP) reduced the voltage operated Ca^{2+} current but increased the amplitude of the delayed rectifier K^+ current in adult rat intracardiac ganglion neurons (Dyavanapalli et al., 2010; Whyte et al., 2009). Nakaya et al. (1992) examined the mechanism of membrane depolarization induced by CHP in guinea-pig papillary muscles, using ion-selective microelectrode and patch clamp techniques. They demonstrated that the depolarization of the resting membrane is, at least in part, due to the inhibition of inward rectifier K^+ channel activity, and may play an important role in the genesis of reperfusion-induced arrhythmias.

There are conflicting descriptions of the current changes induced by ROS, and an incomplete understanding of which is responsible for the observed changes in action potential duration. For example, the inward rectifying K^+ current has been reported to be either unaffected (Cerbai et al., 1991) or decreased (Tarr & Valenzeno, 1991). The electrophysiological effects of ROS generally consist of a reduction in action potential amplitude and an increase in action potential duration followed by a reduction (Tarr and Valenzeno, 1989; Barrington, 1994; Satoh and Matsui, 1997), although either only a reduction (Goldhaber et al., 1989; Hayashi et al., 1989; Coetzee et al., 1990) or only an increase in action potential duration (Barrington, 1994) have also been reported. Nakaya et al. (1991) reported that ROS-induced shortening of the action potential duration of guinea-pig isolated ventricular myocytes. The underlying mechanisms of the action potential shortening are undoubtedly complex, and changes in membrane currents other than the outward current through the ATP-sensitive K^+ channels may also contribute to the action potential shortening. Matsuura and Shattock (1991) demonstrated that oxidant stress induces a decrease in the resting potassium conductance and an increase in Ca^{2+} activated membrane conductance. Both factors may underlie the depolarization of resting membrane potential, prolongation of the action potential and automaticity. Tokube et al. (1996) reported biphasic changes in the action potential duration, with initial lengthening of the action potential and subsequent shortening. In voltage-clamp experiments, ROS suppressed the L-type calcium current, the delayed rectifier K^+ current and the inward rectifier K^+ current. A recent paper reported that relatively low concentrations of CHP (100 μM) led to a significant decrease in the cellular content of ATP and reduced glutathione (Vimard et al., 2010).

K^+ channels are a family of ion channels that govern the intrinsic electrical properties of neurons in the brain (Lujan, 2010). K^+ currents control action potential duration, Ca^{2+} dependent synaptic plasticity, the release of neurotransmitters and epileptiform burst activity. Enhanced excitability of K^+ channels (via downmodulation, or changes in biophysical properties such as inactivation kinetics and voltage dependence), could all result in enhanced Ca^{2+} responses to firing activity (Pongs, 1999). Ca^{2+} activated K^+ channels are a large family of K^+ channels that are found throughout the central nervous system and in many other cell types, but its *in vivo* physiological functions have not been fully defined. Ca^{2+} dependent K^+ channels are activated by both depolarization and increases in intracellular free [Ca^{2+}]. Ca^{2+} dependent K^+ currents contribute to the repolarization of neurons to resting membrane potential (Hille, 2001). Thus, Ca^{2+} dependent K^+ channels determine the shape of the action potential and help in regulating cell excitability (Goodman, 2008). Outward currents play a principal but not a sole role in repolarization in many types of excitable cells. The excitability of neurons is governed by the input they receive from their neighbours and the intrinsic excitability of the neuron. Electrophysiological studies have revealed that the voltage gated ion channels are important in determining the intrinsic excitability of neurons in the CNS. The voltage gated ion channels are critical in producing hyperexcitability such as that associated with seizure discharges (Errington, 2005) and causing epilepsy in humans (Du et al., 2005; Ez-Sampedro et al., 2006; Jorge et al., 2011). Ca^{2+} activated K^+ channels are essential for the production of bursting activity in mammalian cortical neurons (Jin et al., 2000) and they can also influence rhythmic firing patterns and bursting output (Gu et al., 2007). Voltage gated K^+ currents play crucial roles in modifying neuronal cellular and network excitability and activity (Muller & Connor, 1991).

Results of our study demonstrate that SH reducing agent, GSH, incompletely inhibited the effect of CHP on calcium-activated potassium channels in LRNC. The SH groups are known to be important for the function of many membrane transport systems. These include also various potassium channels (Lee et al., 1994; Han et al., 1996). Redox modification of cysteine SH groups may also be an important mechanism of controlling ion channel function. There are several explanations for the incomplete recovery of calcium-activated potassium channels. The simplest could be that CHP treatment must be modifying other amino acid residues, e.g., as methionine or tryptophan, besides cysteine. Cysteine and methionine residues are particularly sensitive to oxidation by almost all forms of ROS. In addition, the localization of the critical SH groups (responsible for the inhibitory action of the oxidative agents), could explain the observed partly protective effects of glutathione against cumene hydroperoxide-induced toxicity. The part of changes in channel properties depend on cysteine residues located on the cytoplasmic domains of the calcium-activated potassium channels in LRNC. The activity of potassium channels is dependent on the redox status of one or more SH groups on the channel protein, or an associated regulatory protein. Of course, it is possible that the oxidant agent affects other components associated to the membrane or to the channel (the target of the oxidizing agent could be a β-subunit or some membrane-bound enzyme able to promote channel phosphorylation).

5. Conclusions and implications

The present data show that the CHP is a more efficient neurotoxin and oxidant than H_2O_2, as well as that the suppression of Ca^{2+} activated outward K^+ currents is responsible for the prolongation of spike potential in leech Retzius nerve cells. Here we discuss the implications that free radicals can have a significant role in the appearance of spontaneous repetitive activity in Retzius nerve cells by interrupting the process of repolarization.

What is the pathophysiological relevance of a block of voltage-gated K^+ channels? In the past few years it has become more appreciated that a block of voltage-gated K^+ channels by ROS contributes to increased neuronal excitability and repetitive firing. These data indicate that a block of voltage gated K^+ channels contributes to an increase in neuronal excitability such as that associated with seizure discharges and causing epilepsy in humans. The interaction of ROS with K^+ channels may cause modifications of membrane currents and potentials thereby leading to neuronal dysfunction. The suppression of Ca^{2+} dependent K^+ currents proposed in this paper might have a broader significance, pertaining not only to leeches, but mammalian neurons as well. Leech ganglia are good models for studying the cellular basis for epileptiform activity. The largest neurons in the leech nervous system are Retzius cells which exhibit stable resting membrane potential and which are non-bursting neurons with a low spontaneous firing rate. An understanding of ion mechanisms epilepsy will provide insight into the molecular events of epileptogenesis, improve molecular diagnostic utility, and identify novel therapeutic targets for improved treatment of human epilepsy.

Electrophysiological analyses showed that oxidative modification of K^+ channels might represent a fundamental pathogenic mechanism in the mammalian brain during normal aging, as well as in neurodegenerative diseases such as Alzheimer's and Parkinson's. Therefore, it is probable that the action of ROS on K^+ channels might play a role in changes in electrical identity of neurons produced by ischemia and of course in neuronal death.

Considering that K^+ channels and ROS are universal players in the biological game, we put forward the hypothesis that the oxidation of voltage-gated K^+ channels may represent a general pathogenic mechanism in biological organisms. Obviously, more work is needed to establish the possible involvement of ion channels and of their modulation by ROS as important mechanisms in several pathological conditions in the brain. In addition, such knowledge may help to explain pathophysiological alterations in neurological diseases and to develop new strategies for therapeutic intervention that aim at preventing oxidative stress in the brain.

6. References

Aoyama, K.; Watabe, M. & Nakaki, T. (2008). Regulation of neuronal glutathione synthesis. *Journal of Pharmacological Sciences,* Vol.108, No.3, pp. 227-238

Axelsen, P.H.; Komatsu, H. & Murray, I.V. (2011). Oxidative stress and cell membranes in the pathogenesis of Alzheimer's disease. Physiology (Bethesda), Vol. 26, No.3, pp. 54-69

Barrington, P.L. (1994). Interactions of H2O2, EGTA and patch pipette recording methods in feline ventricular myocytes. *Journal of Molecular and Cellular Cardiology, Vol.*26, pp. 557–568

Bienert, G.P.; Moller, A.L.; Kristiansen, K.A.; Schulz, A.; Moller, I.M.; Schjoerring, J.K. & Jahn, T.P. (2007). Specific aquaporins facilitate the diffusion of hydrogen peroxide across membranes. *Journal of Biological Chemistry,* Vol.282, No.2, pp. 1183-1192

Beleslin, B.B. (1982). Membrane physiology of excitable cells in annelids. In: *Membrane physiology of invertebrates.* R. B. Podesta, (Ed.), 199-260, Marcel Dekker, ISBN 0824715039, New York, U.S.A

Beleslin, B.B. (1985). Sensitivity of the resting sodium conductivity of leech Retzius nerve cells to tetrodotoxin. *Comparative Biochemistry and Physiology,* Vol.81, No.2, pp. 323-328

Beleslin, B.B.; Ristanovic, D. & Osmanovic, S. (1988). Somatic outward currents in voltage clamp leech Retzius nerve cell. *Comparative Biochemistry and Physiology* Part A: Physiology, Vol.89, No.2, pp. 187-196

Beleslin, B.B.; Dekleva, N.M.; Jovanovic, D.Z.; Beleslin-Cokic, B.B.; Cokic, V. & Cemerikic, D. (1998). Resistivity of different tissues to oxidative stress. *Iugoslavica Physiologica et Pharmacologica Acta,* Vol.34, No.2, pp. 39-45

Bracci, R. (1992). Calcium involvement in free radical effects. *Calcified Tissue International,* Vol.51, No.6, pp. 401-405

Carmeliet, E. (1999). Cardiac ionic currents and acute ischemia: from channels to arrhythmias. Physiological Reviews, Vol.79, No.3, pp. 917–1017

Cerbai, E.; Ambrosio, G.; Porciatti, F.; Chiariello, M.; Giotti, A. & Mugelli, A. (1991). Cellular electrophysiological basis for oxygen radical-induced arrhythmias. A patch-clamp study in Guinea pig ventricular myocytes. *Circulatio,* Vol.84, pp. 1773-1782

Cheng, A.; Wang, S.; Yang, D.; Xiao, R. & Mattson, M.P. (2003). Calmodulin mediates brain-derived neurotrophic factor cell survival signaling upstream of Akt kinase in embryonic neocortical neurons. *Journal of Biological Chemistry*, Vol.278, No.9, pp. 7591–7599

Clark, J. & Simon, D.K. (2009). Transcribe to survive: transcriptional control of antioxidant defense programs for neuroprotection in Parkinson's disease. *Antioxidants and Redox Signaling*, Vol.11, No.3, pp. 509-528

Cohen, G. (1994). Enzymatic/nonenzymatic sources of oxyradicals and regulation of antioxidant defenses. *Annals of the New York Academy of Sciences*, Vol.73, pp. 8–14

Coetzee, W.A.; Owen, P.; Dennis, S.C.; Saman, S. & Opie, L.H. (1990). Reperfusion damage: Free radicals mediate delayed membrane changes rather than early ventricular arrhythmias. *Cardiovascular Research*, Vol. 24, pp. 156–164

Correa, F.; Mallard, C.; Nilsson, M. & Sandberg M. (2011). Activated microglia decrease histone acetylation and Nrf2-inducible anti-oxidant defence in astrocytes: restoring effects of inhibitors of HDACs, p38 MAPK and GSK3β. *Neurobiology of Disease*, Vol.44, No.1, pp. 142-151

Goldhaber, J.I.; Ji, S.; Lamp, S.T. & Weiss, J.N. (1989). Effects of exogenous free radicals on electromechanical function and metabolism in isolated rabbit and guinea pig ventricle. Implications for ischemia and reperfusion injury. *Journal of Clinical Investigation*, Vol.83, No.6, pp. 1800-1809

Goldhaber, J.I. & Liu, E. (1994). Excitation-contraction coupling in single guinea-pig ventricular myocytes exposed to hydrogen peroxide. *Journal of Physiology*, Vol.477, No.1, pp. 135-147

Goodman, B.E. (2008). Channels active in the excitability of nerves and skeletal muscles across the neuromuscular junction: basic function and pathophysiology. *Advances in Physiology Education*, Vol.32, No.2, pp. 127-135

Graham, S.; Ding, M.; Ding, Y.; Sours-Brothers, S.; Luchowski, R.; Gryczynski, Z.; Yorio, T.; Ma, H. & Ma, R. (2010). Canonical transient receptor potential 6 (TRPC6), a redox-regulated cation channel. *Journal of Biological Chemistry*, Vol.285, No.30, pp. 23466-23476

Gu, N.; Vervaeke, K. & Storm, J.F. (2007). BK potassium channels facilitate high-frequency firing and cause early spike frequency adaptation in rat CA1 hippocampal pyramidal cells. *Journal of Physiology*, Vol.580, No.3, pp. 859–882

Gutowicz, M. (2011). The influence of reactive oxygen species on the central nervous system. Postepy Hig Med Dosw (Online), ISSN:1732-2693 (Electronic), Vol.65, pp. 104-113

Del Maestro, R.; Thaw, H.H.; Björk, J.; Planker, M. & Arfors, K.E. (1980). Free radicals as mediators of tissue injury. *Acta Physiologica Scandinavica*, Vol.492, pp. 43-57

Dringen, R. & Gutterer, J.M. (2002). Glutathione reductase from bovine brain. *Methods in Enzymology*, Vol. 348, pp.281-288

Dringen, R. & Hirrlinger, J. (2003). Glutathione pathways in the brain. *Journal of Biological Chemistry*, Vol. 384, No.4, pp. 505-516

Du, W.; Bautista, JF.; Yang, H.; ez-Sampedro, A.; You, SA.; Wang, L.; Kotagal, P.; Lüders, H.O.; Shi, J.; Cui, J.; Richerson, G.B. & Wang, Q.K. (2005). Calcium-sensitive potassium channelopathy in human epilepsy and paroxysmal movement disorder. *Nature Genetics*, Vol.37, No.7, pp. 733–738

Dudek, E.; Yasumura, T. & Rash, J.E. (1998). 'Non-synaptic' mechanisms in seizures and epileptogenesis. *Cell Biology International*, Vol.22, pp. 793–805

Dyavanapalli, J.; Rimmer, K. & Harper, A.A. (2010). Reactive oxygen species alters the electrophysiological properties and raises [Ca2+]i in intracardiac ganglion neurons.

The American Journal of Physiology - Regulatory, Integrative and Comparative Physiology, Vol. 299, No.1, pp. 42-54

Errington, A.C.; Stohr, T. & Lees, G. (2005). Voltage gated ion channels: targets for anticonvulsant drugs. *Current Topics in Medicinal Chemistry*, Vol.5, No.1, pp. 15-30

Ez-Sampedro, A.; Silverman, W.R.; Bautista, J.F. & Richerson, G.B. (2006). Mechanism of increased open probability by a mutation of the BK channel. *Journal of Neurophysiology*, Vol.96, pp. 1507–1516

Facchinetti, F.; Dawson, V.L. & Dawson, T.M. (1998). Free radicals as mediators of neuronal injuri. *Cellular and Molecular Neurobiology*, Vol.18, No.6, pp. 667-682

Forman, H.; Maiorino, M. & Ursini, F. (2010). Signaling Functions of Reactive Oxygen Species. *Biochemistry*, Vol. 49, No.5, pp. 835-842

Hagiwara, S. & Morita, H. (1962). Electrotonic transmission between two nerve cells in leech ganglion. *Journal of Neurophysiology*, Vol.25, pp. 721-731

Halliwell, B. & Gutteridge, J.M.C. (1984). Oxygen toxicity, oxygen radicals, transition metals and disease. *Biochemical Journal*, Vol. 219, pp. 1-14

Han, J.; Kim, E.; Ho, W.K. & Earm, Y.E. (1996). Sulfhydryl redox modulates ATP-sensitive K^+ channels in rabbit ventricular myocytes. *Biochemical and Biophysical Research Communications*, Vol. 219, No.3, pp. 900-903

Hasan, S.M.; Joe, M. & Alshuaib, W.B. (2007). Oxidative stress alters physiological and morphological neuronal properties. *Neurochemical Research*, Vol.32, No.7, pp. 1169-1178

Haskew-Layton, R.E.; Payappilly, J.B.; Smirnova, N.A.; Ma, T.C.; Chan, K.K.; Murphy, T.H.; Guo, H.; Langley, B.; Sultana, R.; Butterfield, D.A.; Santagata, S.; Alldred, M.J.; Gazaryan, I.G.; Bell, G.W.; Ginsberg, S.D. & Ratan, R.R. (2010). Controlled enzymatic production of astrocytic hydrogen peroxide protects neurons from oxidative stress via an Nrf2-independent pathway. *Proceedings of the National Academy of Sciences of the United States of America*, Vol. 107, No.40, pp. 17385-17390

Hayashi, H.; Miyata, H.; Watanabe, H.; Kobayashi, A. & Yamazaki, N. (1989). Effects of hydrogen peroxide on action potentials and intracellular Ca2+ concentration of guinea pig heart. *Cardiovascular Research*, Vol.23, pp. 767–773

Hille, B. (2001). *Ion Channels of Excitable Membranes*, Third edition, Sinauer Associates, Inc. (Ed.), ISBN 0-87893-321-2, Massachussetts, U.S.A

Hool, L.C. (2006). Reactive oxygen species in cardiac signalling: from mitochondria to plasma membrane ion channels. *Clinical and Experimental Pharmacology and Physiology*, Vol.33, pp. 146–151

Hur, W. & Gray, N.S. (2011). Small molecule modulators of antioxidant response pathway. *Current Opinion in Chemical Biology*, Vol.15, No.1, pp. 162-173

Hwang, Y.P.; Yun, H.J.; Chun, H.K.; Chung, Y.C.; Kim, H.K.; Jeong, M.H.; Jeong, M.H.; Yoon, T.R. & Jeong, H.G. (2009). Protective mechanisms of 3-caffeoyl, 4-dihydrocaffeoyl quinic acid from Salicornia herbacea against tert-butyl hydroperoxide-induced oxidative damage. *Chemico-Biological Interactions*, Vol.181, pp. 366–376

Jin, W.; Sugaya, A.; Tsuda, T.; Ohguchi, H. & Sugaya, E. (2000). Relationship between large conductance calcium-activated potassium channel and bursting activity. *Brain Research*, Vol.860, pp. 21–28

Jovanović, Z. & Beleslin, B.B. (1996). Resistivity of leech Retzius nerve cells to long-lasting oxidant. *Journal of Neurochemistry*, Vol.66, pp. S32, ISSN:0022-3042

Jovanović, Z. & Beleslin, B.B. (1997). Resistivity of leech Retzius nerve cells to long-lasting oxidant. In: *Neurochemistry, Cellular, Molecular and Clinical Aspects*, A. Teelken & J. Korf, (Ed.), 983-986, ISBN 0-306-45705-9, New York, U.S.A.

Jovanović, Z. & Beleslin, B.B. (2004). Effects of long lasting oxidants on the electrophysiological properties of leech Retzius nerve cells. *Iugoslavica Physiologica et Pharmacologica Acta*, Vol.40, No.1-3, pp. 55-64

Jovanović, Z. (2010). Neuroprotective effect of the mannitol on oxidative stress induced by cumene hydroperoxide. *Medicinski časopis,* Vol.44, No.3, pp. 9-14, ISSN:0350.1221.UDK.61.

Jorge, B.S.; Campbell, C.M.; Miller, A.R.; Rutte, E.D.; Gurnett, C.A.; Vanoye, C.G.; George, A.L. & Kearney, J.A. (2011). Voltage-gated potassium channel KCNV2 (Kv8.2) contributes to epilepsy susceptibility. *Proceedings of the National Academy of Sciences of the United States of America,* Vol.108, No.13, pp. 5443-5448

Kourie, J.I. (1998). Interaction of reactive oxygen species with ion transport mechanisms. (1998). *American Journal of Physiology - Cell Physiology,* Vol. 275, pp. C1–C24

Lee, M.Y.; Bang, H.W.; Lim, I.J.; Uhm, D.Y. & Rhee, S.D. (1994). Modulation of large conductance calcium-activated K+ channel by membrane-delimited protein kinase and phosphatase activities. *Pflügers Archiv,* Vol.429, No.1, pp. 150-152

Lee, J.W.; Miyawaki, H.; Bobst, E.V.; Hester, J.D.; Ashraf, M. & Bobst, A.M. (1999). Improved functional recovery of ischemic rat hearts due to singlet oxygen scavengers histidine and carnosine. *Journal of Molecular and Cellular Cardiology,* Vol. 31, pp. 113–121

Lent, C.M. (1977). The Retzius cells within the central nervous system of leeches. *Progress in Neurobiology,* Vol. 8, pp. 8l- 117

Limon-Pacheco, J.H. & Gonsebatt, M.E. (2010). The glutathione system and its regulation by neurohormone melatonin in the central nervous system. *Current Medicinal Chemistry - Central Nervous System Agents*, Vol.10, No.4, pp. 287-297

Liu, Y. & Templeton, D.M. (2008). Initiation of caspase-independent death in mouse mesangial cells by Cd2+: involvement of p38 kinase and CaMK-II. *Journal of Cellular Physiology,* Vol.217, pp. 307–318

Lujan, R. (2010). Organisation of potassium channels on the neuronal surface. *Journal of Chemical Neuroanatomy,* Vol.40, No.1, pp. 1-20

Makino, N.; Sasaki, K.; Hashida, K. & Sakakura, Y. (2004). A metabolic model describing the H_2O_2 elimination by mammalian cells including H_2O_2 permeation through cytoplasmic and peroxisomal membranes: comparison with experimental data. *Biochimica et Biophysica Acta,* Vol.1673, No.3, pp. 149-159

Matsuura, H. & Shattock, M.J. (1991). Effects of oxidant stress on steady-state background currents in isilated ventricular myocytes. *American Journal of Physiology,* Vol. 261, pp. H1358-H1365

McCubrey, J.A.; Lahair, M.M. & Franklin, R.A. (2006). Reactive oxygen species-induced activation of the MAP kinase signaling pathways. *Antioxidants and Redox Signaling,* Vol.8, No.9-10, pp. 1775-1789

Muller ,W. & Connor, J.A. (1991). Dendritic spines as individual neuronal compartments for synaptic Ca2+ responses. *Nature,* Vol. 354, pp. 73–76

Nakaya, H.; Takeda, Y.; Tohse, N. & Kanno, M. (1991). Effects of ATP-sensitive K^+ channel blockers on the action potential shortening in hypoxic and ischaemic myocardium. *British Journal of Pharmacology,* Vol.103, pp. 1019-1026

Nakaya, H.; Takeda, Y.; Tohse, N. & Kanno, M. (1992). Mechanism of the membrane depolarization induced by oxidative stress in guinea-pig ventricular cells. *Journal of Molecular and Cellular Cardiology,* Vol.24, No.5, pp. 523-534

Nistico, R.; Piccirilli, S.; Cucchiaroni, M.L.; Armogida, M.; Guatteo, E.; Giampa, C.; Fusco, FR.; Bernardi, G.; Nistico, G. & Mercuri, N.B. (2008). Neuroprotective effect of hydrogen peroxide on an *in vitro* model of brain ischaemia. *British Journal of Pharmacology,* Vol.153, No.5, pp. 1022-1029

Pongs, O. (1999). Voltage-gated potassium channels: from hyperexcitability to excitement. *FEBS Letters,* Vol.452, pp. 31–35

Racay, P.; Kaplan, P.; Mezesova, V. & Lehotsky, J. (1997). Lipid peroxidation both inhibits $Ca^{(2+)}$-ATPase and increases Ca^{2+} permeability of endoplasmic reticulum membrane. *Biochemistry and Molecular Biology International,* Vol.41, No.4, pp. 647-655

Ruffels, J.; Griffin, M. & Dickenson, J.M. (2004). Activation of ERK1/2, JNK and PKB by hydrogen peroxide in human SH-SY5Y neuroblastoma cells: role of ERK1/2 in H2O2-induced cell death. *European Journal of Pharmacology,* Vol.483, No.2-3, pp. 163-173

Satoh, H. & Matsui, K. (1997). Electrical and mechanical modulations by oxygen-derived free-radical generating systems in Guinea-pig heart muscles. *Journal of Pharmacy and Pharmacology,* Vol.49, pp. 505–510

Shih, A.Y.; Johnson, D.A.; Wong, G.; Kraft, A.D.; Jiang, L.; Erb, H.; Johnson, J.A. & Murphy, T.H. (2003). Coordinate regulation of glutathione biosynthesis and release by Nrf2-expressing glia potently protects neurons from oxidative stress. *Journal of Neuroscience,* Vol.23, pp. 3394–3406

Skaper, S.D.; Floreani, M.; Ceccon, M.; Facci, L. & Giusti, P. (1999). Excitotoxicity, Oxidative Stress, and the Neuroprotective Potential of Melatonin. *Annals of the New York Academy of Sciences,* Vol.890, pp. 107–118

Son, Y.; Cheong, Y.K.; Kim, N.H.; Chung, H.T.; Kang, D.G. & Pae, H.O. (2011). Mitogen-Activated Protein Kinases and Reactive Oxygen Species: How Can ROS Activate MAPK Pathways? *Journal of Receptors and Signal Transduction,* 2011;2011:792639. Epub 2011 Feb 6

Son ,Y.O.; Wang, X.; Hitron, J.A.; Zhang, Z.; Cheng, S.; Budhraja, A.; Ding, S.; Lee, J.C. & Shi, X. (2011). Cadmium induces autophagy through ROS-dependent activation of the LKB1-AMPK signaling in skin epidermal cells. *Toxicology and Applied Pharmacology,* Vol.255, No.3, pp. 287-296

Soto, M.A.; Gonzalez, C.; Lissi, E.; Vergara, C. & Latorre, R. (2002). Ca2+-activated K+ channel inhibition by reactive oxygen species. *American Journal of Physiology - Cell Physiology,* Vol.282, pp. C461-C471

Stepkowski, T.M. & Kruszewski, M.K. (2011). Molecular cross-talk between the NRF2/KEAP1 signaling pathway, autophagy, and apoptosis. *Free Radical Biology & Medicine,* Vol.50, No.9, pp.1186-1195

Stewart, R.R.; Nicholls, J.G. & Adams, W.B. (1989). Na^{+}, K^{+} and Ca^{2+} currents in identified leech neurones in culture. *Journal of Experimental Biology,* Vol.141, pp. 1-20

Stone, J.R. (2004). An assessment of proposed mechanisms for sensing hydrogen peroxide in mammalian systems. *Archives of Biochemistry and Biophysics,* Vol.422, No.2, pp. 119-124

Su, Z.; Limberis, J.; Martin, R.L.; Xu, R.; Kolbe, K.; Heinemann, S.H.; Hoshi, T.; Cox, B.F. & Gintant, G.A. (2007). Functional consequences of methionine oxidation of hERG potassium channels. *Biochemical Pharmacology,* Vol.74, No.5, pp. 702-711

Takeuchi, K. & Yoshii, K. (2008). Superoxide modifies AMPA receptors and voltage-gated K^+ channels of mouse hippocampal neurons. *Brain Research,* Vol.21, No.1236, pp. 49-56

Tarr, M. & Valenzeno, D.P. (1989). Modification of cardiac action potential by photosensitizer-generated reactive oxygen. *Journal of Molecular and Cellular Cardiology,* Vol.21, pp. 539–543

Tarr, M. & Valenzeno, D.P. (1991). Modification of cardiac ionic currents by photosensiter-generated reactive oxygen. *Journal of Molecular and Cellular Cardiology,* Vol.23, pp. 639-649

Tarr, M.; Arriaga, E. & Valenzeno, D. (1995). Progression ofcardiac potassium current modification after brief exposure to reactive oxygen. *Journal of Molecular and Cellular Cardiology,* Vol.27, pp. 1099–1109

Thannickal, V.J. & Fanburg, B.L. (2000). Reactive oxygen species in cell signaling. *American Journal of Physiology: Lung Cellular and Molecular Physiology,* Vol.279, No.6, pp. L1005-1028

Tokube, K.; Kiyosue, T. & Arita, M. (1996). Openings of cardiac K_{ATP} channel by oxygen free radicals produced by xanthine oxidase reaction. *American Journal of Physiology,* Vol.271, No.2, pp. H478-489

Vacher, H.; Mohapatra, D.P. & Trimmer, J.S. (2008). Localization and targeting of voltage-dependent ion channels in mammalian central neurons. Physiological Reviews, Vol.88, No.4, pp. 1407-1447

Van der Vliet, A. & Bast, A. (1992). Effect of oxidative stress on receptors and signal transmission. *Chemico-Biological Interactions,* Vol.85, No.2-3, pp. 95-116

Vega-Saenz de Miera, E. & Rudy, B. (1992). Modulation of K^+ channels by hydrogen peroxide. *Biochemical and Biophysical Research Communications,* Vol.186, No.3, pp. 1681-1687

Vimard, F.; Saucet, M.; Nicole, O.; Feuilloley, M. & Duval, D. (2010). Toxicity induced by cumene hydroperoxide in PC12 cells: Protective role of thiol donors. *Journal of Biochemical and Molecular Toxicology,* Vol.25, No.4, pp.205-215

Ward, C.A. & Giles, W.R. (1997). Ionic mechanism of the effects of hydrogen peroxide in rat ventricular myocytes. *Journal of Physiology,* Vol.500, No.3, pp. 631-642

Wilson, J.X. (1997). Antioxidant defense of the brain: a role for astrocytes. *Canadian Journal of Physiology and Pharmacology,* Vol.7, No.10-11, pp. 1149-1163

Whittemore, E.R.; Loo, D.T.; Watt, J.A. & Cotman, C.W. (1995). A detailed analysis of hydrogen peroxide-induced cell death in primary neuronal culture. *Neuroscience,* Vol.67, No.4, pp. 921-993

Whyte, K.A.; Hogg, R.C.; Dyavanapalli, J.; Harper, A.A. & Adams, D.J. (2009). Reactive oxygen species modulate neuronal excitability in rat intrinsic cardiac ganglia. *Autonomic Neuroscience,* Vol.150, pp. 45–52

Yang, J.L.; Sykora, P.; Wilson, D.M.; Mattson, M.P. & Bohr, V.A. (2011). The excitatory neurotransmitter glutamate stimulates DNA repair to increase neuronal resiliency. *Mechanisms of Ageing and Development,* Vol.132, No.8-9, pp. 405-411

Zou, X.; Feng, Z.; Li, Y.; Wang, Y.; Wertz, K.; Weber, P.; Fu, Y. & Liu, J. (2011). Stimulation of GSH synthesis to prevent oxidative stress-induced apoptosis by hydroxytyrosol in human retinal pigment epithelial cells: activation of Nrf2 and JNK-p62/SQSTM1 pathways. *Journal of Nutritional Biochemistry,* [Epub ahead of print]

16

Circulating Advanced Oxidation Protein Products, Nε-(Carboxymethyl) Lysine and Pro-Inflammatory Cytokines in Patients with Liver Cirrhosis: Correlations with Clinical Parameters

Jolanta Zuwala-Jagiello[1],
Eugenia Murawska-Cialowicz[2] and Monika Pazgan-Simon[3]
[1]*Department of Pharmaceutical Biochemistry, Wroclaw Medical University,*
[2]*Department of Physiology and Biochemistry, University of Physical Education, Wroclaw,*
[3]*Clinic of Infectious Diseases, Liver Diseases and Acquired Immune Deficiency,*
Wroclaw Medical University,
Poland

1. Introduction

Patients with chronic liver disease are characterized by hepatic inflammation and the destruction of hepatocytes. Viral antigen-specific cytotoxic T lymphocytes, polyclonal cytokines, immune modulators, and oxidized biomolecules have been shown to induce damage and destruction of hepatocytes in these patients (Tsutsui *et al.*, 2003). The contribution of oxidative stress *per se* to the chronic inflammatory state has been suggested, and consistent evidence has been afforded that both monocyte/macrophage activation and a defect in antioxidant systems occur early in the course of chronic liver failure and gradually increase with its progression to end-stage liver disease (Kirkham, 2007; Videla, 2009). Oxidative stress lead to formation of glycoxidation products, including advanced glycation endproducts (AGEs - among them Nε-(carboxymethyl)lysine (CML) is best known), and advanced oxidation protein products (AOPPs). AOPPs can be formed *in vitro* by exposure of serum albumin to hypochlorous acid. *In vivo*, plasma AOPPs are mainly carried by albumin and their concentrations are closely correlated with the levels of dityrosine. Within the heterogeneous group of AGEs, Nε-(carboxymethyl)lysine has been identified as a major AGEs *in vivo* (Reddy *et al.*, 1995). Plasma concentrations of AGEs (closely correlating with AOPPs levels) increase with progression of chronic diseases (Witko-Sarsat *et al.*, 1996; 1998), therefore CML has been considered as liver disease-related biomarker for oxidative stress (Sebeková *et al.*, 2002; Yagmur *et al.*, 2006).

The receptor for advanced glycation endproducts (RAGE) is a signal transduction receptor that binds both AGEs and AOPPs. RAGE is expressed by various cell types, including monocytes/macrophages, endothelial cells, smooth muscle cells and renal cells (Miyata *et al.*, 1994). Advanced glycation endproducts have been found to act as pro-inflammatory factors (Sparvero *et al.*, 2009). Nevertheless, AOPPs are believed to be more closely related to inflammation (Alderman *et al.*, 2002; Baskol *et al.*, 2006; Fialova *et al.*, 2006; Witko-Sarsat *et al.*, 2003; Yazici *et al.*, 2004) than AGEs, whose receptor for advanced glycation endproducts participates in AOPPs-mediated signal transduction (Kalousová *et al.*, 2003; 2005). These interactions enhance reactive oxygen species formation, with activation of nuclear factor NF-κB and release of pro-inflammatory cytokines (Bierhaus *et al.*, 2006; Hyogo & Yamagishi, 2008; Saito & Ishii, 2004). Moreover, the monocyte/macrophage RAGE can be up-regulated by tumor necrosis factor-α (TNF-α) (Miyata *et al.*, 1994). Peripheral blood monocytes showed activity and elevated expression of TNF-α which correlated with liver disease severity (Hanck *et al.*, 2000). The concentrations of advanced oxidation protein products are high in liver cirrhosis of various etiologies (Zuwala-Jagiello *et al.*, 2009) and can reflect hemodynamic alterations in the liver (Guo *et al.*, 2008). This is accompanied by the activation of monocytes and increased expression of TNF-α (Giron-González *et al.*, 2004). High serum levels of TNF-α and interleukin-6 (IL-6) have been found in cirrhotic patients with ascites in the absence of demonstrable infection (Tilg *et al.*, 1992; Zeni *et al.*, 1993).

The accumulation of AGEs has been linked to vascular lesions in diabetes, chronic renal insufficiency, and atherosclerosis. Activation of NF-κB, mediated by RAGE, promotes expression of the cytokines, as well as pro-inflammatory adhesion molecules (Basta *et al.*, 2002; Bierhaus *et al.*, 1998; Esposito *et al.*, 1989), what may enhance interaction of cirrhotic vasculature with circulating monocytes (Cybulsky *et al.*, 1991; Li *et al.*, 1993). Recently, it has also been shown that AOPPs activates vascular endothelial cells *via* RAGE-mediated signals (Guo *et al.*, 2008).

Endothelial activation plays an active role in the modifications of circulatory status of cirrhotic patients (Genesca *et al.*, 1999). The circulatory changes are more evident in advanced stages of liver cirrhosis, such as those represented by the presence of ascites or hepatorenal syndrome (Porcel *et al.*, 2002). We have demonstrated that elevated levels of AOPPs modified–albumin (AOPPs-albumin) are related to the severity of liver cirrhosis (Zuwala-Jagiello *et al.*, 2009; 2011). The role of AOPPs-albumin in liver cirrhosis and portal hypertension has not yet been studied. The effects of pro-inflammatory cytokines on the vessels and on liver function would influence the liver cirrhosis, with higher plasma levels of AOPPs indicating a poor prognosis. In the present study, plasma levels of AOPPs-albumin, as well as of Nε (carboxymethyl)lysine modified-albumin (CML-albumin) and pro-inflammatory cytokines, such as TNF-α and IL-6, have been analyzed in cirrhotic patients and were found to be correlated with clinical parameters of liver dysfunction.

2. Patients and methods

2.1 Patients

This study was performed on 129 patients with chronic liver disease admitted to the Clinic of Infectious Diseases, Liver Diseases and Acquired Immune Deficiency for evaluation. The experimental group consisted of 68 men and 61 women with age of 18–74 years (median age was 66). The control group contained 40 healthy subjects (23 men and 17 women) with age of 19–56 (median age was 55). Blood samples were collected in the Department of

Physiology and Biochemistry, University of Physical Education in Wroclaw. Clinical and biochemical characteristics of the study group are reported in detail in Table 1.

	Healthy controls	All patients	Non-cirrhotic patients	Cirrhotic patients
(*n*)	40	129	41	88
Male:Female ratio	23:17	68:61	15:26	53:35
Age (years)	55 (19–56)	66 (18–74)	56 (18–69)	55 (21-74)
Etiology (n)				
Virus hepatitis		62	18	44
Alcohol		54	21	33
Biliary		13	2	11
Albumin (g/L)	45 (36–57)	34 (16–45)	37* (29–49)	30* (16-45)
ALT (U/L)	24 (20-28)	40 (16-79)	28 (24-33)	47** (16-79)
AST (U/L)	27 (23-30)	70 (19-150)	41 (19-64)	79** (19-150)
Bilirubin (mg/dL)	0.7 (0.6-0.9)	0.98 (1.0-3.6)	0.92 (0.90-0.95)	1.6* (1.0-3.6)
γGT (U/L)	26 (25.3-27.8)	70 (41-106)	48 (41-56)	92** (78-106)
AP (U/L)	90 (50-130)	125 (100-163)	105 (100-147)	152** (141-163)
Serum creatinine (mg/dL)	0.8 (0.7-1.0)	1.4 (0.7-2.4)	0.96 (0.9-1.2)	1.39* (0.7-2.4)
Serum sodium (mEq/L)	140 (138-141)	137 (129-142)	136 (129-138)	130** (129-142)

Table 1. Clinical and biochemical characteristics of the study subjects. Statistical significance: *$P < 0.05$; ** $P < 0.01$ vs. healthy controls. AST, aspartate aminotransferase; ALT, alanine aminotransferase; AP, alkaline phosphatase; γGT, γ-glutamyltransferase; INR, normalised international ratio; MELD, model of end-stage liver disease.

The diagnosis of liver cirrhosis was based on clinical, laboratory and ultrasonographic findings or histological criteria. Alcohol-related liver cirrhosis was diagnosed in 33 of patients, primary biliary cirrhosis in 11, cirrhosis caused by hepatitis C virus in 30, whereas cirrhosis caused by hepatitis B virus in 14 patients. The Child-Pugh score was used to assess the severity of liver disease. Three biochemical variables [serum albumin, bilirubin, and prothrombin time (international normalized ratio, INR)] in addition to the two clinical characteristics (presence or absence of ascites and clinical signs of encephalopathy) were determined. Patients were scored as follows: 5–6 as class (group) A, 7–9 as class (group) B and 10–15 as class (group) C. The patients with cirrhosis were divided into compensated (Child-Pugh class A) and decompensated (Child-Pugh classes B and C) groups. At the time of the study no Child-Pugh A patients showed clinical features of decompensated liver cirrhosis (ascites or hepatic encephalopathy). At enrollment, esophageal varices were detected by endoscopy in 88% of patients, ascites and hepatic encephalopathy grade were present by physical examination in 53 (60%) and 23 (26%) patients, respectively.

Exclusion criteria were concurrent use of antioxidant drugs; co-existing diseases like diabetes mellitus, chronic kidney disease, cardiovascular disease, hepatocellular carcinoma; gastrointestinal bleeding, bacterial infection, and blood transfusion within previous two weeks.

Patients had not been receiving diuretic, antibiotic, vasoactive drug (nitrates, β-blockers), and lactulose or lactitiol therapy during the eight days before inclusion in the study. After 2 h of bed rest, blood pressure was determined with an automatic digital sphygmomanometer and blood samples were collected in ice-cooled, ethylenediaminetetraacetic acid (EDTA)-containing tubes for the determination of plasma renin activity, antidiuretic hormone, and plasma AOPPs or Nε-(carboxymethyl)lysine, in tubes with no additive for routine biochemical study and aldosterone and cytokine concentrations. All samples were separated immediately by centrifugation at 4°C and stored at -80°C until further analysis.

The consent of the Bioethics Committee of the Wroclaw Medical University was obtained and all patients were informed about the character of analyses made. Studies were conducted in compliance with the ethical standards formulated in the Helsinki Declaration of 1975 (revised in 1983).

2.2 Determination of circulating AOPPs

In vivo plasma levels of AOPPs closely correlate with levels of dityrosine, a hallmark of oxidized proteins and with pentosidine, a marker of protein glycation closely related to oxidative stress. A new chromogen is found which caused increased absorbance at 340 nm and its spectrophotometric determination is proposed as a novel index of oxidative stress measuring the level of AOPPs (Witko-Sarsat *et al.*, 1996). Two- hundred microliters of plasma diluted 1:5 in 20 mM phosphate buffer pH 7.4 containing 0.9% sodium chloride (PBS), or chloramine-T standard solutions (0 to 100 μmol/L), were placed in each well of a 96-well microtiter plate (Becton Dickinson Labware, Lincoln Park, NJ, USA), followed by 20 μL of 10% acetic acid. Ten microliters of 1.16 M potassium iodide (Sigma-Aldrich Co. LLC, Canada) were then added, followed by 20 μL of 10% acetic acid. The absorbance of the reaction mixture was immediately read at 340 nm in a microplate reader against a blank containing 200 μL of PBS, 10 μL of KI and 20 μL of 10% acetic acid. The chloramine-T absorbance at 340 nm was linear within the range of 0 to 100 μmol/L. The ratio of AOPPs concentration to albumin level (AOPPs-albumin) was expressed in micromoles of AOPPs per gram of albumin (μmol/g). The ratio of AOPPs to albumin content allows the evaluation of whether the proportion of oxidatively modified albumin is altered. Coefficient of variation (CV) served as an indicator of precision. Intra-day and inter-day CV values were <10%.

2.3 Determination of circulating Nε-(carboxymethyl) lysine

Plasma Nε-(carboxymethyl)lysine (CML) levels were determined using a specific competitive ELISA kit [CircuLex CML/Nε-(carboxymethyl)lysine ELISA Kit (CycLex Co., Ltd, Nagano, Japan)]. Measurements were performed in duplicate and the results were averaged. The ratio of CML concentration to albumin level (CML-albumin) was expressed in micrograms of CML per gram of albumin (μg/g).

2.4 Laboratory determinations

Biochemical parameters were measured using routine laboratory methods. Serum high-sensitivity C-reactive protein (hs-CRP) level was determined with a high-sensitivity nephelometric method using the Beckman Image Immunochemistry system (Beckman Instruments, Fullerton, CA), which has a minimum level of detection of 0.2 mg/L. Serum levels of TNF-α and IL-6 were assayed with enzyme-linked immunosorbent assay (ELISA) kits (R&D Systems Inc., Minneapolis, MN, USA) according to the manufacturer's instructions. The minimum levels of detection were 1.6 pg/mL and < 0.70 pg/mL for TNF-α and IL-6, respectively. The intra- and interassay coefficients of variation for measurements of CRP, IL-6, and TNF-α were 2.7%, 4.3%, and 5.0%, respectively, and 3.0%, 5.5, and 6.9%, respectively.

Aldosterone (Aldoctk-2-P2714; Sorin Biomedica Diagnostics, Barcelona, Spain. Normal values, 35-150 pg/mL) and plasma renin activity (Clinical Assays, Baxter, Cambridge, Mass., USA. Normal values, 0.4-2.3 ng mL^{-1} h^{-1}) were measured by specific radioimmunoassays. Antidiuretic hormone was also tested by a commercial radioimmunoassay (Buhlman Laboratories, Basel, Switzerland. Normal values, less than 1 pg/mL).

2.5 Measurement of the total antioxidant status of plasma

The plasma antioxidant capacity was measured using a commercially available total antioxidant status TAS kit (Randox Laboratories, Crumlin, UK). The TAS assay is based on the inhibition by antioxidants of the absorbance of the radical cation of 2,2'-azinobis-(3-ethylbenzothiazoline-6-sulfonate) (ABTS) formed by the interaction of ABTS with ferrylmyoglobin radical species. Upon the addition of a plasma sample, the oxidative reactions initiated by the hydroxyl radicals present in the reaction mix are suppressed by the antioxidant components of the plasma, preventing the color change and thereby providing an effective measure of the total antioxidant capacity of the plasma. The assay has excellent precision values, lower than 3%, and the results are expressed as mmol/L.

2.6 Model for End-stage Liver Disease (MELD) score

The model for end-stage liver disease (MELD) score was calculated from the following equation:

9.57 × $\log_e$ (creatinine mg/dL) + 3.78 × $\log_e$ (total bilirubin mg/dL) + 11.2 × $\log_e$ (international normalized ratio-INR) + 6.43 (constant for liver disease etiology).

The maximal creatinine concentration considered in the MELD score is 4.0 mg/dL (Huo *et al.*, 2006).

2.7 Statistical analysis

Results are expressed as median (25th percentile–75th percentile). Frequency data were compared using the $\chi2$ test or the Fischer's exact test when necessary. Because many of the variables analyzed did not have a normal distribution as determined by the Kolmogorov-Smirnov test, nonparametric tests were used for comparison of data. The Mann- Whitney U test and the Kruskal-Wallis test were used to analyze differences among two or more groups, respectively. Multivariate analysis by conditional logistical regression with a forward stepwise method was performed to find independent variables associated with the presence of ascites and low mean arterial pressure. Regression analysis to determine significant correlations among different parameters was performed using the Spearman correlation coefficient. Statistical significance was established at $P < 0.05$

3. Results

3.1 AOPPs-albumin plasma concentrations in patients with chronic liver disease and healthy controls

We analyzed 129 patients (68 males/61 females, median age 66 years, range 18–74 years) with chronic liver disease. The distribution of the stages of liver cirrhosis as defined according to the Child-Pugh score, and measurements of AOPPs-albumin and CML-albumin plasma concentrations are presented in Fig.1. The concentration of AOPPs-albumin

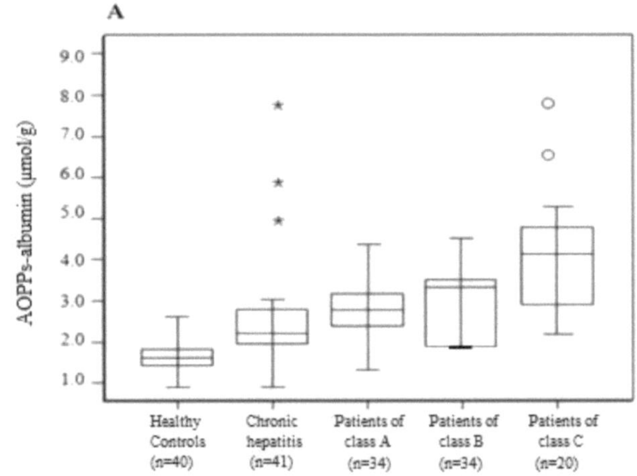

	Healthy Controls	Chronic hepatitis	Patients of class A	Patients of class B	Patients of class C
AOPPs-albumin (µmol/g)	1.7 (0.8-2.7)	2.1* (0.9-3.0)	2.8* (1.3-4.4)	3.2 (1.9-4.5)	4.1**+ (2.3-5.2)

Significance between groups: $^*P < 0.05$; $^{**}P < 0.01$ vs. healthy controls; $^+P < 0.05$ vs. patients of class A

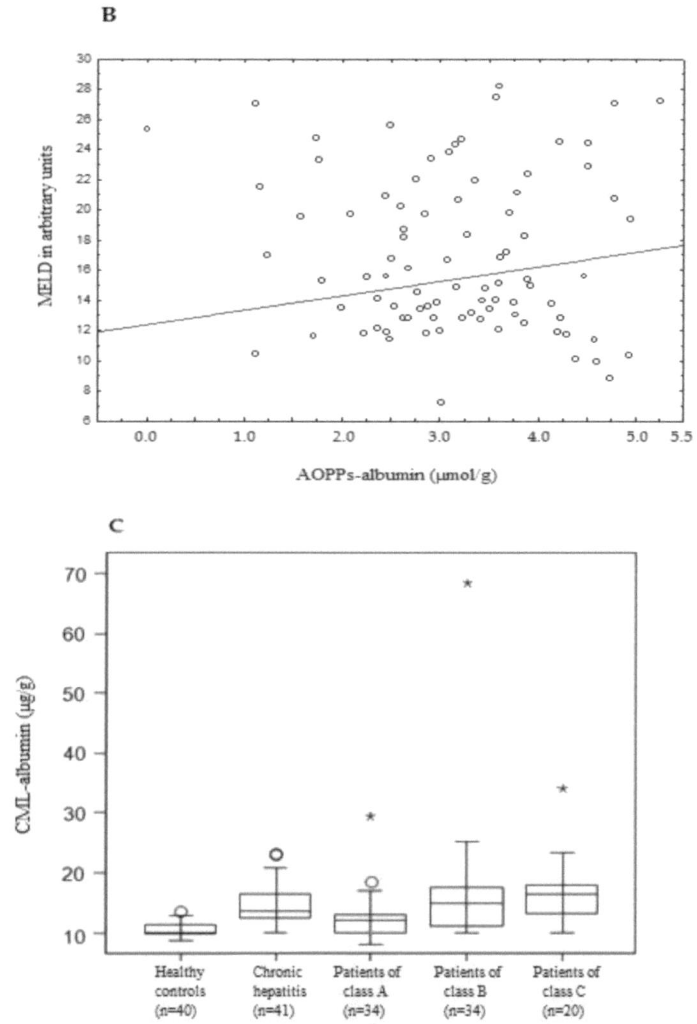

	Healthy Controls	Chronic hepatitis	Patients of class A	Patients of class B	Patients of class C
CML-albumin (μg/g)	10.7 (9.0–13.5)	14.1 (9.8-20.1)	12.6* (8.3-18.2)	15.8** (11.2–25.5)	18.3** (9.7–23.8)

Significance between groups: *$P < 0.05$; ** $P < 0.01$ vs. healthy controls.

Fig. 1. **(A)** AOPPs-albumin serum concentrations in 129 patients with chronic liver disease, according to Child's stage of cirrhosis, and in an control group of 40 healthy blood donors. *P* values are given in the table. Comparisons between subgroups are illustrated with box plot graphics, where the dotted line indicates the median per group, the box represents 50% of the values, and horizontal lines show minimum and maximum values of the calculated non-outlier values; asterisks and open circles indicate outlier values. **(B)** AOPPs-albumin serum concentrations in patients with cirrhosis are correlated with the MELD (model of end-stage liver disease) score ($r = 0.43$, $P < 0.01$, Spearman rank correlation test). **(C)** CML-albumin serum concentrations increase with the stage of liver cirrhosis in patients with chronic liver disease. *P* values are given in the table.

in healthy subjects was 1.7 μmol/g (range 0.8-2.7 μmol/g, $P < 0.05$). In patients with chronic liver disease, AOPPs-albumin plasma concentrations were 1.3-fold higher. In healthy controls, the plasma AOPPs or CML were similar to those in control groups in other studies (Sebeková *et al.*, 2002; Kalousová *et al.*, 2003).

3.2 AOPPs-albumin and liver cirrhosis

AOPPs-albumin plasma concentration was significantly higher in patients with liver cirrhosis (n = 88, median 2.4 μmol/g, range 1.3-5.6 μmol/g) compared to patients with chronic liver disease without cirrhosis (n = 41, median 2.1 μmol/g, range 0.9-3.0 μmol/g) ($P < 0.05$, Fig.1A). Patients with Child-Pugh class C exhibited significantly higher plasma concentrations of AOPPs-albumin than patients with Child-Pugh class A and controls ($P < 0.05$, $P < 0.01$, respectively) (Fig.1A). There was no significant difference in AOPPs concentrations between control subjects and Child-Pugh B cirrhotic patients.

Differences in plasma AOPPs-albumin or CML-albumin were not significant in patients with liver cirrhosis of various etiologies (Table 2). Only in the group with primary biliary cirrhosis AOPPs-albumin were decreased (n = 11, median 1.3 μmol/g, range 0.80-2.2 μmol/g), though it should be consider with caution since small number of subjects included in this group.

	AOPPs-albumin (μmol/g)	CML-albumin (μg/g)	TAS (mmol/L)
Healthy controls (n=40)	1.7 (0.80-2.7)	10.7 (9.0–13.5)	1.31 (1.12-1.5)
Viral hepatitis-related cirrhosis (n=44)	3.09* (1.5-5.2)	13.3* (11.6-18.1)	0.65* (0.48-0.75)
Alcohol-related cirrhosis (n=33)	2.9* (1.6-4.3)	16.3* (13.3-25.5)	0.71* (0.60-0.73)
Primary biliary cirrhosis (n=11)	1.3 (0.80-2.2)	11.8 (8.3-12.5)	0.98 (0.76-0.83)

Biliary etiology shows lower AOPPs-albumin levels compared with other etiologies of liver disease. Significance levels between groups: *$P < 0.05$ vs. healthy controls.
AOPPs, advanced oxidation protein products; CML, Nε-(carboxymethyl)lysine; TAS, total antioxidant status.

Table 2. Plasma AOPPs-albumin, CML-albumin and TAS in liver cirrhosis patients of various etiologies.

The MELD scores were determined in the 88 patients with liver cirrhosis (Table 3). These were higher in the Child-Pugh C cirrhotic patients than in the Child-Pugh A cirrhotic patients (p<0.01). Significant correlations between AOPPs levels and MELD scores (r = 0.43, $P < 0.01$; Fig. 1B) were observed among the cirrhotic patients belonging to all three Child-Pugh classes.

	Healthy controls	Non-cirrhotic patients	Patients of class A	Patients of class B	Patients of class C
(*n*)	40	41	34	34	20
Age (years)	55 (19–56)	56 (18–69)	51 (21–74)	58 (24–71)	56 (29–69)
Albumin (g/L)	45 (36–57)	40 (29–49)	34* (28–45)	30* (20–40)	25* (16–32)
Bilirubin (mg/dL)	0.7 (0.6-0.9)	0.92 (0.90-0.95)	1.01 (1.02-1.03)	1.56* (1.0-2.0)	2.15* (1.1-3.6)
AOPPs-albumin (μmol/g)	1.7 (0.8-2.7)	2.1* (0.9-3.0)	2.8* (1.3-4.4)	3.2 (1.9-4.5)	4.1**+ (2.3–5.2)
CML-albumin (μg/g)	10.7 (9.0–13.5)	14.1 (9.8-20.1)	12.6* (8.3-18.2)	15.8** (11.2–25.5)	18.3** (9.7–23.8)
Uric acid (mmol/L)	0.35 (0.25-0.39)	0.29 (0.21-0.33)	0.31 (0.26-0.34)	0.22 (0.16-0.24)	0.18* (0.19-0.31)
Vitamin C (μmol/L)	54.3 (38.3-70.3)	45.2 (31.9-58.6)	47.1 (28.3-64.0)	33.6 (20.2-45.7)	36.9 (29.2-54.2)
TAS (mmol/L)	1.3 (1.1-1.5)	1.1 (0.9-1.3)	0.9 (0.6-1.0)	0.63 (0.5-0.76)	0.53**+ (0.5-0.8)
INR	0.8-1.1	-	0.9 (0.8-1.09)	1.2 (1.1-1.3)	2.3 (1.6-2.9)
MELD score	6-8	-	7.8 (5.2-10.3)	15.9* (8.7-23.1)	24.1*+ + (14.4-28.4)

Table 3. Plasma concentrations of AOPPs-albumin, CML-albumin and antioxidant parameters in patients with chronic liver disease without cirrhosis and in patients with cirrhosis. Significance between groups: $^*P < 0.05$; $^{**} P < 0.01$ vs. healthy controls; $^+ P < 0.05$; $^{++}P < 0.01$ vs. patients of class A. AOPPs, advanced oxidation protein products; CML, Nε-(carboxymethyl)lysine; TAS, total antioxidant status; MELD, model for end-stage liver disease score.

3.3 CML-albumin plasma concentrations in patients with CLD and healthy controls

In patients with chronic liver disease, CML-albumin had a median value of 14.1 µg/g (range 9.8-20.1 µg/g). Plasma CML-albumin concentrations were higher in Child-Pugh A to C cirrhotic patients (n = 88, median 15.7 µg/g, range 8.3-25.5 µg/g) than in patients without cirrhosis, but this difference was not statistically significant (Fig. 1C). The levels of plasma CML-albumin in all liver cirrhotic patients were higher than those of the controls and this difference was statistically significant (Fig. 1C). Plasma CML-albumin in patients with Child-Pugh class C cirrhosis was only slightly elevated compared with those in Child-Pugh class A cirrhosis ($P = 0.17$) (Fig. 1C). There was no statistically significant correlation between CML-albumin levels and the Child-Pugh score in cirrhotic patients.

3.4 Antioxidant parameters and liver cirrhosis

As it is seen in Table 3, while all individual parameters of the antioxidant status tend to decrease, only the decrease of uric acid was statistically significant. There was a markedly decreased total antioxidant status (TAS) in patients with Child-Pugh class C cirrhosis compared to those with Child-Pugh class A cirrhosis or controls ($P < 0.05$, $P < 0.01$, respectively). Although differences between cirrhosis and chronic liver disease (n = 41, median 1.1, mmol/L, range 0.9-1.3 mmol/L) were not statistically significant, weak but significant correlation was observed between TAS and plasma AOPPs-albumin ($r = -0.31$, $P < 0.05$). We failed to find, however, any relation between circulating CML-albumin levels and TAS ($r = -0.22$, $P = 0.059$).

3.5 Markers of oxidative stress and hepatic function

The serum albumin concentration was determined in all patients (n = 129, median 34 g/L, range 16–45 g/L) and healthy control subjects (n = 40, median 45 g/L, range 36–57 g/L). Level of albumin, the main substrate in both AOPPs and CML formation (Kalousová *et al.*; 2005), was significantly depleted both in chronic liver disease (n = 41, median 37 g/L, range 29–49 g/L) and in cirrhosis (median 30 g/L, range 16-45 g/L) (Table 1). Plasma CML-albumin and foremost AOPPs-albumin showed significant associations with biochemical indices of liver function (albumin, prothrombin time, bilirubin concentration) but not with markers of liver injury - aminotransferases (Table 4). As expected, in patients with cirrhosis, AOPPs-albumin weakly but significantly correlated with the serum albumin ($r = -0.38$, $P < 0.05$).

3.6 AOPPs-albumin, CML-albumin and chronic inflammatory state in cirrhotic patients

We assessed the levels of several inflammatory markers and their association with the levels of AOPPs-albumin and CML-albumin. Serum high-sensitivity C-reactive protein (hs-CRP) levels and white blood cells (WBC) counts were significantly elevated in cirrhotic patients (Table 5). Serum TNF-α levels were higher in the Child-Pugh class C cirrhosis patients than in the Child-Pugh class A cirrhosis patients ($P < 0.05$) (Table 5). Moreover, TNF-α concentrations were weakly but significantly correlated with Child-Pugh score in cirrhotic group ($r = 0.31$, $P < 0.05$). The levels of serum IL-6 in cirrhotic patients were higher than those of the control group and this difference was statistically significant ($P < 0.05$) (Table 5). The levels of serum IL-6 in patients with Child-Pugh class C cirrhosis were higher than those in Child-Pugh class A cirrhosis, but this difference was not statistically significant.

	AOPPs-albumin (μmol/g)	CML-albumin (μg/g)
Albumin (g/L)	r = -0.38, $P < 0.05$	r = - 0.26, $P = 0.07$
ALT (U/L)	r = 0.10, $P = 0.54$	r = -0.14, $P = 0.31$
AST (U/L)	r = -0.20, $P = 0.11$	r = -0.15, $P = 0.26$
Bilirubin (mg/dL)	r = 0.23, $P = 0.07$	r = 0.24, $P = 0.06$
Prothrombin ratio (%)	r = -0.25, $P < 0.05$	r = - 0.43, $P < 0.001$
MELD score	r = 0.43, $P < 0.01$	r = 0.23, $P = 0.07$

Table 4. Correlations between plasma AOPPs-albumin and CML-albumin and selected biochemical indices of liver function and injury. ALT, alanine aminotransferase; AST, aspartate aminotransferase; MELD, model for end-stage liver disease score.

	Healthy controls (n=40)	Overall (n=88)	Patients of class A (n=34)	Patients of class B (n=34)	Patients of class C (n=20)
AOPPs-albumin (μmol/g)	1.7 (0.8-2.7)	2.4* (1.3-5.6)	2.8* (1.3-4.4)	3.2 (1.9-4.5)	4.1*+ (2.3–5.2)
CML-albumin (μg/g)	10.7 (9.0–13.5)	15.7* (8.3-25.5)	12.6* (8.3-18.2)	15.8** (11.2–25.5)	18.3** (9.7–23.8)
Albumin (g/L)	45 (36–57)	31** (16-35.4)	34* (28–45)	30* (20–40)	25* (16–32)
TNF-α (pg/mL)	32.9 (31.0-35.2)	41.5* (37.6-64.0)	36.9* (37.7-45.6)	42.0* (37.6-47.2)	51.7*+ (48.7-58.3)
IL-6 (pg/mL)	5.9 (5.4-6.8)	13.3** (6.4-39.9)	8.8* (6.4-34.6)	12.3* (6.8-33.9)	18.9* (9.0-39.9)
hsCRP (mg/L)	1.5 (0.63-2.0)	5.3** (4.9-11.0)	4.8* (5.5-7.0)	5.2** (4.9-7.7)	6.3*+ (6.8-10.1)

	Healthy controls (n=40)	Overall (n=88)	Patients of class A (n=34)	Patients of class B (n=34)	Patients of class C (n=20)
WBC ($x10^9$/L)	4.0 (4.2-5.0)	5.0 (1.1-8.6)	4.7 (1.1-8.6)	5.2* (3.0-7.8)	5.4**+ (2.7-8.2)
MELD score	6-8	13.5* (5.2-28.4)	7.8 (5.2-10.3)	15.9* (8.7-23.1)	24.1**+ + (14.4-28.4)

Table 5. Plasma concentrations of AOPPs-albumin, CML-albumin and inflammatory markers in healthy controls and in patients with liver cirrhosis. Significance levels between groups: *$P < 0.05$; ** $P < 0.01$ vs. healthy controls; + $P < 0.05$, ++$P < 0.01$ vs. patients of class A. AOPPs, advanced oxidation protein products; CML, Nε-(carboxymethyl)lysine; TNF, tumor necrosis factor; IL, interleukin; CRP, C-reactive protein; WBC, white blood cells; MELD, model for end-stage liver disease score.

The association study revealed only a tendency toward an extremely weak but significant correlation between AOPPs-albumin and WBC in all cirrhotic patients (r = 0.23, $P < 0.05$). In turn, a weak but significant correlation between AOPPs-albumin levels and hs-CRP was observed among the cirrhotic patients belonging to all three Child-Pugh classes (r = 0.33, $P < 0.05$). There was a significant correlation between the IL-6 and the AOPPs-albumin level (r = 0.42, $P < 0.05$) and MELD score (r = 0.38, $P < 0.05$) in cirrhotic patients. As it was expected, a significant correlation between AOPPs-albumin levels and TNF-α (r = 0.48, $P < 0.05$) was observed in Child-Pugh class A cirrhosis patients. In the multivariate analysis the relationship between plasma AOPPs-albumin, TNF-α and Child-Pugh score was independent of age, sex and liver cirrhosis etiology (data not shown).

There was no statistically significant correlation between CML-albumin level and hs-CRP or cytokines levels in all liver cirrhotic patients (data not shown).

The ROC curve analyses are shown in Fig. 2 (sensitivity versus 1-specificity). The cut-off values of plasma AOPPs-albumin, TNF-α and IL-6 to separate cirrhotic patients from healthy controls were 3.71 μmol/g, 37.2 pg/mL, and 8.95 pg/mL, respectively.

3.7 Hemodynamic characteristics of the patients with liver cirrhosis

Hemodynamic characteristics of patients are shown in Tables 1 and 6. Cirrhotic patients had significantly lower values of mean arterial pressure (MAP) when compared with controls (Table 6). Parameters related to hemodynamic disturbances such as decreased mean arterial pressure and increased plasma renin activity and aldosterone levels deteriorated with increasing of Child-Pugh score. However, similar values of antidiuretic hormone were detected in all patients grouped according to the Child-Pugh classification.

Among clinical parameters of liver dysfunction ascites revealed significant association with plasma AOPPs-albumin, TNF-α and IL-6 (Table 6). By contrast, patients presented similar AOPPs-albumin levels when classified according to the presence or absence of encephalopathy grade I (data not shown). Ascitic patients had a more intense alteration of hemodynamic parameters (plasma renin activity, aldosterone), along with higher levels of

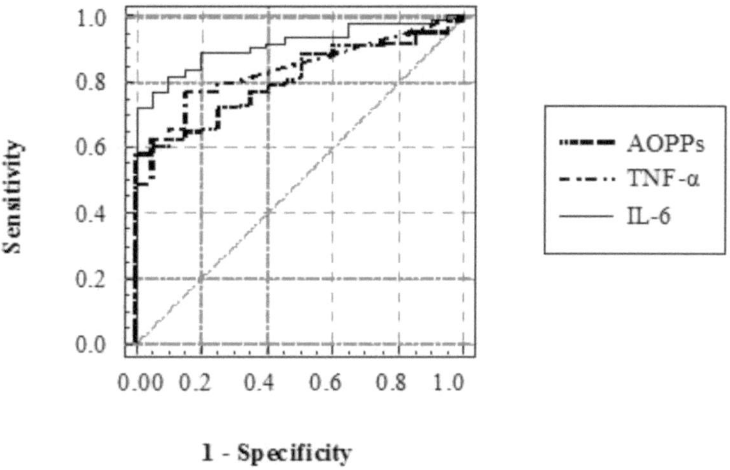

	AUC	Standard error	95% confidence interval	Sensitivity (%)	Specificity (%)	Optimal cut-off
AOPPs-albumin	0.802	0.018	0.766-0.838	57.6	100	3.71 μmol/g
TNF-α	0.902	0.015	0.872-0.932	71.7	100	37.2 pg/mL
IL-6	0.832	0.012	0.808-0.856	76.1	85	8.95 pg/mL

Fig. 2. Receiver operating characteristic (ROC) curve and optimal cut-off levels of advanced oxidation protein products (AOPPs), tumor necrosis factor-α (TNF-α), and interleukin-6 (IL-6) for distinguishing cirrhotic patients from healthy controls; AUC, area under the curve.

AOPPs-albumin, TNF-a, and IL-6, compared with patients without ascites. Cirrhotic patients who had ascites showed higher AOPPs-albumin levels (n = 53, median 3.6 μmol/g, range 1.5-5.3 μmol/g) than patients without ascites (n = 35, median 2.2 μmol/g, range 1.0-3.4 μmol/g) ($P < 0.05$, Table 6). AOPPs-albumin levels were not different between cirrhotic patients without ascites and controls, while patients with ascites had higher AOPPs-albumin levels than controls (median 1.7 μmol/g, range 0.8-2.7 μmol/g) ($P < 0.01$). High IL-6 levels showed an independent association with the presence of ascites.

To differentiate cirrhotic patients with a more intense hemodynamic alteration (vasodilatation), we divided patients according to those with low mean arterial pressure (MAP ≤83 mm Hg) and high mean arterial pressure (MAP >83 mm Hg) (Table 7). Only IL-6 levels were significantly higher in patients with more severe vasodilatation; this association was independent of other factors.

Plasma levels of AOPPs-albumin very weakly but significantly correlated with MAP ($r = -0.25$, $P < 0.01$; Fig.3). Furthermore, IL-6 levels had a significant correlation with several parameters, including plasma renin activity (r = 0.39, $P < 0.05$) and MAP (r = -0.38, $P < 0.01$), in addition to albumin (r = - 0.51, $P < 0.001$). Neither TNF-α levels nor the CML-albumin levels correlated significantly with hemodynamic parameters.

	Overall (n=88)	Patients of class A (n=34)	Patients of class B (n=34)	Patients of class C (n=20)	Cirrhosis without ascites (n=35)	Cirrhosis with ascites n=53)
Mean arterial pressure-MAP (mmHg)	83 (76-93)	89 (85-93)	83 (77-91)	76* (73-81)	88 (85-93)	77+ (73-89)
Plasma renin activity (ng mL^{-1} h^{-1})	0.6 (0.1-7.6)	0.37 (0.1-1.2)	1.9* (0.95-4.8)	6.0** 1.2-7.6)	0.48 (0.13-1.6)	1.9++ (0.51-6.2)
Aldosterone (ng/dL) 20.6 (14.0-51.0)	15.0 (5.0-71.0)	12.0 (5.0-19.0)	20.6 (14.0-/51.0)	30.0* (21.0-71.0)	13.2 (5.5-20.9)	33.0+++ (13.7-52.2)
Antidiuretic hormone (pg/mL)	4.9 (2.5-6.5)	3.8 (2.5-5.7)	4.5 (3.7-6.2)	4.8 (3.8-6.5)	4.6 (3.0-6.8)	4.5 (3.6-6.4)
AOPPs-albumin (µmol/g)	2.4 (1.3-5.2)	2.8 (1.3-4.4)	3.2 (1.9-4.5)	4.1* (2.3-5.2)	2.2 (1.0-3.4)	3.6+ (1.5-5.3)
TNF-α (pg/mL)	41.5 (37.6-64.0)	36.9 (37.7-45.6)	42.0 (37.6-47.2)	51.7* (48.7-58.3)	37.5 (35.4-46.5)	57.5+ (52.1-69.7)
IL-6 (pg/mL)	13.3 (6.4-39.9)	8.8 (6.4-34.6)	12.3 (6.8-33.9)	18.9 (9.0-39.9	6.4 (5.6-7.3)	10.8++ (8.5-12.4)

Significance between groups: $^{*}P < 0.05$; $^{**}P < 0.001$ vs. patients of class A. $^{+}P < 0.05$; $^{++}P < 0.01$, $^{+++}P < 0.001$ vs. liver cirrhosis without ascites. AOPPs, advanced oxidation protein products; TNF, tumor necrosis factor; IL, interleukin.

Table 6. Blood pressure, plasma renin activity and plasma concentrations of aldosterone, antidiuretic hormone and AOPPs-albumin according to the Child–Pugh class or presence of ascites.

	Mean arterial pressure (MAP) ≤ 83 mm Hg (n=51)	Mean arterial pressure (MAP) > 83 mm Hg (n=37)
Plasma renin activity (ng mL^{-1} h^{-1})	1.7 (0.46-5.5)	1.4 (0.37-4.4)
Aldosterone (ng/dL)	25.6 (10.6-40.5)	13.7 (5.7-21.6)
Antidiuretic hormone (pg/mL)	4.7 (3.7-6.7)	4.2 (3.3-5.9)
AOPPs-albumin (µmol/g)	3.3 (1.4-4.8)	3.01 (1.2-4.5)
IL-6 (pg/mL)	11.0^{+} (9.5-12.8)	6.3 (5.4-7.0)
TNF-α (pg/mL)	47.9 (43.4-58.0)	49.8 (45.1-60.3)

Table 7. Comparison between cirrhotic patients classified according to the finding of low (≤ 83 mm Hg) and high (>83 mm Hg) mean arterial pressure (MAP). Significance between groups: $^{+}P < 0.01$ by multivariate analysis.

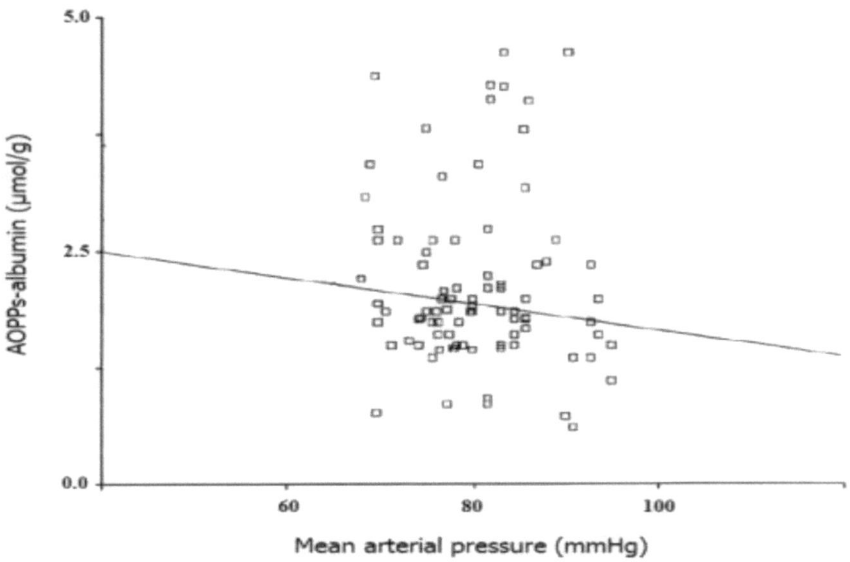

Fig. 3. AOPPs-albumin concentrations are very weakly but significantly correlated with the mean arterial pressure (MAP) in patients with chronic liver disease (r = -0.25, $P < 0.01$).

4. Discussion

Cirrhosis is characterized by inflammation of the liver, often caused by a rise in oxygen-derived free radicals within the liver. Under normal circumstances, the liver maintains a supply of internal antioxidants to neutralize the reactive species generated in response to viral infection and during metabolism of various endo- and exogenous compounds processed in the liver. However, when the liver antioxidants are low, or when the liver is undergone to continued oxidative insults (e.g., long-lasting alcohol abuse or infection with different hepatitis viruses), the damage from reactive species (Halliwell, 2007) may increase, resulting in inflammation and the formation of scar tissue (fibrosis) (Valko *et al.*, 2007). The progressive decrease of antioxidant reserves, the dysfunction of liver microcirculation through nitric oxide-mediated pathways, may determine the shift to liver cirrhosis. Advanced glycation and oxidation endproducts (AGEs and AOPPs, respectively) cause oxidative stress and trigger cytokine driven inflammatory reactions *in vitro*. (reviewed in Yan *et al.*, 2010). The net effects on markers of inflammation and hemodynamic changes in cirrhotic patients are unknown.

Advanced glycation endproducts are formed from the reaction of glucose and other reducing sugars with amino acid groups of proteins. This interaction generates a labile Schiff base followed by rearrangement to more stable Amadori-products, and subsequently these early glycation products may undergo further chemical rearrangements resulting in various irreversibly formed AGEs (Baynes & Thorpe, 1999). Three different mechanisms have been proposed by which AGEs lead to cirrhosis complications: 1) the binding of AGEs to the receptors for advanced glycation endproducts on different cell types including monocytes/macrophages, T lymphocytes, endothelial cells, smooth muscle cells, and activation of cell signaling pathways with subsequent modulation of gene expression, 2) intracellular AGEs formation leading to impaired cell function, and 3) the accumulation of AGEs in the extracellular matrix. CML-albumin levels (as prototype of the AGEs) were higher in cirrhosis groups than in the controls. In agreement with two previous reports (Zuwala-Jagiello *et al.*, 2009; 2011) these results indicate that reactive oxygen species are overproduced in patients with liver cirrhosis. CML may lead to progression of cirrhosis by interaction with receptors that induce production of reactive species followed by a release of inflammatory cytokines in different cell types (Bierhaus *et al.*, 1998; Raj *et al.*, 2000) such as IL-6, ultimately leading to the production of CRP by the liver. A correlation to high sensitive C-reactive protein (hs-CRP) could not be demonstrated, and the suggestion that high levels of CML may activate an inflammatory response was not demonstrated by serum markers (TNF-α and IL-6). It is likely that the blood load of CML resembles only a small fraction of body's AGEs content and that the serum levels reflect particular changes in the body's AGEs pool. Thus, circulating CML-albumin may not be an adequate parameter for demonstrating effects on inflammatory response in cirrhotic patients. Most likely the focus should be on intracellular AGEs (Thornalley *et al.*, 2003).

A role of oxidative stress in the pathogenesis of chronic liver disease has been proposed by several authors (Bandara *et al.*, 2005; Nagata *et al.*, 2007; Nakhjavani *et al.*, 2011; Serejo *et al.*, 2003; Zuwala-Jagiello *et al.*, 2007). Studies have shown increased plasma levels of markers of lipid peroxidation and reduced plasma antioxidant content. Protein oxidation products are increasingly being used as markers instead of lipid peroxidation products in demonstrating oxidative stress (Dalle-Donne *et al.*, 2003). AOPPs measurements reflect the reactive species generation and the degree of protein oxidation (Witko-Sarsat *et al.*, 1996). It was reported that AOPPs generated by different oxidation patterns lead to the production of either hydrogen peroxide or nitric oxide (Servettaz *et al.*, 2007). Nitric oxide can interact with superoxide anion-radical forming reactive nitrogen species such as peroxynitrite. These reactive nitrogen species secondarily promote important reactions such as nitrosation, oxidation or nitration, leading to impaired cellular functions and enhanced inflammatory reactions (Friedman, 2008; Iwakiri & Groszmann, 2007). AOPPs are referred to as markers of oxidative stress as well as markers of neutrophil activation in chronic disease (Witko-Sarsat *et al.*, 2003). It has thus been shown that chlorinated oxidants of neutrophil origin may lead to oxidative stress, notably protein oxidation. Once formed, such AOPPs foci create a nidus for the amplification of oxidative stress. In addition to increased formation, decreased removal/detoxification of AOPPs may contribute to the stress. There is increasing evidence that the liver plays important roles in the elimination of AOPPs (Iwao *et al.*, 2006). In patients with chronic liver diseases, constriction of the sinusoidal blood stream leads to the development of portal hypertension with portocaval shunts (Svistounov & Smedsrød, 2004). The hindrance of substance exchange between hepatocytes and the sinusoidal blood stream could increase plasma level of AOPPs in these patients. Therefore, the liver, especially in cirrhotic patients, cannot prevent the accumulation of AOPPs effectively. Finally, our findings extended the results of Oettl *et al.* (2008) which suggested that albumin is oxidatively modified in patients with advanced liver disease depending on its severity. The present finding that AOPPs-albumin accumulation coexists with decreased TAS, while the plasma concentration of CML-modified albumin remains stable, supports the contention that AOPPs-albumin is more accurate marker of oxidative stress than glycoxidation products in cirrhotic patients. An increase in reactive species formation, manifested by increased hepatic and plasma levels of AOPPs (Gorka *et al.*, 2008; Sebeková *et al.*, 2002; Yagmur *et al.*, 2006; Zuwala–Jagiello *et al.*, 2006;) and as well as decreased antioxidant levels (Jain *et al.*, 2002; Zuwala–Jagiello *et al.*, 2009) have been reported in patients with liver cirrhosis. Finally, our previous study found that the patients with cirrhosis were exposed to oxidative stress and the level of AOPPs was significantly related to the severity of liver cirrhosis of various etiologies (Zuwala-Jagiello *et al.*, 2011).

The adverse effects of oxidative stress on the progression of cirrhosis may be categorized into effects on protein modifications and inflammatory response. Figure 4 presents a summary of the effects of AOPPs or AGEs and oxidative stress on markers of inflammation and hemodynamic changes in cirrhotic patients.

Very recently, advanced glycation endproducts have been found to act as pro-inflammatory factors (Sparvero *et al.*, 2009). Nevertheless, AOPPs are believed to be more closely related to inflammation (Fialova *et al.*, 2006) than AGEs, whose RAGE participates in AOPPs-mediated signal transduction (Kalousová *et al.*, 2005; 2006). These interactions enhance reactive oxygen species formation, with activation of nuclear factor NF-κB and release of pro-inflammatory cytokines (Bierhaus *et al.*, 2006; Hyogo & Yamagishi, 2008; Saito & Ishii, 2004) (Fig. 4). Moreover, the macrophage RAGE can be up-regulated by TNF-α (Miyata *et al.*,

1994). This is accompanied by the activation of macrophages and increased expression of TNF-α (Giron-González *et al.*, 2004). TNF-α production is also stimulated by macrophage sensing of intestinal microflora pathogen associated molecular patterns by toll-like receptors (Riordan *et al.*, 2003). It could therefore be consistent with observed increase levels of both AOPPs-albumin and TNF-α at an early stage of liver cirrhosis.

The hyperdynamic circulatory state associated with liver cirrhosis is characterized by vasodilatation and increased cardiac output; the arterial hypotension and relative hypovolemia caused by vasodilatation activate a number of vasoactive and neurohumoral systems (Wiest & Groszmann, 2002). TNF-α induces an endothelial activation, which can be detected by increased synthesis of nitric oxide (Spitzer, 1994). Endogenous nitric oxide, a powerful endothelium-derived vasodilator, has been implicated in hemodynamic changes present in cirrhotic patients (Garcı'a-Tsao *et al.*, 1998). Treatment with both specific anti-TNF polyclonal antibodies and thalidomide, an inhibitor of TNF-α production, significantly prevent the development of the hyperdynamic circulation and reduces portal pressure (Gatta *et al.*, 2008). TNF-α levels in our patients were clearly different from control group and were much higher in ascitic patients. However, no differences existed between patients with high and low mean arterial pressure, and no significant correlations with hemodynamic values were found. These data suggest that, although TNF-α might be one of the inducers of nitric oxide generation in cirrhotic patients, other factors acting through different pathways probably exist.

AOPPs derived from *in vivo* sources stimulated endothelial cell generation of reactive oxygen species, in particular superoxide anion (Guo *et al.*, 2008), at least in part through NADPH-oxidase (Wautier *et al.*, 2001). However, the exact mechanisms and sources by which reactive oxygen species are generated in the vasculature are not yet known in detail. It has been observed in several experimental animal models, that the endothelium is one of the major sources for the generation of reactive oxygen species. In parallel with the vascular dysfunction the formation of superoxide anions became augmented, and removal of endothelium completely abolished the production of reactive oxygen species. (reviewed in Wright *et al.*, 2006). In another report, Rhee *et al.* (2003) demonstrated that growth factor-induced H_2O_2 production (e.g. PDGF, EGF) requires the activation of phosphoinositide 3-kinase. The essential role of phosphoinositide 3-kinase is likely to provide phosphatidylinositol (3, 4, 5)-trisphosphate that recruits and activates a guanine nucleotide exchange factor of Rac, which is required for the activation of NADPH-oxidase. Thus, the generation of reactive oxygen species is largely dependent on the activation of NADPH-oxidase that is present in endothelial cell. AOPPs stimulated endothelial cell activation of the following signaling mediators: NADPH oxidase and NF-κB, the factors linked to increased expression of pro-inflammatory adhesion molecules, such as intercellular adhesion molecule-1 (ICAM-1) and vascular adhesion molecule-1 (VCAM-1) (Kim *et al.*, 2001; Yan *et al.*, 2010) (Fig. 4). Endothelial activation plays an active role in the modifications of circulatory status of cirrhotic patients (Grangé & Amiot, 2004). Elevated levels of AOPPs-albumin were detected in the early stages of liver dysfunction: plasma concentrations were increased in patients in Child Pugh class A, with higher values found in those in class B or C. Plasma concentrations of AOPPs-albumin were very weakly correlated with hemodynamic alterations (mean arterial pressure).

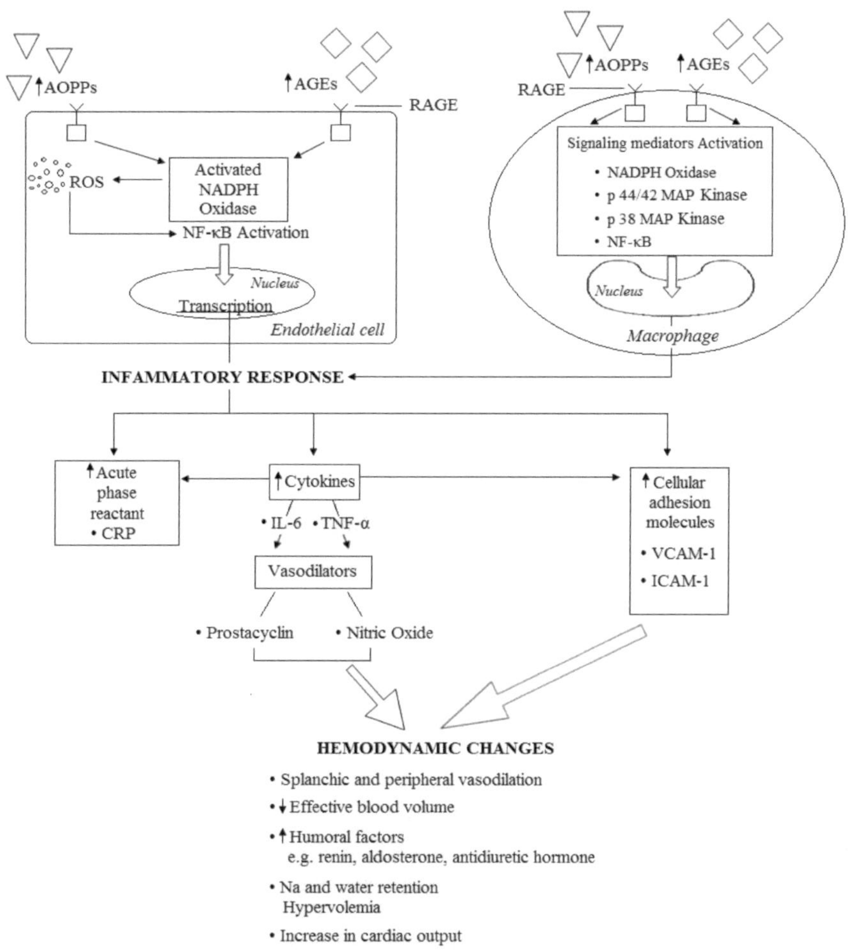

Fig. 4. Summary of the effects of AOPPs or AGEs and oxidative stress on markers of inflammation and hemodynamic changes in cirrhotic patients. AOPPs or AGEs bind with RAGE on the surface of endothelial cells lining blood vessels. AOPPS, AGEs ligands of RAGE sustain stimulation of RAGE. One consequence of RAGE signaling is the activation of NADPH oxidase and production of reactive oxygen species. Once formed, reactive oxygen species activate key transcription factor such as NF-κB, which results in the transcriptional activation of genes relevant for inflammation. Consequences include increased migration and activation of RAGE-expressing macrophages. This results in release of the pro-inflammatory cytokines. In this inflammatory environment, *via* interaction with RAGE on the surface of macrophages, AOPPs or AGEs magnify activation of NF-κB and other factors, thereby amplifying cellular stress and hepatic damage. In the aggregate, these processes may contribute to propagation of inflammation and vascular perturbation in liver cirrhosis. AGEs, advanced glycation endproducts; AOPPs, advanced oxidation protein products; CRP, C-reactive protein; ICAM-1, intercellular adhesion molecule 1; IL, interleukin; MAP, mitogen activated protein; NADPH, nicotinamide adenine dinucleotide phosphate (reduced form); NF-κB, nuclear factor κB; RAGE, receptor for AGEs; ROS, reactive oxygen species; TNF-α, tumour necrosis factor α; VCAM-1, vascular cell adhesion molecule.

These results suggested that this association of AOPPs with hemodynamic disturbances is dependent of the severity of cirrhosis. Additionally, AOPPs levels could be elevated as a result of insufficient renal elimination. However, the precise mechanism by which AOPPs is cleared from plasma is currently unknown. In addition, we found no correlation between AOPPs-albumin and serum creatinine levels. In any case, the values of AOPPs-albumin in patients with a low Child-Pugh score and absence of ascites suggests that AOPPs might have a role in the late stages of cirrhosis by aggravating the already initiated vasodilatation. Indeed, the presence of ascites, one of the major complications of cirrhosis and closely related to the hemodynamic disturbances of cirrhotic patients, was found in patients with higher levels of AOPPs. Finally, the extremely weak correlation between AOPPs-albumin levels and mean arterial pressure may suggest an indirect contribution of AOPPs to arterial vasodilatation through other mediators.

Structure and function of albumin are impaired in advanced liver disease by different mechanisms: plasma levels are decreased due to reduced synthesis and albumin is oxidatively modified. In this context, AOPPs-albumin may shows altered binding capacities for several substances. Decreased bilirubin binding was reported for *in vitro* oxidized albumin (Oettl & Stauber, 2007). As bilirubin is preferentially bound by the fully reduced form of albumin, impaired binding of bilirubin and other ligands (e.g. nitric oxide) is likely to occur in liver cirrhosis. Theoretically, increased circulating AOPPs-albumin may indirectly lead to elevation of nitric oxide which can, in turn, contribute to oxidative stress in cells (La Villa & Gentilini, 2008). Finally, nitric oxide plays a major key role in the development of hyperdynamic circulation and portal hypertension in cirrhosis (Iwakiri & Groszmann, 2007). Infusion of albumin (Garcovich *et al.*, 2009) as well as albumin dialysis has been shown to improve the circulatory dysfunction as evidenced by an increase in mean blood pressure and systemic vascular resistance (Mitzner *et al.*, 2001). This improvement in systemic hemodynamics might be due to a reduction in vasodilation following removal of nitric oxide which results in deactivation of the neurohormonal systems and a decrease in plasma levels of renin, aldosterone, norepinephrine and vasopressin (Chen *et al.*, 2009). However, other findings of the present study imply that AOPPs are not only the factors responsible for the hemodynamic changes observed in cirrhotic patients. The AOPPs-albumin levels did not correlate significantly with the parameters that accompany important hemodynamic alterations in cirrhotic patients, such as plasma renin activity and aldosterone. Finally, when cirrhotic patients in our study were divided according to high and low mean arterial pressure, we found similar AOPPs-albumin levels in both groups.

Portal hypertension and cirrhosis can increase gut permeability to endotoxin and impair reticuloendothelial function of the liver that may result in increased serum endotoxin concentrations (Cariello *et al.*, 2010). This may be a stimulus for the production of pro-inflammatory cytokines, resulting in the increased production of acute phase proteins such as C-reactive protein. In turn, CRP is capable of stimulating IL-6 and TNF-α production by monocytes (Ballou & Lozanski, 1992) and reactive oxygen species formation (Wang *et al.*, 2003). Advanced oxidation protein products, as pro-inflammatory factors, accumulated in cirrhotic patients (Zuwala–Jagiello *et al.*, 2006, 2009, 2011) and played an important role in the occurrence and progression of complications such as dysfunction of endothelial cells (Witko-Sarsat *et al.*, 1998). AOPPs correlate well with certain cytokines (Kalousová *et al.*, 2005) as well as with some markers of inflammation, including fibrinogen, orosomucoid. Even if the correlation between AOPPs-albumin and hs-CRP were poor, other studies demonstrated fair associations with other markers of oxidative stress, such as lipid peroxidation products and F2-isoprostanes. Furthermore, results from a recent study demonstrate that glycosylated and oxidized proteins indirectly up-regulate CRP expression in hepatocytes by stimulating monocytes to produce IL-6 (Li *et al.*, 2007). It seem, based on our study, even though there was functional loss of hepatocytes in patients with hepatic cirrhosis, the serum CRP level was still maintained in high level and dependent of AOPPs-albumin level with its significant correlation. The remaining viable hepatocytes may still contribute to this result. IL-6 is the main stimulant for hepatic production of CRP but also has other important roles leading to increased endothelial cell adhesiveness by up-regulating ICAM-1, and VCAM-1 and releasing inflammatory mediators, including IL-6 itself (Szmitko *et al.*, 2003). Finally, the significant correlation between the levels of AOPPs and IL-6 supports the existence of a link between AOPPs and hemodynamic changes present in cirrhotic patients (Fig. 4).

Portal hypertension is characterized by intrahepatic vascular resistance causing an increase of portal vein pressure, and leads to the development of ascite (Møller *et al.*, 2008). IL-6 levels in our cirrhotic patients were different from those in controls, increased with the severity of liver disease, were independently associated to the presence of ascites. IL-6 increased in serum of patients with ascites compared to compensated (Child-Pugh class A) patients without ascites, and similar results were obtained in a study where serum IL-6 was also analyzed (Zhang *et al.*, 2002). In a simplistic view, portal hypertension leads to the formation of portosystemic collateral veins in liver cirrhosis and the resulting shunting (Cichoz-Lach *et al.*, 2008) also contributes to impaired hepatic uptake of IL-6. It has been convincingly shown that hepatic uptake of IL-6 is significantly impaired in patients with liver cirrhosis, and this may at least in part explain elevated serum levels in these patients (Soresi *et al.*, 2006). In our study, IL-6 levels increase significantly in association with the severity of liver cirrhosis according to the MELD score. Moreover, IL-6 levels in all cirrhotic patients were independently associated to the presence of low mean arterial pressure, and showed significant correlations with parameters related to hemodynamic abnormalities. The mechanism by which IL-6 could cause vasodilatation is unknown. However, the effect appears to be independent of nitric oxide, possibly due to an important role of prostacyclin synthesis (Dagher & Moore, 2001). It is then possible that IL-6 would produces vasodilatation by inducing prostacyclin synthesis; the effect of IL-6 would be potentiated by AOPPs stimulation (Li et al., 2007).

Further, investigators have tried to find more noninvasive biomarkers for cirrhotic patients for years (Schuppan & Afdhal, 2008). We observed good abilities of plasma AOPPs-albumin, TNF-α and IL-6 levels to distinguish cirrhotic patients from healthy controls, with good sensitivities and specificities by ROC analysis. Additionally, these parameters also were found to be elevated in concordance with the severity of cirrhosis. Thereby, it is possible that plasma levels of AOPPs-albumin, TNF-α and IL-6 levels could be evaluated as candidate biomarkers for initial and long-term assessment of liver cirrhosis.

5. Conclusion

In conclusion, there are differences between advanced oxidation protein products modified-albumin (AOPPs-albumin), which act as a pure oxidative stress marker, and Nε (carboxymethyl)lysine modified-albumin (CML-albumin; as prototype of the advanced glycation endproducts-AGEs), which behave as both oxidative and carbonyl stress markers. AOPPs-albumin shows a closer relationship to inflammation than CML-albumin. Because of the relationship of AOPPs-albumin with formation of inflammation, their relationship with certain inflammatory markers and their changes during progression of chronic liver disease, AOPPs may provide a marker of chronic long-lasting liver damage. Oxidative stress not only contributes to the derangement of hemodynamic chronic liver failure, but also gradually increases with its progression to end-stage liver disease.

6. References

Alderman, C.J., Shah, S., Foreman, J.C., Chain, B.M. & Katz, D.R. (2002) The role of advanced oxidation protein products in regulation of dendritic cell function. *Free Radical Biology & Medicine*, Vol.32, No.5, (March 2002), pp. 377-385, ISSN:0891-5849

Ballou, S.P. & Lozanski, G. (1992) Induction of inflammatory cytokine release from cultured human monocytes by C-reactive protein. *Cytokine* Vol.4, No.5, (September 1992), pp. 361-368, ISSN 1043-4666

Bandara, P., George, J., McCaughan, G., Naidoo, D., Lux O., Salonikas, C., Kench, J., Byth, K. & Farrell, G.C. (2005) Antioxidant levels in peripheral blood, disease activity and fibrotic stage in chronic hepatitis C. *Liver International*, Vol.2, No.3, (June 2005), pp. 518-526, ISSN 1478-3223

Baskol, G., Demir, H., Baskol, M., Kilic, E., Ates, F., Karakukcu, C. & Ustdal, M. (2006) Investigation of protein oxidation and lipid peroxidation in patients with rheumatoid arthritis. *Cell Biochemistry and Function*, Vol.24, No.4, (July 2006), pp. 307-311, ISSN 263-6484

Baynes, J.W. & Thorpe, S.R. (1999) Role of oxidative stress in diabetic complications: a new perspective on an old paradigm. *Diabetes*, Vol.48, No.1, (January 1999), pp. 1-9, ISSN 0012-1797

Bierhaus, A., Hofmann, M.A., Ziegler, R. & Nawroth, P.P. (1998) AGEs and their interaction with AGE-receptors in vascular disease and diabetes mellitus. I. The AGE concept. *Cardiovascular Research*, Vol.37, No.3, (March 1998), pp. 586-600, ISSN 0008-6363

Bierhaus, A., Stern, D.M. & Nawroth, P.P. (2006) RAGE in inflammation: a new therapeutic target? *Current Opinion in Investigational Drugs*, Vol.7, No.11, (November 2006), pp. 985-991, ISSN 1472-4472

Cariello, R., Federico, A., Sapone, A., Tuccillo, C., Scialdone, VR., Tiso, A., Miranda, A., Portincasa, P., Carbonara, V., Palasciano, G., Martorelli, L., Esposito, P., Cartenì, M., Del Vecchio Blanco, C. & Loguercio, C. (2010) Intestinal permeability in patients with chronic liver diseases: Its relationship with the aetiology and the entity of liver damage. *Digestive and Liver Disease*, Vol.42, No.3, (March 2010), pp. 200-204, ISSN 1590-8658

Chen, T.A., Tsao, Y.C., Chen, A., Lo, G.H., Lin, C.K., Yu, H.C., Cheng, L.C., Hsu, P.I. & Tsai, W.L. (2009) Effect of intravenous albumin on endotoxin removal., cytokines., and nitric oxide production in patients with cirrhosis and spontaneous bacterial peritonitis. *Scandinavian Journal of Gastroenterology*, Vol.44, No.5, pp. 619-625, ISSN 0036-5521

Cichoz-Lach, H., Celiński, K., Slomka, M. & Kasztelan-Szczerbińska, B. (2008) Pathophysiology of portal hypertension. *Journal of Physiology and Pharmacology Supplement*, Vol.59, Suppl.2, (August 2008), pp. 231-238. ISSN 0867-5910

Cybulsky, M.I., Fries, J.W., Williams, A.J., Sultan, P., Eddy, R., Byers, M., Shows, T., Gimbrone, M.A.Jr. & Collins, T. (1991) Gene structure., chromosomal location., and basis for alternative mRNA splicing of the human VCAM1 gene. *Proceedings of the National Academy of Sciences of the United States of America*, Vol.88, No.17, (September 1991), pp. 7859-7863, ISSN 0027-8424

Dagher, L. & Moore, K. (2001) The hepatorenal syndrome. *Gut*, Vol.49, No.5, (November 2001), pp. 729-737, ISSN 0017-5749

Dalle-Donne, I., Rossi, R., Giustarini, D., Milzani, A. & Colombo, R. (2003) Protein carbonyl groups as biomarkers of oxidative stress. *Clinica Chimica Acta*, Vol.329, No.1-2, (March 2003), pp. 23-38, ISSN 0009-8981

Esposito, C., Gerlach, H., Brett, J., Stern, D. & Vlassara, H. (1989) Endothelial receptor-mediated binding of glucose-modified albumin is associated with increased monolayer permeability and modulation of cell surface coagulant properties. *The Journal of Experimental Medicine*, Vol.170, No.4, (October 1989), pp. 1387-1407, ISSN 0022-1007

Fialová, L., Malbohan, I., Kalousová, M., Soukupová, J., Krofta, L., Stípek, S. & Zima, T. (2006) Oxidative stress and inflammation in pregnancy. *Scandinavian Journal of Clinical and Laboratory Investigation*, Vol.66, No.2, pp. 121-127, ISSN 0036-5513

Friedman, S.L. Mechanisms of hepatic fibrogenesis. (2008) *Gastroenterology*, Vol.134, No.6, (May 2008), pp. 1655-1669, ISSN 0016-5085

Garcia-Tsao, G., Angulo, P., Garcia, JC., Groszmann, RJ. & Cadelina, GW. (1998) The diagnostic and predictive value of ascites nitric oxide levels in patients with spontaneous bacterial peritonitis. *Hepatology*, Vol.28, No.1, (July 1998), pp. 17-21, ISSN 0270-9139

Garcovich, M., Zocco, M.A. & Gasbarrini, A. (2009) Clinical use of albumin in hepatology. *Blood Transfusion*, Vol.7, No.4, (October 2009), pp. 268-77, ISSN 1723-2007

Gatta, A., Bolognesi, M. & Merkel, C. (2008) Vasoactive factors and hemodynamic mechanisms in the pathophysiology of portal hypertension in cirrhosis. *Molecular Aspects of Medicine*, Vol.29, No.1-2, (February-April 2008), pp. 119-129, ISSN 0098-2997

Genesca, J., González, A., Mujal, A., Cereto, F. & Segura, R. (1999) Vascular endothelia growth factor levels in liver cirrhosis. *Digestive Diseases and Sciences*, Vol.44, No.6, (June 1999), pp. 1261-1262, ISSN 0163-2116

Giron-González, JA., Martínez-Sierra, C., Rodriguez-Ramos, C., Macías, M.A., Rendon, P., Díaz, F., Fernández-Gutiérrez, C. & Martín-Herrera, L. (2004) Implication of inflammation-related cytokines in the natural history of liver cirrhosis. *Liver International*, Vol.24, No.5, (October 2004), pp. 437-445, ISSN 1478-3223

Gorka, J., Zuwala-Jagiello, J., Pazgan-Simon, M., Simon, K. & Warwas, M. (2008) [Fluorescence of age in serum in detecting liver cirrhosis and hepatocellular carcinoma among patients with anti-HCV antibodies]. *Przeglad Epidemiologiczny*, Vol.62, No.2, pp. 393-400. Polish. ISSN 0033-210

Grangé, JD. & Amiot, X. (2004) Nitric oxide and renal function in cirrhotic patients with ascites, from physiopathology to practice. *European Journal of Gastroenterology & Hepatology*, Vol.16, No.6, (June 2004), pp. 567-570, ISSN 0954-691X

Guo, ZJ., Niu, H.X., Hou, F.F., Zhang, L., Fu, N., Nagai, R., Lu, X., Chen, B.H., Shan, Y.X., Tian, J.W., Nagaraj, R.H., Xie, D. & Zhang, X. (2008) Advanced oxidation protein products activate vascular endothelial cells via a RAGE-mediated signaling pathway. *Antioxidants & Redox Signaling,* Vol.10, No.10, (October 2008), pp. 1699-1712, ISSN 1523-0864

Halliwell, B. (2007) Oxidative stress and cancer: have we moved forward? *The Biochemical Journal,* Vol.401, No1, (January 2007), pp. 1-11, ISSN 0264-6021

Hanck, C., Glatzel, M., Singer, M.V. & Rossol, S. (2000) Gene expression of TNF-receptors in peripheral blood mononuclear cells of patients with alcoholic cirrhosis. *Journal of Hepatology,* Vol.32, No.1, (January 2000), pp. 51-57, ISSN 0168-8278

Huo, T.I., Lin, H.C., Wu, J.C., Lee, F.Y., Hou, M.C., Lee, P.C., Chang, F.Y. & Lee, S.D. (2006) Proposal of a modified Child-Turcotte-Pugh scoring system and comparison with the model for end-stage liver disease for outcome prediction in patients with cirrhosis. *Liver Transplantation,* Vol.12, No.1, (January 2006), pp. 65-71, ISSN 1527-6465

Hyogo, H. & Yamagishi, S. (2008) Advanced glycation end products (AGEs) and their involvement in liver disease. *Current Pharmaceutical Design,* Vol.14, No.10,(October 2008), pp. 969-972, ISSN 1381-6128

Iwakiri, Y. & Groszmann, R.J. (2007) Vascular endothelial dysfunction in cirrhosis. *Journal of Hepatology,* Vol.46, No.5, (May 2007), pp. 927-934, ISSN 0168-8278

Jain, S.K., Pemberton, P.W., Smith, A., McMahon, R.F., Burrows, P.C., Aboutwerat, A. & Warnes, T.W. (2002) Oxidative stress in chronic hepatitis C, not just a feature of late stage disease. *Journal of Hepatology,* Vol.36, No.6, (June 2002), pp. 805-811, ISSN 0168-8278

Kalousová, M., Sulková, S., Fialová, L., Soukupová, J., Malbohan, IM., Spacek, P., Braun, M., Mikulíková, L., Fortová, M., Horejsí, M., Tesar, V. & Zima, T. (2003) Glycoxidation and inflammation in chronic haemodialysis patients. *Nephrology, Dialysis, Transplantation,* Vol.18, No.12, (December 2003), pp. 2577-2581, ISSN 0931-0509

Kalousová, M., Zima, T., Tesar, V., Dusilová-Sulková, S. & Skrha, J. (2005) Advanced glycoxidation end products in chronic diseases-clinical chemistry and genetic background. *Mutation Research,* Vol.579, No.1-2, (November 2005), pp. 37-46, ISSN 0027-5107

Kim, I., Moon, S.O., Kim, S.H., Kim, H.J., Koh, Y.S. & Koh, G.Y. (2001) Vascular endothelial growth factor expression of intercellular adhesion molecule 1 (ICAM-1)., vascular cell adhesion molecule 1 (VCAM-1)., and E-selectin through nuclear factor-kappa B activation in endothelial cells. *The Journal of Biological Chemistry,* Vol.276, No.10, (March 2001), pp. 7614-7620, ISSN 0021-9258

Kirkham, P. (2007) Oxidative stress and macrophage function, a failure to resolve the inflammatory response. *Biochemical Society Transactions,* Vol.35, No.Pt2 (April 2007), pp. 284-287, ISSN 0300-5127

La Villa, G. & Gentilini, P. (2008) Hemodynamic alterations in liver cirrhosis. *Molecular Aspects of Medicine,* Vol.29, No.1-2, (February-April 2008), pp. 112-118, ISSN 0098-2997

Li, J.T., Hou, F.F., Guo, Z.J., Shan, Y.X., Zhang, X. & Liu, Z.Q. (2007) Advanced glycation end products upregulate C-reactive protein synthesis by human hepatocytes through stimulation of monocyte IL-6 and IL-1 beta production. *Scandinavian Journal of Immunology,* Vol.66, No.5, (November 2007), pp. 555-562, ISSN 0300-9475

Mitzner, S.R., Klammt, S., Peszynski, P., Hickstein, H., Korten, G., Stange, J. & Schmidt, R. (2001) Improvement of multiple organ functions in hepatorenal syndrome during albumin dialysis with the molecular adsorbent recirculating system. *Therapeutic Apheresis*, Vol.5, No.5, (October 2001), pp. 417-422, ISSN 1091-6660

Miyata, T., Inagi, R., Iida, Y., Sato, M., Yamada, N., Oda, O., Maeda, K. & Seo, H. (1994) Involvement of beta 2-microglobulin modified with advanced glycation end products in the pathogenesis of hemodialysis-associated amyloidosis. Induction of human monocyte chemotaxis and macrophage secretion of tumor necrosis factor-alpha and interleukin-1. *The Journal of Clinical Investigation*, Vol.94, No.2, (February 1994), pp. 521-528, ISSN 0021-9738

Møller, S., Henriksen, J.H. & Bendtsen, F. (2008) Pathogenetic background for treatment of ascites and hepatorenal syndrome. *Hepatology International*, Vol.2, No.4, (December 2008), pp. 416-428, ISSN 1936-0533

Nagata, K., Suzuki, H. & Sakaguchi, S. (2007) Common pathogenic mechanism in development progression of liver injury caused by non-alcoholic or alcoholic steatohepatitis. *The Journal of Toxicological Sciences*, Vol.32, No.5, (December 2007), pp. 453-468, ISSN 0388-1350

Nakhjavani, M., Mashayekh, A., Khalilzadeh, O., Asgarani, F., Morteza, A., Omidi, M. & Froutan, H. (2011) Oxidized low-density lipoprotein is associated with viral load and disease activity in patients with chronic hepatitis C. *Clinics and Research in Hepatology & Gastroenterology*, Vol.35, No.2, (February 2011), pp. 111-116, ISSN 2210-7401

Oettl, K. & Stauber, R.E. (2007) Physiological and pathological changes in the redox state of human serum albumin critically influence its binding properties. *British Journal of Pharmacology*, Vol.151, No.5, (July 2007), pp. 580-590, ISSN 0007-1188

Oettl, K., Stadlbauer, V., Petter, F., Greilberger, J., Putz-Bankuti, C., Hallström, S., Lackner, C. & Stauber, R.E. (2008) Oxidative damage of albumin in advanced liver disease. *Biochimica et Biophysica Acta*, Vol.1782, No.7-8, (July-August 2008), pp. 469-473, ISSN 0006-3002

Porcel, J.M. (2002) Unilateral pleural effusion secondary to brachiocephalic venous thrombosis, a rare complication of central vein catheterization. *Respiration,* Vol.69, No.6, pp. 569, ISSN 0025-7931

Raj, D.S., Choudhury, D., Welbourne, T.C. & Levi, M. (2000) Advanced glycation end products, a Nephrologist's perspective. *American Journal of Kidney Diseases,* Vol.35, No.3, (March 2000), pp. 365-380, ISSN 0272-6386

Reddy, S., Bichler, J., Wells-Knecht, K.J., Thorpe, S.R. & Baynes, J.W. (1995) Nepsilon-(carboxymethyl)lysine is a dominant advanced glycation end product (AGE) antigen in tissue proteins. *Biochemistry,* Vol.34, No.34, (August 1995), pp. 10872-10878, ISSN 0006-2960

Rhee, S.G., Chang, T.S., Bae, Y.S., Lee, S.R. & Kang SW. (2003) Cellular regulation by hydrogen peroxide. Journal of the American Society of Nephrology : JASN, Vol.14, No.8 Suppl 3, (August 2003), pp. S211-S215, ISSN 1046-6673

Riordan, S.M., Skinner, N., Nagree, A., McCallum, H., McIver, C.J., Kurtovic, J., Hamilton, J.A., Bengmark, S., Williams, R. & Visvanathan, K. (2003) Peripheral blood mononuclear cell expression of toll-like receptors and relation to cytokine levels in cirrhosis. *Hepatology,* Vol.37, No.5, (May 2003), pp. 1154-1164, ISSN 0270-9139

Saito, H. & Ishii, H. (2004) Recent understanding of immunological aspects in alcoholic hepatitis. *Hepatology Research,* Vol.30, No.4, (December 2004), pp. 193-198, ISSN 1386-6346

Schuppan, D. & Afdhal, N.H. (2008) Liver cirrhosis. *Lancet* Vol.371, No.9615, (March 2008), pp. 838-851, ISSN 0140-6736

Szmitko, P.E., Wang, C.H., Weisel, R.D., de Almeida, J.R., Anderson, T.J. & Verma S. (2003) New markers of inflammation and endothelial cell activation: Part I. *Circulation,* Vol.108, No.16, (October 2003), pp. 1917-1923. ISSN 0009-7322

Sebeková, K., Kupcová, V., Schinzel, R. & Heidland, A. (2002) Markedly elevated levels of plasma advanced glycation end products in patients with liver cirrhosis - amelioration by liver transplantation. *Journal of Hepatology,* Vol.36, No.1, (January 2002), pp. 66-71, ISSN 0168-8278

Serejo, F., Emerit, I., Filipe, P.M., Fernandes, A.C., Costa, M.A., Freitas, J.P. & de Moura, M.C. (2003) Oxidative stress in chronic hepatitis C, the effect of interferon therapy and correlation with pathological features. *Canadian Journal of Gastroenterology,* Vol.17, No.11, (November 2003), pp. 644-650, ISSN 0835-7900

Servettaz, A., Guilpain, P., Goulvestre, C., Chéreau, C., Hercend, C., Nicco, C., Guillevin, L., Weill, B., Mouthon, L. & Batteux, F. (2007) Radical oxygen species production induced by advanced oxidation protein products predicts clinical evolution and response to treatment in systemic sclerosis. *Annals of The Rheumatic Diseases*, Vol.66, No.9, (September 2007), pp. 1202-1209, ISSN 0003-4967

Soresi, M., Giannitrapani, L., D'Antona, F., Florena, A.M., La Spada, E., Terranova, A., Cervello, M., D'Alessandro, N. & Montalto, G. (2006) Interleukin-6 and its soluble receptor in patients with liver cirrhosis and hepatocellular carcinoma. *World journal of gastroenterology,* Vol.12, No.16, (April 2006), pp. 2563-2568, ISSN 1007-9327

Sparvero, L.J., Asafu-Adjei, D., Kang, R., Tang, D., Amin, N., Im, J., Rutledge, R., Lin, B., Amoscato, A.A., Zeh, H.J. & Lotze, M.T. (2009) RAGE (Receptor for Advanced Glycation Endproducts); RAGE ligands., and their role in cancer and inflammation. *Journal of Translational Medicine,* Vol.17, No.7 (March 2007), pp. 17, ISSN 1479-5876

Spitzer, J.A. (1994) Cytokine stimulation of nitric oxide formation and differential regulation in hepatocytes and nonparenchymal cells of endotoxemic rats. *Hepatology,* Vol.19, No.1, (January 1994), pp. 217-228, ISSN 0270-9139

Svistounov, D. & Smedsrød, B. (2004) Hepatic clearance of advanced glycation end products (AGEs)--myth or truth? *Journal of Hepatology,* Vol.41, No.6, (December 2004), pp. 1038-1040, ISSN 0168-8278

Thornalley, PJ., Battah, S., Ahmed, N., Karachalias, N., Agalou, S., Babaei-Jadidi, R. & Dawnay, A. (2003) Quantitative screening of advanced glycation endproducts in cellular and extracellular proteins by tandem mass spectrometry. *The Biochemical Journal,* Vol.375, No.Pt3, (November 2003), pp. 581-592, ISSN 0264-6021

Tilg, H., Wilmer, A., Vogel, W., Herold, M., Nölchen, B., Judmaier, G. & Huber, C. (1992) Serum levels of cytokines in chronic liver diseases. *Gastroenterology,* Vol.103, No.1, (July 1992), pp. 264-274, ISSN 0016-5085

Tsutsui, H., Adachi, K., Seki, E. & Nakanishi, K. (2003) Cytokine-induced inflammatory liver injuries. *Current Molecular Medicine,* Vol.3, No.6, (September 2003), pp. 545-559, ISSN 1566-5240

Valko, M., Leibfritz, D., Moncol, J., Cronin, M.T., Mazur, M. & Telser, J. (2007) Free radicals and antioxidants in normal physiological functions and human disease. *The International Journal of Biochemistry & Cell Biology,* Vol.39, No.1, pp. 44-84, ISSN 1357-2725

Wang, C.H., Li, S.H., Weisel, R.D., Fedak, P.W., Dumont, A.S., Szmitko, P., Li, R.K., Mickle, D.A. & Verma, S. (2003) C-reactive protein upregulates angiotensin type 1 receptors in vascular smooth muscle. *Circulation,* Vol.107, No.13, (April 2003), pp. 1783-1790, ISSN 0009-7322

Wautier, M.P., Chappey, O., Corda, S., Stern, D.M., Schmidt, A.M. & Wautier, J.L. (2001) Activation of NADPH oxidase by AGE links oxidant stress to altered gene expression via RAGE. *American Journal of Physiology. Endocrinology and Metabolism,* Vol.280, No.5, (May 2001), pp.E685-E694, ISSN 0193-1849

Wiest, R. & Groszmann, R.J. (2002) The paradox of nitric oxide in cirrhosis and portal hypertension, too much: not enough. *Hepatology,* Vol.35, No.2, (February 2002), pp. 478-491, ISSN 0270-9139

Witko-Sarsat, V., Friedlander, M., Capeillère-Blandin, C., Nguyen-Khoa, T., Nguyen, A.T., Zingraff, J., Jungers, P. & Descamps-Latscha, B. (1996) Advanced oxidation protein products as a novel marker of oxidative stress in uremia. *Kidney International,* Vol.49, No.5, (May 1996), pp. 1304-1313, ISSN 0085-2538

Witko-Sarsat, V., Friedlander, M., Nguyen, Khoaj T., Capeillère-Blandin, C., Nguyen, A.T., Canteloup, S., Dayer, J.M., Jungers, P., Drüeke, T. & Descamps-Latscha, B. (1998) Advanced oxidation protein products as novel mediators of inflammation and monocyte activation in chronic renal failure. *Journal Immunology,* Vol.161, No.5, (September 5), pp 2524-2532, ISSN 0022-1767

Witko-Sarsat, V., Gausson, V., Nguyen, A., Touam, M., Drüeke, T., Santangelo, F. & Descamps-Latscha, B. (2003) AOPP-induced activation of human neutrophil and monocyte oxidative metabolism, a potential target for N-acetylcysteine treatment in dialysis patients. *Kidney International,* Vol.64, No.1, (July 2003), pp. 82-91, ISSN 0085-2538

Wright, E.Jr, Scism-Bacon, J.L. & Glass, L.C. (2006) Oxidative stress in type 2 diabetes: the role of fasting and postprandial glycaemia. *International Journal of Clinical Practice,* Vol.60, No.3, (March 2006), pp. 308-314. ISSN 1368-5031

Yan, S.F., Ramasamy, R. & Schmidt, A.M. (2010) The RAGE axis: a fundamental mechanism signaling danger to the vulnerable vasculature. *Circulation Research,* Vol.106, No5, (March 2010), pp. 842-853, ISSN 0009-7330

Yagmur, E., Tacke, F., Weiss, C., Lahme, B., Manns, MP., Kiefer, P., Trautwein, C. & Gressner, A.M. (2006) Elevation of Nepsilon-(carboxymethyl)lysine-modified advanced glycation end products in chronic liver disease is an indicator of liver cirrhosis. *Clinical Biochemistry,* Vol.39, No.1, (Jananuary 2006), pp. 39-45, ISSN 0009-9120

Yazici, C., Köse, K., Calis, M., Kuzugüden, S. & Kirnap, M. (2004) Protein oxidation status in patients with ankylosing spondylitis. *Rheumatology (Oxford,* Vol.43, No.10, (October 2004), 1235-1239, ISSN 1462-0324

Zeni, F., Tardy, B., Vindimian, M., Comtet, C., Page, Y., Cusey, I. & Bertrand, J.C. (1993) High levels of tumor necrosis factor-alpha and interleukin-6 in the ascitic fluid of cirrhotic patients with spontaneous bacterial peritonitis. *Clinical Infectious Diseases*, Vol.17, No.2, (August 1993), pp. 218-223, ISSN 1058-4838

Zhang, W., Yue, B., Wang, G.Q. & Lu, S.L. (2002) Serum and ascites levels of macrophage migration inhibitory factor: TNF-alpha and IL-6 in patients with chronic virus hepatitis B and hepatitis cirrhosis. *Hepatobiliary & pancreatic diseases international*, Vol.1, No.4, (November 2002), pp 577-580, ISSN 1499-3872

Zuwala-Jagiello, J., Pazgan-Simon, M., Gorka., J., Simon, K., Milczarska, J. & Warwas, M. (2007) Serum advanced glycation end products and the development of hepatocellular carcinoma among HBV carriers. *Polish Journal of Environmental Studies*, Vol.16, No.5C, pp. 747-751, ISSN 1230-1485

Zuwala-Jagiello, J., Pazgan-Simon, M., Simon, K. & Warwas, M. (2009) Elevated advanced oxidation protein products levels in patients with liver cirrhosis. *Acta Biochimica Polonica* Vol.56(4), 679-85. ISSN, 0001-527X

Zuwala-Jagiello, J., Pazgan-Simon, M., Simon, K. & Warwas, M. (2011) Advanced oxidation protein products and inflammatory markers in liver cirrhosis, a comparison between alcohol-related and HCV-related cirrhosis. *Acta Biochimica Polonica*, Vol.58, No.1, pp. 59-65 ISSN 0001-527X

17

Oxidative Stress in Parkinson's Disease; Parallels Between Current Animal Models, Human Studies and Cells

Anwar Norazit[1,2], George Mellick[1] and Adrian C. B. Meedeniya[1,3*]
[1]Eskitis Institute for Cell and Molecular Therapies, Griffith University, Nathan, Queensland
[2]Department of Molecular Medicine, Faculty of Medicine, University of Kuala Lumpur,
[3]Griffith Health Institute, Griffith University, Gold Coast, Queensland,
[1,3]Australia
[2]Malaysia

1. Introduction

Reactive oxygen species (ROS) are byproducts generated primarily from the breakdown of oxygen during aerobic metabolism. ROS can be found as free radicals containing highly reactive unpaired electrons (super oxide, nitric oxide, hydroxyl radical) or as other molecules (hydrogen peroxide, peroxynitrate). Under normal physiological conditions, ROS are neutralized by antioxidants. However, an increased production of ROS, namely, oxidative stress, can occur under pathophysiological conditions. Oxidative stress can be defined as an imbalance between oxidants and antioxidants where the oxidants are favoured, potentially leading to cellular damage (Sies 1985, Sies 1986, Sies 1991).

The brain is highly susceptible to oxidative stress due to its high metabolic rate and limited regeneration capability (Andersen 2004). Oxidative stress has been implicated in a variety of neurodegenerative disease, including Parkinson's disease (PD), Alzheimer's disease, and amyotrophic lateral sclerosis. However, presence of oxidative stress as a cause or consequence of neurodegeneration, remains to be determined.

This review focuses on the pathogenesis of PD in relation to oxidative stress and the current animal models used to mimic the pathophysiology of human PD. We will also compare the animal and human data for PD like neurodegeneration with cell models of PD. This will also include a review on current experimentation and antioxidant therapies for counteracting oxidative stress.

2. Parkinson's disease

PD was first described in the early 19th century in the monologue "An essay on the shaking palsy" (Parkinson 2002). The three cardinal symptoms of PD are bradykinesia, rigidity, and

* Corresponding Author

postural instability (Gash et al. 1996). The clinical diagnosis of PD is usually based on the United Kingdom Parkinson's Disease Society Brain Research Centre criteria (Gibb and Lees 1988), with the accuracy of this diagnosis being high (90%) (Hughes, Daniel and Lees 2001). During the first 10 years of the disease, patients usually exhibit slowness of movement, mild gait hypokinesia, resting tremor, micrographic handwriting and reduced speech volume (Morris 2000). During the latter stages of the disease, festination, dyskinesia, akinesia, marked hypokinesia, postural instability and falls are usually more pronounced (Morris 2000). The symptoms of this condition only show after 80% of the striatal innervations and 60% of the substantia nigra par compacta dopaminergic neurons are lost, suggestive of a pathological process initiated at the synaptic end of the nigral neurons, with neuronal death as a result from a 'dying back' process (Dauer and Przedborski 2003).

2.1 Parkinson's disease pathology

PD can be defined as a progressive neurodegenerative disorder characterised histopathologically by the degeneration of the dopaminergic nigrostriatal pathway (Watts et al. 1997). Post-mortem analyses of the substantia nigra in PD patients have shown effects of oxidative stress with a decrease in glutathione (GSH) levels, increased levels of iron, neuromelanin associated redox-active iron, lipid peroxidation, protein oxidation and DNA damage (Jenner and Olanow 1998, Faucheux et al. 2003, Dexter et al. 1989). These changes may directly induce nigral cell degeneration via oxidative stress or render neurons susceptible to the actions of toxins.

The neurotrophic factor milieu of the brain is affected in PD patients. A decrease in brain derived neurotrophic factor (BDNF) in the post-mortem brains of clinically and pathologically diagnosed PD patients, compared to normal controls (Mogi et al. 1999, Parain et al. 1999). A decrease in BDNF mRNA expression in the substantia nigra of PD patients has also been demonstrated (Howells et al. 2000). A decrease in glial cell derived neurotrophic factor (GDNF) and ciliary neurotrophic factor (CNTF) also occurs in the brains of PD patients (Chauhan, Siegel and Lee 2001). The resultant inability to up-regulate neurotrophic factors in response to injury or stress may compromised defence mechanisms of the brain, thus contributing to cell degeneration (Olanow and Tatton 1999).

2.2 Pathogenic role of host/exogenous factors

There is increasing evidence of host and /or exogenous factors playing a role in the pathogenesis of PD. Many of these factors negatively impact mitochondrial function.

2.2.1 Age

The incidence of PD is related to increasing age (de Rijk et al. 1997, Mayeux et al. 1992, Van Den Eeden et al. 2003). With age, high levels of mitochondrial DNA deletion (Bender et al. 2006); increase in α-synuclein (Chu and Kordower 2007); decrease in dopamine transporter mRNA (Bannon et al. 1992); decrease in neurotrophic factor gene expression (Lee, Weindruch and Prolla 2000); reduced response to growth factors (Smith 1996); decrease in brain peroxidase and catalase activity (Ambani, Van Woert and Murphy 1975); and a decrease in dopamine binding sites (Severson et al. 1982) are apparent in the neuronal population of the substantia nigra. The relationship between PD and aging includes a superposition of a topographic gradient of neuronal loss in brainstem and basal forebrain structures related to the disease process and an age-related temporal gradient. Clinical progression of PD is determined by advancing age and not by disease duration; and a biological interaction is involved in the effects of the disease process and aging on non dopaminergic structures (Levy 2007).

2.2.2 Environmental toxins

Pesticide exposure is implicated as an environmental risk factor for PD (Herishanu et al. 2001, Le Couteur et al. 1999, Tanner 1989, Ho, Woo and Lee 1989). The susceptibility of humans to these pesticides has been reported to be linked to genetic factors (Menegon et al. 1998, Drozdzik et al. 2003). Many of these pesticides have a major site of action along the mitochondrial electron transport chain (Degli Esposti 1998), which results in increasing oxidative stress.

2.2.3 Genetic determinants

The role of genetic factors in PD has been the subject of intense scrutiny. The first clue of familial PD was provided in 1907 when Gowers reported approximately 15% of his PD patients reported an affected family member (Gowers 1902) Since then many genes have been identified as causing familial PD (Schapira 2008). The products associated with the gene mutations are either mitochondrial proteins or are associated with mitochondria. Namely, proteins that interface with the pathways of oxidative stress and free radical damage.

Gene	Locus	Inheritance	Gene product
PARK1/4	4q21	Autosomal dominant	α-synuclein
PARK2	6q25	Autosomal recessive	Parkin
PARK3	2p13	Autosomal dominant	-
UCH-L1	4p15	Autosomal dominant	Ubiquitin thiolesterase
PINK1	1p35	Autosomal recessive	PTEN-induced putative kinase 1
PARK7	1p36	Autosomal recessive	DJ-1
LRRK2	12p	Autosomal dominant	Leucine-rich repeat kinase 2
ATP13A2	1p36	Autosomal recessive	ATPase type 13A2
PARK10	1p32	Autosomal recessive	-
PARK11	2q36-q37	-	-

Table 1. Genetic causes of PD (modified from Schapira, 2008)

2.2.4 Sporadic Parkinson's disease

The Braak hypothesis suggests that the initial event in sporadic PD may be an infectious assault on susceptible neuronal types in the olfactory or enteric nervous system (Braak et al. 2003a, Hawkes, Del Tredici and Braak 2007, Braak et al. 2003b). The Lewy neuritis and Lewy bodies' progress rostrally in stages into the lower brainstem region (medulla oblongata and pontine tegmentum; stages 1 and 2), followed by the midbrain (substantia nigra; stage 3) and the basal prosencephalon and mesocortex (stage 4), and eventually the neocortex (stage 5 and 6) (Braak et al. 2003a, Braak et al. 2003b). Stages 1 to 3 have been characterised as the pre-symptomatic phase while stage 4 to 6 has been characterised as the symptomatic phase. The sequential ascending topography reported by Braak (2003b) has been reported to be only partially in line with the latest imaging of PD (Brooks 2010). It may instead reflect the more primitive regions of the nervous system (and perhaps the more active) showing a greater susceptibility.

3. Parkinson's disease animal models

There are both toxin and genetic animal models popularly used to represent PD. Both of these models increase ROS production directly or indirectly to induce the degeneration of the nigrostriatal pathway in laboratory animals.

3.1 Neurotoxins

There are four main toxin induced models popularly used to produce PD like symptoms in rodents. The neurotoxins used are 6-OHDA, MPTP, paraquat in combination with Maneb, and rotenone.

3.1.1 6-Hydroxydopamine (6-OHDA)

The neurotoxin 6-OHDA destroys catecholaminergic neurons by the combined effect of reactive oxygen species (ROS) and quinines (Cohen and Heikkila 1984). To specifically induce PD in an animal model, 6-OHDA is injected stereotaxically into the substantia nigra, the medial forebrain bundle, or the striatum (Javoy et al. 1976). 6-OHDA is delivered directly into the brain by stereotaxic means as 6-OHDA does not cross the blood-brain barrier, thus ruling out systemic injections (Bove et al. 2005). The administration of 6-OHDA into the substantia nigra or the medial forebrain bundle mediates its uptake anterogradely, while administration into the striatum causes the uptake of the chemical retrogradely. 6-OHDA is transported into dopaminergic neurons via their high-affinity catecholaminergic uptake system (Zigmond, Hastings and Abercrombie 1992). 6-OHDA is usually administered unilaterally to produce a unilateral lesion, allowing the unlesioned side to act as an internal control and to minimise morbidity and mortality (Betarbet, Sherer and Greenamyre 2002). The 6-OHDA lesioned rat has been extensively characterised behaviourally and pathologically, making it one of the models of choice when investigating PD (Schwarting and Huston 1996). However, the effects of 6-OHDA are acute and do not show the same cellular pathology (Lewy bodies) as seen in PD (Dawson and Dawson 2002).

3.1.2 1-Methyl-4-Phenyl-1,2,5,6-Tetrahydropyridine (MPTP)

MPTP was accidentally produced during the illegal production of 1-methyl-4-phenyl-4-propionoxypiperidine (MPPP), a synthetic opioid drug, causing heroin addicts to display Parkinson-like symptoms (Langston 1996). MPTP readily crosses the blood-brain-barrier and is converted by the enzyme monoamine oxidase B (MAO-B) to 1-methyl-4-phenyl-2, 3-dihydropyridium (MPDP+) that then deprotonates to generate the corresponding pyridium species, MPP+ (Smeyne and Jackson-Lewis 2005). MPP+ has a high affinity to the dopamine transporter, thus it is highly selective to dopaminergic neurons (Javitch et al. 1985). Its selective uptake leads to severe damage to the nigrostriatal dopaminergic system, acting as a neurotoxin that inhibits mitochondrial complex I, producing oxidative stress and disturbing intracellular calcium homeostasis (Sedelis, Schwarting and Huston 2001). When MPTP is delivered systemically, MPTP produces bilateral lesions of the dopamine neurons (Sedelis et al. 2001). Following systemic administration and collateral damage to the ventral tegmental area, an external source of dopamine is needed to stimulate adequate food and water uptake (Petzinger and Langston 1998). Bilateral lesions also have a high morbidity and mortality rate. The other difficulty with using MPTP lesioned animal models is that MPTP has varying effects on different animal models and strains due to differences in visceral functions (Betarbet et al. 2002). These drawbacks in mice are being looked at with the behavioural phenotyping of a MPTP mouse animal model for PD (Sedelis et al. 2001).

3.1.3 Paraquat and Maneb

1,1-dimethyl-4,4-bipyridinium, better known as paraquat is a herbicide that has a similar structure to MPP+, making it a putative risk factor for PD (Dawson and Dawson 2002). Paraquat when delivered systemically can pass the blood brain barrier (Brooks et al. 1999). Paraquat has a high affinity to the nigrostriatal dopaminergic system (Thiruchelvam et al. 2000) and exposure in mice can cause up-regulation and aggregation of α-synuclein, a pathological sign of PD in humans (Manning-Bog et al. 2002). Due to its structural similarity to MPP+, paraquat's mechanism of action is believed to involve oxidative stress and its toxic effect via the mitochondria (Betarbet et al. 2002). A link between paraquat and other types of herbicide/pesticides with a increased incidence of PD has been demonstrated (Liou et al. 1997). The effects of paraquat on the dopaminergic system can be increased when mixed with Maneb (manganese ethylenebisdithiocarbamate) (Thiruchelvam et al. 2000). Maneb is a fungicide that has been implicated in an increased incidence of PD in humans (Ferraz et al. 1988, Meco et al. 1994). This animal model is of use when examining PD like syndromes due to environmental factors.

3.1.4 Rotenone

Rotenone is a naturally occurring root extract of *Lonchocarpus utilis* and *Lonchocarpus urucu* used as an insecticide as well as a piscicide (Caboni et al. 2004). Rotenone is a high-affinity inhibitor of complex 1 of the mitochondrial electron transport chain (Sherer et al. 2003b). Rotenone cytotoxicity is not dependent on the dopamine transporter (Hirata et al. 2008). Complex 1 inhibition by rotenone can cause the production of ROS that causes oxidative damage in dopaminergic neurons (Testa, Sherer and Greenamyre 2005).

When neurons are exposed to rotenone in cell culture, they produce ROS and superoxides, with dopaminergic neurons showing higher susceptibility to rotenone compared to other neurons (Radad, Rausch and Gille 2006, Ahmadi et al. 2003, Moon et al. 2005). Over time, the increase in ROS and superoxides produced by rotenone exposure leads to cell death (Ahmadi et al. 2003, Moon et al. 2005). Thus rotenone is a relevant toxin for developing a rat model of PD.

In general, rotenone blocks the electron transfer between the Complex I-associated iron-sulfur clusters and ubiquinone binding site (Grivennikova et al. 1997) (Figure 1). Specifically, rotenone acts as a semiquinone antagonist and displaces the ubisemiquinone intermediate at the ubiquinone binding site (Degli Esposti 1998). By inhibiting the ubiquinone binding site, rotenone alters the state of complex I, leading to higher superoxide

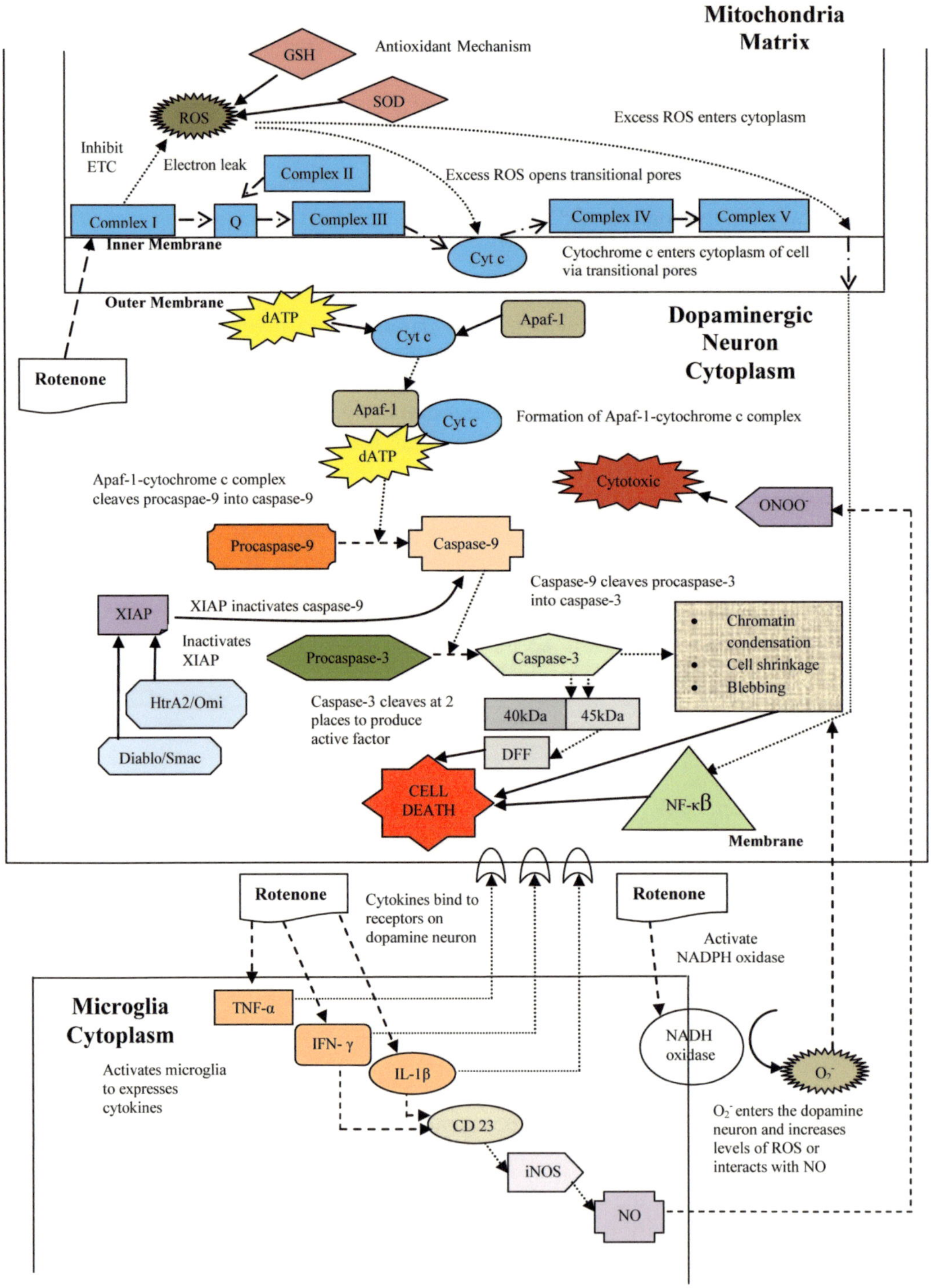

Fig. 1. Mechanism of action of rotenone

production at the same site (Lambert and Brand 2004). The inhibition of Complex I may overwhelm the mitochondria antioxidant system that consist of superoxide dismutase production with manganese (SOD) at the active site and GSH (Fridovich 1995, Betarbet et al. 2002), increasing the ROS concentration in the mitochondrial matrix. The increase of ROS activates the apoptotic intrinsic pathway, which increases the permeability of the outer membrane via the opening of transition pores (Turrens 2003). This allows cytochrome c to move from the intermembrane space into the cells cytoplasm, allowing it to bind with Apaf-1 (apoptopic protease activating factor) (Zou et al. 1997). In the presence of ATP or dATP, the Apaf-1 - cytochrome c complex changes its configuration, exposing the Apaf-1's CARD (caspase recruitment domain) to allow for the recruitment of procaspase-9 (Li et al. 1997). This interaction changes procaspase-9 into caspase-9 that in turn cleaves procaspase-3 into caspase-3. Cells contain an inhibitor of apoptosis (IAP) to prevent accidental caspase-9 activation. XIAP binds to the activated N terminus of caspase-9, making it inactive (Shiozaki et al. 2003). This process can be reversed by the mitochondrial proteins Diablo/Smac and HtrA2/Omi that are released during apoptosis (Vaux and Silke 2003), leading to caspase-3 activation. Caspase-3 cleaves the 45 kDa subunit of a two unit protein in two places producing a DNA Fragmentation Factor (DFF) (Liu et al. 1997). The increase in oxidative stress can also activate nuclear factor kappa β (NF-κβ) (Panet et al. 2001), which has been implicated in the beginning of a pro-apoptopic gene expression programme which may play a role in neurodegenerative disease (Qin et al. 1998, Panet et al. 2001).

Rotenone has the ability to activate microglia *in vivo* (Sherer et al. 2003a). This activation causes the release of tumour necrosis factor α (TNF- α), interleukin 1β (IL-1β), and interferon γ (IFN- γ). These cytokines can bind to their respective receptors and activate transduction pathways, leading to NF-κβ activation and ultimately, apoptosis (Gao, Liu and Hong 2003). It was reported that NF-κβ is present before caspase-3 (Wang et al. 2002), which suggests that superoxides and cytokines produced by the activation of microglia by rotenone play a role in the activation of NF-κβ before complex I inhibition initiates the activation of caspase-3 apoptosis. However, excess ROS from the cytoplasm due to the Complex I inhibition could result in ROS crossing over into the cytoplasm via voltage-dependent anion channels (Han et al. 2003), which could also help activate NF-κβ. Excess ROS in the cytoplasm could also be complemented by the superoxides produced by the activated microglia via NADPH oxidase (Gao et al. 2002). The superoxides produced by NADPH oxidase can also interact with nitric oxide (NO) to produce peroxinitrate (ONOO-), a potent oxidant (Gao et al. 2003) implicated with being cytotoxic and able to damage the neuron's cell membrane (Hirsch 2000, Imao et al. 1998). NO is produced via the inducible nitric oxide synthase that is activated by CD23 which in turn is induced by the presence of TNF- α and IFN- γ (Munoz-Fernandez and Fresno 1998, Hirsch 2000).

Initial studies of the effect of rotenone used systemically in the rat showed a decrease in brain dopamine levels, decreases in tyrosine hydroxylase immunoreactivity in the substantia nigra, and motor deficits similar to those seen in PD (Betarbet et al. 2000, Sherer et al. 2003c, Alam and Schmidt 2002). Rotenone treatment also leads to intracytoplasmic inclusions within dopaminergic neurons thereby mimicking some aspects of PD histopathology (Betarbet et al. 2002). Unfortunately, systemic delivery of rotenone results in high mortality due to the systemic toxicity resulting in liver failure and inconsistent lesions of the substantia nigra (Dawson and Dawson 2002). These problems were alleviated with intra-peritoneal administration of rotenone in a specialised vehicle of a medium-chain triglyceride, although this model developed a debilitating behavioural phenotype in a relatively short time and is not appropriate as a slow onset chronic model (Cannon et al. 2009).

The side effects of peripheral rotenone treatment can be reduced or avoided by the infusion of a lower dose directly into the striatum, medial forebrain bundle or substantia nigra (Ravenstijn et al. 2008, Xiong et al. 2009). Bilateral infusion of rotenone into the medial forebrain bundle causes reductions in striatal dopamine and disruptions in motor behaviours (Alam, Mayerhofer and Schmidt 2004). However, bilateral infusions lead to weight loss and require specialised diets to maintain the animals (Betarbet et al. 2000, Sherer et al. 2003c), possibly due to bilateral lesioning of the ventral tegmental area. These problems are ameliorated by unilateral lesions which reduce dopamine signalling, dopamine level, DOPAC (3,4-dihydroxyphenylacetic acid) level and dopaminergic innervation, while increasing oxidative stress (hydroxyl radicals, GSH level, superoxide dismutase levels), as well as up-regulating α-synuclein expression in the ipsilateral substantia nigra (Sindhu et al. 2006, Antkiewicz-Michaluk et al. 2004, Saravanan, Sindhu and Mohanakumar 2005, Sindhu, Saravanan and Mohanakumar 2005, Ravenstijn et al. 2008, Xiong et al. 2009). Unilateral rotenone lesioned animals have shown differences in several behavioural indices, including rotarod and amphetamine or apomorphine-induced rotation, demonstrating the unilateral functional motor deficits associated with substantia nigra dopamine neuron loss (Sindhu et al. 2006, Sindhu et al. 2005, Ravenstijn et al. 2008, Xiong et al. 2009). Behavioural indices are also influenced by the lesion of the ventral tegmental area, as can occur with larger doses of rotenone in the medial forebrain bundle (Sindhu et al. 2005, Xiong et al. 2009, Thomas et al. 1994).

Our laboratory has recently reported that a low dose of rotenone injected into the medial forebrain pathway in adult rats caused progressive loss of dopaminergic neurons with the remaining neurons displaying pathophysiological hallmark of human PD (Norazit et al. 2010)(Figure 2). Unlike the complete lesion of dopaminergic neurons induced by focal 6-OHDA injection, rotenone injection into the medial forebrain bundle induced the up-regulation of markers of oxidative stress and markers of cell stress in dopaminergic neurons (Sindhu et al. 2005, Norazit et al. 2010). 0.5 μg of rotenone caused negligible necrosis, inflammation and a diffused glial response. A progressive loss of dopaminergic neurons in the substantia nigra and loss of striatal innervation was shown. The low dose of rotenone mediated dopaminergic cell death by oxidative stress as previously demonstrated (Rodrigues, Gomide and Chadi 2004). An increase in astrocytes and microglia occurs in human PD, where they have been ascribed both a neuroprotective and deleterious role (Imamura et al. 2003, Ishida et al. 2006, Vila et al. 2001). The study presented direct support for the hypothesis that rotenone induces a chronic state of oxidative stress in dopaminergic neurons. Rotenone exposure increased SOD2 immunoreactivity within surviving tyrosine hydroxylase positive neurons. The toxin leads to high super-oxide production, activating the apoptotic pathway as shown in the study with increased caspase-3 immunoreactivity (Esposti 1998, Lambert and Brand 2004, Turrens 2003). Under oxidative stress, cells generate G3BP positive cytoplasmic stress granules (Cande et al. 2004, Kedersha and Anderson 2002). This proposal was further validated by the presence of α-synuclein in tyrosine hydroxylase positive neurons 60 days following rotenone exposure (Norazit et al. 2010). α-synuclein is up-regulated in neurons subject to chronic oxidative stress, and plays a neuroprotective role and is expressed sporadically in the substantia nigra 28 days after rotenone infusion into the medial forebrain bundle (Hashimoto et al. 2002, Quilty et al. 2006). This model has now been successfully used to test the neuroprotective properties of chronic exposure to neurotrophic factors (unpublished data).

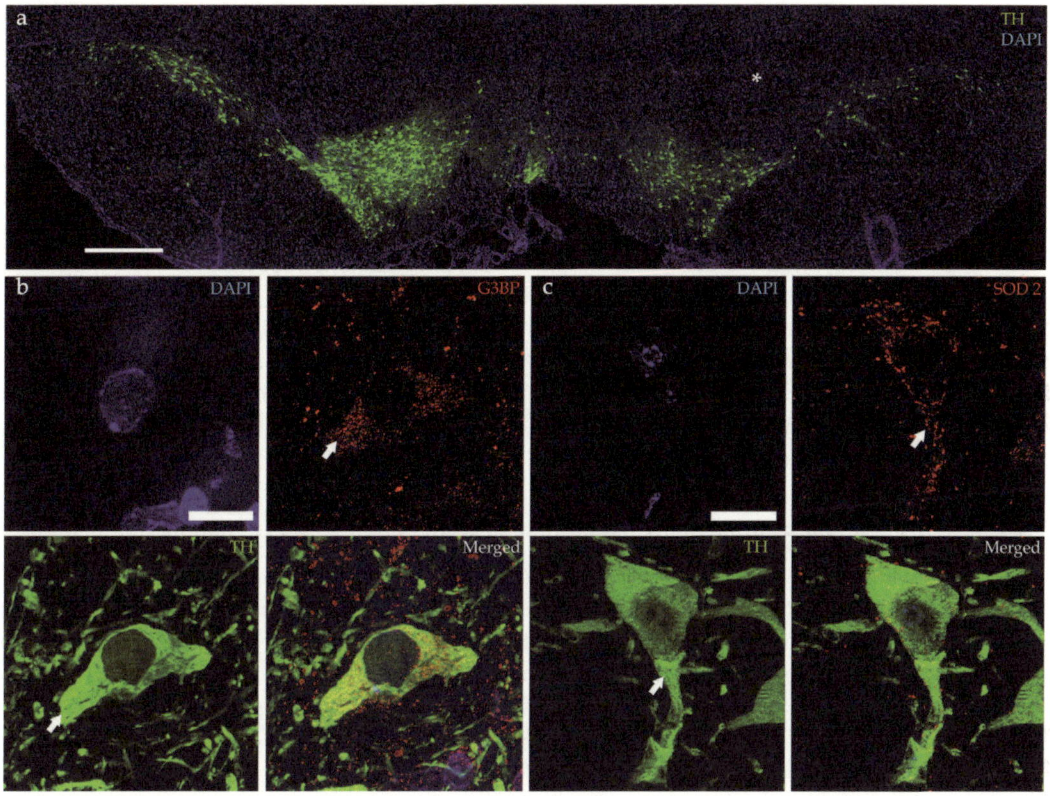

Fig. 2. Dopamine cell pathophysiology of the substantia nigra, induced by 0.5-µg rotenone delivered focally into the medial forebrain bundle and harvested after 14 days. a) The unilateral lesion is manifest as a subtle yet significant reduction in the number of dopaminergic neurons and dendritic arbour within the substantia nigra (asterisk) and a reduction in the dopaminergic innervation of the striatum (data not shown). The nigrostriatal circuitry contralateral to the lesion is uneffected by the rotenone treatment. b) Ras-GAP SH3 domain binding protein (G3BP) immunoreactivity (red, filled arrowhead) was expressed in tyrosine hydroxylase immunoreactive (green, filled arrowhead) dopaminergic neurons located in the rotenone exposed substantia nigra. c) Superoxide dismutase (SOD2) immunoreactivity (red, filled arrowhead) was also expressed in the rotenone exposed tyrosine hydroxylase immunoreactive (green, filled arrowhead) dopaminergic neurons. Nuclei for all sections are counterstained with the nuclear marker DAPI (blue) (scale bar=10 µm)

3.2 Cellular based models

Complete human disease phenotype is rarely observed in animal models introduced with human gene mutations. Thus, relevant human tissue is required to study the disease process and potential therapies for neurodegenerative disorders such as PD. Pathological human samples are often confounded by difficult-to-control artefacts resulting from the disease process itself (Sutherland et al. 2009), biased sampling, and the necessity to process tissue in a timely manner following death (Atz et al. 2007, Marcotte, Srivastava and Quirion 2003, Preece and Cairns 2003). Together with rare foetal derived tissue, patient derived olfactory stem cells and induced pluripotent stem cells are currently used as models for PD.

3.2.1 Patient derived olfactory stem cells

Procuring relevant neural cells from patients with central nervous system disorders is difficult. Therefore, we have developed olfactory stem cells as a model for PD. Neural stem cells from adult human olfactory mucosa may be harvested and expanded to enrich for the stem cells, which are then frozen, banked, thawed, and regrown in quantity for gene and protein expression analyses and functional investigations. Assays on olfactory stem cell function have shown a reduction in gluthathione while pathway analysis has demonstrated significantly dysregulated pathways associated with mitochondrial function and oxidative stress (Matigian et al. 2010). The ease of patient derived olfactory stem cells propagation and banking allows them to be used for extended genomic, proteomic, and functional studies, including drug and biomarker discovery.

3.2.2 Patient derived induced pluripotent stem cells

Induced pluripotent stem (iPS) cells are pluripotent cells derived from differentiated cells, for example by introducing key transcription factor genes, as demonstrated in adult mouse fibroblasts (Takahashi and Yamanaka 2006). iPS cells have successfully been used to generate neurons from patients with sporadic PD (Soldner et al. 2009). Notably, despite these iPS cells being derived from LRRK2 mutation carriers, no phenotypic differences between sporadic PD iPS and control iPS cells were demonstrated (Nguyen et al. 2011). Patient-derived iPS cells have the potential to be used to identify changes in neural cell biology associated with the identified mutations.

3.3 Genetic animal models

Transgenic models have been developed as genetic factors linked to PD have been identified. Several autosomal dominant and recessive genes linked to mitochondrial dysfunction have been identified in humans as reviewed by Schapira (Schapira 2008). This created an opportunity for transgenic animals to mimic familial forms of PD (Fleming, Fernagut and Chesselet 2005).

3.3.1 PARK2 (PARKIN)

PARK 2 (Parkin) is transcribed in the mitochondria (Schapira 2008). The function of parkin remains to be elucidated; however the direct association between parkin and the mitochondria is of interest and warrants further study. In the knockout transgenic mouse model, animals had a decrease in mitochondrial respiratory chain function in the striatum and reductions in specific respiratory chain and antioxidant proteins (Palacino et al. 2004). Midbrain neuronal cultures obtained from PARK2 knockout mice had an increased sensitivity to rotenone, suggesting an effect on the mitochondrial respiratory chain

(Casarejos et al. 2006). In some of the mouse knockout models, subtle abnormalities of the nigrostriatal pathway or the locus coeruleus noradrenergic system have been observed (Goldberg et al. 2003, von Coelln et al. 2006). Conversely, over-expression of mutant parkin produces a progressive loss of dopaminergic neurons in the nigrostriatal pathway in both mice and drosophila (Lu et al. 2009, Sang et al. 2007, Wang et al. 2007). This suggests that some parkin mutants may act in a dominant negative fashion. The parkin animal model exhibits several movement indices in both drosophila and mice (Greene et al. 2003, Whitworth et al. 2005).

3.3.2 PINK1

Similar to parkin knockouts, PINK1 knockouts also have mild mitochondrial defects (Gautier, Kitada and Shen 2008, Palacino et al. 2004).The PINK1 product is transcribed in the nucleus, translated in the cytoplasm, and imported intact into the mitochondria, with subsequent processing and intra mitochondrial sorting (Schapira 2008). The lack of PINK1 in transgenic mice causes enlargement of mitochondria as well as a decrease in mitochondrial numbers in dopaminergic neurons of the nigrostriatal pathway (Gautier et al. 2008, Gispert et al. 2009, Kitada et al. 2007). Although these animals do not exhibit any changes in the nigrostriatal pathway, a deficit in dopamine neurotransmission has been observed (Kitada et al. 2007). Changes in several behavioral indices have also been shown in the PINK1 knockout drosophila animal model (Clark et al. 2006, Park et al. 2006).

It is interesting to point out that while both the knockdown of parkin and PINK1 have been linked to mitochondrial dysfunction, the expression of parkin ameliorates PINK1-related abnormalities but not vice versa (Clark et al. 2006, Park et al. 2006). This suggests that parkin and PINK1 are part of a common pathway with PINK1 functioning upstream from parkin.

3.3.3 α -Synuclein

α -synuclein is a protein aggregate that is the main part of Lewy bodies in human PD. The function of α-synuclein is as yet unclear, however, there appears to be a reciprocal relationship between this protein and oxidative stress (Henchcliffe and Beal 2008). α-synuclein is up-regulated in neurons subject to chronic oxidative stress and expressed sporadically in the substantia nigra (Hashimoto et al. 2002, Quilty et al. 2006, Norazit et al. 2010). The association between the presence of α-synuclein and PD has led to the development of a variety of animal models (Table 1). The over-expression of α-synuclein increased the loss in dopaminergic neurons in both drosophila and C. elegans models. (Feany and Bender 2000, Kuwahara et al. 2006, Lakso et al. 2003). However, only the dopaminergic loss in the drosophila model is progressive. A loss of dopaminergic neurons with the over-expression of α-synuclein has been demonstrated in mice; however the phenotypic outcome depends on the promoters used to drive transgene expression (Chesselet 2008). Transgenic mice presented with several functional abnormalities in the nigrostriatal system, some of which are dopamine responsive (Chesselet 2008). However, the loss of dopaminergic neurons is not progressive. α-synuclein toxicity is induced though mitochondrial dysfunction, proteasomal and lysosomal impairments, and disruption of ER-Golgi trafficking (Cooper et al. 2006, Cuervo et al. 2004, Martin et al. 2006, Tanaka et al. 2001). The link between mitochondrial dysfunction and α-synuclein aggregation suggests a feed-forward loop that has the potential to initiate the progressive loss of dopaminergic neurons in the nigrostriatal system due to oxidative stress.

3.3.4 LRRK2

The LRRK2 protein functions as a serine-thereonine kinase, a known affector of mitochondrial function. A small percentage (10%) of LRRK2 is located in the outer mitochondrial membrane (West et al. 2005). Although the precise function of mitochondrial-located LRRK2 is not known, it has been suggested that it interacts with parkin. The current transgenic LRRK2 animal models are not robust enough to be used as a PD animal model due to the lack of loss of dopaminergic neurons of the nigrostriatal pathway (Li et al. 2010, Li et al. 2009, Lin et al. 2009, Wang et al. 2008, Tong et al. 2009). However, these animals do show several abnormalities in DA neurotransmission or in dopamine responsive behavior. It has been suggested that the mouse LRRK2 transgenic models do not exhibit more substantial pathology as LRRK2 mutations in humans are only partially penetrant, with further genetic and/or environmental insult required to induce the degeneration of dopaminergic neurons (Dawson, Ko and Dawson 2010).

4. Experimental therapies

4.1 Metal chelation therapy

Increased iron levels have been detected in the midbrain of PD patients suggesting that the increased levels of iron may be part of the disease pathology (Andersen 2004). Notably, iron participates as a catalyst to produce ROS.

4.1.1 8-Hydroxyquinolines

Previously the hydroxyquinoline clioquinol had been examined as a metal chelator in a clinical trial for Alzeimer's disease (Ritchie et al. 2003). The use of a variety of hydroxyquinolines to chelate iron into a form that does not catalyze ROS has shown promise in both *in vivo* and *in vitro* models (Table 2).

Hydroxyquinoline	Model	Reference
Clioquinol	MPTP mouse model	(Kaur et al. 2003)
HLA20	P19 cells exposuded to 6-OHDA	(Zheng et al. 2005)
VK-28	6-OHDA rat model	(Tsubaki, Honma and Hoshi 1971)
M30	MPTP mouse model In vitro	(Gal et al. 2005, Gal et al. 2006)
M98 and M99	SH-SY5Y and PC12 exposed to 6-OHDA	(Gal et al. 2006, Zheng, Blat and Fridkin 2006)
M10	PC12 cells exposed to 6-OHDA	(Ritchie et al. 2003)

Table 2. Hydroxyquinolines shown to chelate iron in both *in vivo* and *in vitro* models

Hydroxyquinolines are able to cross the blood brain barrier, allowing for oral administration. Hydroxyquinolines have also shown inhibitory effect on the activity of enzyme MAO-B (Yassin et al. 2000, Youdim, Fridkin and Zheng 2005).

4.1.2 Desferrioxamine

Previously, desferrioxamine was used to treat iron overload disease (Mandel et al. 2007). The use of Desferrioxamine has been reported to be neuroprotective *in vivo* and *in vitro* (Ben-Shachar et al. 1991, Jiang et al. 2006, Sangchot et al. 2002, Youdim, Stephenson and Ben Shachar 2004). Unlike hydroxyquinolines, desferrioxamine does not cross the blood brain barrier, thus removing the option of oral administration (Aouad et al. 2002).

4.2 Plant polyphenols

Polyphenols have been reported to have antioxidant properties, thus making them a candidate for antioxidant therapies (Malesev and Kuntic 2007). Green tea, cranberry, traditional chinese tea, and tumeric are sources of a variety of polyphenols (Reto et al. 2007, Ramassamy 2006, Perez, Wei and Guo 2009, Tan, Meng and Hostettmann 2000). Neuroprotective and neurorescue properties of plant polyphenols have been demonstrated *in vivo* and *in vitro* (Mandel, Maor and Youdim 2004, Mercer et al. 2005, Chen et al. 2006, Zbarsky et al. 2005, Mandel et al. 2006). Polyphenols exert their antioxidant effect via scavenging of free radicals and inhibition of the Fenton reaction (Perez et al. 2009, Pan, Jankovic and Le 2003).

4.3 Antioxidant therapy

The effects of oxidative stress are demonstrated in PD patients who have decreased GSH levels, increased levels of iron, neuromelanin associated redox-active iron, lipid peroxidation, protein oxidation and DNA damage in the substantia nigra (Jenner and Olanow 1998, Faucheux et al. 2003, Dexter et al. 1989). Antioxidant therapy has been suggested to ameliorate these effects.

4.4 Coenzyme Q_{10} (CoQ_{10})

CoQ_{10}, also known as ubiquinone is a cofactor that accepts electrons from Complex I and II of the electron transport chain in the mitochiondria (Beyer 1992, Dallner and Sindelar 2000). CoQ_{10} mediates its antioxidant effect via its interaction with a-tocopherol (Beyer 1992, Noack, Kube and Augustin 1994), inhibiting the activation of mitochondrial permeability, and acting independently of its free radical scavenging activity. Thus it blocks apoptosis (Papucci *et al.*, 2003), acting as a co-factor of mitochondrial uncoupling proteins which reduces mitochondrial-free radical generation (Echtay, Winkler and Klingenberg 2000, Echtay et al. 2002). Neuroprotection has been associated with the ability of CoQ_{10} to induce mitochondrial uncoupling in the substantia nigra of primates, after MPTP toxicity (Horvath et al. 2003). The use of CoQ_{10} as an antioxidant has been translated into phase II clinical trials (Shults et al. 2002) which showed a slowing of disease progression following 16 months of treatment.

4.5 Deprenyl and Tocopherol Antioxidative Therapy of Parkinsonism (DATATOP)

Deprenyl and tocopherol antioxidative therapy have been clinically trialed to explore its potential as therapy for PD (Shoulson et al. 2002). Deprenyl treatment delayed the initiation of levodopa therapy. Continued deprenyl treated subjects exhibited slower motor decline and lower likelihood of developing freezing of gait. However, this treatment increased the likelihood of developing dyskinesia.

5. Conclusion

There is increasing evidence that many factors including age, environmental toxins, genetic determinants, and lifestyle factors influence the risk for PD. Many of these impact on oxidative stress related pathways. Animal and cellular models have been developed to mimic the disease pathology in humans. Currently, antioxidant therapies are being investigated in both animals and human clinical trials, with promising outcomes. Notably, antioxidant therapies appear to delay the onset of disease and disease progression, although they do not prevent or reverse disease progression.

6. Acknowledgment

The authors would like to thank Suzita Mohd Noor, Maria Nguyen, Charlotte Dickson, and Brenton Cavanagh for their technical and editing support.

7. References

Ahmadi, F. A., D. A. Linseman, T. N. Grammatopoulos, S. M. Jones, R. J. Bouchard, C. R. Freed, K. A. Heidenreich & W. M. Zawada (2003) The pesticide rotenone induces caspase-3-mediated apoptosis in ventral mesencephalic dopaminergic neurons. *J Neurochem,* 87, 914-21.

Alam, M., A. Mayerhofer & W. J. Schmidt (2004) The neurobehavioral changes induced by bilateral rotenone lesion in medial forebrain bundle of rats are reversed by L-DOPA. *Behav Brain Res,* 151, 117-24.

Alam, M. & W. J. Schmidt (2002) Rotenone destroys dopaminergic neurons and induces parkinsonian symptoms in rats. *Behav Brain Res,* 136, 317-24.

Ambani, L. M., M. H. Van Woert & S. Murphy (1975) Brain peroxidase and catalase in Parkinson disease. *Arch Neurol,* 32, 114-8.

Andersen, J. K. (2004) Oxidative stress in neurodegeneration: cause or consequence? *Nature medicine,* 10 Suppl, S18-25.

Antkiewicz-Michaluk, L., J. Wardas, J. Michaluk, I. Romaska, A. Bojarski & J. Vetulani (2004) Protective effect of 1-methyl-1,2,3,4-tetrahydroisoquinoline against dopaminergic neurodegeneration in the extrapyramidal structures produced by intracerebral injection of rotenone. *Int J Neuropsychopharmacol,* 7, 155-63.

Aouad, F., A. Florence, Y. Zhang, F. Collins, C. Henry, R. J. Ward & R. Crichton (2002) Evaluation of new iron chelators and their therapeutic potential. *Inorganica Chimica Acta,* 339, 470-480.

Atz, M., D. Walsh, P. Cartagena, J. Li, S. Evans, P. Choudary, K. Overman, R. Stein, H. Tomita, S. Potkin, R. Myers, S. J. Watson, E. G. Jones, H. Akil, W. E. Bunney, Jr. & M. P. Vawter (2007) Methodological considerations for gene expression profiling of human brain. *Journal of neuroscience methods,* 163, 295-309.

Bannon, M. J., M. S. Poosch, Y. Xia, D. J. Goebel, B. Cassin & G. Kapatos (1992) Dopamine transporter mRNA content in human substantia nigra decreases precipitously with age. *Proc Natl Acad Sci U S A,* 89, 7095-9.

Ben-Shachar, D., G. Eshel, J. P. Finberg & M. B. Youdim (1991) The iron chelator desferrioxamine (Desferal) retards 6-hydroxydopamine-induced degeneration of nigrostriatal dopamine neurons. *Journal of neurochemistry,* 56, 1441-4.

Bender, A., K. J. Krishnan, C. M. Morris, G. A. Taylor, A. K. Reeve, R. H. Perry, E. Jaros, J. S. Hersheson, J. Betts, T. Klopstock, R. W. Taylor & D. M. Turnbull (2006) High levels of mitochondrial DNA deletions in substantia nigra neurons in aging and Parkinson disease. *Nat Genet,* 38, 515-7.

Betarbet, R., T. B. Sherer & J. T. Greenamyre (2002) Animal models of Parkinson's disease. *Bioessays,* 24, 308-18.

Betarbet, R., T. B. Sherer, G. MacKenzie, M. Garcia-Osuna, A. V. Panov & J. T. Greenamyre (2000) Chronic systemic pesticide exposure reproduces features of Parkinson's disease. *Nat Neurosci,* 3, 1301-6.

Beyer, R. E. (1992) An analysis of the role of coenzyme Q in free radical generation and as an antioxidant. *Biochemistry and cell biology = Biochimie et biologie cellulaire,* 70, 390-403.

Bove, J., D. Prou, C. Perier & S. Przedborski (2005) Toxin-induced models of Parkinson's disease. *NeuroRx,* 2, 484-94.

Braak, H., K. Del Tredici, U. Rub, R. A. de Vos, E. N. Jansen Steur & E. Braak (2003a) Staging of brain pathology related to sporadic Parkinson's disease. *Neurobiol Aging,* 24, 197-211.

Braak, H., U. Rub, W. P. Gai & K. Del Tredici (2003b) Idiopathic Parkinson's disease: possible routes by which vulnerable neuronal types may be subject to neuroinvasion by an unknown pathogen. *J Neural Transm,* 110, 517-36.

Brooks, A. I., C. A. Chadwick, H. A. Gelbard, D. A. Cory-Slechta & H. J. Federoff (1999) Paraquat elicited neurobehavioral syndrome caused by dopaminergic neuron loss. *Brain Res,* 823, 1-10.

Brooks, D. J. (2010) Examining Braak's hypothesis by imaging Parkinson's disease. *Mov Disord,* 25 Suppl 1, S83-8.

Caboni, P., T. B. Sherer, N. Zhang, G. Taylor, H. M. Na, J. T. Greenamyre & J. E. Casida (2004) Rotenone, deguelin, their metabolites, and the rat model of Parkinson's disease. *Chem Res Toxicol,* 17, 1540-8.

Cande, C., N. Vahsen, D. Metivier, H. Tourriere, K. Chebli, C. Garrido, J. Tazi & G. Kroemer (2004) Regulation of cytoplasmic stress granules by apoptosis-inducing factor. *J Cell Sci,* 117, 4461-8.

Cannon, J. R., V. Tapias, H. M. Na, A. S. Honick, R. E. Drolet & J. T. Greenamyre (2009) A highly reproducible rotenone model of Parkinson's disease. *Neurobiol Dis,* 34, 279-90.

Casarejos, M. J., J. Menendez, R. M. Solano, J. A. Rodriguez-Navarro, J. Garcia de Yebenes & M. A. Mena (2006) Susceptibility to rotenone is increased in neurons from parkin null mice and is reduced by minocycline. *Journal of neurochemistry,* 97, 934-46.

Chauhan, N. B., G. J. Siegel & J. M. Lee (2001) Depletion of glial cell line-derived neurotrophic factor in substantia nigra neurons of Parkinson's disease brain. *J Chem Neuroanat,* 21, 277-88.

Chen, J., X. Q. Tang, J. L. Zhi, Y. Cui, H. M. Yu, E. H. Tang, S. N. Sun, J. Q. Feng & P. X. Chen (2006) Curcumin protects PC12 cells against 1-methyl-4-phenylpyridinium ion-induced apoptosis by bcl-2-mitochondria-ROS-iNOS pathway. *Apoptosis : an international journal on programmed cell death,* 11, 943-53.

Chesselet, M. F. (2008) In vivo alpha-synuclein overexpression in rodents: a useful model of Parkinson's disease? *Experimental neurology,* 209, 22-7.

Chu, Y. & J. H. Kordower (2007) Age-associated increases of alpha-synuclein in monkeys and humans are associated with nigrostriatal dopamine depletion: Is this the target for Parkinson's disease? *Neurobiol Dis,* 25, 134-49.

Clark, I. E., M. W. Dodson, C. Jiang, J. H. Cao, J. R. Huh, J. H. Seol, S. J. Yoo, B. A. Hay & M. Guo (2006) Drosophila pink1 is required for mitochondrial function and interacts genetically with parkin. *Nature,* 441, 1162-6.

Cohen, G. & R. E. Heikkila (1984) Alloxan and 6-hydroxydopamine: cellular toxins. *Methods Enzymol,* 105, 510-6.

Cooper, A. A., A. D. Gitler, A. Cashikar, C. M. Haynes, K. J. Hill, B. Bhullar, K. Liu, K. Xu, K. E. Strathearn, F. Liu, S. Cao, K. A. Caldwell, G. A. Caldwell, G. Marsischky, R. D. Kolodner, J. Labaer, J. C. Rochet, N. M. Bonini & S. Lindquist (2006) Alpha-synuclein blocks ER-Golgi traffic and Rab1 rescues neuron loss in Parkinson's models. *Science,* 313, 324-8.

Cuervo, A. M., L. Stefanis, R. Fredenburg, P. T. Lansbury & D. Sulzer (2004) Impaired degradation of mutant alpha-synuclein by chaperone-mediated autophagy. *Science,* 305, 1292-5.

Dallner, G. & P. J. Sindelar (2000) Regulation of ubiquinone metabolism. *Free radical biology & medicine,* 29, 285-94.

Dauer, W. & S. Przedborski (2003) Parkinson's disease: mechanisms and models. *Neuron,* 39, 889-909.

Dawson, T. M. & V. L. Dawson (2002) Neuroprotective and neurorestorative strategies for Parkinson's disease. *Nat Neurosci,* 5 Suppl, 1058-61.

Dawson, T. M., H. S. Ko & V. L. Dawson (2010) Genetic animal models of Parkinson's disease. *Neuron,* 66, 646-61.

de Rijk, M. C., C. Tzourio, M. M. Breteler, J. F. Dartigues, L. Amaducci, S. Lopez-Pousa, J. M. Manubens-Bertran, A. Alperovitch & W. A. Rocca (1997) Prevalence of parkinsonism and Parkinson's disease in Europe: the EUROPARKINSON Collaborative Study. European Community Concerted Action on the Epidemiology of Parkinson's disease. *J Neurol Neurosurg Psychiatry,* 62, 10-5.

Degli Esposti, M. (1998) Inhibitors of NADH-ubiquinone reductase: an overview. *Biochim Biophys Acta,* 1364, 222-35.

Dexter, D. T., C. J. Carter, F. R. Wells, F. Javoy-Agid, Y. Agid, A. Lees, P. Jenner & C. D. Marsden (1989) Basal lipid peroxidation in substantia nigra is increased in Parkinson's disease. *Journal of neurochemistry,* 52, 381-9.

Drozdzik, M., M. Bialecka, K. Mysliwiec, K. Honczarenko, J. Stankiewicz & Z. Sych (2003) Polymorphism in the P-glycoprotein drug transporter MDR1 gene: a possible link between environmental and genetic factors in Parkinson's disease. *Pharmacogenetics,* 13, 259-63.

Echtay, K. S., D. Roussel, J. St-Pierre, M. B. Jekabsons, S. Cadenas, J. A. Stuart, J. A. Harper, S. J. Roebuck, A. Morrison, S. Pickering, J. C. Clapham & M. D. Brand (2002) Superoxide activates mitochondrial uncoupling proteins. *Nature,* 415, 96-9.

Echtay, K. S., E. Winkler & M. Klingenberg (2000) Coenzyme Q is an obligatory cofactor for uncoupling protein function. *Nature,* 408, 609-13.

Esposti, M. D. (1998) Apoptosis: who was first? *Cell Death Differ,* 5, 719.

Faucheux, B. A., M. E. Martin, C. Beaumont, J. J. Hauw, Y. Agid & E. C. Hirsch (2003) Neuromelanin associated redox-active iron is increased in the substantia nigra of patients with Parkinson's disease. *J Neurochem,* 86, 1142-8.

Feany, M. B. & W. W. Bender (2000) A Drosophila model of Parkinson's disease. *Nature,* 404, 394-8.

Ferraz, H. B., P. H. Bertolucci, J. S. Pereira, J. G. Lima & L. A. Andrade (1988) Chronic exposure to the fungicide maneb may produce symptoms and signs of CNS manganese intoxication. *Neurology,* 38, 550-3.

Fleming, S. M., P. O. Fernagut & M. F. Chesselet (2005) Genetic mouse models of parkinsonism: strengths and limitations. *NeuroRx 2,* 495-503.

Fridovich, I. (1995) Superoxide radical and superoxide dismutases. *Annu Rev Biochem,* 64, 97-112.

Gal, S., M. Fridkin, T. Amit, H. Zheng & M. B. Youdim (2006) M30, a novel multifunctional neuroprotective drug with potent iron chelating and brain selective monoamine oxidase-ab inhibitory activity for Parkinson's disease. *Journal of neural transmission. Supplementum,* 447-56.

Gal, S., H. Zheng, M. Fridkin & M. B. Youdim (2005) Novel multifunctional neuroprotective iron chelator-monoamine oxidase inhibitor drugs for neurodegenerative diseases. In vivo selective brain monoamine oxidase inhibition and prevention of MPTP-induced striatal dopamine depletion. *Journal of neurochemistry,* 95, 79-88.

Gao, H. M., J. S. Hong, W. Zhang & B. Liu (2002) Distinct role for microglia in rotenone-induced degeneration of dopaminergic neurons. *J Neurosci,* 22, 782-90.

Gao, H. M., B. Liu & J. S. Hong (2003) Critical role for microglial NADPH oxidase in rotenone-induced degeneration of dopaminergic neurons. *J Neurosci,* 23, 6181-7.

Gash, D. M., Z. Zhang, A. Ovadia, W. A. Cass, A. Yi, L. Simmerman, D. Russell, D. Martin, P. A. Lapchak, F. Collins, B. J. Hoffer & G. A. Gerhardt (1996) Functional recovery in parkinsonian monkeys treated with GDNF. *Nature,* 380, 252-5.

Gautier, C. A., T. Kitada & J. Shen (2008) Loss of PINK1 causes mitochondrial functional defects and increased sensitivity to oxidative stress. *Proceedings of the National Academy of Sciences of the United States of America,* 105, 11364-9.

Gibb, W. R. & A. J. Lees (1988) The relevance of the Lewy body to the pathogenesis of idiopathic Parkinson's disease. *J Neurol Neurosurg Psychiatry,* 51, 745-52.

Gispert, S., F. Ricciardi, A. Kurz, M. Azizov, H. H. Hoepken, D. Becker, W. Voos, K. Leuner, W. E. Muller, A. P. Kudin, W. S. Kunz, A. Zimmermann, J. Roeper, D. Wenzel, M. Jendrach, M. Garcia-Arencibia, J. Fernandez-Ruiz, L. Huber, H. Rohrer, M. Barrera, A. S. Reichert, U. Rub, A. Chen, R. L. Nussbaum & G. Auburger (2009) Parkinson phenotype in aged PINK1-deficient mice is accompanied by progressive mitochondrial dysfunction in absence of neurodegeneration. *PloS one,* 4, e5777.

Goldberg, M. S., S. M. Fleming, J. J. Palacino, C. Cepeda, H. A. Lam, A. Bhatnagar, E. G. Meloni, N. Wu, L. C. Ackerson, G. J. Klapstein, M. Gajendiran, B. L. Roth, M. F. Chesselet, N. T. Maidment, M. S. Levine & J. Shen (2003) Parkin-deficient mice exhibit nigrostriatal deficits but not loss of dopaminergic neurons. *The Journal of biological chemistry,* 278, 43628-35.

Gowers, W. R. (1902) A lecture on myopathy and a distal form. *British Medical Journal,* 2, 89-92.

Greene, J. C., A. J. Whitworth, I. Kuo, L. A. Andrews, M. B. Feany & L. J. Pallanck (2003) Mitochondrial pathology and apoptotic muscle degeneration in Drosophila parkin mutants. *Proceedings of the National Academy of Sciences of the United States of America*, 100, 4078-83.

Grivennikova, V. G., E. O. Maklashina, E. V. Gavrikova & A. D. Vinogradov (1997) Interaction of the mitochondrial NADH-ubiquinone reductase with rotenone as related to the enzyme active/inactive transition. *Biochimica et biophysica acta*, 1319, 223-32.

Han, D., F. Antunes, R. Canali, D. Rettori & E. Cadenas (2003) Voltage-dependent anion channels control the release of the superoxide anion from mitochondria to cytosol. *The Journal of biological chemistry*, 278, 5557-63.

Hashimoto, M., L. J. Hsu, E. Rockenstein, T. Takenouchi, M. Mallory & E. Masliah (2002) alpha-Synuclein protects against oxidative stress via inactivation of the c-Jun N-terminal kinase stress-signaling pathway in neuronal cells. *J Biol Chem*, 277, 11465-72.

Hawkes, C. H., K. Del Tredici & H. Braak (2007) Parkinson's disease: a dual-hit hypothesis. *Neuropathol Appl Neurobiol*, 33, 599-614.

Henchcliffe, C. & M. F. Beal (2008) Mitochondrial biology and oxidative stress in Parkinson disease pathogenesis. *Nature clinical practice. Neurology*, 4, 600-9.

Herishanu, Y. O., M. Medvedovski, J. R. Goldsmith & E. Kordysh (2001) A case-control study of Parkinson's disease in urban population of southern Israel. *Can J Neurol Sci*, 28, 144-7.

Hirata, Y., H. Suzuno, T. Tsuruta, K. Oh-hashi & K. Kiuchi (2008) The role of dopamine transporter in selective toxicity of manganese and rotenone. *Toxicology*, 244, 249-56.

Hirsch, E. C. (2000) Glial cells and Parkinson's disease. *Journal of neurology*, 247 Suppl 2, II58-62.

Ho, S. C., J. Woo & C. M. Lee (1989) Epidemiologic study of Parkinson's disease in Hong Kong. *Neurology*, 39, 1314-8.

Horvath, T. L., S. Diano, C. Leranth, L. M. Garcia-Segura, M. A. Cowley, M. Shanabrough, J. D. Elsworth, P. Sotonyi, R. H. Roth, E. H. Dietrich, R. T. Matthews, C. J. Barnstable & D. E. Redmond, Jr. (2003) Coenzyme Q induces nigral mitochondrial uncoupling and prevents dopamine cell loss in a primate model of Parkinson's disease. *Endocrinology*, 144, 2757-60.

Howells, D. W., M. J. Porritt, J. Y. Wong, P. E. Batchelor, R. Kalnins, A. J. Hughes & G. A. Donnan (2000) Reduced BDNF mRNA expression in the Parkinson's disease substantia nigra. *Exp Neurol*, 166, 127-35.

Hughes, A. J., S. E. Daniel & A. J. Lees (2001) Improved accuracy of clinical diagnosis of Lewy body Parkinson's disease. *Neurology*, 57, 1497-9.

Imamura, K., N. Hishikawa, M. Sawada, T. Nagatsu, M. Yoshida & Y. Hashizume (2003) Distribution of major histocompatibility complex class II-positive microglia and cytokine profile of Parkinson's disease brains. *Acta Neuropathol*, 106, 518-26.

Imao, K., H. Wang, M. Komatsu & M. Hiramatsu (1998) Free radical scavenging activity of fermented papaya preparation and its effect on lipid peroxide level and superoxide dismutase activity in iron-induced epileptic foci of rats. *Biochemistry and molecular biology international*, 45, 11-23.

Ishida, Y., A. Nagai, S. Kobayashi & S. U. Kim (2006) Upregulation of protease-activated receptor-1 in astrocytes in Parkinson disease: astrocyte-mediated neuroprotection through increased levels of glutathione peroxidase. *J Neuropathol Exp Neurol,* 65, 66-77.

Javitch, J. A., R. J. D'Amato, S. M. Strittmatter & S. H. Snyder (1985) Parkinsonism-inducing neurotoxin, N-methyl-4-phenyl-1,2,3,6 -tetrahydropyridine: uptake of the metabolite N-methyl-4-phenylpyridine by dopamine neurons explains selective toxicity. *Proc Natl Acad Sci U S A,* 82, 2173-7.

Javoy, F., C. Sotelo, A. Herbet & Y. Agid (1976) Specificity of dopaminergic neuronal degeneration induced by intracerebral injection of 6-hydroxydopamine in the nigrostriatal dopamine system. *Brain Res,* 102, 201-15.

Jenner, P. & C. W. Olanow (1998) Understanding cell death in Parkinson's disease. *Ann Neurol,* 44, S72-84.

Jiang, H., Z. Luan, J. Wang & J. Xie (2006) Neuroprotective effects of iron chelator Desferal on dopaminergic neurons in the substantia nigra of rats with iron-overload. *Neurochemistry international,* 49, 605-9.

Kaur, D., F. Yantiri, S. Rajagopalan, J. Kumar, J. Q. Mo, R. Boonplueang, V. Viswanath, R. Jacobs, L. Yang, M. F. Beal, D. DiMonte, I. Volitaskis, L. Ellerby, R. A. Cherny, A. I. Bush & J. K. Andersen (2003) Genetic or pharmacological iron chelation prevents MPTP-induced neurotoxicity in vivo: a novel therapy for Parkinson's disease. *Neuron,* 37, 899-909.

Kedersha, N. & P. Anderson (2002) Stress granules: sites of mRNA triage that regulate mRNA stability and translatability. *Biochem Soc Trans,* 30, 963-9.

Kitada, T., A. Pisani, D. R. Porter, H. Yamaguchi, A. Tscherter, G. Martella, P. Bonsi, C. Zhang, E. N. Pothos & J. Shen (2007) Impaired dopamine release and synaptic plasticity in the striatum of PINK1-deficient mice. *Proceedings of the National Academy of Sciences of the United States of America,* 104, 11441-6.

Kuwahara, T., A. Koyama, K. Gengyo-Ando, M. Masuda, H. Kowa, M. Tsunoda, S. Mitani & T. Iwatsubo (2006) Familial Parkinson mutant alpha-synuclein causes dopamine neuron dysfunction in transgenic Caenorhabditis elegans. *The Journal of biological chemistry,* 281, 334-40.

Lakso, M., S. Vartiainen, A. M. Moilanen, J. Sirvio, J. H. Thomas, R. Nass, R. D. Blakely & G. Wong (2003) Dopaminergic neuronal loss and motor deficits in Caenorhabditis elegans overexpressing human alpha-synuclein. *Journal of neurochemistry,* 86, 165-72.

Lambert, A. J. & M. D. Brand (2004) Inhibitors of the quinone-binding site allow rapid superoxide production from mitochondrial NADH:ubiquinone oxidoreductase (complex I). *J Biol Chem,* 279, 39414-20.

Langston, J. W. (1996) The etiology of Parkinson's disease with emphasis on the MPTP story. *Neurology,* 47, S153-60.

Le Couteur, D. G., A. J. McLean, M. C. Taylor, B. L. Woodham & P. G. Board (1999) Pesticides and Parkinson's disease. *Biomed Pharmacother,* 53, 122-30.

Lee, C. K., R. Weindruch & T. A. Prolla (2000) Gene-expression profile of the ageing brain in mice. *Nat Genet,* 25, 294-7.

Levy, G. (2007) The relationship of Parkinson disease with aging. *Arch Neurol,* 64, 1242-6.

Li, P., D. Nijhawan, I. Budihardjo, S. M. Srinivasula, M. Ahmad, E. S. Alnemri & X. Wang (1997) Cytochrome c and dATP-dependent formation of Apaf-1/caspase-9 complex initiates an apoptotic protease cascade. *Cell,* 91, 479-89.

Li, X., J. C. Patel, J. Wang, M. V. Avshalumov, C. Nicholson, J. D. Buxbaum, G. A. Elder, M. E. Rice & Z. Yue (2010) Enhanced striatal dopamine transmission and motor performance with LRRK2 overexpression in mice is eliminated by familial Parkinson's disease mutation G2019S. *The Journal of neuroscience : the official journal of the Society for Neuroscience,* 30, 1788-97.

Li, Y., W. Liu, T. F. Oo, L. Wang, Y. Tang, V. Jackson-Lewis, C. Zhou, K. Geghman, M. Bogdanov, S. Przedborski, M. F. Beal, R. E. Burke & C. Li (2009) Mutant LRRK2(R1441G) BAC transgenic mice recapitulate cardinal features of Parkinson's disease. *Nature neuroscience,* 12, 826-8.

Lin, X., L. Parisiadou, X. L. Gu, L. Wang, H. Shim, L. Sun, C. Xie, C. X. Long, W. J. Yang, J. Ding, Z. Z. Chen, P. E. Gallant, J. H. Tao-Cheng, G. Rudow, J. C. Troncoso, Z. Liu, Z. Li & H. Cai (2009) Leucine-rich repeat kinase 2 regulates the progression of neuropathology induced by Parkinson's-disease-related mutant alpha-synuclein. *Neuron,* 64, 807-27.

Liou, H. H., M. C. Tsai, C. J. Chen, J. S. Jeng, Y. C. Chang, S. Y. Chen & R. C. Chen (1997) Environmental risk factors and Parkinson's disease: a case-control study in Taiwan. *Neurology,* 48, 1583-8.

Liu, X., H. Zou, C. Slaughter & X. Wang (1997) DFF, a heterodimeric protein that functions downstream of caspase-3 to trigger DNA fragmentation during apoptosis. *Cell,* 89, 175-84.

Lu, X. H., S. M. Fleming, B. Meurers, L. C. Ackerson, F. Mortazavi, V. Lo, D. Hernandez, D. Sulzer, G. R. Jackson, N. T. Maidment, M. F. Chesselet & X. W. Yang (2009) Bacterial artificial chromosome transgenic mice expressing a truncated mutant parkin exhibit age-dependent hypokinetic motor deficits, dopaminergic neuron degeneration, and accumulation of proteinase K-resistant alpha-synuclein. *The Journal of neuroscience : the official journal of the Society for Neuroscience,* 29, 1962-76.

Malesev, D. & V. Kuntic (2007) Investigation of metal-flavonoid chelates and the determination of flavonoids via metal-flavonoid complexing reactions. *Journal of the Serbia Chemical Society* 72, 921-939.

Mandel, S., T. Amit, O. Bar-Am & M. B. Youdim (2007) Iron dysregulation in Alzheimer's disease: multimodal brain permeable iron chelating drugs, possessing neuroprotective-neurorescue and amyloid precursor protein-processing regulatory activities as therapeutic agents. *Progress in neurobiology,* 82, 348-60.

Mandel, S., G. Maor & M. B. Youdim (2004) Iron and alpha-synuclein in the substantia nigra of MPTP-treated mice: effect of neuroprotective drugs R-apomorphine and green tea polyphenol (-)-epigallocatechin-3-gallate. *Journal of molecular neuroscience : MN,* 24, 401-16.

Mandel, S., O. Weinreb, L. Reznichenko, L. Kalfon & T. Amit (2006) Green tea catechins as brain-permeable, non toxic iron chelators to "iron out iron" from the brain. *Journal of neural transmission. Supplementum,* 249-57.

Manning-Bog, A. B., A. L. McCormack, J. Li, V. N. Uversky, A. L. Fink & D. A. Di Monte (2002) The herbicide paraquat causes up-regulation and aggregation of alpha-synuclein in mice: paraquat and alpha-synuclein. *J Biol Chem,* 277, 1641-4.

Marcotte, E. R., L. K. Srivastava & R. Quirion (2003) cDNA microarray and proteomic approaches in the study of brain diseases: focus on schizophrenia and Alzheimer's disease. *Pharmacology & therapeutics,* 100, 63-74.

Martin, L. J., Y. Pan, A. C. Price, W. Sterling, N. G. Copeland, N. A. Jenkins, D. L. Price & M. K. Lee (2006) Parkinson's disease alpha-synuclein transgenic mice develop neuronal mitochondrial degeneration and cell death. *The Journal of neuroscience : the official journal of the Society for Neuroscience,* 26, 41-50.

Matigian, N., G. Abrahamsen, R. Sutharsan, A. L. Cook, A. M. Vitale, A. Nouwens, B. Bellette, J. An, M. Anderson, A. G. Beckhouse, M. Bennebroek, R. Cecil, A. M. Chalk, J. Cochrane, Y. Fan, F. Feron, R. McCurdy, J. J. McGrath, W. Murrell, C. Perry, J. Raju, S. Ravishankar, P. A. Silburn, G. T. Sutherland, S. Mahler, G. D. Mellick, S. A. Wood, C. M. Sue, C. A. Wells & A. Mackay-Sim (2010) Disease-specific, neurosphere-derived cells as models for brain disorders. *Disease models & mechanisms,* 3, 785-98.

Mayeux, R., J. Denaro, N. Hemenegildo, K. Marder, M. X. Tang, L. J. Cote & Y. Stern (1992) A population-based investigation of Parkinson's disease with and without dementia. Relationship to age and gender. *Arch Neurol,* 49, 492-7.

Meco, G., V. Bonifati, N. Vanacore & E. Fabrizio (1994) Parkinsonism after chronic exposure to the fungicide maneb (manganese ethylene-bis-dithiocarbamate). *Scand J Work Environ Health,* 20, 301-5.

Menegon, A., P. G. Board, A. C. Blackburn, G. D. Mellick & D. G. Le Couteur (1998) Parkinson's disease, pesticides, and glutathione transferase polymorphisms. *Lancet,* 352, 1344-6.

Mercer, L. D., B. L. Kelly, M. K. Horne & P. M. Beart (2005) Dietary polyphenols protect dopamine neurons from oxidative insults and apoptosis: investigations in primary rat mesencephalic cultures. *Biochemical pharmacology,* 69, 339-45.

Mogi, M., A. Togari, T. Kondo, Y. Mizuno, O. Komure, S. Kuno, H. Ichinose & T. Nagatsu (1999) Brain-derived growth factor and nerve growth factor concentrations are decreased in the substantia nigra in Parkinson's disease. *Neurosci Lett,* 270, 45-8.

Moon, Y., K. H. Lee, J. H. Park, D. Geum & K. Kim (2005) Mitochondrial membrane depolarization and the selective death of dopaminergic neurons by rotenone: protective effect of coenzyme Q10. *J Neurochem,* 93, 1199-208.

Morris, M. E. (2000) Movement disorders in people with Parkinson disease: a model for physical therapy. *Phys Ther,* 80, 578-97.

Munoz-Fernandez, M. A. & M. Fresno (1998) The role of tumour necrosis factor, interleukin 6, interferon-gamma and inducible nitric oxide synthase in the development and pathology of the nervous system. *Progress in neurobiology,* 56, 307-40.

Nguyen, H. N., B. Byers, B. Cord, A. Shcheglovitov, J. Byrne, P. Gujar, K. Kee, B. Schule, R. E. Dolmetsch, W. Langston, T. D. Palmer & R. R. Pera (2011) LRRK2 mutant iPSC-derived DA neurons demonstrate increased susceptibility to oxidative stress. *Cell stem cell,* 8, 267-80.

Noack, H., U. Kube & W. Augustin (1994) Relations between tocopherol depletion and coenzyme Q during lipid peroxidation in rat liver mitochondria. *Free radical research,* 20, 375-86.

Norazit, A., A. C. Meedeniya, M. N. Nguyen & A. Mackay-Sim (2010) Progressive loss of dopaminergic neurons induced by unilateral rotenone infusion into the medial forebrain bundle. *Brain Res,* 1360, 119-29.

Olanow, C. W. & W. G. Tatton (1999) Etiology and pathogenesis of Parkinson's disease. *Annu Rev Neurosci,* 22, 123-44.

Palacino, J. J., D. Sagi, M. S. Goldberg, S. Krauss, C. Motz, M. Wacker, J. Klose & J. Shen (2004) Mitochondrial dysfunction and oxidative damage in parkin-deficient mice. *The Journal of biological chemistry,* 279, 18614-22.

Pan, T., J. Jankovic & W. Le (2003) Potential therapeutic properties of green tea polyphenols in Parkinson's disease. *Drugs & aging,* 20, 711-21.

Panet, H., A. Barzilai, D. Daily, E. Melamed & D. Offen (2001) Activation of nuclear transcription factor kappa B (NF-kappaB) is essential for dopamine-induced apoptosis in PC12 cells. *Journal of neurochemistry,* 77, 391-8.

Parain, K., M. G. Murer, Q. Yan, B. Faucheux, Y. Agid, E. Hirsch & R. Raisman-Vozari (1999) Reduced expression of brain-derived neurotrophic factor protein in Parkinson's disease substantia nigra. *Neuroreport,* 10, 557-61.

Park, J., S. B. Lee, S. Lee, Y. Kim, S. Song, S. Kim, E. Bae, J. Kim, M. Shong, J. M. Kim & J. Chung (2006) Mitochondrial dysfunction in Drosophila PINK1 mutants is complemented by parkin. *Nature,* 441, 1157-61.

Parkinson, J. (2002) An essay on the shaking palsy. 1817. *J Neuropsychiatry Clin Neurosci,* 14, 223-36; discussion 222.

Perez, C. A., Y. Wei & M. Guo (2009) Iron-binding and anti-Fenton properties of baicalein and baicalin. *Journal of inorganic biochemistry,* 103, 326-32.

Petzinger, G. M. & J. W. Langston. 1998. The MPTP-lesioned non-human primate: a model for Parkinson's disease. In *Advances in Neurodegenerative Disorders. Parkinson's Disease,* eds. J. Marwah & H. Teitelbaum, 113-148. Scottsdale: Prominent Press.

Preece, P. & N. J. Cairns (2003) Quantifying mRNA in postmortem human brain: influence of gender, age at death, postmortem interval, brain pH, agonal state and inter-lobe mRNA variance. *Brain research. Molecular brain research,* 118, 60-71.

Qin, Z. H., Y. Wang, M. Nakai & T. N. Chase (1998) Nuclear factor-kappa B contributes to excitotoxin-induced apoptosis in rat striatum. *Molecular pharmacology,* 53, 33-42.

Quilty, M. C., A. E. King, W. P. Gai, D. L. Pountney, A. K. West, J. C. Vickers & T. C. Dickson (2006) Alpha-synuclein is upregulated in neurones in response to chronic oxidative stress and is associated with neuroprotection. *Exp Neurol,* 199, 249-56.

Radad, K., W. D. Rausch & G. Gille (2006) Rotenone induces cell death in primary dopaminergic culture by increasing ROS production and inhibiting mitochondrial respiration. *Neurochem Int,* 49, 379-86.

Ramassamy, C. (2006) Emerging role of polyphenolic compounds in the treatment of neurodegenerative diseases: a review of their intracellular targets. *European journal of pharmacology,* 545, 51-64.

Ravenstijn, P. G., M. Merlini, M. Hameetman, T. K. Murray, M. A. Ward, H. Lewis, G. Ball, C. Mottart, C. de Ville de Goyet, T. Lemarchand, K. van Belle, M. J. O'Neill, M. Danhof & E. C. de Lange (2008) The exploration of rotenone as a toxin for inducing Parkinson's disease in rats, for application in BBB transport and PK-PD experiments. *J Pharmacol Toxicol Methods,* 57, 114-30.

Reto, M., M. E. Figueira, H. M. Filipe & C. M. Almeida (2007) Chemical composition of green tea (Camellia sinensis) infusions commercialized in Portugal. *Plant foods for human nutrition,* 62, 139-44.

Ritchie, C. W., A. I. Bush, A. Mackinnon, S. Macfarlane, M. Mastwyk, L. MacGregor, L. Kiers, R. Cherny, Q. X. Li, A. Tammer, D. Carrington, C. Mavros, I. Volitakis, M. Xilinas, D. Ames, S. Davis, K. Beyreuther, R. E. Tanzi & C. L. Masters (2003) Metal-protein attenuation with iodochlorhydroxyquin (clioquinol) targeting Abeta amyloid deposition and toxicity in Alzheimer disease: a pilot phase 2 clinical trial. *Archives of neurology*, 60, 1685-91.

Rodrigues, R. W., V. C. Gomide & G. Chadi (2004) Astroglial and microglial activation in the wistar rat ventral tegmental area after a single striatal injection of 6-hydroxydopamine. *Int J Neurosci*, 114, 197-216.

Sang, T. K., H. Y. Chang, G. M. Lawless, A. Ratnaparkhi, L. Mee, L. C. Ackerson, N. T. Maidment, D. E. Krantz & G. R. Jackson (2007) A Drosophila model of mutant human parkin-induced toxicity demonstrates selective loss of dopaminergic neurons and dependence on cellular dopamine. *The Journal of neuroscience : the official journal of the Society for Neuroscience*, 27, 981-92.

Sangchot, P., S. Sharma, B. Chetsawang, J. Porter, P. Govitrapong & M. Ebadi (2002) Deferoxamine attenuates iron-induced oxidative stress and prevents mitochondrial aggregation and alpha-synuclein translocation in SK-N-SH cells in culture. *Developmental neuroscience*, 24, 143-53.

Saravanan, K. S., K. M. Sindhu & K. P. Mohanakumar (2005) Acute intranigral infusion of rotenone in rats causes progressive biochemical lesions in the striatum similar to Parkinson's disease. *Brain Res*, 1049, 147-55.

Schapira, A. H. (2008) Mitochondria in the aetiology and pathogenesis of Parkinson's disease. *Lancet Neurol*, 7, 97-109.

Schwarting, R. K. & J. P. Huston (1996) The unilateral 6-hydroxydopamine lesion model in behavioral brain research. Analysis of functional deficits, recovery and treatments. *Prog Neurobiol*, 50, 275-331.

Sedelis, M., R. K. Schwarting & J. P. Huston (2001) Behavioral phenotyping of the MPTP mouse model of Parkinson's disease. *Behav Brain Res*, 125, 109-25.

Severson, J. A., J. Marcusson, B. Winblad & C. E. Finch (1982) Age-correlated loss of dopaminergic binding sites in human basal ganglia. *J Neurochem*, 39, 1623-31.

Sherer, T. B., R. Betarbet, J. H. Kim & J. T. Greenamyre (2003a) Selective microglial activation in the rat rotenone model of Parkinson's disease. *Neurosci Lett*, 341, 87-90.

Sherer, T. B., R. Betarbet, C. M. Testa, B. B. Seo, J. R. Richardson, J. H. Kim, G. W. Miller, T. Yagi, A. Matsuno-Yagi & J. T. Greenamyre (2003b) Mechanism of toxicity in rotenone models of Parkinson's disease. *J Neurosci*, 23, 10756-64.

Sherer, T. B., J. H. Kim, R. Betarbet & J. T. Greenamyre (2003c) Subcutaneous rotenone exposure causes highly selective dopaminergic degeneration and alpha-synuclein aggregation. *Exp Neurol*, 179, 9-16.

Shiozaki, E. N., J. Chai, D. J. Rigotti, S. J. Riedl, P. Li, S. M. Srinivasula, E. S. Alnemri, R. Fairman & Y. Shi (2003) Mechanism of XIAP-mediated inhibition of caspase-9. *Molecular cell*, 11, 519-27.

Shoulson, I., D. Oakes, S. Fahn, A. Lang, J. W. Langston, P. LeWitt, C. W. Olanow, J. B. Penney, C. Tanner, K. Kieburtz & A. Rudolph (2002) Impact of sustained deprenyl (selegiline) in levodopa-treated Parkinson's disease: a randomized placebo-controlled extension of the deprenyl and tocopherol antioxidative therapy of parkinsonism trial. *Annals of neurology*, 51, 604-12.

Shults, C. W., D. Oakes, K. Kieburtz, M. F. Beal, R. Haas, S. Plumb, J. L. Juncos, J. Nutt, I. Shoulson, J. Carter, K. Kompoliti, J. S. Perlmutter, S. Reich, M. Stern, R. L. Watts, R. Kurlan, E. Molho, M. Harrison & M. Lew (2002) Effects of coenzyme Q10 in early

Parkinson disease: evidence of slowing of the functional decline. *Archives of neurology*, 59, 1541-50.

Sies, H. 1985. *Oxidative stress: introductory remarks.* London: Academic Press.--- (1986) Biochemistry of oxidative stress. *Angewaudte Chemie, International Edition in English*, 28, 1058-1071.---. 1991. *Oxidative stress: introduction.* London: Academic Press.

Sindhu, K. M., R. Banerjee, K. S. Senthilkumar, K. S. Saravanan, B. C. Raju, J. M. Rao & K. P. Mohanakumar (2006) Rats with unilateral median forebrain bundle, but not striatal or nigral, lesions by the neurotoxins MPP+ or rotenone display differential sensitivity to amphetamine and apomorphine. *Pharmacol Biochem Behav*, 84, 321-9.

Sindhu, K. M., K. S. Saravanan & K. P. Mohanakumar (2005) Behavioral differences in a rotenone-induced hemiparkinsonian rat model developed following intranigral or median forebrain bundle infusion. *Brain Res*, 1051, 25-34.

Smeyne, R. J. & V. Jackson-Lewis (2005) The MPTP model of Parkinson's disease. *Brain Res Mol Brain Res*, 134, 57-66.

Smith, M. A. (1996) Hippocampal vulnerability to stress and aging: possible role of neurotrophic factors. *Behav Brain Res*, 78, 25-36.

Soldner, F., D. Hockemeyer, C. Beard, Q. Gao, G. W. Bell, E. G. Cook, G. Hargus, A. Blak, O. Cooper, M. Mitalipova, O. Isacson & R. Jaenisch (2009) Parkinson's disease patient-derived induced pluripotent stem cells free of viral reprogramming factors. *Cell*, 136, 964-77.

Sutherland, G. T., N. A. Matigian, A. M. Chalk, M. J. Anderson, P. A. Silburn, A. Mackay-Sim, C. A. Wells & G. D. Mellick (2009) A cross-study transcriptional analysis of Parkinson's disease. *PloS one*, 4, e4955.

Takahashi, K. & S. Yamanaka (2006) Induction of pluripotent stem cells from mouse embryonic and adult fibroblast cultures by defined factors. *Cell*, 126, 663-76.

Tan, R. X., J. C. Meng & K. Hostettmann (2000) Phytochemical investigation of some traditional Chinese medicines and endophyte cultures. *Pharmaceutical Biology*, 38, 25-32.

Tanaka, K., T. Suzuki, T. Chiba, H. Shimura, N. Hattori & Y. Mizuno (2001) Parkin is linked to the ubiquitin pathway. *Journal of molecular medicine*, 79, 482-94.

Tanner, C. M. (1989) The role of environmental toxins in the etiology of Parkinson's disease. *Trends Neurosci*, 12, 49-54.

Testa, C. M., T. B. Sherer & J. T. Greenamyre (2005) Rotenone induces oxidative stress and dopaminergic neuron damage in organotypic substantia nigra cultures. *Brain Res Mol Brain Res*, 134, 109-18.

Thiruchelvam, M., E. K. Richfield, R. B. Baggs, A. W. Tank & D. A. Cory-Slechta (2000) The nigrostriatal dopaminergic system as a preferential target of repeated exposures to combined paraquat and maneb: implications for Parkinson's disease. *J Neurosci*, 20, 9207-14.

Thomas, J., J. Wang, H. Takubo, J. Sheng, S. de Jesus & K. S. Bankiewicz (1994) A 6-hydroxydopamine-induced selective parkinsonian rat model: further biochemical and behavioral characterization. *Exp Neurol*, 126, 159-67.

Tong, Y., A. Pisani, G. Martella, M. Karouani, H. Yamaguchi, E. N. Pothos & J. Shen (2009) R1441C mutation in LRRK2 impairs dopaminergic neurotransmission in mice. *Proceedings of the National Academy of Sciences of the United States of America*, 106, 14622-7.

Tsubaki, T., Y. Honma & M. Hoshi (1971) Neurological syndrome associated with clioquinol. *Lancet,* 1, 696-7.

Turrens, J. F. (2003) Mitochondrial formation of reactive oxygen species. *J Physiol,* 552, 335-44.

Van Den Eeden, S. K., C. M. Tanner, A. L. Bernstein, R. D. Fross, A. Leimpeter, D. A. Bloch & L. M. Nelson (2003) Incidence of Parkinson's disease: variation by age, gender, and race/ethnicity. *Am J Epidemiol,* 157, 1015-22.

Vaux, D. L. & J. Silke (2003) Mammalian mitochondrial IAP binding proteins. *Biochemical and biophysical research communications,* 304, 499-504.

Vila, M., V. Jackson-Lewis, C. Guegan, D. C. Wu, P. Teismann, D. K. Choi, K. Tieu & S. Przedborski (2001) The role of glial cells in Parkinson's disease. *Curr Opin Neurol,* 14, 483-9.

von Coelln, R., B. Thomas, S. A. Andrabi, K. L. Lim, J. M. Savitt, R. Saffary, W. Stirling, K. Bruno, E. J. Hess, M. K. Lee, V. L. Dawson & T. M. Dawson (2006) Inclusion body formation and neurodegeneration are parkin independent in a mouse model of alpha-synucleinopathy. *The Journal of neuroscience : the official journal of the Society for Neuroscience,* 26, 3685-96.

Wang, C., R. Lu, X. Ouyang, M. W. Ho, W. Chia, F. Yu & K. L. Lim (2007) Drosophila overexpressing parkin R275W mutant exhibits dopaminergic neuron degeneration and mitochondrial abnormalities. *The Journal of neuroscience : the official journal of the Society for Neuroscience,* 27, 8563-70.

Wang, L., C. Xie, E. Greggio, L. Parisiadou, H. Shim, L. Sun, J. Chandran, X. Lin, C. Lai, W. J. Yang, D. J. Moore, T. M. Dawson, V. L. Dawson, G. Chiosis, M. R. Cookson & H. Cai (2008) The chaperone activity of heat shock protein 90 is critical for maintaining the stability of leucine-rich repeat kinase 2. *The Journal of neuroscience : the official journal of the Society for Neuroscience,* 28, 3384-91.

Wang, X., Z. H. Qin, Y. Leng, Y. Wang, X. Jin, T. N. Chase & M. C. Bennett (2002) Prostaglandin A1 inhibits rotenone-induced apoptosis in SH-SY5Y cells. *Journal of neurochemistry,* 83, 1094-102.

Watts, R. L., T. Subramanian, A. Freeman, C. G. Goetz, R. D. Penn, G. T. Stebbins, J. H. Kordower & R. A. Bakay (1997) Effect of stereotaxic intrastriatal cografts of autologous adrenal medulla and peripheral nerve in Parkinson's disease: two-year follow-up study. *Exp Neurol,* 147, 510-7.

West, A. B., D. J. Moore, S. Biskup, A. Bugayenko, W. W. Smith, C. A. Ross, V. L. Dawson & T. M. Dawson (2005) Parkinson's disease-associated mutations in leucine-rich repeat kinase 2 augment kinase activity. *Proceedings of the National Academy of Sciences of the United States of America,* 102, 16842-7.

Whitworth, A. J., D. A. Theodore, J. C. Greene, H. Benes, P. D. Wes & L. J. Pallanck (2005) Increased glutathione S-transferase activity rescues dopaminergic neuron loss in a Drosophila model of Parkinson's disease. *Proceedings of the National Academy of Sciences of the United States of America,* 102, 8024-9.

Xiong, N., J. Huang, Z. Zhang, J. Xiong, X. Liu, M. Jia, F. Wang, C. Chen, X. Cao, Z. Liang, S. Sun, Z. Lin & T. Wang (2009) Stereotaxical infusion of rotenone: a reliable rodent model for Parkinson's disease. *PLoS One,* 4, e7878.

Yassin, M. S., J. Ekblom, M. Xilinas, C. G. Gottfries & L. Oreland (2000) Changes in uptake of vitamin B(12) and trace metals in brains of mice treated with clioquinol. *Journal of the neurological sciences,* 173, 40-4.

Youdim, M. B., M. Fridkin & H. Zheng (2005) Bifunctional drug derivatives of MAO-B inhibitor rasagiline and iron chelator VK-28 as a more effective approach to treatment of brain ageing and ageing neurodegenerative diseases. *Mechanisms of ageing and development,* 126, 317-26.

Youdim, M. B., G. Stephenson & D. Ben Shachar (2004) Ironing iron out in Parkinson's disease and other neurodegenerative diseases with iron chelators: a lesson from 6-hydroxydopamine and iron chelators, desferal and VK-28. *Annals of the New York Academy of Sciences,* 1012, 306-25.

Zbarsky, V., K. P. Datla, S. Parkar, D. K. Rai, O. I. Aruoma & D. T. Dexter (2005) Neuroprotective properties of the natural phenolic antioxidants curcumin and naringenin but not quercetin and fisetin in a 6-OHDA model of Parkinson's disease. *Free radical research,* 39, 1119-25.

Zheng, H., D. Blat & M. Fridkin (2006) Novel neuroprotective neurotrophic NAP analogs targeting metal toxicity and oxidative stress: potential candidates for the control of neurodegenerative diseases. *Journal of neural transmission. Supplementum,* 163-72.

Zheng, H., L. M. Weiner, O. Bar-Am, S. Epsztejn, Z. I. Cabantchik, A. Warshawsky, M. B. Youdim & M. Fridkin (2005) Design, synthesis, and evaluation of novel bifunctional iron-chelators as potential agents for neuroprotection in Alzheimer's, Parkinson's, and other neurodegenerative diseases. *Bioorganic & medicinal chemistry,* 13, 773-83.

Zigmond, M. J., T. G. Hastings & E. D. Abercrombie (1992) Neurochemical responses to 6-hydroxydopamine and L-dopa therapy: implications for Parkinson's disease. *Ann N Y Acad Sci,* 648, 71-86.

Zou, H., W. J. Henzel, X. Liu, A. Lutschg & X. Wang (1997) Apaf-1, a human protein homologous to C. elegans CED-4, participates in cytochrome c-dependent activation of caspase-3. *Cell,* 90, 405-13.

18

The Relationship Between Thyroid States, Oxidative Stress and Cellular Damage

Cano-Europa, Blas-Valdivia Vanessa,
Franco-Colin Margarita and Ortiz-Butron Rocio
Escuela Nacional de Ciencias
Biológicas del Instituto Politécnico Nacional,
México

1. Introduction

The thyroid hormones play an important role in many physiological processes, such as differentiation, growth, development, and the physiology of all cells. One of the most studied effects of the thyroid hormone is the control of the basal metabolic rate. Modifications in its levels can produce several alterations including modifications in the ROS steady-state and the REDOX environment in the cells. There is much evidence that show both hyperthyroidism and hypothyroidism are related to oxidative stress and cellular damage. For hypothyroidism, there are other findings that point to its protective effects. In this chapter we show both findings and propose that hypothyroidism is a protective state against toxic agents.

2. Thyroid hormones

Thyroid hormones (THs) T_4 (thyroxine or 3´,5´,3,5-L-tetra-iodothyronine) and T_3 (3´,3,5-triiodothyronine) are synthesized in the thyroid gland located in the anterior part of the trachea, just below the larynx. It consists of two lobes joined in the middle by a narrow portion of the gland. The major thyroid-secretor cells, known as follicular cells, are arranged into hollow spheres, each of which it forms a functional unit called a follicle. On a microscopic section, rings of follicular cells enclosing an inner lumen filled with colloid form the follicles (figure 1).

The principal constituent of the colloid is a large protein molecule, thyroglobulin, where thyroid hormones are incorporated in their various stages of synthesis. The follicular cells produce the two iodine-containing hormones derived from the amino acid tyrosine; T_4 and $T_{3,}$ the thyroid hormones. The mechanism involved in thyroid hormone syntheses and their release from thyrolobulin are shown in figure 2. Iodine, an essential element of the thyroid molecule, is actively transported by the Na^+-I^- symporter (NIS, encoded by the *SLC5A5* gene) at the basolateral membrane of the thyrocyte and it diffuses by an exchanger, known as pendrin (PDS, encoded by the *SLC26A4* gene) to the lumen at the apical membrane. At the extracellular apical membrane, thyroperoxidase (TPO, EC 1.11.1.8) with hydrogen peroxide (H_2O_2), generated by dual oxidase 2 (DUOX2, EC 1.6.3.1), oxidizes and binds iodine

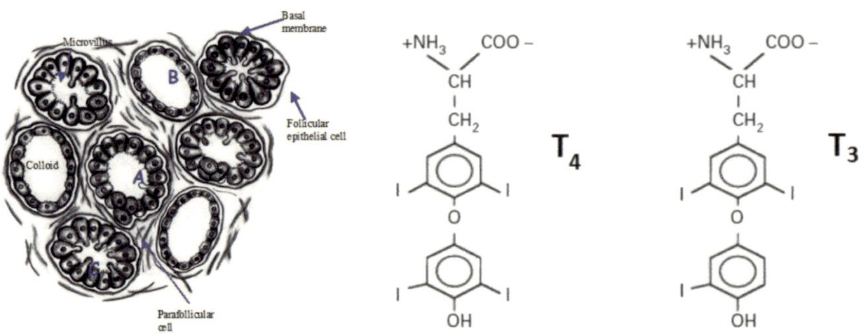

Fig. 1. Histological thyroid and the thyroid hormone structure. There are thyroid follicles with different activity. A: Thyroid follicle resting. B: Follicle with high activity.

covalently to tyrosyl residues, producing monoiodotyrosine (MIT) and diiodotyrosine (DIT) within the thyrogloblin macromolecule. The enzyme thyroperoxidase catalyzes the coupling of two iodotyrosine residues to produce the prohormone T_4 and smaller amounts of the active hormone T_3. After endocytosis, iodinated thyroglobulin is hydrolyzed in the lysosomes by cathepsins and the thyroid hormone is released from the thyroglobulin backbone. The released MIT and DIT are deiodinated by a specific iodotyrosine deiodinase (IYD, or DEHAL1, EC 1.22.1.1), and the released iodine is recycled within the cell. The mechanism involved in the last step in the process, the thyroid hormone secretion, remains unknown (Di Cosmo et al., 2010). About 90% of the secretory product released from the thyroid gland is in the form of T_4 though T_3 is about four times more potent in its biologic activity. Most of the secreted T_4 is converted into T_3 by a group of enzymes known as iodothyronine deiodinases (D1 and D2, EC 1.97.1.10), which also include an inactivating deiodinase, the type 3 deiodinase (D3), that inactivates both T_4 and T_3 (Bianco et al., 2002)(table 1).

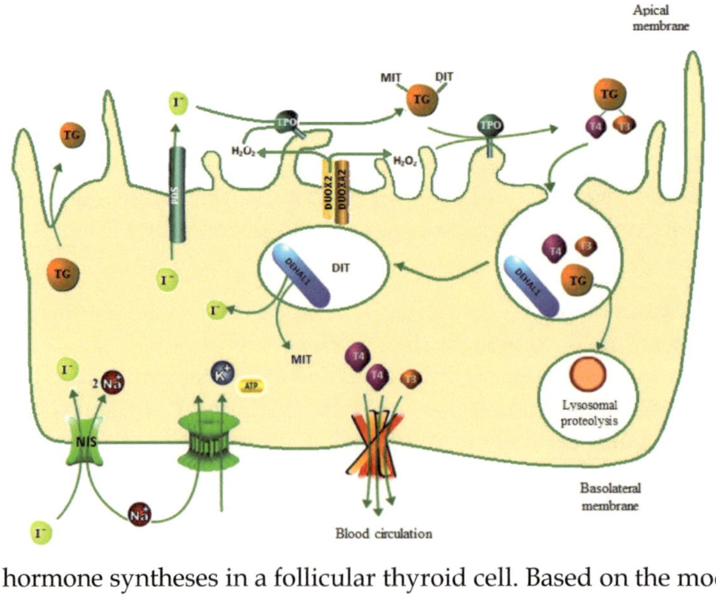

Fig. 2. Thyroid hormone syntheses in a follicular thyroid cell. Based on the model proposed by Di Cosmo (Di Cosmo et al., 2010)

The role played by the deiodinases is physiologically relevant. They have a role in various aspects of mammalian physiology, such as the maintenance of plasma T_3 concentration (Bianco et al., 2002), TSH and TRH feedback regulation (Christoffolete et al., 2006; Larsen, 1982), and the clearance of sulfated iodothyronines (Schneider et al., 2006).

Deiodinase	Tissue
D1	Liver, thyroid, kidney
D2	Brain, pituitary gland, BAT, thyroid, muscle
D3	Developing tissues and placenta, adult skin, brain

Table 1. Tissue distribution of deiodinases in humans (St.Germain et al., 2009).

2.1 Thyroid hormone regulation levels

Because the thyroid hormones have a crucial role in the function of every tissue in the body, their levels must be maintained relatively constant around an optimum level. This homeostatic-control mechanism primarily operates on the principle of negative feedback (figure 3). In this homeostatic-control mechanism, the hypothalamic thyrotropin-releasing hormone (TRH), the thyroid-stimulating hormone (TSH), and thyroid hormone all together form the hypothalamus-pituitary-thyroid axis. Thus, TRH in trophic fashion turns on the TSH secretion by the anterior pituitary, whereas thyroid hormone, in negative feedback fashion, turns off the TSH secretion. In the hypothalamus-pituitary-thyroid axis, inhibition is exerted primarily at the level of the anterior pituitary. As with other negative feedback loops, the one between thyroid hormone and TSH tends to maintain a stable thyroid hormone output (Hulbert, 2000).

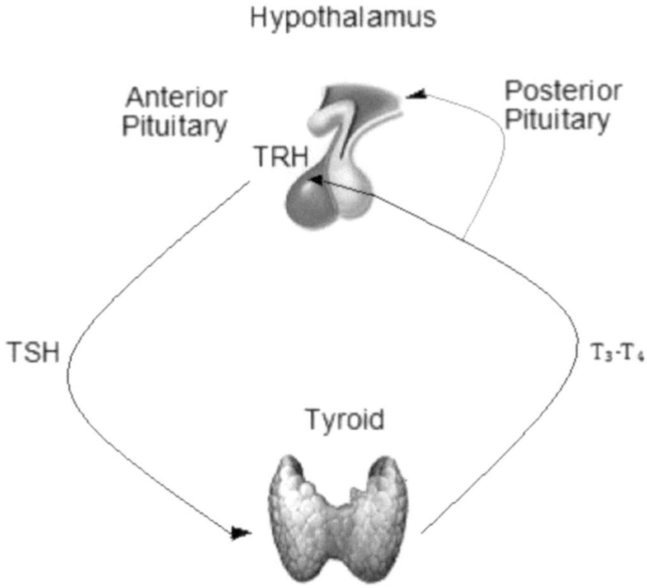

Fig. 3. Hypothalamus-pituitary-thyroid axes. In this image is shown the negative feedback exerted by a high T_3 concentration.

2.2 Mechanism of action of the thyroid hormones

Because thyroid hormones have been considered as lipophilic in their intracellular action, passive hormone diffusion through the lipid bilayer has been accepted. Because of the existence of nuclear receptors for thyroid hormones, it has long been believed that the THs caused effects only via genomic effects, however since the late 1980s it has been proposed that the THs may cause effects independently of genetic mechanisms, affecting membrane lipid composition or activation of enzymes (Lazar, 1993). Receptors for thyroid hormones (TRs) are proteins that act as transcription factors that belong to the superfamily of nuclear receptors, which includes steroids, vitamin D, retinoic acid, fatty acids, prostaglandins, and orphan receptors (Zhang & Lazar, 2000). The TRs have regions; the DNA binding domain (DBD), ligand binding domain (LBD), hinge region (HR), and amino terminal domain (A-B) (Sap et al., 1986). The THs cross the lipid membrane because of their hydrophobic nature. In the cytoplasm they can bind to newly synthesized TRs, however most THs bind to nuclear receptors. The TRs bound to the THs may regulate the transcription process by modifying the structure of chromatin, allowing other factors to exert their action on elements of the TH responses (figure 4). In addition, the THs interact, directly or indirectly, through bridge or coactivator molecules, with the transcriptional machinery of the process. A critical aspect in regulating the transcription process by the TRs is the conformational change that T_3 exerts on the receiver itself. The T_3 decreases the ability of the hydrophobic TRs and can modify the way in which the TRs, either as dimer or heterodimer, bind to DNA. The TRs bind to regulate transcription as a monomer, homodimer, heterodimer, or heteromultimer. The thyroid hormones binding to the TRs cause changes in the structure of these complexes thus modulating the interaction with other elements of the transcriptional apparatus to determine the type of response, enhancing or inhibiting (Cheng et al., 2010; Yen, 2001).

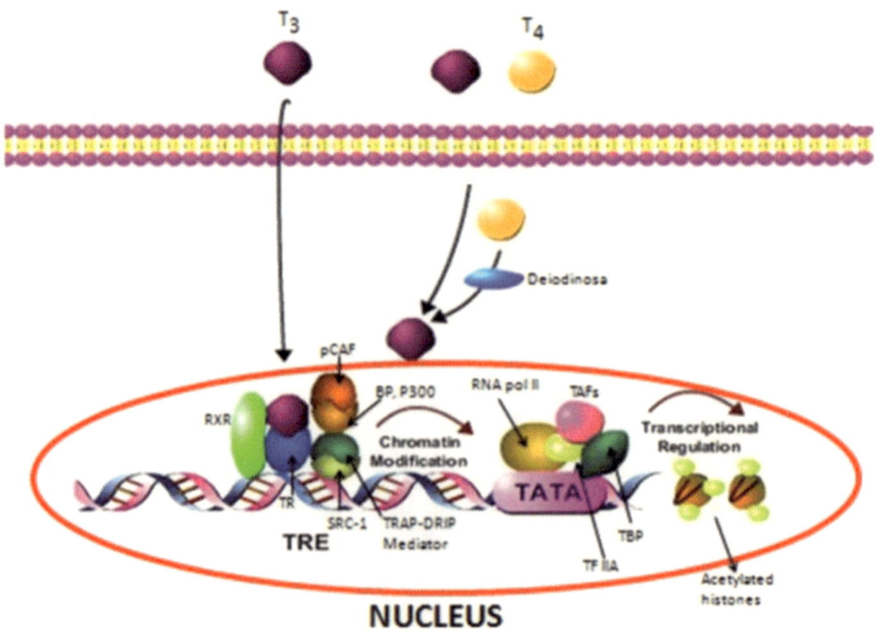

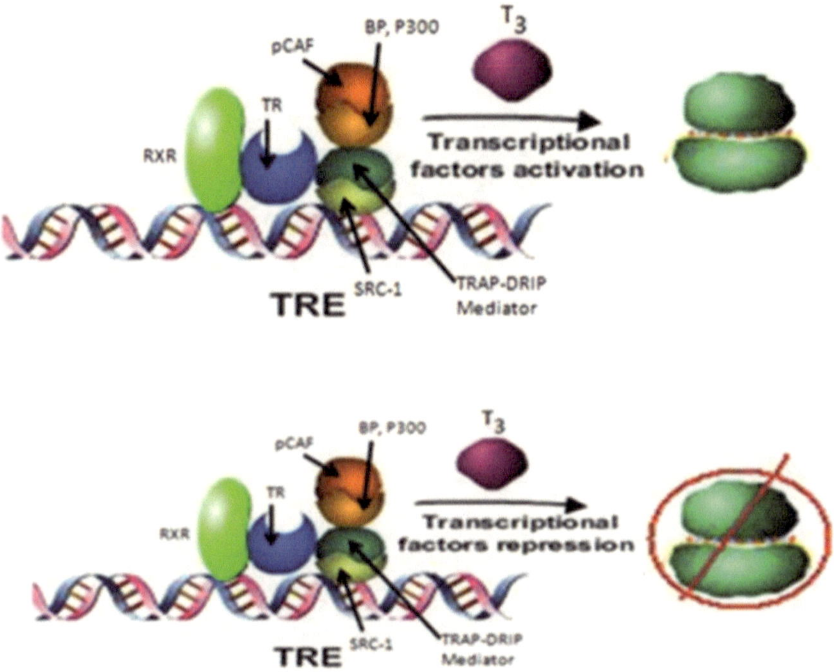

Fig. 4. Nuclear gene expressions by T_3 to the thyroid hormone receptors TRα and TRβ. Heterodimers must bind to specific thyroid response elements (TREs) in the promoters of T_3-target genes and activate or repress transcription in response to hormone.

The existence of cell-surface receptors for thyroid hormones has been acknowledged. The presence of binding sites for thyroid hormones on the cell surface has been known for many years in the red blood-cell membrane (Davis et al., 1983) and in the synaptosome (Giguere et al., 1996; Giguere et al., 1992). The identity of the proteins involved in membrane binding of hormones was not established in these studies and there has been a reluctance to believe that integrin avβ3, containing a binding site for the thyroid hormones, is an initiation site for complex hormone-directed cellular events, such as cell division and angiogenesis (Davis et al., 2005).

Integrins are ubiquitous heterodimeric structural proteins of the cell membrane that convey signals from the cell interior to the extracellular matrix (ECM) (inside-out) and from the ECM to the cell (outside-in). The integrin purified from the plasma membrane bound radiolabeled thyroid hormones and with high affinity. This integrin contains a binding site for thyroid hormones caused by the functional consequences of the binding activation of MAPK (figure 5). The receptor has been located at the Arg-Gly-Asp (RGD) recognition site on the integrin that is important to the binding of a number of extracellular-matrix proteins and growth factors. From this site, the thyroid hormone signals are transduced by MAPK (ERK1-2) in angiogenesis in endothelial cells and the cell proliferation of tumor cell lines. The T_4 in concentrations that are physiological (10^{-10} M free T_4) and T_3 in supraphysiological concentrations cause ERK-dependent cell proliferation. It is now clear that the hormone receptor domain on the integrin is more complex than initially thought. There is a T_3-specific

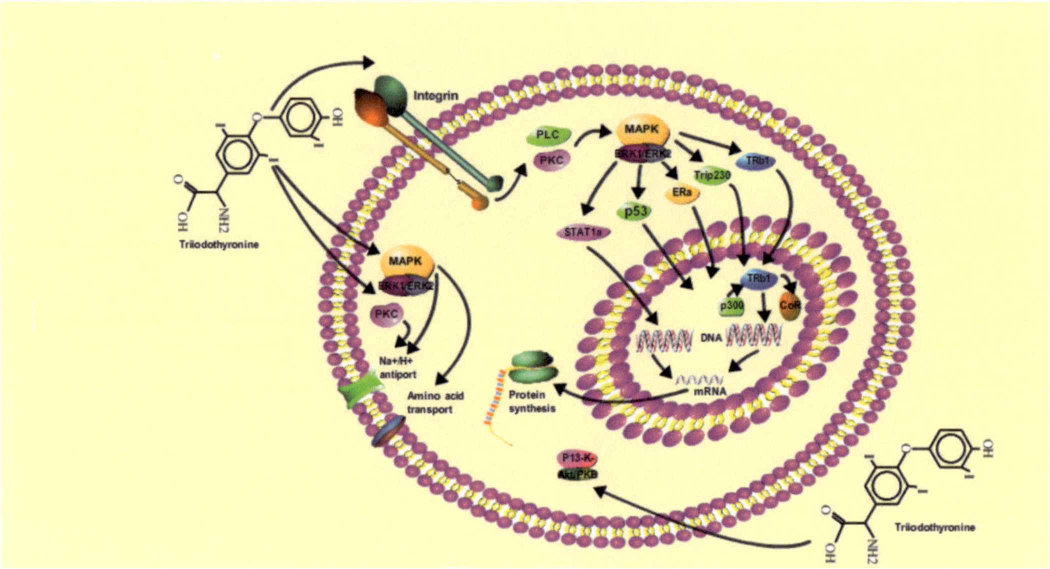

Fig. 5. Nongenomic mechanisms of action of thyroid hormones mediated by integrine-type membranal receptors.

site in the domain and a site at which both T_4 and T_3 may act. The T_3-specific site activates PI3K and is linked not to cell proliferation, but to trafficking of certain intracellular proteins such as shuttling of TRs from the cytoplasm to nucleus and to the transcription of specific genes, such as hypoxia-inducible factor-1 (HIF-1). T_4 is unable to activate PI3K (Cheng et al., 2010).

2.3 Thyroid hormone actions

The T_3 is recognized as a key metabolic hormone of the body. It has many physiological actions and it modulates all metabolic pathways through alterations in oxygen consumption and changes in protein, lipid, carbohydrate, and vitamin metabolism. Through its direct manipulation of protein expression associated with such pathways, T_3 affects the synthesis and degradation of many other hormones and growth factors and indirectly influences additional endocrine signaling. To see more details of the thyroid hormone action, check the review of Hulbert (Hulbert, 2000).

2.4 Abnormalities of the thyroid function

Abnormalities of the thyroid function are among the most common of all endocrine disorders. They fall into two categories, hypothyroidism and hyperthyroidism, reflecting deficient and excess thyroid hormone secretion. There are many causes that generate these conditions. Whatever the cause, the consequences of too little or too much thyroid hormone secretion are largely predictable, given the knowledge of the functions of the thyroid hormones.

3. Relationship between alterations of the thyroid hormones and the ROS-steady state

It has been proposed that the thyroid hormones influence the ROS steady-state and REDOX environment in the cell. The most common idea is that hyperthyroidism enhances the ROS production that perturbs the ROS steady-state and changes the REDOX environment to facilitate cell damage. A hypometabolic state caused by hypothyroidism could be a protective state. In the next part of this chapter we show the evidence for this.

3.1 Hyperthyroidism and the ROS-steady state

Because thyroid hormones modulate many functions, if thyroid hormone levels change, many cellular processes could be altered, including modifications in the REDOX environment. Related to this issue we can ask what happens in a hyperthyroid condition?. Because one of the most studied effects of the thyroid hormone is the control of the basal metabolic rate, a hypermetabolic state produces a modification of the REDOX environment (Venditti & Di Meo, 2006). It is well-known that a higher T_3 level, a hypermetabolic state, causes calorigenesis in two ways. The first is a short-term signaling mechanism with the allosteric activation of cytochrome-C oxidase and the second is a long-term pathway producing nuclear and mitochondrial gene transcription through T_3 signaling, thus stimulating basal thermogenesis (Oppenheimer et al., 1994). This last mechanism causes the synthesis of the enzymes involved in energy metabolism and the components of the respiratory-chain apparatus, leading to a higher capacity of oxidative phosphorylation (Videla, 2000; Soboll, 1993). These short- and long-term pathways are mainly responsible for the increased cellular respiration caused by the hyperthyroid state. Other processes may also play a role, namely 1) energy expenditure caused by a higher active cation transport, 2) loss of energy from futile cycles caused by increases in catabolic and anabolic pathways of intermediary metabolism, 3) higher activity of membrane-bound enzymes associated with electron transfer and metabolite carriers caused by changes in the lipid composition of mitochondrial membranes (Soboll, 1993), and 4) O_2 equivalents related to oxidative stress (Videla, 2000), a REDOX imbalance that leads to various pathological events in several organs as the liver (Jaeschke et al., 2002). In these pathologies, the cellular damage occurs when the balance between oxidant and antioxidants is disturbed and the antioxidant system does not balance the oxidants, thus altering the ROS steady-state level (Lushchak, 2011). An enhanced ROS causes lipid peroxidation, enhancement of reactive oxygen species, nitration, carbonylation, or glutathionylation of proteins, and fragmentation of DNA.

Fernandez et al. found that thyroid calorigenesis is a hormonal stimulus for the REDOX activation of NFκB, a response that is triggered in Kupffer cells having higher respiratory-burst activities (Fernandez et al., 2006). These findings are in agreement with studies showing that the NFκB activation can be achieved by physiological levels of the ROS, which are produced during the respiratory burst after stimulation of isolated or cultured macrophages (Kaul & Forman, 1996) and in carbon-stimulated Kupffer cells in the isolated, perfused rat liver (Romanque et al., 2003). This may be caused by the damage produced by the oxidative stress generated by an excess of thyroid hormones. There are data indicating that excess thyroid hormones act at multiple levels to cause apoptosis, because this higher level enhances the expression of several death receptors and their ligands, such as TNF-α,

FasL, proNGF, and proBDNF, resulting in activation of apical caspase-8, which is further amplified through the activation of the p75NRT-mediated pathways (Kumar et al., 2007). Hyperthyroid animals appear to have a shorter lifespan and, at an advanced age, have a myelin deficit (Carageorgiou et al., 2005). It is known that hyperthyroidism increases hepatic protein oxidation, as evidenced by a significant 88% increase in the content of protein hydrazone derivatives 3 days after a T_3 treatment. This effect may be caused by the increased generation of ROS generated by T_3 (Fernández et al., 1985; Fernandez & Videla, 1993) leading to the formation of carbonyl derivatives mainly occurring at the arginyl, prolyl, lysyl, and histidyl residues in proteins (Stadtman, 1990; Reznick & Packer, 1994). The T_3-caused ROS formation can cause the conversion of cysteinyl residues to protein-protein disulfide conjugates or to mixed-disulfide derivatives (Stadtman, 1990), whereas T_3-caused NO generation (Fernandez et al., 1997) may lead to protein oxidation or nitration through peroxynitrite formation (Alvarez & Radi, 2001). The biological significance of the oxidative modification of proteins in T_3-caused liver oxidative stress can be visualized on two levels; 1) loss of protein function and 2) increased protein degradation. Under high rates of ROS and RNS input, the oxidative modification of enzymes can occur with the consequent reduction in enzyme activity (Stadtman, 1990; Lissi et al., 1991). The inactivation of hepatic antioxidant enzymes has been described in several conditions in vivo involving oxidative stress in the tissue, including hyperthyroidism (Lissi et al., 1991), which determines a decrease in the activity of superoxide dismutase and catalase (Fernandez et al., 1988) and in the content of cytochrome P450 (Fernández et al., 1985). In agreement with this contention, inactivation of superoxide dismutase by H_2O_2 (Bray et al., 1974) and of catalase by $O_2^{\cdot-}$ (Kono & Fridovich, 1982) has been reported in conditions in vitro. In addition to enzyme inactivation, thyrotoxicosis in mammals results in the stimulation of both synthesis and degradation of protein, with a predominance of degradation, as shown by the increase in protein catabolism, negative nitrogen balance, and the loss of protein from muscle and other body stores (Loeb, 1996). These findings are in accordance with those of Tapia et al. who found a higher oxidation of the liver protein and an increase in lipid peroxidation levels in hyperthyroid rats (Tapia et al., 2010).

Interestingly, the activities of both GPx-1 and GR are decreased in hyperthyroid rats. It is remarkable that both enzymatic activities are strongly GSH-dependent. The GPx-1 catalyzes the reduction of H_2O_2 and lipid hydroperoxides coupled with oxidation of GSH into GSSG whereas the GR replenishes the GSH pool with the help of NADPH principally provided by the pentose-phosphate pathway. The intracellular GSH status appears to be a sensitive indicator of the cellular ability to resist ROS. Furthermore, it has been found that total GSH equivalents and the GSH and GSSG pools were increasingly depleted by T_3 over time (Chattopadhyay et al., 2007). The liver is especially rich in GST that metabolizes xenobiotics by conjugating with GSH. In fact, the GST-catalyzed conjugation of GSH with exogenous compounds and endogenous metabolites such as 4-hydroxynonenal is regarded as a major cellular-defense mechanism against toxicity (Cheng et al., 2001). The activities of GST were considerably impaired with the progression of the T_3 treatment (Chattopadhyay et al., 2007). Because recycling of oxidized glutathione consumes NADPH, the cellular levels of NADPH and its synthesis represent the rate limiting factors of H_2O_2 consumption by catalase-deficient tissues (Ho et al., 2004). Moreover, prolonged hyperthyroidism diminishes GR but elevated G6PD activity indicates that severe hyperthyroidism may compromise the cellular ability to maintain the redox state. Lombardi et al. have demonstrated that injection of T_3 into hypothyroid rats caused an increase in both enzyme activity and mRNA expression of G6PD in the liver. Nevertheless, the reduced activities of GPx, GR, and GST in the hyperthyroid liver prevent optimum GSH use and recycling. Accumulation of GSSG can lead to protein modifications because of interactions with –SH groups (Reed, 1990). Though the T_3 exerted a positive stimulatory effect on the NADPH supply, it was not sufficient to compensate for the massive GSH depletion and this probably explains the negative regulatory impact of T_3 on activities of GSH-dependent enzymes such as GPx and GR in the rat liver. Under such conditions, the cellular redox-status is disturbed, as reflected in the high oxidative-stress index of hyperthyroid rats.

In brief, thyroid calorigenesis resulting from acceleration of energy metabolism and secondary electron-transfer processes lead to a higher generation of ROS in the target tissue. This prooxidant condition enhances the oxidative-stress status of the organs when the decrease in the antioxidant potential is not adequately compensated for, leading to

a) substantial oxidative deterioration of biomolecules, with loss of their functions that may compromise cell viability, b) activities of GPx, GR, GST, catalase, and superoxide dismutase are considerably impaired, c) total GSH equivalents and GSH and GSSG pools were increasingly depleted, d) a higher susceptibility of the liver to toxic stimuli that exacerbate liver injury, e) upregulation of gene expression, f) apoptosis, g) shorter lifespan, and h) myelin deficit.

3.2 Hypothyrodism and the ROS-steady state

Hypothyroidism has been related to some diseases because it causes a hypometabolic state. This condition can be beneficial. Why can we make this assertion? There are many findings to support this suggestion. It is well-known that a deficiency of the thyroid hormones results in decreased metabolism and lowering of the basal metabolic rate (BMR). There is evidence that supports the lower cell stress in the hypothyroidism condition. Tenorio-Velázquez et al. have demonstrated that hypothyroidism attenuates oxidative stress and renal injury caused by ischemia-reperfusion, produced by an increase in the ROS and reactive nitrogen species (Tenorio-Velásquez et al., 2005). Most research has been done in the kidney and liver models of ischemia (Swaroop & Ramasarma, 1985; Paller, 1986). The postulated mechanism in such organs has been either a decrease in the general metabolic rate or a reduced free radical scavenging response after ischemia. The lipid peroxidation in hypothyroid animals with renal ischemia was decreased (Paller, 1986). The content of malondialdehyde, which is an indirect measure of the generation of oxygen free radicals, was decreased and the cortical content of glutathione, a free radical scavenger, was increased in the hypothyroid, ischemic animals. Similarly, in the liver model of hypothyroid-ischemic injury, lipid peroxidation and free-radical generation were decreased in the hypothyroid animals (Swaroop & Ramasarma, 1985). These investigators have shown a significant decrease in hydrogen peroxide, a measure of the oxygen free-radical status, in the liver mitochondrion in the hypothyroid animals. Hypothyroidism attenuates not only renal but also cardiac damage caused by ischemia and reperfusion. Bobadilla et al. have shown that hypothyroidism conferred protection against reperfusion arrhythmias and the cardiac release of creatine kinase and aspartate amino transferase and preserved the normal structure of the myocardial tissue (Bobadilla et al., 2002). It has been proposed that hypothyroidism protects against pore opening and heart reperfusion (Chávez et al., 1998). This may be relevant to the protective effect of hypothyroidism in ischemia and reperfusion because it has been recognized that the mitochondria play a key role in cell-death pathways by activating the mitochondrial-permeability transition pore and causing the release of cytochrome C, proapoptotic factors, and the Ca^{2+} overload that causes a nonselective permeability of the inner membrane. The prolonged opening of the membrane-permeability transition pore during the first few minutes of reperfusion is a critical determinant of cell death, and pharmacological inhibition of the pore at the time of reperfusion protects the cell (Halestrap et al., 2004). It has been found that there is a decreased glutamate release during hypothyroidism and this is correlated to a protection in cerebral ischemia (Shuaib et al., 1994). The reason why hypothyroidism results in a decreased release of glutamate is as yet unknown. It is possible that the hypothyroidism affects the release mechanisms in the presynaptic receptors. It is also possible that the hypothyroid state results in an increase in the reuptake mechanism for glutamate.

We have noted the protector effect of hypothyroidism, but many investigators use methimazole to cause it. There are some indications that antithyroid-caused hypothyroidism can produce cellular damage. Although, some results indicate that this drug causes cellular protection because of its chemical structure (Bruck et al., 2007; Tutuncu et al., 2007). In addition, there is evidence of extrathyroidal effects of antithyroid drugs, such as thionamides, in humans and animals (Bandyopadhyay et al., 2002). One of the effects of thionamides is the contribution to oxidative stress and cellular damage. These effects can produce an increase of oxidant species that causes lipid peroxidation, nitration, carbonylation, or glutathionylation of proteins, and fragmentation of DNA (Halliwell & Gutteridge, 2007; Valko et al., 2007). Because of this, we determined if methimazole or hypothyroidism causes cellular damage in several organs. After producing a hypothyroid animal caused by thyroidectomy or methimazole administration, the spleen, heart, liver, lung, and kidney were obtained. A portion of these tissues was processed for histological study and another portion was used for the biochemical assay for determining oxidative stress. Histologically, we demonstrated that only methimazole-caused hypothyroidism causes cellular damage in the kidney, lung, liver, heart, and spleen. Animals with methimazole and with T_4 supplementation showed cellular damage in the lung, spleen, and renal medulla with lesser damage in the liver, renal cortex, and heart. Hypothyroidism did not produce cellular damage in any organs except the lung. The thyroidectomy group showed no other tissue alterations (Cano-Europa et al., 2011). These results are in accordance with what others have observed in animals and humans. Five percent of patients with hyperthyroidism treated with antithyroid drugs, including methimazole, are reported to have liver (Casallo Blanco et al., 2007; Woeber, 2002), lung (Tsai et al., 2001) and kidney damage (Calañas-Continente et al., 2005). The methimazole-caused hypothyroidism in animals has tumorigenic effects (Jemec, 1977) and modifies the pulmonary function (Liu & Ng, 1991). No tissue damage was seen in a model of hypothyroidism caused by a thyroidectomy (Tenorio-Velásquez et al., 2005). We also compared, over a time-course, markers of oxidative stress, the REDOX environment, and the antioxidant enzymatic system in the liver and the spleen of rats with methimazole- or thyroidectomy-caused hypothyroidism. We found that the cell damage was related with an increase of oxidative stress markers (ROS and lipid peroxidation) that were not compensated for by the antioxidant system. The catalase activity is reduced in hepatic tissue and this allows H_2O_2-caused hepatic damage (Cano-Europa et al., 2010). The increase of the glutathione-cycle enzymes was insufficient to prevent oxidative-stress markers (Ortiz-Butron et al., 2011). All these findings together pointed out that methimazole and not the hypothyroidism is responsible for the cell damage. The tissues evaluated, especially the kidney and liver, have a high metabolic activity that generates ROS. Under physiological conditions the presence of antioxidant enzymes, in particular peroxidases and dismutases, prevent oxidative stress and tissue damage (Halliwell & Gutteridge, 2007; Angermuller et al., 2009). Some drugs, such as methimazole, disturb the physiological steady state. Methimazole alters the intracellular REDOX environment and causes cellular damage because of oxidant generation and ROS, and consequently the lipid peroxidation is not completely neutralized by the antioxidant system. We suggest that the central mechanism of the methimazole-caused cell damage is based on the reduction of catalase activity caused by a methimazole-inactivated catalytic center (Bandyopadhyay et al., 1995; Bandyopadhyay et al., 2002).

Other investigators, like Bergman and Brittebo, have demonstrated this anthytiroid-caused damage in other models, i.e. an olfactory mucosa model. They found that this drug covalently binds to the tissue, and pretreatment with the cytochrome-P450 inhibitor metyrapone prevented both the covalent binding and the toxicity of methimazole in this tissue. They suggest a cytochrome P450-dependent metabolic activation of methimazole to a reactive and toxic intermediate at this site (Bergman & Brittebo, 1999). The pretreatment with thyroxin did not protect against the methimazole-caused necrosis, suggesting that this lesion is not related to a transient decrease in thyroid hormone levels. The covalent binding shown by methimazole in this tissue has been found in other tissues, such as the bronchial epithelium and the centrilobular parts of the liver. It is possible that methimazole suffers activation at these sites. Further, this drug is metabolized stepwise to the corresponding sulfenic and sulfinic acids with a concurrent formation of reactive intermediates (Poulsen et al., 1974). It is known that methimazole produces a decrease of P450 at the hepatic level (Decker & Doerge, 1992). In rodents given the methimazole analogs 1-methy-imidazole, 4-methylimidazol, or methyl pyrrole, which are devoid of a thiol group, no morphological changes were observed in the olfactory mucosa (Brittebo, 1995). The thiol group in methimazole seems to be important for the methimazole-caused toxicity, suggesting that enzyme-catalyzed changes of the thiol group will give rise to an intermediate toxin in the tissue.

Other methimazole-caused damage mechanisms are associated with its chemical structure and its biotransformation. Some investigators suggest that this drug binds covalently to the hepatocytes, mainly those next to the hepatic triad (Decker & Doerge, 1992; Lee & Neal, 1978). For biotransformation, methimazole may be oxidized by the P450 enzymes to form the 4,5-epoxide. The enzymatic or nonenzymatic hydrolysis of the epoxide formed would produce an unstable hemiketal-like intermediate, which it is expected to undergo spontaneous ring cleavage to form glyoxal and N-methylthiourea. The metabolism of N-methylthiourea is complex, but it is believed that sulfur oxidation, mediated mainly by flavin-monooxigenase (FMO, EC.EC 1.14.13.8), proceeds primarly to the sulfenic acids and then possibly to the sulfinic acids. It is known that this step is necessary in the bioactivation of thioureas resulting in protein binding, enzyme inactivation, and organ toxicity (Mizutani et al., 1994; Neal & Halpert, 1982).

The thyroidectomy group examinee showed no other tissue alterations, except for the lung. There is some evidence that demonstrates molecular mechanisms by which hypothyroidism itself may produce a protected state of the tissues, such as reducing the enzyme activity associated with the mitochondrial-respiratory chain (Paradies et al., 1994), the decrease in adenine nucleotide translocase (Schonfeld et al., 1997), reduced activity of cytochrome-C oxidase (Paradies et al., 1997), and the resistance to forming the permeability transition-pore formation of the inner mitochondrial membrane (Chávez et al., 1998).

With all this evidence it is important to develop other therapies or antithyroid drugs with fewer side effects. We suggest that hypothyroidism is a protective state against toxic agents and it is related to an increase of reduced glutathione or γ–L-glutamyl- cysteinyl-glycine (GSH) synthesis and a mild immunosuppression.

3.3 Enhanced GSH synthesis in the hypothyroid state, a mechanism of cell protection

Before we show evidence of the relationship between hypothyroidism and high γ –L-glutamyl- cysteinyl-glycine (GSH) concentration, we need to know more about GSH. The synthesis of reduced glutathione or GSH involves two ATP-dependent enzymatic steps made in the cell cytoplasm. Figure 6 shows the cycle of GSH.

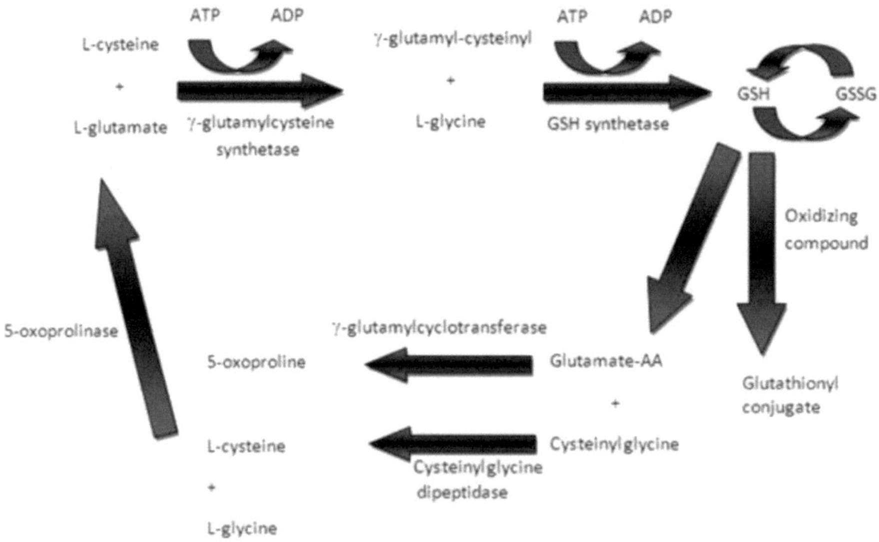

Fig. 6. GSH cycle. GR is glutathione reductase; GST glutathione S-transferase, and GSSG oxidized glutathione.

The synthesis of GSH starts with the entry into the cells of its amino acid precursors: glutamate, cysteine, and glycine. Glutamate and glycine can enter the cell by secondary active transport. Some of the glutamate cotransport carriers transfer cysteine. For the cysteine, entry into the cell may also be caused by the transporters of the neutral amino acid system. It is believed that cysteine is the limiting amino acid for the synthesis of GSH because it occurs in lower concentrations in plasma and has a lower Km (Aoyama et al., 2008). Once the amino acids have entered the cell, the g-glutamylcysteine synthetase (γ-GCS, EC 6.3.2.2) forms the g-glutamylcysteine. The formation of the product involves two steps. The first is the interaction between glutamate and ATP in the presence of Mg^{+2} to form g - glutamylphosphate and the second involves the interaction of this intermediate with the cysteine and with ADP release (Griffith & Mulcahy, 1999; Griffith, 1999). This first step is the most important in the formation of GSH because γ-GCS is the limiting enzyme in the synthesis of GSH. The γ-GCS is an heterodimeric enzyme composed of a catalytic subunit known as the heavy subunit (γ-GCS_H Mr, ≈ 73 kDa) and a regulatory or light subunit (γ-GCS_L Mr, ≈ 31 kDa). The γ-GCS activity depends primarily on the substrates and is inhibited by GSH. The γ-GCS_L activity is under the control of kinases such as protein kinase A (PKA) and PKC (Griffith, 1999)

Two processes can occur thermodynamically once γ-glutamyl-cysteinyl is formed. The compound may be used by the GSH synthetase (GS, EC 6.3.2.3) to form GSH when conjugated with glycine or it may interact with g -glutamyl cyclotransferase to form 5-oxo-L-proline and L-cysteine. The pathway that prevails depends of the Km of each enzyme. Under physiological conditions the Km of GS is 12 times greater than the γ-glutamyl cyclotransferase so it favors the formation of GSH in more than 95% (Weber, 1999). Once GSH has been synthesized there are different processes in which it participates;

1. In the hydrolysis of plasma GSH to synthesize GSH de novo for another cell. For example, if a hepatocyte secretes GSH, another cell can hydrolyze such a compound into its precursors (cysteinylglycine and glutamate) by the g-glutamyl transpeptidase (γ-GT, EC 2.3.2.2) expressed on the outside of the plasmatic membrane. The cysteinylglycine compounds or their S-conjugates can be hydrolyzed by dipeptidases to yield free amino acids that can be introduced into the cell and start the formation of GSH (Weber, 1999).
2. In the detoxification of electrophiles by conjugating these with a-carbonyls and by b-unsaturation by glutathion-S transferase (GST, EC. 2.5.1.18). This reaction results in the elimination of the electrophile by the consequent metabolism of the glutathione S-conjugate by the γ-GT enzymes and the cysteinylglycine dypeptidase. This process is not always in the favor for the cell, because it can sometimes create more toxic species (Weber, 1999).
3. In the detoxification of hydrogen peroxide by the action of the glutathione peroxidase enzymes (GPX, EC 1.11.1.19) (Beckett & Arthur, 2005).
4. In maintaining ascorbic acid and vitamin E (Van Acker et al., 1993).
5. In intracellular communication processes as a modulator of diverse signaling pathways (Cruz et al., 2003).
6. In the modulation of membrane receptors as for NMDA receptors in the central nervous system (Oja et al., 2000).
7. In the transport of metals such as Cu^{+2}, Hg^{+2}, Pb^{+2}, and Zn^{+2} (Filomeni et al., 2002).

The mitochondrial concentration of GSH is approximately 11-15 mM. The entry of GSH into the mitochondria depends on the electroneutral transporters, such as the tricarboxylic or dicarboxylic acids (Lash, 2006). In general, the ratio GSH/GSSG is greater than 10 for the cells and organelles, such as mitochondria and nucleus, whereas the endoplasmic reticulum has the lowest GSH/GSSG ratio of 1 to 3. The best indicator of the REDOX environment is the $GSH^2/GSSG$ ratio because the REDOX environment involves the transfer of electrons, for which the theoretical model of Schafer and Buettner uses the Nernst equation (Schafer & Buettner, 2001). These authors proposed that other REDOX couples can participate in the REDOX environment maintaining the ratios of $NADPH/NADP^+$, reduced thioredoxin/oxidized thioredoxin ($TrxSH_2/TrxSS$), and $GSH^2/GSSG$. These REDOX couples could participate in the maintaining of the REDOX environment because their pKas are above the physiological pH and the ratio of the reduced pair to its oxidized counterpart is 1:100, 1:1000, or greater. The $GSH^2/GSSG$ ratio is the most important couple in the REDOX environment because their chemical structures are not susceptible to any peptidase and their use is in the cell, particularly for cell antioxidant protection, and not in essential biosynthetic pathways. Also, the $GSH^2/GSSG$ ratio has the highest concentration of the three REDOX ratios mentioned, and this one best buffers the REDOX potential changes between -300 and -100 mV, despite varying the concentration of the GSH. The change in the half-cell reduction potential of this REDOX couple is related to the processes such as cell proliferation, differentiation, apoptosis, and necrosis in biological experiments (Cai & Jones, 1998; Cai et al., 2000; Hwang et al., 1992; Jones et al., 1995; Kirlin et al., 1999).

In our group we are studying the effect of the hypothyroid state and the GSH synthesis in various organs, with special interest in the liver and kidney. For that we used thyroidectomyzed rats with a parathyroid gland reimplant (only to affect thyroid hormone system). Two weeks postsurgery we determined the GSH content by a fluorometric method and the γ-GCS by a spectophotometric method as described (Cano-Europa et al., 2010; Ortiz-Butron et al., 2011). Figure 7 shows that hypothyroid animals have a higher GSH content than euthyroid animals because they have an enhanced γ -GCS activity.

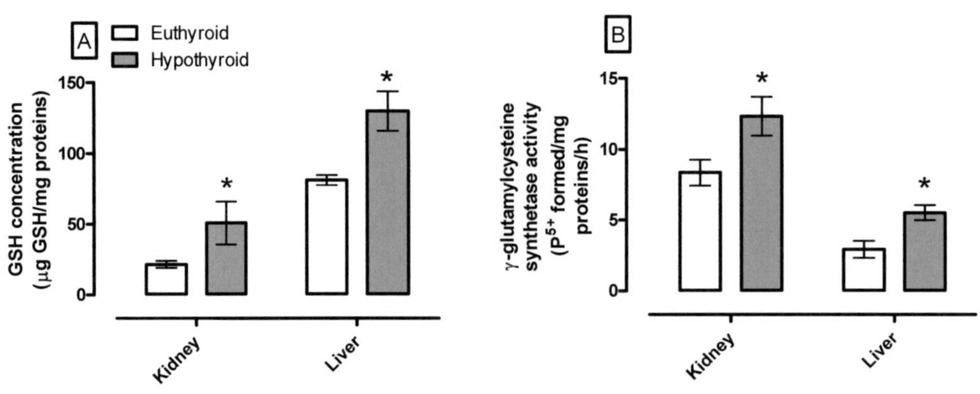

Fig. 7. Effect of hypothyroidism on GSH content (A) and γ-GCS activity in liver and kidney. Values are the mean ± SE. (*) $P < 0.05$ vs. euthyroid ($n = 5$ for each group).

It is possible that some intracellular signals modify the γ-GCS activity. It is also probable that the thyroid hormone-receptor complex acts as a negative regulator for γ-GCS because the putative thyroid-hormone response-element sequences in the promoter regions of both the catalytic and modulator subunit of γ-GCS genes have been seen. However, we need to do further experiments to demonstrate this. If this does occur then hypothyroidism could be a protective state against chemical- or physical-caused oxidative stress and cell damage. At present, we are evaluated if the hypothyroid state protects against ethylene glycol-caused oxidative stress and renal damage. At this respect, the results are in accordance with the idea that the hypothyroidism-enhanced REDOX environment (unpublished data).

3.4 Thyroid hormone alteration levels and the immune response

There is evidence of the thyroid hormones and immune systems and their development and function from amphibious animals to mammals (Rollins-Smith & Blair, 1990; Lam et al., 2005; Watanabe et al., 1995; Nakamura et al., 2007).

In zebra fish the thyroid state participates in thymus development and lymphopoiesis (Lam et al., 2005). In humans and other mammals, clinical hyperthyroidism increased the size and cellularity of the thymus, particularly a larger number of thymus nurse cells, $Thy1^+$ thymocytes, and the CD4-CD8- and CD44-positive cells (Villa-Verde et al., 1993; Scheiff et al., 1977). Hyperthyroidism increases T cells in the spleen and thymus with high levels of NK cells only in the spleen (Watanabe et al., 1995). Hypothyroidism reduces the cellularity in the spleen and thymus (Bendyug et al., 2003). In neonatal hypothyroidism, it has been observed that the NK cells and regulatory T cells ($CD4^+CD25^+$) are enhanced in thymus, spleen, and peripheral blood. The dendritic cells integrate signals from several pathways and receptors, including those arising from engagement of uptake and pattern recognition receptors, proinflammatory and antiinflammatory cytokines, chemokines, and hormones like THs. The T_3 promotes the dendritic-cell maturation and Th1-type cytokine secretion (Mascanfroni et al., 2008). The dendritic cells are modulated by the THs because theT_3-TRβ1 causes Akt signaling-pathway activation and NFκB-dependence, but a PI3K-independent pathway (Mascanfroni et al., 2010).

There are reports that hypothyroidism decreases immune system activity and increases infection in humans (Schoenfeld et al., 1995; Amadi et al., 2008).

All this evidence suggests the proposal that the hypothyroid condition decreases the immune response. This could be protective in the case of toxicant-caused oxidative stress and cell damage caused by the immune system activation by a substance like aniline. Aniline is a toxic, aromatic amine and it is an extensively used industrial chemical. Exposure to aniline is known to cause toxicity to the hematopoietic system. Aniline toxicity is generally characterized by methemoglobinemia, hemolysis, and hemolytic anemia and by the development of splenic hyperplasia, fibrosis, and a variety of primary sarcomas after chronic exposure in rats. The immunological system participates actively in aniline-caused oxidative stress and spleen damage (Wang et al., 2011; Wang et al., 2010; Wang et al., 2008).

In our laboratory, we evaluated the participation of hypothyroidism and aniline-caused oxidative stress and spleen damage. We used male Wistar rats weighing 240 to 260 g divided into four groups; 1) euthyroid, 2) euthyroid + aniline, 3) hypothyroid, and 4) hypothyroid + aniline. The hypothyroidism was produced by thyroidectomy with implantation of the parathyroid gland. Two weeks after surgery, the animals were treated with 1 mmol/kg/d ig aniline for five days. On the fifth day, the animals were killed, the blood obtained to determine the lymphocyte count and the spleen was dissected to assess lipid peroxidation and the quantification of reactive oxygen species as preliminary results. In figure 8 are the results. It was shown that hypothyroid rats had decreased ROS concentration, lipid peroxidation, and the lymphocyte counts in aniline-treated rats compared with euthyroid rats.

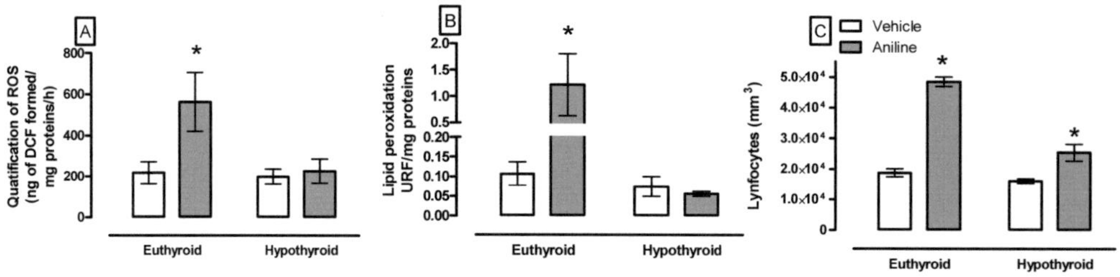

Fig. 8. Effect of hypothyroidism on ROS concentration (A), lipid peroxidation (B), and lymphocyte count (C) in the spleen of rats treated with aniline. Values are the mean ± SE. (*) $P < 0.05$ vs. euthyroid ($n = 5$ for each group).

The hypothyroid state can be protective in this situation because it decreased the ROS production, increased the GSH, and decreased the lymphocyte count. Although we need to do more experiments to demonstrate the idea of a mild immunosuppression participating in cell protection, these preliminary results suggest it.

4. Final remarks

In earlier years it was believed that the hypo- and hyperthyroid conditions modifying the ROS steady state caused cell damage. Presently, there is much evidence that only hyperthyroidism does this. Hypothyroidism is believed to be a protective state because scientists did not believe the drug-caused hypothyroidism modified the ROS steady state. On this point, by studying hypothyroidism in animal models that modify only TH concentrations, such as thyroidectomy, we can observe cell protection against chemical- and physical-caused oxidative stress. Right now, we can describe two different pathways by which the hypothyroid state can protect: GSH synthesis and mild immunosuppression. This is now an open field in which to study these possibilities.

5. Acknowledgement

This study was partially supported by SIP-IPN 20110283 y 20110336. Thanks to Dr. Ellis Glazier for editing this English-language text.

6. References

Alvarez,B. & Radi,R. (2001). Peroxynitrite decay in the presence of hydrogen peroxide, mannitol and ethanol: a reappraisal. *Free Radical Research* Vol. 34, No. 5, pp. 467-475 (2001) ISSN 1071-5762

Amadi,K., Sabo,A.M., Ogunkeye,O.O. & Oluwole,F.S. (2008). Thyroid hormone: a "prime suspect" in human immunodeficiency virus (HIV/AIDS) patients? *Physiological Society of Nigeria* Vol. 23, No. 1-2, pp 61-66 (Jun-Dec, 2008) ISSN 0794-859X

Angermuller,S., Islinger,M. & Volkl,A. (2009). Peroxisomes and reactive oxygen species, a lasting challenge. *Histochemistry and Cell Biology* Vol. 131, No. 4, pp 459-463 (April, 2009) ISSN

Aoyama,K., Watabe,M. & Nakaki,T. (2008). Regulation of neuronal glutathione synthesis. *Journal of Pharmacology Sciences* Vol. 108, No. 3, pp 227-238 (November, 2008) ISSN 1347-8648

Bandyopadhyay,U., Bhattacharyya,D.K., Chatterjee,R. & Banerjee,R.K. (1995). Irreversible inactivation of lactoperoxidase by mercaptomethylimidazole through generation of a thiyl radical: its use as a probe to study the active site. *Biochemical Journal* Vol. 306 (Pt 3), pp 751-757 (March, 2005) ISSN 0264-6021

Bandyopadhyay,U., Biswas,K. & Banerjee,R.K. (2002). Extrathyroidal actions of antithyroid thionamides. *Toxicology Letters* Vol. 128, No. 1-3, pp 117-127 (March, 2008) ISSN 0378-4274

Beckett,G.J. & Arthur,J.R. (2005). Selenium and endocrine systems. *Journal of Endocrinology* Vol. 184, No. 3, pp 455-465 (March, 2005) ISSN 0022-0795

Bendyug,G.D., Grinevich,Y.A., Khranovskaya,N.N., Fil'chakov,F.V., Yugrinova,L.G. & Kad'kalenko,A.G. (2003). The state of the immune system in thyroidectomized rats. *Bulletin of Experimental Biology and* Medicine Vol. 135, No. 2, pp 154-157 (February, 2003) ISSN 0007-4888

Bergman,U. & Brittebo,E.B. (1999). Methimazole toxicity in rodents: covalent binding in the olfactory mucosa and detection of glial fibrillary acidic protein in the olfactory bulb. *Toxicology and Applied Pharmacology* Vol. 155, No. 2, pp 190-200 (March, 1999) ISSN 0041-008X

Bianco,A.C., Salvatore,D., Gereben,B., Berry,M.J. & Larsen,P.R. (2002). Biochemistry, cellular and molecular biology, and physiological roles of the iodothyronine selenodeiodinases. *Endocrine Reviews* Vol. 23, No. 1, *pp* 38-89 (February, 2002) ISSN 0163-769X

Bobadilla,I., Franco,M., Cruz,D., Zamora,J., Robles,S.G. & Chavez,E. (2002). Hypothyroidism protects the myocardium against ischemia-reperfusion injury. Archivos de cardiología de México Vol. 72 Suppl 1, pp S27-S30 (January, 2002) ISSN 1405-9940

Bray,R.C., Cockle,S.A., Fielden,E.M., Roberts,P.B., Rotilio,G. & Calabrese,L. (1974). Reduction and inactivation of superoxide dismutase by hydrogen peroxide. *Biochemical Journal* Vol. 139, No.1, pp 43-48 (April, 1974) ISSN 0264-6021

Brittebo,E.B. (1995). Metabolism-dependent toxicity of methimazole in the olfactory nasal mucosa. *Pharmacology & Toxicology* Vol. 76, No. 1, pp 76-79 (January, 1995) ISSN 0901-9928

Bruck,R., Weiss,S., Traister,A., Zvibel,I., Aeed,H., Halpern,Z. & Oren,R. (2007). Induced hypothyroidism accelerates the regression of liver fibrosis in rats. *Journal of Gastroenterology and Hepatology* Vol. 22, No. 12, pp 2189-2194 (December, 2007) ISSN 1440-1746

Cai,J. & Jones,D.P. (1998). Superoxide in Apoptosis. Mitocondrial generation triggered by cytocrome c loss. *Journal of* Biological *Chemistry* Vol. 273, No. 19, pp 11401-11404 (May, 1998) ISSN 1083-351X

Cai,J., Wallace,D.C., Zhivotovsky,B. & Jones,D.P. (2000). Separation of cytochrome c-dependent caspase activation from thiol-disulfide redox change in cells lacking mitochondrial DNA. *Free Radical Biology & Medicine* Vol. 29, No. (3-4), pp 334-342 (Ausgut, 2000) ISSN 0891-5849

Calañas-Continente,A., Espinosa,M., Manzano-García,G., Santamaría,R., López-Rubio,F. & Aljama,P. (2005). Necrotizing glomerulonephritis and pulmunary hemorrhage associated with carbimazole therapy. *Thyroid* Vol. 15, No. 3, pp 285-288 (March, 2005) ISSN 1050-7256

Cano-Europa,E., Blas-Valdivia,V., Franco-Colin,M., Gallardo-Casas,C.A. & Ortiz-Butron,R. (2011). Methimazole-induced hypothyroidism causes cellular damage in the spleen, heart, liver, lung and kidney. *Acta Histochemica* Vol. 113, No. 1, pp 1-5 (January, 2011) ISSN 0044-5991

Cano-Europa,E., Blas-Valdivia,V., Lopez-Galindo,G.E., Franco-Colin,M., Pineda-Reynoso,M., Hernandez-Garcia,A. & Ortiz-Butron,R. (2010). Methimazole-induced hypothyroidism causes alteration of the REDOX environment, oxidative stress, and hepatic damage; events not caused by hypothyroidism itself. *Annals of hepatology* Vol. 9, No.1, pp 80-88 (January, 2010) ISSN 1665-2681

Carageorgiou,H., Pantos,C., Zarros,A., Mourouzis,I., Varonos,D., Cokkinos,D. & Tsakiris,S. (2005). Changes in antioxidant status, protein concentration, acetylcholinesterase, (Na^+,K^+)-, and Mg^{2+}-ATPase activities in the brain of hyper- and hypothyroid adult rats. *Metabolic Brain Disease* Vol. 20, No. 2, pp 129-139 (June, 2005) ISSN 0885-7490

Casallo Blanco,S., Valero,M.A., Marcos Sanchez,F., de Matias Salces,L., Blanco Gonzalez,J.J. & Martin Barranco,M.J. (2007). [Methimazole and propylthiouracil induced acute toxic hepatitis]. *Journal of Gastroenterology and Hepatology* Vol. 30,No. 5, pp 268-270 (May, 2007) ISSN 1440-1746

Chattopadhyay,S., Sahoo,D.K., Subudhi,U. & Chainy,G.B. (2007). Differential expression profiles of antioxidant enzymes and glutathione redox status in hyperthyroid rats: a temporal analysis. *Comparative Biochemistry and Physiology - Part C: Toxicology & Pharmacology* Vol. 146, No. 3,pp 383-391 (September, 2007) ISSN 0742-8413

Chávez,E., Franco,M., Reyes-Vivas,H., Zazueta,C., Ramirez,J. & Carrillo,R. (1998). Hypothyroidism renders liver mitochondria resistant to the opening of membrane permeability transition pore. *Biochimica et biophysica acta* Vol. 1407, No. 3, pp 243-248 (September, 1998) ISSN 0006-3002

Cheng,J.Z., Singhal,S.S., Sharma,A., Saini,M., Yang,Y., Awasthi,S., Zimniak,P. & Awasthi,Y.C. (2001). Transfection of mGSTA4 in HL-60 cells protects against 4-hydroxynonenal-induced apoptosis by inhibiting JNK-mediated signaling. *Archives of Biochemistry and Biophysics* Vol. 392, No. 2, pp 197-207 (August, 2001) ISSN 0003-9861

Cheng,S.Y., Leonard,J.L. & Davis,P.J. (2010). Molecular aspects of thyroid hormone actions. *Endocrine Reviews* Vol. 31, No.2, pp 139-170 (April, 2010) ISSN 0163-769X

Christoffolete,M.A., Ribeiro,R., Singru,P., Fekete,C., da Silva,W.S., Gordon,D.F., Huang,S.A., Crescenzi,A., Harney,J.W., Ridgway,E.C., Larsen,P.R., Lechan,R.M. & Bianco,A.C. (2006). Atypical expression of type 2 iodothyronine deiodinase in thyrotrophs explains the thyroxine-mediated pituitary thyrotropin feedback mechanism. *Endocrinology* Vol. 147, No. 4, pp 1735-1743 (April, 2006) ISSN 0013-7227

Cruz,R., Almaguer-Melian,J.A. & Bergado-Rosado,J.A. (2003). El glutatión en la función cognitiva y la neurodegeneración. Revista *de Neurología* Vol. 36, No. 9, pp 877-886 (May, 2003) ISSN 0210-0010

Davis,F.B., Davis,P.J. & Blas,S.D. (1983). Role of calmodulin in thyroid hormone stimulation in vitro of human erythrocyte Ca^{2+}-ATPase activity. *The Journal of Clinical Investigation* Vol. 71, No. 3, pp 579-586 (March, 1983) ISSN 0021-9738

Davis,P.J., Davis,F.B. & Cody,V. (2005). Membrane receptors mediating thyroid hormone action. *Trends in* Endocrinology *and Metabolism* Vol. 16, No. 9, pp 429-435 (November, 2005) ISSN 1043-2760

Decker,C.J. & Doerge,D.R. (1992). Covalent binding of 14C- and 35S-labeled thiocarbamides in rat hepatic microsomes. *Biochemical pharmacology* Vol. 43, No. 4, pp 881-888 (February, 1992) ISSN 0006-2952

Di Cosmo,C., Liao,X.H., Dumitrescu,A.M., Philp,N.J., Weiss,R.E. & Refetoff,S. (2010). Mice deficient in MCT8 reveal a mechanism regulating thyroid hormone secretion. *The Journal of Clinical Investigation* Vol. 120, No. 9, pp 3377-3388 (September, 2010) ISSN 0021-9738

Fernandez,V., Cornejo,P., Tapia,G. & Videla,L.A. (1997). Influence of hyperthyroidism on the activity of liver nitric oxide synthase in the rat. *Nitric Oxide* Vol. 1, No. 6, pp 463-468 (1997) ISSN 1089-8603

Fernandez,V., Llesuy,S., Solari,L., Kipreos,K., Videla,L.A. & Boveris,A. (1988). Chemiluminescent and respiratory responses related to thyroid hormone-induced liver oxidative stress. *Free Radical Research Communications* Vol. 5, No.2, pp 77-84 (1988) ISSN 8755-0199

Fernandez,V., Tapia,G., Varela,P., Romanque,P., Cartier-Ugarte,D. & Videla,L.A. (2006). Thyroid hormone-induced oxidative stress in rodents and humans: a comparative view and relation to redox regulation of gene expression. *Comparative Biochemistry and Physiology. Toxicology & Pharmacology* Vol. 142, No. 4-3, pp 231-239 (March-April, 2006) ISSN 1532-0456

Fernandez,V. & Videla,L.A. (1993). Influence of hyperthyroidism on superoxide radical and hydrogen peroxide production by rat liver submitochondrial particles. *Free Radical Research Communications* Vol. 18, No. 6, pp 329-335 (1993) ISSN 8755-0199

Fernández,V.I.R.G., BARRIENTOS,X.I.M.E., KIPREOS,K.A.T.I., VALENZUELA,A.L.F.O. & Videla,L.A. (1985). Superoxide Radical Generation, NADPH Oxidase Activity, and Cytochrome P-450 Content of Rat Liver Microsomal Fractions in an Experimental Hyperthyroid State: Relation to Lipid Peroxidation. *Endocrinology* Vol. 117, No. 2, pp 496-501 (August, 1985) ISSN 0013-7227

Filomeni,G., Rotilio,G. & Ciriolo,M.R. (2002). Cell signalling and the glutathione redox system. *Biochemical Pharmacology* Vol. 64, No. 5-6, pp 1057-1064 (September, 2002) ISSN 0006-2952

Giguere,A., Fortier,S., Beaudry,C., Gallo-Payet,N. & Bellabarba,D. (1996). Effect of thyroid hormones on G proteins in synaptosomes of chick embryo. *Endocrinology* Vol. 137, No. 6, pp 2558-2564 (June, 1996) ISSN 0013-7227

Giguere,A., Lehoux,J.G., Gallo-Payet,N. & Bellabarba,D. (1992). 3,5,3'-Triiodothyronine binding sites in synaptosomes from brain of chick embryo. Properties and ontogeny. *Brain Research. Developmental Brain Research* Vol. 66, No. 2,pp 221-227 (April, 1992) ISSN 0165-3806

Griffith,O.W. (1999). Biologic and pharmacologic regulation of mammalian glutathione synthesis. *Free Radical Biology &* Medicine Vol. 27, No.9-10, pp 922-935 (November, 1999) ISSN 0891-5849

Griffith,O.W. & Mulcahy,R.T. (1999). The enzymes of glutathione synthesis: gamma-glutamylcysteine synthetase. Advances *in Enzymology and Related Areas of Molecular Biology* Vol. 73, pp 209-67, xii (1999) ISSN 0065-258X

Halestrap,A.P., Clarke,S.J. & Javadov,S.A. (2004). Mitochondrial permeability transition pore opening during myocardial reperfusionGÇöa target for cardioprotection. *Cardiovascular Research* Vol. 61, No.3, pp 372-385 (February, 2004) ISSN 0008-6363

Halliwell,B. & Gutteridge,J.M.C. (2007). Free radicals in biology and medicine. UK: Oxford University Press.

Ho,Y.S., Xiong,Y., Ma,W., Spector,A. & Ho,D.S. (2004). Mice Lacking Catalase Develop Normally but Show Differential Sensitivity to Oxidant Tissue Injury. *Journal of Biological Chemistry* Vol. 279, No. 31, pp 32804-32812 (Juliy, 2000) ISSN 0021-9258

Hulbert,A. (2000). Thyroid hormones and their effects: a new perspective. *Biological Reviews of the Cambridge Philosophical* Society Vol. 75, No. 4, pp 519-621 (November, 2000) ISSN 1464-7931

Hwang,C., Sinskey,A.J. & Lodish,H.F. (1992). Oxidized redox state of glutathione in the endoplasmic reticulum. *Science* Vol. 257, No. 5076, pp 1496-1502 (September, 1992) ISSN 0036-8075

Jaeschke,H., Gores,G.J., Cederbaum,A.I., Hinson,J.A., Pessayre,D. & Lemasters,J.J. (2002). Mechanisms of Hepatotoxicity. *Toxicological Sciences* Vol. 65, No. 2, pp 166-176 (February, 2002) ISSN 1096-6080

Jemec,B. (1977). Studies of the tumorigenic effect of two goitrogens. *Cancer* Vol. 40, No. 5, pp 2188-2202 (November, 1977) ISSN 0008-543X

Jones,D.P., Maellaro,E., Jiang,S., Slater,A.F. & Orrenius,S. (1995). Effects of N-acetyl-L-cysteine on T-cell apoptosis are not mediated by increased cellular glutathione. *Immunology Letters* Vol. 45, No. 3, pp 205-209 (March, 1995) ISSN 0165-2478

Kaul,N. & Forman,H.J. (1996). Activation of NF kappa B by the respiratory burst of macrophages. *Free Radical Biology & Medicine* Vol. 21, No. 3, pp 401-405 (1996) ISSN 0891-5849

Kirlin,W.G., Cai,J., Thompson,S.A., Diaz,D., Kavanagh,T.J. & Jones,D.P. (1999). Glutathione redox potential in response to differentiation and enzyme inducers. *Free Radical Biology & Medicine* Vol. 27, No. 11-12, pp 1208-1218 (December, 1999) ISSN 0891-5849

Kono,Y. & Fridovich,I. (1982). Superoxide radical inhibits catalase. *Journal of Biological Chemistry* Vol. 257, No. 10, pp 5751-5754 (May, 1982) ISSN 0021-9258

Kumar,A., Sinha,R.A., Tiwari,M., Singh,R., Koji,T., Manhas,N., Rastogi,L., Pal,L., Shrivastava,A., Sahu,R.P. & Godbole,M.M. (2007). Hyperthyroidism induces apoptosis in rat liver through activation of death receptor-mediated pathways. *Journal of Hepatology* Vol. 46, No. 5, pp 888-898 (May, 2007) ISSN 0168-8278

Lam,S.H., Sin,Y.M., Gong,Z. & Lam,T.J. (2005). Effects of thyroid hormone on the development of immune system in zebrafish. *General and Comparative Endocrinology* Vol. 142, No. 33, pp 325-335 (July, 1995) ISSN 0016-6480

Larsen,P.R. (1982). Thyroid-pituitary interaction: feedback regulation of thyrotropin secretion by thyroid hormones. *The New England Journal of Medicine* Vol. 306, No. 1, pp 23-32 (Janu, 1982) ISSN 0028-4793

Lazar,M.A. (1993). Thyroid hormone receptors: multiple forms, multiple possibilities. *Endocrine Reviews* Vol. 14, No. 2, pp 184-193 (April, 1993) ISSN 0163-769X

Lee,P.W. & Neal,R.A. (1978). Metabolism of methimazole by rat liver cytochrome P-450-containing monoxygenases. *Drug Metabolism and Disposition: the biological fate of chemicals* Vol. 6, No. 5, pp 591-600 (October, 1978) ISSN 0090-9556

Lissi,E.A., Salim-Hanna,M., Faure,M. & Videla,L.A. (1991). 2,2'-Azo-bis-amidinopropane as a radical source for lipid peroxidation and enzyme inactivation studies. *Xenobiotica* Vol. 21, No. 8, pp 995-1001 (August, 1991) ISSN 0049-8254

Liu,W.K. & Ng,T.B. (1991). Effect of methimazole-induced hypothyroidism on alveolar macrophages. *Virchows Archiv. B, Cell Pathology Including Molecular Pathology* Vol. 60, No. 1, pp 21-26 (1991) ISSN 0340-6075

Lushchak,V.I. (2011). Adaptive response to oxidative stress: Bacteria, fungi, plants and animals. *Comparative Biochemistry and Physiology. Toxicology & Pharmacology* Vol. 153, No. 2, pp 175-190 (March, 2011) ISSN 1532-0456

Mascanfroni,I.D., del Mar Montesinos,M., Alamino,V.A., Susperreguy,S., Nicola,J.P., Ilarregui,J.M., Masini-Repiso,A.M., Rabinovich,G.A. & Pellizas,C.G. (2010). Nuclear factor (NF)-kB-dependent thyroid hormone receptor b1 expression controls dendritic cell function via Akt signaling. *Journal of Biological Chemistry* Vol. 285, No.13, pp 9569-9582 (March, 2010) ISSN 0021-9258

Mascanfroni,I., Montesinos,M.d.M., Susperreguy,S., Cervi,L., Ilarregui,J.M., Ramseyer,V.D., Masini-Repiso,A.M., Targovnik,H.M., Rabinovich,G.A. & Pellizas,C.G. (2008). Control of dendritic cell maturation and function by triiodothyronine. *The FASEB journal : official publication of the Federation of American Societies for Experimental Biology* Vol. 22, No. 4, pp 1032-1042 (April, 2008) ISSN 0892-6638

Mizutani,T., Yoshida,K. & Kawazoe,S. (1994). Formation of toxic metabolites from thiabendazole and other thiazoles in mice. Identification of thioamides as ring cleavage products. *Drug Metabolism and Disposition: the biological fate of chemicals* Vol. 22, No. 5, pp 750-755 (September-October, 1994) ISSN 0090-9556

Nakamura,R., Teshima,R., Hachisuka,A., Sato,Y., Takagi,K., Nakamura,R., Woo,G.H., Shibutani,M. & Sawada,J. (2007). Effects of developmental hypothyroidism induced by maternal administration of methimazole or propylthiouracil on the immune system of rats. *International Immunopharmacology* Vol.7, No.13 (December 2007), pp.1630-1638, ISSN 1567-5769

Neal,R.A. & Halpert,J. (1982). Toxicology of thiono-sulfur compounds. *Annual Review of Pharmacology and Toxicology* Vol.22, pp.321-339, ISSN 0362-1642

Oja,S.S., Janaky,R., Varga,V. & Saransaari,P. (2000). Modulation of glutamate receptor functions by glutathione. *Neurochemestry International* Vol.37, No. 2-3 (August 2000) pp.299-306, ISSN 0197-0186

Oppenheimer,J.H., Schwartz,H.L. & Strait,K.A. (1994). Thyroid hormone action 1994: the plot thickens. *European Journal of Endocrinology* Vol.130, No.1 (January 1994) Pp.15-24, ISSN 0804-4643

Ortiz-Butron,R., Blas-Valdivia,V., Franco-Colin,M., Pineda-Reynoso,M. & Cano-Europa,E. (2011). An increase of oxidative stress markers and the alteration of the antioxidant enzymatic system are associated with spleen damage caused by methimazole-induced hypothyroidism. *Drug and Chemical Toxicology* Vol.34, No.2 (April 2011), pp.180-188, ISSN 0148-0545

Paller,M.S. (1986). Hypothyroidism protects against free radical damage in ischemic acute renal failure. *Kidney International* Vol.29, No.6 (June 1986), pp.1162-1166, ISSN 0085-2538

Paradies,G., Petrosillo,G. & Ruggiero,F.M. (1997). Cardiolipin-dependent decrease of cytochrome c oxidase activity in heart mitochondria from hypothyroid rats. *Biochimica et Biophysica Acta* Vol.1319, No.1 (March 1997), pp.5-8, ISSN 0006-3002

Paradies,G., Ruggiero,F.M., Petrosillo,G. & Quagliariello,E. (1994). Enhanced cytochrome oxidase activity and modification of lipids in heart mitochondria from hyperthyroid rats. *Biochimica et Biophysica Acta* Vol.1225, No. 2(January 1994), pp.165-170, ISSN 0006-3002

Poulsen,L.L., Hyslop,R.M. & Ziegler,D.M. (1974). S-oxidation of thioureylenes catalyzed by a microsomal flavoprotein mixed-function oxidase. *Biochemical Pharmacology* Vol.23, No. 24 (December 1974), pp.3431-3440, ISSN 006-2952

Reed,D.J. (1990). Glutathione: toxicological implications. *Annual Review Of Pharmacology and Toxicology* Vol.30, pp.603-631, ISSN 0362-1642

Reznick,A.Z. & Packer,L. (1994). Oxidative damage to proteins: spectrophotometric method for carbonyl assay. *Methods in Enzymology* Vol.233, No.233, pp.357-363, ISSN 0076-6879

Rollins-Smith,L.A. & Blair,P. (1990). Expression of class II major histocompatibility complex antigens on adult T cells in *Xenopus* is metamorphosis-dependent. *Developmental and comparative Immunology* Vol.1, No.2, pp.97-104, ISSN

Romanque,P., Tapia,G. & Videla,L.A. (2003). Kupffer cell stimulation in the isolated perfused rat liver triggers nuclear factor-kappaB DNA binding activity. *Redox Report* Vol.8, No.6 (December 2003) pp.341-346, ISSN 1351-0002

Sap,J., Munoz,A., Damm,K., Goldberg,Y., Ghysdael,J., Leutz,A., Beug,H. & Vennstrom,B. (1986). The c-erb-A protein is a high-affinity receptor for thyroid hormone. *Nature* Vol.324, No.6098 (December 1986), pp.635-640, ISSN 0028-0836

Schafer,F.Q. & Buettner,G.R. (2001). Redox environment of the cell as viewed through the redox state of the glutathione disulfide/glutathione couple. *Free Radical Biology and Medicine* Vol.30, No.11 (June 2001), pp.1191-1212, ISSN 0891-5849

Scheiff,J.M., Cordier,A.C. & Haumont,S. (1977). Epithelial cell proliferation in thymic hyperplasia induced by triiodothyronine. *Cliical and Experimental Immunology* Vol.27, No. 3 (March 1977), pp.516-521, ISSN 1365-2249

Schneider,M.J., Fiering,S.N., Thai,B., Wu,S.Y., St.Germain,E., Parlow,A.F., St.Germain,D.L. & Galton,V.A. (2006). Targeted disruption of the type 1 selenodeiodinase gene (Dio1) results in marked changes in thyroid hormone economy in mice. *Endocrinology* Vol.147, No.1 (January 2006), pp.580-589, ISSN 0013-7227

Schoenfeld,P.S., Myers,J.W., Myers,L. & LaRocque,J.C. (1995). Suppression of cell-mediated immunity in hypothyroidism. *Southern Medical Journal* Vol.88, No.3 (March 1995), pp.347-349, ISSN 0038-4348

Schonfeld,P., Wieckowski,M.R. & Wojtczak,L. (1997). Thyroid hormone-induced expression of the ADP/ATP carrier and its effect on fatty acid-induced uncoupling of oxidative phosphorylation. *FEBS Letters* Vol.416, No.1 (October 1997), pp.19-22, ISSN 0014-5793

Shuaib,A., Ijaz,S., Hemmings,S., Galazka,P., Ishaqzay,R., Liu,L., Ravindran,J. & Miyashita,H. (1994). Decreased glutamate release during hypothyroidism may contribute to protection in cerebral ischemia. *Experimental Neurology* Vol.128, No.2 (August 1994), pp.260-265, ISSN 0014-4886

Soboll,S. (1993). Thyroid hormone action on mitochondrial energy transfer. *Biochimica et Biophysica Acta* Vol.1144, No.1 (August 1993), pp.1-16, ISSN 0006-3002

St.Germain,D.L., Galton,V.A. & Hernandez,A. (2009). Defining the roles of the iodothyronine deiodinases: current concepts and challenges. *Endocrinology* Vol.150, No.3 (March 2009), pp.1097-1107, ISSN 0013-7227

Stadtman,E.R. (1990). Metal ion-catalyzed oxidation of proteins: biochemical mechanism and biological consequences. Free *Radical Biology and Medicine* Vol.9, No.4, pp.315-325, ISSN 0891-5849

Swaroop,A. & Ramasarma,T. (1985). Heat exposure and hypothyroid conditions decrease hydrogen peroxide generation in liver mitochondria. *Biochemical Journal* Vol.226, No.2 (March 1985), pp.403-408, ISSN 0264-6021

Tapia,G., Santibanez,C., Farias,J., Fuenzalida,G., Varela,P., Videla,L.A. & Fernandez,V. (2010). Kupffer-cell activity is essential for thyroid hormone rat liver preconditioning. *Mollecular and Cellular Endocrinology* Vol.323, No.2 (July 2010), pp.292-297, ISSN 0303-7207

Tenorio-Velásquez,V.M., Barrera,D., Franco,M., Tapia,E., Hernández-Pando,R., Medina-Campos,O.N. & Pedraza-Chaverri,J. (2005). Hypothyroidism attenuates protein tyrosine nitration, oxidative stress and renal damage induced by ischemia and reperfusion: effect unrelated to antioxidant enzymes activities. *BMC Nephrology* Vol.7, pp.6-12, ISSN 1471-2369

Tsai,M.H., Chang,Y.L., Wu,V.C., Chang,C.C. & Huang,T.S. (2001). Methimazole-induced pulmonary hemorrhage associated with antimyeloperoxidase-antineutrophil cytoplasmic antibody: a case report. *Journal of the Formosan Medical Association* Vol.100, No.11 (November 2001), pp.772-775, ISSN 0929-6646

Tutuncu,T., Demirci,C., Gozalan,U., Yuksek,Y.N., Bilgihan,A. & Kama,N.A. (2007). Methimazole protects lungs during hepatic ischemia-reperfusion injury in rats: an effect not induced by hypothyroidism. *Journal of Gastroenterology and Hepatology* Vol.22, No.5 (May 2007), pp.704-709, ISSN 1440-1746

Valko,M., Leibfritz,D., Moncol,J., Cronin,M.T., Mazur,M. & Telser,J. (2007). Free radicals and antioxidants in normal physiological functions and human disease. *International Journal of Biochemestry and Cell Biology* Vol.39, No.1 (January 2007), pp.44-84, ISSN 1357-2725

Van Acker,S.A.B.E., Koymans,L.M.C. & Bast,A. (1993). Molecular pharmacology of vitamin E: structural aspects of antioxidant activity. *Free Radical Biology and Medicine* Vol.15, No.3 (September 1993), pp.311-328, ISSN 0891-5849

Venditti,P. & Di Meo,S. (2006). Thyroid hormone-induced oxidative stress. *Cellular and Molecular Life Sciences* Vol.63, No.4 (February 2006), pp.414-434, ISSN1420-682X

Videla,L.A. (2000). Energy metabolism, thyroid calorigenesis, and oxidative stress: functional and cytotoxic consequences. *Redox Report* Vol.5, No.5 (October 2000), pp.65-275, ISSN 1351-0002

Villa-Verde,D.M., de Mello-Coelho,V., Farias-de-Oliveira,D.A., Dardenne,M. & Savino,W. (1993). Pleiotropic influence of triiodothyronine on thymus physiology. *Endocrinology* Vol.133, No.2 (August 1993) 867-875, ISSN 0013-7227

Wang,J., Ma,H., Boor,P.J., Ramanujam,V.M., Ansari,G.A. & Khan,M.F. (2010). Up-regulation of heme oxygenase-1 in rat spleen after aniline exposure. *Free Radical Biology and Medicine* Vol.48, No.4 (February 2010), pp.513-518, ISSN 0891-5849

Wang,J., Wang,G., Ansari,G.A. & Khan,M.F. (2008). Activation of oxidative stress-responsive signaling pathways in early splenotoxic response of aniline. *Toxicology and Applied Pharmacology* Vol.230, No.2 (July 2008), pp.227-234, ISSN 0041-008X

Wang,J., Wang,G., Ma,H. & Khan,M.F. (2011). Enhanced expression of cyclins and cyclin-dependent kinases in aniline-induced cell proliferation in rat spleen. *Toxicology and Applied Pharmacology* Vol.250, No.2 (January 2011), pp.213-220, ISSN 0041-008X

Watanabe,K., Iwatani,Y., Hidaka,Y., Watanabe,M. & Amino,N. (1995). Long-term effects of thyroid hormone on lymphocyte subsets in spleens and thymuses of mice. *Endocrine Journal* Vol.42, No.5 (October 1995), pp.661-668, ISSN 1348-4540

Weber,G.F. (1999). Final common pathways in neurodegenerative diseases: regulatory role of the glutathione cycle. *Neuroscience and Biobehavioral Rev*iews 23, No.8 (December 1999), pp.1079-1086, ISSN 0149-7634

Woeber,K.A. (2002). Methimazole-induced hepatotoxicity. *Endocrine Practice* Vol.8, No.3 (May 2002), pp.222-224, ISSN 1530-891X

Yen,P.M. (2001). Physiological and molecular basis of thyroid hormone action. *Physiological Reviews* Vol. 81, No.3 (July 2001) , pp.1097-1142, ISSN 0031-9333

Zhang,J. & Lazar,M.A. (2000). The mechanism of action of thyroid hormones. *Annual Revew of Physiology* Vol.62, No.62 (March 2000), pp.439-466, ISSN 0066-4278

19

Oxidative Stress in Human Autoimmune Joint Diseases

Martina Škurlová

Department of Normal, Pathological, and Clinical Physiology, Third Faculty of Medicine, Charles University in Prague, Czech Republic

1. Introduction

Living with oxygen is basically unsafe, but vital. During evolution, oxygen originally a waste product of the metabolism in primitive unicellular organisms became normal product of the metabolism in higher animal species involving humans. Even when oxidative reactions are toxic, and destructive, they are tolerated by all organisms to some extent. The fact has opened the discussion about efficiency of antioxidant mechanisms. The classical enzyme antioxidant defence alone does not explain high tolerance of the organism for oxygen. Moreover, enzyme antioxidant mechanisms are not hundred percent effective in preventing oxidation what allows oxidative damage to continue.

The pathogenesis of autoimmune joint inflammatory diseases is related to activation of native immune system. At site of inflammation, activated neutrophils and macrophages consume large amounts of oxygen, whose corollary is the increase of reactive oxygen species (ROS) production. There are several mechanisms how oxidative stress is involved into the pathogenesis of autoimmune joint inflammatory diseases. Excess production of ROS in the joint area encourages process of re-oxygenation, which then promotes joint inflammation. ROS further inhibit connective tissue cell proliferation, in some cases ROS have been shown to induce cell death to these cells inducing apoptosis.

2. Oxidative stress

2.1 Biology of oxidative stress

Cellular responses to oxidative stress depend on the cellular redox status. When the oxidants' level does not exceed the redox capacities in a cell, oxidants are beneficial to the cell controlling cellular functions such as signal transduction. In contrast, when the cellular antioxidant capacity is insufficient, the production of oxidants exceeds the capacity to neutralize them (Hitchon & El- Gabalawy, 2004). Insufficient oxidative defence mechanisms shift the balance between oxidants and antioxidants in the direction of oxidants leading to oxidative stress. Insufficient oxidative defence mechanisms result from depletion of enzymatic (e.g., superoxide dismuthase, catalase, glutathione peroxidase), and non-enzymatic (e.g., glutathione, vitamins A, C, and E, and selenium) antioxidants (Hovatta et al., 2010). The pro-oxidant conditions of the *´internal milieu´*, due to low redox status of the cell led to a new definition of oxidative stress. Oxidative stress is defined as " disruption between ROS production and elimination leading to their enhanced steady- state in the body " (Lushchak, 2011).

Reactive oxygen species destroy not only intracellular components, but also cell membranes, and extracellular components. ROS modify proteins by oxidation, nitrosylation, nitration or chlorination of specific amino acids, leading to their impaired biological activity, changes in protein structure and accumulation of damaged proteins in the tissue. During lipid peroxidation, which is a marker of oxidative stress, polyunsaturated fatty lipids are oxidized and produce lipid peroxyl radicals that in turn up-regulate oxidation, and cell membrane damage (Hitchon & El- Gabalawy, 2004). Genotoxic effects of oxidative stress involve direct breakage of DNA and DNA repair mechanisms. Oxidative stress may also cause cell death. Cellular content containing oxidized molecules when released into the extracellular environment may contribute to the exacerbation of synovial inflammation as newly formed ROS and degradation products form a vicious inflammatory circle (Henrontin et al., 2003).

3. Reactive oxidant species

Free radicals are very reactive chemical species that have unpaired valence shell electrons in their outer orbitals (Afonso et al., 2007). Highly reactive and partly reduced oxygen metabolites are a by-product of oxidative phosphorylation process, which takes part in mitochondria. These metabolites called ROS include oxygen radicals [superoxide ($O_2^{\bullet-}$), hydroxyl ($HO^{\bullet}$), peroxyl ($O_2R^{\bullet}$), and alkoxyl ($OR^{\bullet}$)] and certain non radicals that are either oxidizing agents or are easily converted into radicals, such as hypochlorous acid (HOCl), ozone (O_3), singlet oxygen ($^1O_2$), and hydrogen peroxide (H_2O_2). Other oxidants, generated by interactions with these molecules, include reactive nitrogen species (RNS), as an example nitric oxide (NO), peroxynitrite ($ONOO^-$).

3.1 Generation of reactive oxidant species

Generation of ROS is generally cascade of reactions that starts with the production of $O_2^{\bullet-}$. Superoxide rapidly dismutates to H_2O_2 either spontaneously, particularly at low pH, or catalyzed by superoxide dismutase (SOD) enzyme. Other steps in the cascade of ROS generation include the reaction of $O_2^{\bullet-}$ with $ON^{\bullet}$ to form $ONOO^-$, the peroxidase-catalyzed formation of HOCl from H_2O_2, and the iron-catalyzed Fenton reaction leading to the generation of $HO^{\bullet}$. Hydroxyl radical is one of the most reactive oxygen radicals. In biologic systems, the $HO^{\bullet}$ is formed by the reaction between H_2O_2 and iron or copper in a low valence state. The oxidized halogens are almost as diverse group of reactive oxidants as are the free radicals. They consist of HOCl and the vast number of chloramines. Chloramines can be produced from the reaction of HOCl with the many amines that are found in biological systems. Like HOCl, the chloramines are oxidizing species. Chloramine (NH_2Cl) is formed by the reaction of HOCl with ammonia (NH_3). The reaction of HOCl with amino acids leads through chloramines to aldehydes. Altogether, the oxidized halogens represent probably the most important microbicidal oxidants produced by neutrophils. Oxygen (O_2) alone is a diradical with two unpaired electrons. There is also a much more reactive form of oxygen known as $^1O_2$, in which those two electrons are paired. The $^1O_2$ is produced by neutrophils, which manufacture it by the reaction between H_2O_2 and an oxidized halogen.

Reactive nitrogen species are produced by phagocytes during the reaction of NO with $O_2^{\bullet-}$, and other oxidizing species. The first characterized of these species is $ONOO^-$, formed in a reaction between $ON^\bullet$ and $O_2^{\bullet-}$, both of which are free radicals. Peroxynitrite then undergoes a secondary reaction to produce an agent that is able to nitrate tyrosine. The precise composition of the agent is not known, but several candidates have been proposed. Among them are various derivatives of $ONOO^-$. Major cellular sites of ROS generation include the mitochondria, and non- mitochondrial membrane bound enzyme systems (Babior, 2000).

3.2 Reactive oxidant species in the joint tissue

Articular cartilage is a unique tissue for its constituent cells, the chondrocytes, which maintain the cartilage matrix through their continual synthesis and degradation. The environment is avascular, hyperosmotic and acidic. Cartilage cells are synoviocytes, and chondrocytes. Chondrocytes display a metabolism adapted to anaerobic conditions. Synoviocytes supply the avascular cartilage tissue with nutrients via synovial fluid. Because cartilage is an avascular environment, the oxygen tension in the area is usually low. In pathological conditions, like inflammation, oxygen tension is subject of fluctuations. These variations of oxygen tension force chondrocytes to produce reactive species. The main reactive species produced by chondrocytes are $O_2^{\bullet-}$ radical, and NO that generate other derivative radicals, including $ONOO^-$ and H_2O_2 (Hiran et al., 1997; Stefanovic- Racic et al., 1997). The effects of free radicals on articular cartilage are dual. "Chondrocyte- derived" free radical levels are important for the maintenance of ion homeostasis. Natrium hydrogen (Na^+ - H^+) - exchanger (NHE- activity) and free radical levels exhibit a significant positive correlation. How exactly highly reactive species alter ion transport is not known, although interference with protein phosphorylation is possible (Gibson et al., 2008).

Except beneficial effect free radicals may have on articular cartilage when exceed in a cell, free radicals damage both chondrocytes, and extracellular matrix (ECM) components of articular cartilage. Free radicals shift the redox balance in articular cartilage in direction of oxidants. Hypochlorous acid, singlet oxygen, and peroxynitrite radicals balance the ascorbate, an antioxidant vitamin, from cartilage (Hajdigogos et al., 2003).

ROS and RNS damage articular cartilage directly or indirectly by up- regulating the mediators of the ECM degradation. Reactive oxygen/ nitrogen species, e.g. $ONOO^-$, also have been shown to degrade aggrecan, a major component of ECM, and this degradation is one of the initial events in the process of cartilage destruction (Billinghurst *et al.,* 1997). The incidence of sulfated glycosaminoglycans (GAGs) reflects the ratio of aggrecan degradation in the cartilage.

In seeking for a role of oxidative radicals in cartilage metabolism, it has been noted that endogenously generated NO suppresses the biosynthesis of aggrecan, a major macromolecular component of the cartilaginous matrix (Cao et al., 1997). Furthermore, it was discovered that oxygen radicals fragment hyaluronan and chondroitin sulphate (Kennett & Davies, 2009).

Collagen, which provides tensile strength and forms a network that resists the swelling pressure of aggrecan- hyaluronate aggregates, can be altered directly by oxygen radicals. Free radicals prime collagen to proteolytic enzymes. Incubation of cartilage slices with xanthine-oxidase- generated $O_2^{\bullet -}$ anion degrades type I collagen and fibril formation by this collagen. Hydroxyl radical in the presence of oxygen fragments collagen into small peptides. The cleavage seems to be specific to proline or 4- hydroxyproline residues (Monboisse & Borel, 1992). Interestingly, free radicals may destruct collagen synthesis indirectly. NO inhibits collagen synthesis via interleukin-1 (IL-1) (Cao et al., 1997). H_2O_2 inhibits cartilage proteoglycan synthesis interfering with adenosine triphosphate (ATP) synthesis, in part by inhibiting the glycolytic enzyme glyceraldehyde-3-phosphate dehydrogenase in chondrocytes. $ONOO^-$ and HOCl may facilitate cartilage damage by inactivating tissue inhibitor of metalloproteinases (TIMPs). TIMP-1 inhibits stromelysins, collagenases and gelatinases (Henrontin et al., 2003). Moreover it was observed, that treatment of chondrocytes with the NO-producing agent, S-nitroso-N-acetylpenicillamine, up- regulates the collagenase mRNA levels, which is one of MMPs (Lo et al., 1998).

Exposure of the chondrocytes to H_2O_2 inhibits proteoglycan synthesis (Henrontin et al., 2003). Chondrocytes in arthritic cartilage respond poorly to insulin- like growth factor 1 (IGF-1) what may lead to abrogation of cartilage repair. In this context, ROS may participate in reducing the capacity of chondrogenic precursor cells to migrate and proliferate within joint area. Nitric oxide radical was also demonstrated to inhibit chondrocyte migration and attachment to fibronectin via modification of the actin cytoskeleton. Chondrocytes produce high levels of NO, which is a mediator of anti- proliferative effects of IL-1 in these articular cells (Blanco & Lotz, 1994). In addition, it was discovered that IL-1 induces apoptosis to chondrocytes via NO. Combination of IL-1 with the radical scavengers like N-acetyl cysteine, dimethyl sulfoxide, or 5, 5'-dimetylpyrroline 1-oxide induced apoptosis, which was inhibited in a dose dependent manner by the NO synthase inhibitor N-monomethyl L-arginine (Blanco et al., 1995). Chondrocyte death, determined as the percentage of empty lacunae in articular cartilage, was completely blocked in p47phox-/- mice confirming the "Nicotinamide adenine dinucleotide phosphate" (NADPH)- oxidase" driven oxygen radical production in mediating these effects (Lem van Lent et al., 2005).

Synoviocytes are the second kind of articular cells. These cells consume larger amount of oxygen when compared to chondrocytes (Schneider et al., 2005). An indirect evidence of oxidative stress in synoviocytes is the incidence of antioxidant enzymes such as superoxide dismutase, glutathione peroxidase and catalase in these cells (Mattey et al., 1993). Oxidative stress makes synoviocytes to undergo a cell death of an apoptotic nature (Galleron et al., 1999). The ROS scavenger system of synoviocytes protects chondrocytes from toxic effects of free radicals. In a co-culture of these cells synoviocytes reduced toxic effects of H_2O_2 on chondrocyte cell damage (Kurz et al., 1999). NO is the primary inducer of apoptosis in human articular chondrocytes (Blanco et al., 1995). NO^- mediated chondrocyte cell death requires generation of additional reactive species like $ONOO^-$ and $O_2^{\cdot -}$ (Del Carlo Jr. & Loeser, 2002).

Joint fluid is produced as a transudate of plasma from synovial cells and provides nutrition to the articular cartilage by diffusion of oxygen and other molecules. The primary catalytic antioxidant of the joint fluid is the extracellular SOD (Regan et al., 2008). SOD type III accounts for 80% of the enzyme's activity in the joint fluid (Afonso et al., 2007). Glycosaminoglycans (long-chain polysaccharides) are major components of the extracellular matrix, glycocalyx, and synovial fluid. Modifications to these materials are linked to multiple human pathologies including autoimmune diseases. Hyaluronan and chondroitin sulfate are extensively depolymerized by hydroxyl and carbonyl radicals, which may be formed from ONOO-. Polymer fragmentation is shown to be dependent on the radical flux (Kennett & Davies, 2009). NO, and O_{2}- inhibit type II collagen and proteoglycans synthesis and the sulfation of newly synthesized GaGs (Hickery & Bayliss, 1998).

4. Inflammatory synovitis: May oxidative stress be a cause?

4.1 ROS in inflammatory synovium

In autoimmune joint diseases systemic inflammation exists long before it exerts local effects on synovial membrane. At one point, systemic inflammation is translocated into synovium where it initiates the inflammatory response often leading to oxidative burst. Oxidative burst in rheumatoid joints is a result of the activation of innate immune system cells. Activated phagocytic cells such as neutrophils, and macrophages both produce free radicals in the joint area. Activated phagocytes produce reactive oxidants by enzymes: the NADPH- oxidase, and the nitric oxide synthase (NOS). Mechanism of free radicals production differs between these cell groups. While macrophages are stimulated by the "NADPH- oxidase" system to produce free radicals, the presence of NOS accompanied by the NADPH- oxidase is necessary for neutrophils to secrete free radicals. RA neutrophils also generate enhanced amount of $ONOO^-$ by NOS (El Benna et al., 2002). Chemiluminescence assays demonstrated significant activation of the neutrophil myeloperoxidase H_2O_2 system in synovial fluids from patients with RA further suggesting that oxidative stress may contribute to the cyclic, self- perpetuating nature of rheumatoid inflammation. ROS, produced by activated phagocytes alters the antigenic behaviour of immunoglobulin G (IgG). Radical-exposed IgG is able to bind rheumatoid factor and results in the generation of C3alpha complement component. This reaction may be self-perpetuating within the rheumatoid joint, suggesting that free radicals play a role in the chronicity of rheumatoid inflammation (Newkirk et al., 2002).

Pro-inflammatory cytokines´ presence and activity undoubtedly subjects to rheumatoid synovitis governing a variety of pathological processes including cell activation, cell proliferation, tissue resorption and chemotaxis (Schett et al., 2000). Experimental evidence confirms cytokine- induced oxidative stress in rheumatoid synovium. Thioredoxin, a cellular catalyst induced by oxidative stress, is found in high amounts in RA synovial cells and tissue. Thioredoxin acts as a co- factor for tumor necrosis factor- alpha (TNF- α) - induced synthesis of interleukins (IL-6 and IL-8) in synovial fibroblastlike cells (Yoshida et al., 1999). Edaravone, which is a clinically available antioxidant, suppresses IL-1β- induced synovial cells proliferation and migration under *in vitro* conditions (Arii et al., 2006). N-acetylcytein, a known thiol antioxidant, abrogated L-6 - induced proliferation of RA patients synovial fibroblasts (Ji-Yeon et al., 2000).

ROS are documented as mediators of synovial inflammation. Excessive production of ROS at the site of inflammation contributes to the inflammatory process in general, by induction of the expression of adhesion molecules, pro-inflammatory cytokines, and chemoattractants. Furthermore, ROS can directly increase tissue destruction through inactivation of the major inhibitor of degrading enzymes, α1-antiproteinase, which subsequently leads to the activation of extracellular matrix-degrading metalloproteinases (MMPs) (Maurice et al., 1997). 3-nitrotyrosine (3- NT) has been identified as a stable end product and marker of inflammation and RNS production. Nitrated proteins are generated in inflamed tissues by inflammatory cells producing $ONOO^-$, a naturally occurring nitrating agent. A study by Khan & Siddiqui (2006) further investigated the binding characteristics of naturally occurring antibodies to 3- NT present in synovial fluid. Antibodies to 3- NT were found higher in the synovial fluid of RA patients.

Ex-vivo cultured rheumatoid synovium produces a significant amount of nitrite, and the addition of N- methylarginine (L-NMMA) significantly inhibits NO production. *In vitro* study revealed that NO production from freshly isolated synovial cells was up- regulated by stimulation with a combination of IL-1β, TNF-α and lipopolysaccharide. Inducible NOS expression was induced when human chondrocytes were stimulated with IL-1β, TNF-α or endotoxin in a dose- and time-dependent manner. Inflammatory reaction in the synovium of RA patients could be augmented by the autocrine or other cytokine-induced production of IL-6 with subsequent generation of ROS in the synoviocytes. Fibroblast- like synoviocytes proliferation by IL-6 was inhibited by N- acetylcysteine. Oxidative stress of RA synovial tissue can cause DNA damage and suppress the DNA mismatch repair (MMR) system in cultured synoviocytes. DNA MMR enzyme expression is greatest in the synovial intimal lining layer, where maximal oxidative stress in RA occurs (Šimelyte et al., 2004).

4.2 Cycles of hypoxia/ reoxygenation in inflammatory synovium

Angiogenesis in the synovial membrane is an important early step in pathogenesis of RA, in the perpetuation of the disease and may precede other pathological features. Elevated levels of pro-angiogenic factor, the vascular endothelial growth factor VEGF, are expressed in synovium, synovial fluids, and serum of RA patients. An increased VEGF level in RA is responsible for subsequent joint destruction. The synovium of RA is hypoxic as a result of synovial tissue proliferation outpacing in angiogenesis. Hypoxia is a potent inducer of cytokines, matrix degrading enzymes, angiogenic factors that play a central role in the inflammatory response. Hypoxia- inducible factor- 1α (HIF-1α) is a key transcription factor which is highly inducible by hypoxia and expressed predominantly in synovium of RA. Expression of HIF-1α is critical for joint inflammation. RA synovial fluids are hypoxic, acidic with low glucose and elevated lactate concentrations. This biochemical profile is indicative of a chronically hypoxic microenvironment that compensates by anaerobic metabolism. The oxygen partial pressure (pO_2) is extremely low in RA synovial fluids, and correlates with elevated plasma levels of lactate. Inflamed synovitis is a hallmark of RA which is hypoxic in nature (Shankar et al., 2009). The biological basis of this process relates to hypoxia- inducible factor (HIF). The response of mammalian cells to hypoxia is mediated partly through stabilization of certain transcription factors including HIF-1 and HIF-2. These oxygen sensitive transcription factors are multifunctional. Firstly, they program the cells to anaerobic metabolism, secondly, they enhance cell survival by inhibiting apoptosis, and thirdly they improve the supply of oxygen by promoting angiogenesis and increase oxygen-carrying capacity. In view of the crucial role of HIF-1 in cellular adaptation to hypoxia, its regulation needs to be rapidly responsive to changes in the cellular oxygen supply. Inhibition of degradation is the primary mechanism by which hypoxia directly regulates HIF- 1α. In the absence of oxygen critical step of degradation process of HIF-1α, the hydroxylation of proline and asparagine residues, becomes rate limiting, thus preventing HIF-1α from being degraded and leaving it free to bind to its constitutively expressed partner HIF-1β. In rheumatic patients, joint movement in a ratio of normally functional joint increases the pO_2 leading to re-oxygenation. In RA cycling transient episodes of hypoxia/re-oxygenation increase levels of ROS. Increased mitochondrial ROS levels stabilize the transcription factor HIF- 1α (Chandel et al., 2000). Of particular relevance to RA was the marked attenuation of synovitis and articular damage in an adjuvant arthritis model when HIF- 1α was absent. In RA synovitis, HIF-1a protein accumulates and translocates to the nucleus and directly activates transcription of pro-angiogenic factor like VEGF. VEGF is highly inducible by hypoxia which occurs in the inflamed joints of RA. The HIF-1α translocates and binds to core DNA motif in the hypoxia responsive elements (HRE) which are associated with target genes such as VEGF and induces its gene expression and thereby angiogenesis. HIF-1α is expressed abundantly by macrophages in most rheumatoid synovia, predominantly close to the intimal layer but also in the subintimal zone (Hollander et al., 2001). The synovial expression of HIF-1α also showed a mixed nuclear and cytoplasmic pattern mostly seen in lining cells, stromal cells, mononuclear cells, and blood vessels (Giatromanolaki et al., 2002). The number of HIF-1α -positive cells correlated strongly with the number of blood vessels in RA synovial tissue and with inflammatory endothelial cell infiltration (blood vessels), cell proliferation (Ki67) and the synovitis score (Brouwer et al., 2009). Reduction in the degradation rate of HIFs (HIF-1α, and HIF-2α) as occurs under hypoxic stress throughout arthritis, results in increased steady- state level of HIFs proteins and up-regulation of the neo- angiogenic process. Neo-angiogenic VEGF/ KDR pathway was shown persistently increased in RA, as indeed was microvessel density and the expression of PD- ECGF, irrespective of the extent of HIF expression (Giatromanolaki et al., 2002). The direct link exists between accumulation of HIFs and overexpression of VEGF in RA. Neo-angiogenesis contributes to pathogenesis of RA encouraging synovitis, pannus formation and articular cartilage destruction. Concluding, the HIF seems to be a promising factor that targets both synovitis and angiogenesis in RA.

5. Oxidative stress in human autoimmune joint diseases

5.1 Rheumatoid arthritis

Rheumatoid arthritis (RA) is a systemic autoimmune inflammatory disease primarily affecting synovial membranes of joints. Pathogenesis of RA is a multistep process where cellular and humoral interactions mediated by lymphocytes (T and B cells) and non hematopoietic cells like fibroblasts, connective tissue cells, and bone cells play a role. At site of inflammation, activation of T cells and macrophages leads to a large increase in oxygen consumption, whose corollary is increased release of ROS (Afonso et al., 2007). Both, hematopoietic, and connective tissue cells are subject of oxidative stress process in arthritis.

5.1.1 Hematopoietic cells and tissue as oxidative stress targets in RA

Activity of NADPH- oxidase is enhanced in circulating neutrophils and monocytes of RA patients. These phagocytic cells synthesize two- to eight- fold higher amounts of $O_2^{\bullet-}$ when compared to healthy controls. Production rates of $O_2^{\bullet-}$ in neutrophils and monocytes from rheumatic patients positively correlate with the plasma levels of TNF- α (Miesel et al., 1996). Other parameters of oxidative stress like decrease in neutrophil SOD activity and an increase in the levels of "loose" iron in the plasmalemma of RA neutrophils and monocytes were also observed (Ostrakhovitch & Afanas´ev, 2001). A characteristic feature of RA ROS-producing neutrophils is their functional state. The production of $O_2^{\bullet-}$ by blood neutrophils from RA patients in response to N-formyl-methionylleucyl-phenylalanine, a stimulatory agent, was greater in arthritic than control blood neutrophils (Eggleton et al., 1995). The study suggested that stimulated sub-population of neutrophils are source of ROS in arthritis.

5.1.2 Connective cells and tissue as oxidative stress targets in RA

Studies of RA synovial fluid (SF) and tissue have demonstrated oxidative damage to the tissue. Signs of oxidative stress such as DNA oxidative damage, and lipid peroxidation are present in the inflammatory synovium of RA patients. Immunohistochemical analysis revealed increased staining of 8- oxo- 7,8- dihydro- 2´- deoxyguanine, a marker of DNA oxidative damage, and increased staining of 4-hydroxy-2-nonenal in the lining and sublining layers of the RA inflammatory synovium (Šimelyte et al., 2004). Furthermore, it was shown that increased lipid peroxidation damage in RA inflammatory synovium is proportional to the levels of hypoxia in the joint, disease activity and angiogenic marker expression (Biniecka et al., 2009). Synovial fluids macrophages produce increased amounts of $O_2^{\bullet-}$. Also neutrophils from synovial fluids of rheumatic patients generate increased amounts of $O_2^{\bullet-}$ possibly because of their exposure to cytokines present in synovial fluids (Hitchon & El-Gabalawy, 2004). Chronic oxidative stress contributes to functional hyporesponsiveness of synovial T lymphocytes. The impaired mitogenic responses of SF T lymphocytes correlated with a significant decrease in the levels of the intracellular redox-regulating agent glutathione (GSH) (Maurice et al., 1997).

Indirect evidence for ROS implication in cartilage degradation comes from the presence of lipid peroxidation products, nitrite, nitrotyrosine, a nitrated type II collagen peptide, modified low-density lipoprotein (LDL) and oxidized IgG in the biological fluids of patients with arthritis. Furthermore, nitrotyrosine, nitrated proteins and oxidized LDL (ox-LDL) have been found to be accumulated in cartilage of arthritic patients demonstrating the direct implication of ROS in some joint diseases. Rheumatoid arthritis is characterized by irreversible damage to the cartilage matrix caused by enzymatic degradation of the proteins, e.g., collagen type II (CII), and proteoglycans of cartilage (e.g., aggrecan) (Billinghurst et al., 1997). As a result of the breakdown of the proteins and proteoglycans, CII degradation products and sulfated glycosaminoglycans (GAGs) appear in SFs of the affected joints. The level of GAGs in SF indicates the extent of proteoglycan degradation (Lark et al., 1997). Hydrogene peroxide, and singlet oxygen accelerate bone resorption by osteoclasts. Osteoclasts generate ROS through "NADPH- oxidase dependent mechanisms". Studies involving assays of nitrotyrosine residues in synovial tissues from patients with RA or exposure of chondrocytes to synthetic peroxynitrite *in vitro* have established that combination of the O_2^{-} anion to nitric oxide (NO) causes cartilage damage (Abramson et al., 2001).

The cytokine network is involved in the pathogenesis of RA. IL-1 is a key mediator of bone resorption and cartilage destruction in arthritis. The cytokine activates bone resorption through its effects on osteoclast differentiation and activation. IL-1 destructs cartilage by stimulating release of MMPs from fibroblasts and chondrocytes. Neutralizing ROS activity significantly attenuated IL-1- induced collagenase gene expression in bovine chondrocytes (Lo et al., 1998).

In RA oxidative stress also features by oxidation of low- density lipoproteins (LDL). Oxidized LDLs promote inflammatory changes including local up- regulation of adhesion molecules and chemokines.

RA tissue has evidence of microsatellite instability reflecting ongoing mutagenesis. Such mutagenesis is normally corrected by DNA repair systems including the mismatch repair system, which is defective in RA, probably due to oxidative stress.

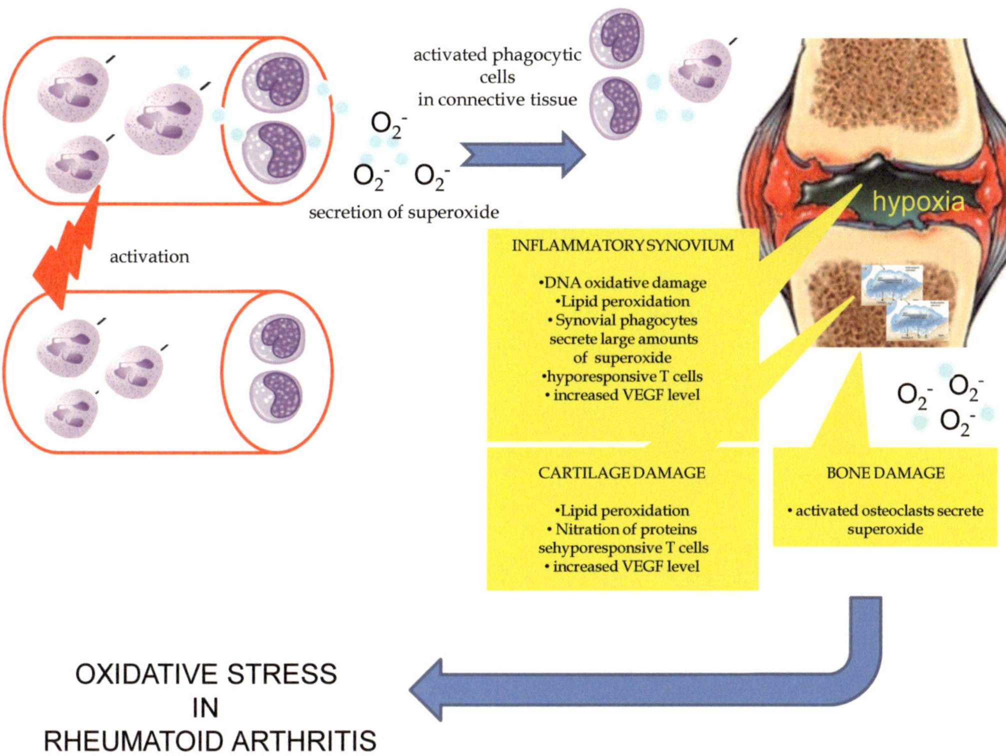

Fig. 1. Connective tissue and cells as targets of oxidative stress in rheumatoid arthritis.

6. Systemic lupus erythematosus

Systemic lupus erythematosus (SLE) is a prototype autoimmune, multisystem and multifactorial disease characterized by the presence of auto-antibodies to a variety of nuclear antigens such as DNA and histones, as well as protein antigens and protein–nucleic acid complexes. The initial immunizing antigen(s) that drive the development of SLE are unknown, but characteristics of the immune response in SLE suggest that it is an antigen-driven condition. Multiorgan inflammatory lesions also involve the joints. Immune complex deposits in the synovium are associated with mild inflammation and cartilage destruction is seldom severe. The arthritis of SLE is described as non-destructive and non-deforming. Immune complex deposits in the synovium trigger inflammatory reaction, which led continuously to cartilage destruction (Khan & Siddiqui, 2006). Free radicals synthesize autoantigens, which contribute to disease development. Oxidative stress and inflammation are interrelated in SLE. Malondialdehyd (MDA) levels positively correlated with levels of interferon- γ (INF-γ), and interleukin- 12 (IL- 12) in lupus disease (Shah et al., 2010).

6.1 Hematopoietic cells and tissue as oxidative stress targets in SLE

Oxidative damage to red blood cells and leukocytes are hallmarks of oxidative stress in SLE. Lipid peroxidation, in SLE erythrocytes, and generation of $O_2^{\cdot-}$ and H_2O_2 in leukocytes were increased in SLE patients when compared to healthy controls (Tewthanom et al., 2008). Destroying effects of free radicals in lupus disease are apparent on the reactions with serum proteins. Oxidation makes the proteins more fragile. Modified proteins become autoantigens, and more, their presence enhances oxidative stress in serum. 4-hydroxy-2-nonenal (4- HNE), which is a marker of lipid peroxidation in SLE, after binding protein forms dangerous protein adducts. The target of 4- HNE modification reported was catalase, a membrane protein of red blood cells (D'Souza et al., 2008). Hydroxyl radical binds human serum albumin. The increase in total serum protein carbonyl levels in the SLE patients was largely due to an increase in oxidized albumin (Shjekh et al., 2007).

In lupus disease, oxidative stress presents by lipid peroxidation mostly. Moreover it was discovered that lipid peroxidation influences pathogenesis of the disease. The disease activity score (SLEDAI) positively correlates with serum levels of MDA. T-lymphocyte apoptosis and MDA were positively associated with disease activity (Shah et al., 2011). MDA- modified proteins as the catalase, and SOD are targets of IgG circulated autoantibodies promoting disease development. On the other hand, SLEDAI score correlates negatively with serum antioxidant enzymes as SOD, and glutathione peroxidase (GPx) (Taysi et al., 2002 b). Auto- antibodies against plasma lipoproteins have been reported in SLE patients (Batuca et al., 2007). The study further documented incidence of antibodies toward high density lipoproteins (HDL) in patients with SLE, and identified Apo A-I as a target of oxidative damage. The incidence of auto-antibodies against lipid particles correlated with reduced activity of paraoxonase (PON), which is the most active antioxidant enzyme in lipids, and also prevents lipid peroxidation of low density lipoproteins (LDL).

6.2 Connective cells and tissue as oxidative stress targets in SLE

The arthritis of SLE is described as non- destructive and non- deforming. Immune complex deposits in the synovium are associated with mild inflammation and cartilage destruction is seldom severe. In SLE patients, NO and its intermediates may be mediators of inflammatory arthritis. Antibodies against 3- nitrotyrosine (3- NT) were found elevated in sera, and synovial fluid of SLE patients. Interestingly, the sera levels were much higher than in synovial fluid (Khan & Siddiqui, 2006).

7. Markers of oxidative stress in human autoimmune joint diseases

A short lifetime of free radicals in body fluids restricts their direct estimation instead effects of oxygen on lipids, proteins, and nucleic acids molecules are used. There are many chemical modifiers of protein, and lipid structures, whose activity is accelerated by oxidative stress. *N*-carboxymethyllysine (CML) represents a chemically modified amino acid and originates *in vivo* from carbohydrate as well as from lipid derived precursors. Oxidative damage to proteins is also reflected by increased levels of advanced oxidation protein products (AOPP), which form by the reaction between chlorinated oxidants (HOCl/OCl-) and proteins. AOPP are defined as dityrosine-containing cross-linked proteins. MDA is one of the end products of lipid peroxidation induced by ROS and marker of oxidative stress in lipids. 8-Hydroxy-2′-deoxyguanosine (8-OHdG) has been recognized as a biomarker of oxidative DNA damage by endogenously generated oxygen radicals. In addition, oxidative stress may be estimated by levels of enzymes like thioredoxin, a protein with reduction / oxidation active disulfide / dithiol groups in its active site. Signs of oxidative stress are apparent on cells and tissue affected by arthritis. Advanced glycation end products (AGEs), which are formed during the Maillard reaction by non-enzymatic glycation, and oxidation of proteins were detected in the synovial lining, sublining, and endothelium in RA patiens. CML showed positive immunostaining in some RA macrophages (CD68+) and T cells (CD45RO+) (Drinda et al., 2002). High levels of protein carbonyl (PCO), and AGE products were found in serum of collagen - induced arthritis mice (Choi, 2007). Plasma MDA concentrations are significantly higher in RA patients (Sarban et al., 2005). An excessive degree of oxidative stress in RA patients confirm decline of protein thiol levels and lower activity of antioxidant enzymes like glutathione (GSH), GPx, and CuZn SOD in blood of these patients (Seven et al., 2008). The study by Jikimoto (Jikimoto et al., 2001) discovered elevated levels of TRX in plasma, and synovial fluid of RA patients. Plasma TRX correlated with urinary excretion of 8-hydroxy-29-deoxyguanosine (8-OHdG). Serum MDA levels were increased in SLE patients, while serum antioxidant levels were decreased in these patients what confirms oxidative stress in the pathology of SLE (Taysi et al., 2002 a).

8. Oxidative stress in autoimmune joint diseases: Beneficial or harmful?

The recent research describes dual role of ROS in autoimmune- joint diseases. The ROS production by the activated NOX- family (NADPH) of oxidases has a principal function throughout the priming phase of the development of autoimmune joint diseases. The NADPH oxidase- deficient knockout mice developed a serious inflammatory arthritis with extensive bone erosions and a massive osteolysis (van de Loo et al., 2003). ROS might reduce arthritis development influencing circulating inflammatory cells before they reach the joint. ROS limit T cell responses to self- antigens inducing their apoptosis, what inhibits disease development (Olofsson et al., 2003). Arthritis development correlates with functionality of NADPH- oxidase complex, which is determined by the neutrophil cytosolic factor 1 (Ncf 1), a phagocytic oxidase. The naturally occurring polymorphism of Ncf1 allele limiting the NADPH functionality promotes activation of arthritogenic CD4+ cells. An expansion of arthritogenic T cells owing to the lower activity of the NADPH- oxidase complex was observed in the DA Ncf 1 allele (Olofsson et al., 2003). An increased severity of arthritis was observed in animals with either loss of function mutations or deletions in components of the phagocyte NADPH- oxidase like the p47phox (van de Loo et al., 2003). Furthermore, the effect of NOX-derived ROS might depend on the arthritis model: in IFN-gamma (INF- γ) enhanced imine complex arthritis, the p47phox-deficient animals showed a less severe joint destruction and decreased chondrocyte death (Lem van Lent et al., 2005).

The NADPH- oxidase- derived superoxide is not exclusive effector molecule in arthritis. Superoxide dismuthase (SOD) catalyses the dismutation of superoxide anion to oxygen and hydrogen peroxide. Three SOD enzyme isoforms have been characterized in humans. SOD I, and SOD III are copper, zinc, enzyme isoforms. SOD II is a manganese enzyme isoform.

Whereas type I SOD is found mostly in the cytoplasm, nucleus, and intermembrane space of mitochondria, type III of SOD is extracellular. Manganese is cofactor for SOD type II, which is a mitochondrial enzyme. The enzyme is involved in the pathogenesis of inflammatory joint disease. In adjuvant model of arthritis the enzyme suppressed swelling, and retarded bone destruction (Shingu et al., 1994). An intra-articular injection of SOD significantly reduced synovitis in streptococcal wall cell (SWC)- model of arthritis. Intra- aricular injection of native SOD (bovine orgotein) produced greater clinical improvements than did intra- articular aspirin in patients with RA involving the knee (Afonso et al., 2007). Available data suggest a protective role of SOD in inflammatory joint disease. In mice that are genetically deficient in SOD III, both the severity of collagen-induced arthritis and the production of pro-inflammatory cytokines are increased. SODIII gene transferred subcutaneously or intra- articularly decreased the severity of experimental arthritis in rodents.

9. Antioxidants as therapeutic possibilities in human autoimmune joint diseases

9.1 Antioxidant enzymes

SODs exert protective effects in animal models of inflammation. In mice, genetically deficient in SOD III, both the severity of collagen- induced arthritis and the production of pro- inflammatory cytokines are increased (Ross et al., 2004). SOD III gene transfer into the knee decreased the severity of experimental arthritis in rodents. In humans, serum SOD III levels correlated negatively with disease activity. Despite conflicting results of native SOD (orgotein) in RA patients, SOD mimetics have shown beneficial effects. Until now, the most promising are nitroxide (tempol) and Mn (II) pentaazamacrocyclic ligand (M40403). *In vitro*, tempol diminishes hydroxyl radical production, and decreases the cytotoxic effects of hydrogen peroxide and peroxynitrite. Tempol decreased collagen- induced arthritis in rats (Cuzzocrea et al., 2001). The anti-inflammatory effects of M40403 ligand are related to superoxide elimination, and restraint of nitration of tyrosine residues in proteins. M40403 ligand diminishes the expression of adhesion molecules such as integrins or selectins decreasing influx of neutrophils to inflammatory site. M40403 ligand inhibits TNF-α via blocking the nuclear factor kappa B (NF- κB). Its beneficial effects have been reported in rats with collagen- induced arthritis (Cuzzocrea et al., 2005).

9.2 Vitamins

Micronutrient supplementation has been recommended to arthritic patients based on findings that the antioxidant status is very low in these patients. It has been documented that the mean synovial fluid concentrations of α-tocopherol are significantly decreased in arthritic patients compared to healthy controls. Also, levels of vitamin E in peripheral blood cell were significantly decreased in patients with active arthritis than in healthy subjects (Vasanthi et al., 2009). Concentrations of other antioxidant vitamins such as A, C are of lower order in RA and SLE patients than in normal subjects too. Based on animal studies, there is evidence that antioxidant vitamins may prevent arthritis, and increase antioxidant status. Daily oral administration of vitamin E to male arthritic rats restored levels of thiol (-SH) groups to pre- arthritic levels (Kheir- Eldin et al., 1992). High doses of vitamin C (1-

2g/kg body weight) applied to arthritic Lewis rats, delayed incidence of paw oedema in these rats. Histological studies revealed a decreased inflammatory cells infiltration of superficial layer of synovium, and decreased synovial SOD activity in these rats (Sakai et al., 1999). In addition, administration of rutin (vitamin P) strongly inhibited spontaneous ROS production in RA neutrophils (Ostrakhovitch & Afanas´ev, 2001). Vitamin E exerts analgetic effects. The results from a double blind clinical trials suggested that a dose of 400–1200 mg of α-tocopherol daily was effective with respect to various pain parameters such as pain on pressure, pain at rest, and pain on movement. The postulated analgesic properties of vitamin E seem to be correlated to vitamin E plasma concentrations. Patients with active RA supplemented with a combination of conjugated fatty acids and vitamin E improved their disease activity score. The diet in these patients relieved from night and activity pain, and morning stiffness (Aryaeian et al., 2009). The analgesic effect of vitamin E is independent of a peripheral anti-inflammatory action, thereby suggesting a central rather than peripheral action. Dietary antioxidant micronutrients act as scavengers of reactive oxygen radicals and may protect against free radical mediated tissue damage in an inflamed joint. Vitamin E supplemented in soyabean oil reduced anti- double- stranded DNA IgG antibodies (Chia-Chien & Bi- Fong, 2005).

9.3 Fatty acids

Eicosapentaenoic acid and docosahexaenoic acid (EPA and DHA respectively) exert potent antioxidant properties. Supplementation with these acids to lupus patients restored levels of antioxidant enzymes as the GPx, and SOD to baseline levels (Mohan, & Das, 1997). Lupus autoimmune female mice fed with fish oil exhibited significantly higher liver of catalase, SOD, and GPx. The diet was shown to be beneficial against oxidative damage of hepatic tissue (Bhattacharya et al., 2003). Sera of lupus mice treated with conjugated linoleic acid (CLA) contained higher concentrations of total GSH which were negatively correlated with the levels of oxidative stress markers. Moreover, increased GSH, gammaGCL, glutathione S-transferase (GSTs), and NAD(P)H:quinone oxidoreductase (NQO1) activities were measured in liver and spleen of CLA-treated animals. The activation of detoxifying enzymes may be one of the mechanisms whereby dietary CLA down-regulates oxidative stress in lupus mice (Bergamo et al., 2007).

10. Conclusions and future perspectives

In all cell types, oxygen metabolism can lead to the production of reactive oxygen / nitrogen species. Reactive species are known for their dual role as both beneficial and harmful. Deleterious effects of oxidative stress on cell components (proteins, lipids, DNA) include changes in their structure, and function. On the other hand, beneficial effects of ROS/RNS involve physiological cellular responses to noxious agents, e.g., in defense against infectious agents, in a number of cellular signaling pathways and in the induction of a mitogenic response. Oxidants even protect cells against oxidative stress and re-establish or maintain redox homeostasis (Ortona et al., 2008).

Oxygen metabolism has an important role in the pathogenesis of autoimmune joint diseases. Reactive oxygen/nitrogen species are documented as mediators of synovial inflammation. Their excessive production at the site of inflammation contributes to inflammatory process in general, by induction of local production of chemoattractants, adhesion molecules, and pro- inflammatory cytokines. In addition, oxidative stress may contribute to the cyclic, self-perpetuating nature of autoimmune inflammation. Immune cells when "affected" by oxidants became auto- antigens intensifying auto- immune responses. Persisting auto-inflammation, and oxidative stress in joint area leads to damages of connective tissue and the ECM directly or indirectly. *In vitro,* lipid peroxidation, $ONOO^-$ formation is associated with decreased production of type II collagen and aggrecan, and with diminished chondrocyte responses to growth factors. Moreover, $ONOO^-$ interferes with metabolism of matrix enhancing the expression of matrix degrading enzymes inhibiting the production and activity of tissue inhibiting enzymes. Hydrogen peroxide and singlet oxygen accelerate bone resorption. Level of oxidative stress in rheumatoid synovium is proportional to the levels of hypoxia and angiogenesis in the joint area.

Oxidative stress generated within an inflammatory joint can produce autoimmune phenomena and connective tissue destruction in rheumatoid synovitis (Vasanthi et al., 2009). Swelling stiffness pain in rest immobility are common symptoms of autoimmune joint diseases. Rationale of antioxidant therapy should relieve from objective complications. Polyunsaturated fatty acids (PUFA) can modulate oxidative stress and may have a role as regulators in the synthesis of antioxidant enzymes (Mohan & Das, 1997). Arthritic patients taking these acids showed biochemical and chemical improvement. Dietary supplementation significantly decreased joint pain index. In combination with other dietary modifications modest improvement in morning stiffness and in the number of painful joints were reported. Clinical improvements were connected with anti- inflammatory effects as a decreased synthesis of leukotriens by neutrophils and lower synthesis of IL-1β by macrophages. Significant clinical benefit has been claimed in SLE patients given a low- fat diet with PUFA (reviewed in Darlington & Stone, 2001). The clinical work with diets containing PUFA has clearly demonstrated their anti-inflammatory effects, but it was also shown that these effects were attributed to omega- 3 (ω-3) rather than ω-6 PUFA. As there is no doubt about dietary fatty acids do decrease the generation of inflammatory agents, opposite results have been obtained on free radical formation. PUFA are especially potent at increasing levels of oxidative stress. On the other hand, EPA increases mitochondrial Mn-SOD mitochondrial activity.

The hypothesis about oxidative stress promotes arthritic process was challenged when oxidants were shown to decrease disease severity in mouse and rat arthritis models. Certain oils with an alkane structure such as phytol besides its oxidative effects protect against arthritis development. Its subcutaneous administration prevented development of pristane-induced arthritis (Hultqvist et al., 2006). Rats treated with phytol in acute phases of pristane arthritis showed no signs of inflammation. A decrease in COMP, a measurement of ongoing cartilage destruction, was prevented during chronic phases of the disease. The efficiency of phytol in preventing arthritis was compared to methotrexate and/or etanecerpt. Etanecerpt, TNF-α blocker, was highly effective in reducing collagen- induced arthritis. In pristane-induced arthritis, the preventive effects of phytol was more pronounced than that of etanecerpt. Also, in comparison to MTX, phytol was valid as a potential therapeutic agent. Concluded, ROS-promoting substances such as phytol represent a promising class of therapeutics for treatment of autoimmune joint inflammatory diseases what needs further research.

11. Acknowledgements

The work was supported by VZ 0021620816 and by 262708/SVV/2011 and by CN LC 554.

12. References

Abramson, S.B.; Amin, A.R.; Clancy, R.M. & Attur, M. (2001). The role of nitric oxide in tissue destruction. *Best Practice & Research Clinical Rheumatology,* Vol. 15, No.5, pp. 831-845.

Arii, K.; Kumon, Y.; Ikeda, Y; Suehiro, T. &Hashimoto, K. (2006). Edaravone inhibits rheumatoid synovial cell proliferation and migration. *Free Radic Res,* Vol. 40, No. 2, pp. 121-125.

Aryaeian, N.; Shahram, F.; Djalali, M.; Eshragian, M.R.; Djazayeri, A.; Sarrafnejad, A.; Salimzadeh, A.; Naderi, N.; Maryam, Ch. (2009). Effect of conjugated linoleic acids, vitamin E and thein combination on the clinical outcome of Iranian adults with active rheumatoid arthritis. *International Journal of Rheumatic Diseases,* Vol. 12, pp. 20–28.

Afonso, V.; Champy, R.; Mitrovic, D.; Collin, P. & Lomri, A. (2007). Reactive oxygen species and superoxide dismutases: Role in joint diseases. *Joint Bone Spine,* Vol. 74, No. 4 , pp. 324- 329.

Babior, B.M. (2000). Phagocytes and oxidative stress. *Am J Med,* Vol. 109, No. 1, pp. 33-44.

Batuca, J.R.; Ames, P.R.J.; Isenberg, D.A. & Delgado Aves, J. (2007). Antibodies toward high/densitz lipoprotein components inhibit paraoxonase activity in patients with systemic lupus erythematosus. *Ann. N.Y.Acad. Sci.* Vol. 1108, No. 1, pp. 137- 146.

Bergamo, P.; Maurano, F. & Rossi, M. (2007). Phase 2 enzyme induction by conjugated linoleic acid improves lupus- associated oxidative stress. *Free Radic Biol Med,* Vol. 43, No. 1, pp. 71-79.

Bhattacharya, A. & Lawrence, R.A. (2003). Effect of dietary n-3 and n-6 oils with and without food restriction on activity of antioxidant enzymes and lipid peroxidation in livers of cyclophosphamide treated autoimmune- prone NZB/W female mice. *J Am Coll Nutr,* Vol. 22, No. 5, pp. 388-399.

Billinghurst, R.C.;Dahlberg, L.; Ionescu, M., Reiner, A.; Bourne, R.; Rorabeck, C.; Mitchell, P.; Hambor, J.; Diekmann, O.; Tischesche, H.; Chen, J.; Van Wart, H.& Poole, A.R.. (1997). Enhanced cleavage of type ll collagen by collagenases in osteoarthritic articular cartilage. *J Clin Invest,* Vol. 99, No. 7, pp.1534–1545.

Biniecka, M. ; Kennedy, A. ; Fearon, U. ; Ng, Ch. T.. ; Veale, D.J. & O' Sullivan. (2009). Oxidative damage in synovial tissue is associated with in vivo hypoxic status in the arthritic joint. *Ann Rheum Dis,* Vol. 69, No.6 , pp. 1172- 1178.

Blanco, F. & Lotz, M. (1994). IL-1-induced nitric oxide inhibits chondrocyte proliferation via PGE2. *FASEB J,* Vol. 8, pp. A365.

Blanco, F.J. ; Ochs, R.L. ; Schwarz, H. & Lotz, M. (1995). Chondrocyte apoptosis induced by nitric oxide. *Am J Pathol,* Vol. 146, No. 1, pp.75-85.

Brouwer, E. ; Gouw, A.S. ; Posthumus, M.D. ; van Leeuwen, M.A. ; Boerboom, A.L. ; Bijzet, J. ; Bos, R. ; Limburg, P.C. ; Kallenberg, C.G. & Westra J. (2009). Hypoxia inducible factor- 1- alpha (HIF- 1alpha) is related to both angiogenesis and inflammation in rheumatoid arthritis. *Clin Exp Rheumatol,* Vol. 27, No. 6, pp. 945-951.

Cao, M. ; Westerhausen-Larson, A. ; Niyibizi, C. ; Kavalkovich, H.I. ; Georgescu, H.I. ; Riyyo, C. F. ; Hebda, P.A. ; Stefanovic-Racic, M. & Evans, C.H. (1997). Nitric oxide inhibits the synthesis of type II collagen without altering Col2A1 mRNA abundance : prolyl hydroxylase as a possible target. *Biochem. J*, Vol. 324, No. Pt1 , pp. 305- 310.

Chandel, N.S.; Maltepe, E.; Goldwasser, E.; Mathieu, C.E.; Simon, M.C. & Schumacker, P.T. (1998). Mitochondrial reactive oxygen species trigger hypoxia- induced transcription. *Cell Biology*, Vol. 95, No. 20, pp. 11715- 11720.

Chia- Chien, H. & Bi- Fong, L. (2005). The effects of vitamin E supplementation of autoimmune- prone New Zeland black 3 New Yeland white F1 mice fed an oxidized oil diet. *Br J Nutr*, Vol. 93, No. , pp. 655- 662.

Choi, E-M. (2007). Oxidative status of DBA/ 1J mice with type II collagen induced arthritis. *J Appl Toxicol*, Vol. 27, No.5, pp. 472- 481.

Cuzzocrea, S. ; Riley, D.P. ; Achille, P.C. & Salvemini, D. (2001). Antioxidant therapy : A new pharmacological approach in shock, inflammation, and ischemia / reperfusion injury. *Pharmacol Rev*, Vol. 53, No. 1, pp. 135- 159.

Cuzzocrea, S.; Mazzon, E.; di Paola, R.; Genovese, T.; Muia, C.; Caputi, A.P. (2005). Synergistic interaction between methotrexate and a superoxide dismutase mimetic: pharmacologic and potential clinical significance. *Arthritis Rheum*, Vol. 52, No. pp. 3755-3760.

Darlington, L.G & Stone, T.W. (2001). Antioxidants and fatty acids in the amelioration of rheumatoid arthritis and related disorders. *Br J Nutr*. Vol. 85, No. , pp. 251- 269.

Del Carlo Jr, M. & Loeser, R.F. (2002). Nitric oxide- mediated chondrocyte cell death requires the generation of additional reactive oxygen species. *Arthritis & Rheumatism*, Vol. 46, No. 2, pp/ 394- 403.

Drinda, S. ; Franke, S. ; Canet, C.C ; Petrow, P. ; Bräuer, R. ; Hüttich, C. ; Stein, G. & Hein, G. (2002). Identification of the advanced glycation end products N-carboxymethyllysine in the synovial tissue of patients with rheumatoid arthritis. *Ann Rheum Dis*, Vol. 61, No. 6, pp. 488-492.

D' Souza, A. ; Kurien, B. T. ; Ridgers, R. ; Shenoi, J. ; Kurono, S. ; Matsumo, H. ; Hensley. ; Nath, S.K. & Scofield, R.H. (2008). Detection of catalase as a major protein target of the lipid peroxidation product 4-HNE and the lack of its genetic association as a risk factor in SLE. *BMC Medical Genetics*, Vol. 9, pp.62.

Eggleton, P. ; Wang, L. ; Penhallow, J. ; Crawford, N. & Brown, K.A. (1995). Differences in oxidative response of subpopulations of neutrophils from healthy subjects and patients with rheumatoid arthritis. Ann Rheum Dis, Vol. 54, No. 11, pp. 916- 923.

El Benna, J. ; Hayem, G. ; My-Chan Dang, P. ; Fay, M. ; Chollet- Martin, S. ; Elbim, C. ; Meyer, O. & Gougerot- Pocidalo, M-A. (2002). NADPH oxidase priming and p47phox phosphorylation in neutrophils from synovial fluid of patients with rheumatoid arthritis and spondylarthropathy. *Inflammation*, Vol. 26, No. 6, pp. 273- 278.

Galleron, S.; Borderie, D.; Ponteziere, C.; Lemarechal, H.; Jambou, M.; Roch- Arveiller, M.; Ekindjan, O.G. & Calls, M.J. (1999). Reactive oxygen species induce apoptosis of synoviocytes in vitro. Alpha tocopherol provides no protection. *Cell Biol Int*, Vol. 23, No. 9, pp. 637- 642.

Giatromanolaki, A.; Sivridis, E.; Maltezos, E.; Athanassou, N.; Papazoglou, D.; Gatter, K.C.; Harris, A.L. & Koukourakis, M.I. (2003). Upregulated hypoxia inducible factor- 1α and -2α pathway in rheumatoid arthritis and osteoarthritis. *Arthritis Res Ther*, Vol. 5, No. 4, pp. R193- R201.

Gibson, J.S.; Milner, P.I.; White, R.; Fairfax, T.P.A. & Wilkins, R.J. (2008). Oxygen and reactive oxygen species in articular cartilage: modulators of ionic homeostasis. *Pflugers Arch - Eur J Physiol, Vol.* 455, No. 4, pp.563–573.

Hadjigogos, K. (2003). The role of free radicals in the pathogenesis of rheumatoid arthritis. *Panminerva Med,* Vol. 45, No. 1, pp. 7-13.

Henrotin,Y. E.; Bruckner, P.; Pujol, J.P.L. (2003). The role of reactive oxygen species in homeostasis and degradation of cartilage, *OsteoArthritis and Cartilage,* Vol. 11, No. 10, pp. 747–755.

Hickery, M.S. & Bayliss, M.T. (1998). Interleukin-1 induced nitric oxide inhibic sulphation of glycosaminoglycan chaos in human articular cartilage chondrocytes. Biochimica et Biophysica Acta, Vol. 1425, No.2 , pp. 282- 290.

Hiran, T. S.; Moulton, P.J. ; Hancoc, J.T. (1997). Detection of superoxide and NADPH oxidase in porcine articular chondrocytes. *Free Radical Biology & Medicine,* Vol. 23, No. 5, pp. 736–743.

Hitchon, C. A. & El- Gabalawy, H.S. (2004). Oxidation in rheumatoid arthritis. *Arthritis Res Ther,* Vol. 6, No. 6, pp. 265- 278.

Hollander, A.P.; Corke, K.P.; Freemont, A.J. & Lewis, C.E. (2001). Expression of hypoxia-inducible factor 1 a by macrophages in the rheumatoid synovium. Implications for targeting genes to the inflammaed joint. Arthritis *& Rheumatism,* Vol. 44, No. 7, pp. 1540-1544.

Hovatta, I.; Juhila, J.; Donner, J. (2010). Oxidative stress in anxiety and comorbid disorders. *Neurosci Res,* Vol. 68, No. 4, pp.261-275.

Hultqvist, M.; Olofsson, P.; Gelderman, K. A.; Holmberg, J.; Holmdahl, R. (2006). A New Arthritis Therapy with Oxidative Burst Inducers. *Plos Medicine,* Vol 3, No. 9, pp.1625-1636.

Jikimoto, T.; Nishikubo, Y.; Kanagawa, S.; Morinobu, S.; Saura, R.; Miyuno, K,; Kondo, S.; Toyokuni, S.; Nakamurad, H.; Yodoi, J. & Kumagai, S. (2001). Thioredoxin as a biomarker for oxidative stress in patients with rheumatoid arthritis. *Mol Immunol,* Vol. 38, No. 10 ,pp. 765- 772.

Ji-Yeon, S.; Jang- Hee, H.; Hyung-Sik, K.; Inpyo, Ch.; Sang-Deok, L.; June- Kyu, L.; Jeong-Ho, S.; Jae-Heun, L. & Gang- Min, H. (2000). Methotrexate suppresses the interleukin-6 induced generation of reactive oxygen species in the synoviocytes of rheumatoid arthritis. *Immunopharmacology,* Vol. 47, No. , pp. 35- 44.

Kennett, E.C. & Davies, M.J. (2009). Glycosaminoglycans are fragmented by hydroxy L carbonate and nitrogen dioxide radicals in a site- selective manner: implications for peroxynitrite- mediated damage at sites of inflammation. *Free Radical Biology & Medicine,* Vol. 47, No. 4 , pp. 389- 400.

Khan, F. & Siddiqui, A.A. (2006). Prevalence of anti- 3- nitrotyrosine antibodies in the joint synovial fluid of patients with rheumatoid arthritis, osteoarthritis and systemic lupus erythematosus. *Clin Chim Acta,* Vol. 370, No. 1-2, pp. 100-107.

Kheir- Eldin, A.A; Hamdy, M.A.; Motawi, T.K.; Shaheen, A.A. & Abd El Gawad, H.M. (1992). Biochemical changes in arthritic rats under the influence of vitamin E. *Agents Actions,* Vol. 36, No. 3-4, pp. 300-305.

Kurz, B.; Steinhagen, J. & Schünke, M. (1999). Articular chondrocytes and synoviocytes in a co-culture system: influence on reactive oxygen species- induced cytotoxicity and lipid peroxidation. *Cell Tissue Res,* Vol. 295, No. 3, pp. 555-563.

Lark, M.W.; Bayne, E.K.; Flanagan, J.; Harper, C.F.; Hoerner, L.A.; Hutchinson, N.I.; Singer, I.I.; Donatelli, S,A.; Weidner, J.R.; Williams,H.R.; Mumford, R.A.; Lohmander, L.S. (1997) Aggrecan degradation in human cartilage. Evidence for both matrix metalloproteinase and aggrecanase activity in normal, osteoarthritic, and rheumatoid joints. *J Clin Invest,* Vol. 100, No. , pp.93–106.

Lem van Lent, P.; Nabbe, K.C.; Blom, A.B.; Sloetjes, A.; Holthuysen, A.E.M.; Kolls, J.; Van De Loo, F. A.J.; Holland, S.M. & Van Den Berg, W.B. (2005). (NADPH)-oxidase- driven oxygen radical production determines chondrocyte death and partly regulates metalloproteinase- mediated cartilage matrix degradation during interferon- γ-stimulated immune complex arthritis. *Arth Res & Ther,* Vol. 7, No. 4, pp. 2005.

Lo, Y. C.L.; Wong, J.M.S. & Cruz, T.F. (1998). Reactive oxygen species mediate cytokine activation of c- Jun NH2- terminal kinases. *J Biol Chem,* Vol. 271, No. 26, pp. 15703-15707.

Lushchak, V. (2011). Adaptive response to oxidative stress: Bacteria, fungi, plants and animals. *Comp Biochem Physiol,* Vol. , No. pp. 175- 190.

Mattey, D.L.; Nixon, N.; Alldersea, J.E.; Cotton, W.; Fryer, A.A.; Zhao, L.; Jones, P. & Strange, R.C. (1993). Alpha, mu and pi class glutathione S- transferases in human synovium and cultured synovial fibroblasts: effects of interleukin-1 alpha, hydrogen peroxide and inhibition of eicosanoid synthesis. *Free Radic Res Commun,* Vol. 19, No. 3, pp. 159- 617.

Maurice, M.M.; Nakamura, H.; van der Voort, E.A.; van Vliet, A.I.; Staal, F.J.; Tak, P.P; Breedveld, F.C.& Verweij, C.L. (1997). Evidence for the role of an altered redox state in hyporesponsiveness of synovial T cells in rheumatoid arthritis. *J Immunol,* Vol. 158, No.3, pp. 1458- 1465.

Miesel, R.; Kurpisz, M. & Kröger, H. (1996). Suppression of inflammatory arthritis by simultaneous inhibition of nitric oxide synthase and NADPH oxidase. *Free Radical Biology & Medicine,* Vol. 20, No. 1, pp. 75-81.

Mohan, I.K. & Das, U.N. (1997). Oxidant stress, anti-oxidants and essential fatty acids in systemic lupus erythematosus. *Prostag Leu Ess Fatty Acid,* Vol. 56, No.3, pp. 193- 198.

Monboisse, J.C. & Borel, J.P. (1992). Oxidative damage to collagen. *EXS,* Vol. 62, pp. 323-327.

Newkirk, M.M.; Goldbach- Mansky, R.; Lee, J.; Hoxworth, J.; McCoy, A,; Yarboro, Ch.; Klippel, J. & El- Gabalawy, H.S. (2003). Advanced glycation end-product (AGE)-damaged IgG and IgM autoantibodies to IgG AGE in patients with early synovitis. *Arthritis Res Ther,* Vol. 5, No. 2 , pp. R82- R90.

Olofsson, P.; Holmberg, J.; Tordsson, J.; Lu, S.; Akerström, B. & Holmdahl, R. (2003). Positional identification of Ncf 1 as a gene that regulates arthritis severity in rats. *Nat Genet,* Vol. 33, No. 2 , pp. 25-32.

Ortona, E.; Margutti, P.; Matarrese, P.; Franconi, F.; Malorni, W. (2008). Redox state, cell death and autoimmune diseases: a gender perspective. *Autoimmun Rev,* Vol. 7, No. 7, pp. 579- 584.

Ostrakhovitch, E.A. & Afanas' ev, L.B. (2001). Oxidative stress in rheumatoid arthritis leukocytes: suppression by rutin and other antioxidants and chelators. *Biochemical Pharmacology,* Vol. 62, No. 6, pp. 743-746.

Regan, E.A.; Bowler, R.P. & Crapo, J.D. (2008). Joint fluid antioxidants are decreased in osteoarthritic joints compared to joints with macroscopically intact cartilage and subacute injury. *Osteoarthritis & Cartilage,* Vol. 16, No. 4 , pp. 515- 521.

Ross, A.D.; Banda, N.K.; Muggli, M.; Arend, W.P.(2004). Enhancement of collagen induced arthritis in mice genetically deficient in extracellular superoxide dismuthase. *Arthritis Rheum,* Vol. 50, No. , pp. 3702- 3711.

Sakai, A.; Hirano, T.; Okayaki, R.; Okimoto, N.; Tanaka, K. & Nakamura, T. (1999). Large-dose ascorbic acid administration suppresses the development of arthritis in adjuvant- injected rats. Arch Orthop Trauma Surg, Vol. 119, No. 3-4, pp. 121- 126.

Sarban, S.; Kocyigit, A.; Yazar, M. & Isikan, U.E. (2005). Plasma total antioxidant capacity, lipid peroxidation, and erythrocyte antioxidant enzyme activities in patients with rheumatoid arthritis and osteoarthritis. Clin Bioch, Vol. 38, No.11 , pp. 981- 986.

Seven, A.; Güzel, S.; Aslan, M. & Hamuryudan, V. (2008). Lipid, protein, DNA oxidation and antioxidant status in rheumatoid arthritis. Clin Bioch, Vol. 41, No. 7-8, pp. 538-543.

Shah, D.; Kiran, R.; Wanchu, A. & Bhatnagar, A. (2010). Oxidative stress in systemic lupuys erythematosus: relationship to Th1 cytokine and disease activity. *Immunol Lett,* Vol. 129, pp. 7-12.

Shah, D.; Wanchu, A. & Bhatnagar, A. (2011). Interaction between oxidative stress and chemokines: Possible pathogenic role in systemic lupus erythematosus and rheumatoid arthritis. doi: 10. 1016/ j.imbio. 2001. 04. 001.

Shankar, J.; Thippegowda, P.B. & Kanum, S.A. (2009). Inhibition of HIF-1a activity by BP-1 ameliorates adjuvant induced arthritis in rats. *Biochemical and Biophysical Research Communications,* Vol. 387, No. 2 , pp. 223- 228.

Shingu, M.; Takahashi, S.; Ito, M.; Hamamatu, N.; Suenaga, Y.; Ichibangase, Y.; Nobunaga, M. (1994). Anti- inflammatory effects of recombinant human manganese superoxide dismuthase on adjuvant arthritis in rats. *Rheumatol Int,* Vol. 14, No. 2, pp. 77-81.

Shejkh, Z.; Ahmad, R.; Shejkh, N.; Ali, R. (2007). Enhanced recognition of reactive oxygen species damaged human serum albumin by circulating systemic lupus erythematosus autoantibodies. *Autoimmunity,* Vol. 40, No. 7, pp. 512- 520.

Schett, G.; Tohidast- Akrad, M.; Steiner, G. & Smolen, J. (2001). Commentary. The stressed synovium. *Arthritis Res,* Vol. 3, No. 2, pp. 80-86.

Schneider, N.; Mouithys- Mickalad, A.L.; Lejeune, J.- P.; Deby-Dupont, G.P.; Hoebeke, M. & Serteyn, D.A. (2005). Synoviocytes, not chondrocytes, release free radical after cycles of anoxia/ re-oxygenation. Biochimical *and Biophysical Research Communications,* Vol. 334, No. , pp. 669- 673.

Stefanovic- Racic, M.; Mollers, M.O.; Miller, M.A.& Evans, C.H. (1997). Nitric oxide and proteoglycan turnover in rabbit articular cartilage. *J Orthop Res,* Vol. 15, No. 3, pp. 442- 449.

Šimelyte, E.; Boyle, D. L. & Firestein, G.S. (2004). DNA mismatch repair enzyme expression in synovial tissue. *Ann Rheum Dis,* Vol. 63, No. 12, pp. 1695-1699.

Vasanthi, P.; Nalini, G.; Rajasekhar, R. (2009). Status of oxidative stress in rheumatoid arthritis. *Int J Rheum Dis,* Vol. 12, No., pp. 29- 33.

Taysi, T.; Gul, M.; Saris, R.A.; Akcay, F. & Bakan, N. (2002 a). Serum oxidant/ antioxidant status of patients with systemic lupus erythematosus. *Clin Chem Lab Med,* Vol. 40, No. 7, pp. 684- 688.

Taysi, T.; Polat, F.; Gul, M.; Saris, R.A. Bakan, N. (2002 b). Lipid peroxidation, some extracellular antioxidants, and antioxidant enzymes in serum of patients with rheumatoid arthritis. *Rheumatol Int,* Vol. 21, No. 5, pp. 200- 204.

Tewthanom, K.; Janwityanuchit, S.; Totemchockchyakarn, K. & Panomvana, D. (2008). Correlation of lipid peroxidation and glutatione levels with severity of systemic lupus erythematosus: A pilot study from single center. *J Pharm Pharmaceut Sci,* Vol. 11, No. 3, pp. 30-34.

Van de Loo, F.A.J.; Bennink, M.B.; Arntz, O.J.; Smeets, R.L.; Lubberts, E.; Joosten, L.A.B.; van Lent, P.L.E.M.; Coenen- de Roo, Ch. J.J.; Cuzzocrea, S,; Segal, B.H.; Holland, S.M. & van den Berg, W. B. (2003). Deficiency of NADPH oxidase components p47phox and gp91phox caused granulomatosus synovitis and increased tissue destruction in experimental arthritis model. *Am J Pathol,* Vol. 163, No. 4, pp. 1525- 1536.

Vasanthi, P.; Nalini, G. & Rajasekhar, G. (2009). Status of oxidative stress in rheumatoid arthritis. *Int J Rheum Dis,* Vol. 12, No. 1 , pp. 29- 33.

Yoshida, S.; Katoh, T.; Tetsuka, T.; Uno, K.; Matsui, N. & Okamoto, T. (1999). Involvement of thioredoxin in rheumatoid arthritis: its costimulatory roles in the TNF- α- induced production of IL-6 and IL-8 from cultured synovial fibroblasts. *Immunol,* Vol. 163, No. 1, pp. 351-358.

20

Oxidative Stress in Multiple Organ Damage in Hypertension, Diabetes and CKD, Mechanisms and New Therapeutic Possibilities

Tatsuo Shimosawa* et al.
Department of Clinical Laboratory, Faculty of Medicine, University of Tokyo
Japan

1. Introduction

Hypertension, diabetes, hypercholesterolemia and chronic kidney disease (CKD) lead to cardiovascular (CV) events and cardiovascular death consists of main cause in mortality of those diseases. Understanding of pathophysiology that links them and CV events has been vigorously studied and several factors are believed to play roles such as NO, renin-angiotensin system, and oxidative stress. It has been shown that those factors affect endothelial function and consequently organ circulation as well as function and viability of cells and organs. Despite overwhelming evidences in the consequences of experimental models of ROS-induced organ damage, large-scale clinical trials of former antioxidant therapies, such as vitamin C, vitamin E or β-carotene, could not demonstrate satisfactory benefit to patients and they seemed to be harmful in some cases (Hennekens *et al.*, 1996; Omenn *et al.*, 1996; Virtamo *et al.*, 1998; Hercberg *et al.*, 1999; Lee *et al.*, 1999; Yusuf *et al.*, 2000; de Gaetano, 2001; Heart, 2002; Vivekananthan *et al.*, 2003; Hercberg *et al.*, 2004; Kris-Etherton *et al.*, 2004; Lonn *et al.*, 2005). Several studies concluded that β-carotene supplementation increased the relative risk of death in patients with some types of cancer and had no benefit on patients with cardiovascular disease. Another study said vitamin E increased hemorrhagic stroke. Even antioxidant cocktails increased in all-cause motality (Omenn *et al.*, 1996; Rosen *et al.*, 2001a). So far, supplementation with vitamins C and E, either alone or in combination with each other or with other antioxidant vitamins, does not appear to be efficacious for the treatment of cardiovascular disease (Lonn *et al.*, 2005). We investigated role of oxidative stress in consequences of multiple organ damages in mouse and possible new therapeutic agent.

---

* Tomoyo Kaneko[2], Xu Qingyou[1], Yusei Miyamoto[3], Mu Shengyu[2], Hong Wang[2], Sayoko Ogura[2], Rika Jimbo[2], Bohumil Majtan[2], Yuzaburo Uetake[2], Daigoro Hirohama[2], Fumiko Kawakami-Mori[2], Toshiro Fujita[2] and Yutaka Yatomi[1]
[1] *Department of Clinical Laboratory, Faculty of Medicine, University of Tokyo, Japan*
[2] *Department of Endocrinology and Nephrology, Faculty of Medicinem, Japan*
[3] *Department of Integrated Biosciences, Graduate School of Frontier Sciences, University of Tokyo, Japan*

2. Adrenomedullin

2.1 Cardiovascular effects

Adrenomedullin is a 52-amino-acid peptide and was originally isolated from pheochromocytoma cell but is also produced and secreted in endothelial cells and potent hypotensive peptide (Shimosawa & Fujita, 2005). We generated its deficient mice and proved that it is an endogenous antioxidants.

We examined the antioxidant properties of AM in both angiotensin II-salt (Shimosawa *et al.*, 2002) and pulmonary hypertension models (Matsui *et al.*, 2004). We showed that AM-knockout mice had higher oxidative stress through 3 ways: the urinary excretion of oxidative stress markers, such as 8-hydroxydeoxyguanosine (Fig. 1a) and isoprostane (Fig. 1b) by ELISA method, the immunostaining of 3-nitrotyrosine to localize oxidative stress (Fig. 1c), and real-time oxidant production measurement by the electron spin resonance (ESR) method (Fig. 1d). Pathological changes in the heart, such as periarterial fibrosis and coronary artery occlusion, were prominent in the knockout mice, and further investigation revealed that high oxidative stress caused coronary artery damage in this model.

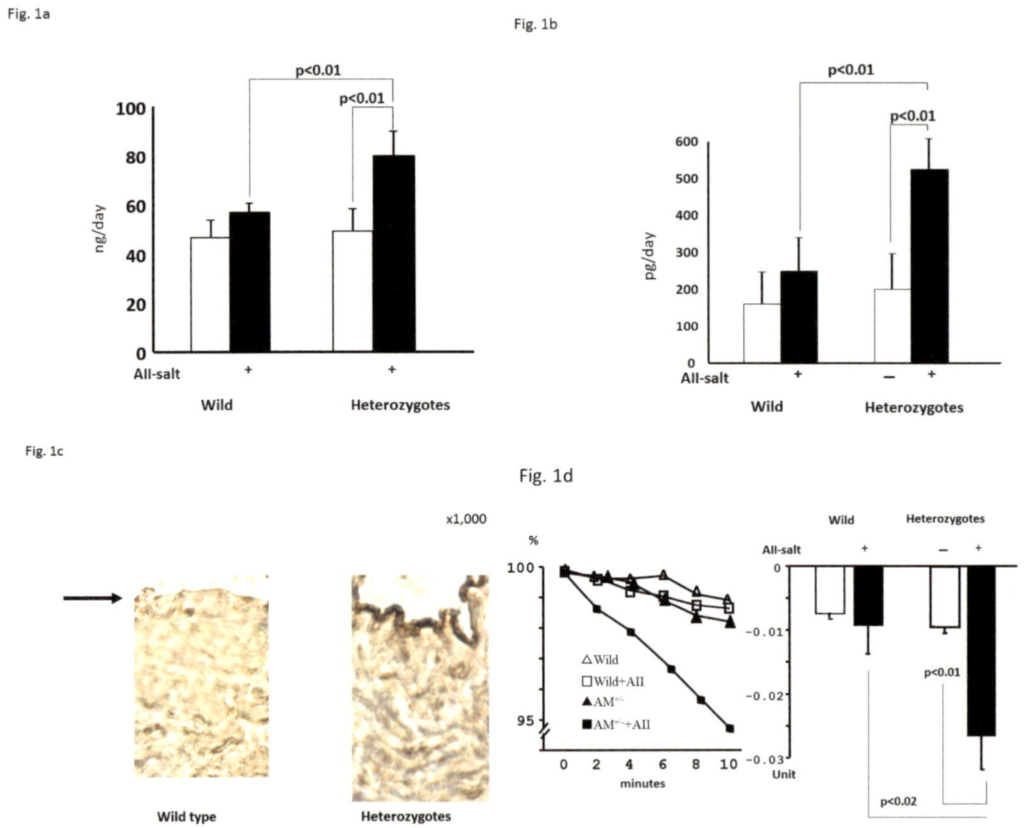

Fig. 1. Evaluation of oxidative stress in $AM^{+/-}$ mice after angiotensin II and salt loading.

We measured urinary excretion of 8-OHdG (a) and isoprostane (b) as footsteps of oxidative stress in whole body. As for confirming local oxidative stress, we immunostained coronary artery with 3-nitrotyrosine (c) that reflects NO-related oxidative stress and is a good marker for oxidative stress at the endothelial layer (arrow). For evaluation of real time production of oxidative stress, we measured ESR signal in the heart (d). On the left of panel d, time dependent of decay of ESR signal were plotted and on the right panel, the decay ratio of ESR signal that reflects production of oxidative stress was calculated. All these data suggest angiotensin II and salt-loaded $AM^{+/-}$ mice has higher oxidative stress than wild type mice. Modified from Shimosawa *et al.* 2002.

Hypoxia is known to cause pulmonary hypertension and pulmonary vascular remodeling. With this model, evidence is accumulating that ROS are the upstream signals of chronic hypoxia-induced pulmonary vasoconstriction and the development of vascular remodeling. It has been reported that ROS generated by hypoxia can induce calcium release from sarcoplasmic reticulum stores, which is followed by pulmonary vasoconstriction (Waypa *et al.*, 2002). Moreover, ROS activated several growth factors such as vascular endothelial growth factor and platelet-activating factor (PAF) (Hartung *et al.*, 1983; Ono *et al.*, 1992; Chandel *et al.*, 1998), which induce vascular remodeling. In the early phase of hypoxic conditions, ROS may act as a trigger of this signaling cascade in the process of vascular remodeling. In our experiments, 10% O_2 conditions caused higher ROS in AM-knockout mice compared with wild-type mice. Concomitant with increased oxidative stress in the pulmonary artery, AM-knockout mice showed marked vascular remodeling and higher mortality (Matsui *et al.*, 2004), which were reversed by AM supplementation or by treatment with 4-Hydroxy-2,2,6,6-tetramethyl-piperidine-N-oxyl (hydroxyl-TEMPO), a mimetic of superoxide dismutase. Based on this basic research, translational research studies have been conducted in patients with pulmonary hypertension, and potent therapeutic effects of inhaling AM have been reported (Nagaya *et al.*, 2004). As the mortality among patients with pulmonary hypertension is high even treatment with nitric oxide and prostaglandins, AM, or other agents may be novel and promising agents for the treatment of these patients.

2.2 Renal effects and possible role in CKD and diabetic kidney disease

Renal dysfunction or chronic kidney disease (CKD) draws high interests among nephrologists as well as cardiologists and other specialities. There are several factors implicated to connect renal dysfunction and cardiovascular events, endothelial dysfunction, renin-angiotensin-aldosterone axis, oxidative stress, and unknown toxic agents. In order to investigate if renin-angiotensin axis and oxidative stress can be therapeutical target in CKD, we used AM knockout mice. We found increased oxidative stress and local renin-angiotensin system in the ureter-obstructed kidney of AM knockout mice. Concordance with the increase of oxidative stress and renin-angiotensin system, severe interstitial fibrosis, and cell proliferation were prominent in AM-knockout mice. The interstitial fibrosis can be partly reversed by hydroxyl-TEMPO, angiotensin receptor blockers, or the systemic replacement of AM (unpublished observation). When dual treatment with angiotensin receptor blocker and hydroxyl-TEMPO were given, pathological changes are more effectively reversed compared with that by each agent alone. Angiotensin II is known to induce oxidative stress via activating NADPH oxidase and AM can block this pathway via c-Src (Liu *et al.*, 2007). In the kidney, oxidative stress is generated not only by NADPH oxidase but from mitochondria and xanthine oxidase and thus AM or angiotensin II blocker alone therapy is not sufficient and together with hydroxyl-TEMPO that can totally block oxidative stress is effective.

Multiple lines of study have shown that diabetic patients have increased oxidative stress and the resultant organ damage (Rosen *et al.*, 2001b). In turn, it is hypothesized that oxidative stress can induce diabetes by series of studies; oxidative stress impairs insulin internalization (Bertelsen *et al.*, 2001), blocks insulin receptor substrate phosphorylation, impairs phosphoinositide-3 kinase activity (Najib & Sanchez-Margalet, 2001), induces protein glycation and as a consequence of advanced glycation end-products-receptor binding that leads to cytotoxicity in pancreatic beta cells and reduces the translocation of glucose transporter type-4 (Rudich *et al.*, 1997; Rudich *et al.*, 1998). An in vivo study also showed that the administration of oxidative stress aggravated diabetes in diabetes-prone obese-Zucker rats (Laight *et al.*, 2000). Antioxidan supplementation studies have shown conflicting resuts; some reported beneficial effects in endothelial function, retinal blood flow and renal function outcomes (Blum *et al.*; Ziegler *et al.*, 2004; Lopes de Jesus *et al.*, 2008), in contrast, the recent metaanalysis of antioxidants, vitamin C and E, supplementation trials revealed ineffectiveness in glycemic control (Akbar *et al.*, 2011). On the other hand, in clinical settings, diabetics have higher oxidative stress and AM levels (Hayashi *et al.*, 1997), which led us to assume that AM is upregulated in order to antagonize oxidative stress. In fact, aged or angiotensin II-treated AM-knockout mice showed insulin resistance, and this was reversed by AM supplementation (Shimosawa *et al.*, 2003; Xing *et al.*, 2004) (Fig. 2). In this experiment, we showed that oxidative stress directly impaired insulin signaling by interfering with insulin receptor substrate 1 and 2 phosphorylations. By in vitro experiments, we found that oxidative stress not only impairs insulin signaling, but also reduces glucose transporter 4 transcription (unpublished observation).

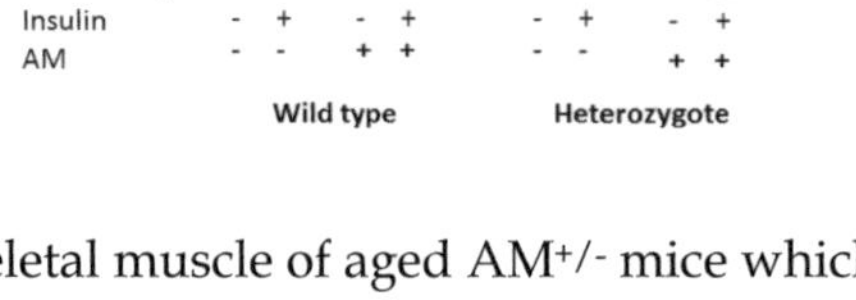

Fig. 2. Insulin resistance in skeletal muscle of aged $AM^{+/-}$ mice which was recovered by AM supplement.

Insulin resistance was measured by ex vivo experiments. Isolated soleus muscle was incubated with insulin and ^{12}C-deoxyglucose. Deoxyglucose uptake was evaluated as insulin sensitivity. Aged male $AM^{+/-}$ mice (55 weeks old) showed insulin resistance and AM supplementation for a month successfully reversed insulin resistant state. Modified from Shimosawa *et al.* 2003.

Recent clinical trial in diabetic CKD patients revealed bardoxolone methyl effectively improved in the estimated GFR independent from blood pressure which is the most important risk in CKD (Pergola *et al.*, 2011). Also, it improved insulin resistance by increasing glucose uptake in skeletal muscle (Saha *et al.*), which is compatible with our findings in AM knockout mice as described above. Bardoxolone methyl is an oral antioxidant inflammation modulator and activates the Keap1–Nrf2 pathway. Keap1-Nrf2 pathway regulates inflammation and oxidative stress (Dinkova-Kostova *et al.*, 2005) via increased expression of heme oxygenase 1 (Wu *et al.*, 2011). This compound is so far the only clinically available antioxidants that show organ protective effect, however, it requires further assessment if bardoxolone methyl can prevent hard end-point such as cardiovascular events or mortality in CKD patients.

3. Platinum nanoparticle

In diabetic-CKD, possible clinical usefulness of bardoxolone methyl was shown as mentioned above, so far few antioxidant agents are proved to be effective in cardiovascular protection. Although in pulmonary hypertension AM showed its clinical usefulness by inhaling, AM is a peptide and its clinical use is limited due to its short half life. We next investigated the possible therapeutic effect of platinum-nano-particle.

In recent years, a few reports about new drug delivery system using nanotechnology have been released (Muro *et al.*, 2006; Kajita *et al.*, 2007; Shimizu et al., 2010). Among them platinum nanoparticles as both superoxide dismutase (SOD) mimetic and catalase mimetic (Kajita *et al.*, 2007; Watanabe *et al.*, 2009). In vivo experiments shows its effectiveness in smoking-induced lung damage (Onizawa *et al.*, 2009) or stroke model mice (Takamiya et al.*et al.*, 2011). Platinum nanoparticles (PAA-Pt) was administered intranasally, which were then exposed to cigarette smoking for 3 days. Cigarette smoking induced NFkappaB activation, and neutrophilic inflammation in the lungs of mice, and intranasal administration of PAA-Pt inhibited these changes. Moreover in in vitro experiments, treatment of alveolar-type-II-like A549 cells with PAA-Pt inhibited cell death after exposure to a cigarette smoke extract. Transient middle cerebral artery occlusion (tMCAO) and reperfusion model was used in this study. PAA-Pt was administered intravenously. PAA-Pt dramatically reduced oxidative stress in the brain and significantly improved the motor function and greatly reduced the infarct volume, especially in the cerebral cortex with preserved collagen IV and a remarkable suppression of MMP-9. By these acute models the antioxidant effect and concomitant organ protection by PAA-Pt were established. We investigated the chronic effect of PAA-Pt and studied if PAA-Pt reverse cardiovascular damage in metabolic syndrome model by eliminating ROS.

Metabolic syndrome model was established by angiotensin II and high salt diet on diabetic 8-week-old male db/db mice. 10 μM platinum nanoparticles were given orally. The oxidative stress was measured in two ways. First, the urinary excretion of isoprostane reflects the state of systemic oxidative stress. Ang II and salt loading increased isoprostane excretion in db/db mice. PAA-Pt reduced isoprostane excretion, suggesting that PAA-Pt would be an effective antioxidant (Fig 3). Blood pressure was elevated by angiotensin II and high salt diet and PAA-Pt treatment did not have any effects on blood pressure and other metabolic biomarkers of mice.

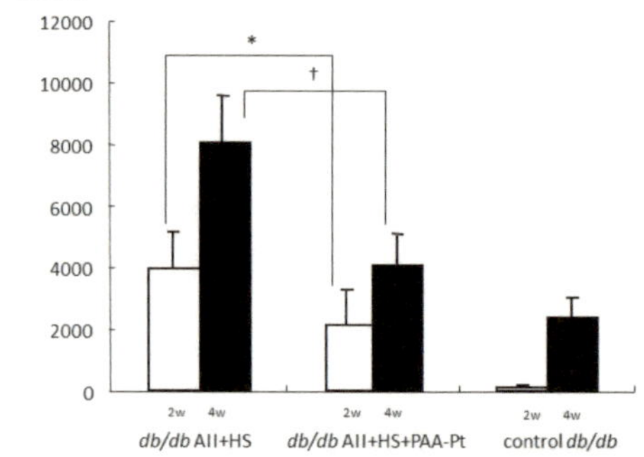

Fig. 3. PAA-Pt effect on oxidative stress

Db/db mice were treated with angiotensin II and high salt diet and urinary isoprostane was measured as a marker of oxidative stress. PAA-Pt effectively reduced oxidative stress.

Consistent with AM knockout mice, angiotensin II and high salt diet induced pericoronary fibrosis in db/db mice (Fig. 4a). The degree of deterioration of vascular damage was much severer in the db/db mice than wild type mice. PAA-Pt therapy reversed the vascular damage in angiotensin II/salt loaded db/db mice. The area of fibrous changes was calculated for each group (Fig 4b). The results of RT-PCR supported the aforesaid

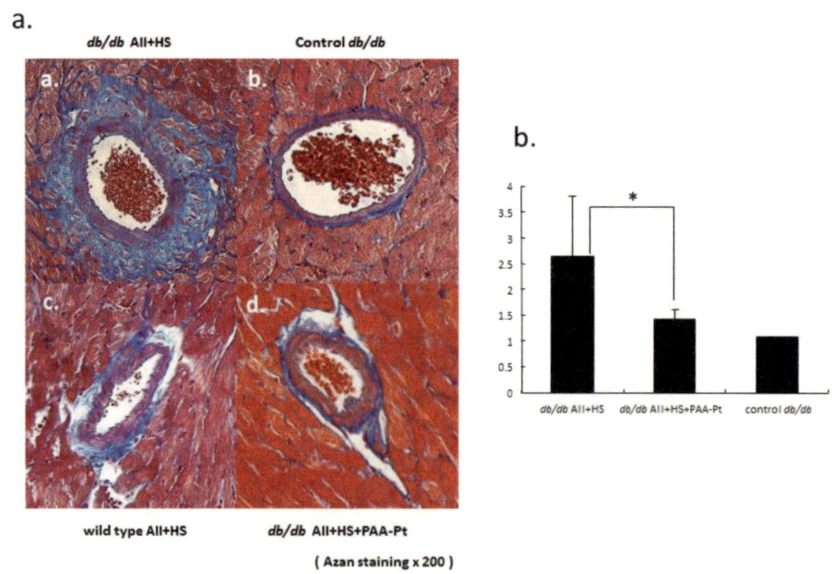

Fig. 4. Histopathological changes of db/db mice by angiotensin II/high salt diet and effect of PAA-Pt.

histopathological findings. We examined mRNA expression of ANP and procollagen type Iα in the heart as molecular markers of cardiac damage and we found that those molecular markers were apparently up-regulated by angiotensin II and salt loading (Fig 5). PAA-Pt reduced these markers expressions to the almost same extent with the control db/db mice and these results support our findings in the histopathological examinations.

Pericoronary fibrosis were evaluated by Azan staining. Fibrosis was robust by angiotensin II and high salt diet and was reversed by PAA-Pt.

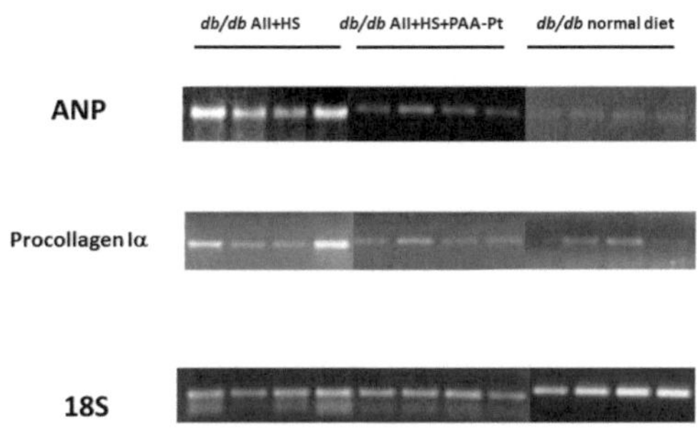

Fig. 5. Molecular markers for cardiac damage and fibrosis.

mRNA expression of ANP and procollagen type I were evaluated. Concomitant with figure 4, angiotensin II and high salt diet aggravated cardiac damage and it was reversed by PAA-Pt.

PAA-Pt behaves as an SOD mimetic and possesses a catalase activity, then its efficacy can last longer than vitamin C (Kajita *et al.*, 2007). It is mainly because the catalytic property of PAA-Pt which is distinguished from vitamin C that is quickly consumed. Therefore we examined the effect of PAA-Pt in metabolic syndrome model mice to reduce oxidative stress and protect the cardiovascular system. Concordance with in vitro study, PAA-Pt effectually reduced ROS and prevented cardiovascular damage in hypertensive db/db mice.

We found the extension of cardiovascular damages was much severer and the level of systemic oxidative stress, which was evaluated by urinary excretion of isoprostane, was much higher in db/db mice. Then, it is indicated that the 'metabolic-syndrome-status' is equal to 'high-oxidative-stress-status' and this status seems to be the trigger of the vicious cycle of organ damage. Thus, the scavenging ROS would be a promising approach to preventing organ damage in metabolic syndrome.

PAA-Pt also has the possibility to solve the problems of former antioxidants as vitamin C, E or β-carotene. It is said the one of the reasons why those former antioxidants would have failed to be effective against organ damage that they are short-acting and could not eliminate intracellular ROS, including mitochondrial ROS. PAA-Pt possesses long-lasting activity (means catalytic effect) and dual properties as SOD and catalase mimetics. The pharmacokinetics of PAA-Pt in detail have not been revealed yet that PAA-Pt should enter to systemic circulation from digestive apparatus, and be excreted from urine. Also we suggestively expect the novel antioxidant PAA-Pt enables to eliminate intracellular ROS. Further studies in pharmacokinetics and safety of PAA-Pt in chronic use are required. Specially, PAA-Pt contains platinum, which is sometimes toxic to the kidney, we must be careful about its nephrotoxicity before clinical applications. In site of some assignments such as its safety or full internal dynamism must be proven before clinical use, this novel agent will be certain way to open the door to interdisciplinary treatments between nanotechnology and medicine.

4. Perspectives

Piles of evidence accumulated that oxidative stress is a new therapeutic targets in preventing cardiovascular events and its risks. Among risks, hypertension, glucose metabolism and lipid accumulation in the vasculature are closely related with oxidative stress, however, some but not all antioxidant lower blood pressure or prevent atherosclerosis. Blood pressure is regulated by both circulating blood volume and vascular resistance and most of the data suggest that oxidative stress may affect vascular resistance but not blood volume, which can explain antioxidant therapy is not consistent in lowering blood pressure. For lipid disorders and consecutive atherosclerosis, oxidized LDL as well as its receptor is important. In mice LDL level are almost negligible however, oxidized LDL receptor such as LOX-1 overexpression leads to vascular damage (Inoue *et al.*, 2005). It suggests that ligand regulation by targeting oxidative stress is not sufficient but we should consider receptor regulation as well. On the other hand, insulin resistance or glucose metabolism can be a good target of antioxidant therapy. Insulin signaling is impaired by oxidative stress and it is reversed by antioxidants. Our and others' basic trials as well as recent data by bardoxolone methyl are promising, although the optimal glucose regulation level to prevent cardiovascular complications in diabetes are still under debate. The 'lower the better' of blood glucose is controversial because of hypoglycemia induces poor prognosis in cardiovascular event, however, targeting oxidative stress recovers impaired-insulin resistance and does not stimulate insulin release, therefore, it would be safer than insulin replacement or insulin secretion stimulating agents such as sulphonylurea. Further clinical trials are required.

5. Conclusion

AM, PAA-PT or bardoxolone are possibly promising antioxidants in treating or reducing risks for chronic metabolic disease and organ damages. Other possible agents are also under investigations and novel technology will lead us to invent antioxidants with more efficacy and less side effect. Oxidative stress is indispensable for host defence and appropriate reduction of oxidative stress is required when considering antioxidants in clinical use.

6. References

Akbar S, Bellary S & Griffiths HR. (2011). Dietary Antioxidant Interventions in Type 2 Diabetes Patients A Meta-analysis. *Br J Diabetes Vasc Dis* 11, 62-68.

Bertelsen M, Anggard EE & Carrier MJ. (2001). Oxidative stress impairs insulin internalization in endothelial cells in vitro. *Diabetologia* 44, 605-613.

Blum S, Vardi M, Brown JB, Russell A, Milman U, Shapira C, Levy NS, Miller-Lotan R, Asleh R & Levy AP. Vitamin E reduces cardiovascular disease in individuals with diabetes mellitus and the haptoglobin 2-2 genotype. *Pharmacogenomics* 11, 675-684.

Chandel NS, Maltepe E, Goldwasser E, Mathieu CE, Simon MC & Schumacker PT. (1998). Mitochondrial reactive oxygen species trigger hypoxia-induced transcription. *Proc Natl Acad Sci U S A* 95, 11715-11720.

de Gaetano G. (2001). Low-dose aspirin and vitamin E in people at cardiovascular risk: a randomised trial in general practice. Collaborative Group of the Primary Prevention Project. *Lancet* 357, 89-95.

Dinkova-Kostova AT, Liby KT, Stephenson KK, Holtzclaw WD, Gao X, Suh N, Williams C, Risingsong R, Honda T, Gribble GW, Sporn MB & Talalay P. (2005). Extremely potent triterpenoid inducers of the phase 2 response: correlations of protection against oxidant and inflammatory stress. *Proc Natl Acad Sci U S A* 102, 4584-4589.

Hartung HP, Parnham MJ, Winkelmann J, Englberger W & Hadding U. (1983). Platelet activating factor (PAF) induces the oxidative burst in macrophages. *Int J Immunopharmacol* 5, 115-121.

Hayashi M, Shimosawa T, Isaka M, Yamada S, Fujita R & Fujita T. (1997). Plasma adrenomedullin in diabetes. *Lancet* 350, 1449-1450.

Heart P, Study, Collaborative, Group. (2002). MRC/BHF Heart Protection Study of antioxidant vitamin supplementation in 20,536 high-risk individuals: a randomised placebo-controlled trial. *Lancet* 360, 23-33.

Hennekens CH, Buring JE, Manson JE, Stampfer M, Rosner B, Cook NR, Belanger C, LaMotte F, Gaziano JM, Ridker PM, Willett W & Peto R. (1996). Lack of effect of long-term supplementation with beta carotene on the incidence of malignant neoplasms and cardiovascular disease. *N Engl J Med* 334, 1145-1149.

Hercberg S, Galan P, Preziosi P, Bertrais S, Mennen L, Malvy D, Roussel AM, Favier A & Briancon S. (2004). The SU.VI.MAX Study: a randomized, placebo-controlled trial of the health effects of antioxidant vitamins and minerals. *Arch Intern Med* 164, 2335-2342.

Hercberg S, Preziosi P, Galan P, Faure H, Arnaud J, Duport N, Malvy D, Roussel AM, Briancon S & Favier A. (1999). "The SU.VI.MAX Study": a primary prevention trial using nutritional doses of antioxidant vitamins and minerals in cardiovascular diseases and cancers. SUpplementation on VItamines et Mineraux AntioXydants. *Food Chem Toxicol* 37, 925-930.

Inoue K, Arai Y, Kurihara H, Kita T & Sawamura T. (2005). Overexpression of lectin-like oxidized low-density lipoprotein receptor-1 induces intramyocardial vasculopathy in apolipoprotein E-null mice. *Circ Res* 97, 176-184.

Kajita M, Hikosaka K, Iitsuka M, Kanayama A, Toshima N & Miyamoto Y. (2007). Platinum nanoparticle is a useful scavenger of superoxide anion and hydrogen peroxide. *Free Radic Res* 41, 615-626.

Kris-Etherton PM, Lichtenstein AH, Howard BV, Steinberg D & Witztum JL. (2004). Antioxidant vitamin supplements and cardiovascular disease. *Circulation* 110, 637-641.

Laight DW, Desai KM, Anggard EE & Carrier MJ. (2000). Endothelial dysfunction accompanies a pro-oxidant, pro-diabetic challenge in the insulin resistant, obese Zucker rat in vivo. *Eur J Pharmacol* 402, 95-99.

Lee IM, Cook NR, Manson JE, Buring JE & Hennekens CH. (1999). Beta-carotene supplementation and incidence of cancer and cardiovascular disease: the Women's Health Study. *J Natl Cancer Inst* 91, 2102-2106.

Liu J, Shimosawa T, Matsui H, Meng F, Supowit SC, Dipette DJ, Ando K & Fujita T. (2007). Adrenomedullin Inhibits Angiotensin II-Induced Oxidative Stress Via Csk-Mediated Inhibition of Src Activity. *Am J Physiol Heart Circ Physiol* 292, H1714-H1721.

Lonn E, Bosch J, Yusuf S, Sheridan P, Pogue J, Arnold JM, Ross C, Arnold A, Sleight P, Probstfield J & Dagenais GR. (2005). Effects of long-term vitamin E supplementation on cardiovascular events and cancer: a randomized controlled trial. *Jama* 293, 1338-1347.

Lopes de Jesus CC, Atallah AN, Valente O & Moca Trevisani VF. (2008). Vitamin C and superoxide dismutase (SOD) for diabetic retinopathy. *Cochrane Database Syst Rev*, CD006695.

Matsui H, Shimosawa T, Itakura K, Guanqun X, Ando K & Fujita T. (2004). Adrenomedullin Can Protect Against Pulmonary Vascular Remodeling Induced by Hypoxia. *Circulation* 109, 2246-2251.

Muro S, Mateescu M, Gajewski C, Robinson M, Muzykantov VR & Koval M. (2006). Control of intracellular trafficking of ICAM-1-targeted nanocarriers by endothelial Na+/H+ exchanger proteins. *Am J Physiol Lung Cell Mol Physiol* 290, L809-817.

Nagaya N, Kyotani S, Uematsu M, Ueno K, Oya H, Nakanishi N, Shirai M, Mori H, Miyatake K & Kangawa K. (2004). Effects of adrenomedullin inhalation on hemodynamics and exercise capacity in patients with idiopathic pulmonary arterial hypertension. *Circulation* 109, 351-356.

Najib S & Sanchez-Margalet V. (2001). Homocysteine thiolactone inhibits insulin signaling, and glutathione has a protective effect. *J Mol Endocrinol* 27, 85-91.

Omenn GS, Goodman GE, Thornquist MD, Balmes J, Cullen MR, Glass A, Keogh JP, Meyskens FL, Valanis B, Williams JH, Barnhart S & Hammar S. (1996). Effects of a combination of beta carotene and vitamin A on lung cancer and cardiovascular disease. *N Engl J Med* 334, 1150-1155.

Onizawa S, Aoshiba K, Kajita M, Miyamoto Y & Nagai A. (2009). Platinum nanoparticle antioxidants inhibit pulmonary inflammation in mice exposed to cigarette smoke. *Pulm Pharmacol Ther* 22, 340-349.

Ono S, Westcott JY & Voelkel NF. (1992). PAF antagonists inhibit pulmonary vascular remodeling induced by hypobaric hypoxia in rats. *J Appl Physiol* 73, 1084-1092.

Pergola PE, Raskin P, Toto RD, Meyer CJ, Huff JW, Grossman EB, Krauth M, Ruiz S, Audhya P, Christ-Schmidt H, Wittes J & Warnock DG. (2011). Bardoxolone methyl and kidney function in CKD with type 2 diabetes. *N Engl J Med* 365, 327-336.

Rosen P, Nawroth PP, King G, Moller W, Tritschler HJ & Packer L. (2001a). The role of oxidative stress in the onset and progression of diabetes and its complications: a summary of a Congress Series sponsored by UNESCO-MCBN, the American Diabetes Association and the German Diabetes Society. *Diabetes Metab Res Rev* 17, 189-212.

Rosen P, Nawroth PP, King G, Moller W, Tritschler HJ & Packer L. (2001b). The role of oxidative stress in the onset and progression of diabetes and its complications: a summary of a Congress Series sponsored by UNESCO-MCBN, the American Diabetes Association and the German Diabetes Society. *Diabetes Metab Res Rev* 17, 189-212.

Rudich A, Kozlovsky N, Potashnik R & Bashan N. (1997). Oxidant stress reduces insulin responsiveness in 3T3-L1 adipocytes. *Am J Physiol* 272, E935-940.

Rudich A, Tirosh A, Potashnik R, Hemi R, Kanety H & Bashan N. (1998). Prolonged oxidative stress impairs insulin-induced GLUT4 translocation in 3T3-L1 adipocytes. *Diabetes* 47, 1562-1569.

Saha PK, Reddy VT, Konopleva M, Andreeff M & Chan L. (2010). The triterpenoid 2-cyano-3,12-dioxooleana-1,9-dien-28-oic-acid methyl ester has potent anti-diabetic effects in diet-induced diabetic mice and Lepr(db/db) mice. *J Biol Chem* 285, 40581-40592.

Shimizu H, Hori Y, Kaname S, Yamada K, Nishiyama N, Matsumoto S, Miyata K, Oba M, Yamada A, Kataoka K & Fujita T. (2010). siRNA-based therapy ameliorates glomerulonephritis. *J Am Soc Nephrol* 21, 622-633.

Shimosawa T & Fujita T. (2005). Adrenomedullin and its related peptide. *Endocr J* 52, 1-10.

Shimosawa T, Ogihara T, Matsui H, Asano T, Ando K & Fujita T. (2003). Deficiency of adrenomedullin induces insulin resistance by increasing oxidative stress. *Hypertension* 41, 1080-1085.

Shimosawa T, Shibagaki Y, Ishibashi K, Kitamura K, Kangawa K, Kato S, Ando K & Fujita T. (2002). Adrenomedullin, an Endogenous Peptide, Counteracts Cardiovascular Damage. *Circulation* 105, 106-111.

Takamiya M, Miyamoto Y, Yamashita T, Deguchi K, Ohta Y, Ikeda Y, Matsuura T & Abe K. (2011). Neurological and pathological improvements of cerebral infarction in mice with platinum nanoparticles. *J Neurosci Res* 89, 1125-1133.

Virtamo J, Rapola JM, Ripatti S, Heinonen OP, Taylor PR, Albanes D & Huttunen JK. (1998). Effect of vitamin E and beta carotene on the incidence of primary nonfatal myocardial infarction and fatal coronary heart disease. *Arch Intern Med* 158, 668-675.

Vivekananthan DP, Penn MS, Sapp SK, Hsu A & Topol EJ. (2003). Use of antioxidant vitamins for the prevention of cardiovascular disease: meta-analysis of randomised trials. *Lancet* 361, 2017-2023.

Watanabe A, Kajita M, Kim J, Kanayama A, Takahashi K, Mashino T & Miyamoto Y. (2009). In vitro free radical scavenging activity of platinum nanoparticles. *Nanotechnology* 20, 455105.

Waypa GB, Marks JD, Mack MM, Boriboun C, Mungai PT & Schumacker PT. (2002). Mitochondrial reactive oxygen species trigger calcium increases during hypoxia in pulmonary arterial myocytes. *Circ Res* 91, 719-726.

Wu QQ, Wang Y, Senitko M, Meyer C, Wigley WC, Ferguson DA, Grossman E, Chen J, Zhou XJ, Hartono J, Winterberg P, Chen B, Agarwal A & Lu CY. (2011). Bardoxolone methyl (BARD) ameliorates ischemic AKI and increases expression of protective genes Nrf2, PPARgamma, and HO-1. *Am J Physiol Renal Physiol* 300, F1180-1192.

Xing G, Shimosawa T, Ogihara T, Matsui H, Itakura K, Qingyou X, Asano T, Ando K & Fujita T. (2004). Angiotensin II-induced insulin resistance is enhanced in adrenomedullin-deficient mice. *Endocrinology* 145, 3647-3651. Epub 2004 Apr 3622.

Yusuf S, Dagenais G, Pogue J, Bosch J & Sleight P. (2000). Vitamin E supplementation and cardiovascular events in high-risk patients. The Heart Outcomes Prevention Evaluation Study Investigators. *N Engl J Med* 342, 154-160.

Ziegler D, Nowak H, Kempler P, Vargha P & Low PA. (2004). Treatment of symptomatic diabetic polyneuropathy with the antioxidant alpha-lipoic acid: a meta-analysis. *Diabet Med* 21, 114-121.

21

Retinal Vein Occlusion Induced by a MEK Inhibitor – Impact of Oxidative Stress on the Blood-Retinal Barrier

Amy H. Yang and Wenhu Huang
Drug Safety Research & Development, Pfizer Inc., La Jolla Laboratories, USA

1. Introduction

The retina is a highly specialized sensory organ that transduces light energy into neural signal. It also has high energy requirement and an extensive vascular network. Reactive oxygen species (ROS) generated via light exposure, normal energy production, phagocytosis of spent photoreceptor membranes by retinal pigment epithelium (RPE) cells, and circulating toxins render retina at an increased risk for oxidative stress (Hardy et al., 2005; Siu et al., 2008). To cope with the high oxidant load, the retina is equipped with various antioxidant defense mechanisms, such as the expression of glutathione peroxidase and superoxide dismutase, the production of glutathione by Müller cells, high levels of vitamins C and E, and the presence of free radical scavenger melanin in RPE cells (Siu et al., 2008). However, when the redox balance is disrupted, retinal pathologies could result, and one of the consequences is impairment of the blood retinal barrier (BRB). Indeed, several retinal diseases have been shown or postulated to be linked to a state of oxidative stress and resulting BRB dysfunction.

Previously, we investigated the molecular mechanisms towards the development of retinal vein occlusion (RVO) in cancer patients treated with a mitogen-activated protein kinase kinase (MEK) inhibitor, PD0325901 (LoRusso et al., 2010). Through gene expression profiling analysis, we identified several mechanisms relevant to the development of RVO, including oxidative stress response, acute phase and inflammatory response, blood-retinal barrier (BRB) breakdown, leukostasis, and coagulation cascade (Huang et al., 2009).

This chapter aims to provide an overview of BRB structures and functions, the role of oxidative stress in BRB disruption and development of retinal pathologies, a detailed overview of RVO, and finally, a description of proposed mechanisms of PD0325901-induced RVO, highlighting several important cellular and molecular processes relevant to this pathology.

2. Blood-retinal barrier

The BRB has an endothelial and an epithelial component, namely the tight junctions between the endothelial cells of the inner retinal vessels, and those between cells of the RPE;

these cell types comprise integral components of the inner and outer BRB, respectively (Siu et al., 2008; Fig. 1A). The BRB regulates the transport of fluid and molecules between the retinal tissue and vasculature, hence playing an important role in maintaining the homeostatsis of the retinal microenvironment (Kaur et al., 2008; Siu et al., 2008).

2.1 Inner blood-retinal barrier

The inner BRB is composed of endothelial cells, astrocytes, Müller cells, and pericytes (Fig. 1A). Tight junctions between capillary endothelial cells form the basis of the inner BRB (Fig. 1B). Astrocytes, Müller cells and pericytes, all closely associated with the endothelial cells of the inner BRB, contribute to proper BRB functions.

The endothelial cells of inner retinal capillaries are not fenestrated, contributing to their low permeability. Solutes traverse the retinal endothelium via both the transcellular and paracellular pathways: the former involves vesicle-mediated transport of macromolecules, and the latter, passage through minute intercellular space safeguarded by junctional proteins (Vandenbroucke et al., 2008; Fig. 1B). Tight junctions consist of occludins, claudins, and junctional adhesion molecules (JAMs), all of which form complexes between adjacent endothelial cells. Zonula occludens (ZO) proteins link occludins and claudins to the endothelial actin cytoskeleton via cingulin. In addition to tight junctions, adherens junctions (AJ) also contribute to the endothelial barrier, where vascular endothelial (VE) cadherins on adjacent endothelial cells form a homophilic complex (Garrido-Urbani et al., 2008; Vandenbroucke et al., 2008). The C-terminal domain of VE-cadherin binds β-catenins and α-catenins, linking the AJs to the actin cytoskeleton. Several lines of evidence show that the regulation of actin cytoskeletal dynamics is central to the proper functioning of the endothelial barrier (Houle and Huot, 2006; Houle et al., 2003; Huot et al., 1998; Lum and Roebuck, 2001). It has also been reported that retinal endothelial cells are more susceptible to oxidative damage, leading to increased permeability, than endothelial cells at other sites. Indeed, ROS are also known to induce the expression of vascular endothelial growth factor (VEGF), a well-known endothelial mitogen and permeability factor, which contributes to the breakdown of BRB in experimental diabetes models (Chua et al., 1998; El-Remessy et al., 2003).

Pericytes line the outer surface of endothelial cells (Fig. 1A) and are contractile in nature, expressing actin, myosin, and tropomyosin (Kaur et al., 2008). They contract in response to signals such as hypoxia, endothelin-1, and angiontensin II, and relax on exposure to carbon dioxide, nitric oxide and adenosine. Therefore, pericytes regulate the vascular tone and blood flow. Under normoxia, they maintain the integrity of the inner BRB by inducing mRNA and protein expression of occludin and ZO-1, and by partially reversing the occludin decrease under hypoxia. Loss of pericytes and disruption of inner BRB are early events in diabetes.

Müller cells are the principal glial cells of the retina, and a functional link between neurons and vessels (Reichenbach et al., 2007). They span the inner and outer limiting membranes of the retina, with their foot processes in close contact with the retinal endothelial cells (Fig. 1A). Under physiological conditions, Müller cells contribute to the integrity of the BRB; however, when exposed to cellular stress they impair the barrier function. Under normoxia, Müller cells secrete pigment epithelium-derived factor (PEDF),

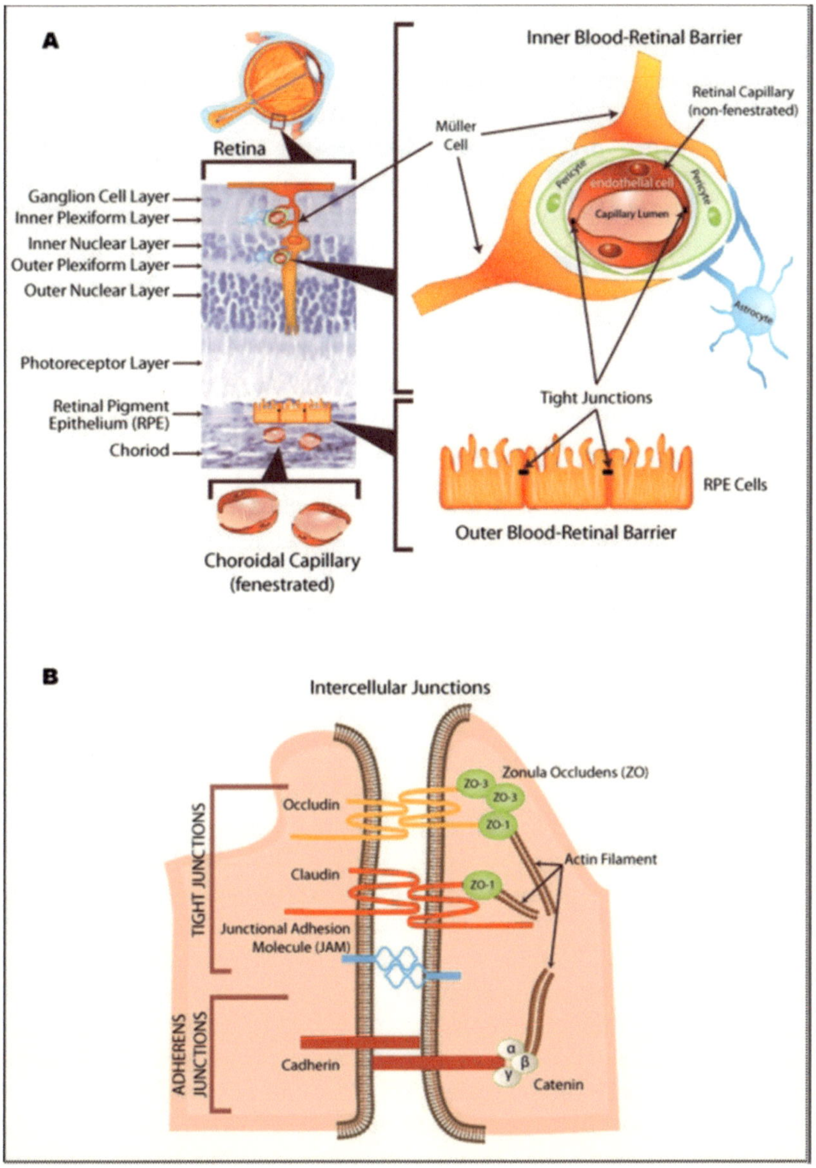

Fig. 1. The blood-retinal barrier (A) The retina is a multi-layered tissue in the posterior segment of the eye, and is shown by the H&E stained micrograph on the left. The cell types comprising the inner BRB (endothelial cells, pericytes, astrocytes, and Müller cells) and outer BRB (retinal pigment epithelial cells) are overlaid on the retinal micrograph, and are magnified on the right. Tight junctions between retinal capillary endothelial cells and retinal pigment epithelial cells form the basis of the inner and outer BRB, respectively. The endothelial cells of inner retinal capillaries are not fenestrated, whereas those of the choroidal capillaries are (depicted below the retinal micrograph). (B) Protein components of the intercellular junctions. Sources: Kaur et al., 2008; Niessen, 2007; http://www.landesbioscience.com/curie/images/chapters/Hosoya1.jpg

which downregulates VEGF expression and decreases vascular permeability (Yafai et al., 2007). Under hypoxia (Kaur et al., 2008) and oxidative stress (Yoshida et al., 2009), PEDF expression is decreased in Müller cells, thus favoring the secretion of VEGF and breakdown of the inner BRB. In addition, Müller cells are a source of matrix metalloproteinases, which proteolytically degrade the tight junction protein occludin, impairing the barrier function of retinal endothelial cells under cellular stress conditions. Müller cells also play a vital role in maintaining the retinal fluid balance (Reichenbach et al., 2007). Under physiological conditions, Müller cells carry out transcellular water transport from the retinal interstitial space into the blood, thus preventing excess fluid buildup within the retina. The transcellular water transport is osmotically coupled to the transport of potassium ions. When exposed to oxidative stress and inflammation, Müller cells have been shown to contribute to retinal edema through a disturbed intracellular fluid transport. Finally, Müller cells also respond to oxidative stress by increasing their production of the antioxidant glutathione (Siu et al., 2008).

Similar to pericytes and Müller cells, astrocytes are closely associated with the retinal vessels (Fig. 1A). They help maintain the BRB integrity by increasing the expression of the tight junction protein ZO-1 and modifying endothelial morphology (Kaur et al., 2008). Dysfunction of astrocytes has been linked to inner BRB breakdown and vasogenic edema.

2.2 Outer blood-retinal barrier

The outer BRB consists of tight junctions between RPE cells (Fig. 1A). The RPE is a monolayer of cells between the neuroretina and the choroid, and regulates access of blood components to the retina. Similar to the endothelium, movement across RPE is both transcellular and paracellular. The RPE cells exhibit a polarized morphology, with apical microvilli in contact with photoreceptor outer segments, and basal infoldings adjacent to the Bruch's membrane that separates the retina from choroidal capillaries called choriocapillaris (Kaur et al., 2008). Unlike the capillaries of the inner retina, the choroidal capillaries are fenestrated (Fig. 1A) and therefore do not contribute to the outer BRB (Kaur et al., 2008; Siu et al., 2008). Na+,K+-ATPase and aquaporin 1 (AQP1) expressed on the apical surface regulate movement of sodium, potassium, and water molecules across the RPE. Tight junctions, located at the apical side of the lateral membrane of the RPE cells, restrict paracellular movement between neighboring RPE cells. In addition to its function to regulate molecular transport integral to the outer BRB, RPE is responsible for phagocytizing photoreceptor outer segment membranes, which are digested by an extensive lysosome system, whose waste products are removed by the adjacent choriocapillaris (Burke, 2008; Siu et al., 2008). In pigmented animals, RPE cells also express melanin, a free radical scavenger that is also capable of absorbing stray light, and is thought to contribute to the retinal antioxidant mechanisms (Siu et al., 2008).

3. Oxidative stress, BRB dysfunction and ocular diseases

3.1 Sources of ROS in the Retina

In addition to the mitochondria, cellular sources of ROS in retina include endothelial cell xanthine oxidase, NAD(P)H oxidase, cyclooxygenase (COX), nitric oxide synthase (NOS), and lipoxygenase pathways (Frey and Antonetti, 2011; Hardy et al., 2005; Kunsch and Medford, 1999). ROS can also act as intracellular second messengers and activate various signaling transduction pathways.

3.2 Ocular pathologies associated with oxidative stress and BRB dysfunction

3.2.1 Diabetic retinopathy

Diabetic retinopathy is a significant cause of blindness. Tissue hypoxia and hyperglycemia are generally regarded as contributors to diabetic retinopathy, but how these lead to the disease state is unclear. Current hypotheses, which are not mutually exclusive, for pathogenic mechanisms leading to diabetic retinopathy include oxidative stress, hemodynamic changes, inflammation and the activation of microglia, and increased leukocyte adhesion to the endothelial cells and entrapment (leukostasis) (Chibber et al., 2007). Many of these processes in fact have an association with excessive production of ROS (Yang et al., 2010b). For instance, growing evidence supports an important role for leukostasis in the development of diabetic retinopathy, with downstream consequences including capillary occlusion and localized production of ROS, resulting in endothelial cell damage, BRB breakdown, and increased vascular permeability (Chibber et al., 2007). Inflammatory cytokines interact with cell surface receptors in various cell types to activate signaling pathways that mediate responses of cell adhesion, permeability and apoptosis; they also increase the production of ROS by mitochondria (Busik et al., 2008; Sprague and Khalil, 2009). There are several models that recapitulate various aspects of diabetic retinopathy, including streptozotocin-induced diabetes and ischemia-reperfusion injury.

3.2.2 Retinopathy of prematurity

Retinopathy of prematurity (ROP) is a vasoproliferative disease that often develops when premature infants are given supplemental oxygen, and is a leading cause of blindness in children (Hardy et al., 2005; Uno et al., 2010). The developing eye is at an increased risk for oxidative injury from hyperoxia, as the retinal vasculature in premature infants lacks fully-developed mechanisms to auto-regulate oxygen tension (Hardy et al., 2005). ROP develops in two phases (Hardy et al., 2005). Hyperoxia in the retina leads to cessation of vascular development, resulting in endothelial cell death, vaso-obliteration and consequently, ischemia. To re-establish retinal perfusion, the retina mounts an exaggerated intravitreal preretinal neovascularization, which may ultimately result in retinal detachment and vision loss. Many features of ROP are recapitulated in oxygen induced retinopathy (OIR) (Brafman et al., 2004; Gu et al., 2002; Uno et al., 2010), in which neonatal animals are exposed to hyperoxia, leading to the generation of ROS, which have been postulated to be causal for vaso-obliteration, death of endothelial cells, and consequently, impairment of the BRB.

3.2.3 Age-related macular degeneration

One of the major causes of blindness in the elderly population, age-related macular degeneration (AMD) is characterized by regional degeneration of photoreceptors and the RPE, lipofuscin accumulation in RPE cells, chronic inflammation, and drusen formation. Chronic oxidative stress has also been suggested to be an important factor to the pathogenesis of AMD. As alluded to earlier, RPE may be at a high risk for oxidative stress due to its location and function. The RPE is in an oxygen-rich environment adjacent to the choriocapillaris, is continuously exposed to light, sometimes at phototoxic wavelengths, and is responsible for the renewal of photoreceptor outer segments via phagocytosis (Burke, 2008). The high content of polyunsaturated fatty acids of these membrane segments make them susceptible to lipid peroxidation and subsequent free radical formation. Experimental evidence supporting a role of oxidative stress in AMD showed that supplementation of antioxidants in AMD patients has a protective effect, and that cigarette smoking, known to be a source of exogenous free radicals, is a risk factor for AMD (Burke, 2008). Given the central role RPE plays in AMD pathogenesis, a commonly used experimental model to study the link between oxidative stress and AMD involves the use of cultured human RPE (ARPE-19) cells. Common endpoints include cell survival, morphology, activation of signaling cascades, and cytokine production (Chan et al., 2008; Dong et al., 2011; Glotin et al., 2006; Jiang et al., 2009; Klettner and Roider, 2009; Qin et al., 2006; Tsao et al., 2006; Wang et al., 1998; Wu et al., 2010).

4. Retinal vein occlusion

Retinal vein occlusion is a vascular disorder of the retina that occurs when one or more of the retinal veins are blocked and the circulation of retinal blood becomes obstructed. This ocular pathology can be a primary lesion or secondary to other retinal diseases. With the blockage, poor venous drainage and increased retinal capillary pressure and permeability ultimately lead to retinal ischemia and edema. Retinal ischemia could lead to the generation of ROS, impacting the integrity of the BRB. Diabetic retinopathy and RVO are the two most common causes of inner BRB breakdown. Among complications found in the clinical examination are hemorrhages, edema, ischemia, neovascularization of the retina as well as increased intraocular pressure. Depending on the location and severity, loss of visual acuity can range from very mild to severe. While some patients with RVO may not have any symptoms, some patients may complain of blurred vision or visual field defects. In severe cases, RVO can lead to vision loss in the affected eye. The most common cause of decreased vision is macular degeneration secondary to RVO, which occurs when leakage within macula leads to macular edema and ischemia. Neovascularization and neovascular glaucoma are the other vision-threatening complications that are devastating for patients with RVO and that should be promptly diagnosed and treated. Vein occlusion is commonly diagnosed by examining the fundus with ophthalmoscope for characteristic morphological changes such as venous tortuosity, cotton-wool spots, dot and flame hemorrhage, and edematous optic nerves, and by fluorescein angiography for vasculature blood flow obstruction, leakage in the retina, retinal ischemia, aneurysm, neovascularization, and macular edema. Sometimes optical coherence tomography (OCT) is used to measure retinal thickness for the determination of the presence of macular edema. Central and peripheral visual disturbance should be evaluated by functional tests in the physical examination.

4.1 Classification of RVO

Retinal vein occlusion is primarily classified into central retinal vein occlusion (CRVO) and branch retinal vein occlusion (BRVO) based on the location of obstruction. In CRVO, the occlusion of the central retinal vein can slow or stop blood from leaving the retina and therefore most of the retina is affected. In BRVO, when macular venules are occluded, a vision decrease can occur depending on the amount of ischemia and edema. When one of the vein's two trunks is blocked and half of the retina is affected, it is called hemi-central retinal vein occlusion (HRVO). According to several RVO epidemiology studies, the prevalence of both CRVO and BRVO increases significantly with age, more in middle-aged and elderly populations and uncommon in young adults under the age of 40. Most patients with CRVO are male and over 65 years of age, but there seems to be no gender difference for BRVO. Most CRVO cases are unilateral and painless and only 6-14% of cases are found to be bilateral (Cheung et al., 2008; Klein et al., 2008; Lim et al., 2008; Marcucci et al., 2011; Xu et al., 2007). A recent combined world-wide data pool, containing 68,751 individuals with ages ranging from 30 to 101 years, suggested that approximately 16 million people are affected by RVO with 5.2 per 1000 for any RVO, 4.42 per 1000 for BRVO and 0.8 per 1000 for CRVO. The incidence of CRVO was lower than that of BRVO in all ethnic populations (Rogers et al., 2010). However, CRVO is the most clinically relevant RVO as it is associated with severe vision loss, especially for the ischemic (non-perfused or hemorrhagic retinopathy) RVO. Among the complications of RVO, the devastating neovascular glaucoma resulting from anterior segment neovascularization is seen only in ischemic CRVO. Fortunately, most cases (81%) (Hayreh et al., 1994) are of the non-ischemic type that rarely develops blindness-causing complications.

4.2 Risk factors of RVO

CRVO and BRVO have different symptoms, risk factors, pathogenesis, and therefore treatment. The pathogenesis for RVO is multifactorial and still under investigation. Anatomical positions of retinal veins play an important role in the pathogenesis of RVO (Fraenkl et al., 2010). The central retinal artery and vein share a common adventitial sheath in the optic nerve head. In CRVO, the tract of central retinal vein passing through the narrowing lamina cribrosa is the most frequent site of occlusion. In BRVO, vein occlusions occur at the junction of retinal vein and artery crossings in the retina. The mechanical compression of the veins at the narrowing passage or arteriovenous crossings predispose retinal veins to thrombus formation by various factors, including slowed or disturbed blood flow, endothelial damage in the vessel wall, changes in the blood viscosity, perivascular changes such as in lamina cribrosa (Albon et al., 1995), and sclerotic changes in the retinal arteries. Ocular risk factors associated with RVO include glaucoma or ocular hypertension. In glaucoma, increased intraocular pressure causes mechanical compression of retinal veins, which may induce RVO.

RVO has often been associated with a variety of systemic vascular disorders including arterial hypertension, arteriosclerosis, diabetes mellitus, dyslipidemia, and systemic vasculitis (The Eye Disease Case-Control Study Group, 1993, 1996; Koizumi et al., 2007; Mitchell et al., 1996; Sperduto et al., 1998). The increased rigidity of arterial wall affiliated with these diseases may result in compression of retinal veins.

Abnormal blood viscosity, platelets, and coagulation have also been suggested to be involved in RVO pathogenesis (Trope et al., 1983). Hematological dysfunction, such as increased plasma fibrinogen and disruption of the thrombosis-fibrinolysis balance, have been implicated in the development of RVO (Rehak and Rehak, 2008). Increased fibrinogen has been associated with RVO in several clinical reports (Lip et al., 1998; Patrassi et al., 1987; Peduzzi et al., 1986). An increasing number of studies have sought to establish an association between RVO and thrombophilic abnormalities. Thrombophilic risk factors related to RVO include hyperhomocysteinemia, methylenetetrahydrofolate reductase (MTHFR) gene mutation, factor V Leiden mutation, protein C and S deficiency, antithrombin deficiency, prothrombin gene mutation, anticardiolipin antibodies and lupus anticoagulant. High levels of circulating homocysteine may damage the vascular endothelium by releasing free radicals, creating a hypercoagulable environment (Angayarkanni et al., 2008). It appears that there is an association between RVO and hyperhomocysteinaemia and anti-phospholipid antibodies. However, for the other thrombophilic risk factors, there is a lack of consistency among the studies and the association with RVO is inconclusive (Fegan, 2002; Janssen et al., 2005; Rehak and Rehak, 2008). More recently, elevated levels of soluble endothelial protein C receptor (sEPCR) emerged an important candidate risk factor especially for CRVO (Gumus et al., 2006).

Significantly increased concentrations of growth factors, cytokines, and chemokines such as VEGF, interleukin (IL)-6, IL-8, interferon-inducible 10-kDa protein (IP-10), monocytochemotactic protein-1 (MCP-1), and platelet-derived growth factor (PDGF)-AA were observed in vitreous or aqueous humor samples of patients with RVO (Funk et al., 2009; Noma et al., 2009; Yoshimura et al., 2009). Excessive production of VEGF and inflammatory cytokines can be induced by ischemic conditions. The levels of VEGF and inflammatory cytokines are correlated with severity of retinal ischemia and macular edema (Noma et al., 2006), as well as neovascularization. A close correlation between aqueous VEGF levels and iris neovascularization and vascular permeability in CRVO patients has been found (Boyd et al., 2002).

4.3 Oxidative stress and RVO

Retinal ischemia that occurs in some cases of RVO could lead to the generation of ROS, and compromise the integrity of the BRB. In fact, RVO is a common complication of diabetic retinopathy, in which hypoxia-ischemia is thought to play a role in its pathogenesis. Many of the risk factors for RVO described above, such as alterations in blood flow, systemic vascular disorders, hypercoagulability, and elevated levels of pro-inflammatory cytokines, may also be associated with a state of oxidative stress (Simoncini et al., 2005). Indeed, in a case-control prospective study in young adult CRVO patients, serum levels of paraoxonase-1 arylesterase (PON1-ARE) activity, reported to have antioxidant potential, were found to be negatively correlated with hyperhomocysteinemia and lipid peroxidation, an indicator of oxidative stress (Angayarkanni et al., 2008). Decreased levels of PON1-ARE activity as well as increased levels of the lipid peroxidation marker were shown to be risk factors for CRVO. In another case study, an individual with glucose-6-phosphate dehydrogenase(G6PD) deficiency was exposed to an oxidative stressor, and later developed CRVO (Kotwal et al., 2009). G6PD deficiency is known to increase erythrocyte vulnerability to oxidative stress, which may precipitate hemolysis, increased erythrocyte aggregation and erythrocyte-endothelium interaction, leading to thrombosis (Kotwal et al., 2009). Anti-phospholipid antibodies have been associated with the development of RVO, and shown to induce oxidative stress in endothelial cells (Simoncini et al., 2005). Taken together, these lines of evidence suggest that a state of oxidative stress may predispose individuals to RVO.

4.4 Therapeutics associated with the clinical presentation of RVO

In addition to RVO that arises due to pathophysiological causes described above, this ocular disorder can also develop as an adverse event from treatment with certain therapeutics.

4.4.1 Interferon-α

Interferon-α (IFN-α) is used for the treatment of many cancers and chronic hepatitis C. Interferon-associated retinopathy has been documented since the 1990s, most commonly characterized by hemorrhage and cotton-wool spots, and sometimes by macular edema, retinal vascular occlusion, and retinal ischemia. The RVO could involve either the vein or artery, or both, and in most cases is reversible. The exact pathophysiological mechanism of interferon-induced retinopathy is unknown, although there are similarities with early stages of diabetic retinopathy (Bajaire et al., 2011; Esmaeli et al., 2001). Several risk factors have been suggested, including hypertension, hyperlipidemia, a hypercoagulable state, and diabetes (Nadir et al., 2000). In addition, IFN-α is known to cause the development of autoantibodies in 10% of the patients receiving treatment, and to exacerbate certain systemic autoimmune diseases. It is speculated that IFN-α therapy might cause deposition of immune complexes in retinal vasculature, with sequelae of retinal ischemia, hemorrhages and cotton wool spots.

4.4.2 Tumor necrosis factor

Tumor necrosis factor (TNF) is a proinflammatory cytokine that has been implicated in various diseases, including autoimmune diseases, diabetes, and cancer. In a phase II trial of recombinant TNF in patients with advanced colon cancer, TNF was administered by i.v. infusions twice daily for 5 consecutive days every other week for 8 weeks (Kemeny et al., 1990). Two out of 16 patients developed retinal vein thrombosis several weeks following completion of therapy. This finding is consistent with the known role of TNF in vascular leakage and blood-retinal barrier breakdown in diabetic retinopathy (Frey and Antonetti, 2011). In support of this, a patient with macular edema secondary to BRVO saw an improvement in visual acuity and cessation of macular edema during treatment with infliximab, a TNF-α antibody, administered for rheumatoid arthritis (Kachi et al., 2010). Paradoxically, infliximab therapy has also been linked in several case studies to the development of retinal vein thrombosis/occlusion in a patient being treated for ulcerative colitis (Veerappan et al., 2008), psoriasis (Vergou et al., 2010), or Crohn's disease (Puli and Benage, 2003). The temporal relationship between infliximab infusion and retinopathy suggested the two may be causally related. In two of the three cases, a medical history of myocardial infarction or hyperlipidemia was noted, both of which considered risk factors for RVO. Moreover, all three of these diseases are inflammatory in nature, and may predispose patients to weakened BRB.

4.4.3 MEK inhibitor PD0325901

PD0325901 is a potent and selective MEK inhibitor, developed for the treatment of advanced cancer. MEK is a key molecule in the Ras-mitogen-activated protein kinase (MAPK) pathway, which has roles including cellular proliferation and survival, and its only known substrate is the extracellular signal-regulated kinase (ERK), which in turn phosphorylates and activates downstream molecules in the pathway (Fig. 2). In the phase I dose escalation clinical trial of PD0325901, dose-limiting RVO was observed, characterized by the presence of cotton wool spots, hemorrhages, and vein occlusion. RVO developed in 2 patients after 3.5-4 months of 10 or 15 mg BID continuous treatment schedule, and in 1 patient after 9 months of 10 mg BID on a 5 days on/2 days off schedule, and was reversible upon treatment discontinuation (LoRusso et al., 2010). It was noted that at doses >= 4 mg BID, the systemic exposure of PD0325901 was equivalent to that in animal models that resulted in 90% phosphorylated ERK (pERK) suppression (LoRusso et al., 2010). Therefore, the ocular lesions could be related to the prolonged and/or significant levels of pERK suppression.

Two other MEK inhibitors, CI-1040 and selumetinib (AZD6244), also progressed to the clinic, but did not cause RVO. CI-1040 is a structural analogue of PD0325901. Insufficient clinical efficacy was reported due to poor bioavailability and metabolic instability (Rinehart et al., 2004). Selumetinib caused blurred vision in 12% of patients at >=100 mg BID in a Phase I trial (Adjei et al., 2008); this finding was not reported in subsequent Phase II trials at the 100 mg BID dose (Bekaii-Saab et al., 2011; Bodoky et al., 2011). Compared to PD0325901, selumetinib is approximately 10-fold less potent, and has a relatively poor bioavailability. Taken together, even though it is at present unclear whether PD0325901 caused RVO due to its deep inhibition of pERK, or to its chemotype, the above evidence suggests that the incidence of ocular lesions correlates with the efficacy of MEK inhibition.

5. Molecular mechanisms of MEK inhibitor PD0325901-Induced RVO

To develop an animal model of RVO to investigate mechanisms of toxicity, an in-life study was performed in rabbits, in which PD0325901 was administered by intravitreal injection at doses of 0.5 and 1 mg/eye, with an observation period of 2 weeks (Huang et al., 2009). The high dose was extrapolated to be a potentially toxic dose, while the low dose was chosen as a subtoxic dose, based on in vitro cytotoxicity data (Huang et al., 2009). As early as 1 day after treatment, the high dose produced hemorrhages and vascular leakage with branch occlusion. These lesions progressed to retinal detachment, edema, abnormal kinetic blood flow, and retinal vessel occlusion after 7 days. At the low dose, retinal vascular leakage was observed without vascular occlusion. Therefore, the rabbit model provided evidence that PD0325901 at sufficient ocular concentrations could lead to similar retinal lesions seen in the clinic.

The retinal vascular toxicity was not observed in preclinical safety studies where PD0325901 was administered orally in rats and dogs for up to 13 weeks (Huang et al., 2009). The difference in the level of ocular toxicity between rabbits and rats/dogs could be attributed to ocular drug concentration differences arising from local vs. systemic routes of administration. Since molecular events could precede overt signs of tissue injury, an investigative study was conducted in which rats were dosed orally for 3 or 5 days at 45 mg/kg/day, estimated to be at 70% maximal tolerated dose (Huang et al., 2009). No retinal toxicity was observed by ophthalmic examinations or fundus fluorescein angiography. Despite the absence of overt injury, global gene expression profiling on vehicle and PD0325901-treated retinas revealed several mechanisms relevant to the development of RVO, including oxidative stress response, acute phase and inflammatory response, BRB

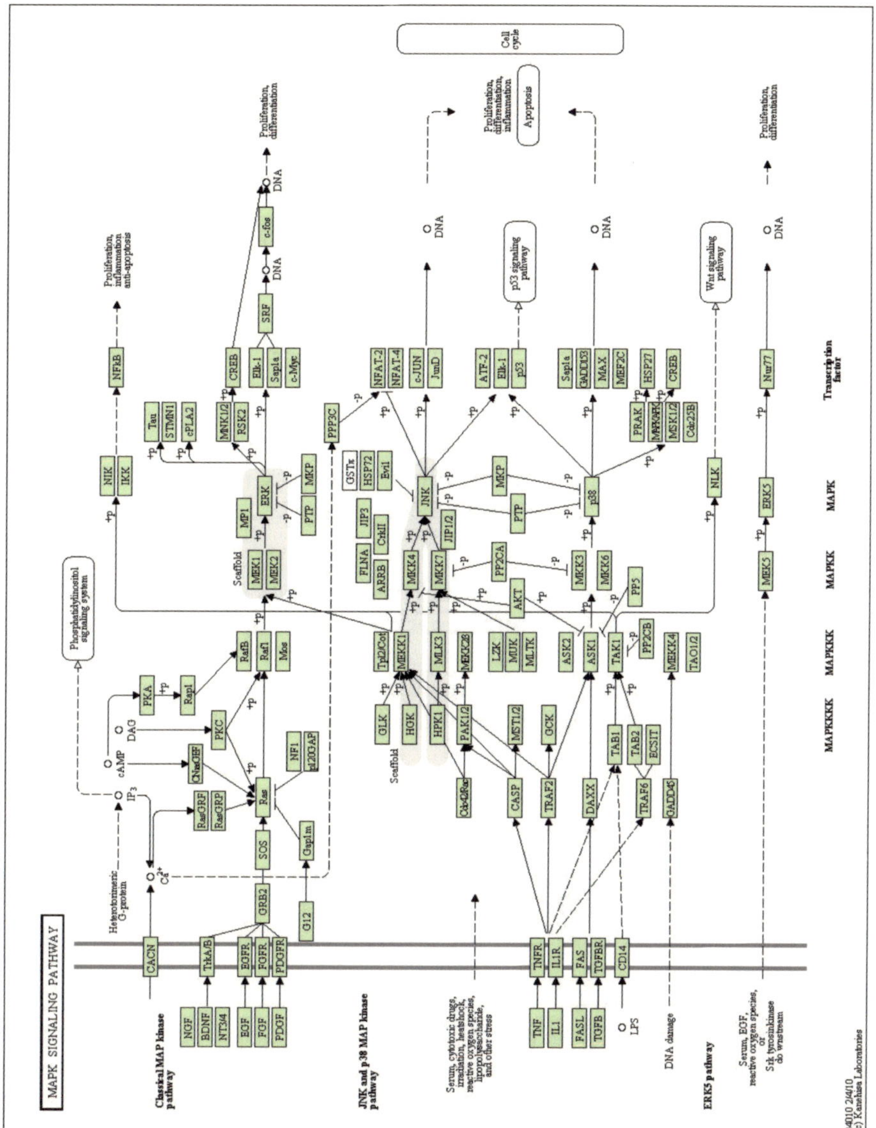

Fig. 2. MAPK signaling pathway The MAPK cascade is a highly conserved module that is involved in various cellular functions, including cell proliferation, differentiation and migration. Mammals express at least four distinctly regulated groups of MAPKs, ERK1/2, JNK1/2/3, p38alpha/beta/gamma/delta and ERK5, that are activated by specific MAPKKs: MEK1/2 for ERK1/2, MKK3/6 for the p38, MKK4/7 (JNKK1/2) for the JNKs, and MEK5 for ERK5. Each MAPKK, however, can be activated by more than one MAPKKK, increasing the complexity and diversity of MAPK signalling. Presumably each MAPKKK confers responsiveness to distinct stimuli. For example, activation of ERK1/2 by growth factors depends on the MAPKKK c-Raf, but other MAPKKKs may activate ERK1/2 in response to pro-inflammatory stimuli. Source: KEGG (http://www.genome.jp/dbget-bin/www_bget?map04010) (Kanehisa, 2000, 2012)

breakdown, leukostasis, and activation of coagulation cascade (Huang et al., 2009). Progressive induction of oxidative stress response genes was observed over time, suggesting the tissue was mounting a response against ongoing oxidative stress. The induced genes encoding for antioxidant proteins include heat shock protein 27 (HSP27), αβ-crystalline, and those involved in glutathione synthesis/metabolism (GCLM, GSS, GSTs), and adhesion molecules; the only repressed genes were glutaredoxin 2 and peroxiredoxins. Of the oxidative stress response genes induced in this study, HSP27 and αβ-crystalline show some of the greatest magnitude of induction. These are small heat shock proteins that have diverse cytoprotective functions, including modulation of ubiquitin-proteosome pathway, inhibition of apoptosis, and increased resistance to oxidative stress and inflammation (Arrigo et al., 2007). Notably, the ubiquitin-proteosome pathway was significantly perturbed on both day 3 and day 5, which could be a response to misfolded proteins arising from oxidative stress. Antigen presentation by retinal cells is also a cited response to oxidative stress (Tezel et al., 2007; Zhang et al., 2005), consistent with the induction of β-2-microglobulin gene of the major histocompatibility complex (MHC) class I on both day 3 and day 5. MHC class I molecules are normally expressed in the vascular endothelium and RPE (Zhang et al., 1997).

Multiple lines of evidence demonstrate that ROS mediate activation of the MAPK signaling pathway, which in turn modulates inflammation, intercellular junction assembly, actin cytoskeleton reorganization, and water transport, all of which are of critical importance to the maintenance of the BRB integrity. Disruption of one of the key MAPK pathways by PD0325901 could contribute to impaired BRB integrity, ultimately leading to retinal edema and RVO.

5.1 MAPK activation and oxidative stress response in the retina

Three main MAPK groups have been identified – ERKs, p38 MAPKs, and c-Jun N-terminal kinases (JNK). Typically, activation of ERKs are associated with growth-related signals, whereas p38 MAPKs and JNKs become activated in response to stress stimuli, including inflammation and oxidative stress (Fig. 2). However, the exact responses of these kinases in different cell types and tissue microenvironment under various experimental stimuli have proven to be more dynamic and less dichotomous than characterized above. Some degree of cross-talk also exist between these pathways (Houle and Huot, 2006). In the retina, the dynamic balance and cross-talk of these MAPK signaling pathways in cell types comprising the BRB, chiefly RPE, endothelial, and Müller cells, has been shown in experimental systems to be critical for modulating the integrity of the BRB.

The role of the MAPK pathway has been extensively investigated in cultured RPE cells (ARPE-19) following experimentally induced oxidative stress. In response to oxidants such as hydrogen peroxide or tert-butyl hydroperoxide, MAPK (most notably ERKs and p38 MAPK) activation has been shown to either protect against or exacerbate oxidative injury, differentiated by the amount of RPE cell death (Chan et al., 2008; Dong et al., 2011; Glotin et al., 2006; Jiang et al., 2009; Klettner and Roider, 2009; Qin et al., 2006; Tsao et al., 2006; Wang et al., 1998; Wu et al., 2010). These findings also raise questions as to the impact of oxidative stress on the outer BRB when the MAPK pathway is modulated pharmacologically by a MEK inhibitor. In endothelial cells, ROS are known to modulate the expression of redox-sensitive signaling pathways, including the MAPK cascades (Kunsch and Medford, 1999;

Ushio-Fukai and Alexander, 2004), and inhibition of the ERK1/2 has been shown to lead to endothelial apoptosis (Huot et al., 1998). In a porcine model of retinal ischemia-reperfusion, Müller cells exhibited increased levels of glial fibrillary acidic protein (GFAP) and phosphorylated ERK proteins, implicating ERK in the process of glial activation in response to oxidative/ischemic stress (Wurm et al., 2011).

The following sections highlight specific MAPK-mediated molecular and cellular events in response to oxidative stress that are important for the maintenance of BRB function. The published data at times reveal contradictory findings with regards to whether the MAPKs are protective or disruptive in modulating these cellular processes following oxidative stress, underscoring the complexicity of these signaling pathways. In each section, literature review is followed by a discussion of relevant gene expression profiling data from the rat investigative study in which PD0325901 was administered orally for 3 or 5 days at 45 mg/kg/day.

5.1.1 MAPK activation and Inflammation in the retina

Inflammation is a non-specific response to injury, and involves a plethora of cellular and molecular mediators. Chronic inflammatory processes are also an important source of ROS in the retina, and have been implicated in ocular diseases such as diabetic retinopathy and AMD. Both oxidative stress and inflammation negatively impact the integrity of the BRB. MAPKs mediate some of the downstream effects of proinflammatory cytokines such as IL-1, IL-6 and TNF-α (Du et al., 2010; Larrayoz et al., 2010; Wang et al., 2010).

In the 5-day rat investigative study involving PD0325901, hematology analysis revealed an increased number of phagocytes (neutrophils and monocytes) and increased plasma fibrinogen levels, indicating a mild inflammation in the compound treated animals. Consistently, the gene expression of many acute phase response proteins, such as lipocalin 2, fibronectin, fibrinogen, ferritin light chain, complement proteins, and coagulation factors, are significantly induced on day 5. In addition to being an acute phase response protein, fibrinogen is also a key player in the coagulation cascade; as alluded in Section 4.2, it has been associated with the development of RVO in several clinical reports. Notably, some studies show that fibrinogen may increase endothelial permeability and mediate vasoconstriction through activation of ERK1/2 (Sen et al., 2009; Tyagi et al., 2008). Though the expression levels of IL-1, IL-6, IL-8, and TNF-α genes were not affected, induction of downstream genes within these signaling pathways, including TRAF6 (TNF receptor associated factor 6), TNF receptor, IκB kinase, signal transducer and activator of transcription (STAT) 3, c-Jun, collagen type I, intracellular adhesion molecule (ICAM-1), vascular cell adhesion molecule (VCAM)-1, and cyclooxygenase (Cox)-2, suggests pathway activation downstream of these cytokines. TNF-α has been shown to increase vascular permeability via modulation of tight junction proteins in diabetic retinopathy (Aveleira et al., 2010). IL-1β may have a role in mediating retinal capillary degradation in diabetic retinopathy (Frey and Antonetti, 2011). Intravitreal levels of IL-6 are correlated with macular edema in branch retinal vein occlusion (Noma et al., 2006). ICAM-1, VCAM-1 and Cox-2 are downstream effectors of NF-κB in the IL-8 signaling pathway. ICAM-1 and VCAM-1 are adhesions molecules expressed on vascular endothelial cells and their induction play a critical role in leukostasis and inflammation. Cox-2 mediates the production of proinflammatory prostaglandins. NF-κB, c-Jun and STAT3 are important regulators of many genes mediating mammalian inflammatory and immune responses. In addition, the expression of GFAP was induced on day 5, suggesting activation of Müller cells in response to retinal stress such as inflammation.

Conversely, glucocorticoids, which have anti-inflammatory properties, have been shown to have a positive impact on promoting barrier integrity. In a porcine model of RVO, triamcinolone treatment, a widely used glucocorticoid in ocular applications, reduced VEGF and increased tight junction occludin levels in the retina, suggesting increased BRB integrity (McAllister et al., 2009). A study conducted to examine the impact of Streptococcus suis infection on blood-CSF (cerebral spinal fluid) barrier showed that the glucocorticoid dexamethasone improved the barrier function by preventing tight junction protein reorganization and degradation, and attenuated ERK activation and matrix metalloproteinase 3 (MMP3) expression (Tenenbaum et al., 2008). Paradoxically, dexamethasone has also been shown to activate ERK and JNK, which in turn induce the expression of the anti-inflammatory mediator MAPK phosphatase 1 (MKP-1) in human umbilical vein endothelial cells (Furst et al., 2008). Activated MKP-1 is then able to terminate the activity of activated MAPKs in a negative feedback loop (Furst et al., 2008). These data further demonstrate the complex spatiotemporal signaling network in which the MAPKs participate.

In our gene expression analysis, the glucocorticoid receptor signaling pathway was one of the few pathways significantly perturbed on day 3 following PD0325901 administration at 45 mg/kg/day, and many genes within the pathway were induced. On day 5, many of the same pathway genes became repressed. This could indicate an adaptive response to ongoing inflammation in the retina. As alluded to earlier, HSP27 and αβ-crystallin levels were also induced following PD0325901 administration. Their gene products have the ability to interfere with inflammatory signaling, such as attenuation of TNF-α, NF-κB signaling pathways, and may represent another cellular response to inflammation.

5.1.2 MAPK-mediated modulation of intercellular junctions in response to oxidative stress

Intercellular junctions are of critical importance to the integrity of the BRB function (Fig. 1). Oxidative stress is known to disrupt the structure and function of tight junctions and adherens junctions through MAPK activation, in both endothelial cells (Niwa et al., 2001; Simoncini et al., 2005; Usatyuk and Natarajan, 2004; Usatyuk et al., 2006; Yuan, 2002) and epithelial cells (Basuroy et al., 2006; Gonzalez et al., 2009), and these adverse effects on the junctional complexes could be ameliorated with the application of specific MAPK inhibitors. The presence of ROS could also induce the expression of the vascular permeability factor VEGF in endothelial cells (Chua et al., 1998; El-Remessy et al., 2003), often associated with downstream MAPK activation (Yang et al., 2010a; Zheng et al., 2010). In Müller cells, oxidative stress leads to decreased PEDF expression (Yoshida et al., 2009), thus relieving its antagonistic effect on VEGF action and subsequent MAPK activation in endothelial cells (Yafai et al., 2007), contributing to increased vascular permeability and breakdown of the inner BRB.

In our 5-day rat investigative study, the expression of myosin light chain kinase (MLCK) was significantly increased as a result of NF-κB signaling. Phosphorylation of myosin light chain by MLCK leads to actin-mediated endothelial cell contraction and increases permeability of endothelial junctional barrier. Activation of phosphatidylinositol 3-kinase (PI3K), whose expression was induced on both day 3 and day 5, has also been shown to increase vascular permeability (Abid et al., 2004; Lee et al., 2006; Serban et al., 2008). In addition, induction of MMP14 was observed on day 5. Under inflammatory conditions, Müller cells are a source of matrix metalloproteinases which impair the barrier function of retinal endothelial cells by degradation of the tight junction protein occludin (Reichenbach et al., 2007). Taken together, these data suggest increased retinal endothelial cell permeability and impaired BRB function as a result of PD0325901 administration. On the other hand, our data set also uncovered induction of genes important for maintaining the vascular endothelial barrier function, presumably as feedback mechanism to counteract permeability increases, such as repression of RhoA and induction of Rac1 to facilitate reannealing of adherens junctions (Vandenbroucke et al., 2008); induction of tight junction components claudin 11 and JAM-2; and induction of PEDF, likely in Müller cells, which represses expression of VEGF and decreases vascular permeability (Reichenbach et al., 2007).

5.1.3 Regulation of actin dynamics by MAPK in response to oxidative stress

The remodeling of actin cytoskeleton is an important response in endothelial cells exposed to oxidative stress, and contributes to increased permeability of the endothelial barrier (Houle and Huot, 2006; Lum and Roebuck, 2001). Under physiological and pathological stress conditions, endothelial cells undergo cell shape change, intercellular gap formation, and remodeling of the actin cytoskeleton, characterized by stress fiber formation and reduced cortical actin band. The formation of stress fibers is dependent on actin polymerization, and increases the endothelial cells' capacity to resist stress. On the other hand, stress fibers also pull apart intercellular junctions, likely contributing to their disruption and impaired endothelial barrier integrity.

ROS-induced MAPK activation plays an important role in actin remodeling. ERKs, p38 and JNK have all been shown to regulate actin dynamics induced by oxidative stress in endothelial cells (El-Remessy et al., 2011; Houle and Huot, 2006; Houle et al., 2003; Huot et al., 1998; Schweitzer et al., 2011; Usatyuk and Natarajan, 2004). p38 MAPK activation leads to phosphorylation of HSP27, which promotes actin polymerization. ERK activation results in phosphorylation of tropomyosin-1, which contributes to focal adhesion assembly and stress fiber formation, and modulates cell contractility. Inhibition of ERK activity by the MEK inhibitor PD098059 led to misassembly of focal adhesions and membrane blebbing, ultimately resulting in apoptosis (Huot et al. 1998). Physio-pathological consequence of surface blebbing of endothelial cells includes narrowing of vascular lumen associated with increased vascular resistance. Bleb shedding may also contribute to obstruction of blood vessels. Consistent with this interplay of MAPKs and actin dynamics, treatment with PD0325901 in the 5-day rat investigative study led to induction of genes in actin cytoskeleton and focal adhesion signaling pathways on study day 5, supporting perturbation of actin dynamics, likely downstream of oxidative stress. These data also raise the possibility of membrane blebbing in retinal vasculature following PD0325901 treatment, contributing to the development of RVO.

5.1.4 MAPK pathway and water permeability in response to oxidative stress

Macular edema was observed in our animal model administered with PD0325901. Two factors contribute to the development of chronic edema in the retina: increased vascular permeability leading to excessive fluid buildup, and reduced fluid absorption from the retina back into the blood. Müller and RPE cells play an integral role in transcellular fluid equilibrium (Reichenbach et al., 2007). Aquaporin 4 (AQP4) expressed on Müller cells and AQP1 expressed on RPE cells facilitate bidirectional water movements to maintain the osmotic and hydrostatic equilibrium in the retina. The Müller cell-specific AQP4 is co-localized with the inwardly rectifying potassium channel Kir4.1. Together they mediate the co-transport of water and potassium ions from the retinal tissue into the blood under normal conditions. In various animal models of retinopathy, characterized by inflammatory or oxidative stress conditions, Kir4.1 channel becomes mislocalized, and its expression is decreased in some cases (Reichenbach et al., 2007). This may lead to an intracellular potassium overload, increased osmotic pressure, and consequently, Müller cell swelling. In a study employing a rat model of RVO, downregulation of AQP1, AQP4, and Kir4.1 were observed, in addition to an altered distribution of Kir4.1 protein. Consequently, Müller cells displayed a decrease in potassium currents and increased in size (Rehak et al., 2008).

Application triamcinolone, a glucocorticoid frequently used for diabetic macular edema due to its anti-inflammatory properties (Felinski and Antonetti, 2005), reduced Müller cell swelling in animal models of ischemia-reperfusion and diabetic retinopathy (Reichenbach et al., 2007). In a porcine model of RVO, triamcinolone treatment reduced the glial activation marker GFAP expression in Müller cells, and also increased BRB integrity, as evidenced by reduced VEGF and increased tight junction occludin levels, potentially contributing to the resolution of edema in the retina (McAllister et al., 2009).

MAPKs are known to play an important role in cellular osmotic stress regulation (Cowan and Storey, 2003; de Nadal et al., 2002). In RPE cells, ultraviolet radiation (UVB) and hydrogen peroxide treatment, both of which are oxidative stress inducers, resulted in AQP1 downregulation which was mediated by MEK/ERK activation (Jiang et al., 2009). In the brain, astrocyte swelling often accompanies vascular edema (Reichenbach et al., 2007). In astrocytes exposed to the oxidative stressor manganese or glial reactive injury, there was an altered expression of AQPs, mediated by the MEK/ERK and p38 MAPKs (McCoy and Sontheimer, 2010; Rao et al., 2010).

In our 5-day rat investigative study, the repression of the Müller cell-specific water channel AQP4 on both day 3 and day 5, coupled with the repression of the inwardly rectifying potassium channels (Kcnj5, Kcnj6), and sodium channels on day 5, signals impaired transcellular fluid transport. Given the evidence for inflammation, intercellular junction disruption and actin cytoskeleton changes in the retina following PD0325901 treatment, this fluid imbalance would contribute to the observed retinal edema in the study and further weaken BRB integrity. The documented involvement of MAPKs in regulating transcellular fluid balance in the retina and the brain raises the possibility that MEK inhibition may play a role in perturbing this equilibrium.

5.2 MAPK, IFN-α and RVO

Given the complex signaling cascades and cross-talk between various MAPK pathways in multiple cell types comprising the BRB, it is conceivable that inhibition of ERK activation by a MEK inhibitor could lead to dysregulated BRB integrity and subsequent development of RVO. Intriguingly, IFN-α treatment, which is also associated with the development of RVO in the clinic (see Section 4.4.1), has been shown to inhibit the activation of ERK and the associated survival effects, and that MEK and ERK inhibitors enhance the anti-proliferative effect of IFN-α in tumor cells or transformed epithelial cells (Battcock et al., 2006; Caraglia et al., 2005; Caraglia et al., 2003; Christian et al., 2009; Li et al., 2004; Romerio et al., 2000; Romerio and Zella, 2002). Cross-talk between the IFN-α and Ras-MAPK pathways converge on the STAT family of transcription factors. STAT proteins are involved in cytokine, hormone, and growth factor signal transduction, mediating biological processes as diverse as cell proliferation, differentiation, apoptosis, transformation, inflammation and immune response (Caraglia et al., 2005). Activated Ras/MEK has been shown to inhibit the antiviral response of IFN-α by reducing STAT2 levels (Christian et al., 2009). It is conceivable that clinical IFN-α usage may perturb the balance of MAPK signaling pathways in the retina, disrupt BRB function, and ultimately contribute to the development of RVO. That both IFN-α therapy and PD0325901 inhibit ERK activation and are linked to clinical development of RVO lends further support to the hypothesis that modulation of the Ras-MAPK pathway and subsequently BRB permeability changes play a role in the pathogenesis of this ocular adverse event.

6. Conclusion

The BRB, consisting of an endothelial and an epithelial barrier, serves to regulate the bidirectional passage of macromolecules through the retina. Oxidative stress can negatively impact the equilibrium across the BRB, leading to cellular disruption and ocular disorders. MAPK pathways involving ERK, p38 and JNK play a central role in the oxidative stress response of the BRB, modulating inflammatory response, actin cytoskeletal dynamics, water transport, as well as inter-epithelial and inter-endothelial adhesion molecule expression and redistribution. Disruption of the ERK signaling pathway by the MEK inhibitor PD0325901 may disrupt the balance and cross-talk between interconnected signaling networks and produce unexpected cellular sequalae. PD0325901-induced RVO could arise as a consequence of disruption of these tightly regulated molecular processes vital for proper functioning of the BRB. The animal models employed in our study serves as an investigative or screening paradigm for pre-clinical compounds suspected of RVO-inducing potential. Finally, while a firm connection between MEK inhibition and the development of RVO has not been established, it would be prudent for clinicians to monitor patients on MEK inhibitor therapy for signs of ocular adverse events.

7. Acknowledgements

The authors would like to thank Patrick Lappin for critical reading of the manuscript, and Constance Benedict for preparation of Fig. 1.

8. References

Abid, M.R., Guo, S., Minami, T., Spokes, K.C., Ueki, K., Skurk, C., Walsh, K., and Aird, W.C. (2004). Vascular endothelial growth factor activates PI3K/Akt/forkhead signaling in endothelial cells. Arterioscler Thromb Vasc Biol *24*, 294-300.

Adjei, A.A., Cohen, R.B., Franklin, W., Morris, C., Wilson, D., Molina, J.R., Hanson, L.J., Gore, L., Chow, L., Leong, S., *et al.* (2008). Phase I pharmacokinetic and pharmacodynamic study of the oral, small-molecule mitogen-activated protein kinase kinase 1/2 inhibitor AZD6244 (ARRY-142886) in patients with advanced cancers. J Clin Oncol *26*, 2139-2146.

Albon, J., Karwatowski, W.S., Avery, N., Easty, D.L., and Duance, V.C. (1995). Changes in the collagenous matrix of the aging human lamina cribrosa. Br J Ophthalmol *79*, 368-375.

Angayarkanni, N., Barathi, S., Seethalakshmi, T., Punitham, R., Sivaramakrishna, R., Suganeswari, G., and Tarun, S. (2008). Serum PON1 arylesterase activity in relation to hyperhomocysteinaemia and oxidative stress in young adult central retinal venous occlusion patients. Eye (Lond) *22*, 969-974.

Arrigo, A.P., Simon, S., Gibert, B., Kretz-Remy, C., Nivon, M., Czekalla, A., Guillet, D., Moulin, M., Diaz-Latoud, C., and Vicart, P. (2007). Hsp27 (HspB1) and alphaB-crystallin (HspB5) as therapeutic targets. FEBS Lett *581*, 3665-3674.

Aveleira, C.A., Lin, C.M., Abcouwer, S.F., Ambrosio, A.F., and Antonetti, D.A. (2010). TNF-alpha signals through PKCzeta/NF-kappaB to alter the tight junction complex and increase retinal endothelial cell permeability. Diabetes *59*, 2872-2882.

Bajaire, B.J., Paipilla, D.F., Arrieta, C.E., and Oudovitchenko, E. (2011). Mixed vascular occlusion in a patient with interferon-associated retinopathy. Case Report Ophthalmol *2*, 23-29.

Basuroy, S., Seth, A., Elias, B., Naren, A.P., and Rao, R. (2006). MAPK interacts with occludin and mediates EGF-induced prevention of tight junction disruption by hydrogen peroxide. Biochem J *393*, 69-77.

Battcock, S.M., Collier, T.W., Zu, D., and Hirasawa, K. (2006). Negative regulation of the alpha interferon-induced antiviral response by the Ras/Raf/MEK pathway. J Virol *80*, 4422-4430.

Bekaii-Saab, T., Phelps, M.A., Li, X., Saji, M., Goff, L., Kauh, J.S., O'Neil, B.H., Balsom, S., Balint, C., Liersemann, R., *et al.* (2011). Multi-institutional phase II study of selumetinib in patients with metastatic biliary cancers. J Clin Oncol *29*, 2357-2363.

Bodoky, G., Timcheva, C., Spigel, D.R., La Stella, P.J., Ciuleanu, T.E., Pover, G., and Tebbutt, N.C. (2011). A phase II open-label randomized study to assess the efficacy and safety of selumetinib (AZD6244 [ARRY-142886]) versus capecitabine in patients with advanced or metastatic pancreatic cancer who have failed first-line gemcitabine therapy. Invest New Drugs.

Boyd, S.R., Zachary, I., Chakravarthy, U., Allen, G.J., Wisdom, G.B., Cree, I.A., Martin, J.F., and Hykin, P.G. (2002). Correlation of increased vascular endothelial growth factor with neovascularization and permeability in ischemic central vein occlusion. Arch Ophthalmol *120*, 1644-1650.

Brafman, A., Mett, I., Shafir, M., Gottlieb, H., Damari, G., Gozlan-Kelner, S., Vishnevskia-Dai, V., Skaliter, R., Einat, P., Faerman, A., *et al.* (2004). Inhibition of oxygen-induced retinopathy in RTP801-deficient mice. Invest Ophthalmol Vis Sci *45*, 3796-3805.

Burke, J.M. (2008). Epithelial phenotype and the RPE: is the answer blowing in the Wnt? Prog Retin Eye Res *27*, 579-595.

Busik, J.V., Mohr, S., and Grant, M.B. (2008). Hyperglycemia-induced reactive oxygen species toxicity to endothelial cells is dependent on paracrine mediators. Diabetes *57*, 1952-1965.

Caraglia, M., Marra, M., Pelaia, G., Maselli, R., Caputi, M., Marsico, S.A., and Abbruzzese, A. (2005). Alpha-interferon and its effects on signal transduction pathways. J Cell Physiol *202*, 323-335.

Caraglia, M., Tagliaferri, P., Marra, M., Giuberti, G., Budillon, A., Gennaro, E.D., Pepe, S., Vitale, G., Improta, S., Tassone, P., *et al.* (2003). EGF activates an inducible survival response via the RAS-> Erk-1/2 pathway to counteract interferon-alpha-mediated apoptosis in epidermoid cancer cells. Cell Death Differ *10*, 218-229.

Chan, C.M., Huang, J.H., Lin, H.H., Chiang, H.S., Chen, B.H., Hong, J.Y., and Hung, C.F. (2008). Protective effects of (-)-epigallocatechin gallate on UVA-induced damage in ARPE19 cells. Mol Vis *14*, 2528-2534.

Cheung, N., Klein, R., Wang, J.J., Cotch, M.F., Islam, A.F., Klein, B.E., Cushman, M., and Wong, T.Y. (2008). Traditional and novel cardiovascular risk factors for retinal vein occlusion: the multiethnic study of atherosclerosis. Invest Ophthalmol Vis Sci *49*, 4297-4302.

Chibber, R., Ben-Mahmud, B.M., Chibber, S., and Kohner, E.M. (2007). Leukocytes in diabetic retinopathy. Curr Diabetes Rev *3*, 3-14.

Christian, S.L., Collier, T.W., Zu, D., Licursi, M., Hough, C.M., and Hirasawa, K. (2009). Activated Ras/MEK inhibits the antiviral response of alpha interferon by reducing STAT2 levels. J Virol *83*, 6717-6726.

Chua, C.C., Hamdy, R.C., and Chua, B.H. (1998). Upregulation of vascular endothelial growth factor by H2O2 in rat heart endothelial cells. Free Radic Biol Med *25*, 891-897.

Cowan, K.J., and Storey, K.B. (2003). Mitogen-activated protein kinases: new signaling pathways functioning in cellular responses to environmental stress. J Exp Biol *206*, 1107-1115.

de Nadal, E., Alepuz, P.M., and Posas, F. (2002). Dealing with osmostress through MAP kinase activation. EMBO Rep *3*, 735-740.

Dong, X., Li, Z., Wang, W., Zhang, W., Liu, S., and Zhang, X. (2011). Protective effect of canolol from oxidative stress-induced cell damage in ARPE-19 cells via an ERK mediated antioxidative pathway. Mol Vis *17*, 2040-2048.

Du, Y., Tang, J., Li, G., Berti-Mattera, L., Lee, C.A., Bartkowski, D., Gale, D., Monahan, J., Niesman, M.R., Alton, G., *et al.* (2010). Effects of p38 MAPK inhibition on early stages of diabetic retinopathy and sensory nerve function. Invest Ophthalmol Vis Sci *51*, 2158-2164.

El-Remessy, A.B., Behzadian, M.A., Abou-Mohamed, G., Franklin, T., Caldwell, R.W., and Caldwell, R.B. (2003). Experimental diabetes causes breakdown of the blood-retina barrier by a mechanism involving tyrosine nitration and increases in expression of vascular endothelial growth factor and urokinase plasminogen activator receptor. Am J Pathol *162*, 1995-2004.

El-Remessy, A.B., Rajesh, M., Mukhopadhyay, P., Horvath, B., Patel, V., Al-Gayyar, M.M., Pillai, B.A., and Pacher, P. (2011). Cannabinoid 1 receptor activation contributes to vascular inflammation and cell death in a mouse model of diabetic retinopathy and a human retinal cell line. Diabetologia *54*, 1567-1578.

Esmaeli, B., Koller, C., Papadopoulos, N., and Romaguera, J. (2001). Interferon-induced retinopathy in asymptomatic cancer patients. Ophthalmology *108*, 858-860.

Fegan, C.D. (2002). Central retinal vein occlusion and thrombophilia. Eye (Lond) *16*, 98-106.

Felinski, E.A., and Antonetti, D.A. (2005). Glucocorticoid regulation of endothelial cell tight junction gene expression: novel treatments for diabetic retinopathy. Curr Eye Res *30*, 949-957.

Fraenkl, S.A., Mozaffarieh, M., and Flammer, J. (2010). Retinal vein occlusions: The potential impact of a dysregulation of the retinal veins. EPMA J *1*, 253-261.

Frey, T., and Antonetti, D.A. (2011). Alterations to the blood-retinal barrier in diabetes: cytokines and reactive oxygen species. Antioxid Redox Signal *15*, 1271-1284.

Funk, M., Kriechbaum, K., Prager, F., Benesch, T., Georgopoulos, M., Zlabinger, G.J., and Schmidt-Erfurth, U. (2009). Intraocular concentrations of growth factors and cytokines in retinal vein occlusion and the effect of therapy with bevacizumab. Invest Ophthalmol Vis Sci *50*, 1025-1032.

Furst, R., Zahler, S., and Vollmar, A.M. (2008). Dexamethasone-induced expression of endothelial mitogen-activated protein kinase phosphatase-1 involves activation of the transcription factors activator protein-1 and 3',5'-cyclic adenosine 5'-monophosphate response element-binding protein and the generation of reactive oxygen species. Endocrinology *149*, 3635-3642.

Garrido-Urbani, S., Bradfield, P.F., Lee, B.P., and Imhof, B.A. (2008). Vascular and epithelial junctions: a barrier for leucocyte migration. Biochem Soc Trans *36*, 203-211.

Glotin, A.L., Calipel, A., Brossas, J.Y., Faussat, A.M., Treton, J., and Mascarelli, F. (2006). Sustained versus transient ERK1/2 signaling underlies the anti- and proapoptotic effects of oxidative stress in human RPE cells. Invest Ophthalmol Vis Sci *47*, 4614-4623.

Gonzalez, J.E., DiGeronimo, R.J., Arthur, D.E., and King, J.M. (2009). Remodeling of the tight junction during recovery from exposure to hydrogen peroxide in kidney epithelial cells. Free Radic Biol Med *47*, 1561-1569.

Gu, X., Samuel, S., El-Shabrawey, M., Caldwell, R.B., Bartoli, M., Marcus, D.M., and Brooks, S.E. (2002). Effects of sustained hyperoxia on revascularization in experimental retinopathy of prematurity. Invest Ophthalmol Vis Sci *43*, 496-502.

Gumus, K., Kadayifcilar, S., Eldem, B., Saracbasi, O., Ozcebe, O., Dundar, S., and Kirazli, S. (2006). Is elevated level of soluble endothelial protein C receptor a new risk factor for retinal vein occlusion? Clin Experiment Ophthalmol *34*, 305-311.

Hardy, P., Beauchamp, M., Sennlaub, F., Gobeil, F., Jr., Tremblay, L., Mwaikambo, B., Lachapelle, P., and Chemtob, S. (2005). New insights into the retinal circulation: inflammatory lipid mediators in ischemic retinopathy. Prostaglandins Leukot Essent Fatty Acids *72*, 301-325.

Hayreh, S.S., Zimmerman, M.B., and Podhajsky, P. (1994). Incidence of various types of retinal vein occlusion and their recurrence and demographic characteristics. Am J Ophthalmol *117*, 429-441.

Houle, F., and Huot, J. (2006). Dysregulation of the endothelial cellular response to oxidative stress in cancer. Mol Carcinog *45*, 362-367.

Houle, F., Rousseau, S., Morrice, N., Luc, M., Mongrain, S., Turner, C.E., Tanaka, S., Moreau, P., and Huot, J. (2003). Extracellular signal-regulated kinase mediates phosphorylation of tropomyosin-1 to promote cytoskeleton remodeling in response to oxidative stress: impact on membrane blebbing. Mol Biol Cell *14*, 1418-1432.

Huang, W., Yang, A.H., Matsumoto, D., Collette, W., Marroquin, L., Ko, M., Aguirre, S., and Younis, H.S. (2009). PD0325901, a mitogen-activated protein kinase kinase inhibitor, produces ocular toxicity in a rabbit animal model of retinal vein occlusion. J Ocul Pharmacol Ther *25*, 519-530.

Huot, J., Houle, F., Rousseau, S., Deschesnes, R.G., Shah, G.M., and Landry, J. (1998). SAPK2/p38-dependent F-actin reorganization regulates early membrane blebbing during stress-induced apoptosis. J Cell Biol *143*, 1361-1373.

Janssen, M.C., den Heijer, M., Cruysberg, J.R., Wollersheim, H., and Bredie, S.J. (2005). Retinal vein occlusion: a form of venous thrombosis or a complication of atherosclerosis? A meta-analysis of thrombophilic factors. Thromb Haemost *93*, 1021-1026.

Jiang, Q., Cao, C., Lu, S., Kivlin, R., Wallin, B., Chu, W., Bi, Z., Wang, X., and Wan, Y. (2009). MEK/ERK pathway mediates UVB-induced AQP1 downregulation and water permeability impairment in human retinal pigment epithelial cells. Int J Mol Med *23*, 771-777.

Kachi, S., Kobayashi, K., Ushida, H., Ito, Y., Kondo, M., and Terasaki, H. (2010). Regression of macular edema secondary to branch retinal vein occlusion during anti-TNF-alpha therapy for rheumatoid arthritis. Clin Ophthalmol *4*, 667-670.

Kanehisa, M. and Goto, S. (2000). KEGG: Kyoto Encyclopedia of Genes and Genomes. Nucleic Acids Res *28*, 27-30.

Kanehisa, M., Goto, S., Sato, Y., Furumichi, M., and Tanabe, M. (2012). KEGG for integration and interpretation of large-scale molecular datasets. Nucleic Acids Res *40*, D109-D114.

Kaur, C., Foulds, W.S., and Ling, E.A. (2008). Blood-retinal barrier in hypoxic ischaemic conditions: basic concepts, clinical features and management. Prog Retin Eye Res *27*, 622-647.

Kemeny, N., Childs, B., Larchian, W., Rosado, K., and Kelsen, D. (1990). A phase II trial of recombinant tumor necrosis factor in patients with advanced colorectal carcinoma. Cancer *66*, 659-663.

Klein, R., Moss, S.E., Meuer, S.M., and Klein, B.E. (2008). The 15-year cumulative incidence of retinal vein occlusion: the Beaver Dam Eye Study. Arch Ophthalmol *126*, 513-518.

Klettner, A., and Roider, J. (2009). Constitutive and oxidative-stress-induced expression of VEGF in the RPE are differently regulated by different Mitogen-activated protein kinases. Graefes Arch Clin Exp Ophthalmol *247*, 1487-1492.

Koizumi, H., Ferrara, D.C., Brue, C., and Spaide, R.F. (2007). Central retinal vein occlusion case-control study. Am J Ophthalmol *144*, 858-863.

Kotwal, R.S., Butler, F.K., Jr., Murray, C.K., Hill, G.J., Rayfield, J.C., and Miles, E.A. (2009). Central retinal vein occlusion in an Army Ranger with glucose-6-phosphate dehydrogenase deficiency. J Spec Oper Med *9*, 59-63.

Kunsch, C., and Medford, R.M. (1999). Oxidative stress as a regulator of gene expression in the vasculature. Circ Res *85*, 753-766.

Larrayoz, I.M., Huang, J.D., Lee, J.W., Pascual, I., and Rodriguez, I.R. (2010). 7-ketocholesterol-induced inflammation: involvement of multiple kinase signaling pathways via NFkappaB but independently of reactive oxygen species formation. Invest Ophthalmol Vis Sci *51*, 4942-4955.

Lee, K.S., Park, S.J., Kim, S.R., Min, K.H., Jin, S.M., Puri, K.D., and Lee, Y.C. (2006). Phosphoinositide 3-kinase-delta inhibitor reduces vascular permeability in a murine model of asthma. J Allergy Clin Immunol *118*, 403-409.

Li, C., Chi, S., He, N., Zhang, X., Guicherit, O., Wagner, R., Tyring, S., and Xie, J. (2004). IFNalpha induces Fas expression and apoptosis in hedgehog pathway activated BCC cells through inhibiting Ras-Erk signaling. Oncogene *23*, 1608-1617.

Lim, L.L., Cheung, N., Wang, J.J., Islam, F.M., Mitchell, P., Saw, S.M., Aung, T., and Wong, T.Y. (2008). Prevalence and risk factors of retinal vein occlusion in an Asian population. Br J Ophthalmol *92*, 1316-1319.

Lip, P.L., Blann, A.D., Jones, A.F., and Lip, G.Y. (1998). Abnormalities in haemorheological factors and lipoprotein (a) in retinal vascular occlusion: implications for increased vascular risk. Eye *12 (Pt 2)*, 245-251.

LoRusso, P.M., Krishnamurthi, S.S., Rinehart, J.J., Nabell, L.M., Malburg, L., Chapman, P.B., DePrimo, S.E., Bentivegna, S., Wilner, K.D., Tan, W., *et al.* (2010). Phase I pharmacokinetic and pharmacodynamic study of the oral MAPK/ERK kinase inhibitor PD-0325901 in patients with advanced cancers. Clin Cancer Res *16*, 1924-1937.

Lum, H., and Roebuck, K.A. (2001). Oxidant stress and endothelial cell dysfunction. Am J Physiol Cell Physiol *280*, C719-741.

Marcucci, R., Sofi, F., Grifoni, E., Sodi, A., and Prisco, D. (2011). Retinal vein occlusions: a review for the internist. Intern Emerg Med *6*, 307-314.

McAllister, I.L., Vijayasekaran, S., Chen, S.D., and Yu, D.Y. (2009). Effect of triamcinolone acetonide on vascular endothelial growth factor and occludin levels in branch retinal vein occlusion. Am J Ophthalmol *147*, 838-846, 846 e831-832.

McCoy, E., and Sontheimer, H. (2010). MAPK induces AQP1 expression in astrocytes following injury. Glia *58*, 209-217.

Mitchell, P., Smith, W., and Chang, A. (1996). Prevalence and associations of retinal vein occlusion in Australia. The Blue Mountains Eye Study. Arch Ophthalmol *114*, 1243-1247.

Nadir, A., Amin, A., Chalisa, N., and van Thiel, D.H. (2000). Retinal vein thrombosis associated with chronic hepatitis C: a case series and review of the literature. J Viral Hepat *7*, 466-470.

Niessen, C.M. (2007) Tight junctions/adherens junctions: basic structure and function. J Invest Dermatol *127*, 2525-32.

Niwa, K., Inanami, O., Ohta, T., Ito, S., Karino, T., and Kuwabara, M. (2001). p38 MAPK and Ca2+ contribute to hydrogen peroxide-induced increase of permeability in vascular endothelial cells but ERK does not. Free Radic Res *35*, 519-527.

Noma, H., Funatsu, H., Mimura, T., Harino, S., and Hori, S. (2009). Vitreous levels of interleukin-6 and vascular endothelial growth factor in macular edema with central retinal vein occlusion. Ophthalmology *116*, 87-93.

Noma, H., Minamoto, A., Funatsu, H., Tsukamoto, H., Nakano, K., Yamashita, H., and Mishima, H.K. (2006). Intravitreal levels of vascular endothelial growth factor and interleukin-6 are correlated with macular edema in branch retinal vein occlusion. Graefes Arch Clin Exp Ophthalmol *244*, 309-315.

Patrassi, G.M., Mares, M., Piermarocchi, S., Santarossa, A., Viero, M., and Girolami, A. (1987). Fibrinolytic behavior in long-standing branch retinal vein occlusion. Ophthalmic Res *19*, 221-225.

Peduzzi, M., Debbia, A., Guerrieri, F., and Bolzani, R. (1986). Abnormal blood rheology in retinal vein occlusion. A preliminary report. Graefes Arch Clin Exp Ophthalmol *224*, 83-85.

Puli, S.R., and Benage, D.D. (2003). Retinal vein thrombosis after infliximab (Remicade) treatment for Crohn's disease. Am J Gastroenterol *98*, 939-940.

Qin, S., McLaughlin, A.P., and De Vries, G.W. (2006). Protection of RPE cells from oxidative injury by 15-deoxy-delta12,14-prostaglandin J2 by augmenting GSH and activating MAPK. Invest Ophthalmol Vis Sci *47*, 5098-5105.

Rao, K.V., Jayakumar, A.R., Reddy, P.V., Tong, X., Curtis, K.M., and Norenberg, M.D. (2010). Aquaporin-4 in manganese-treated cultured astrocytes. Glia *58*, 1490-1499.

Rehak, J., and Rehak, M. (2008). Branch retinal vein occlusion: pathogenesis, visual prognosis, and treatment modalities. Curr Eye Res *33*, 111-131.

Rehak, M., Hollborn, M., Iandiev, I., Pannicke, T., Karl, A., Wurm, A., Kohen, L., Reichenbach, A., Wiedemann, P., and Bringmann, A. (2008). Retinal Gene Expression and Muller Cell Responses after Branch Retinal Vein Occlusion in the Rat. Invest Ophthalmol Vis Sci.

Reichenbach, A., Wurm, A., Pannicke, T., Iandiev, I., Wiedemann, P., and Bringmann, A. (2007). Muller cells as players in retinal degeneration and edema. Graefes Arch Clin Exp Ophthalmol *245*, 627-636.

Rinehart, J., Adjei, A.A., Lorusso, P.M., Waterhouse, D., Hecht, J.R., Natale, R.B., Hamid, O., Varterasian, M., Asbury, P., Kaldjian, E.P., *et al.* (2004). Multicenter phase II study of the oral MEK inhibitor, CI-1040, in patients with advanced non-small-cell lung, breast, colon, and pancreatic cancer. J Clin Oncol *22*, 4456-4462.

Rogers, S., McIntosh, R.L., Cheung, N., Lim, L., Wang, J.J., Mitchell, P., Kowalski, J.W., Nguyen, H., and Wong, T.Y. (2010). The prevalence of retinal vein occlusion: pooled data from population studies from the United States, Europe, Asia, and Australia. Ophthalmology *117*, 313-319 e311.

Romerio, F., and Zella, D. (2002). MEK and ERK inhibitors enhance the anti-proliferative effect of interferon-alpha2b. Faseb J *16*, 1680-1682.

Romerio, F., Riva, A., and Zella, D. (2000). Interferon-alpha2b reduces phosphorylation and activity of MEK and ERK through a Ras/Raf-independent mechanism. Br J Cancer *83*, 532-538.

Schweitzer, K.S., Hatoum, H., Brown, M.B., Gupta, M., Justice, M.J., Beteck, B., Van Demark, M.J., Gu, Y., Presson, R.G., Jr., Hubbard, W.C., *et al.* (2011). Mechanisms of lung endothelial barrier disruption induced by cigarette smoke: role of oxidative stress and ceramides. Am J Physiol Lung Cell Mol Physiol.

Sen, U., Tyagi, N., Patibandla, P.K., Dean, W.L., Tyagi, S.C., Roberts, A.M., and Lominadze, D. (2009). Fibrinogen-induced endothelin-1 production from endothelial cells. Am J Physiol Cell Physiol *296*, C840-847.

Serban, D., Leng, J., and Cheresh, D. (2008). H-ras regulates angiogenesis and vascular permeability by activation of distinct downstream effectors. Circ Res *102*, 1350-1358.

Simoncini, S., Sapet, C., Camoin-Jau, L., Bardin, N., Harle, J.R., Sampol, J., Dignat-George, F., and Anfosso, F. (2005). Role of reactive oxygen species and p38 MAPK in the induction of the pro-adhesive endothelial state mediated by IgG from patients with anti-phospholipid syndrome. Int Immunol *17*, 489-500.

Siu, T.L., Morley, J.W., and Coroneo, M.T. (2008). Toxicology of the retina: advances in understanding the defence mechanisms and pathogenesis of drug- and light-induced retinopathy. Clin Experiment Ophthalmol *36*, 176-185.

Sperduto, R.D., Hiller, R., Chew, E., Seigel, D., Blair, N., Burton, T.C., Farber, M.D., Gragoudas, E.S., Haller, J., Seddon, J.M., *et al.* (1998). Risk factors for hemiretinal vein occlusion: comparison with risk factors for central and branch retinal vein occlusion: the eye disease case-control study. Ophthalmology *105*, 765-771.

Sprague, A.H., and Khalil, R.A. (2009). Inflammatory cytokines in vascular dysfunction and vascular disease. Biochem Pharmacol *78*, 539-552.

Tenenbaum, T., Matalon, D., Adam, R., Seibt, A., Wewer, C., Schwerk, C., Galla, H.J., and Schroten, H. (2008). Dexamethasone prevents alteration of tight junction-associated proteins and barrier function in porcine choroid plexus epithelial cells after infection with Streptococcus suis in vitro. Brain Res *1229*, 1-17.

Tezel, G., Yang, X., Luo, C., Peng, Y., Sun, S.L., and Sun, D. (2007). Mechanisms of immune system activation in glaucoma: oxidative stress-stimulated antigen presentation by the retina and optic nerve head glia. Invest Ophthalmol Vis Sci *48*, 705-714.

The Eye Disease Case-Control Study Group. (1993). Risk factors for branch retinal vein occlusion. Am J Ophthalmol 116, 286-296

The Eye Disease Case-Control Study Group. (1996). Risk factors for central retinal vein occlusion. Arch Ophthalmol 114, 545-554.

Trope, G.E., Lowe, G.D., McArdle, B.M., Douglas, J.T., Forbes, C.D., Prentice, C.M., and Foulds, W.S. (1983). Abnormal blood viscosity and haemostasis in long-standing retinal vein occlusion. Br J Ophthalmol *67*, 137-142.

Tsao, Y.P., Ho, T.C., Chen, S.L., and Cheng, H.C. (2006). Pigment epithelium-derived factor inhibits oxidative stress-induced cell death by activation of extracellular signal-regulated kinases in cultured retinal pigment epithelial cells. Life Sci *79*, 545-550.

Tyagi, N., Roberts, A.M., Dean, W.L., Tyagi, S.C., and Lominadze, D. (2008). Fibrinogen induces endothelial cell permeability. Mol Cell Biochem *307*, 13-22.

Uno, K., Prow, T.W., Bhutto, I.A., Yerrapureddy, A., McLeod, D.S., Yamamoto, M., Reddy, S.P., and Lutty, G.A. (2010). Role of Nrf2 in retinal vascular development and the vaso-obliterative phase of oxygen-induced retinopathy. Exp Eye Res *90*, 493-500.

Usatyuk, P.V., and Natarajan, V. (2004). Role of mitogen-activated protein kinases in 4-hydroxy-2-nonenal-induced actin remodeling and barrier function in endothelial cells. J Biol Chem *279*, 11789-11797.

Usatyuk, P.V., Parinandi, N.L., and Natarajan, V. (2006). Redox regulation of 4-hydroxy-2-nonenal-mediated endothelial barrier dysfunction by focal adhesion, adherens, and tight junction proteins. J Biol Chem *281*, 35554-35566.

Ushio-Fukai, M., and Alexander, R.W. (2004). Reactive oxygen species as mediators of angiogenesis signaling: role of NAD(P)H oxidase. Mol Cell Biochem *264*, 85-97.

Vandenbroucke, E., Mehta, D., Minshall, R., and Malik, A.B. (2008). Regulation of endothelial junctional permeability. Ann N Y Acad Sci *1123*, 134-145.

Veerappan, S.G., Kennedy, M., O'Morain, C.A., and Ryan, B.M. (2008). Retinal vein thrombosis following infliximab treatment for severe left-sided ulcerative colitis. Eur J Gastroenterol Hepatol *20*, 588-589.

Vergou, T., Moustou, A.E., Maniateas, A., Stratigos, A.J., Katsambas, A., and Antoniou, C. (2010). Central retinal vein occlusion following infliximab treatment for plaque-type psoriasis. Int J Dermatol *49*, 1215-1217.

Wang, X., Martindale, J.L., Liu, Y., and Holbrook, N.J. (1998). The cellular response to oxidative stress: influences of mitogen-activated protein kinase signalling pathways on cell survival. Biochem J *333 (Pt 2)*, 291-300.

Wang, Y., Bian, Z.M., Yu, W.Z., Yan, Z., Chen, W.C., and Li, X.X. (2010). Induction of interleukin-8 gene expression and protein secretion by C-reactive protein in ARPE-19 cells. Exp Eye Res *91*, 135-142.

Wu, W.C., Hu, D.N., Gao, H.X., Chen, M., Wang, D., Rosen, R., and McCormick, S.A. (2010). Subtoxic levels hydrogen peroxide-induced production of interleukin-6 by retinal pigment epithelial cells. Mol Vis *16*, 1864-1873.

Wurm, A., Iandiev, I., Uhlmann, S., Wiedemann, P., Reichenbach, A., Bringmann, A., and Pannicke, T. (2011). Effects of ischemia-reperfusion on physiological properties of Muller glial cells in the porcine retina. Invest Ophthalmol Vis Sci *52*, 3360-3367.

Xu, L., Liu, W.W., Wang, Y.X., Yang, H., and Jonas, J.B. (2007). Retinal vein occlusions and mortality: the Beijing Eye Study. Am J Ophthalmol *144*, 972-973.

Yafai, Y., Lange, J., Wiedemann, P., Reichenbach, A., and Eichler, W. (2007). Pigment epithelium-derived factor acts as an opponent of growth-stimulatory factors in retinal glial-endothelial cell interactions. Glia *55*, 642-651.

Yang, J., Duh, E.J., Caldwell, R.B., and Behzadian, M.A. (2010a). Antipermeability function of PEDF involves blockade of the MAP kinase/GSK/beta-catenin signaling pathway and uPAR expression. Invest Ophthalmol Vis Sci *51*, 3273-3280.

Yang, Y., Hayden, M.R., Sowers, S., Bagree, S.V., and Sowers, J.R. (2010b). Retinal redox stress and remodeling in cardiometabolic syndrome and diabetes. Oxid Med Cell Longev *3*, 392-403.

Yoshida, Y., Yamagishi, S., Matsui, T., Jinnouchi, Y., Fukami, K., Imaizumi, T., and Yamakawa, R. (2009). Protective role of pigment epithelium-derived factor (PEDF) in early phase of experimental diabetic retinopathy. Diabetes Metab Res Rev *25*, 678-686.

Yoshimura, T., Sonoda, K.H., Sugahara, M., Mochizuki, Y., Enaida, H., Oshima, Y., Ueno, A., Hata, Y., Yoshida, H., and Ishibashi, T. (2009). Comprehensive analysis of inflammatory immune mediators in vitreoretinal diseases. PLoS One *4*, e8158.

Yuan, S.Y. (2002). Protein kinase signaling in the modulation of microvascular permeability. Vascul Pharmacol *39*, 213-223.

Zhang, C., Lam, T.T., and Tso, M.O. (2005). Heterogeneous populations of microglia/macrophages in the retina and their activation after retinal ischemia and reperfusion injury. Exp Eye Res *81*, 700-709.

Zhang, J., Wu, G.S., Ishimoto, S., Pararajasegaram, G., and Rao, N.A. (1997). Expression of major histocompatibility complex molecules in rodent retina. Immunohistochemical study. Invest Ophthalmol Vis Sci *38*, 1848-1857.

Zheng, Z., Chen, H., Wang, H., Ke, B., Zheng, B., Li, Q., Li, P., Su, L., Gu, Q., and Xu, X. (2010). Improvement of retinal vascular injury in diabetic rats by statins is associated with the inhibition of mitochondrial reactive oxygen species pathway mediated by peroxisome proliferator-activated receptor gamma coactivator 1alpha. Diabetes *59*, 2315-2325.

Section 6

Cancer

22

Oxidative Therapy Against Cancer

Manuel de Miguel and Mario D. Cordero
Departamento de Citología e Histología Normal y Patológica,
Facultad de Medicina, Universidad de Sevilla, Sevilla
Spain

1. Introduction

Although a moderate increase of reactive oxygen species (ROS) may induce cell proliferation, excessive amounts of ROS can cause oxidative damage to lipids, proteins, and DNA, provoking oncogenic transformation, increased metabolic activity, and mitochondrial dysfunction (Dreher and Junod, 1996; Behrend et al., 2003; Pelicano et al, 2003). Many reports suggest that cancer cells are under a continuous oxidative stress (Pervaiz and Clement, 2004; Schumacker et al., 2006; Kryston et al., 2011). Studies with human tumor cell lines clearly show that these cells produce ROS at a much higher rate than healthy cells (Oberley and Buettner, 1979; Lu et al., 2007). ROS have been established as important molecules involved in the multistage process of carcinogenesis (Klaunig and Kamendulis, 2004). Mitochondria are the major consumers of molecular oxygen in cells, representing an important source of ROS. It is well accepted that cancer cells present mitochondrial alterations which result in respiration injury. This mitochondrial dysfunction may induce a low coupling efficiency of the mitochondrial electron chain, increasing electron leakage and leading to enhanced ROS formation. The resulting oxidative stress may cause further damage to both mitochondrial DNA (mtDNA) and the respiratory chain, amplifying the ROS generation (Zorov et al., 2006).

The higher oxidative stress observed in cancer cells can also result from a decrease or inactivation of antioxidants (Huang et al., 2003; Conklin, 2004). The majority of tumor cells usually present very few antioxidative enzymes, such as catalase, superoxide dismutase, and glutathione peroxidase, which are known to play a protective role against ROS in normal cells (Sato et al., 1992; Hasegawa et al., 2002; Pelicano et al., 2004). The lack of proper antioxidant defences makes tumor cells very vulnerable to oxidative stress. Nevertheless, some studies have revealed increased expression of antioxidants, probably as a consequence of selective pressure towards stress adaptation. The sources of ROS in cancer cells and the consequences of oxidative stress in the carcinogenesis process are still under debate.

What seems accepted is that cancer cells have increased ROS steady state level and are likely to be more vulnerable to damage by further ROS insults induced by exogenous agents. Thus, manipulating ROS levels by redox modulation could be a way to selectively kill cancer cells without causing significant toxicity to normal cells. A promising anticancer strategy named "oxidation therapy" has been developed by inducing cytotoxic oxidative stress for cancer treatment. This could be achieved by two different methods: inducing the generation of cytotoxic levels of ROS, and inhibiting the antioxidant system of tumor cells (Fang et al., 2007; Trachootham et al., 2009).

It is well known that ROS, such as hydrogen peroxide (H_2O_2) and superoxide anion, induce apoptosis to a wide range of tumor cells through the activation of the caspase cascade. It has been described that mitochondrial damage induced by the use of certain drugs provokes an increment of oxidative stress and cell death (Chandra et al., 2000; Conklin, 2004). Major ROS-modulating agents are based on the capacity to induce high ROS generation or to reduce the antioxidant defence machinery of cancer cells.

An interesting drug for oxidative cancer therapy is amitriptyline, a tricyclic antidepressant commonly prescribed for depression and therapeutic treatments of several neuropathic and inflammatory illnesses. Chlorimipramine, another tricyclic antidepressant, has been already proposed as a novel anticancer agent targeted to mitochondria as it induces caspase-3-dependent apoptosis (Daley et al., 2005). Several reports showed that the toxicity of this drug is due to an increase in oxidative stress by the generation of high amounts of ROS (Daley et al., 2005; Moreno-Fernández et al., 2008; Cordero et al., 2009). Therefore, amitriptyline has being proposed to be used for anticancer oxidant therapy against tumors that present significant oxidative stress and/or low antioxidant defences (Cordero et al., 2010).

2. Mitochondria and Reactive Oxygen Species (ROS)

Mitochondria are dynamic organelles that play a central role in many cellular functions including the generation of chemical energy (adenosine triphosphate, ATP), heat, and intracellular calcium homeostasis. They are also responsible for the formation of ROS and for triggering the programmed cell death or apoptosis (Turrens, 2003). The primary metabolic function of mitochondria is oxidative phosphorylation, an energy-generating process that couples oxidation of respiratory substrates to the synthesis of ATP (Pieczenik & Neustadt, 2007). The mitochondrial respiratory chain (MRC) is composed of five multisubunit enzyme complexes. Both the mtDNA and the nuclear DNA (nDNA) encode for polypeptide components of these complexes. Electron transport between MRC complexes I–IV is coupled to the extrusion of protons across the inner mitochondrial membrane by proton pump components of the respiratory chain. This movement of protons creates an electrochemical gradient ($\Delta\Psi m$) across the inner mitochondrial membrane. Protons return to the mitochondrial matrix by flowing through ATP synthase (complex V), which utilizes the energy thus produced to synthesize ATP from adenosine diphosphate (ADP) and inorganic phosphate. Both the mtDNA and the nDNA encode for polypeptide components of these complexes. As a consequence, mutations in either genome can cause MRC dysfunction that impairs transport of electrons and/or protons and decreases ATP synthesis. Primary or secondary genetic diseases affecting MRC or secondary mitochondrial dysfunctions usually affect brain and skeletal muscle because of their energy requirements. Besides MRC enzyme complexes, two electron carriers, coenzyme Q_{10} (CoQ) and cytochrome c, are essential for mitochondrial synthesis of ATP. CoQ transports electrons from complexes I and II to complex III and is essential for the stability of complex III. CoQ is a lipid-soluble component of virtually all cell membranes. CoQ also functions as an antioxidant that protects cells both by direct ROS scavenging and by regenerating other antioxidants such as vitamins C and E (Turunen et al., 2004). Given the critical role of CoQ in mitochondria function, it has been suggested that CoQ levels could be a useful biological marker of mitochondrial function (Haas et al., 2008). CoQ deficiency induces decreased mitochondrial respiratory enzymes activity, reduced expression of mitochondrial proteins involved in oxidative phosphorylation, decreased mitochondrial membrane potential, increased production of ROS, mitochondrial permeabilization, mitophagy of dysfunctional mitochondria, reduced growth rates and cell death (Rodriguez-Hernandez et al., 2009, Cotan et al, 2011).

In addition to energy, mitochondrial oxidative phosphorylation also generates ROS. When the MRC becomes highly reduced, the excess electrons from complex I or complex III may increase substantially, passing directly to O_2 to generate high amounts of superoxide anion ($O_2^{\bullet-}$). Superoxide is transformed to hydrogen peroxide (H_2O_2) by the detoxification enzymes manganese superoxide dismutase (MnSOD) or copper/zinc superoxide dismutase (Cu/Zn SOD), and then to water by catalase, glutathione peroxidase (GPx) or peroxiredoxin III (PRX III). However, when these enzymes cannot convert ROS such as the superoxide radical to water fast enough, oxidative damage occurs and accumulates in the mitochondria. If H_2O_2 encounters a reduced transition metal or is mixed with $O_2^{\bullet-}$, the H_2O_2 can be further reduced to hydroxyl radical ($HO^{\bullet}$), the most potent oxidizing agent among ROS. Additionally, nitric oxide ($^{\bullet}NO$) is produced within the mitochondria by mitochondrial nitric oxide synthase (mtNOS) and also freely diffuses into the mitochondria from the cytosol. $^{\bullet}NO$ reacts with $O_2^{\bullet-}$ to produce peroxynitrite ($ONOO^-$). Together, these two radicals as well as others can do great damage to mitochondria and other cellular components (Turrens, 2003).

Under normal physiological conditions, ROS production is highly regulated. However, if the MRC is inhibited, or key mitochondrial components, such as CoQ, are deficient, then, electrons accumulate on the MRC carriers, greatly increasing the rate of a single electron being transferred to O_2 to generate $O_2^{\bullet-}$. An excessive mitochondrial ROS production can exceed the cellular antioxidant defense and the cumulative damage can ultimately destroy the cell by necrosis or apoptosis.

Mitochondria play an important role in cell bioenergetics and life signaling. Mitochondria are necessary for cell survival but they can also trigger cell death, thus exerting decisive control over the biochemistry of several cascades that lead to cell death, specifically the intrinsic pathway of apoptosis. The particular biochemical properties of these organelles are closely related to their segmented structures, which provide an optimal environment for multiple pathways of biosynthesis and bioenergetics. Consequently, it is possible that these organelles are involved in the process of carcinogenesis through alterations in cell metabolism and cell death pathways (Pilkington et al., 2008). Cancer cells show alterations in mtDNA, in oxidative phosphorylation and in energetic metabolism, all triggered by a pro-oxidative change (Indo et al., 2007). The "respiratory damage" in cancer cells predicts low coupling efficiency in electron transfer at the inner membrane of mitochondria and, consequently, greater loss of electrons, leading to the formation of more $O_2^{\bullet-}$ (Pelicano et al., 2003). The superoxide anion will thus generate more free radicals. Generated ROS can be released into cytosol and trigger "ROS-induced ROS-release" (RIRR) in neighbouring mitochondria. This mitochondrion-to-mitochondrion ROS-signaling constitutes a positive feedback mechanism for enhanced ROS production potentially leading to significant mitochondrial injury (Zorov et al., 2006). Recent studies by a number of groups have demonstrated that ROS can directly modify signaling proteins through different modifications, for example by nitrosylation, carbonylation, disulphide bond formation and glutathionylation. Moreover, redox modification of proteins permits further regulation of cell signaling pathways (England and Cotter, 2005).

3. Oxidative stress and cancer

3.1 ROS and carcinogenesis

In general, oxidative/nitrosative stress could be defined as an imbalance between the presence of high levels of ROS and reactive nitrogen species (RNS), and the antioxidative defense mechanisms. These toxic molecules are formed via oxidation-reduction reactions and are highly reactive since they have an odd number of electrons. ROS generated under physiological conditions are essential for life, as they are involved in bactericidal activity of phagocytes, and in signal transduction pathways, regulating cell growth and reduction–oxidation (redox) status (Davies, 1995). ROS includes free radicals, such as hydroxyl and superoxide radicals, and non-radicals, including hydrogen peroxide and singlet oxygen. Oxidative stress and generation of free radicals, as primary or secondary event, have been related in a great number of diseases, including cancer (Floyd, 1990).

At the beginning of the carcinogenic process, tumor cells accumulate mutations that allow them to proliferate in an uncontrolled way. Moreover, these alterations contribute to increase the susceptibility to accumulate additional genetic modifications, facilitating tumor progression and cancer development. Cancer could be defined as a cell-cycle desease, where its misregulation is considered an essential step (Sandhu et al., 2000). Carcinogenesis is a complex process of different sequencies that allow a cell to evolve from a healthy state into a pre-cancerous state and eventually reach a cancerous state. In this sense, there are several theories about the process of carcinogenesis. For instance, an increase of DNA synthesis and mitosis triggered by non-genotoxic agents could induce mutations in new cells. These mutations could spread through new cell divisions, evolving from an initial pre-neoplastic state into a neoplastic state. Another theory explains the existence of an imbalance between proliferation and cell death, where proliferation is favoured. If DNA damage is too high, there are important mechanisms, such as apoptosis, by which the altered cells are selectively eliminated. Protein p53 plays a fundamental role in this process, as it initiates mechanisms that eliminate, for example, those oxidized DNA bases that could cause mutations. If cell damage is too high, p53 initiates the mechanisms of apoptosis, although uncontrolled processes of apoptosis can be harmful for the organism, since healthy cells could also be eliminated. Therefore, there are systems for regulating apoptosis that consist of both pro-apoptotic and anti-apoptotic factors. Alterations that affect the function of gene p53 have been found in more than half of all types of cancer. This fact supports the idea that carcinogenesis would be caused by an imbalance between proliferation and cell death, in favour of proliferation.

Studies of epidemiology and animal experimentation have shown that carcinogenesis could occur in several stages characterized by different mechanisms. Thus, the model of carcinogenesis based on the hypothesis of three stages: initiation, promotion and progression, should be highlighted. Genotoxic agents are mainly chemical substances that damage DNA directly, inducing the generation of a mutation and/or a set of structural changes. On the other hand, there is a second category of non-genotoxic carcinogenic agents, whose role in the carcinogenic process is not related directly to DNA damage. These compounds modulate mechanisms of cell growth and death. Thus, the development process of a cancer would consist of the accumulation of multiple events, and the ROS could act at different levels and in all stages (Klauning and Kamendulis, 2004). Thereby, ROS can induce both genomic instability, caused by DNA damage, and alterations in cell signaling processes related to survival, proliferation, resistance to apoptosis, angiogenesis and metastasis, thus contributing to cancer initiation, promotion and progression.

Initiation involves a DNA mutation that is not lethal, but it produces a cell alteration followed by at least one round of DNA synthesis that allows fixing the damage done. At this point, the cell can stop its cycle temporally to undo DNA damage and then resume cell division. DNA damage may be done by ROS, like hydroxyl radicals formed by the Fenton´s reaction. Several studies have revealed an interesting correlation between tumor size and the amount of 8-OHdG (8-hydroxy-2'-desoxyguanosine; also known as 8-oxo-deoxyguanosine, 8-oxo-dG), a nucleotide modified by the activity of free radicals (Kennedy et al., 1998; Yano et al., 2009). The promotion stage is characterized by the expansion of initiated cells, stimulating cell proliferation and/or apoptosis inhibition. As a result of this process, an identificable lesion is formed, thus requiring the constant presence of an agent that stimulates promotion. However, it is a reversible process. Many promoter agents have a strong inhibitory capacity against antioxidants like catalases, glutathione, SOD, etc. While a high level of oxidative stress is cytotoxic for cells and stops proliferation inducing apoptosis or even necrosis, moderate levels of oxidative stress may stimulate cell division and, therefore, stimulate tumor growth and promotion (Dreher and Junod, 1996). Progression is the third and last stage of the carcinogenic process. This stage involves cellular and molecular changes that occur from a pre-neoplastic state to a neoplastic state. This stage is irreversible and it is characterized by the accumulation of genetic damage that allows the cell evolving from benign to malignant.

ROS are considered as carcinogenic potentials that facilitate cancer promotion and progression (Pelicano et al., 2004). The DNA molecule is one of the main targets of free radicals activity in the cell, and the modifications performed as a consequence of this activity are relevant for the loss of cell homeostasis. This loss may be extended in time due to the DNA functions of information reservoir. This is why the agents and mechanisms of damage by ROS are studied in depth, because its clarification would lead to elucidate the pathogeny of great morbidity and mortality diseases like cancer. There are different types of oxidative damage to DNA, like modifications and depurinations of DNA bases, DNA chain ruptures, and mutations, which tend to accumulate in an environment with high concentrations of ROS. It is known that DNA damage by ROS occurs spontaneously and there is a normal level of bases modified by ROS in cellular DNA (Okamoto, 2000). The most frequent modification of DNA linked to ROS is the formation of 8-OH-dG, resulting from attack of either a hydroxyl radical or singlet oxygen on deoxyguanosine. 8-OH-dG has a highly mutagenic potential, as 5-hydroxymethyl-2-deoxyuridine (Retel et al., 1993). With relative frequency, the cell will evade DNA damage using specific DNA polymerases and enter DNA replication creating mutations and chromosomal lesions. Alternatively, the presence of unrepaired DNA lesions can induce cell death through the apoptotic pathway. Chronic exposure to DNA lesions can lead to mutations and genomic instability (pre-cancerous state) and eventually to malignant transformations (cancerous state) (Kryston et al., 2011).

3.2 Sources of oxidative stress

Cells from all organisms are exposed to several oxidizing and harmful agents. These attacks can be divided into two groups: exogenous and endogenous. Exogenous sources are related to environmental, medical, diagnostic ionizing and non-ionizing radiations (X- or γ-rays, α-particles from radon decay, UVA radiation) or chemical agents. Endogenous (intracelullar) sources of reactive species are primarily produced by O_2 metabolism, immune responses and inflammation. These processes may result in the production of ROS and RNS that react with DNA and produce several lesions and indirect effects. Ionizing radiations can damage DNA also by direct energy deposition and ionizations (Kryston et al., 2011).

Oxygen metabolism is the major source of ROS in tumor tissues. ROS are continously formed in mitochondria as respiration byproducts. Cancerous cells are metabolically very active and require a great supply of ATP in order to maintain proliferation and cell growth under control. This high energy demand in the mitocondrial respiratory chain contributes to the generation of ROS. Usually, ATP is produced with high efficiency through oxidative phosphorylation in mitochondria. However, a malfunction of mitochondrial respiration is usually observed in neoplastic cells due to deletions/mutations in mtDNA, to the aberrant expression of some enzymes involved in energy metabolism and to hypoxia (Xu et al., 2005; Verrax et al., 2008). On the other hand, the increase of glycolysis in tumor cells has been shown to be related to the aggressiveness of the tumor (Cuezva et al., 2002). Acquiring a glycolytic phenotype represents a key element for cancer survival and progression, while glycolysis inhibition could be proposed as a goal in antitumor therapy (Pelicano et al., 2004). In this sense, glucose deprivation in laboratory models has been shown to be related to an increase of oxidative stress in tumor cells (Spitz et al., 2000). In cell lines of breast carcinoma, glucose deprivation leads to an intracellular increase of pro-oxidants, a decrease of free radical neutralization, and pyruvate depletion, which leads to an increase of oxidative stress (Spitz et al., 2000; Lee et al., 1999). As a compensation mechanism, glucose deprivation induces the expression of heme oxigenase-1 (HO-1), an enzyme that plays an important role in the antioxidant defense system of the organism and in Fe homeostasis. Chang and collegues (Chang et al., 2003) showed that the generation of ROS in mitochondria induces the overexpression of HO-1, which demonstrates that this is a common mechanism of regulation with the aim of protecting cells against oxidative damage.

As already mentioned, immune response and inflamation are other sources of ROS. It is known that oxidative stress activates inflammatory pathways leading to transformation of a normal cell to tumor cell, tumor cell survival, proliferation, insensitivity to anti-growth signaling, invasion, sustained angiogenesis, and stem cell survival (Reuter et al., 2010). Chronic inflammation is triggered by environmental (extrinsic) factors (eg, infection, tobacco, asbestos) and host mutations (intrinsic) factors (eg, Ras, Myc, p53). Activation of Ras, Myc, and p53 cause mitochondrial dysfunction, resulting in mitochondrial ROS production and downstream signaling (eg, NFkappaB, STAT3, etc.) that promote inflammation-associated cancer (Kamp at al., 2011).

On the other hand, during immune responses of many carcinogenetic processes, several immune-related cells play their roles, like intratumoral lymphocytes killing malignant cells and macrophages and neutrophils degrading cells by using oxidants and enzymes. One of these enzymes is NADPH oxidase, which activity produces ROS. The increased intensity of oxidative stress helps tumor to go on to malignancy. As an example, *in vitro* data suggest that in environments with certain levels of oxidative stress some cytokines, such as interleukin-2 (IL-2) or interferon α (IFNα), induce a decrease of T-lymphocytes or *natural killer* cells, which could suposse a tumor evasion to the immune response (Mantovani et al., 2003). Another source of free radical generation, usually underestimated but highlighted by Kryston et al. (2011), is the chronic exposure to viral infections; as in the case of hepatitis viruses, where there is a connection between chronic infection and induction of oxidative stress. There is a variety of viruses associated with increased ROS levels, DNA damage and mutagenic rate. The high intracellular oxidation status in viral infections consists of decreased antioxidant enzymes like catalase, glutathione peroxidase, glutathione reductase as well as high level of hydroxyl radicals (Kryston et al., 2011).

3.3 Influence of ROS in the cell cycle

Since some time already, an increase of ROS and an altered redox state has been observed in cancerous cells (Trachootham et al., 2009). It is known that ROS may serve as cellular messengers in the signal translation pathway and also an increase of ROS may trigger cell growth and proliferation, contributing to cancer development (Filomeno et al., 2005). Uncontrolled tumor cell proliferation requires the up-regulation of multiple intracellular signaling pathways, including cascades involved in survival, proliferation, and cell cycle progression. The most significant effects of oxidants on signaling pathways have been observed in the MAPK/AP-1 and NF-κB pathways (Muller et al., 2010). At the advanced stage of the disease, cancerous cells usually show genetic instability and a sharp increase of ROS, which induces to genetic mutations and failures in metabolic functioning, provoking a greater generation of ROS (Pelicano et al., 2004). Several mechanisms may lead to oxidative stress in cancer patients, such as altered energy metabolism, overproduction of cytokines, which in turn may increase ROS production, and the use of anti-neoplastic drugs. Altered energy metabolism in cancer may explain symptoms such as anorexia/cachexia, nausea and vomiting, which prevent normal nutrition. This deficit in the normal supply of nutrients like glucose, proteins, antioxidants and vitamins, leads eventually to the lack of antioxidant defenses for controlling free radical production.

Protein p53 is known as "the guardian of the genome" because it is essential for maintaining its integrity. This tumor suppressor protein has a fundamental role at detecting and eliminating oxidative damage in nuclear and mitochondrial DNA, at preventing mutations and at genetic instability. On the other hand, p53 acts also as a transcription factor that regulates the expression of many pro-oxidants and antioxidant genes. The functional loss of p53 is related to redox disequilibrium, increase of ROS, greater mutagenesis and tumor growth (Attardi and Donehower, 2005). This loss of p53 function is observed in many human cancers, especially in advanced stages (Bourdon, 2007).

There is evidence that the increase of ROS in tumor cells has a fundamental role in the acquisition of cancer characteristics (Hanahan and Weinberg, 2011): immortalization and transformation, cell proliferation and mitogenic signals, and cell survival and interruption of apoptotic death. Interestingly, in contrast to the effect of tumor promotion, recent studies suggest that the high ROS level has a role in the induction and maintenance of the senescence induced by tumor suppression, through the supported activation of the cell cycle inhibitor p16 (Ramsey and Sharpless, 2006; Takahashi et al., 2006). On the other hand, if the

ROS level increases up to a specific threshold that is incompatible with cell survival, ROS can exert cytotoxic effects that lead to the death of malignant cells and, therefore, limit cancer progression. This double game of ROS effect on cancerous cells may be used for developing new antitumor drugs that provide an increase of lethal oxidative stress in tumor cells, which are more sensitive to this type of attack than normal cells.

3.4 Angiogenesis induced by ROS

In addition to alterations in the cell cycle, an important event in the growth of any tumor is the generation of a new blood supply system that feeds the malignant cells. Migration, proliferation and tubular formation by endothelial cells are essential events in the process of angiogenesis. It has been suggested that ROS play an important role in angiogenesis, although their molecular mechanism remains unknown (Ushio-Fukai, 2004). The vascular endothelial growth factor (VEGF) triggers angiogenesis by stimulating the proliferation of endothelial cells and their migration through the receptor 2 (Flk1/KDR) of VEGF, which has tyrosine kinase activity. ROS derived from NAD(P)H oxidase are important for in vitro VEGF signaling and for in vivo angiogenesis. Arbiser and collegues (Arbiser et al., 2002) showed that ROS increased the expression of the VEGF, triggering the promotion of vascularization mechanisms and the fast expansion of tumors. On the other hand, greater metastatic capacity has been associated with high ROS levels in most tumors (Ishikawa et al., 2008). So, exogenous administration of ROS could increase certain metastatic states, while a treatment with antioxidants could slow down the metastatic progression (Ferraro et al., 2006).

Hypoxia seems to be the most important mechanism for tumor progression through the activation of angiogenesis, which is essential for the tumor growth (Harris, 2002). The neoplastic cells respond to hypoxia with an increase of ROS level; this occurs in the first stages of tumor development as a consequence of the blood supply deficit (Denko et al., 2003). It was shown that despite hypoxia there was a greater production of ROS, a paradox, since the oxygen availability for the formation of $O_2^{\bullet -}$ would be limited. Perhaps the generation of ROS occurs later, throughout tumor development, at the first stages of angiogenesis. When the hypoxia of a tumor is followed by blood supply reperfusion, high levels of ROS are generated; something similar occurs in a myocardial infarction or a brain ischemia.

3.5 ROS and tumor cell invasion

Tumor invasion and metastasis are two important events in cancer in which oxidative stress has shown to have an important role. When mammalian carcinoma cells are treated with hydrogen peroxide before intravenous injection into mice, an increase in lung metastasis formation is observed (Kundu et al., 1995), probably due to a decreased attachment of tumor cells to the basal lamina or it could alternatively be due to the increased activity or expression of proteins that regulate cellular motility.

On the other hand, the matrix metalloproteinases (MMPs) have been involved in the invasion and metastasis of malignant tumors of various histogenetic origins, and are capable of cleaving most components of the basement membrane and extracellular matrix (Westermarck et al., 1999). The activation of MMPs, such as MMP-2, probably occurs by the reaction of ROS with thiol groups in the protease catalytic domain, being also ROS involved in MMP gene expression (Rajagopalan et al., 1996).

Recently, a number of steps in the progression of metastatic disease have been shown to be regulated by redox signaling (Diers et al., 2010). One such redox signaling molecule is the electrophilic cyclopentenone prostaglandin, 15-deoxy-Δ12,14-prostaglandin J2 (15d-PGJ2), which can affect redox signaling through the posttranslational modification of critical cysteine residues in proteins such as actin, vimentin, and tubulin. The fact that 15d-PGJ2 can alter the cytoskeleton coincides with decreased migration and increased focal-adhesion disassembly, which might have important implications in the inhibition of metastatic processes such as invasion, intravasation, and extravasation (Diers et al., 2010).

3.6 ROS adaptation by cancer cells

There is sufficient evidence that cancer cells are under greater oxidative stress (Pervaiz and Clement, 2004; Kryston et al., 2011). High levels of oxidative stress have been found in cancer patients (McEligot et al., 2005; Lu et al., 2007), and it has been reported that different biomarkers of oxidative-stress-mediated events are elevated in cancer-prone tissues (Bartsch and Nair, 2000). *In vitro* studies clearly show that human tumor cell lines produce ROS at a much higher rate than non-transformed cells (Oberley and Buettner, 1979; Lu et al., 2007). In cancerous cells, a high level of oxidative stress is observed, which may result not only from the overproduction of ROS, but also from low levels or inactivation of antioxidants (Huang et al., 2003). Antioxidants are molecules capable of slowing down or even preventing the oxidation of other molecules and play an essential role at protecting cells against ROS aggression. Inhibition of these enzymes seriously endangers the capability of cells to face ROS activity. The first frontier of cellular defense against ROS damage consists of endogenous non-enzymatic radical scavengers like glutathione (GSH) and vitamins like C, E, antioxidant enzymes like SOD, catalase and GPx, as well as specific repair pathways (Kryston et al., 2011).

A decrease of mitochondrial activity and an overexpression of Mn-SOD with a greater production of $O_2^{\bullet -}$ have been detected in some colorectal carcinomas and tumor cells of the pancreas (Van-Driel et al., 1997; Cullen et al., 2003). The accumulation of anion $O_2^{\bullet -}$ stimulates cell growth by altering the redox states of transcription factors and regulators of the protein cell cycle. The increase of ROS in tumor cells may induce an increase of endogenous antioxidants in order to avoid intracellular lesions. On the contrary, a decrease of SOD activity was detected in blood cells of patients with cervical cancer. The decrease of SOD activity observed could be related to the generation of free radicals that cause direct damage to the enzyme by reticulation or mutation induction (Manoharan et al., 2004; Naidu et al., 2007). Besides, this decrease may be caused by an alteration of the oligoelements (essential trace elements) that act as cofactors of this enzyme, which may be considered as a risk factor of tumor growth or carcinogenesis (Naidu et al., 2007). On the other hand, it was observed that the increase in the intensity of oxidative stress in the blood of patients with ovarian cancer is accompained by a decrease of antioxidants like SOD, catalase, vitamin C and vitamin E (Senthil et al., 2004). A high percentage of tumors show low catalase activity, which means an advantageous adaptation for the tumor, which continues to benefit from the high levels of ROS. Although oxidant agents can be toxic to normal cells, the moderate increase of ROS contributes to the growth and survival of many cancers.

The strategy adopted by each type of tumor to increase the intensity of oxidative stress may vary from an increase of ROS to a decrease of antioxidants, going through a combination of both. The concentration of ROS in the tumor cell must be compensated with that of antioxidants in order to obtain an increase of ROS steady state level without reaching lethal levels. However, alterations in the mechanisms of antioxidant production are considered as indicators of oxidative stress in several types of cancer (Schumacker, 2006). Cancerous cells may adapt to survive at certain levels of oxidative stress. For example, greater levels of $O_2^{\bullet-}$ and H_2O_2 were observed in cells transformed with H-ras, showing high levels of antioxidants like peroxiredoxin-3 and thioredoxin peroxidase, compared to normal cells (Young et al., 2004). These adaptive mechanisms keep ROS levels in a distribution space that allows cancerous cells to avoid serious oxidative damage and to survive ROS-mediated stress and mutations. Redox adaptation may be crucial not only for cancer development, but also for drug resistance (Pervaiz and Clement, 2004; Sullivan and Graham, 2008). Redox adaptation, through the increase of endogenous antioxidants and the activation of the cell survival pathway, may confer greater capacity for tolerating the action of exogenous stress, with capacity for increasing DNA repair and decreased apoptosis. Thus, although cancerous cells are under chronic oxidative stress, they possess remodeled antioxidant system which let them to avoid deleterious ROS effects.

4. Antitumor oxidative therapy

4.1 The strategy

The therapeutic selectivity and avoiding resistance to drugs are two important issues in the therapy against cancer. Strategies for improving therapeutic selectivity depend largely on understanding the biological difference between cancerous and normal cells. Tumor cells, compared to normal cells, are under greater oxidative stress related to the oncogenic transformation, to alterations in metabolic activity and to an increase of ROS generation (Toyokuni et al., 1995; Hileman et al., 2003; Behrend et al., 2003). The high concentration of ROS in cancerous cells may have beneficial consequencies, like the stimulation of cell proliferation, mutation multiplication, genetic instability and alterations in the sensitivity to agents against cancer. However, because ROS are chemically active and may inflict serious cell damage, the very fact that cancerous cells usually show greater intrinsic oxidative stress may itself provide a unique opportunity to kill tumor cells according to the vulnerability of ROS action.

In this sense, the high concentration of ROS could function as a double-edged sword. A moderate increase of ROS could trigger both proliferation and differentiation, as well as other tumor characteristics. However, when ROS levels increase up to the lethal threshold it may break through the antioxidant capacity of the cell and trigger its death, by apoptosis or necrosis, depending on the degree of oxidative damage. Under physiological conditions, normal cells maintain redox homeostasis with a low level of basal ROS by controlling the equilibrium between the generation of ROS (pro-oxidant) and their elimination (antioxidant capacity). Exogenous agents that increase the generation of ROS or decrease the antioxidant capacity of cancerous cells will move the redox equilibrium and induce a general increase of ROS levels, which will cause cell death when exceeding the tolerance threshold (Figure 1).

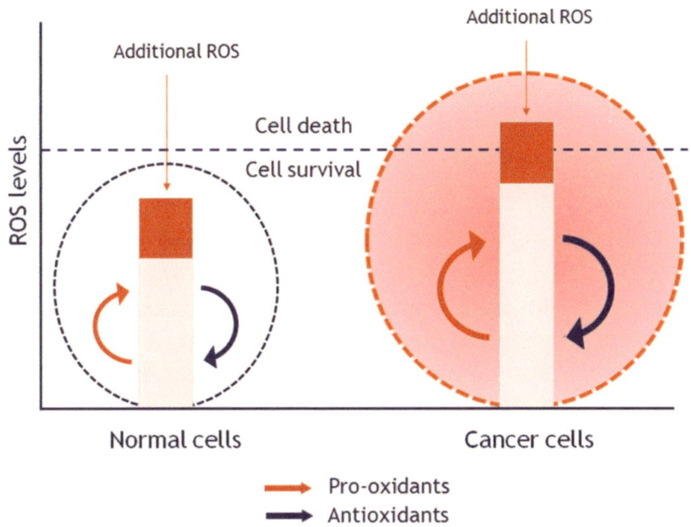

Fig. 1. Biological basis for therapeutic selectivity in oxidative therapy against cancer cells. Adapted from Gupte et al., 2009 and Trachootham et al., 2009.

Anticancer therapies aimed at the mitochondria of tumor cells are being developed in present years, since these organelles are involved in cell death (Daley et al., 2005; Nguyen and Hussain, 2007; Ozben, 2007; Pilkington et al., 2008). Mitochondria are the greatest oxygen consumers in the cell and they are an important source of reactive oxygen mediators. A drug that damages these organelles would cause an increase in ROS production and cell death. Currently, there is an anticancer strategy at its peak known as "oxidative therapy", which consists of inducing high ROS steady state levels in tumor cells. This therapy may be carried out in two different ways: causing the generation of high levels of ROS in solid tumors and inhibiting the antioxidant system of tumor cells (Fang et al., 2007; Trachootham et al., 2009). It is well established that high levels of ROS, like H_2O_2 and $O_2^{\bullet-}$, induce apoptosis in a wide variety of tumor cells activating the caspase cascade (Matsura et al., 1999; Yamakawa et al., 2000).

4.2 Cell death by ROS increment

Neoplastic cells are metabolically more active and require a high supply of ATP in order to keep cell growth and proliferation under control. This high energy demand in the MRC leads to the increase of ROS generation (Behrend et al., 2003). The excessive production of ROS may damage several cellular components like DNA, proteins, lipids and cell membranes. The oxidation of mitochondrial lipids and proteins causes the permeabilization of the mitochondrial membrane, which leads to an alteration of the coupling efficiency of the electron transport chain, resulting in the generation of more free radicals, and the release of cytochrome *c*, activating the process of programmed cell death (apoptosis) which depends on caspases (Conklin, 2004). There is evidence that the main mechanism by which oxidant agents may kill cells is the activation of apoptosis. In some cases, the high levels of ROS generated may inhibit apoptosis at a caspase level and divert the process toward necrosis (Chandra et al., 2000). The change from apoptosis to necrosis is critical in solid tumors and requires considerable amounts of ROS, a decrease of ATP and alterations in the mitochondrial electron-transport chain (Lee et al., 1999). The harmful consequences of this change lie in the inflammation caused by the rupture of necrotic cells and later release of enzymes that degrade the tissues. Thereby, death by apoptosis is preferred in antineoplastic therapies. Apoptotic cells cause the least damage to nearby tissues, since they do not release their content and are phagocytosed by macrophages.

Cancerous cells evolve with the mediation of endogenous and exogenous oxidative agents, depending on the cell type and the evolution state of the tumor. Tumors adapt to these conditions through the development of powerful antioxidant mechanisms and even by the use of endogenous ROS for proliferation. When ROS levels increase above the tolerance threshold, death of tumor cells is induced. Therefore, the fact that an excess of ROS causes cell damage and even death by apoptosis provides us with a strategy for eliminating cancerous cells, which are more sensitive to exogenous oxidative stress than normal cells, through the generation of free radicals, induced by oxidant pharmacological agents. In some cases, tumor cells attacked with antineoplastic therapies may gain resistance to oxidative stress, which is why combined therapies are promising, and are intended to converge toward improving the oxidative action above the critical threshold, or gathering different cytotoxic mechanisms.

Unfortunately, antitumor therapies may exert harmful effects on normal tissues, partially caused by ROS, which limits the application dose and its antitumor activity. Overcoming these secondary effects, without altering the therapy efficiency, is a priority and a challenge in biomedical research. In this sense, great importance is given to targeted therapies, using vehicles (liposomes, nanoparticles) that recognize specific molecules expressed in tumor cells.

4.3 Antioxidants in oxidative therapy against cancer

Antioxidants play an essential role in cell protection against ROS. The oxidation of antioxidant enzymes reduces the capacity of cells to eliminate free radicals. An important approach in the antitumor therapeutic strategies is to inhibit the antioxidant systems, like catalase, SOD and GPx, which are the main defense lines of the cell. The inhibitors of different antioxidant enzymes have been characterized by their capacity for eliminating neoplastic cells, alone or combined. It has also been described that many pharmacological agents may have more than one mechanism of action and affect multiple biological processes. There are agents that induce apoptosis which are oxidant and others that stimulate cell metabolism. On the other hand, there are apoptosis inhibitors that have antioxidant activities. In the absence of adequate antioxidant defenses, the damage from oxidative stress leads to the activation of the genes responsible for apoptosis.

There are conflicting data in the results obtained by different researchers regarding the levels of antioxidants in tumor tissue and in blood from cancer patients. In some cases, there are differences between different antioxidants in the same patient; some increase and others decrease (Ray et al., 2000). In breast cancer, for example, several studies describe an increase of lipid peroxidation and a decrease of antioxidants (Khanzode et al., 2004; Sener et al., 2007). However, other studies performed in neoplastic tissues have shown a greater presence of ROS and a high expression of antioxidants (Oltra et al., 2001; Gönenç et al.,

2006). So, for instance, an increase in the expression of Mn-SOD has been observed in breast cancer and in blood samples from patients with different types of leukemia (Nishiura et al., 1992; Devi et al., 2000; Ray et al., 2000). This fact may reflect an adaptive mechanism by which cancerous cells respond to an increase of ROS levels produced in mitochondria. ROS can induce the over-regulation of Mn-SOD through the modulation of the redox states of the transcription factors (AP- 1, NF-kappaB). Due to its high expression in certain types of cancer, Mn-SOD has been considered as a tumor marker (Schadendorf et al., 1995). This expression of SOD protects tumor cells against a lethal increase of ROS levels. In fact, it has been demonstrated that the inhibition of SOD with 2-methoxyestradiol would induce apoptosis in leukemia cells through a mechanism mediated by free radicals, without showing significant toxicity in normal lymphocytes (Zhou et al., 2003).

Antitumor therapies mediated by ROS show a promising therapeutic activity in clinical studies (Trachootham et al., 2009). However, some tumor cells, especially in advanced stages of the disease, have adapted to oxidative stress due to their antioxidant capacity. This redox adaptation does not only allow tumor cells surviving under high levels of ROS, it also provides an increase of survival molecules and a greater capacity for drug inactivation. Moreover, it has been suggested that resistance to the agents that induce intracellular ROS production, such as paclitaxel, doxorubicin or other drugs, is correlated to the increase of antioxidants (Glorieux et al., 2011). Thereby, the capability of certain drugs to inhibit or reduce the antioxidant machinery is very useful in oxidative therapy. These drugs could be used in combination with oxidant agents for greater efficiency in antitumor therapies.

5. Amitriptyline as an anti-cancer agent

Amitriptyline is a commonly prescribed tricyclic antidepressant drug that is well known to death investigators, forensic pathologists, and toxicologists. Amitriptyline has sedative effects and is frequently prescribed for patients experiencing symptoms of depression. Amitriptyline, have also been used for therapeutic treatment of neuropathic and inflammatory diseases such as fibromyalgia, chronic fatigue syndrome, migraine, irritable bowel syndrome, and atypical facial pain (Gruber et al., 1996). Besides its anxiolytic properties, amitriptyline has central anticholinergic effects. Amitriptyline inhibits serotonin and noradrenaline uptake in presynaptic nerve ending (Maubach et al., 1999). However, toxicity of amitriptyline has been observed during standard treatments, and frequently during suicidal or accidental overdosage. Tricyclic antidepressant overdosage has toxic effects over cardiovascular, autonomous nervous, and central nervous systems, and may result in cardiotoxicity, cardiac conduction delays, dysrhythmia, hypotension, altered mental status, and seizures (Thanacoody and Thomas, 2005; Kiyan et al., 2006).

In vitro administration of amitriptyline to cell cultures induces several signs of toxicity. Amitriptyline treatment induces alteration of cellular permeability based on its detergent nature (Kitagawa et al., 2006). Furthermore, amitriptyline causes alterations in the glucidic metabolism of neurons resulting in a decrease of both uptake and transport of glucose (Mannerstrom and Tahti, 2004). Additionally, amitriptyline provokes an increase of intracellular lipid peroxidation in mouse 3T3 fibroblasts (Viola et al., 2000) and some mouse tissues (Bautista-Ferrufino et al., 2011), and many of these toxic effects are prevented by antioxidants (Slamon and Pentreath, 2000). Recently, our group has shown that amitriptyline induced toxicity is caused through a mitochondrial dysfunction, and increased ROS level (Moreno-Fernandez et al., 2008; Cordero et al., 2009). Amitriptyline reduced significantly the number of cultured cells; enhanced the production of stimulated lipid peroxidation, inverting the lipid reduced/oxidized ratio; decreased catalase protein levels, cytochrome *c*, ΔΨm, and citrate synthase activity; revealing mitochondrial damage. So, amitriptyline-induced toxicity is caused through mitochondrial dysfunction, and increased mitochondrial ROS production. Moreover, CoQ level was decreased by amitriptyline treatment and CoQ and alpha-tocopherol supplementation ameliorated amitriptyline-induced toxicity in both cultured human primary fibroblasts and zebrafish embryos (Cordero et al., 2009).

Other toxic effects attributed to amitriptyline lie in the alteration of neuron carbohydrate metabolism, which results in a decrease of glucose absorption and transport; causing a total loss of neuron viability in a cell line of neuroblastoma (Mannestrom et al., 2004).

Recent studies have shown that some antidepressants can kill cancerous cells. In fact, tricyclic antidepressants have shown to cause cell death in human normal lymphocytes (Karlson et al., 1998), Hodgkin´s lymphoma cells (Serafeim et al., 2003), neurons (Lirk et al., 2006), glioma cells (Xia et al., 1999; Daley et al., 2005; Levkovitz et al., 2005) and colorectal cancer cells (Arimochi y Morita, 2006). Chlorimipramine exerts its effect via the inhibition of complex III of the MRC (Daley et al., 2005). The same is valid for amitriptyline, as we have already reported (Cordero et al., 2009). We showed in fibroblasts treated with amitriptyline a decrease of expression level of proteins of complex I, complex III, cytochrome c, and reduced CoQ_{10} levels. Deficient mitochondrial protein expression levels and reduced levels of CoQ_{10} may impair normal mitochondrial electron flow and proton pumping, inducing a drop in respiratory complexes activity, and mitochondrial membrane potential. Our data showed that amitriptyline-treated fibroblasts have reduced NADH:cytochrome c reductase (complex I+III) activity, and lower mitochondrial membrane potential, which may contribute to impaired mitochondrial protein import and aggravate mitochondrial dysfunction, ROS production, and oxidative stress. It has been proposed that ROS damage can induce the mitochondrial permeability transition (MPT) by the opening of non-specific high conductance permeability transition (PT) pores in the mitochondrial inner membrane (England and Cotter, 2005). This, in turn, leads to a simultaneous collapse of mitochondrial membrane potential. The activation of MPTcauses mitochondria to become permeable to all solutes up to a molecular mass of about 1500 Da (Forte and Bernardi, 2005). After MPT, mitochondria undergo a dramatic swelling driven by colloid osmotic forces, which culminates in the rupture of the outer membrane and release of proapoptotic mitochondrial intermembrane proteins into the cytosol, such as cytochrome c, apoptosis inducing factor, Smac/Diablo, and others (Cordero et al.,2009).

We have also studied the effect of amitriptyline on tumor cell lines (Cordero et al., 2010). We observed that this drug induced important mitochondrial damage in tumor cell lines (H460: non-small cell lung cancer, HeLa: epithelial cervical cancer, and HepG2: hepatoma), generating high amounts of ROS and provoking apoptotic cell death. Moreover, amitriptyline effects have been compared with three antitumor drugs frequently used in cancer therapy: camptothecin (CPT), doxorubicin (Doxo), and methotrexate (Metho). Interestingly, amitriptyline induced significantly higher ROS generation in comparison with the other drugs, producing a dose-dependent increase of apoptosis in human cancer cells through a mechanism dependent on caspase-3 activation. Apoptosis percentage was significally higher in those cells treated with amitriptyline than in cells treated with CPT, Doxo or Metho (Figure 2A). Moreover, when the cell cycle of synchronized cultures was stopped at the G0/G1 phase by depriving cells from serum, the difference of apoptosis percentage among amitriptyline and the remaining drugs was significantly higher than in normal cultures (Figure 2B). These results suggest that the effect of amitriptyline does not depend on cell cycle stage, whereas CPT, Doxo, and Metho are more harmful in dividing cells, as most chemotherapeutic drugs. These data are of special interest for cancer treatment during the nongrowing phases of certain tumors.

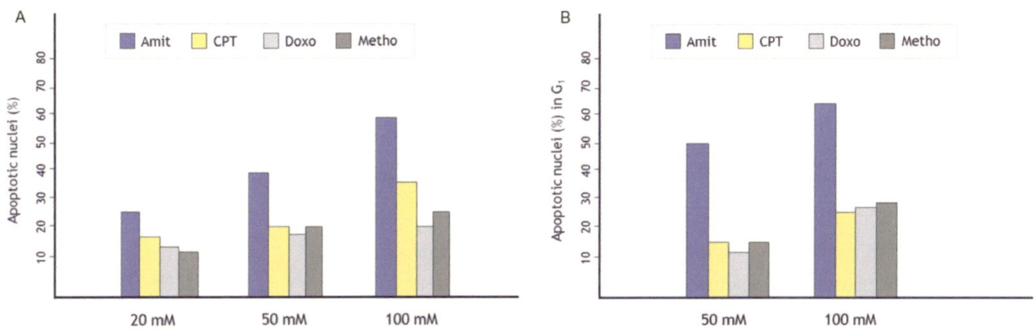

Fig. 2. Comparative study of amitriptyline and different chemotherapeutic drugs for the evaluation of apoptosis. (A) Percentages of apoptotic cells in H460 cell cultures 24 h after administration of drugs at different concentration. (B) Apoptosis assessment in synchronized cultures stopped at the G0/G1 phase. Adapted from Cordero et al., 2010.

After treating cancer cells with amitriptyline, we have found increased ROS level and several signs of mitochondrial damage, as attenuated complex I+III activity, decreased protein levels of complex III, decreased membrane potential, and a significant reduction of the number of this organelle, shown by cytochrome c and citrate synthase determination, and electron microscopy (Figure 3). So, this tricyclic compound provokes oxidative stress in cancer cells, being mitochondria the target of its toxicity. None of the chemotherapeutic drugs tested seemed to damage mitochondria seriously. However, the chemotherapeutic drugs induced apoptosis and increased ROS production in tumor cells, although not with the intensity of amitriptyline.

According to our data, amitriptyline induces a mitochondrial damage characterized by a decrease of the expression levels of complexes I and III of the MRC as well as of cytochrome *c* and of CoQ levels, which suggests an alteration in the activity, organization and assembly of the mitochondrial complexes, being this reflected in a decrease of the electron flow as well as a decrease of the mitochondrial membrane potential and, therefore, an increase of intramitochondrial ROS prodution. The damage caused by the increase of mitochondrial ROS induces the opening of the mitochondrial permeability transition pore (MPT), thus increasing mitochondrial permeability with the consequent release of proapoptotic proteins to the cytosol such as cytochrome c, Smac/Diablo, etc., initiating the intrinsic pathway of apoptosis dependent on caspase-3 (Figure 4).

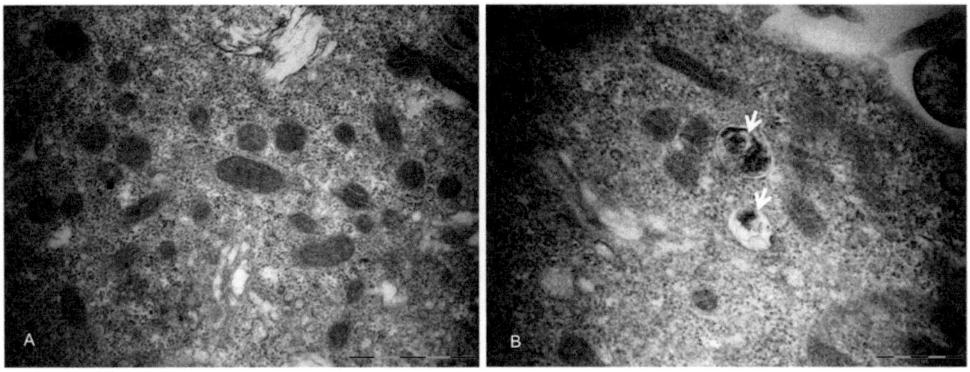

Fig. 3. Transmission electron microscopy showing damage and fewer mitochondria in H460 cells treated with 50 mmol/l of amitriptyline. Degenerating mitochondria (arrows) are observed in treated tumor cells. (A) Nontreated tumor cells. (B) Amitriptyline-treated tumor cells (Cordero et al., 2010).

In general, the increase of ROS production causes, as a response, an increase of the antioxidants activities. However, under the high input rate of ROS, enzyme inactivation prevails, which leads to the reduction of antioxidant enzymes activity and to the process of oxidative damage. Thus, tumor cells frequently possess very little antioxidative enzymes, such as catalase, SOD, and glutathione peroxidase, which are known to play a protective role against ROS in normal cells. We have observed in normal fibroblast treated with amitriptyline a decrease in protein expression of antioxidant enzymes (catalase and MnSOD) 16 h after the treatment, followed by restored levels after 24h, as a mechanism of antioxidant defense (Moreno-Fernández et al., 2008). Interestingly, in cancer cells, the same concentration of amitriptyline provoked an unrestorable decrease of catalase (Cordero et al., 2010). The difference of the antioxidant status observed in cancer cells, in comparison with healthy fibroblasts, may be caused by the lower antioxidant level present in the cancer cell lines used. Besides the decrease of catalase and MnSOD, amitriptyline also produces a significant decrease of CoQ level in tumor cells (Cordero et al., 2010). CoQ plays a critical protective role by either acting as an antioxidant or by the noncompetitive inhibition of the neutral sphingomyelinase of plasma membrane, preventing ceramide production (Mates et al., 1999). Most chemotherapeutic drugs do not provoke any decrement of antioxidants. Instead, they frequently induce an increase of antioxidants as a protecting mechanism against ROS generation, leading to lower cell death (Brea-Calvo et al., 2006). The fact that amitriptyline downregulates both catalase and CoQ activity is very interesting since it destroys the already decreased antioxidant defenses present in cancer cells, making the oxidative stress produced by the amitriptyline-induced ROS generation a more effective weapon.

Thus, amitriptyline promotes enhanced oxidative damage to cancer cells as this drug attacks cells by two different mechanisms: by the production of a high amount of ROS, provoking apoptosis; and by a significant decrease in antioxidant levels, seriously limiting cell reaction to oxidative stress. Therefore, amitriptyline could be used for anticancer oxidant therapy against tumors that present significant oxidative stress and/or low antioxidant defenses. For anticancer therapeutics on those tumors with a similar redox status than normal cells, a drug delivery vehicle should be used.

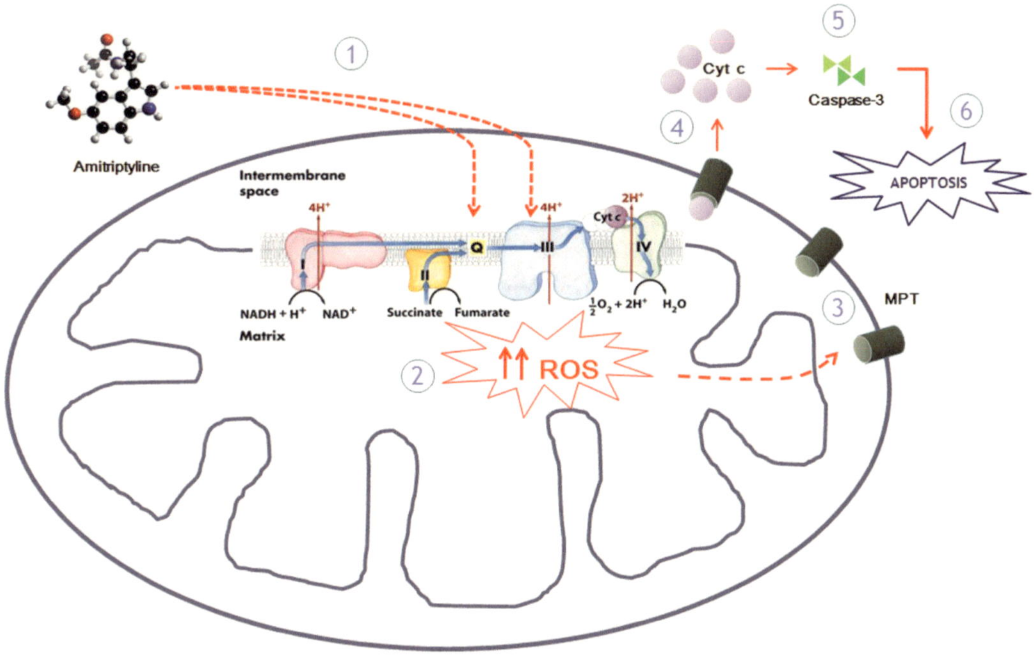

Fig. 4. Mechanism of apoptosis induction by amitriptyline.

6. Conclusion

Evidence exists that cancer cells are under a continuous oxidative stress, facilitating ROS to act as carcinogen, as they were shown to be involved in mutagenesis, cancer promotion and progression. On the other hand, ROS may promote either cell proliferation or cell death, depending on the rate of ROS production and the activity of the antioxidant system. Accordingly, oxidative therapy against cancer arises as a ROS-generating strategy which increase oxidative status above the critical threshold required for cell survival.

In our studies, the tricyclic antidepressant amitriptyline induced high ROS generation as a result of mitochondrial dysfunction, provoking a higher level of apoptosis of tumor cells than common chemotherapeutic drugs. Moreover, it inhibits important antioxidants of the cell-defense machinery, dramatically limiting tumor cell response to ROS production. Thus, amitriptyline, as well as other tricyclic compounds, is being assayed as an anti-cancer drug in oxidative therapy.

Unfortunately, oxidative anti-cancer therapy may exert harmful effects on normal tissues, limiting the applicable dose of drugs and anti-tumor activity. So, differences in ROS-induced cell death and oxidative status between normal and neoplastic cells from different cancer types must be thoroughly investigated, taking into account the complexity of physiological and pathological pathways involved in redox balance. On the other hand, it is not strange that after ROS-generating therapies cancer cells achieve further resistance to oxidative stress. In consequence, combination therapies could be achieved in order to either increase the intensity of oxidative stress above the critical threshold, or to perform different cytotoxic mechanisms.

Nevertheless, although greater efforts must be made, oxidative therapy against cancer is a promising strategy that is worthy of being investigated.

7. References

Arbiser, J.L.; Petros, J.; Klafter R.; Govindajaran, B.; McLaughlin E.R.; Brown L.F.; et al. (2002). Reactive oxygen generated by Nox1 triggers the angiogenic switch. *Proc Natl Acad Sci USA*. 99 (Jan) (715-720), ISSN 0027-8424.

Arimochi, H. & Morita, K. (2006). Characterization of cytotoxic actions of tricyclic antidepressants on human HT29 colon carcinoma cells. *Eur J Pharmacol.* 10,541, (Jul) (17- 23), ISSN 0014-2999.

Attardi, L. D. & Donehower, L. A. (2005). Probing p53 biological functions through the use of genetically engineered mouse models. *Mutat. Res.* 576 (Aug) (4-21), ISSN 0027-5107.

Bartsch, H. & Nair, J. (2000). New DNA-based biomarkers for oxidative stress and cancer chemoprevention studies. *Eur J. Cancer* 36,10, *(*Jun*)* (1229-1234), ISSN 0959-8049.

Bautista-Ferrufino, M.R.; Cordero M.D.; Sánchez-Alcázar, J.A.; Illanes, M.; Fernández-Rodríguez, A.; Navas, P. & de Miguel, M. (2011). Amitriptyline induces coenzyme Q deficiency and oxidative damage in mouse lung and liver. *Toxicol Lett.* 204 (Jul) (32-37), ISSN 0378-4274.

Behrend, L.; Henderson, G. & Zwacka, R. M. (2003). Reactive oxygen species in oncogenic transformation. *Biochem. Soc. Trans.* 31, (Dec.) (1441–1444), ISSN 0300-512.

Bourdon, J. C. (2007). p53 and its isoforms in cancer. *Cancer* 97 *(Aug)* (277–282), ISSN 0007-0920.

Brea-Calvo, G.; Rodriguez-Hernandez, A.; Fernandez-Ayala, D. J.; Navas, P.; & Sanchez-Alcazar, J.A. (2006). Chemotherapy induces an increase in coenzyme Q10 levels in cancer cell lines. *Free Radic Biol Med* 40 (Apr) (1293–1302), ISSN 0891- 5849.

Chandra, J.; Samali, A.; & Orrenius, S. (2000). Triggering and modulaton of apoptosis by oxidative stress. *Free Radic Biol Med;* 29 (Aug) (323–333), ISSN 0891-5849.

Chang, E.F.; Wong, R.J.; Vreman, H.J.; Igarashi, T.; Galo, E.; Sharp, F.R.; Stevenson, D.K.; &Noble-Haeusslein, L.J. (2003). Heme oxygenase-2 protects against lipid peroxidation-mediated cell loss and impaired motor recovery after traumatic brain injury. *J Neurosci.* 23, 9, (May) (3689-3696), ISSN 0270-6474.

Conklin, K. A. (2004). Free radicals: the pros and cons of antioxidants. Cancer chemotherapy and antioxidants *J. Nutr;* 134 (Nov) (3201-3204), ISSN 0022-3166.

Cordero, M.D.; Moreno-Fernández, A.M.; Gomez-Skarmeta, J.L.; De Miguel, M.; Garrido-Maraver, J.; Oropesa-Ávila, M.; et al. (2009). Coenzyme Q10 and alpha tocopherol protect against amitryptyline toxicity. Toxicol Appl Pharmacol 15 (Mar) (329-337), ISSN 00410-008X.

Cordero, M.D.; Sánchez- Alcázar, J.A.; Bautista-Ferrufino, M.R.; Carmona-Lopez, M.I.; Illanes, M.; Rios, M. J.; et al. (2010). Acute oxidant damage promoted on cancer cells by amitriptyline in comparison with some common chemotherapeutic drugs. *Anticancer drugs* 10 *(Nov)* (932-944), ISSN 0959-4973.

Cotan, D.; Cordero, M.D.; Garrido-Maraver, J.; Oropesa-Ávila, M.; Rodríguez-Hernández, A.; Gómez Izquierdo, L.; et al. (2011). Secondary coenzyme Q10 deficiency triggers mitochondria degradation by mitophagy in MELAS fibroblasts. *FASEB J*. 25 (Aug) (2669-2687), ISSN 0892-6638.

Cuezva, J.M.; Krajewska, M.; de Heredia M.L.; Krajewski, S.; Santamaría, G.; Kim, H.; et al. (2002). The bioenergetic signature of cancer: a marker of tumor progression. *Cancer Res*; 62 (6674-6681), ISSN 0008- 5472.

Cullen, J.J.; Mitros, F.A.; & Oberley, L.W. (2003). Expression of antioxidant enzymes in diseases of the human pancreas: another link between chronic pancreatitis and pancreatic cancer. *Pancreas* 26, 1, (Jan) (23-27), ISSN 0885-3177.

Daley, E.; Wilkie, D.; Loesch, A.; Hargreaves, I.P.; Kendall, D.A.; & Pilkington G. J, et al. (2005); Clomipramine: a novel anticancer agent with a mitochondrial target. *Biochem Biophys Res Commun* 328 (Mar) (623–632), ISSN 0006-291X.

Davies, K. (1995). Breast cancer genes. Further enigmatic variations. *Nature* 378 (Dec) (362-363), ISSN 0028-0836.

Denko, N.C.; Fontana, L.A. Hudson, K.M. *et al.* (2003). Investigating hypoxic tumor physiology through gene expression patterns. *Oncogene* 22 (Sep) (5907-14), ISSN 0950-9232.

Devi, G.S.; Prasad, M.H.; Saraswathi, I.; Raghu, D.; Rao, D.N. & Reddy, P.P. (2000). Free radicals, antioxidant enzymes and lipid peroxidation in different types of leukemias. *Clin Chim Acta* 293 (Marz) (53-62), ISSN 0009-8981.

Diers, A.R.; Higdon, A.N.; Ricart, K.C.; Johnson, M.S.; Agarwal, A.; Kayanaraman, B.; et al. (2010). Mitochondrial targeting of the electrophilic lipid 15-deoxy-Delta prostaglandin J2 increases apoptotic efficacy via redox cell signalling mechanisms. *Biochem J*. 426, (Jan) (31-41), ISSN 0264-6021.

Dreher, D.; & Junod, A.F. (1996). Role of oxygen free radicals in cancer development. *European Journal of Cancer,* 32A *(Jan)* (30-38), ISSN 0959-8049.

England, K. & Cotter, T.G. (2005). Direct oxidative modifications of signalling proteins in mammalian cells and their effects on apoptosis. *Redox Rep* 10 (237-245), ISSN 1351-0002.

Fang, J.; Nakamura, H.; & Iyer, A. K. (2007). Tumor-targeted induction of oxystress for cancer therapy. *J. Drug Target*. 15 (Aug) (475-486), ISSN 1061-186X.

Ferraro, D.; Corso, S.; Fasano, E.; Panieri, E.; Santangelo, R.; Borrello, S.; et al. (2006). Pro-metastatic signaling by c-Met through RAC- 1 and reactive oxygen species (ROS). *Oncogene* 25 (3689-3698), ISSN 0950-9232.

Filomeno, G.; Rotilio, G. & Ciriolo, M.R. (2005) Disulfide relays and phosphorylative cascades: partners in redox-mediated signalling patways. *Cell Death Differ* 12 (Dic) (1555-1563), ISSN 1350-9047.

Floyd, R.A. (1990). Role of oxygen free radicals in carcinogenesis and brain ischemia. *FASEB J*. 4 (Jun) (2587–2597), ISSN 0892-6638.

Forte, M. & Bernardi, P. (2005). Genetic dissection of the permeability transition pore. J. *Bioenerg. Biomembr*. 37, 3 (Jun) (121- 128), ISSN 0145-479X.

Glorieux C, Dejeans N, Sid B, Beck R, Calderon PB, Verrax J. (2011). Catalase overexpression in mammary cancer cells leads to a less aggressive phenotype and an altered response to chemotherapy. *Biochem Pharmacol*. Jun 13. PMID: 21689642, ISSN 0006-2952.

Gönenç, A.; Erten, D.; Aslan, S.; Akinci, M.; Simşek, B.; & Torun, M. (2006). Lipid peroxidation and antioxidant status in blood and tissue of malignant breast tumor and benign breast disease. *Cell Biol Int.* 30, 4, (Apr) (376-380), ISSN 1065-6995.

Gruber, A.J.; Hudson, J.I. & Pope, G. (1996). The management of treatment-resistant depression in disorders on the interface of psychiatry and medicine. Fibromyalgia, chronic fatigue syndrome, migrañe, irritable bowel syndrome, atypical facial pain, and premenstrual dysphoric disorder. *Psychiatr Clin North Am,* 19,2, (351-359), ISSN 0193-953X.

Gupte, A. & Mumper, R.J. (2009). Elevated copper and oxidative stress in cancer cells as a target for cancer treatment. *Cancer Treat rev.* 35(Feb) (32-46), ISSN 0305-7372.

Haas, R.H.; Parikh, S.; Falk, M.J.; Saneto, R.P.; Wolf, N.I.; Darin, N. et al. (2008). The in-depth evaluation of suspected mitochondrial disease. *Mol Genet Metab.* 94, (May) (16-37), ISSN 1096-7193.

Hanahan, D. & Weinberg, R.A. (2011).The hallmarks of cancer. *Cell.* 144, (Mar) (209-219), ISSN 0092-8674.

Harris, A.L. (2002). Hypoxia- A key regulatory factor in tumor growth. *Nat Rev Cancer.* 2, 1, (Jan) (38-47), ISSN 1474-175X.

Hasegawa, Y.; Takano, T.; Miyauchi, A.; Matsuzuka, F.; Yoshida, H. & Kuma K. (2002). Decreased expression of glutathione peroxidase mRNA in thyroid anaplastic carcinoma. Cancer Lett; 182, (Aug) (69–74) ISSN 0304-3835.

Hileman, E.O.; Liu, J.; Albitar, M.; Keating, M.J. & Huang, P. (2003). Intrinsic oxidative stress in cancer cells a biochemical basis for therapeutic selectivity. *Cancer Chemother. Pharmacol.* 53, 3 (Mar) (209-219), ISSN 0344-5704.

Huang, P.; Feng, L.; Oldham, E.A.; Keating, M.J. & Plunkett, W. (2003). Superoxide dismutase as a target for the selective killing of cancer cells. *Nature* 407,5, (Dic) (390-395), ISSN 0028-0836.

Indo, H.P.; Davidson, M.; et al. (2007). Evidence of ROS generation by mitochondria in cells with impaired electron transport chain and mitochondrial DNA damage. *Mitochondrion.* 7, 2, (106-118), ISSN 1567-7249.

Ishikawa, K. *et al.* (2008). ROS-generating mitochondrial DNA mutations can regulate tumor cell metástasis. *Science.* 320, (May) (661–664), ISSN 0036-8075.

Kamp, D.W.; Shacter E. & Weitzman, S.A. (2011). Chronic inflammation and cancer: The role of the mitochondria. *Oncology.* 25 (Apr) (400-410), ISSN 0890-9091.

Karlsson, H.; Gu, Y.; DePierre, J.; Nassberger, L. (1998). Induction of apoptosis in proliferating lymphocytes by tricyclic antidepressants. *Apoptosis.* 3, 4 (Sep) (255–260), ISSN 1360-8185.

Kennedy, C. H.; Cueto, R.; Belinsky, S.A.; Lechner, J.F. & Pryor, W. A. (1998). Overexpression of hMTH1 mRNA: a molecular marker of oxidative stress in lung cancer cells. *FEBS Lett.* 429, 1, (Jun) (17-20), ISSN 0014-5793.

Khanzode, S.S.; Muddeshwar, M.G. & Dakhale, G.N. (2004). Antioxidant enzymes and lipid peroxidation in different stages of breast cancer. *Free Radic. Res.* 38, 1, (Jan) (81-85), ISSN 1071-5762.

Kitagawa, N., Oda, M., Nobutaka, I., Satoh, H., Totoki, T. & Morimoto, M., (2006). A proposed mechanism for amitriptyline neurotoxicity based on its detergent nature. *Toxicol. Appl. Pharmacol.* 15, 217, (Nov) (100–106), ISSN 0041-008X.

Kiyan, S.; Aksay, E.; Yanturali, S.; Atilla, R.; & Ersel, M.; (2006). Acute myocardial infarction associated with amitriptyline overdose. *Basic Clin. Pharmacol. Toxicol.* 98, 45, (May) (462–466), ISSN 1742-7835.

Klauning, J.E. & Kamendulis, L.M. (2004). The role of oxidative stress in carcinogenesis. *Annu Rev Pharmacol Toxicol.* 44, (239-267), ISSN 0362- 1642.

Kryston, T.B.; Georgiev, A.B.; Pissis, P. & Georgakilas, A.G. (2011). Role of oxidative stress and DNA damage in human carcinogenesis. *Mutat Res* 3, 711, (Jun) (193-201), ISSN 0027-5107.

Kundu, N.; Zhang, S. & Fulton, A. M. (1995). Sublethal oxidative stress inhibits tumor cell adhesion and enhances experimental metastasis of murine mammary carcinoma. *Clin. Exp. Metastasis* 13, 1, (Nov) (16–22), ISSN 0262-0898.

Lee, Y.J.; Galaforo, S.S.; Sim, J.E.; et al. (1999). Dominant negative Jun Nterminal protein kinase (JNK-1) inhibits metabolic oxidative stress during glucose deprivation in a human breast carcinoma cell line. *Free Radic Biol Med.* 274, 28, (Feb) (575-584) ISSN 0891-0895.

Levkovitz, Y.; Gil-Adl.; Zeldich, E.; Dayag, M. & Weizman, A. (2005). Differential induction of apoptosis by antidepressants in glioma and neuroblastoma cell lines: evidence for p-c-Jun, cytochrome c, and caspase-3 involvement. *J. Mol Neurosci.* 27, 3, (29-42), ISSN 0895-8696.

Lirk, P.; Haller, I.; Hausott, B.; Ingorokva, S.; Deibl, M.; Gerner, P. & Klimaschewski, L. (2006). The neurotoxic effects of amitriptyline are mediated by apoptosis and are effectively blocked by inhibition of caspase activity. *Anesth Analg.* 102, (Jun) (1728-33), ISSN 0003-2999.

Lu, W.; Ogasawara, M. A. & Huang, P. (2007). Models of reactive oxygen species in cancer. *Drug Discov.* 4, (67–73), ISSN 1740-6757.

Mannerstrom, M. & Tahti, H. (2004). Modulation of glucose uptake in glial and neuronal cell lines by selected neurological drugs. *Toxicol. Lett.* 15, 151, (Jun) (87-97), ISSN 0378-4274.

Manoharan, S.; Klanjiappan, K. & Kayalvizi, M. (2004). Enhanced lipid peroxidation and impaired enzimatic antioxidant activities in the erythrocytes of the patients with cervical carcinoma. *Cell Mol Biol Lett.* 9, 4 A (699-707), ISSN 1425-8153.

Mantovani, G.; Maccio, A.; Madeddu, C. & Massa, E. (2003). Cancer-related cachexia and oxidative stress: beyond current therapeutic options. *Expert Rev Anticancer Ther.* 3,3 (Jun) (381-392), ISSN 1473- 7140.

Mates, J.M.; Perez-Gómez, C. & Nuñez de Castro, I. (1999). Antioxidant enzymes and Human diseases. *Clin Biochem;* 32 (Nov) (595–603), ISSN 0009-9120.

Matsura, T.; Kai, M.; Fujii, Y.; Ito H. & Yamada, K. (1999). Hydrogen peroxide-induced apoptosis in HL-60 cells requires caspase-3 activation. *Free Radic Res.* 30 (Jan) (73-83), ISSN 1071-5762.

Maubach, K.A.; Rupniak, N.M.; Kramer, M.S. & Hill, R.G. (1999). Novel strategies for pharmacotherapy of depression. *Curr. Opin. Chem.* Biol. 3, 4 (Aug) (481–488), ISSN 1367-5931.

McEligot, A. J., Yang, S. & Meyskens, F. L. Jr. (2005). Redox regulation by intrinsic species and extrinsic nutrients in normal and cancer cells. *Annu. Rev. Nutr.* 25 (261–295), ISSN 0199-9885.

Moreno-Fernández, A.M.; Cordero, M.D.; De Miguel, M.; Delgado-Rufino, M.D; Sanchez-Alcazar, J.A.; Navas, P. (2008). Cytotoxic effects of amitriptyline in human fibroblasts. *Toxicology;* 243 (Jan) (51-58), ISSN 0300-483X.

Naidu, M.S.K.; Suryakar, A.N.; Sanjay, C.; Swami, S.C.; Katkam. R.V. & Kumbar, K.M. (2007). Oxidative stress and antioxidant status in cervical cancer patients. *Indian J Clin Biochem.* 22, 5 (140-144), ISSN 0200-423.

Nguyen, D.M.; Hussain, M. (2007). The role of the mitochondria in mediating cytotoxicity of anti-cancer therapies. *J Bioenerg Biomembr.* 39, 1, (Feb) (13–21), ISSN 0145-479X.

Nishiura, T.; Suzuki, K. & Kawaguchi, T. et al. (1992). Elevated serum manganese superoxide dismutase in acute leukemias. *Cancer Lett.* 15, 62 (Mar) (211-215), ISSN 0304-3835.

Oberley, L. W. & Buettner, G. R. (1979). Role of superoxide dismutase in cancer: a review. *Cancer Res.* 39, 4, (Apr) (1141–1149), ISSN 0008-5472.

Okamoto, K.; Kondo-Okamoto, N. & Ohsumi, Y. (2009). Mitochondria-anchored receptor Atg32 mediates degradation of mitochondria via selective autophagy. *Dev. Cell.* 17,1 (Jul) (87-97), ISSN 1534-5807.

Oltra, A. M.; Carbonell, F.; Tormos, C.; Iradi, A. & Saez, G. T. (2001). Antioxidant enzyme activities and the production of MDA and 8-oxo-dG in chronic lymphocytic leukemia. *Free Radic. Biol. Med.* 30 (Jun) (1286–1292), ISSN 0891-5849.

Ozben, T. (2008). Oxidative stress and apoptosis: Impact on cancer therapy. *J Pharm Sci.* 96, 9, (Sep) (2181-2196), ISSN 0022-3549.

Pelicano, H.; Feng, L.; Zhou, Y.; Carew, J.S.; Hileman, E.O.; Plunkett, W.; et al. (2003). Inhibition of mitochondrial respiration: a novel strategy to enhance drug-induced apoptosis in human leukemia cells by a reactive oxygen species-mediated mechanism. *J. Biol. Chem.* 278, (Sep) (37832–37839), ISSN 0021-9258.

Pelicano, H.; Carney, D.; & Huang, P. (2004). Ros stress in cancer cells and therapeutic implications. *Drug Resist Updat.* 7, 2, (Apr) (97-110), ISSN 1368-7646.

Pervaiz, S. & Clement, M. V. (2004). Tumor intracellular redox status and drug resistance serendipity or a causal relationship? *Curr. Pharm. Des.* 10, (1969–1977), ISSN 1381-6128.

Pieczenik, S.R. & Neustadt, J. (2007). Mitochondrial dysfunction and molecular pathways of disease. *Exp Mol Pathol.* 83, 1, (Aug) (84-92), ISSN 0014-4800.

Pilkington, G.J.; Parker, K. & Murray, S.A. (2008). Approaches to mitochondrially mediated cancer therapy *Semin Cancer Biol.* 18, (Jun) (226-235), ISSN 1368-7646.

Rajagopalan, S.; Meng, X.P.; Ramasamy, S.; Harrison D.G.; & Galis, Z. S. (1996). Reactive oxygen species produced by macrophage-derived foam cells regulate the activity of vascular matrix metalloproteinases in vitro. Implications for atherosclerotic plaque stability. J Clin Invest. 98, (Dec) (2572-2579), ISSN 0021-9738.

Ramsey, M. R. & Sharpless, N. E. (2006). ROS as a tumour suppressor? *Nature Cell Biol.* 8,11, (1213–1215), ISSN 1465-7392.

Ray, G.; Batra, S.; Shukla, N.K.; Deo, S.; Raina, V.; Ashok, S.; Husain, S.A. (2000). Lipid peroxidation, free radical production and antioxidant status in breast cancer. *Breast Cancer Res. Treat.* 59, 2, (Jan) (163–170) ISSN 0167-6806.

Retel, J.; Hoebee, B. Braun, J.E.; *et al* (1993). Mutational specificity of oxidative DNA damage. *Mutat Res.* 299, (May) (165-182), ISSN 0027-5107.

Reuter, S.; Gupta, S.C.; Chaturvedi, M.M.; & Aggarwal, B.B. (2010). Oxidative stress, inflammation, and cancer: how are they linked? *Free Radic Biol Med.* 49, 11, (Dic) (1603-1616), ISSN 0891-5849.

Sandhu, C. & Slingerland, J. (2000). Desregulación of the cell cycle in cancer. *Cancer Detection and Prevention.* 24, (107-118), ISSN 0361-090X.

Sato, K.; Ito, K.; Kohara, H.; Yamaguchi, Y.; Adachi, K. & Endo, H. (1992). Negative regulation of catalase gene expression in hepatoma cells. *Mol Cell Biol.* 12, (Jun) (2525–2533), ISSN 0270-7306.

Schadendorf, D.; Zuberbier, T.; Diehl, S.; Schadendorf, C.; & Czarnetzki, B.M. (1995). Serum manganese superoxide dismutase is a new tumour marker for malignant melanoma. *Melanoma Res.* 5, (Oct) (351-353), ISSN 8960-8981.

Schumacker, P.T. (2006). Reactive oxygen species in cancer cells: live by the sword, die by the sword. *Cancer cell.* 10, (Sep.) (175-176), ISSN 1535-6108.

Sener, D.E.; Gonenc, A.; Akmer, M. & Torun, M. (2007). Lipid peroxidation and total antioxidant status in patients with breast cancer. *Cell Biochem Func.* 25, (Jul) (377–382), ISSN 0263-6484.

Senthil, K.; Aranganathan, S. & Nalini, N. (2004). Evidence of oxidative stress in the circulation of ovarian cancer patients. *Clin Chim Acta.* 339, (Jan) (27-32), ISSN 0009-8981.

Serafeim, A.; Holder, M.J.; Grafton, G.; Chamba, A.; Dravson, M.T. & Luonq, Q.T, et al. (2003). Selective serotonin reuptake inhibitors directly signal for apoptosis in biopsy-like Burkitt lymphoma cells. *Blood.* 101, (Apr) (3212–3219), ISSN 0006-4971.

Slamon, N.D. & Pentreath, V.W. (2000). Antioxidant defense against antidepressants in C6 and 1321N1 cells. *Chem Biol Interact.* 14, 127, (Jul) (181–199), ISSN 0009-2797.

Spitz, D.R.; Sim, J.E.; Ridnour, L.A.; Galoforo, S.S. & Lee, Y.J. (2000). Glucose deprivation-induced oxidative stress in human tumor cells. A fundamental defect in metabolism? Ann N Y *Acad Sci.* 899, (349-362), ISSN 0077-8923.

Sullivan, R. & Graham, C. H. (2008). Chemosensitization of cancer by nitric oxide. *Curr. Pharm. Des.* 14, (1113–1123), ISSN 1381-6128.

Takahashi, A.; Ohtani, N.; Yamakoshi, K.; Iida, S.; Tahara, H.; Nakayama, K.; et al. (2006). Mitogenic signalling and the p16INK4a-Rb pathway cooperate to enforce irreversible cellular senescence. *Nature Cell Biol.* 8, (Nov) (1291– 1297), ISSN 1465-7392.

Thanacoody, H.K. & Thomas, S.H. (2005). Tricyclic antidepressant poisoning: cardiovascular toxicity. *Toxicol.* 24, 3, (205–214), ISSN 1176-2551.

Toyokuni, S.; Okamoto, K.; Yodoi, J.; & Hiai, H. (1995). Persistent oxidative stress in cancer. *FEBS Lett.* 358, (Jan) (1–3), ISSN 0014-5793.

Trachootham, D.; Alexandre, J. & Huang, P. (2009). Targeting cancer cells by ROS mediated mechanisms: a radical therapeutic approach? *Nat Rev.* 8, (Jul) (579–591), ISSN 1474-1776.

Turrens, J.F. (2003). Mitochondrial formation of reactive oxygen species. *J Physiol.* 552, 2, (Oct) (335-44), ISSN 0022-3751.

Turunen, M.; Olsson, J. & Dallner, G. (2004). Metabolism and function of coenzyme Q. *Biochim Biophys Acta.* 1660, 1, (Jan) (171-99), ISSN 0006-3002.

Ushio-Fukai, M. & Nakamura, Y. (2008). Reactive oxygen species and angiogenesis: NADPH oxidase as target for cancer therapy. *Cancer Lett.* 266, (Jul) (37–52), ISSN 0304-3835.

Van-Driel, B.E.; Lyon, H.; Hoogenraad, D.C.; Anten, S. & Hansen, U. (1997). Expression of CuZn- and Mn-superoxide dismutase in human colorectal neoplasms. *Free Radic Biol Med.* 23, (435- 344), ISSN 0891-5849.

Verrax, J.; Taper, H. & Calderon, P.B. (2008). Targeting cancer cells by an oxidant based-therapy. *Curr Mol Pharmacol.* 1, (Jan) (80-92), ISSN 1874-4672.

Viola, G.; Miolo, G. Vedaldi, D. Dall'Acqua F. (2000). In vitro studies of the phototoxic potential of the antidepressant drugs amitriptyline and imipramine. *Il Farmaco.* 55, 3, (Mar) (211–218), ISSN 0014-827X.

Vousden, K. H. & Lane, D. P. (2007). p53 in health and disease. *Nature Rev. Mol. Cell Biol.* 8 (Apr) (275–283), ISSN 1471-0072.

Westermarck, J.; Kahari, V.M. (1999). Regulation of matrix metalloproteinase expression in tumor invasion. *FASEB J.* 13, 8, (May) (781-792), ISSN 0892-6638.

Xia, Z.; Bergstrand, A.; DePierre, J.W. & Nassberger, L., (1999). The antidepressants imipramine, clomipramine, and citalopram induce apoptosis in human acute myeloid leukemia HL-60 cells via caspase-3 activation. *J. Biochem biol Toxicol.* 13, 6, (338-347), ISSN 1095-6670.

Xu, R.; Pelicano, H.; Zhou, Y.; Carew, J.S.; Feng, L.; Bhalla, K.N.; et al. (2005). Inhibition of glycolysis in cancer cells: a novel strategy to overcome drug-resistance associated with mitochondrial respiratory defect and hypoxia. *Cancer Res.* 65, 2, (Jan) (613-621), ISSN 0008-5472.

Yamakawa, H.; Ito, Y.; Naganawa, T.; Banno, Y.; Nakashima. S. & Yoshimura, S. et al. (2000) Activation of caspase 9 and 3 during H2O2-induced apoptosis of PC12 cells independent of ceramide formation. *Neurol Res.* 22, 6, (Sept) (556–564), ISSN 0161-6412.

Yano, M.; Ikea, M.; Abe, K.; Kawai, Y.; Kuroki, M.; Mori, K.; et al. (2009).Oxidative stress induces anti-hepatitis C virus status via the activation of extracellular signal-regulated kinase. *Hepathology.* 50, 3, (Sep) (556-564), ISSN 0270-9139.

Young, T. W.; Mei, F.C.; Yang, G.; Thompson-Lanza, J.A.; Liu, J.; & Cheng, X. (2004). Activation of antioxidant pathways in ras-mediated oncogenic transformation of human surface ovarian epithelial cells revealed by Functional proteomics and mass spectrometry. *Cancer Res.* 1, 64, (4577–4584), ISSN 0008-5472.

Zhou, Y.; Hileman, E.O.; Plunkett. W.; Keating, M.J. & Huang, P. (2003). Free radical stress in chronic lymphocytic leukemia cells and its role in cellular sensitivity to ROS generating anticancer agents. *Blood. 15,* 101, (May) (4098-104), ISSN 0006-4971.

Zorov,D.B.; Juhaszova, M.; & Sollott, S.J. (2006). Mitochondrial ROS-induced ROS release: An update and review. *Biochimica et Biophysica Acta (BBA)–Bioenergetics.* 1757, (May) (509-517), ISSN 0006-4971.

23

Monensin Induced Oxidative Stress Reduces Prostate Cancer Cell Migration and Cancer Stem Cell Population

Kirsi Ketola[1], Anu Vuoristo[2], Matej Orešič[2],
Olli Kallioniemi[3] and Kristiina Iljin[1]
[1]*Medical Biotechnology, VTT Technical Research Centre of Finland and University of Turku, Turku,*
[2]*VTT Technical Research Centre of Finland, Espoo,*
[3]*Institute for Molecular Medicine, Finland (FIMM), University of Helsinki, Finland*

1. Introduction

Prostate cancer is the most common malignancy and second leading cause of cancer related death in males in developed countries (Jemal et al. 2011). Patients with localized and metastatic prostate cancer are treated with anti-androgens. Although prostate cancer cell proliferation is initially blocked or slowed down with anti-androgen therapy, eventually castration-resistant disease develops (Sharifi, Gulley & Dahut 2010). Therapeutic options for castration-resistant prostate cancer are limited and treatment responses to currently existing therapies are often unsatisfactory (Bracarda et al. 2011). For example, the cytotoxic therapy often causes severe toxicity and eventually leads also to the development of chemo-resistance (Tannock et al. 2004, Berthold et al. 2008, Bracarda et al. 2011). Thus, there is an urgent need for novel agents to block the proliferation and to inhibit the progression of the primary prostate cancer cells to the advanced stage as well as to target advanced and metastatic prostate cancer. Therefore, understanding of disease progression and drug resistance mechanisms may provide valuable insights into the development of novel treatment options to improve the survival of prostate cancer patients.

We have recently performed a high-throughput cell-based screening of 4,910 known drugs and drug-like molecules in four prostate cancer cell models and two non-tumorigenic prostate epithelial cell lines to identify prostate cancer cell growth selective inhibitors (Iljin et al. 2009). Only four compounds, antibiotic ionophore monensin, aldehyde dehydrogenase (ALDH) inhibitor disulfiram, histone deacetylase inhibitor trichostatin A and fungicide thiram inhibited selectively cancer cell growth at nanomolar concentrations. The mechanistic studies indicated that monensin and disulfiram inhibited prostate cancer cell growth by inducing oxidative stress (Iljin et al. 2009, Ketola et al. 2010). In contrast to disulfiram, monensin induced apoptosis, reduced androgen receptor signalling and showed a synergistic anti-proliferative effect with anti-androgens in prostate cancer cells. Moreover, monensin increased the amount of reactive oxygen species (ROS) and induced an oxidative stress signature in prostate cancer cells (VCaP and LNCaP), but not in the non-malignant prostate epithelial cells (RWPE-1, EP156T) (Ketola et al. 2010). Furthermore, antioxidant vitamin C partially rescued the monensin induced growth inhibition, indicating that oxidative stress plays a key role in the antineoplastic effect of monensin in cultured prostate cancer cells (Ketola et al. 2010).

Oxidative stress occurs in the cell when redox regulation is imbalanced. Redox balance depends on the level of intracellular free radicals and reactive oxygen species as well as on the antioxidative capacity of the cell. Figure 1 illustrates the connection between the malignant progression and increase in intracellular ROS (Fig. 1).

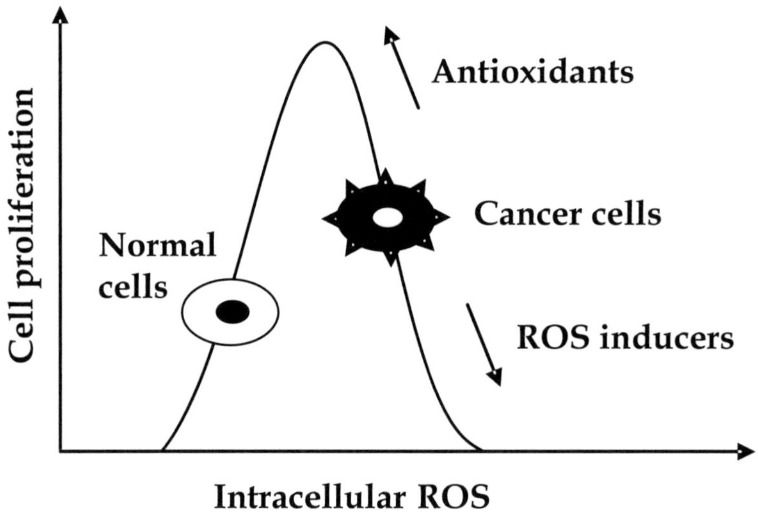

Fig. 1. The balance between cell proliferation and intracellular reactive oxygen species (ROS). The malignant progression and the effects of ROS inducers and antioxidants depend on the intracellular levels of ROS. In cancer cells, intracellular ROS levels are higher than in normal cells making them more vulnerable to agents inducing ROS. Figure idea adapted from Gupte & Mumper 2009.

Cancer cells benefit from the increased mutation rate induced via oxidative stress (Shibutani, Takeshita & Grollman 1991). Therefore, cancer cells need also an active antioxidative mechanism to be able to survive under high oxidative stress. The oxidative stress level is elevated in prostate cancer cells compared to non-malignant prostate epithelial cells (Khandrika et al. 2009, Yossepowitch et al. 2007, Kumar et al. 2008). Many oncogenes are known to protect cells from oxidative stress e.g. androgen receptor (AR), ERG and MYC are known to have antioxidative properties in cancer cells (Pinthus et al. 2007, Tam et al. 2003, Benassi et al. 2006, Swanson et al. 2011, DeNicola et al. 2011). Monensin may sensitize prostate cancer cells to oxidative stress via reducing the expression of these genes (Ketola et al. 2010). In addition, many other anti-neoplastic agents such as vinblastine, cisplatin, mitomycin C, doxorubicin, camptothecin, inostamycin, neocarzinostatin, etoposide, arsenic trioxide and nonsteroidal anti-inflammatory drugs are known to mediate their apoptotic effect by inducing oxidative stress (Fang, Nakamura & Iyer 2007, Rigas, Sun 2008, Sun et al. 2011). The increased sensitivity to oxidative stress combined with dependency on anti-oxidative system may provide a way to selectivity inhibit cancer cell proliferation (Iljin et al. 2009, Ketola et al. 2010).

Recently, redox control including antioxidative defence mechanisms and ROS-scavenging systems has been identified as an important regulator of cancer stem cell potential, metastasis and chemoresistance (Kobayashi, Suda 2011b, Cairns, Harris & Mak 2011, Pani, Galeotti & Chiarugi 2010). Aldehyde dehydrogenase activity is widely used as a marker for cancer stem cells and its activity has been shown to correlate with poor outcome in several cancers such as in prostate cancer (Davydov, Dobaeva & Bozhkov 2004, Burger et al. 2009, Li et al. 2010, Yu et al. 2011, Zhang et al. 2009a). Aldehyde dehydrogenases are detoxifying enzymes that are responsible for the oxidation of intracellular aldehydes (Duester 2000, Magni et al. 1996, Sophos, Vasiliou 2003, Yoshida et al. 1998). Moreover, ALDH oxidize retinol to retinoic acid (vitamin A) known to reduce oxidative stress whereas retinoic acid depletion induces oxidative stress and mitochondrial dysfunction (Ahlemeyer, Krieglstein 1998, Ahlemeyer et al. 2001, Chiu, Fischman & Hammerling 2008, Duester 2000, Chute et al. 2006). Thus, ALDH increases the antioxidative capacity in cells and protects cells from oxidative stress induction. Moreover, the inhibition of ALDH activity has recently been linked to reduced chemotherapy and radiation resistance in cancer stem cells (Croker, Allan 2011). These results suggest that not only cancer cells, but also cancer stem cells could be targeted by oxidative stress induction and/or reduction of antioxidative capacity. Interestingly, the results from mechanistic studies of prostate cancer selective compounds indicated that both disulfiram and monensin reduced the ALDH activity in prostate cancer cells (Iljin et al. 2009, Ketola et al., 2010).

In this study, we explored further the molecular mechanism of monensin induced growth inhibition in cultured prostate cancer cells. Cancer pathway reporter assays and steroid profiling was performed to get insights into altered signalling and metabolite levels in monensin exposed prostate cancer cells. Since monensin reduces ALDH activity, the putative effect on cancer stem cells was evaluated. Furthermore, we studied the effect of monensin on prostate cancer cell differentiation and motility.

2. Materials and methods

2.1 Cells

VCaP prostate carcinoma cells (TMPRSS2-ERG positive, received from Drs. Adrie van Bokhoven, University of Colorado Health Sciences Center, Denver, Colorado and Kenneth Pienta, University of Michigan, Michigan) were grown in Dulbecco's Modified Eagle's Medium (Korenchuk et al. 2001b, Korenchuk et al. 2001a). LNCaP prostate carcinoma cells (received from Dr. Marco Cecchini, University of Bern, Bern, Switzerland) were grown in T-Medium (Invitrogen). PC-3 prostate carcinoma cells were purchased from American Type Culture Collection (LGC Promochem AB) and grown according to provider's instructions. All cells were cultured in appropriate growth media described above including 10% fetal bovine serum (FBS), 2 mM L-glutamine, 100 U/ml penicillin, and 100 μg/ml streptomycin in an incubator with a humidified atmosphere of 95% air and 5% CO_2 at 37°C.

2.2 Compounds

Monensin was purchased from Sigma-Aldrich and diluted in ethanol.

2.3 Cancer 10-pathway reporter array

Cancer 10-pathway Reporter Luciferase Kit (Wnt (TCF/LEF), Notch (RBP-Jκ), p53/DNA damage, TGF-β (SMAD2/3/4), Cell cycle/pRb-E2F (E2F/DP1), NF-κB, Myc/Max, Hypoxia (HIF1A), MAPK/ERK (Elk-1/SRF) and MAPK/JNK (AP-1) was used to study the monensin modulated signalling (SABiosciences, Frederick, MD). The assay was performed according to manufacturer's instructions. In brief, inducible transcription factor responsive firefly luciferase reporters with constitutively expressing Renilla construct transcription factor reporters were plated onto 96-well plates with transfection reagent (siLentFect, Bio-Rad Laboratories), followed by addition of cells and incubation for 24 hours. A mixture of non-inducible firefly luciferase reporter and constitutively expressing Renilla construct was used as the negative control. After 24 hours of transfection, monensin (100 nM) and control treatment were added onto the cells and plates were incubated for 18 hours. The Dual-LuciferaseReporter (DLR™) Assay System (Promega) was utilized in quantitation of reporters and results according to the manufactorer's instructions. The change in the activity of each signalling pathway was determined by comparing the normalized luciferase activity of the reporters in monensin or solvent exposed cells.

2.4 Wound healing assay

The effect of monensin (10 nM, 100 nM and 1 μM) on prostate cancer cell migration was studied using a scratch wound assay. PC-3 cells were plated on 96-well plates (Essen ImageLock, Essen Instruments, UK) and a wound was scratched with wound scratcher (Essen Instruments). Compounds and appropriate controls were added immediately after wound scratching and wound confluence was monitored with Incucyte Live-Cell Imaging System and software (Essen Instruments). Wound closure was calculated for every hour for 24 hours by comparing the mean relative wound density of three biological replicates in each experiment.

2.5 Cell viability assay

Cell viability was determined with CellTiter-Glo (CTG) cell viability assay (Promega, Madison, WI) according to the manufacturer's instructions. Briefly, 2,000 cells per well were plated in 35 μl of their respective growth media and left to attach overnight. Monensin (100 nM) was added to the cells and incubated for 12 or 24 hours. CTG reagent was added and the signals were quantified using Envision Multilabel Plate Reader (Perkin-Elmer, Massachusetts, MA).

2.6 RNA extraction and quantitative real-time PCR

VCaP cells were exposed to monensin for 6 hours, total RNA was extracted and quantitative real-time PCR was done as previously described (Ketola et al. 2010). TaqMan gene expression probes and primers from the Universal Probe Library (Roche Diagnostics, Espoo, Finland) were used to study E-cadherin (5´-cccgggacaacgtttattac-3´ and 5´-gctggctcaagtcaaagtcc-3´) and β-actin (5´-ccaaccgcgagaagatga -3´ and 5´-ccagaggcgtacagggatag -3´) mRNA expression. Three replicate samples were studied.

2.7 Fluorescence-Activated Cell Sorting analysis (FACS)

VCaP and LNCaP cells were exposed to monensin (1 μM) for 6 hours, samples were fixed with 2% paraformaldehyde, and stained with CD44 (FITC-conjugated mouse monoclonal anti-human, BD Pharmingen™ 555478) and CD24 (PE-conjugated rat monoclonal anti-human, Abcam ab25281) antibodies for 45 minutes at 4°C in the dark. Cells were washed and the fluorescence intensity was measured using Accuri C6 Flow Cytometer.

2.8 Immuofluorescence staining

For immunofluorescence stainings, VCaP cells were grown on cover slip slides and exposed to monensin for 6 hours. Cells were fixed with 4 % paraformaldehyde in PBS, permeabilized with 0.2% Triton X-100 in PBS for 15 min, and blocked with 2 % BSA/PBS for 30 min. Cells were stained with E-cadherin antibody (1:100 dilution, polyclonal rabbit anti-human, Cell Signaling Technology, MA, USA) and Alexa-conjugated polyclonal donkey anti-rabbit antibody was used for secondary staining (1:300 dilution, Invitrogen, Molecular Probes, Carlsbad, CA). Cell nuclei were stained with DAPI present in Vectashield mounting medium (Vector Labs) and images were taken with Zeiss Axiovert 200M Microscope with the spinning disc confocal unit Yokogawa CSU22 and a Zeiss Plan-Neofluar 63× oil/1.4 NA objective. Z-stacks with 1 airy unit optical slices were acquired with a step size of 0.5 μm between slices, and the maximum intensity projections were created with SlideBook 4.2.0.7 software (Intelligent Imaging Innovations Inc., CO, USA).

2.9 Statistical analyses

Stars in the figures indicate the significance of the experiments calculated using Student's t-test (*P<0.05, **P<0.01, *** P<0.001).

2.10 Steroid quantification

VCaP cells (1x10^7 cells) were exposed to 1 μM monensin for 6 hours, harvested and counted. An internal standard (labeled C16:0) and chloroform:methanol (2:5) mixture were added, the samples were homogenized with Retsch system (5 min, 20 Hz), centrifuged and the supernatants were collected and evaporated. MOX (25 μl, TS-45950, Thermo Scientific, Helsinki, Finland) was added and the mixture was incubated at 45°C for 60 minutes. Next, 100 μl of MSTFA with 1% trimethylchlorosilane (Fluka, St. Louis, MO) was added and the mixture was incubated at 70°C for 60 minutes. Injection standard was added to the mixture before gas chromatography-mass spectrometry analysis (GC-MS, Agilent 6890 gas chromatograph (GC) combined with Agilent 5973 mass selective detector (MSD)). The injector (injection volume 1 μl with pulsed splitless injection) and MSD temperatures were 230°C (MS Source) and 150°C (MS Quad). The analyses were performed on Supelco 38499-02C capillary column. Selective ion monitoring using specific masses for each target analyte was used in the detection. The following steroids were quantified: 7-ketocholesterol, aldosterone, progesterone, pregnenolone, estrone, 17B-estradiol, 4B-hydroxycholesterol,

25-hydroxycholesterol, 5a,6a-epoxycholesterol (Mono-TMS), dihydrotestosterone and testosterone (the standards were from Steraloids, Newport, RI)).

3. Results

3.1 Monensin reduces NF-κB pathway activity in prostate cancer cells

Here, we studied the effect of monensin exposure on the activities of ten cancer signalling pathways using Cancer pathway Reporter Array in prostate cancer cells. Inducible transcription factor responsive firefly luciferase reporters were transfected to VCaP and LNCaP cells with constitutively active Renilla reporters and incubated for 24 hours. Monensin (100 nM) or solvent control was added onto the transfected cells for 18 hours followed by measure of luciferase activities. The results are presented in Fig. 2. Comparison of the basal pathway activities in VCaP prostate cancer cells indicated that NF-κB was

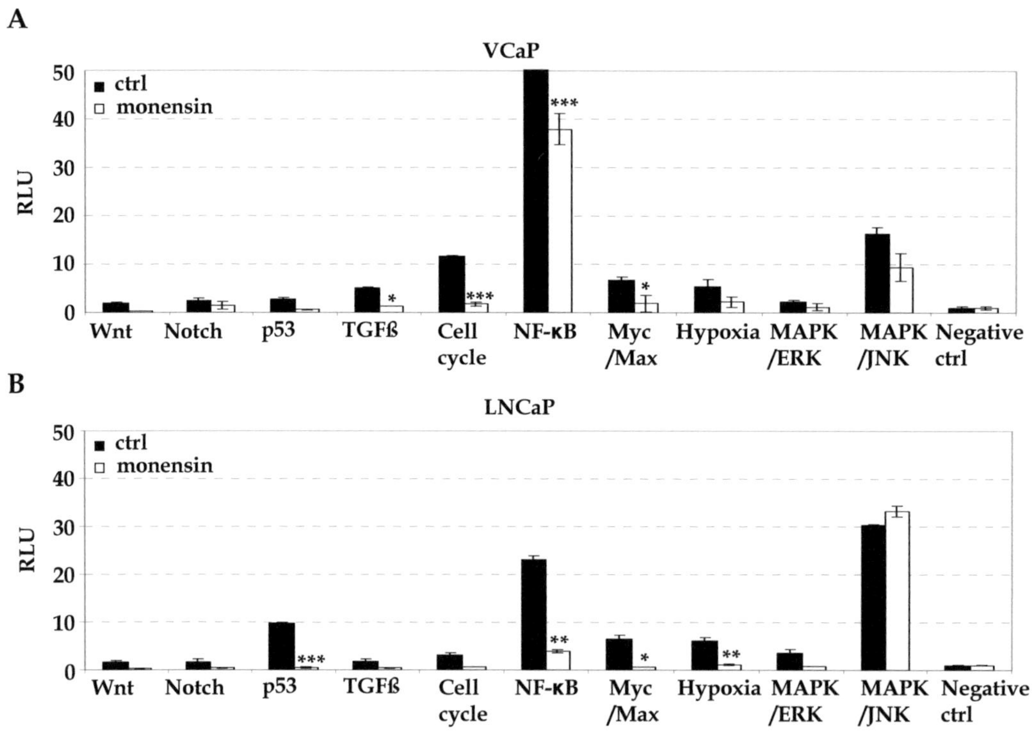

Fig. 2. Cancer pathway activities in VCaP and LNCaP prostate cancer cells. A) VCaP and B) LNCaP cells were exposed to ethanol or 100 nM monensin for 24 hours and pathway activities were measured as described in the text. Results with negative control measuring the background firefly luciferase activity (non-inducible firefly luciferase reporter and constitutively expressing Renilla construct) are indicated and used to determine the basal pathway activities in VCaP and LNCaP cells. The y-axis was set to 50 to allow direct comparison of relative luciferase units (RLU) in VCaP and LNCaP cells, although the basal NK-κB activity in VCaP cells extended RLU 324. Statistical significance of monensin induced changes are shown for the active pathways *P<0.05, **P<0.01, ***P<0.001.

clearly the most active pathway (fold change FC > 300, compared to the negative control). In addition, TGF-ß (FC = 5), cell cycle (FC = 12), Myc/Max (FC = 7) and hypoxia (FC = 5) were active in VCaP cells. In LNCaP cells, MAPK/JNK was the most active pathway (FC = 30 compared to the negative control), followed by NF-κB (FC = 23), p53 (FC = 10), Myc/Max (FC = 7) and hypoxia (FC = 6). Interestingly, NF-κB pathway was 14 times more active in TMPRSS2-ERG fusion positive VCaP cells than in ERG negative LNCaP cells. These results are in agreement with previous data indicating that ERG induces NF-κB activity in prostate cells *in vitro* and *in vivo* (Wang et al. 2010). The results with p53 pathway are also in accordance with the previous literature since VCaP cells are known to have an inactivating mutation in p53 (Trp-248) whereas LNCaP cells express the active form, supporting further the overall functionality of the assay (van Bokhoven et al. 2003).

Monensin exposure inhibited NF-κB activity in both VCaP (by 88%) and LNCaP (by 83%) cells. NF-κB is a transcription factor that regulates various cellular processes such as cellular antioxidant defence capacity (Gloire, Legrand-Poels & Piette 2006). These results suggest that monensin induced oxidative stress may result from reduced NF-κB signalling. In addition, monensin reduced TGF-ß (by 75%), cell cycle (by 85%) and Myc/Max (by 71%) activities in VCaP cells and p53 (by 94%), hypoxia (by 82%) and Myc/Max (by 90%) activities in LNCaP cells. The reduced Myc/Max signalling is supported by reduced MYC mRNA expression seen in monensin exposed VCaP and LNCaP cells (Ketola et al. 2010). Taken together, monensin reduced the activities of multiple signalling pathways such as NF-κB, TGF-ß, hypoxia and Myc/Max, all associated with cancer cell survival, oxidative stress, stem cell potential and metastasis (Jones, Pu & Kyprianou 2009, Blum et al. 2009, Mimeault, M. & Batra, S.K. 2011, Benassi et al. 2006, Koh et al. 2010).

3.2 Monensin reduces the cancer stem cell population in prostate cancer cell cultures

Monensin exposure reduced the activities of multiple pathways maintaining antioxidative capacity and promoting the growth and survival of cancer stem cells such as NF-κB, HIF1A, MYC and ALDH, in cultured prostate cancer cells. Therefore, the effect of monensin on prostate cancer stem cell population was studied. Prostate cancer stem cells can be identified by high expression of CD44 and low expression of CD24 antigens (Klarmann et al. 2009). Interestingly, CD44 cell surface glycoprotein has recently been shown to increase antioxidative capacity in cancer cells, indicating that cancer initiating cells could be targeted by impairing oxidative stress defence mechanisms (Ishimoto et al. 2011). Thus, we analyzed the effect of monensin exposure to the fraction of $CD44^{+}/CD24^{-}$ cells in cultured prostate cancer cells. VCaP and LNCaP cells exposed to monensin (1 μM) for 6 hours were stained with CD44 and CD24 recognizing antibodies and the samples were analyzed using FACS. The results showed that monensin reduced the fraction of $CD44^{+}/CD24^{-}$ cells in both VCaP (from 3 to 1.3%) and LNCaP (3.1 to 2.6%) cells (Fig. 3). In agreement with these results, genome-wide gene expression analysis indicated that monensin decreased CD44 (by 20%) and induced CD24 (by 30%) mRNAs compared to the levels in ethanol control at 6-hour time point (Ketola et al. 2010). Taken together, these results indicate that monensin reduces the fraction of cancer stem cells in prostate cancer cell cultures.

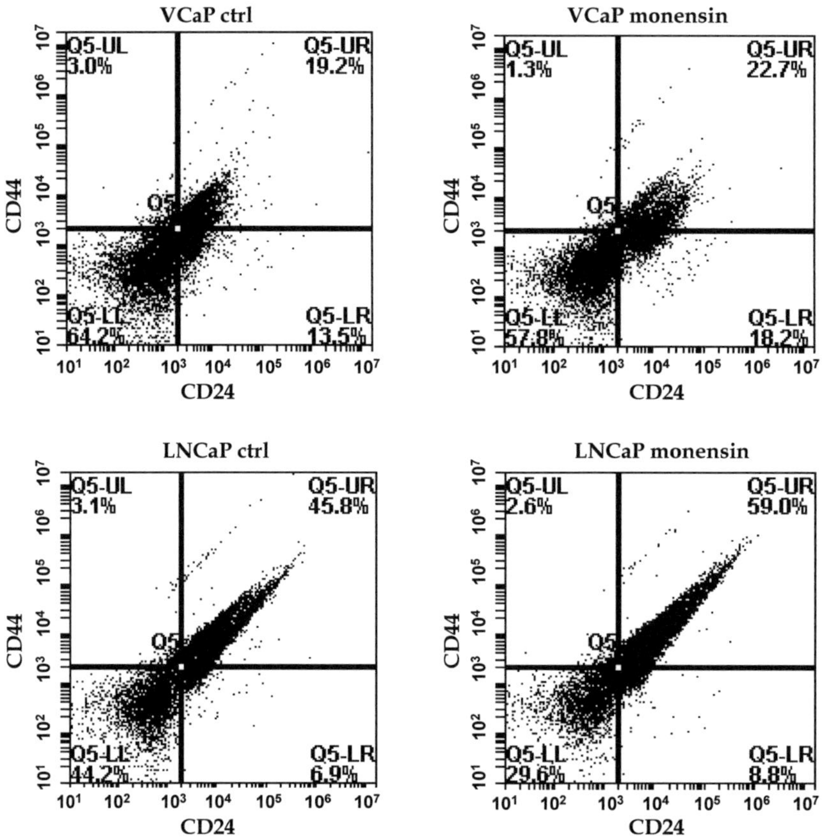

Fig. 3. FACS analysis of CD44 and CD24 immunostained VCaP and LNCaP prostate cancer cells. Monensin reduces the fraction of CD44+/CD24- cells in cultured prostate cancer cells. VCaP and LNCaP cells were stained with CD44 and CD24 antibodies in response to six hour monensin or ethanol exposure. Representative images from one out of four replicates are shown.

3.3 Monensin induces cell differentiation in prostate cancer cells

Cancer stem cells have been hypothesized to arise intrinsically through oncogenic transformation of normal tissue stem or progenitor cells in the early stage of the tumorigenesis or through induction of epithelial-to-mesenchymal transition (EMT) at later stages (Chaffer, Weinberg 2011). The expression of E-cadherin is considered as a marker of epithelial differentiation and it is lost during EMT. Interestingly, ERG knock-down in VCaP cells has been shown to induce E-cadherin expression (Gupta et al. 2010). Moreover, our previous results indicated that monensin reduced ERG expression in VCaP cells (Ketola et al. 2010). Thus, to study whether monensin affects prostate cancer cell differentiation, E-cadherin expression was analysed in monensin exposed VCaP cells. The results from immunochemical staining and quantitative RT-PCR showed that monensin induced E-cadherin expression in VCaP cells (Fig. 4A and B), indicating that monensin promotes cell differentiation in cultured prostate cancer cells.

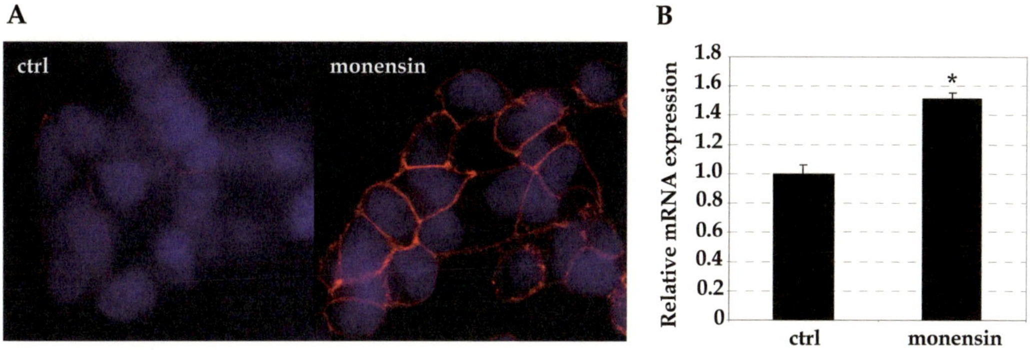

Fig. 4. Monensin induces E-cadherin expression in VCaP prostate cancer cells. A) Immunofluorescence staining of E-cadherin (red) in response to 1 μM monensin or ethanol (ctrl) for 6-hour in VCaP cells. Nuclei are stained with DAPI (blue). B) Relative mRNA expression of E-cadherin in response to 1 μM monensin or ethanol (ctrl) exposure for 6-hour in VCaP cells.

3.4 Monensin reduces migration in cultured prostate cancer cells

Epithelial-to-mesenchymal transition is a perquisite for cancer cell migration (Baum, Settleman & Quinlan 2008). Moreover, in addition to the role in promoting cancer stem cell growth and survival, NF-κB and ALDH activities as well as high CD44 and low CD24 expressions are known to enhance prostate cancer cell migration (van den Hoogen et al. 2010, Klarmann et al. 2009). Since monensin induced cell differentiation, the effect of monensin exposure on prostate cancer cell migration was studied. VCaP and LNCaP cells do not migrate and therefore PC-3 prostate cancer cells were used as a model in migration assay. The results are presented in Fig. 5. Interestingly, already at 10 nM concentration, monensin significantly reduced cell migration. The anti-migratorial effect was stronger at higher concentrations (100 nM and 1 μM) (Fig. 5A). Thus, monensin was able to reduce cell migration at nanomolar concentrations in PC-3 cells although the same concentrations did not significantly decrease cell viability in these cells even at 24 hour time point (Fig. 5B). Pictures showing the decrease in wound closure in monensin exposed PC-3 cells in comparison to control are shown at 12 and 24 hour time points in Fig. 5C.

3.5 Monensin increases oxidative stress inducing steroids as well as reduces the level of androgen precursor and antioxidative steroid

Our previous results indicated that monensin induced oxidative stress and altered the expression of genes involved in cholesterol and steroid biosynthesis (Ketola et al. 2010). Moreover, monensin reduced androgen receptor (AR) signalling and showed synergistic growth inhibitory effects with anti-androgens in prostate cancer cells. To validate the monensin induced changes in cellular steroid levels, steroid profiling was performed in VCaP prostate cancer cells. Cells were exposed to ethanol or monensin (1 μM) for six hours and steroid profiles were studied using gas chromatocraphy - mass spectrometry (GC-MS). The results presented as a heat-map in Fig. 6 show that the most prominent changes in response to monensin exposure were the induction of 7-ketocholesterol and aldosterone

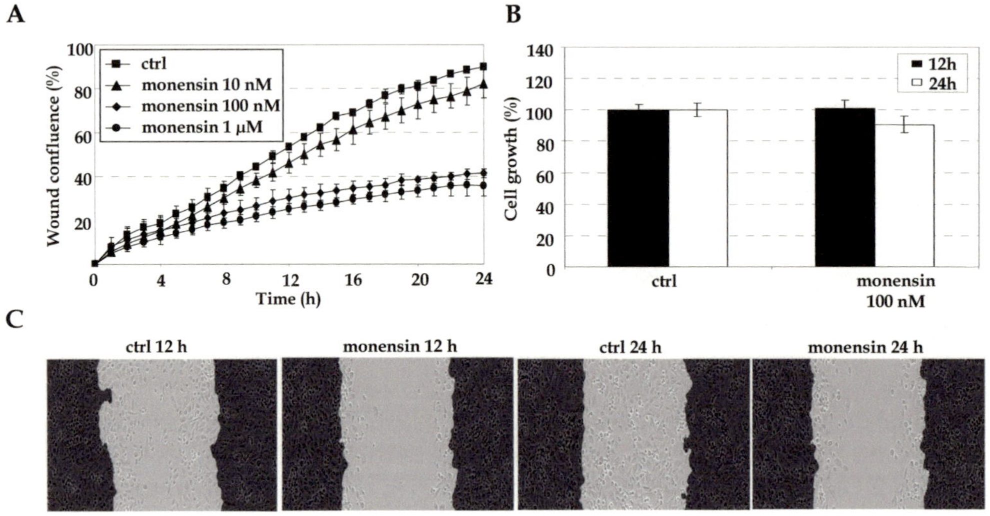

Fig. 5. The effect of monensin exposure on PC-3 prostate cancer cell migration. A) Relative wound confluency in response to monensin (10 nM, 100 nM and 1 µM) or control (ethanol) was monitored for 24 hours. B) Results from cell viability assay in response to monensin exposure (100 nM) for 12 and 24 hours in PC-3 cells. C) Pictures of scratch-wounded wells in response to 100 nM monensin or ethanol exposure at 12- and 24-hour time points. The wound margin in the beginning of the experiment is coloured in dark grey.

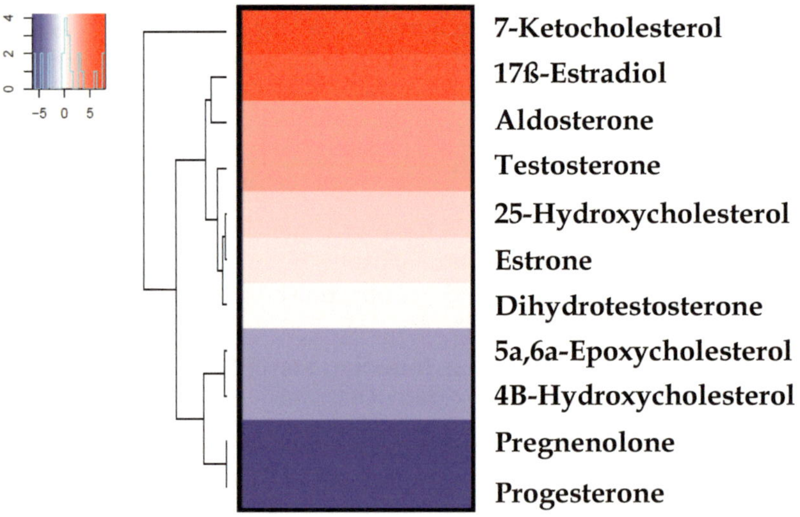

Fig. 6. Steroid profiling heat-map of monensin exposed VCaP prostate cancer cells. The cells were exposed to monensin (1 µM) for 6 hours and the steroid profile was measured with gas chromatography-mass spectrometry (GC-MS). The levels of individual steroids in monensin exposed cells were compared to ethanol exposed samples (presented as fold change, red: induction, blue: reduction).

levels as well as decrease in progesterone and pregnenolone levels. Aldosterone and 7-ketocholesterol are known oxidative stress inducers whereas progesterone has antioxidant properties (Leonarduzzi et al., 2006, Gramajo et al., 2010, Lee et al., 2009, Calo et al., 2010, Queisser et al., 2011, Ozacmak et al., 2009). Moreover, progesterone and pregnenolone are androgen precursors which have been suggested to play a major role in prostate cancer cell survival (Locke et al. 2008). Interestingly, progesterone has also been shown to promote mammary stem cell expansion (Joshi et al. 2010). The steroid profiling validates also the previous Connectivity Map results which indicated that monensin has opposite effects to progesterone and pregnenolone (Ketola et al. 2010). Taken together, monensin induced alterations in cellular steroid profile indicated that monensin induced oxidative stress results from increased aldosterone and 7-ketocholesterol levels as well as decreased progesterone and pregnenolone levels.

4. Conclusion

In this study, we explored the molecular consequences of monensin exposure in cultured prostate cancer cells. Our previous study indicated that monensin inhibited selectively prostate cancer cell viability at nanomolar concentrations by inducing oxidative stress. Cancer cells are constantly under pro-oxidative state (Szatrowski, Nathan 1991, Toyokuni et al. 1995). Long-term oxidative stress stimulates cell growth and proliferation, contributes to metastatic process and promotes cancer cell invasiveness and migration (Mori, Shibanuma & Nose 2004, Sung et al. 2006). Therefore, cancer cells need strong antioxidant mechanisms to survive and profit from these oxidative stress induced changes. Interfering redox balance has been suggested as a potential mean to selectively target cancer cells for example by increasing the cellular ROS level or reducing the expression of antioxidative enzymes (Pelicano, Carney & Huang 2004). Our results with monensin support this hypothesis.

Our previous Connectivity Map results indicated that monensin has agonistic effects to NF-κB inactivator and oxidative stress inducer niclosamide supporting monensin as a potent NF-κB inhibitor. Here, we showed that although monensin reduced the activities of several pathways known to play a role in tumourigenesis, the strongest reduction was seen in NF κB signalling. NF-κB activity promotes cell viability, tumorigenesis and metastasis as well as correlates with poor prognosis in prostate cancer patients (Blum et al. 2009, Sarkar et al. 2008). Importantly, NF-κB regulates the expression of genes responsible for antioxidant defence capacity and its inhibition induces oxidative stress as well as reduces tumourigenesis, metastasis and cancer stem cell potential (Gloire, Legrand-Poels & Piette 2006, Sarkar et al. 2008, Gluschnaider et al. 2010). NF-κB inhibitors are known to decrease AR signalling *in vitro* and reduce the growth of androgen deprivation-resistant prostate cancer xenografts *in vivo* (Jin et al. 2008, Zhang et al. 2009b). However, at present no specific NF-κB inhibitors have reached the stage of clinical trials for prostate cancer treatment (Mahon et al. 2011). Our results support NF-κB as the main mediator of monensin induced oxidative stress, which may also contribute to the reduced androgen signalling and induction of apoptosis in monensin exposed prostate cancer cells.

Recently, cancer stem cell targeting has raised a lot of interest as a prominent way to target cancer drug resistance and metastasic growth (Mimeault, Batra 2011, Clayton, Mousa 2011). In comparison to cancer cells, ROS levels in cancer stem cells are lower due to controlled redox balance system such as high ALDH and CD44 expression protecting cancer stem cells from oxidative stress (Kobayashi, Suda 2011a, Croker, Allan 2011, Ishimoto et al. 2011). Interestingly, NF-κB inhibition induces apoptosis in prostate cancer stem cells and thus NF-κB is considered as an attractive chemotherapeutic target also against cancer stem cells (Jin et al. 2008, Birnie et al. 2008). Since monensin reduced ALDH and NF-κB activities, we studied the fraction of $CD44^{+}/CD24^{-}$ cells in prostate cancer cell cultures in response to monensin exposure. The results confirmed that monensin reduced the amount of prostate cancer stem cells. Moreover, monensin induced epithelial cell differentiation and reduced motility in cultured prostate cancer cells, suggesting that monensin inhibits prostate tumorigenesis by multiple ways. Cancer stem cell inhibitor and cell differentiation inducer salinomycin shares a similar structure as monensin, supporting the functional similarities between these two compounds (Gupta et al. 2009).

Steroidogenic enzymes as well as stem cell markers are induced in castration-resistant prostate cancer both *in vitro* and *in vivo* (Blum et al. 2009, Pfeiffer et al. 2011). Several studies have shown that steroidogenesis is inhibited by ROS (Tsai et al. 2003, Stocco, Wells & Clark 1993, Kodaman, Aten & Behrman 1994, Lee et al. 2009, Abidi et al. 2008). Our previous results indicated that monensin reduced androgen receptor signalling. Here, we showed that monensin increases the levels of oxidative stress inducing steroids, 7-ketocholesterol and aldosterone, and reduces androgen precursor and antioxidative steroid progesterone in cultured prostate cancer cells. Interestingly, 7-ketocholesterol is a ligand for aryl hydrocarbon receptor (AhR) and acts as AhR antagonist (Savouret et al. 2001). AhR expression is elevated in malignant prostate cells and its signalling is activated in prostate cancer stem cells (Blum et al. 2009, Gluschnaider et al. 2010). AhR pathway increases the expression of ALDH proteins and protects cells against oxidative stress and foreign chemicals (Lindros et al. 1998, Vrzal, Ulrichova & Dvorak 2004, Nebert et al. 2000, Kohle, Bock 2007). Interestingly, AhR binds to NF-κB, induces MYC activation and reduces E-cadherin expression in breast cancer cells (Kim et al. 2000, Dietrich, Kaina 2010). Moreover, AhR can form a complex with androgen receptor and protect prostate cancer cells during androgen ablation (Ohtake, Fujii-Kuriyama & Kato 2009, Gluschnaider et al. 2010). Thus, our results indicate that monensin induced oxidative stress is potentially transmitted via reduced AhR signalling. This hypothesis is further supported by our previous gene expression results indicating that although AhR itself was not altered, the expression of AhR target gene mRNAs were decreased in response to monensin exposure (Ketola et al. 2010).

Taken together, we hypothesize that monensin induced anti-neoplastic effects result mainly due to increase in oxidative stress. The overview figure 7 illustrates the various changes occurring in prostate cancer cells in response to monensin exposure. The cancer selectiveness could be explained by increased intracellular ROS due to reduced antioxidative capacity sensitizing prostate cancer cells to oxidative stress. Since normal prostate epithelial cells are not under intensive oxidative stress and therefore, are less dependent on the function of antioxidative genes, they are not as sensitive to monensin exposure as cancer cells. In conclusion, our results support the idea that impairing the redox control, which has a crucial role in cancer cells enabling survival in high intracellular ROS, is a potent way to target prostate cancer cells.

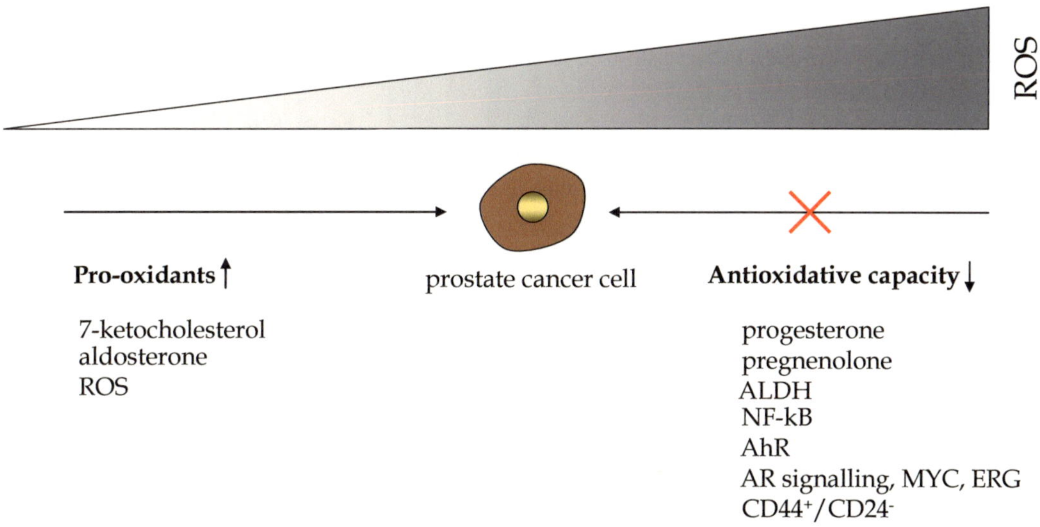

Fig. 7. Overview of monensin induced changes in prostate cancer cells. The figure idea adapted from Cairns, R.A., Harris, I.S. & Mak, T.W. 2011.

5. Acknowledgement

We thank Mika Hilvo, Tuulia Hyötyläinen, Anna-Liisa Ruskeepää (VTT Technical Research Centre of Finland, Espoo, Finland) for their contribution in steroid profiling part of this study.

6. References

Abidi, P., Zhang, H., Zaidi, S.M., Shen, W.J., Leers-Sucheta, S., Cortez, Y., Han, J. & Azhar, S. 2008, "Oxidative stress-induced inhibition of adrenal steroidogenesis requires participation of p38 mitogen-activated protein kinase signaling pathway", *The Journal of endocrinology,* vol. 198, no. 1, pp. 193-207.

Ahlemeyer, B., Bauerbach, E., Plath, M., Steuber, M., Heers, C., Tegtmeier, F. & Krieglstein, J. 2001, "Retinoic acid reduces apoptosis and oxidative stress by preservation of SOD protein level", *Free radical biology & medicine,* vol. 30, no. 10, pp. 1067-1077.

Ahlemeyer, B. & Krieglstein, J. 1998, "Retinoic acid reduces staurosporine-induced apoptotic damage in chick embryonic neurons by suppressing reactive oxygen species production", *Neuroscience letters,* vol. 246, no. 2, pp. 93-96.

Baum, B., Settleman, J. & Quinlan, M.P. 2008, "Transitions between epithelial and mesenchymal states in development and disease", *Seminars in cell & developmental biology,* vol. 19, no. 3, pp. 294-308.

Benassi, B., Fanciulli, M., Fiorentino, F., Porrello, A., Chiorino, G., Loda, M., Zupi, G. & Biroccio, A. 2006, "c-Myc phosphorylation is required for cellular response to oxidative stress", *Molecular cell,* vol. 21, no. 4, pp. 509-519.

Berthold, D.R., Pond, G.R., Soban, F., de Wit, R., Eisenberger, M. & Tannock, I.F. 2008, "Docetaxel plus prednisone or mitoxantrone plus prednisone for advanced prostate cancer: updated survival in the TAX 327 study", *Journal of clinical oncology : official journal of the American Society of Clinical Oncology,* vol. 26, no. 2, pp. 242-245.

Birnie, R., Bryce, S.D., Roome, C., Dussupt, V., Droop, A., Lang, S.H., Berry, P.A., Hyde, C.F., Lewis, J.L., Stower, M.J., Maitland, N.J. & Collins, A.T. 2008, "Gene expression profiling of human prostate cancer stem cells reveals a pro-inflammatory phenotype and the importance of extracellular matrix interactions", *Genome biology,* vol. 9, no. 5, pp. R83.

Blum, R., Gupta, R., Burger, P.E., Ontiveros, C.S., Salm, S.N., Xiong, X., Kamb, A., Wesche, H., Marshall, L., Cutler, G., Wang, X., Zavadil, J., Moscatelli, D. & Wilson, E.L. 2009, "Molecular signatures of prostate stem cells reveal novel signaling pathways and provide insights into prostate cancer", *PloS one,* vol. 4, no. 5, pp. e5722.

Bracarda, S., Logothetis, C., Sternberg, C.N. & Oudard, S. 2011, "Current and emerging treatment modalities for metastatic castration-resistant prostate cancer", *BJU international,* vol. 107 Suppl 2, pp. 13-20.

Burger, P.E., Gupta, R., Xiong, X., Ontiveros, C.S., Salm, S.N., Moscatelli, D. & Wilson, E.L. 2009, "High aldehyde dehydrogenase activity: a novel functional marker of murine prostate stem/progenitor cells", *Stem cells (Dayton, Ohio),* vol. 27, no. 9, pp. 2220-2228.

Cairns, R.A., Harris, I.S. & Mak, T.W. 2011, "Regulation of cancer cell metabolism", *Nature reviews.Cancer,* vol. 11, no. 2, pp. 85-95.

Chaffer, C.L. & Weinberg, R.A. 2011, "A perspective on cancer cell metastasis", *Science (New York, N.Y.),* vol. 331, no. 6024, pp. 1559-1564.

Chiu, H.J., Fischman, D.A. & Hammerling, U. 2008, "Vitamin A depletion causes oxidative stress, mitochondrial dysfunction, and PARP-1-dependent energy deprivation", *The FASEB journal : official publication of the Federation of American Societies for Experimental Biology,* vol. 22, no. 11, pp. 3878-3887.

Chute, J.P., Muramoto, G.G., Whitesides, J., Colvin, M., Safi, R., Chao, N.J. & McDonnell, D.P. 2006, "Inhibition of aldehyde dehydrogenase and retinoid signaling induces the expansion of human hematopoietic stem cells", *Proceedings of the National Academy of Sciences of the United States of America,* vol. 103, no. 31, pp. 11707-11712.

Clayton, S. & Mousa, S.A. 2011, "Therapeutics formulated to target cancer stem cells: Is it in our future?", *Cancer cell international,* vol. 11, pp. 7.

Croker, A.K. & Allan, A.L. 2011, "Inhibition of aldehyde dehydrogenase (ALDH) activity reduces chemotherapy and radiation resistance of stem-like ALDH(hi)CD44 (+) human breast cancer cells", *Breast cancer research and treatment,* .

Dakhova, O., Ozen, M., Creighton, C.J., Li, R., Ayala, G., Rowley, D. & Ittmann, M. 2009, "Global gene expression analysis of reactive stroma in prostate cancer", *Clinical cancer research : an official journal of the American Association for Cancer Research,* vol. 15, no. 12, pp. 3979-3989.

Davydov, V.V., Dobaeva, N.M. & Bozhkov, A.I. 2004, "Possible role of alteration of aldehyde's scavenger enzymes during aging", *Experimental gerontology,* vol. 39, no. 1, pp. 11-16.

DeNicola, G.M., Karreth, F.A., Humpton, T.J., Gopinathan, A., Wei, C., Frese, K., Mangal, D., Yu, K.H., Yeo, C.J., Calhoun, E.S., Scrimieri, F., Winter, J.M., Hruban, R.H., Iacobuzio-Donahue, C., Kern, S.E., Blair, I.A. & Tuveson, D.A. 2011, "Oncogene-induced Nrf2 transcription promotes ROS detoxification and tumorigenesis", *Nature,* vol. 475, no. 7354, pp. 106-109.

Dietrich, C. & Kaina, B. 2010, "The aryl hydrocarbon receptor (AhR) in the regulation of cell-cell contact and tumor growth", *Carcinogenesis,* vol. 31, no. 8, pp. 1319-1328.

Duester, G. 2000, "Families of retinoid dehydrogenases regulating vitamin A function: production of visual pigment and retinoic acid", *European journal of biochemistry / FEBS,* vol. 267, no. 14, pp. 4315-4324.

Fang, J., Nakamura, H. & Iyer, A.K. 2007, "Tumor-targeted induction of oxystress for cancer therapy", *Journal of drug targeting,* vol. 15, no. 7-8, pp. 475-486.

Gloire, G., Legrand-Poels, S. & Piette, J. 2006, "NF-kappaB activation by reactive oxygen species: fifteen years later", *Biochemical pharmacology,* vol. 72, no. 11, pp. 1493-1505.

Gluschnaider, U., Hidas, G., Cojocaru, G., Yutkin, V., Ben-Neriah, Y. & Pikarsky, E. 2010, "beta-TrCP inhibition reduces prostate cancer cell growth via upregulation of the aryl hydrocarbon receptor", *PloS one,* vol. 5, no. 2, pp. e9060.

Gupta, P.B., Onder, T.T., Jiang, G., Tao, K., Kuperwasser, C., Weinberg, R.A. & Lander, E.S. 2009, "Identification of selective inhibitors of cancer stem cells by high-throughput screening", *Cell,* vol. 138, no. 4, pp. 645-659.

Gupta, S., Iljin, K., Sara, H., Mpindi, J.P., Mirtti, T., Vainio, P., Rantala, J., Alanen, K., Nees, M. & Kallioniemi, O. 2010, "FZD4 as a mediator of ERG oncogene-induced WNT signaling and epithelial-to-mesenchymal transition in human prostate cancer cells", *Cancer research,* vol. 70, no. 17, pp. 6735-6745.

Gupte, A. & Mumper, R.J. 2009, "Elevated copper and oxidative stress in cancer cells as a target for cancer treatment", *Cancer treatment reviews,* vol. 35, no. 1, pp. 32-46.

Iljin, K., Ketola, K., Vainio, P., Halonen, P., Kohonen, P., Fey, V., Grafstrom, R.C., Perala, M. & Kallioniemi, O. 2009, "High-throughput cell-based screening of 4910 known drugs and drug-like small molecules identifies disulfiram as an inhibitor of prostate cancer cell growth", *Clinical cancer research : an official journal of the American Association for Cancer Research,* vol. 15, no. 19, pp. 6070-6078.

Ishimoto, T., Nagano, O., Yae, T., Tamada, M., Motohara, T., Oshima, H., Oshima, M., Ikeda, T., Asaba, R., Yagi, H., Masuko, T., Shimizu, T., Ishikawa, T., Kai, K., Takahashi, E., Imamura, Y., Baba, Y., Ohmura, M., Suematsu, M., Baba, H. & Saya, H. 2011, "CD44 variant regulates redox status in cancer cells by stabilizing the xCT subunit of system xc(-) and thereby promotes tumor growth", *Cancer cell,* vol. 19, no. 3, pp. 387-400.

Jemal, A., Bray, F., Center, M.M., Ferlay, J., Ward, E. & Forman, D. 2011, "Global cancer statistics", *CA: a cancer journal for clinicians,* vol. 61, no. 2, pp. 69-90.

Jin, R.J., Lho, Y., Connelly, L., Wang, Y., Yu, X., Saint Jean, L., Case, T.C., Ellwood-Yen, K., Sawyers, C.L., Bhowmick, N.A., Blackwell, T.S., Yull, F.E. & Matusik, R.J. 2008, "The nuclear factor-kappaB pathway controls the progression of prostate cancer to androgen-independent growth", *Cancer research,* vol. 68, no. 16, pp. 6762-6769.

Jones, E., Pu, H. & Kyprianou, N. 2009, "Targeting TGF-beta in prostate cancer: therapeutic possibilities during tumor progression", *Expert opinion on therapeutic targets*, vol. 13, no. 2, pp. 227-234.

Joshi, P.A., Jackson, H.W., Beristain, A.G., Di Grappa, M.A., Mote, P.A., Clarke, C.L., Stingl, J., Waterhouse, P.D. & Khokha, R. 2010, "Progesterone induces adult mammary stem cell expansion", *Nature*, vol. 465, no. 7299, pp. 803-807.

Ketola, K., Vainio, P., Fey, V., Kallioniemi, O. & Iljin, K. 2010, "Monensin is a potent inducer of oxidative stress and inhibitor of androgen signaling leading to apoptosis in prostate cancer cells", *Molecular cancer therapeutics*, vol. 9, no. 12, pp. 3175-3185.

Khandrika, L., Kumar, B., Koul, S., Maroni, P. & Koul, H.K. 2009, "Oxidative stress in prostate cancer", *Cancer letters*, vol. 282, no. 2, pp. 125-136.

Kim, D.W., Gazourian, L., Quadri, S.A., Romieu-Mourez, R., Sherr, D.H. & Sonenshein, G.E. 2000, "The RelA NF-kappaB subunit and the aryl hydrocarbon receptor (AhR) cooperate to transactivate the c-myc promoter in mammary cells", *Oncogene*, vol. 19, no. 48, pp. 5498-5506.

Klarmann, G.J., Hurt, E.M., Mathews, L.A., Zhang, X., Duhagon, M.A., Mistree, T., Thomas, S.B. & Farrar, W.L. 2009, "Invasive prostate cancer cells are tumor initiating cells that have a stem cell-like genomic signature", *Clinical & experimental metastasis*, vol. 26, no. 5, pp. 433-446.

Kobayashi, C.I. & Suda, T. 2011a, "Regulation of reactive oxygen species in stem cells and cancer stem cells", *Journal of cellular physiology*, .

Kobayashi, C.I. & Suda, T. 2011b, "Regulation of reactive oxygen species in stem cells and cancer stem cells", *Journal of cellular physiology*, .

Kodaman, P.H., Aten, R.F. & Behrman, H.R. 1994, "Lipid hydroperoxides evoke antigonadotropic and antisteroidogenic activity in rat luteal cells", *Endocrinology*, vol. 135, no. 6, pp. 2723-2730.

Koh, C.M., Bieberich, C.J., Dang, C.V., Nelson, W.G., Yegnasubramanian, S. & De Marzo, A.M. 2010, "MYC and Prostate Cancer", *Genes & cancer*, vol. 1, no. 6, pp. 617-628.

Kohle, C. & Bock, K.W. 2007, "Coordinate regulation of Phase I and II xenobiotic metabolisms by the Ah receptor and Nrf2", *Biochemical pharmacology*, vol. 73, no. 12, pp. 1853-1862.

Korenchuk, S., Lehr, J.E., MClean, L., Lee, Y.G., Whitney, S., Vessella, R., Lin, D.L. & Pienta, K.J. 2001a, "VCaP, a cell-based model system of human prostate cancer", *In vivo (Athens, Greece)*, vol. 15, no. 2, pp. 163-168.

Korenchuk, S., Lehr, J.E., MClean, L., Lee, Y.G., Whitney, S., Vessella, R., Lin, D.L. & Pienta, K.J. 2001b, "VCaP, a cell-based model system of human prostate cancer", *In vivo (Athens, Greece)*, vol. 15, no. 2, pp. 163-168.

Kumar, B., Koul, S., Khandrika, L., Meacham, R.B. & Koul, H.K. 2008, "Oxidative stress is inherent in prostate cancer cells and is required for aggressive phenotype", *Cancer research*, vol. 68, no. 6, pp. 1777-1785.

Lee, S.Y., Gong, E.Y., Hong, C.Y., Kim, K.H., Han, J.S., Ryu, J.C., Chae, H.Z., Yun, C.H. & Lee, K. 2009, "ROS inhibit the expression of testicular steroidogenic enzyme genes via the suppression of Nur77 transactivation", *Free radical biology & medicine,* vol. 47, no. 11, pp. 1591-1600.

Leonarduzzi, G., Vizio, B., Sottero, B., Verde, V., Gamba, P., Mascia, C., Chiarpotto, E., Poli, G. & Biasi, F. 2006, "Early involvement of ROS overproduction in apoptosis induced by 7-ketocholesterol", *Antioxidants & redox signaling,* vol. 8, no. 3-4, pp. 375-380.

Li, T., Su, Y., Mei, Y., Leng, Q., Leng, B., Liu, Z., Stass, S.A. & Jiang, F. 2010, "ALDH1A1 is a marker for malignant prostate stem cells and predictor of prostate cancer patients' outcome", *Laboratory investigation; a journal of technical methods and pathology,* vol. 90, no. 2, pp. 234-244.

Lindros, K.O., Oinonen, T., Kettunen, E., Sippel, H., Muro-Lupori, C. & Koivusalo, M. 1998, "Aryl hydrocarbon receptor-associated genes in rat liver: regional coinduction of aldehyde dehydrogenase 3 and glutathione transferase Ya", *Biochemical pharmacology,* vol. 55, no. 4, pp. 413-421.

Locke, J.A., Guns, E.S., Lubik, A.A., Adomat, H.H., Hendy, S.C., Wood, C.A., Ettinger, S.L., Gleave, M.E. & Nelson, C.C. 2008, "Androgen levels increase by intratumoral de novo steroidogenesis during progression of castration-resistant prostate cancer", *Cancer research,* vol. 68, no. 15, pp. 6407-6415.

Magni, M., Shammah, S., Schiro, R., Mellado, W., Dalla-Favera, R. & Gianni, A.M. 1996, "Induction of cyclophosphamide-resistance by aldehyde-dehydrogenase gene transfer", *Blood,* vol. 87, no. 3, pp. 1097-1103.

Mahon, K.L., Henshall, S.M., Sutherland, R.L. & Horvath, L.G. 2011, "Pathways of chemotherapy resistance in castration-resistant prostate cancer", *Endocrine-related cancer,* vol. 18, no. 4, pp. R103-23.

Mimeault, M. & Batra, S.K. 2011, "Frequent Gene Products and Molecular Pathways Altered in Prostate Cancer- and Metastasis-Initiating Cells and their Progenies and Novel Promising Multitargeted Therapies", *Molecular medicine (Cambridge, Mass.)* .

Mori, K., Shibanuma, M. & Nose, K. 2004, "Invasive potential induced under long-term oxidative stress in mammary epithelial cells", *Cancer research,* vol. 64, no. 20, pp. 7464-7472.

Nebert, D.W., Roe, A.L., Dieter, M.Z., Solis, W.A., Yang, Y. & Dalton, T.P. 2000, "Role of the aromatic hydrocarbon receptor and [Ah] gene battery in the oxidative stress response, cell cycle control, and apoptosis", *Biochemical pharmacology,* vol. 59, no. 1, pp. 65-85.

Ohtake, F., Fujii-Kuriyama, Y. & Kato, S. 2009, "AhR acts as an E3 ubiquitin ligase to modulate steroid receptor functions", *Biochemical pharmacology,* vol. 77, no. 4, pp. 474-484.

Pani, G., Galeotti, T. & Chiarugi, P. 2010, "Metastasis: cancer cell's escape from oxidative stress", *Cancer metastasis reviews,* vol. 29, no. 2, pp. 351-378.

Pelicano, H., Carney, D. & Huang, P. 2004, "ROS stress in cancer cells and therapeutic implications", *Drug resistance updates : reviews and commentaries in antimicrobial and anticancer chemotherapy,* vol. 7, no. 2, pp. 97-110.

Pfeiffer, M.J., Smit, F.P., Sedelaar, J.P. & Schalken, J.A. 2011, "Steroidogenic Enzymes and Stem Cell Markers Are Upregulated during Androgen Deprivation in Prostate Cancer", *Molecular medicine (Cambridge, Mass.),* vol. 17, no. 7-8, pp. 657-664.

Pinthus, J.H., Bryskin, I., Trachtenberg, J., Lu, J.P., Singh, G., Fridman, E. & Wilson, B.C. 2007, "Androgen induces adaptation to oxidative stress in prostate cancer: implications for treatment with radiation therapy", *Neoplasia (New York, N.Y.),* vol. 9, no. 1, pp. 68-80.

Rigas, B. & Sun, Y. 2008, "Induction of oxidative stress as a mechanism of action of chemopreventive agents against cancer", *British journal of cancer,* vol. 98, no. 7, pp. 1157-1160.

Sarkar, F.H., Li, Y., Wang, Z. & Kong, D. 2008, "NF-kappaB signaling pathway and its therapeutic implications in human diseases", *International reviews of immunology,* vol. 27, no. 5, pp. 293-319.

Savouret, J.F., Antenos, M., Quesne, M., Xu, J., Milgrom, E. & Casper, R.F. 2001, "7-Ketocholesterol is an Endogenous Modulator for the Arylhydrocarbon Receptor", *The Journal of biological chemistry,* vol. 276, no. 5, pp. 3054-3059.

Sharifi, N., Gulley, J.L. & Dahut, W.L. 2010, "An update on androgen deprivation therapy for prostate cancer", *Endocrine-related cancer,* vol. 17, no. 4, pp. R305-15.

Shibutani, S., Takeshita, M. & Grollman, A.P. 1991, "Insertion of specific bases during DNA synthesis past the oxidation-damaged base 8-oxodG", *Nature,* vol. 349, no. 6308, pp. 431-434.

Sophos, N.A. & Vasiliou, V. 2003, "Aldehyde dehydrogenase gene superfamily: the 2002 update", *Chemico-biological interactions,* vol. 143-144, pp. 5-22.

Stocco, D.M., Wells, J. & Clark, B.J. 1993, "The effects of hydrogen peroxide on steroidogenesis in mouse Leydig tumor cells", *Endocrinology,* vol. 133, no. 6, pp. 2827-2832.

Sun, Y., Huang, L., Mackenzie, G.G. & Rigas, B. 2011, "Oxidative stress mediates through apoptosis the anticancer effect of phospho-NSAIDs: Implications for the role of oxidative stress in the action of anticancer agents", *The Journal of pharmacology and experimental therapeutics,* .

Sung, S.Y., Kubo, H., Shigemura, K., Arnold, R.S., Logani, S., Wang, R., Konaka, H., Nakagawa, M., Mousses, S., Amin, M., Anderson, C., Johnstone, P., Petros, J.A., Marshall, F.F., Zhau, H.E. & Chung, L.W. 2006, "Oxidative stress induces ADAM9 protein expression in human prostate cancer cells", *Cancer research,* vol. 66, no. 19, pp. 9519-9526.

Swanson, T.A., Krueger, S.A., Galoforo, S., Thibodeau, B.J., Martinez, A.A., Wilson, G.D. & Marples, B. 2011, "TMPRSS2/ERG fusion gene expression alters chemo- and radio-responsiveness in cell culture models of androgen independent prostate cancer", *The Prostate,* .

Szatrowski, T.P. & Nathan, C.F. 1991, "Production of large amounts of hydrogen peroxide by human tumor cells", *Cancer research,* vol. 51, no. 3, pp. 794-798.

Tam, N.N., Gao, Y., Leung, Y.K. & Ho, S.M. 2003, "Androgenic regulation of oxidative stress in the rat prostate: involvement of NAD(P)H oxidases and antioxidant defense machinery during prostatic involution and regrowth", *The American journal of pathology,* vol. 163, no. 6, pp. 2513-2522.

Tannock, I.F., de Wit, R., Berry, W.R., Horti, J., Pluzanska, A., Chi, K.N., Oudard, S., Theodore, C., James, N.D., Turesson, I., Rosenthal, M.A., Eisenberger, M.A. & TAX 327 Investigators 2004, "Docetaxel plus prednisone or mitoxantrone plus prednisone for advanced prostate cancer", *The New England journal of medicine,* vol. 351, no. 15, pp. 1502-1512.

Toyokuni, S., Okamoto, K., Yodoi, J. & Hiai, H. 1995, "Persistent oxidative stress in cancer", *FEBS letters,* vol. 358, no. 1, pp. 1-3.

Tsai, S.C., Lu, C.C., Lin, C.S. & Wang, P.S. 2003, "Antisteroidogenic actions of hydrogen peroxide on rat Leydig cells", *Journal of cellular biochemistry,* vol. 90, no. 6, pp. 1276-1286.

Vainio, P., Gupta, S., Ketola, K., Mirtti, T., Mpindi, J.P., Kohonen, P., Fey, V., Perala, M., Smit, F., Verhaegh, G., Schalken, J., Alanen, K.A., Kallioniemi, O. & Iljin, K. 2011, "Arachidonic acid pathway members PLA2G7, HPGD, EPHX2, and CYP4F8 identified as putative novel therapeutic targets in prostate cancer", *The American journal of pathology,* vol. 178, no. 2, pp. 525-536.

van Bokhoven, A., Varella-Garcia, M., Korch, C., Johannes, W.U., Smith, E.E., Miller, H.L., Nordeen, S.K., Miller, G.J. & Lucia, M.S. 2003, "Molecular characterization of human prostate carcinoma cell lines", *The Prostate,* vol. 57, no. 3, pp. 205-225.

van den Hoogen, C., van der Horst, G., Cheung, H., Buijs, J.T., Lippitt, J.M., Guzman-Ramirez, N., Hamdy, F.C., Eaton, C.L., Thalmann, G.N., Cecchini, M.G., Pelger, R.C. & van der Pluijm, G. 2010, "High aldehyde dehydrogenase activity identifies tumor-initiating and metastasis-initiating cells in human prostate cancer", *Cancer research,* vol. 70, no. 12, pp. 5163-5173.

Vrzal, R., Ulrichova, J. & Dvorak, Z. 2004, "Aromatic hydrocarbon receptor status in the metabolism of xenobiotics under normal and pathophysiological conditions", *Biomedical papers of the Medical Faculty of the University Palacky, Olomouc, Czechoslovakia,* vol. 148, no. 1, pp. 3-10.

Wang, J., Cai, Y., Shao, L.J., Siddiqui, J., Palanisamy, N., Li, R., Ren, C., Ayala, G. & Ittmann, M.M. 2010, "Activation of NF-kB by TMPRSS2/ERG fusion isoforms through Toll-like receptor-4", *Cancer research,* .

Yoshida, A., Rzhetsky, A., Hsu, L.C. & Chang, C. 1998, "Human aldehyde dehydrogenase gene family", *European journal of biochemistry / FEBS,* vol. 251, no. 3, pp. 549-557.

Yossepowitch, O., Pinchuk, I., Gur, U., Neumann, A., Lichtenberg, D. & Baniel, J. 2007, "Advanced but not localized prostate cancer is associated with increased oxidative stress", *The Journal of urology,* vol. 178, no. 4 Pt 1, pp. 1238-43; discussion 1243-4.

Yu, C., Yao, Z., Dai, J., Zhang, H., Escara-Wilke, J., Zhang, X. & Keller, E.T. 2011, "ALDH Activity Indicates Increased Tumorigenic Cells, But Not Cancer Stem Cells, in Prostate Cancer Cell Lines", *In vivo (Athens, Greece),* vol. 25, no. 1, pp. 69-76.

Zhang, M., Shoeb, M., Goswamy, J., Liu, P., Xiao, T.L., Hogan, D., Campbell, G.A. & Ansari, N.H. 2009a, "Overexpression of aldehyde dehydrogenase 1A1 reduces oxidation-induced toxicity in SH-SY5Y neuroblastoma cells", *Journal of neuroscience research*, .

Zhang, Q., Helfand, B.T., Jang, T.L., Zhu, L.J., Chen, L., Yang, X.J., Kozlowski, J., Smith, N., Kundu, S.D., Yang, G., Raji, A.A., Javonovic, B., Pins, M., Lindholm, P., Guo, Y., Catalona, W.J. & Lee, C. 2009b, "Nuclear factor-kappaB-mediated transforming growth factor-beta-induced expression of vimentin is an independent predictor of biochemical recurrence after radical prostatectomy", *Clinical cancer research : an official journal of the American Association for Cancer Research*, vol. 15, no. 10, pp. 3557-3567.

Section 7

Antioxidants as Therapeutics

24

Compounds with Antioxidant Capacity as Potential Tools Against Several Oxidative Stress Related Disorders: Fact or Artifact?

P. Pérez-Matute[1*], A.B. Crujeiras[2],
M. Fernández-Galilea[3] and P. Prieto-Hontoria[3]
[1]*HIV and Associated Metabolic Alterations Unit,*
Infectious Diseases Area,
Center for Biomedical Research of La Rioja (CIBIR)
[2]*Laboratory of Molecular and Cellular Endocrinology,*
Instituto de Investigación Sanitaria,
Complejo Hospitalario de Santiago and Santiago de Compostela University
[3]*Department of Nutrition, Food Science,*
Physiology and Toxicology, University of Navarra,
Spain

1. Introduction

Oxidative stress has been generating much recent interest primarily because of its accepted role as a major contributor to the aetiology of both normal senescence and severe pathologies with serious public health implications such as obesity, diabetes, atherosclerosis, metabolic syndrome, cancer etc. However, 'Living with the risk of oxidative stress is a price that aerobic organisms must pay for more efficient bioenergetics' (quoted from V. P. Skulachev).

The term oxidative stress is vaguely defined. In essence, it refers to a serious imbalance between production of reactive species and antioxidant defenses. Thus, oxidative stress can result from diminished levels of antioxidants but can also result from increased production of reactive species (Lushchak, 2011). The consequences of oxidative stress can include: firstly, adaptation of the cell or organism by upregulation of defence systems, which may first, completely protect against damage; second, protect against damage to some extent but not completely; or third, 'overprotect' (e.g. the cell is then resistant to higher levels of oxidative stress imposed subsequently). Secondly, cell injury, which involves damage (oxidative damage) to any or all molecular targets: lipids, DNA, proteins, carbohydrates, etc. Thirdly, cell death as the cell may first, recover from the oxidative damage by repairing it or replacing the damaged molecules, or second, it may survive with persistent oxidative damage or third, oxidative damage, especially to DNA, that may trigger cell death, by apoptosis or necrosis (reviewed by Perez-Matute et al., 2009). There are different types of

* Corresponding Author

reactive species: reactive oxygen species (ROS, thus, oxygen-containing molecules that are highly reactive), reactive chlorine species (RCN) and reactive nitrogen species (RNS). All these reactants contain free radicals as well as nonradicals. Low concentrations of these reactive species are necessary for normal cell redox status, cell function and intracellular signalling (Droge, 2002; Valko et al., 2007; Perez-Matute et al., 2009). However, in some disease states, free radicals are produced in excess and can damage DNA, proteins, carbohydrates and lipid constituents and compromise cell function leading to the development of type 2 diabetes, atherosclerosis, obesity, arthritis etc. Thus, it is clear that excessive production of free radicals causes damage to biological material and is an essential event in the aetiopathogenesis of various diseases. However, the question that has risen in the past years is whether uncontrolled formation of ROS is a primary cause or a downstream consequence of the pathological processes. In other words, it is still not clear what comes first, the chicken or the egg. However, what is clear is that there must be a balance between these reactive species and the antioxidants, whose main function is to counteract the deleterious effects of these reactive species. In fact, antioxidant is defined as any substance that when present at low concentrations compared with those of an oxidizable substrate, significantly delays or prevents oxidation of that substrate (Halliwell & Gutteridge, 1999). These defences include both enzymatic (superoxide dismutases, glutathione peroxidase, catalase, thioredoxin) and non-enzimatic systems (vitamins such as vitamin C, E, A, minerals such as selenium, zinc, cooper, bilirrubine, uric acid, some aminoacids etc).

Several studies have demonstrated an increased oxidative state (either caused by an increased ROS production or diminished levels of antioxidants) in serious pathologies such as obesity, cardiovascular diseases, metabolic syndrome, cancer etc. Thus, oxidative stress actually may be related with the mentioned processes. In this context, it is tempting to suggest that if oxidative damage significantly contributes to disease pathology, then, actions that decrease it (via decreasing ROS production or increasing endogenous levels of antioxidants) might be therapeutically beneficial. In fact, attenuation or complete suppression of oxidative stress as a way to improve several diseases has flourished as one of the main challenges of research in the last years. Thus, several approaches have been carried out in order to either decrease the high levels of ROS generated or boost the endogenous levels of antioxiants. Inhibition of ROS production through the development of inhibitors (natural or chemical) against the main sources of ROS generation offers an interesting approach. Thus, NADPH oxidase and mitochondria have been postulated as the main targets to reduce ROS production (reviewed by Pérez-Matute et al., 2009). Another strategy to decrease the consequences of an increased oxidative state is the investigation that is being carried out in the last years to prove the benefits from usage of antioxidant vitamins, minerals or drinks and foods with bioactive compounds to prevent these oxidative-stress-related diseases. Thus, this chapter will focus on the potential beneficial effects of modulating oxidative stress by several bioactive compounds with antioxidant properties.

2. Counteracting oxidative stress to improve health: Role of antioxidants

As previously mentioned, increasing amount of evidence suggests that oxidative stress is linked to pathophysiological mechanisms concerning multiple acute and chronic human diseases (Dalle-Donne et al., 2006; Halliwell & Gutteridge, 2007). In this context, different strategies have been developed in order to counteract oxidative stress to improve health. We will focus on the modulation antioxidant status through a nutritional approach. Thus, and concerning the conventional antioxidant therapies that have been carried out in the last years, we can underline that there are two main ways to deal with this issue: to promote the ingestion of diets rich in several micro and macronutrients with antioxidant properties that could be beneficial for health (such as the well known Mediterranean diet) or to supplement the diet with specific bioactive compounds with antioxidant properties. In this sense, many diseases have been reported to benefit from antioxidant therapy and covering all of them in one chapter is not possible. However, it is important to note that those pathologies that may benefit the most from this antioxidant therapy are neurodegenerative diseases, Alzheimer disease, Parkinson disease, amyotrophic lateral sclerosis, cancer, stroke, obesity and diabetes (reviewed by Firuzi et al., 2011).

2.1 Diets with recognized benefits on oxidative stress and health: Diets rich in antioxidants

Epidemiological and experimental studies have demonstrated that plant-food intake decreases the risk of chronic diseases and therefore significantly contributes to the maintenance of health. For instance, the lower occurrence of cancer and cardiovascular diseases in the population around the Mediterranean basin has been linked to the dietary habits of this region. This so-called Mediterranean diet is essentially different from the diets consumed in Western and Northern European countries and is rich in nuts, fruits, vegetables, legumes, whole-wheat bread, fish, and olive oil, with moderate amounts of red wine, which is mainly consumed during meals. The components of this diet contain an ample source of molecules with antioxidant and anti-inflammatory actions, among which we can find omega-3 fatty acids, oleic acid, and phenolic compounds (Pauwels, 2011). There are several studies where the health benefits of consuming this diet have been demonstrated. Thus, the study of Dai et al. (2008) has demonstrated that the association between the Mediterranean diet and plasma oxidative stress is robust and is not confounded by genetic or shared environmental factors. Moreover, they demonstrated that a decreased oxidative stress is a plausible mechanism linking the Mediterranean diet ingestion to reduced cardiovascular disease risk (Dai et al., 2008). Moreover, it has been shown that subjects following a Mediterranean diet present low oxidised LDL levels, which seems to be one of the protective effects against cardiovascular events according to a PREDIMED (*Prevención Con Dieta Mediterránea*) cohort trial (Fito et al., 2007). Furthermore, the *French Paradox* is the observation that French people suffer a relatively low incidence of coronary heart diseases, despite having a diet relatively rich in saturated fats along with fruits, vegetables and red wine. In fact, this paradox has been attributed to the consumption of red wine and more specifically to polyphenols (antioxidants such as resveratrol) present in red wine. These effects underline the hypothesis that the Mediterranean diet may also neutralize the deleterious effects caused by the consumption of relatively high amounts of animal fats.

The dietary patterns based on the DASH (Dietary Approaches to Stop Hypertension) emphasizes the consumption of fruits, vegetables, and low-fat dairy products and the reduced ingestion of saturated fat, total fat, and cholesterol (as in the Mediterranean diet) as it has been demonstrated that these patterns substantially lowered blood pressure and low-density lipoprotein cholesterol (Miller et al., 2006). Participants from the SU.VI.MAX (*Supplementation en Vitamines et Minéraux Antioxydants*) cohort who achieved the current daily fruit and vegetable intake recommendations within the DASH diet guidelines presented a lower increase in blood pressure with aging (Dauchet et al., 2007). In addition, a prospective study in the EPIC (European Prospective Investigation into Cancer and Nutrition) cohort evidenced that a high vegetables, legumes, and fruit diet was associated with a reduced risk of all-cause mortality, especially deaths due to cardiovascular disease underling the recommendation for the diabetic population to eat large amounts of vegetables, legumes, and fruit (Nothlings et al., 2008). Furthermore, fruit-enriched hypocaloric diets appear to be more effective against oxidative stress according to the study of Crujeiras et al. (2006). In fact, consumption of antioxidant substances contained in fruit could be a useful strategy in the design of hypocaloric diets that, with the weight reduction, could increase the improvement of cardiovascular risk factors related to obesity. Finally, in a case-control study, an inverse association has been found between the first acute myocardial infarction and the consumption of fruits among the Spanish Mediterranean diet (Martinez-Gonzalez et al., 2002).

Among all the foods included in these healthy diets (such as the Mediterranean diet), legumes have also been suggested to contribute to prevent cardiovascular disease and diabetes mellitus. Indeed, epidemiological studies have shown that Asian people consuming soy in their staple diet present much lower mortality and morbidity from cardiovascular disease than their counterparts in Western counties (Heneman et al., 2007). However, lentils, chickpeas, peas, and beans are the legumes more commonly consumed in Western countries but it has also been demonstrated that a non soybean legumes-based hypocaloric diet induced a higher decrease in blood lipids concentrations as well as lower lipid peroxidation markers related to obesity comorbidities as compared to a conventional and balanced hypocaloric diet (Crujeiras et al., 2007a).

All these studies mentioned above are examples that evidenced the beneficial effects of plant-food intake in promoting health and life-span in part attributed to their high level of antioxidant compounds, which contribute to decrease oxidative stress (Crujeiras et al., 2009). Some studies have also attributed antioxidative properties to fiber-enriched diets, since these compounds enhance the capacity to detoxify free radicals (Diniz et al., 2005). Fiber alters fat absorption from the diet by impairing lipid hydrolysis, resulting in increased fat excretion and as consequence, decreased lipid peroxidation probability. Moreover, fiber secondary metabolites that arise from bacterial fermentation in the colon may have antioxidant properties (Diniz et al., 2005). Reinforcing this idea, a significant correlation between antioxidant power in plasma and dietary fiber plus fructose evidenced the beneficial effects of fruit intake on antioxidant capacity in obese women (Crujeiras et al., 2006). In addition, the fruit (Crujeiras et al., 2006) or legumes (Crujeiras et al., 2007a) hypocholesterolemic effects were in parallel with oxidative stress improvement when evaluated by means of the prooxidant and antioxidant ratio in plasma (Crujeiras et al., 2006) or lipid peroxidation biomarkers (Crujeiras et al., 2007a), suggesting an indirect antioxidant effect of these plant-foods intake mediated by the hypocholesterolemic induction.

The antioxidant effect of plant-food could be also produced by the action of lesser known compounds or by the combination of different compounds occurring in the foods with direct or indirect antioxidant effects (Crujeiras et al., 2007b). In this context, fructose has been proposed to produce specific effects on oxidative stress. Animal models fed with a high content of fructose have shown a significant increase in antioxidant capacity and prevention of lipid peroxidation (Girard et al., 2005). This fruit monosaccharide stimulates uric acid synthesis due to its rapid metabolism by fructokinase (Heuckenkamp & Zollner, 1971). Uric acid has been widely recognized in the scientific literature as a metabolic compound with high antioxidant power participating as an *in vivo* scavenger (Glantzounis et al., 2005). Thus, it has been suggested that urate is responsible for the increase in antioxidant capacity after consuming apples as fruit in healthy subjects (Lotito & Frei, 2004) and after following a fruit-based hypocaloric diet in obese women (Crujeiras et al., 2006). However, the role of uric acid on oxidative stress and health is not clear enough and conflicting results have been provided in different studies, as will be discussed later on in the vitamins section. Taking together these observations, it is conceivable that besides of the direct effect of the antioxidant compounds of plant-foods present in the Mediterranean and other healthy diets, some reported antioxidant health effects can be also associated with the metabolic effect of these foods that indirectly reduces the oxidative damage probability in presence of free radicals. Thus and despite the fact that the Mediterranean diet along with other diets enriched in fruits, fiber or legumes are beneficial for health, it is very difficult to identify which component of the diet is responsible for the positive effects (in fact, in many cases is the association of several compounds). Thus and although the presence of antioxidants has been claimed by many to be responsible for the beneficial effect of vegetables and fruits, it has also been postulated that low content of fat in these foods may be the responsible cause (reviewed by Firuzi et al., 2011). Because of that, several investigations have been carried out to analyze the effects of specific compounds with antioxidant properties more than a food which contains plenty of compounds. In this sense, the most potent antioxidants with beneficial effects on health are presented in the following part of this chapter. It is important to note that we here present a brief review of the most important antioxidants found in foods more than in antioxidants that are currently in clinical use and that have been extensively reviewed elsewhere (Firuzi et al., 2011). Indeed, we have focused the chapter on a nutritional approach of oxidative stress related diseases more than on a pharmacological approach. However, a list with the main antioxidant drugs approved for clinical use is provided in table 1.

Antioxidant	**Clinical Use**
Edaravone	Ischemic stroke
Idebenone	Alzheimer disease (?)
N-Aceylcysteine	Acetaminophen overdose, mucolytic, dry eye syndrome
α-Lipoic acid*	Diabetic neuropathy
Micronized purified flavonoids fraction (MPFF, Daflon 500®)	Persistent venous ulcers
0-β-hydroxyethyl-rutosides (Venoruton®)	Chronic venous insufficiency
Silibinin (Leaglon®)	Hepatoprotective (?), chemopreventive
Baicalein and catechins (flavocoxid)	Osteoarthritis

*Lipoic acid, due to its dietary source will be deeply discussed in this chapter

Table 1. Antioxidant drugs approved for clinical use in various diseases (Firuzi et al., 2011).

2.2 Supplementation with specific bioactive compounds with antioxidant properties

2.2.1 Lipoic acid

α-Lipoic acid (LA), also known as 1,2-dithiolane-3-pentanoic acid or thioctic acid, is a promising dietary bioactive molecule because of its recognized therapeutic potential on several diseases such as diabetes, vascular disease, hypertension, alzheimer and inflammation (Shay et al., 2009; Firuzi et al., 2011). In fact, LA (dexlipotam) has been clinically approved and used for diabetic neuropathy as pointed out in table 1. In fact, it has been used in Germany for treatment of symptomatic diabetic neuropahty since several years ago.

The two enantiomers of this acid are the R form and the S form. Both R-LA and its reduced form, dihydrolipoic acid or 6,8-dimercaptooctanoic acid (DHLA) exert powerful antioxidant properties although DHLA seems to be more effective (Packer & Suzuki, 1993). Their antioxidant functions involve: quenching ROS (reactive oxygen species), regeneration of endogenous and exogenous antioxidants involving vitamin C, vitamin E and glutathione, chelation of redox metal including Cu(II) and Fe (II) and repair of oxidized proteins.

Lipoic Acid can be found in different foods such as spinach and cabbage, liver and meat, whole wheat and yeast of beer, but it is also endogenously produced by the liver through the lipoic acid synthase (LASY) machinery. Deficiency of LASY results in an overall disturbance in the antioxidant defence network, leading to increased inflammation, insulin resistance and mitochondrial dysfunction (Padmalayam et al., 2009).

Lipoic Acid is also an essential cofactor for mitochondrial bioenergetic enzymes (Smith et al., 2004). In fact, it is well known the intimate connection of LA with cell metabolism and redox state (Packer et al., 1997) as LA is essential for normal oxidative metabolism and plays a vital role as a cofactor in mitochondrial dehydrogenase reactions (Gilgun-Sherki et al., 2002).

Oxidative stress has been linked to different pathologies such as endothelial dysfunction. In this context, several studies noted that LA plays an important role in the activation of endothelial nitric oxide synthase (eNOS), which is one enzyme responsible for nitric oxide (NO) release/production, which, in turn, is an important regulator and mediator of numerous processes in the nervous, immune and cardiovascular systems. These actions include vascular smooth muscle relaxation resulting in arterial vasodilation and increasing blood flow (Federici et al., 2002; Montagnani et al., 2002). An *in vitro* study in human endothelial cells showed that treatment with LA potentate endothelial NO synthesis and bioactivity by mechanisms that appear to be independent of cellular GSH levels (Visioli et al., 2002). Furthermore, one trial demonstrated that the administration of LA improved vasodilation in patients with metabolic syndrome (Sola et al., 2005), corroborating its positive effects in endothelial dysfunction.

Recent studies also suggest that chronic oxidative stress plays an important role in the aetiology of human obesity (Vincent et al., 2007; Wang et al., 2011). Inadequacy of antioxidant defences probably begins with a low dietary intake of bioactive compounds with antioxidant capacity (Taylor et al., 2006). In fact, it has been demonstrated that obese individuals have a lower intake of bioactive compounds compared with non-obese persons. Based on that, different studies suggest a possible nutritional intervention with antioxidants eg. LA for treating obesity which has been associated with an increased oxidative state caused by either an increase in ROS production or a decrease in the antioxidant levels

(Prieto-Hontoria et al., 2009; Carbonelli et al., 2011; Koh et al., 2011). In this context, it has been demonstrated that LA reduces body weight and adiposity in rodents (Kim et al., 2004; Prieto-Hontoria et al., 2009) and humans (Carbonelli et al., 2011). Several mechanisms may contribute to the anti-obesity effects of LA including the suppression of hypothalamic AMPK (adenosine monophosphate-activated protein kinase) activity (Shen et al., 2005), which, in turn, leads to a reduction in food intake. Other mechanism that could also contribute to the anti-obesity effects of LA is the stimulation of energy expenditure by increasing Ucp-1 mRNA levels in brown adipose tissue (Kim et al., 2004). A very recent study has also demonstrated that LA increases energy expenditure by enhancing AMPK in skeletal muscle, a cellular energy sensor that can regulate peroxisome proliferator-activated receptor-gamma coactivator-1alpha (PGC-1alpha), which is a master regulator of mitochondrial biogenesis. Thus, this study demonstrated that LA improves skeletal muscle energy metabolism in aged mice possibly through enhancing AMPK-PGC-1alpha-mediated mitochondrial biogenesis and function (Wang et al., 2010). Furthermore, the inhibitory actions of LA on intestinal sugar transport could also contribute to a lower feed efficiency observed in LA-treated animals (Prieto-Hontoria et al., 2009). Another mechanism that could also contribute in reducing adiposity is the ability of LA to inhibit adipocyte differentiation, as described by Cho et al., (2003). These inhibitory effects of LA on adipocyte differentiation appear to be mediated by reduced levels of PPARγ and C/EBPα, as well as by the activation of MAPK. Another study suggests that the anorexigenic effect of LA are mediated by inhibition the activity of various liver enzymes involved in fatty acid synthesis and desaturation such as glucose 6 - phosphate dehydrogenase, malic enzyme, pyruvate kinase enzyme, ATP-citrate lyase and fatty acid synthase (Huong & Ide, 2008).

In addition, LA has also beneficial actions in both glucose and lipid metabolism and, it has been proposed, as mentioned before, as a potential therapy for insulin resistance and type 2 diabetes. LA positively interacts with the insulin pathway and glucose handling in muscle and adipocytes, by modulating the IR/PI3K/Akt pathway and GLUT4 translocation (Shay et al., 2009). LA also promotes mitochondrial biogenesis in adipocytes and muscle through a stimulation of PGC-1α, contributing to improve the defective mitochondrial function associated to diabetes/obesity (Shen et al., 2008a; Shen et al., 2008b). Furthermore, a very recent study has demonstrated that LA treatment over a period of 2 months improves fasting blood glucose (FBG), insulin resistance (IR), and glutathione peroxidase (GH-Px) activity in type 2 diabetes (T2DM) patients (Ansar et al., 2011).

Furthremore, LA treatment in rats with thioacetamide-induced liver fibrosis, inhibited the development of liver cirrhosis, as indicated by reductions in cirrhosis incidence, hepatic fibrosis, and AST/ALT activities (Foo et al., 2011). Several studies from our group have also demonstrated the beneficial effects of LA supplementation on fatty liver in a diet-induced obesity rat model (Valdecantos et al., 2010b, 2011a,b).

Finally, several trials have also suggested the potential use of LA in cancer therapy (Novotny et al., 2008) due to its ability to induce apoptosis in cancer cells (Shi et al., 2008; Choi et al., 2009). However, the molecular mechanisms underlying the anti-carcinogenic actions of LA are not well understood.

To sum up, LA seems to be a promising candidate against not only diabetes (in fact is one antioxidant approved for clinical use in diabetic neuropathy) but also against obesity and its comorbidities (glucose and lipid impairments) as well as against cardiovascular events, some cancers and liver injuries.

2.2.2 Polyphenolic compunds: Resveratrol

Grapes (*Vitis vinifera L.*) contain high concentrations of polyphenols, especially flavonoids. The amount and composition of biologically active compounds presented in grapes and grape products vary greatly according to the species, variety, maturity, seasonal conditions, production area and yield of the fruit. The main grape polyphenols are anthocyanins in red grapes and flavan-3-ols in the case of white grapes. Red grapes contain more total polyphenols than white grapes. Grape seeds and skins are also an important dietary source of flavonoids, and seeds contain significant amounts of proanthocyanidins or condensed tannins. The most common commercial product derived from grapes is wine, a moderately alcoholic drink made by fermentation of juice extracted from fresh, ripe grapes. Its moderate consumption is suggested in the Mediterranean diet as cited before. The processing of grapes to yield wine transforms the polyphenols present in grapes and as a result the main polyphenols in wine are flavan-3-ols, flavan-3,4-diols, anthocyanins and anthocyanidins, flavonols, flavones, condensed tannins and a characteristic biologically active compound, resveratrol - a stilbene whose concentration can range from 1·5 to 3 mg/l (reviewed by Perez-Jimenez & Saura-Calixto, 2008). Resveratrol (trans-3,5,4'-trihydroxystilbene) is also found in various plants, including berries and peanuts. Moreover, this compound is now available in tablets on the market as a dietary supplement (not for clinical use).

A remarkable range of biological functions have been ascribed to this molecule. For example, resveratrol has shown cardioprotective actions (Hung et al., 2000), anti-cancer effects (Vanamala et al.) and anti-inflammatory and antioxidant properties (de la Lastra & Villegas, 2007). Its cardiovascular properties, including inhibition of platelet aggregation and promotion of vasodilation by enhancing the production of nitric oxide, have also been described (Cucciolla et al., 2007). It has also been reported to have many biological activities and protect against several neurodegenerative disorders such as Alzheimer's disease (Sun et al., 2010), but also to protect against oxidative stress in liver as well as steatosis in obese rats (Sebai et al., 2010; Gomez-Zorita et al., 2011) and against other diseases including AIDS (James, 2006; Zhang et al., 2009; Touzet & Philips, 2010), age-related illnesses and, more recently, obesity (Macarulla et al., 2009; Alberdi et al., 2011; Lasa et al., 2011). In fact, it seems to mimic the effects of energy restriction, thus leading to reduced body fat and improved insulin sensitivity. The mechanisms underlying these positive effects on obesity include: inhibition of preadipocyte proliferation and adipogenic differentiation, stimulation of basal and insulin-stimulated glucose uptake and inhibition of *de novo* lipogenesis (Fischer-Posovszky et al.). Resveratrol may also influence the secretion and plasma concentrations of some adipokines such as adiponectin and TNF-α and inhibits leptin secretion from rat adipocytes (Baur et al., 2006; Szkudelska et al., 2009). Resveratrol also regulates lipolysis via adipose triglyceride lipase (Lasa et al., 2011).

Several studies have suggested that activation of SIRT1 and AMPK plays a key role in the metabolic effects of resveratrol (Feige et al., 2008; Um et al., 2010). Sirtuins may provide novel targets for treating some diseases associated with oxidative stress. More specifically, SIRT1 has been shown to regulate metabolism and stress response by acting on several transcription factors and cofactors, histones and other chromatin proteins and components of DNA repair machinery. A recent research has also shown that resveratrol modulates tumor cell proliferation and protein translation via SIRT1-dependent AMPK activation (Lin et al.). In this context, resveratrol has been proposed as a potential dietary compound against various cancers including breast and colon tumors. Resveratrol may affect all three discrete stages of carcinogenesis (initiation, promotion, and progression) by modulating signal transduction pathways that control cell division and growth, apoptosis, inflammation, angiogenesis, and metastasis (Bishayee, 2009). Recently, it has been shown that resveratrol suppresses IGF-1 induced cell proliferation and elevates apoptosis in human colon cancer cells, via suppression of IGF-1R/Wnt and activation of p53 signaling pathways (Vanamala et al., 2010).

Tat protein plays a pivotal role in both the human immunodeficiency virus type 1 (HIV-1) replication cycle and the pathogenesis of HIV-1 infection. A very recent study has demonstrated that resveratrol, a SIRT1 activator, attenuates the transactive effects of Tat in HeLA-CD4-long terminal repeat-β-gal cells (MAGI) via NAD(+)-dependent SIRT1 activity suggesting that this antioxidant, through the regulation of different pathways such as SIRT1 activation, could be a novel therapeutic approach in anti-HIV-1 therapy (Zhang et al., 2009).

In addition, resveratrol also induces the activation of genes that encode for proteins involved in oxidative phosphorylation and mitochondrial biogenesis processes (reviewed by Szkudelska & Szkudelski, 2010). In this context, it has been shown that resveratrol improves the functioning of mitochondria in cells. In fact, the capacity of this antioxidant to reduce mitochondrial ROS levels and to induce the biosynthesis of antioxidant molecules, like MnSOD, along with its ability to increase the activity of these antioxidant defences, has been previously demonstrated (Valdecantos et al. 2010a). These actions could also explain the protective role of this antioxidant against situations with an imbalance in the oxidative status such as steatosis, obesity etc.

2.2.3 Vitamins with antioxidant properties: Vitamin E and Vitamin C

Vitamin E is the nature´s most effective lipid-soluble antioxidant, with an important role protecting unsaturated fatty acids residues in cells membranes, which are important for membrane function and structure (Van Gossum et al., 1988). Vitamin E is only produced by photosynthetic organisms. It refers to a group of eight naturally occurring compounds α-, β-, γ-, δ- tocopherols and tocotrienols. α-tocopherol, especially the naturally occurring D-α-tocopherol, is the one with the highest biological activity (Brigelius-Flohe & Traber, 1999). This variant of vitamin E can be found most abundantly in vegetable oils such as wheat germ oil, sunflower, and safflower oils (Reboul et al., 2006). Vitamin E is also found in many foods, mainly of plant origin, especially in leafy green (broccoli, spinach), seeds, including soybeans, wheat germ, some breakfast cereals and yeast beer. It can also be found in animal foods such as egg yolk.

The role of the vitamin E has emerged as a possible therapy for decreasing ROS production or increasing the endogenous levels of antioxidants and for protecting cell membranes at an early stage of free radical attack (Horwitt, 1986). Thus, vitamin E down-regulates NADPH oxidase (Calvisi et al., 2004), which is the major source of ROS in the vascular wall and it also up-regulates eNOS activity which leads to an increase in NO production (Ulker et al., 2003). As vitamin E is a potent antioxidant with anti-inflammatory properties, several lines of evidence suggest that α-tocopherol has also potential beneficial effects with regard to cardiovascular disease (Singh et al., 2005; Rodrigo et al., 2008). A recent study has also demonstrated that natural vitamin E analog alpha-tocopheryl phosphate (alphaTP) modulates atherosclerotic and inflammatory events through the regulation of certain genes (Zingg et al., 2010). However, it is also important to point out that the non-antioxidant activities of tocopherols may also represent the main biological reason for the selective retention of alpha-tocopherol in the body, or vice versa, for the metabolic conversion and consequent elimination of the other tocopherols (Zingg et al., 2004).

Several studies have demonstrated the beneficial effects of vitamin E on obesity and its related disorders such as diabetes. In fact, plasma vitamin E reflects the amount of α-tocopherol in the body. It is interesting to note that lower plasma vitamin E levels have been observed in type 2 diabetic patients (Skrha et al., 1999). In addition, the study from Botella-Carretero et al., (2010) demonstrated that alpha-tocopherol concentrations are inversely associated with body mass index in morbid obesity. Other study has demonstrated that vitamin E intervention increased the plasma activity of several antioxidant enzymes such as superoxide dismutase (SOD), glutathione peroxidase (GPx) and T-AOC (total anti-oxidative capacity) whereas it is able to decrease the levels of Isoprostane 8-epi PGF2alpha, which is a product of oxidative stress that causes potent smooth muscle contraction. The same study demonstrated that vitamin E intervention also decreased plasma glucose, insulin and triglycerides level in obese rats. Therefore, this study demonstrated that vitamin E has positive effects for improvement of oxidative stress status and glucose metabolism in an animal model of diet-induced obesity (Shen et al., 2009). In this context, Manning et al., (2004) showed that vitamin E supplementation decreased plasma peroxide concentration in obese individuals. Other study showed that antioxidant supplementation with vitamin E, C and β-carotene reduced exercise-induced lipid hidroperoxide (ΔPEROX) in overweight young adults. Possible collective mechanisms to explain this finding include a shift in the cytokine profile from a pro-inflammatory to a less inflammatory profile (lowered IL-6, increased adiponectin), an attenuation of cholesterol and triglyceride levels during exercise and a small increase in total antioxidant status (Vincent et al., 2006). On the other hand, vitamin E supplementation decreased concentrations of both 8-isoprostane and lipid peroxides in overweight subjects, indicating a decrease in systemic oxidative stress (Sutherland et al., 2007). Vitamin E supplementation in patients with diabetes decreased the levels of proinflammatory adipokines, such as IL-1, TNF-α, IL-6, and reactive C protein in serum and stimulated monocytes (Devaraj & Jialal, 2000; Upritchard et al., 2000). A recent study demonstrated that supplementing alpha-tocopherol (vitamin E) and vitamin D3 in high fat diet decreases IL-6 production in murine epididymal adipose tissue and 3T3-L1 adipocytes following LPS stimulation (Lira et al., 2011). Thus, this study suggested that vitamin E and D3 supplementation can be used as an adjunctive therapy to reduce the proinflammatory cytokines present in obese patients. A significant role played by oxidative stress and lipid peroxidation in the cascade of events involved in hepatic necroinflammatory damage is supported by an experimental study, which also showed that antioxidant vitamin E reduces fatty liver in obese Zucker rats (Soltys et al., 2001). In this context, the study from Vajro et al., (2004) strengthens the view that antioxidants, and especially vitamin E, may represent a relevant therapeutic tool for the treatment of children with obesity-related dysfunction who are unable to adhere to low-calorie diets (Vajro et al., 2004).

Finally, a very recent study concludes that MitoVES, a mitochondrially targeted analog of α-tocopheryl succinate, is an efficient anti-angiogenic agent of potential clinical relevance, exerting considerably higher activity than its untargeted counterpart. MitoVES may be helpful against cancer but may compromise wound healing (Neuzil et al., 2011). However, it is important to state that there are several controversial effects of vitamin E on cancer and diabetes that will be discuss later.

Vitamin C (Vit C) or ascorbic acid is one of the non-enzymatic antioxidants that can eliminate ROS, thus preventing tissue damage (Fetoui et al., 2008). Moreover, Vitamin C is the most abundant water-soluble antioxidant in the body and acts primarily in cellular fluid having the potential to protect both cytosolic and membrane components of cells from oxidant damage (Talaulikar & Manyonda, 2011). Vit C exerts its antioxidant effects in both direct and indirect ways. In the direct way, Vit C scavenges free radicals formed (Dawson et al., 1990) or interacts with reduced glutathione (Dudek et al., 2005). As an indirect way, it helps recycling vitamin E, thus, supplying active vitamin E (Netke et al., 1997).

Vit C is present in several fruits and vegetables such as citrus fruits, tomato, strawberry, pepper, cabbage, and leafy greens. Vit C can not be stored in the body, and excess Vit C is excreted in urine (Alpsoy & Yalvac, 2011).

Over the years, it has been suggested the usage of Vit C as a remedy against many diseases ranging from common colds to several types of cancers. Moreover, it is known that there is a close relationship between Vit C supply and immune cell activity, especially phagocytosis activity and T-cell function (Strohle et al., 2011) It also contributes to the formation and health of blood vessels, tendons, ligaments, bones, teeth and gums, it helps the body to absorb iron and to recover from wounds and burns, and serious deficiency of this vitamin can lead to scurvy, which is now a rare condition in the Western world (Garriguet, 2010; Strohle et al., 2011).

It has been described that obese patients have lower mean serum concentration of Vit C being even in an inadequate Vit C status, which leads to lower serum antioxidant capacity and greater inflammatory responses (Mah et al., 2011; Aasheim et al., 2008). Thus and regarding its effects on obesity, several studies demonstrated that Vit C dietary supplementation reduced body weight in a cafeteria diet-induced obese rat model, without affecting food intake (Campion et al., 2008; Boque et al., 2009). Moreover, it has been described that Vit C increases lipolysis and decreases triglicerides accumulation by decreasing the activity of glycerophosphate dehydrogenase, a marker of adipose conversion (Hasegawa et al., 2002; Senen et al., 2002). It also has been observed that Vit C supplementation is negatively associated with the occurrence of obesity suggesting that higher waist-to-hip ratios were associated with lower plasma ascorbic acid concentrations and that Vit C depleted individuals may be more resistant to fat mass loss.

Interestingly, these beneficial effects of Vit C seem to be due to a decrease observed in uric acid levels. In fact, it is known that hominoids during the Miocene could not biosynthesize Vit C, as a key gene involved in Vit C production: L-gulono-lactone oxidase had mutated. Hence, this mutation has been proposed to increase uric acid as an antioxidant that could replace the decrease in Vit C availability that may have occurred during this period (Johnson et al., 2009). Moreover, uric acid helps to raise blood pressure, stimulate salt-sensitivity, and induce insulin resistance and mild obesity, and thereby it helps to promote survival during a period of famine or stress which also leads to de development of obesity and its related comorbidities nowadays. Uric acid has been shown to be involved in metabolic pathways that lead to oxidative stress, endothelial dysfunction, and to a vascular and systemic inflammatory response. Moreover, the elevation in uric acid levels observed after fructose ingestion, with a consequent reduction in nitric oxide may lead to a reduced glucose uptake in the skeletal muscle, hyperinsulinemia, and insulin resistance. Thus, several clinical studies showed the beneficial effects of lowering uric acid therapies on several markers of cardiovascular and renal disease (Stellato et al. 2011). In this context and supporting this idea, Hunter et al., (2011) concluded that dietary supplementation with Vit C may confer health benefits because of increased antioxidant potential or through mechanisms resulting from increased endogenous Vit C generation or decreased serum uric acid concentrations.

In summary, Vit C is a potent antioxidant that might prevent and improve obesity and several comorbidities by different mechanisms. Besides its antioxidant power, Vit C can also exert its beneficial effects by regenerating other antioxidants such as reduced glutation or vitamin E as well as by lowering uric acid levels.

2.2.4 Selenium

Selenium (Se) is an essential trace element consumed in submilligram amounts. It is primarily found in organically bound forms in the diet. Selenium is naturally found in plants, seafood, meat and meat products. The amount of selenium that is needed to ingest to maximize plasma glutathione peroxidase (GSHPX) activity is established between 55-75 μg/d in the EU (Rayman, 2005). The element exists in both organic form of selenium, as part of selenoproteins (selenomethionine and methylated selenocompounds) as well as in inorganic forms such as selenites and selenates (Gromadzinska et al., 2008).

Selenium is required for the function of a number of key selenium-dependent enzymes (selenoproteins). Many of the known selenoproteins, in which selenium is the active site, are necessary for a wide range of metabolic processes, including thyroid hormone regulation, immune function and reproduction and they catalyze redox reactions (Kryukov et al., 2003). Because of the potential of selenoproteins to protect against oxidative stress, selenium functions as a dietary antioxidant and because of that it has been studied for its potential role in chronic diseases such as hypertension, cardiovascular disease, cancer and diabetes mellitus, as well as aging and mortality (Boosalis, 2008). In this context, experimental studies have shown that selenium has carcinostatic effects when added in high levels to the diet of animals treated with carcinogenic chemicals (Gromadzinska et al., 2008). In this context, evaluation of health claims by the FDA in the U.S. concerning the purportedly positive effects of selenium provided certain evidence for permitting a qualified health claim (Trumbo, 2005). Recent results of the SUVIMAX study showed that supplementation with vitamin C, vitamin E, β-carotene, selenium and zinc is able to reduce the rate of prostate cancer in men having normal levels of prostate-specific antigen in their plasma (Meyer et al., 2005).

Observational and interventional studies in humans have demonstrated the beneficial effect of selenium dietary intake. Thus, antioxidant supplementation contained selenium (100 mg) combined with vitamin C (500 mg), vitamin E (200 IU) and co-enzyme Q10 (60 mg) significantly alleviated the atherosclerotic damage caused by excessive production of ROS in patients with multiple cardiovascular risk factors. This beneficial vascular effect was associated with an improvement in glucose and lipid metabolism as well as with a decrease in blood pressure (Shargorodsky et al. 2010). It has also been demonstrated that the selenium supplementation is able to decrease lipid hydroperoxides (LH) post-exercise in overweight subjects, providing preliminary evidence for a potential role of selenium as an effective antioxidant therapy to reduce oxidant stress at rest and following high-intensity exercise in high-risk population groups (Savory et al. 2011).

The mechanisms responsible for the link between selenium and prevention of diseases associated or induced by an excessive production of reactive oxygen species are currently under-known. However, there are experimental evidence of selenium compounds affecting cell growth, cell cycle, DNA repair, gene expression, signal transduction and regulation of the redox status (Gromadzinska et al., 2008). On the other hand and as mentioned before, selenium functions as part of the selenoproteins which are involved in a wide range of metabolic processes. The cellular form of glutathione peroxidase (GPx 1) was the first selenoprotein identified. Several other GPxs containing the amino acid selenocysteine (Sec; analogous to cysteine in which sulfur is replaced by selenium) have been found since then. The glutathione (GSH)-Px system is found in almost all tissues and is believed to play a part in the body's antioxidant defence protecting polyunsaturated fatty acids and proteins from the damaging effects of peroxides and lipid hydroperoxide (LH) (Halliwell B, 2007). The other two major groups of known selenoprotein enzymes are the iodothyronine deiodinases that regulate operation of thyroid hormones, and the thioredoxin reductases (TrxR), involved in catalyzing the reduction of oxidized thioredoxin and other substrates. Additional selenoprotein is the selenoprotein P, the major form of selenium in the plasma and it also acts as an antioxidant in the extracellular space by reducing peroxynitrite and phospolipid hydroperoxides and forming complexes with mercury and cadmium (Gromadzinska et al., 2008).

Therefore and to sum up, there is strong evidence that selenium and the selenoproteins play a regulatory role in the following processes, which underlines its positive effects on health (Gromadzinska et al., 2008):

- ROS-activation of protein kinases in the cytoplasm and nucleus;
- ROS-activated modification of the thiol and hydroxyl groups in the Cys and Tyr;
- Controlling changes in the cell redox potential through inducing activation of the transcriptional factors and initiating *de novo* gene expression;
- Regulating the expression of membrane and nuclear receptors responsible for cell maintenance, intercellular communication, and changes in cell growth;
- Affecting apoptosis, necrosis and cell survival processes.

2.2.5 Green tea

Green tea, a product made from the leaves and buds of the plant *Camellia sinensis*, is, after water, the second most popular beverage worldwide, and a mayor source of dietary polyphenols that are known to render a myriad of health benefits (Rietveld & Wiseman, 2003). Green tea polyphenols are generally known as catechins. These group of compounds includes epicatechin, epigallocatechin, epicatechin gallate and epigallocatechin-3-gallate (EGCG) which is the most active of the major polyphenols and primarily responsible for the effects of green tea (Stewart et al., 2005).

EGCG has a four ring structure with eight hydroxyl groups being, therefore, highly hydrophilic, exhibiting good solubility in aqueous media (Zhong & Shahidi, 2011). EGCG is also a powerful antioxidant, possessing the highest antioxidant potency among all tea catechins, and it plays a protective role against oxidative stress in biological environments. For example, EGCG induced enzymes that play important roles as cellular antioxidant defenses such as SOD and catalase. It also lowers Malonil dialdehide (a product of lipid peroxidation and, therefore, a marker of oxidative stress) and it has also the ability of interacting with singlet molecular-oxygen, superoxide, peroxyl radicals, hydroxyl radicals, and peroxynitrite (Wei & Meng, 2010). Thus, green tea consumption may also show potential preventive effects against several oxidative stress-related disorders such as cardiovascular diseases (Rickman et al., 2010; Plutner et al., 1990; Nantz et al., 2009) and several types of cancer such as breast, prostate, lung, skin, gastric and colon cancer. It also shows neuroprotective effects in Parkinson and Alzeimer's disease (Zhao, 2009), ameliorates several autoimmune diseases such as autoimmune arthritis (Kim, H. R. et al., 2008), and immune-mediated liver injury (Wang et al., 2006) or even it seems to prevent skin cell damage (Jorge et al. 2011). Furthermore, green tea (or its active biomolecule EGCG) could be one potential anti-obesogenic agent (Stefanovic et al., 2008) and might be used in the prevention and treatment of this disease. Moreover, several "*in vivo*" studies demonstrated that green tea extracts or EGCG dietary supplementation decreased both body and adipose tissue weights (Park et al., 2011; Choo, 2003; Hasegawa et al., 2003), improved insulin sensitivity and glucose tolerance (Cao et al., 2007; Serisier et al., 2008) and had beneficial effects on prevention of hypertension (Ihm et al., 2009) and modulation of plasma cholesterol (Bursill et al., 2007), conditions linked to metabolic syndrome. In addition, it lowers the incidence of streptozotocin-induced diabetes (Song et al., 2003) and reduces body weight, body fat, and blood levels of glucose and lipid in leptin receptor-defective obese rats (Kao et al., 2000).

Several mechanisms have been proposed to explain the beneficial effects of EGCG in obesity and diabetes. Thus, EGCG protects pancreatic cells (Song et al., 2003), enhances insulin activity (Dhawan et al., 2002), represses hepatic glucose production (Waltner-Law et al., 2002), reduces food uptake and absorption (Kao et al., 2000), stimulates thermogenesis by increasing the uncoupling protein 2 (UCP2) and lipid excretion (Dulloo et al., 1999; Liao, 2001), and modulates insulin-leptin endocrine systems (Kao et al., 2000). Moreover, EGCG inhibits the sodium-dependent glucose transporter (Kobayashi et al., 2000) and represses various enzymes related to lipid metabolism, such as acetyl-CoA carboxylase, fatty acid synthase, pancreatic lipase, gastric lipase, and lipooxygenase (Liao, 2001; Wang & Tian, 2001) as well as lipolytic genes such as hormone sensitive lipase (HSL) and adipose triglyceride lipase (ATGL) in adipose tissue (Lee et al., 2009). It also reduces serum- or insulin-induced increases in the cell number and the triacylglycerol content of 3T3-L1 adipocytes during a 9-day period of differentiation (Sakurai et al., 2009) and also reviewed by Liu et al. (2006). It also inhibits adipocyte proliferation (Hung et al., 2005). Moreover, EGCG suppressed the differentiation of adipocytes through the inactivation of the forkhead transcription factor class O1 (FoxO1) and sterol regulatory element-binding protein-1 (SREBP1c) which are involved in adipocyte differentiation and lipid synthesis respectively in 3T3-L1 adipocytes (Freise et al. 2010). Regarding adipocytes hyperplasia it has been described that green tea EGCG may act at different concentrations in regulating mitogenesis and apoptosis of 3T3-L1 preadipocytes by inducing a decrease in the phosphorylated

ERK1/2, which are signal elements found to modulate the mitogenic and adipogenic signaling in 3T3-L1 (Wu et al., 2005), as well as decreasing ciclin dependent kinase 2 (Cdk2) activity and protein levels. Moreover, it has also been described that EGCG inhibited the mitogenic effect of insulin on preadipocytes in a dose and time-dependent manner, and that this inhibition might be due to its suppressive effects on the activities of the insulin receptor (Ku et al., 2009). Thus, the traditional knowledge about the anti-obesity effects of green tea can be confirmed and validated by scientific evidence.

It is important to point out that the beneficial effects of EGCG in cancer, but also in obesity and related disorders, are not always due to its antioxidant nature. In fact, it has been demonstrated that EGCG contribute to the beneficial effects of green tea on diabetes, obesity, and cancer by modulating gene expression. In fact, one of the possible mechanisms by which EGCG can inhibit cancer progression is through the modulation of angiogenesis signaling cascade as EGCG treatment leads to the downregulation of genes involved in the stimulation of proliferation, adhesion and motility as well as invasion processes, but also to the upregulation of several genes known to have antagonist effects (Tudoran et al., 2011). Very recent studies have also suggested the ability of EGCG to prevent several types of cancer through epigenetic mechanisms (Berner et al., 2010; Li Y et al., 2010; Nandakumar et al., 2011).

Concerning its effects on obesity, it has been reported that EGCG reduced them RNA levels of several gluconeogenic enzymes, glucose-6-phosphatase (G6Pase) and phosphoenolpyruvate carboxykinase (PEPCK) in the normal mouse liver as well as in the intestine (Yasui et al., 2011a, b). EGCG also improves cholesterol metabolism through the up-regulation of LDL receptor and also reduces extracellular apoB levels (Goto et al., 2011). Finally, it appears that EGCG modulates body weight gain in high fat-fed mice both by increasing the expression of genes related to fat oxidation in skeletal muscle and by modulating fat absorption from the diet (Sae-Tan et al., 2011).

3. However, not everything is positive: Side effects of antioxidants

Despite the initial positive and beneficial effects observed in many studies (some of them mentioned in the first part of this chapter), not all that glitters is gold. Thus, other clinical studies investigating antioxidant effects have been often disappointing given the consistent and promising findings from experimental investigations, clinical observations and epidemiological data. In this context, there are some controversial results, especially in the field of antioxidant supplementation, cancer and cardiovascular events (and mortality associated with these events) as well as when assessing the direct effects of antioxidants on mitochondria which are the main sources of reactive species in the organism apart from NADPH oxidase in the vascular walls. In this context, clinical trials of antioxidant therapeutics in human volunteers have produced negative or inconclusive results or have shown very little benefit. The inability of clinical trials to prove the usefulness of antioxidant therapies shows the failure in translating our knowledge of molecular and cellular mechanisms into efficient clinical remedies (Firuzi et al., 2011). The reason of clinical failure of many antioxidants despite the existence of overwhelming evidence on the involvement of oxidative damage in various pathologies still remains elusive although it is interesting to note that most of these studies generally agree on the notion that antioxidants are much more effective in prevention of disease rather than in the treatment of an already established active pathology (reviewed by Firuzi et al., 2011). In this context, we will review in the following part of the chapter some of these studies where no positive effects where found with the aforementioned antioxidants (lipoic acid, resveratrol, vitamins etc) and we will summarize some potential explanations for these controversial data.

3.1 Neutral or even deleterious effects of antioxidants

3.1.1 Lipoic acid

Some studies concerning the prooxidant potential of LA and DHLA have been performed in recent years. In fact, DHLA exerts prooxidant actions by accelerated iron-dependent hydroxyl radical generation and lipid peroxidation in liposomes, probably by reducing Fe^{3+} to Fe^{2+} (Scott et al., 1994). A study also concluded that LA and DHLA have prooxidant properties on markers of protein oxidation such as protein thiol and carbonyl in heart muscle of aging rat (Cakatay et al., 2005). In addition, DHLA stimulates MPT (mitochondrial permeability transition) by increasing production of ROS in isolated rat liver mitochondria and bovine heart submitochondrial particles (Morkunaite-Haimi et al., 2003). In this sense, Valdecantos et al. (2010a) also found that LA inhibited glutathione peroxidase activity and induced the uncoupling of the electron transport chain suggesting prooxidant actions of this antioxidant under the experimental conditions established in this study (Valdecantos et al., 2010a).

It is also very interesting to know that the beneficial role of LA supplementation in Type 2 diabetes is controversial. In one way, it has been postulated that the beneficial effects could be manifested by a mild prooxidant activity of the compound, leading to cellular adaptation against oxidative stress in addition to the attenuation of reductive stress in diabetes (Roy et al., 1997). In fact, the results derived from the study of Moini et al. (2002) pointed to the fact that the oxidized form of LA activates the insulin signal transduction pathway by acting as a prooxidant (Moini et al., 2002). Lipoic Acid increased tyrosine phosphorylation of immunoprecipitated insulin receptors, presumably by oxidation of critical thiol groups present in the insulin receptor β-subunit. Furthermore, it has been demonstrated that short-term incubation of LA in 3T3-L1 adipocytes induced glucose uptake by facilitating oxidative stress (Krieger-Brauer et al., 2000). However, long-term incubation of 3T3-L1 adipocytes with LA increased intracellular glutathione levels and inhibited the rate of glucose uptake (Mottley & Mason, 2001; Moini et al., 2002), which suggests that the duration of LA treatment is a critical step when analyzing the effects of LA on glucose uptake and insulin sensitivity. In addition, the effects of LA on adiponectin, a key adipokine involved in insulin sensitivity are also controversial, which does not help to postulate if LA beneficial actions on insulin sensitivity are mediated through this adipokine. Thus, Cummings et al. (2010) did not observe any significant change in fasting plasma adiponectin levels in fructose-fed University of California, Davis-Type 2 diabetes mellitus (UCD-T2DM) rats after dietary LA supplementation (Cummings et al., 2010). But not only the effects of LA on adiponectin are controversial, but also its actions on diabetes and obesity are questionable since several studies have not found any positive effects of this antioxidant on these disorders. Thus, supplementation with LA did not exhibit any effect on the lipid profile or insulin sensitivity of patients with diabetes type 2, with no changes in the concentrations of total cholesterol, cholesterol fractions, TG, and HOMA index (de Oliveira et al., 2011). Furthermore, LA administered orally at this dose for 2 weeks did not protect against lipid-induced insulin resistance in overweight and obese humans (Xiao et al., 2011). In a pilot study with adolescents with type 1 diabetes mellitus LA was not an effective treatment for decreasing oxidative damage, total antioxidant status HbA1c or microalbuminuria in type 1 diabetes mellitus (Huang & Gitelman, 2008). In addition, other studies did not even observe the ability of LA to induce weight loss in obese subjects (Koh et al., 2011).

The experiment design is also another point to take into account when describing the actions of LA, as it can influence the sense of the data obtained. Thus, Volchegorskii et al. (2011) studied the correlation between the effect of α-lipoic acid, emoxipin, reamberin, and mexidol on LPO *in vitro* and the action of these drugs on insulin sensitivity and tolerance to glucose load *in vivo*. They found that the preparations producing prooxidant effect *in vitro* (α-lipoic acid and reamberin) are characterized by pronounced insulin-potentiating activity, but only slightly increase (α-lipoic acid) or even decrease (reamberin) tolerance to glucose load suggesting controversial effects depending on experimental procedure: *in vitro vs. in vivo* (Volchegorskii et al., 2011). In this sense, we have also found that LA exerted direct effects on mitochondria oxidative status in a prooxidant manner (Valdecantos et al., 2010a) whereas we also observed that LA increases hepatic mitochondrial defenses through Foxo3a in a diet-induced obesity rat model (Valdecantos et al., 2011a) corroborating the controversial actions found for this fatty acid depending on the experimental procedures.

Finally, it is important to state that the ability of LA and/or DHLA to function as either anti- or prooxidants, at least in part, is also determined by the type of oxidant stress and the physiological circumstances. These prooxidant actions suggest that LA and DHLA act by multiple mechanisms, many of which are only now being explored and it is interesting to declare that prooxidant actions does not necessary mean deleterious effects as previously described for this antioxidant. In fact, α-Lipoic acid was shown to stimulate glucose uptake into 3T3-L1 adipocytes by increasing intracellular oxidant levels and/or facilitating insulin receptor autophosphorylation presumably by oxidation of critical thiol groups present in the insulin receptor β-subunit. Thus, the real meaning of the antioxidant or prooxidant effects of LA as well as the compounds described in this chapter warrants further investigation.

Lipoic Acid has been reported to have a number of potentially beneficial effects in both prevention and treatment of oxygen- related diseases. Selection of appropriate pharmacological doses of LA for use in oxygen-related diseases is also critical apart from experimental design and duration of treatment as previously described. Thus, in further studies, careful evaluation will be necessary for the decision in the biological system whether LA administration is beneficial or harmful (Cakatay, 2006).

3.1.2 Resveratrol

As mentioned before, many beneficial effects on health have been ascribed to this molecule. However, it should be emphasised that a great deal of work has been developed in isolated cells thus limiting the extrapolation of the results to the *in vivo* situation. In this context, Pérez-Jiménez and Saura-Calixto (2008) have reviewed the *in vivo* trials published during the last 13 years (seventy five trials) were the effects of different grape products on different CVD risk factors have been evaluated (Perez-Jimenez & Saura-Calixto, 2008). Most published studies have dealt with some specific aspects of mechanisms of grape flavonoid action or have focused only on one product, such as wine. Thus, it is important to point out that not only resveratrol actions have been evaluated in these trials but also polyphenols, alcohol and dietary fibre have been tested. In animal and human studies, grape products have been shown to produce hypotensive, hypolipidaemic and anti-atherosclerotic effects, and also to improve antioxidant status as measured in terms of plasma antioxidant capacity, oxidation biomarkers, antioxidant compounds or antioxidant enzymes. However, there are several studies where neutral and even negative effects were found regarding its effects on lipid profile and markers of oxidative stress (reviewed by Pérez-Jiménez & Saura-Calixto, 2008). It is important to underline that differences in the design of the studies and in the composition of the tested products (not always provided) could explain the different results observed and therefore these results can not been strictly extrapolated to resveratrol actions.

Despite its potential as an anti-obesity compound, data regarding the effects of resveratrol on adipokines are still insufficient to be conclusive. Adipokines are bioactive peptides produced by adipose tissue and involved in the physiological regulation of fat storage, energy metabolism, food intake, insulin sensitivity, and immune function among others. Several trials have observed that oxidative stress caused dysregulated production of adipokines (Soares et al., 2005; Kamigaki et al., 2006), therefore, it could be very important in the future to analyze the effects of resveratrol on these adipokines in an attempt to restore the optimal concentrations of those which, in turn, could lead to an improvement in obesity and related disorders.

Finally and although long-term effects of using resveratrol are still unknown, it is fair to state that this antioxidant shows a very good profile and could be a potential therapy against a wide range of diseases related to oxidative stress and aging (through SIRT1 actions), although more studies are needed in this field.

3.1.3 Vitamins E and C

Vitamins were selected for antioxidant therapy in several studies in the past decades because they were cheap and available, but they are not the best antioxidant molecules in terms of efficacy. In fact, many studies agree on the lack of evidence on the beneficial effects of antioxidant vitamins and in some cases even point to harmful effects. Thus, observational studies have reported an inverse association between vitamin E and cardiometabolic risk, but also, results from trials studying supplementation with this antioxidant failed to confirm any protective effect of them on cardiovascular disease (Devaraj et al., 2007; Wu et al., 2007).

In the review of Bjelakovic et al. (2007), 68 randomized trials conducted on 232,606 adults who were randomized to receive commonly used antioxidants including β-carotene, selenium, vitamins A, C and E were analyzed for the effect of antioxidant on all cause mortality (Bjelakovic et al., 2007). This review followed the Cochrane Collaboration method and included primary (healthy subjects) and secondary (diseased individuals) prevention studies. When all trials were considered, antioxidants did not seem to significantly affect mortality. However, when 47 "low-bias" trials were separately analyzed, β -carotene, vitamin A and vitamin E administered alone or in combination, significantly enhanced all-cause mortality whereas Vitamin C and selenium did not have any significant effect on mortality. Another meta-analysis performed on 7 large trials of vitamin E involving 81,788 individuals showed that there was no significant difference in cardiovascular mortality when individuals receiving vitamin E were compared to control (Vivekananthan et al., 2003). In another large meta-analysis including 19 trials and 135,967subjects, it was shown that high dose intake of vitamin E (>400IU/day) may increase all-cause mortality (Miller et al., 2005). However, other authors have claimed that the increase in mortality caused by vitamin E is questionable. Large secondary prevention trials of vitamin E including Secondary Prevention with Antioxidants of Cardiovascular Disease in Endstage Renal Disease (SPACE), the Cambridge Heart AntioxidantStudy (CHAOS), the Heart Outcomes Prevention Evaluation (HOPE), Gruppo Italiano per lo Studio de lla Sopravvianzan ell'Infarto Miocardico (GISSI) have evaluated the effects of vitamin E on mortality rates. In a meta-analysis of these trials and other primary and secondary prevention trials, it was concluded that vitamin E supplementation did not significantly affect mortality or risk of cardiovascular diseases (reviewed by Firuzi et al., 2011).

Numerous assays demonstrated that vitamin E decreased atherosclerotic formation (Fruebis et al., 1995; Parker et al., 1995), however, other studies showed no effects on plasma lipids (Nagyova et al., 2002; Cyrus et al., 2003; Hasty et al., 2007) or even an increase in plasma lipids after vitamin E treatment was also observed (Crawford et al., 1998). Mechanistic studies demonstrated that the role of α-tocopherol during the early stages of lipoprotein lipid peroxidation is complex and that the vitamin does not act as a chain-breaking antioxidant (Stocker & Keaney, 2005). It is tempting to suggest that the positive or deleterious effects of vitamin E supplementation or treatment on lipid profile also depend on the population chosen, the study design, types and dosages of antioxidant, and their duration of use. All these factors make the comparison and interpretation of the studies difficult. In addition, in a very recent study, it was demonstrated that vitamin E did not perform any positive effect on heat stress in Japanese quails (Halici et al., 2011). Moreover, there are conflicting results regarding the effects of this vitamin on blood pressure (Plantinga et al., 2007; Ward et al., 2007; Rodrigo et al., 2008).

Apart from the ambiguous effects observed after vitamin E treatment on cardiovascular events and mortality, its effects on cancer are not very clear either. Thus, the Alpha-Tocopherol Beta-Carotene Cancer Prevention Study (ATBC) and the β-Caroteneand Retinol Efficacy Trial, especially on lung cancers did not observe reduction in the incidence of lung cancer among male smokers after five to eight years of dietary supplementation with alpha-tocopherol or β-carotene. In fact, these trials raise the possibility that these supplements may actually have harmful as well as beneficial effects.

Finally, the evidence also suggests no beneficial effect of vitamin E supplementation in improving glycaemic control in unselected patients with type 2 diabetes whereas haemoglobin $A_{(1c)}$ ($HbA_{(1c)}$) (deeply involved in microvascular complications of diabetes and possibly macrovascular disease) may decrease with vitamin E supplementation in patients with inadequate glycaemic control or low serum levels of vitamin E. This shows the importance of targeting therapy. Due to the limitations of the available evidence, further studies are warranted in the field of vitamin E actions on diabetes and obesity (Suksomboon et al. 2011). On the other way and despite the beneficial effects previously described for vitamin E in obesity, there are also different studies where no significant effects of vitamin E on obesity have been found. Thus, body mass index remained unchanged in patients after 3 months of vitamin E treatment (Skrha et al., 1999; Nagyova et al., 2002; Vincent et al., 2007). Different research groups have examined de effect of vitamin E on F_2-isoprostanes (markers of oxidative stress which are increased in obesity), and whereas some of these research groups found statistically significant reductions in F_2-isoprostanes (Kaikkonen et al., 2001; Block et al., 2008), other studies did not find any effect (Meagher & Rader, 2001; Weinberg et al., 2001). Factors that could influence these conflicting results could be the sample size, the degree of obesity and/or presence of elevated F_2-isoprostanes at baseline.

Concerning vitamin C, several studies have also showed controversial results. Thus, the National Health and Nutrition Examination Surveys (NEHENES) reported that low serum levels of Vit C were marginally associated with an increased risk of fatal cardiovascular disease and significantly associated with risk of fatal cardiovascular disease (Schleicher et al., 2009). In contrast, several studies did not find evidence for a protective effect of vitamin C against cardiovascular disease. Thus, Ramos and Martinez-Castelao., (2008) (Ramos & Martinez-Castelao, 2008) failed to demonstrate significant differences on lipoprotein oxidation between vitamin C-treated and not treated patients under haemodialysis. Moreover, other studies found that Vit C further than having benefitial effects it also could have negative effects. Thus, The Physician Health Study (Gaziano et al., 2009) illustrated that vitamin C showed neither health benefits nor safety issues, and Moyad et al., (2008) reported that increased vitamin C intake had adverse effects, such as kidney stones and iron-related disorders. Other reports suggest that it may accelerate atherosclerosis in some people with diabetes, and fail to confer benefit in patients with advanced cancer (Talaulikar & Manyonda, 2011). In fact, vitamin C also seems to have a controversial role in cancer. Thus, many papers have described that millimolar concentrations of ascorbate have a deep inhibitory effect on the growth of several cancer cell lines in vitro. Actually, it seems that such cytotoxic activity of vitamin C relies on its ability to generate reactive oxygen species rather than its popular antioxidant action. This is paradoxical but, the fact is that ascorbic acid may have also prooxidant and even mutagenic effects in the presence of transition metals (reviewed by Verrax & Calderon, 2008). In this sense, Podmore et al., (1998) discovered an increase in a potentially mutagenic lesion, following a typical Vit C supplementation suggesting that prooxidant effects might occur at doses up to 500 mg per day, although at lower doses the antioxidant effect may predominate. In this sense, it is important to mention that the type, dosage and matrix of exogenous antioxidants seem to be determinant in the balance between beneficial or deleterious effects of vit. C. Briefly, the antioxidants in fruit and vegetables may be tightly bound within the tough fibrous material of these foodstuffs and may exert their antioxidant activity not in the blood or tissues but in the gastrointestinal tract where free radicals are constantly generated from food (Kelly et al., 2008) and on the contrary, vitamins ingested as food supplements are probably digested too quickly to replicate these effects. Moreover, in many cases, the equivalent serum levels of vitamin C cannot be achieved if the supplement is given orally since there is an upper limit for absorption of vitamin C of about 500 mg, which is why this is normally the highest dose given (Monsen, 2000). No acute toxic dose has been established but chronic toxicity can occur in those with hereditary glucose-6-phosphate dehydrogenase deficiency given doses of 2 g/day of this vitamin and some of the problems that can occur include kidney stones, diarrhoea, nausea, and red blood hemolysis. There is also the possibility of dental decalcification and rebound scurvy in infants born to women consuming large concentrations of vitamin C and estrogens changes in women (Soni et al., 2010).

Table 2 (modified from Firuzi et al., 2011) shows large meta analysis of randomized controlled clinical trials exploring the efficancy of vitamins E and C in prevention of various diseases (Alkhenizan & Hafez, 2007; Polyzos et al., 2007; Bardia et al., 2008; Evans, 2008; Arain & Qadeer, 2010; Myung et al., 2010). It is important to highlight that only large studies that included at least 4000 subjects were included in this table. Based on the studies summarized in this table and putting all the former findings together, we can led to the conclusion that vitamins cannot be used as effective antioxidant therapeutics for human diseases unless more definitive and comparative studies will be carried out.

Publication	Antioxidants studied	Number of randomized participants	Illness	Results	Conclusions
Arain et al., 2010	Vitamin E	94,069	Prevention of colorectal cancer	No significant effect on prevention of cancer.	No conclusive evidence on the benefit of treatment
Myung et al., 2010	Vitamin E, vitamin C, vitamin A, β-carotene, selenium (alone and in combination)	161,045	Prevention of cancer	No significant effect on prevention of cancer. No significant effect according to the type of antioxidant or type of cancer. Significant increase in the risk of bladder cancer in a subgroup meta-analysis of 4 trials.	No conclusive evidence on the benefit of treatment
Evans et al., 2008	B-carotene and α-tocopherol	23,099	Prevention of age related macular Degeneration (AMD)	No significant effect on prevention or delaying the onset of AMD (all trialsincluded). No significant effect when the analyses were restricted to either β-carotene or α-tocopherol.	No conclusive evidence on the benefit of treatment
Bardia et al., 2008	β-carotene, vitamin E, selenium	104,196	Prevention of cancer and mortality	Significant increase in cancer incidence and cancer mortality among smokers by β-carotene.	Selenium may be beneficial

Publication	Antioxidants studied	Number of randomized participants	Illness	Results	Conclusions
				Vitamin E supplementation had no effect. Selenium supplementation might have anticarcinogenic effects in men and thus requires further research.	
Alkhenizan et al., 2007	Vitamin E	167,025	Prevention of cancer	No significant difference in all-cause mortality, cancer incidence and cancer mortality. Significant reduction in the incidence of prostate cancer.	Beneficial for prostate cancer prevention. Not beneficial for other causes
Polyzos et al., 2007	Combination of vitamin C and vitamin E	4,680	Prevention of preeclampsia	No significant effect on the risk of preeclampsia, fetal or neonatal loss, or small for gestational age infant.	No conclusive evidence on the benefit of treatment

Table 2. Large meta analysis of randomized controlled clinical trials exploring the efficancy of vitamins E and C in prevention of various diseases.

3.1.4 Selenium

Despite the beneficial effects previously mentioned regarding this antioxidant, it is important to note that only selenium-deficient individuals may benefit from selenium supplementation, because such supplementation in selenium-replete individuals may even cause higher risk of diseases such as cancer (Brozmanova et al., 2010). Selenium has a narrow therapeutic window and there is considerable inter-individual variability in terms of metabolic sensitivity and optimal selenium intake. In fact, optimal intake for any individual is likely to depend on polymorphisms in selenoprotein genes that may also affect the risk of disease. Moreover, the baseline levels of each subject could determine the beneficial effect of the selenium intake (Stranges et al., 2010). For instance, no additional benefit of supplementation (even up to 300 μg/d) was found in an elderly population with mild hypothyroidism where selenium status was adequate prior to the start of supplementation (Rayman et al., 2008). High-selenium diets may stimulate the release of glucagon, promoting hyperglycaemia, or may induce over-expression of GPx-1 and other antioxidant selenoproteins resulting in insulin resistance and obesity (Stranges et al., 2010). Moreover, the increase in developing diabetes or adverse lipid profile among the participants in the NHANES 2003-2004 study could be associated to their high plasmatic selenium levels (137 mg/L) (Laclaustra et al., 2009).

Although the underlying mechanisms that could explain the detrimental effects of high selenium are not fully understood yet, they could involve DNA damage and oxidative stress induction resulting in apoptosis (Brozmanova et al., 2010). Therefore, due to a broad interest to exploit the positive effects of selenium on human health, studies investigating the negative effects such as toxicity and DNA damage induction resulting from high selenium intake are also highly required (Brozmanova et al., 2010). Moreover, urgent need for personalized risk prediction with regard to cancer and other diseases prevention and treatment activities of selenium supplementation is highly suggested (Platz & Lippman, 2009).

3.1.5 Green tea

EGCG is regarded as the most active catechin in green tea, but, in spite of its reported favorable effects, conflicting results have been reported from epidemiological studies (Boehm et al., 2009) and EGCG appears to act both as an anti-oxidant as well as a prooxidant agent as previously described for lipoic acid.

In this context, Elbling et al., (2005) concluded that excessive EGCG concentrations induced toxic levels of ROS *in vivo*, and moreover, they found *in vitro* DNA-damaging effects at pharmacological concentrations. Thus, hepatic and intestinal toxicities associated with the consumption of high doses of green tea preparations were reported in animal studies. Furthermore, EGCG mediated mitochondrial toxicity and ROS formation was implicated as the possible mechanism for the cytotoxicity to isolated rat hepatocytes and hepatotoxicity in mice (Galati et al., 2006). Another study found that higher intake of green tea might cause oxidative DNA damage of hamster pancreas and liver and also found that the major cytotoxic mechanism found with hepatocytes was mitochondrial membrane potential collapse and ROS formation (Takabayashi et al., 2004). Moreover, Yun et al. (2006) clarified that EGCG acts as a prooxidant, rather than an antioxidant, in pancreatic β cells *in vivo,* suggesting that consumption of green tea and green tea extracts should be monitored in certain patients. Thus, it should be considered that the effects of green tea and its constituents may be beneficial up to a certain dose, and higher doses may cause some unknown adverse effects similarly as what has been observed with selenium.

The harmful effects of tea overconsumption are due to three main factors: its caffeine content, the presence of aluminum, and the effects of tea polyphenols on iron bioavailability. Caffeine is the world's most popular drug and can be found in many beverages including tea. One reason for the popularity of caffeine-containing beverages is the stimulation of the central nervous system that they provide (MacKenzie et al., 2007). However, caffeine may have other effects, including metabolic and hormonal ones. With short-term dosing, caffeine has been shown to impair glucose metabolism in nondiabetic persons (Greer et al., 2001; Johnston et al., 2003) and in persons with type 2 diabetes mellitus (Lane et al., 2004; Robinson et al., 2004). The effects on other hormonal systems have not been as well investigated. However, cortisol levels may increase after short-term administration of caffeine in healthy subjects or in those with elevated blood pressure (Lovallo et al., 1996). Regarding green tea aluminium content, several studies described that the negative effect of green tea decoction, arises from the high absorption of aluminium released in the decoction. Some analogies in the competition mechanism between aluminium and iron will be obtained in human nutritional conditions; the regular green tea decoction consumption could constitute an important additional source of dietary aluminium. Then, it could have, in a long term, a negative consequence on iron status and erythropoiesis toxicity, particularly in patients with high iron requirements or with chronic renal failure like hemodialysis (Marouani et al., 2007). It is also interesting to mention that an iron–catechin complex formation can cause a significant decrease of the iron bioavailability from the diet (Hamdaoui et al., 2003). Moreover, it has been shown that bioactive dietary polyphenols inhibit heme and non-heme iron absorption in human intestinal cells mainly by reducing basolateral release of iron (Kim, E. Y. et al., 2008).

3.2 Why many antioxidants have failed to show efficacy in interventional human studies? Some explanations

The most simple explanation for the controversial studies found is that not all antioxidants behave in the same way or with the same intensity, at least when their direct actions on mitochondria are analyzed as demonstrated in the study from Valdecantos et al. (2010a). Thus, the outcomes found with different antioxidants should be carefully examined since the physical properties of the assayed molecules are different and could affect their ability to enter the mitochondria and, therefore, to affect their functionality, although other mechanisms different from pure physical characteristics of the compounds can not be rule out.

Some of the antioxidants are ineffective and nonspecific and dosage regimen or duration of therapy was inefficient. Thus, several points should be taken into account before making general conclusions. Thus, the fact that the antioxidant molecule could have low bioavailability should also be considered when planning a trial. In this context, some polyphenolics, especially green tea catechins, may have very low bioavailability (Williamson &; Manach, 2005). Thus, optimization of these molecules has been suggested to improve this outcome, but, it is still under investigation. Other point that should also be taken into account is that the antioxidant could have poor target specificity, that the reaction products of the antioxidant could be toxic, that a single antioxidant is not enough to overcome oxidative stress and therefore a combination of several antioxidant compounds is needed or the fact that certain antioxidants are not effective in well-nourished populations (deeply reviewed by Firuzi et al., 2011).

Other possible reasons relate to patient cohort included in trials, that patients do not equally benefit from antioxidant therapy, the trial design itself and the usage of inappropriate or insensitive methodologies to evaluate oxidative state which underlines the urgent need for the development of sensitive and specific biomarkers to correctly assess the oxidant status of patients. Furthermore, oxidative stress is not always the primary cause of the disease and, therefore, it is not the only cause of the disease (reviewed by Firuzi et al., 2011).

4. Conclusion

There has been much enthusiasm in the field of oxidative-stress related disorders and nutritional approaches to improve health. Antioxidants have been advocated for therapy of a vast range of serious diseases in the 1980s and 1990s. Furthermore, the tendency to add bioactive compounds such as antioxidant molecules in foods to improve consumer health, which has been very strong during the past decade, will increase significantly in the future, in parallel with a growing awareness of the impact of food components on human health. However, in the light of recent negative findings, many doubts have now been raised about the usefulness of administration of single antioxidants. What seems to be clear is that although there are many dietary antioxidants and all of them can act as "antioxidant" molecules, not all behave in the same way. Thus and as described in this chapter, some of them seem to have potential as therapy against several diseases (resveratrol) whereas there are other molecules whose results are not very promising (vitamins C and/or E). Thus, once we apply our experience to select the right disease and the right population, design optimized and highly bioavailable antioxidants directed at specific and appropriate targets and choose optimal treatment times, duration and doses, useful therapeutics could emerge for various diseases. On the other hand, as possible negative interactions with antioxidants may rely on the dose consumed by each person, natural antioxidants from natural foods in a balanced diet such as the Mediterranean diet arise as the best way to implement these substances in regular nutrition instead of consuming them as supplements.

Since there are not yet adequately validated markers of the onset, progression and/or regression of any oxidative stress associated chronic diseases there is the urgent need in sorting out which markers or combinations of markers are predictive of human diseases. Ideally one would wish to demonstrate that modulation of a biomarker by a specific antioxidant intervention is predictive of modulation of incidence of some major chronic disease endpoint in humans. To accomplish this, further investigation is also needed.

Furthermore, inhibition of ROS production through the development of inhibitors against the main sources of ROS generation offers an alternative approach to conventional antioxidant therapies due to their controversial results. Thus, NADPH oxidase, as the main source of ROS production in endothelial cells and directly involved in hypertension and cardiovascular disease, has been suggested as a potential target for decreasing ROS generation. A number of clinically important drugs used for the treatment of hypertension, hypercholesterolaemia and coronary artery disease such as the statins, AT1 (angiotensin II receptor type 1) antagonists and ACE inhibitors have been shown to decrease NADPH oxidase-derived superoxide and ROS production. In this context, one area of investigation that has been the focus of much recent interest in the past years is to address mitochondria, and more specifically, to analyze the potential beneficial effects of modulating mitochondrial ROS generation in order to treat or prevent the development of several oxidative-stress associated disorders (reviewed by Pérez-Matute et al., 2009). Again, more studies are needed in this regard.

Finally, and as described in the review from Prieto-Hontoria et al. (2010), the mechanisms by which antioxidant components modulate obesity, cancer and other oxidative stress related disorders are not fully understood, partly because of the lack of appropriate research tools to identify the complex mechanisms involve. With the emergence of Nutrigenomics, it is now possible to exploit genome-wide changes in gene expression profiles related to molecular nutrition. Evolution of `omics´ such as epigenomics, transcriptomics, proteomics and metabolomics will allow a better understanding of how dietary antioxidants may affect both energy metabolism, carcinogenesis etc leading to healthier foods and, in turn, healthier people and lifestyles.

5. References

Aasheim, E.T., et al. (2008). Vitamin status in morbidly obese patients: a cross-sectional study. *Am J Clin Nutr*, 87(2), 362-9.

Alberdi, G., et al. (2011). Changes in white adipose tissue metabolism induced by resveratrol in rats. *Nutr Metab (Lond)*, 8(1), 29.

Alpsoy, L. & Yalvac, M.E. (2011). Key roles of vitamins A, C, and E in aflatoxin B1-induced oxidative stress. *Vitam Horm*, 86287-305.

Ansar, H., et al. (2011). Effect of alpha-lipoic acid on blood glucose, insulin resistance and glutathione peroxidase of type 2 diabetic patients. *Saudi Med J*, 32(6), 584-8.

Baur, J.A., et al. (2006). Resveratrol improves health and survival of mice on a high-calorie diet. *Nature*, 444(7117), 337-42.

Berner, C., et al. (2011). Epigenetic control of estrogen receptor expression and tumor suppressor genes is modulated by bioactive food compounds. *Ann Nutr Metab*, 57(3-4), 183-9.

Bishayee, A. (2009). Cancer prevention and treatment with resveratrol: from rodent studies to clinical trials. *Cancer Prev. Res. (Phila Pa.)* 2 409–418.

Bjelakovic, G., et al. (2007). Mortality in randomized trials of antioxidant supplements for primary and secondary prevention: systematic review and meta-analysis. *Jama*, 297(8), 842-57.

Block, G., et al. (2008). The effect of vitamins C and E on biomarkers of oxidative stress depends on baseline level. *Free Radic Biol Med*, 45(4), 377-84.

Boehm, K., et al. (2009). Green tea (Camellia sinensis) for the prevention of cancer. *Cochrane Database Syst Rev*, (3), CD005004.

Boosalis, M.G. (2008). The role of selenium in chronic disease. *Nutr Clin Pract*, 23(2), 152-60.

Boque, N., et al. (2009). Some cyclin-dependent kinase inhibitors-related genes are regulated by vitamin C in a model of diet-induced obesity. *Biol Pharm Bull*, 32(8), 1462-8.

Botella-Carretero, J.I., et al. (2010). Retinol and alpha-tocopherol in morbid obesity and nonalcoholic fatty liver disease. *Obes Surg*, 20(1), 69-76.

Brigelius-Flohe, R. & Traber, M.G. (1999). Vitamin E: function and metabolism. *Faseb J*, 13(10), 1145-55.

Brozmanova, J., et al. Selenium: a double-edged sword for defense and offence in cancer. *Arch Toxicol*, 84(12), 919-38.

Bursill, C.A., et al. (2007). A green tea extract lowers plasma cholesterol by inhibiting cholesterol synthesis and upregulating the LDL receptor in the cholesterol-fed rabbit. *Atherosclerosis*, 193(1), 86-93.

Cakatay, U. (2006). Pro-oxidant actions of alpha-lipoic acid and dihydrolipoic acid. *Med Hypotheses*, 66(1), 110-7.

Cakatay, U., et al. (2005). Prooxidant activities of alpha-lipoic acid on oxidative protein damage in the aging rat heart muscle. *Arch Gerontol Geriatr*, 40(3), 231-40.

Calvisi, D.F., et al. (2004). Vitamin E down-modulates iNOS and NADPH oxidase in c-Myc/TGF-alpha transgenic mouse model of liver cancer. *J Hepatol*, 41(5), 815-22.

Campion, J., et al. (2008). Vitamin C supplementation influences body fat mass and steroidogenesis-related genes when fed a high-fat diet. *Int J Vitam Nutr Res*, 78(2), 87-95.

Cao, H., et al. (2007). Green tea polyphenol extract regulates the expression of genes involved in glucose uptake and insulin signaling in rats fed a high fructose diet. *J Agric Food Chem*, 55(15), 6372-8.

Carbonelli, M.G., et al. (2011). Alpha-lipoic acid supplementation: a tool for obesity therapy? *Curr Pharm Des*, 16(7), 840-6.

Crawford, R.S., et al. (1998). Dietary antioxidants inhibit development of fatty streak lesions in the LDL receptor-deficient mouse. *Arterioscler Thromb Vasc Biol*, 18(9), 1506-13.

Crujeiras, A.B., et al. (2009). Fruit, vegetables and legumes consumption: Role in preventing and treating obesity. Bioactive foods in promoting health. Fruits and vegetables. R. R. Watson and B. R. Preedy. Oxford, Academic Press: 359-380.

Crujeiras, A.B., et al. (2007a). A hypocaloric diet enriched in legumes specifically mitigates lipid peroxidation in obese subjects. *Free Radic Res*, 41(4), 498-506.

Crujeiras, A.B., et al. (2007b). Functional properties of fruit. *Food*, 30-35.

Crujeiras, A.B., et al. (2006). A role for fruit content in energy-restricted diets in improving antioxidant status in obese women during weight loss. *Nutrition*, 22(6), 593-9.

Cucciolla, V., et al. (2007). Resveratrol: from basic science to the clinic. *Cell Cycle*, 6(20), 2495-510.

Cummings, B.P., et al. (2010). Dietary fructose accelerates the development of diabetes in UCD-T2DM rats: amelioration by the antioxidant, alpha-lipoic acid. *Am J Physiol Regul Integr Comp Physiol*, 298(5), R1343-50.

Cyrus, T., et al. (2003). Vitamin E reduces progression of atherosclerosis in low-density lipoprotein receptor-deficient mice with established vascular lesions. *Circulation*, 107(4), 521-3.

Cho, K.J., et al. (2003). Alpha-lipoic acid inhibits adipocyte differentiation by regulating pro-adipogenic transcription factors via mitogen-activated protein kinase pathways. *J Biol Chem*, 278(37), 34823-33.

Choi, S.Y., et al. (2009). Mechanism of alpha-lipoic acid-induced apoptosis of lung cancer cells. *Ann N Y Acad Sci*, 1171149-55.

Choo, J.J. (2003). Green tea reduces body fat accretion caused by high-fat diet in rats through beta-adrenoceptor activation of thermogenesis in brown adipose tissue. *J Nutr Biochem*, 14(11), 671-6.

Dai, J., et al. (2008). Association between adherence to the Mediterranean diet and oxidative stress. *Am J Clin Nutr*, 88(5), 1364-70.

Dalle-Donne, I., et al. (2006). Biomarkers of oxidative damage in human disease. *Clin Chem*, 52(4), 601-23.

Dauchet, L., et al. (2007). Dietary patterns and blood pressure change over 5-y follow-up in the SU.VI.MAX cohort. *Am J Clin Nutr*, 85(6), 1650-6.

Dawson, E.B., et al. (1990). Relationship between ascorbic acid and male fertility. *World Rev Nutr Diet*, 621-26.

de la Lastra, C.A. & Villegas, I. (2007). Resveratrol as an antioxidant and pro-oxidant agent: mechanisms and clinical implications. *Biochem Soc Trans*, 35(Pt 5), 1156-60.

de Oliveira, A.M., et al. (2011). The effects of lipoic acid and alpha-tocopherol supplementation on the lipid profile and insulin sensitivity of patients with type 2 diabetes mellitus: a randomized, double-blind, placebo-controlled trial. *Diabetes Res Clin Pract*, 92(2), 253-60.

Devaraj, S. & Jialal, I. (2000). Alpha tocopherol supplementation decreases serum C-reactive protein and monocyte interleukin-6 levels in normal volunteers and type 2 diabetic patients. *Free Radic Biol Med*, 29(8), 790-2.

Devaraj, S., et al. (2007). Effect of high-dose alpha-tocopherol supplementation on biomarkers of oxidative stress and inflammation and carotid atherosclerosis in patients with coronary artery disease. *Am J Clin Nutr*, 86(5), 1392-8.

Dhawan, A., et al. (2002). Evaluation of the antigenotoxic potential of monomeric and dimeric flavanols, and black tea polyphenols against heterocyclic amine-induced DNA damage in human lymphocytes using the Comet assay. *Mutat Res*, 515(1-2), 39-56.

Diniz, Y.S., et al. (2005). Monosodium glutamate in standard and high-fiber diets: metabolic syndrome and oxidative stress in rats. *Nutrition*, 21(6), 749-55.

Droge, W. (2002). Free radicals in the physiological control of cell function. *Physiol Rev*, 82(1), 47-95.

Dudek, H., et al. (2005). [Concentration of glutathione (GSH), ascorbic acid (vitamin C) and substances reacting with thiobarbituric acid (TBA-rs) in single human brain metastases]. *Wiad Lek*, 58(7-8), 379-81.

Dulloo, A.G., et al. (1999). Efficacy of a green tea extract rich in catechin polyphenols and caffeine in increasing 24-h energy expenditure and fat oxidation in humans. *Am J Clin Nutr*, 70(6), 1040-5.

Elbling, L., et al. (2005). Green tea extract and (-)-epigallocatechin-3-gallate, the major tea catechin, exert oxidant but lack antioxidant activities. *Faseb J*, 19(7), 807-9.

Federici, M., et al. (2002). Insulin-dependent activation of endothelial nitric oxide synthase is impaired by O-linked glycosylation modification of signaling proteins in human coronary endothelial cells. *Circulation*, 106(4), 466-72.

Feige, J.N., et al. (2008). Specific SIRT1 activation mimics low energy levels and protects against diet-induced metabolic disorders by enhancing fat oxidation. *Cell Metab*, 8(5), 347-58.

Fetoui, H., et al. (2008). Oxidative stress induced by lambda-cyhalothrin (LTC) in rat erythrocytes and brain: Attenuation by vitamin C. *Environ Toxicol Pharmacol*, 26(2), 225-31.

Firuzi, O., et al. (2011). Antioxidant Therapy: Current Status and Future Prospects. *Curr Med Chem*,

Fischer-Posovszky, P., et al. (2010). Resveratrol regulates human adipocyte number and function in a Sirt1-dependent manner. *Am J Clin Nutr*, 92(1), 5-15.

Fito, M., et al. (2007). Effect of a traditional Mediterranean diet on lipoprotein oxidation: a randomized controlled trial. *Arch Intern Med*, 167(11), 1195-203.

Foo, N.P., et al. (2011). alpha-Lipoic acid inhibits liver fibrosis through the attenuation of ROS-triggered signaling in hepatic stellate cells activated by PDGF and TGF-beta. *Toxicology*, 282(1-2), 39-46.

Freise, C., et al. (2010). An active extract of Lindera obtusiloba inhibits adipogenesis via sustained Wnt signaling and exerts anti-inflammatory effects in the 3T3-L1 preadipocytes. *J Nutr Biochem*, 21(12), 1170-7.

Fruebis, J., et al. (1995). Effect of vitamin E on atherogenesis in LDL receptor-deficient rabbits. *Atherosclerosis*, 117(2), 217-24.

Galati, G., et al. (2006). Cellular and in vivo hepatotoxicity caused by green tea phenolic acids and catechins. *Free Radic Biol Med*, 40(4), 570-80.

Garriguet, D. (2010). The effect of supplement use on vitamin C intake. *Health Rep*, 21(1), 57-62.

Gaziano, J.M., et al. (2009). Vitamins E and C in the prevention of prostate and total cancer in men: the Physicians' Health Study II randomized controlled trial. *Jama*, 301(1), 52-62.

Gilgun-Sherki, Y., et al. (2002). Antioxidant therapy in acute central nervous system injury: current state. *Pharmacol Rev*, 54(2), 271-84.

Girard, A., et al. (2005). Changes in lipid metabolism and antioxidant defense status in spontaneously hypertensive rats and Wistar rats fed a diet enriched with fructose and saturated fatty acids. *Nutrition*, 21(2), 240-8.

Glantzounis, G.K., et al. (2005). Uric acid and oxidative stress. *Curr Pharm Des*, 11(32), 4145-51.

Gomez-Zorita, S., et al. (2011). Resveratrol attenuates steatosis in obese Zucker rats by decreasing fatty acid availability and reducing oxidative stress. *Br J Nutr*, 1-9.

Goto, T., et al. (2011). Epigallocatechin gallate changes mRNA expression level of genes involved in cholesterol metabolism in hepatocytes. *Br J Nutr*, 1-5.

Greer, F., et al. (2001). Caffeine ingestion decreases glucose disposal during a hyperinsulinemic-euglycemic clamp in sedentary humans. *Diabetes*, 50(10), 2349-54.

Gromadzinska, J., et al. (2008). Selenium and cancer: biomarkers of selenium status and molecular action of selenium supplements. *Eur J Nutr*, 47 Suppl 229-50.

Halici, M., et al. (2011). Effects of alpha-lipoic acid, vitamins E and C upon the heat stress in Japanese quails. *J Anim Physiol Anim Nutr (Berl)*,

Halliwell B, G.J. (2007). Free radicals in biology and medicine. Oxford, UK, Clarendon Press.

Halliwell, B. & Gutteridge, J.M. (1999). Free Radicals in Biology and Medicine. Oxford, Oxford University Press.

Halliwell, B. & Gutteridge, J.M. (2007). Free radicals in biology and medicine. Oxford, UK, Clarendon Press.

Hamdaoui, M.H., et al. (2003). Iron bioavailability and weight gains to iron-deficient rats fed a commonly consumed Tunisian meal 'bean seeds ragout' with or without beef and with green or black tea decoction. *J Trace Elem Med Biol*, 17(3), 159-64.

Hasegawa, N., et al. (2002). Vitamin C is one of the lipolytic substances in green tea. *Phytother Res*, 16 Suppl 1S91-2.

Hasegawa, N., et al. (2003). Powdered green tea has antilipogenic effect on Zucker rats fed a high-fat diet. *Phytother Res*, 17(5), 477-80.

Hasty, A.H., et al. (2007). Effects of vitamin E on oxidative stress and atherosclerosis in an obese hyperlipidemic mouse model. *J Nutr Biochem*, 18(2), 127-33.

Heneman, K.M., et al. (2007). Soy protein with and without isoflavones fails to substantially increase postprandial antioxidant capacity. *J Nutr Biochem*, 18(1), 46-53.

Heuckenkamp, P.U. & Zollner, N. (1971). Fructose-induced hyperuricaemia. *Lancet*, 1(7703), 808-9.

Horwitt, M.K. (1986). Interpretations of requirements for thiamin, riboflavin, niacin-tryptophan, and vitamin E plus comments on balance studies and vitamin B-6. *Am J Clin Nutr*, 44(6), 973-85.

Huang, E.A. & Gitelman, S.E. (2008). The effect of oral alpha-lipoic acid on oxidative stress in adolescents with type 1 diabetes mellitus. *Pediatr Diabetes*, 9(3 Pt 2), 69-73.

Hung, L.M., et al. (2000). Cardioprotective effect of resveratrol, a natural antioxidant derived from grapes. *Cardiovasc Res*, 47(3), 549-55.

Hung, P.F., et al. (2005). Antimitogenic effect of green tea (-)-epigallocatechin gallate on 3T3-L1 preadipocytes depends on the ERK and Cdk2 pathways. *Am J Physiol Cell Physiol*, 288(5), C1094-108.

Hunter, D.C., et al. (2011). Changes in markers of inflammation, antioxidant capacity and oxidative stress in smokers following consumption of milk, and milk supplemented with fruit and vegetable extracts and vitamin C. *Int J Food Sci Nutr*,

Huong, D.T. & Ide, T. (2008). Dietary lipoic acid-dependent changes in the activity and mRNA levels of hepatic lipogenic enzymes in rats. *Br J Nutr*, 100(1), 79-87.

Ihm, S.H., et al. (2009). Catechin prevents endothelial dysfunction in the prediabetic stage of OLETF rats by reducing vascular NADPH oxidase activity and expression. *Atherosclerosis*, 206(1), 47-53.

James, J.S. (2006). Resveratrol: why it matters in HIV. *AIDS Treat News*, (420), 3-5.

Johnson, R.J., et al. (2009). Lessons from comparative physiology: could uric acid represent a physiologic alarm signal gone awry in western society? *J Comp Physiol B*, 179(1), 67-76.

Johnston, K.L., et al. (2003). Coffee acutely modifies gastrointestinal hormone secretion and glucose tolerance in humans: glycemic effects of chlorogenic acid and caffeine. *Am J Clin Nutr*, 78(4), 728-33.

Jorge, A.T., et al. A new potent natural antioxidant mixture provides global protection against oxidative skin cell damage. *Int J Cosmet Sci*, 33(2), 113-9.

Kaikkonen, J., et al. (2001). Supplementation with vitamin E but not with vitamin C lowers lipid peroxidation in vivo in mildly hypercholesterolemic men. *Free Radic Res*, 35(6), 967-78.

Kamigaki, M., et al. (2006). Oxidative stress provokes atherogenic changes in adipokine gene expression in 3T3-L1 adipocytes. *Biochem Biophys Res Commun*, 339(2), 624-32.

Kao, Y.H., et al. (2000). Modulation of endocrine systems and food intake by green tea epigallocatechin gallate. *Endocrinology*, 141(3), 980-7.

Kelly, R.P., et al. (2008). Lack of effect of acute oral ingestion of vitamin C on oxidative stress, arterial stiffness or blood pressure in healthy subjects. *Free Radic Res*, 42(5), 514-22.

Kim, E.Y., et al. (2008). Bioactive dietary polyphenolic compounds reduce nonheme iron transport across human intestinal cell monolayers. *J Nutr*, 138(9), 1647-51.

Kim, H.R., et al. (2008). Green tea protects rats against autoimmune arthritis by modulating disease-related immune events. *J Nutr*, 138(11), 2111-6.

Kim, M.S., et al. (2004). Anti-obesity effects of alpha-lipoic acid mediated by suppression of hypothalamic AMP-activated protein kinase. *Nat Med*, 10(7), 727-33.

Kobayashi, Y., et al. (2000). Green tea polyphenols inhibit the sodium-dependent glucose transporter of intestinal epithelial cells by a competitive mechanism. *J Agric Food Chem*, 48(11), 5618-23.

Koh, E.H., et al. (2011). Effects of alpha-lipoic Acid on body weight in obese subjects. *Am J Med*, 124(1), 85 e1-8.

Krieger-Brauer, H.I., et al. (2000). Basic fibroblast growth factor utilizes both types of component subunits of Gs for dual signaling in human adipocytes. Stimulation of adenylyl cyclase via Galph(s) and inhibition of NADPH oxidase by Gbeta gamma(s). *J Biol Chem*, 275(46), 35920-5.

Kryukov, G.V., et al. (2003). Characterization of mammalian selenoproteomes. *Science*, 300(5624), 1439-43.

Ku, H.C., et al. (2009). Green tea (-)-epigallocatechin gallate inhibits insulin stimulation of 3T3-L1 preadipocyte mitogenesis via the 67-kDa laminin receptor pathway. *Am J Physiol Cell Physiol*, 297(1), C121-32.

Laclaustra, M., et al. (2009). Serum selenium concentrations and diabetes in U.S. adults: National Health and Nutrition Examination Survey (NHANES) 2003-2004. *Environ Health Perspect*, 117(9), 1409-13.

Lane, J.D., et al. (2004). Caffeine impairs glucose metabolism in type 2 diabetes. *Diabetes Care*, 27(8), 2047-8.

Lasa, A., et al. (2011). Resveratrol regulates lipolysis via adipose triglyceride lipase. *J Nutr Biochem*,

Lee, M.S., et al. (2009). Green tea (-)-epigallocatechin-3-gallate reduces body weight with regulation of multiple genes expression in adipose tissue of diet-induced obese mice. *Ann Nutr Metab*, 54(2), 151-7.

Li, W., et al. (2011). Synergistic effects of tea polyphenols and ascorbic acid on human lung adenocarcinoma SPC-A-1 cells. *J Zhejiang Univ Sci B*, 11(6), 458-64.

Liao, S. (2001). The medicinal action of androgens and green tea epigallocatechin gallate. *Hong Kong Med J*, 7(4), 369-74.

Lin, J.N., et al. (2010). Resveratrol modulates tumor cell proliferation and protein translation via SIRT1-dependent AMPK activation. *J Agric Food Chem*, 58(3), 1584-92.

Lira, F.S., et al. (2011). Supplementing alpha-tocopherol (vitamin E) and vitamin D3 in high fat diet decrease IL-6 production in murine epididymal adipose tissue and 3T3-L1 adipocytes following LPS stimulation. *Lipids Health Dis*, 1037.

Liu, H.S., et al. (2006). Inhibitory effect of green tea (-)-epigallocatechin gallate on resistin gene expression in 3T3-L1 adipocytes depends on the ERK pathway. *Am J Physiol Endocrinol Metab*, 290(2), E273-81.

Lotito, S.B. & Frei, B. (2004). The increase in human plasma antioxidant capacity after apple consumption is due to the metabolic effect of fructose on urate, not apple-derived antioxidant flavonoids. *Free Radic Biol Med*, 37(2), 251-8.

Lovallo, W.R., et al. (1996). Stress-like adrenocorticotropin responses to caffeine in young healthy men. *Pharmacol Biochem Behav*, 55(3), 365-9.

Lushchak, VI. (2011). Adaptive response to oxidative stress: Bacteria, fungi, plants and animals. Comp *Biochem Physiol C Toxicol Pharmacol*, 153(2), 175-90.

Macarulla, M.T., et al. (2009). Effects of different doses of resveratrol on body fat and serum parameters in rats fed a hypercaloric diet. *J Physiol Biochem*, 65(4), 369-76.

MacKenzie, T., et al. (2007). Metabolic and hormonal effects of caffeine: randomized, double-blind, placebo-controlled crossover trial. *Metabolism*, 56(12), 1694-8.

Mah, E., et al. (2011). Vitamin C status is related to proinflammatory responses and impaired vascular endothelial function in healthy, college-aged lean and obese men. *J Am Diet Assoc*, 111(5), 737-43.

Manning, P.J., et al. (2004). Effect of high-dose vitamin E on insulin resistance and associated parameters in overweight subjects. *Diabetes Care*, 27(9), 2166-71.

Marouani, N., et al. (2007). Both aluminum and polyphenols in green tea decoction (Camellia sinensis) affect iron status and hematological parameters in rats. *Eur J Nutr*, 46(8), 453-9.

Martinez-Gonzalez, M.A., et al. (2002). Mediterranean diet and reduction in the risk of a first acute myocardial infarction: an operational healthy dietary score. *Eur J Nutr*, 41(4), 153-60.

Meagher, E. & Rader, D.J. (2001). Antioxidant therapy and atherosclerosis: animal and human studies. *Trends Cardiovasc Med*, 11(3-4), 162-5.

Meyer, F., et al. (2005). Antioxidant vitamin and mineral supplementation and prostate cancer prevention in the SU.VI.MAX trial. *Int J Cancer*, 116(2), 182-6.

Miller, E.R., 3rd, et al. (2006). The effects of macronutrients on blood pressure and lipids: an overview of the DASH and OmniHeart trials. *Curr Atheroscler Rep*, 8(6), 460-5.

Miller, E.R., 3rd, et al. (2005). Meta-analysis: high-dosage vitamin E supplementation may increase all-cause mortality. *Ann Intern Med*, 142(1), 37-46.

Moini, H., et al. (2002). Antioxidant and prooxidant activities of alpha-lipoic acid and dihydrolipoic acid. *Toxicol Appl Pharmacol*, 182(1), 84-90.

Monsen, E.R. (2000). Dietary reference intakes for the antioxidant nutrients: vitamin C, vitamin E, selenium, and carotenoids. *J Am Diet Assoc*, 100(6), 637-40.

Montagnani, M., et al. (2002). Insulin receptor substrate-1 and phosphoinositide-dependent kinase-1 are required for insulin-stimulated production of nitric oxide in endothelial cells. *Mol Endocrinol*, 16(8), 1931-42.

Morkunaite-Haimi, S., et al. (2003). Reactive oxygen species are involved in the stimulation of the mitochondrial permeability transition by dihydrolipoate. *Biochem Pharmacol*, 65(1), 43-9.

Mottley, C. & Mason, R.P. (2001). Sulfur-centered radical formation from the antioxidant dihydrolipoic acid. *J Biol Chem*, 276(46), 42677-83.

Moyad, M.A., et al. (2008). Vitamin C metabolites, independent of smoking status, significantly enhance leukocyte, but not plasma ascorbate concentrations. *Adv Ther*, 25(10), 995-1009.

Nagyova, A., et al. (2002). Serum ex vivo lipoprotein oxidizability in patients with ischemic heart disease supplemented with vitamin E. *Physiol Res*, 51(5), 457-64.

Nandakumar, V., et al. (2011). (-)-Epigallocatechin-3-gallate reactivates silenced tumor suppressor genes, Cip1/p21 and p16INK4a, by reducing DNA methylation and increasing histones acetylation in human skin cancer cells. *Carcinogenesis*, 32(4), 537-44.

Nantz, M.P., et al. (2009). Standardized capsule of Camellia sinensis lowers cardiovascular risk factors in a randomized, double-blind, placebo-controlled study. *Nutrition*, 25(2), 147-54.

Netke, S.P., et al. (1997). Ascorbic acid protects guinea pigs from acute aflatoxin toxicity. *Toxicol Appl Pharmacol*, 143(2), 429-35.

Neuzil, J., et al. (2011). Mitochondrially targeted -tocopheryl succinate is antiangiogenic: Potential benefit against tumor angiogenesis but caution against wound healing. *Antioxid Redox Signal*,

Nothlings, U., et al. (2008). Intake of vegetables, legumes, and fruit, and risk for all-cause, cardiovascular, and cancer mortality in a European diabetic population. *J Nutr*, 138(4), 775-81.

Novotny, L., et al. (2008). alpha-Lipoic acid: the potential for use in cancer therapy. *Neoplasma*, 55(2), 81-6.

Packer, L., et al. (1997). Alpha-lipoic acid: a metabolic antioxidant and potential redox modulator of transcription. *Adv Pharmacol*, 3879-101.

Packer, L. & Suzuki, Y.J. (1993). Vitamin E and alpha-lipoate: role in antioxidant recycling and activation of the NF-kappa B transcription factor. *Mol Aspects Med*, 14(3), 229-39.

Padmalayam, I., et al. (2009). Lipoic acid synthase (LASY): a novel role in inflammation, mitochondrial function, and insulin resistance. *Diabetes*, 58(3), 600-8.

Park, H.J., et al. (2011). Green tea extract attenuates hepatic steatosis by decreasing adipose lipogenesis and enhancing hepatic antioxidant defenses in ob/ob mice. *J Nutr Biochem*, 22(4), 393-400.

Parker, R.A., et al. (1995). Relation of vascular oxidative stress, alpha-tocopherol, and hypercholesterolemia to early atherosclerosis in hamsters. *Arterioscler Thromb Vasc Biol*, 15(3), 349-58.

Pauwels, E.K. (2011). The protective effect of the Mediterranean diet: focus on cancer and cardiovascular risk. *Med Princ Pract*, 20(2), 103-11.

Perez-Jimenez, J. & Saura-Calixto, F. (2008). Grape products and cardiovascular disease risk factors. *Nutr Res Rev*, 21(2), 158-73.

Perez-Matute, P., et al. (2009). Reactive species and diabetes: counteracting oxidative stress to improve health. *Curr Opin Pharmacol*, 9(6), 771-9.

Plantinga, Y., et al. (2007). Supplementation with vitamins C and E improves arterial stiffness and endothelial function in essential hypertensive patients. *Am J Hypertens*, 20(4), 392-7.

Platz, E.A. & Lippman, S.M. (2009). Selenium, genetic variation, and prostate cancer risk: epidemiology reflects back on selenium and vitamin E cancer prevention trial. *J Clin Oncol*, 27(22), 3569-72.

Plutner, H., et al. (1990). Synthetic peptides of the Rab effector domain inhibit vesicular transport through the secretory pathway. *Embo J*, 9(8), 2375-83.

Podmore, I.D., et al. (1998). Vitamin C exhibits pro-oxidant properties. *Nature*, 392(6676), 559.

Prieto-Hontoria, P.L., et al. (2009). Lipoic acid prevents body weight gain induced by a high fat diet in rats: effects on intestinal sugar transport. *J Physiol Biochem*, 65(1), 43-50.

Prieto-Hontoria, P.L., et al. (2010). Role of obesity-associated dysfunctional adipose tissue in cancer: a molecular nutrition approach. *Biochim Biophys Acta*, 1807(6), 664-78.

Ramos, R. & Martinez-Castelao, A. (2008). Lipoperoxidation and hemodialysis. *Metabolism*, 57(10), 1369-74.

Rayman, M.P. (2005). Selenium in cancer prevention: a review of the evidence and mechanism of action. *Proc Nutr Soc*, 64(4), 527-42.

Rayman, M.P., et al. (2008). Randomized controlled trial of the effect of selenium supplementation on thyroid function in the elderly in the United Kingdom. *Am J Clin Nutr*, 87(2), 370-8.

Reboul, E., et al. (2006). Bioaccessibility of carotenoids and vitamin E from their main dietary sources. *J Agric Food Chem*, 54(23), 8749-55.

Rickman, C., et al. (2010). Green tea attenuates cardiovascular remodelling and metabolic symptoms in high carbohydrate-fed rats. *Curr Pharm Biotechnol*, 11(8), 881-6.

Rietveld, A. & Wiseman, S. (2003). Antioxidant effects of tea: evidence from human clinical trials. *J Nutr*, 133(10), 3285S-3292S.

Robinson, L.E., et al. (2004). Caffeine ingestion before an oral glucose tolerance test impairs blood glucose management in men with type 2 diabetes. *J Nutr*, 134(10), 2528-33.

Rodrigo, R., et al. (2008). Decrease in oxidative stress through supplementation of vitamins C and E is associated with a reduction in blood pressure in patients with essential hypertension. *Clin Sci (Lond)*, 114(10), 625-34.

Roy, S., et al. (1997). Modulation of cellular reducing equivalent homeostasis by alpha-lipoic acid. Mechanisms and implications for diabetes and ischemic injury. *Biochem Pharmacol*, 53(3), 393-9.

Sae-Tan, S., et al. (2011). (-)-Epigallocatechin-3-gallate increases the expression of genes related to fat oxidation in the skeletal muscle of high fat-fed mice. *Food Funct*, 2(2), 111-6.

Sakurai, N., et al. (2009). (-)-Epigallocatechin gallate enhances the expression of genes related to insulin sensitivity and adipocyte differentiation in 3T3-L1 adipocytes at an early stage of differentiation. *Nutrition*, 25(10), 1047-56.

Savory, L.A., et al. (2011). Selenium Supplementation and Exercise: Effect on Oxidant Stress in Overweight Adults. *Obesity (Silver Spring)*,

Scott, B.C., et al. (1994). Lipoic and dihydrolipoic acids as antioxidants. A critical evaluation. *Free Radic Res*, 20(2), 119-33.

Schleicher, R.L., et al. (2009). Serum vitamin C and the prevalence of vitamin C deficiency in the United States: 2003-2004 National Health and Nutrition Examination Survey (NHANES). *Am J Clin Nutr*, 90(5), 1252-63.

Sebai, H., et al. (2010). Resveratrol, a red wine polyphenol, attenuates lipopolysaccharide-induced oxidative stress in rat liver. *Ecotoxicol Environ Saf*, 73(5), 1078-83.

Senen, D., et al. (2002). Contribution of vitamin C administration for increasing lipolysis. *Aesthetic Plast Surg*, 26(2), 123-5.

Serisier, S., et al. (2008). Effects of green tea on insulin sensitivity, lipid profile and expression of PPARalpha and PPARgamma and their target genes in obese dogs. *Br J Nutr*, 99(6), 1208-16.

Shargorodsky, M., et al. (2010). Effect of long-term treatment with antioxidants (vitamin C, vitamin E, coenzyme Q10 and selenium) on arterial compliance, humoral factors and inflammatory markers in patients with multiple cardiovascular risk factors. *Nutr Metab (Lond)*, 755.

Shay, K.P., et al. (2009). Alpha-lipoic acid as a dietary supplement: molecular mechanisms and therapeutic potential. *Biochim Biophys Acta*, 1790(10), 1149-60.

Shen, Q.W., et al. (2005). Effect of dietary alpha-lipoic acid on growth, body composition, muscle pH, and AMP-activated protein kinase phosphorylation in mice. *J Anim Sci*, 83(11), 2611-7.

Shen, W., et al. (2008a). A combination of nutriments improves mitochondrial biogenesis and function in skeletal muscle of type 2 diabetic Goto-Kakizaki rats. *PLoS One*, 3(6), e2328.

Shen, W., et al. (2008b). R-alpha-lipoic acid and acetyl-L-carnitine complementarily promote mitochondrial biogenesis in murine 3T3-L1 adipocytes. *Diabetologia*, 51(1), 165-74.

Shen, X., et al. (2009). Effect of vitamin E supplementation on oxidative stress in a rat model of diet-induced obesity. *Int J Vitam Nutr Res*, 79(4), 255-63.

Shi, D.Y., et al. (2008). Alpha-lipoic acid induces apoptosis in hepatoma cells via the PTEN/Akt pathway. *FEBS Lett*, 582(12), 1667-71.

Singh, U., et al. (2005). Vitamin E, oxidative stress, and inflammation. *Annu Rev Nutr*, 25151-74.

Skrha, J., et al. (1999). Insulin action and fibrinolysis influenced by vitamin E in obese Type 2 diabetes mellitus. *Diabetes Res Clin Pract*, 44(1), 27-33.

Smith, A.R., et al. (2004). Lipoic acid as a potential therapy for chronic diseases associated with oxidative stress. *Curr Med Chem*, 11(9), 1135-46.

Soares, A.F., et al. (2005). Effects of oxidative stress on adiponectin secretion and lactate production in 3T3-L1 adipocytes. *Free Radic Biol Med*, 38(7), 882-9.

Sola, S., et al. (2005). Irbesartan and lipoic acid improve endothelial function and reduce markers of inflammation in the metabolic syndrome: results of the Irbesartan and Lipoic Acid in Endothelial Dysfunction (ISLAND) study. *Circulation*, 111(3), 343-8.

Soltys, K., et al. (2001). Oxidative stress in fatty livers of obese Zucker rats: rapid amelioration and improved tolerance to warm ischemia with tocopherol. *Hepatology*, 34(1), 13-8.

Song, E.K., et al. (2003). Epigallocatechin gallate prevents autoimmune diabetes induced by multiple low doses of streptozotocin in mice. *Arch Pharm Res*, 26(7), 559-63.

Soni, M.G., et al. 2010. Safety of vitamins and minerals: controversies and perspective. *Toxicol Sci*, 118(2), 348-55.

Stefanovic, A., et al. (2008). The influence of obesity on the oxidative stress status and the concentration of leptin in type 2 diabetes mellitus patients. *Diabetes Res Clin Pract*, 79(1), 156-63.

Stellato, D., et al. (2011). Uric acid: a starring role in the intricate scenario of metabolic syndrome with cardio-renal damage? *Intern Emerg Med*,

Stewart, A.J., et al. (2005). On-line high-performance liquid chromatography analysis of the antioxidant activity of phenolic compounds in green and black tea. *Mol Nutr Food Res*, 49(1), 52-60.

Stocker, R. & Keaney, J.F., Jr. (2005). New insights on oxidative stress in the artery wall. *J Thromb Haemost*, 3(8), 1825-34.

Stranges, S., et al. (2010). Selenium status and cardiometabolic health: state of the evidence. *Nutr Metab Cardiovasc Dis*, 20(10), 754-60.

Strohle, A., et al. (2011). Micronutrients at the interface between inflammation and infection--ascorbic acid and calciferol: part 1, general overview with a focus on ascorbic acid. *Inflamm Allergy Drug Targets*, 10(1), 54-63.

Suksomboon, N., et al. (2011). Effects of vitamin E supplementation on glycaemic control in type 2 diabetes: systematic review of randomized controlled trials. *J Clin Pharm Ther*, 36(1), 53-63.

Sun, A.Y., et al. (2010). Resveratrol as a therapeutic agent for neurodegenerative diseases. *Mol Neurobiol*, 41(2-3), 375-83.

Sutherland, W.H., et al. (2007). Vitamin E supplementation and plasma 8-isoprostane and adiponectin in overweight subjects. *Obesity (Silver Spring)*, 15(2), 386-91.

Szkudelska, K., et al. (2009). The inhibitory effect of resveratrol on leptin secretion from rat adipocytes. *Eur J Clin Invest*, 39(10), 899-905.

Takabayashi, F., et al. (2004). Effect of green tea catechins on oxidative DNA damage of hamster pancreas and liver induced by N-Nitrosobis(2-oxopropyl)amine and/or oxidized soybean oil. *Biofactors*, 21(1-4), 335-7.

Talaulikar, V.S. & Manyonda, I.T. (2011). Vitamin C as an antioxidant supplement in women's health: a myth in need of urgent burial. *Eur J Obstet Gynecol Reprod Biol*, 157(1), 10-3.

Taylor, A.G., et al. (2006). Inflammation and oxidative stess are associated with a novel dietary "phytochemical Index" in obese young adults. *North American Research Conference on Complementary and Alternative Medicine*, 24-27.

Touzet, O. & Philips, A. (2010). Resveratrol protects against protease inhibitor-induced reactive oxygen species production, reticulum stress and lipid raft perturbation. *Aids*, 24(10), 1437-47.

Trumbo, P.R. (2005). The level of evidence for permitting a qualified health claim: FDA's review of the evidence for selenium and cancer and vitamin E and heart disease. *J Nutr*, 135(2), 354-6.

Tudoran, O., et al. (2011). Early transcriptional pattern of angiogenesis induced by EGCG treatment in cervical tumor cells. *J Cell Mol Med*, (In press).

Ulker, S., et al. (2003). Vitamins reverse endothelial dysfunction through regulation of eNOS and NAD(P)H oxidase activities. *Hypertension*, 41(3), 534-9.

Um, J.H., et al. (2010). AMP-activated protein kinase-deficient mice are resistant to the metabolic effects of resveratrol. *Diabetes*, 59(3), 554-63.

Upritchard, J.E., et al. (2000). Effect of supplementation with tomato juice, vitamin E, and vitamin C on LDL oxidation and products of inflammatory activity in type 2 diabetes. *Diabetes Care*, 23(6), 733-8.

Vajro, P., et al. (2004). Vitamin E treatment in pediatric obesity-related liver disease: a randomized study. *J Pediatr Gastroenterol Nutr*, 38(1), 48-55.

Valdecantos, M.P., et al. (2010a). Vitamin C, resveratrol and lipoic acid actions on isolated rat liver mitochondria: all antioxidants but different. *Redox Rep*, 15(5), 207-16.

Valdecantos, M.P., et al. (2010b). Lipoic acid improves hepatic mitochondrial function in a model of obesity. *4th International Congress of Nutrigenetics and Nutrigenomics*, Pamplona, Spain.

Valdecantos, M., P., et al. (2011a). Lipoic acid increases hepatic mitochondrial defenses through Foxo3a deacetylation by SIRT3 in a diet-induced obesity rat model. *8th MiPconference on Mitochondrial Physiology and Pathology*, Bordeaux, France.

Valdecantos, M.P., et al. (2011b). Lipoic acid prevents fatty liver in a diet-induced obesity rat model. *19th European Congress of Obesity*, Istambul (Turkey).

Valko, M., et al. (2007). Free radicals and antioxidants in normal physiological functions and human disease. *Int J Biochem Cell Biol*, 39(1), 44-84.

Van Gossum, A., et al. (1988). Increased lipid peroxidation after lipid infusion as measured by breath pentane output. *Am J Clin Nutr*, 48(6), 1394-9.

Vanamala, J., et al. (2010). Resveratrol suppresses IGF-1 induced human colon cancer cell proliferation and elevates apoptosis via suppression of IGF-1R/Wnt and activation of p53 signaling pathways. *BMC Cancer*, 10238.

Verrax, J. & Calderon, PB. (2008). The controversial place of vitamin C in cancer treatment. *Biochem Pharmacol*, 76(12),1644-52.

Vincent, H.K., et al. (2006). Antioxidant supplementation lowers exercise-induced oxidative stress in young overweight adults. *Obesity (Silver Spring)*, 14(12), 2224-35.

Vincent, H.K., et al. (2007). Oxidative stress and potential interventions to reduce oxidative stress in overweight and obesity. *Diabetes Obes Metab*, 9(6), 813-39.

Visioli, F., et al. (2002). Lipoic acid and vitamin C potentiate nitric oxide synthesis in human aortic endothelial cells independently of cellular glutathione status. *Redox Rep*, 7(4), 223-7.

Vivekananthan, D.P., et al. (2003). Use of antioxidant vitamins for the prevention of cardiovascular disease: meta-analysis of randomised trials. *Lancet*, 361(9374), 2017-23.

Volchegorskii, I.A., et al. (2011). Effect of pro- and antioxidants on insulin sensitivity and glucose tolerance. *Bull Exp Biol Med*, 150(3), 327-32.

Waltner-Law, M.E., et al. (2002). Epigallocatechin gallate, a constituent of green tea, represses hepatic glucose production. *J Biol Chem*, 277(38), 34933-40.

Wang, H., et al. (2011). Obesity Modifies the Relations Between Serum Markers of Dairy Fats and Inflammation and Oxidative Stress Among Adolescents. *Obesity (Silver Spring)*, doi: 10.1038/oby.2011.234.

Wang, X. & Tian, W. (2001). Green tea epigallocatechin gallate: a natural inhibitor of fatty-acid synthase. *Biochem Biophys Res Commun*, 288(5), 1200-6.

Wang, Y., et al. (2010). alpha-Lipoic acid increases energy expenditure by enhancing adenosine monophosphate-activated protein kinase-peroxisome proliferator-activated receptor-gamma coactivator-1alpha signaling in the skeletal muscle of aged mice. *Metabolism*, 59(7), 967-76.

Wang, Y., et al. (2006). (-)-Epigallocatechin-3-gallate protects mice from concanavalin A-induced hepatitis through suppressing immune-mediated liver injury. *Clin Exp Immunol*, 145(3), 485-92.

Ward, N.C., et al. (2007). The effect of vitamin E on blood pressure in individuals with type 2 diabetes: a randomized, double-blind, placebo-controlled trial. *J Hypertens*, 25(1), 227-34.

Wei, H. & Meng, Z. (2010). Protective effects of epigallocatechin-3-gallate against lead-induced oxidative damage. *Hum Exp Toxicol*,

Weinberg, R.B., et al. (2001). Pro-oxidant effect of vitamin E in cigarette smokers consuming a high polyunsaturated fat diet. *Arterioscler Thromb Vasc Biol*, 21(6), 1029-33.

Williamson, G. & Manach, C. (2005). Bioavailability and bioefficacy of polyphenols in humans. II. Review of 93 intervention studies. *Am J Clin Nutr*, 81(1 Suppl), 243S-255S.

Wu, B.T., et al. (2005). The apoptotic effect of green tea (-)-epigallocatechin gallate on 3T3-L1 preadipocytes depends on the Cdk2 pathway. *J Agric Food Chem*, 53(14), 5695-701.

Wu, J.H., et al. (2007). Effects of alpha-tocopherol and mixed tocopherol supplementation on markers of oxidative stress and inflammation in type 2 diabetes. *Clin Chem*, 53(3), 511-9.

Xiao, C., et al. (2011). Short-term oral {alpha}-lipoic acid does not prevent lipid-induced dysregulation of glucose homeostasis in obese and overweight non-diabetic men. *Am J Physiol Endocrinol Metab*,

Yasui, K., et al. (2011a). Effects of a catechin-free fraction derived from green tea on gene expression of gluconeogenic enzymes in rat hepatoma H4IIE cells and in the mouse liver. *Biomed Res*, 32(2), 119-25.

Yasui, K., et al. (2011b). Effects of (-)-epigallocatechin-3-O-gallate on expression of gluconeogenesisrelated genes in the mouse duodenum. *Biomed Res*, 32(5), 313-20.

Yun, S.Y., et al. (2006). Effects of (-)-epigallocatechin-3-gallate on pancreatic beta-cell damage in streptozotocin-induced diabetic rats. *Eur J Pharmacol*, 541(1-2), 115-21.

Zhang, H.S., et al. (2009). Resveratrol inhibited Tat-induced HIV-1 LTR transactivation via NAD(+)-dependent SIRT1 activity. *Life Sci*, 85(13-14), 484-9.

Zhao, B. (2009). Natural antioxidants protect neurons in Alzheimer's disease and Parkinson's disease. *Neurochem Res*, 34(4), 630-8.

Zhong, Y. & Shahidi, F. (2011). Lipophilized epigallocatechin gallate (EGCG) derivatives as novel antioxidants. *J Agric Food Chem*, 59(12), 6526-33.

Zingg, JM., et al. (2010). Modulation of gene expression by alpha-tocopherol and alpha-tocopheryl phosphate in THP-1 monocytes. *Free Radic Biol Med*, 49(12), 1989-2000.

Zingg, JM., & Azzi A. (2004). Non-antioxidant activities of vitamin E. *Curr Med Chem*, 11(9), 1113-33.

References from table 2

Alkhenizan, A. & Hafez, K. (2007). The role of vitamin E in the prevention of cancer: a meta-analysis of randomized controlled trials. *Ann Saudi Med*, 27(6), 409-14.

Arain, M.A. & Abdul Qadeer, A. (2010). Systematic review on "vitamin E and prevention of colorectal cancer". *Pak J Pharm Sci*, 23(2), 125-30.

Bardia, A., et al. (2008). Efficacy of antioxidant supplementation in reducing primary cancer incidence and mortality: systematic review and meta-analysis. *Mayo Clin Proc*, 83(1), 23-34.

Evans, J. (2008). Antioxidant supplements to prevent or slow down the progression of AMD: a systematic review and meta-analysis. *Eye (Lond)*, 22(6), 751-60.

Myung, S.K., et al. (2010). Effects of antioxidant supplements on cancer prevention: meta-analysis of randomized controlled trials. *Ann Oncol*, 21(1), 166-79.

Polyzos, N.P., et al. (2007). Combined vitamin C and E supplementation during pregnancy for preeclampsia prevention: a systematic review. *Obstet Gynecol Surv*, 62(3), 202-6.

Microalgae of the Chlorophyceae Class: Potential Nutraceuticals Reducing Oxidative Stress Intensity and Cellular Damage

Blas-Valdivia Vanessa, Ortiz-Butron Rocio,
Rodriguez-Sanchez Ruth, Torres-Manzo Paola,
Hernandez-Garcia Adelaida and Cano-Europa Edgar
Escuela Nacional de Ciencias Biológicas,
Instituto Politécnico Nacional Departamento de Fisiología,
México

1. Introduction

Nutraceutical is a term combining the words nutrition and pharmaceutical. It is a food or food product that provides health and medical benefits, including the prevention and treatment of disease. A nutraceutical has beneficial effects because it possesses many compounds with antioxidant and intracellular signalling-pathway modulator effects. In recent years, it has been demonstrated that microalgae of the Chlorophyceae class could be excellent nutraceuticals because they contain polyphenols, chlorophyll, β-carotene, ascorbic acid, lycopene, α-tocopherol, xanthophylls, and PUFAs. For this reason, some research groups, including ours, have studied the nutraceutical properties of the genera *Dunalliela*, *Haematococcus*, and *Chlorella*. However, our research group has put special emphasis on the genera *Chlorella* and *Chlamydomonas*. For these genera, we present new results that reveal antioxidant effects in different models of oxidative stress and cell damage

2. Nutraceuticals

For a long time, natural products obtained from plants have been used as prominent sources of prophylactic agents for the prevention and treatment of disease in humans, animals, and in plants. Hippocrates (460-370 BC) started "let food be your medicine and medicine be your food". Now, the relationship between food and drugs is getting closer.

As we enter the third millennium, with increased life expectancy and greater media coverage of the health care issue, consumers are understandably more interested in the potential benefits of nutritional support for disease control or prevention. A recent survey in Europe concluded that diet is rated more highly by consumers than exercise or the hereditary factor for achieving good health (Hardy, 2000). For that reason, many entrepreneurs seek to introduce different products into the health and nutritional market. Marketing strategies have exploited the words "functional food" and "nutraceuticals" in their advertisements. Nutraceuticals and functional foods are the fastest growing segment of today´s food industry, although nutraceuticals should be treated as pharmaceutical products as we will detail. Nutraceuticals and functional foods are a market estimated at between $6 billion US and $60 billion US and it is growing at 5% per annum. Unfortunately, entrepreneurs in an effort to make money attract, as irresponsible market entrants, products that do not comply with biosafety tests. This is because there are few laws that regulate the production and sale of such products. Because the products are not submitted for standardized toxicology testing, sometimes they may be toxic for human consumption. There are no specific regulation in any country to control nutraceuticals, and they need to be established and should be considered under the same laws that regulate pharmaceuticals and food (Bernal et al., 2011). For our purposes, we will first define "nutraceuticals" and "functional foods" and how the microalgae could be excellent nutraceuticals.

The term nutraceutical was first mentioned in 1989 to describe the union between nutrition and pharmaceuticals, both key contributors to human wellness. Stephen DeFelice MD is the founder and chairman of the Foundation for Innovation in Medicine (FIM) and he defined a nutraceutical as a food (or part of the food) that provides medicinal health benefits, including the prevention or treatment of a disease. It was proposed that a nutraceutical is not a drug, which is a pharmacologically active substance that potentiates, antagonizes, or otherwise modifies any physiological function. A nutraceutical may be a single natural nutrient in powder, tablet, capsule, or liquid form. It is not necessarily a complete food but equally not a drug (Hardy, 2000). Also, it was proposed that a nutraceutical is a product that delivers a concentrated form of a presumed bioactive agent from a food, presented in a nonfood matrix, and it is used with the purpose of enhancing health in a dosage that exceeds those that could be obtained from normal food (Zeisel, 1999).

Functional food and nutraceutical are terms used incorrectly and indiscriminately for nutrients or nutrient-enriched food that can prevent or treat disease. Functional food is a product that resembles traditional food but it possesses demonstrated physiological benefits (Shahidi, 2009). For example a functional food could be a lutein-rich food as chicken, spinach, tomatoes, or oranges, or the omega-3 fatty acids found in fish oil. All functional foods are processed and consumed as food. A nutraceutical is not a nutritional supplement because the latter are nutrients that are added to the diet to correct or prevent deficiencies of vitamins, minerals, and proteins, and often used in the recovery of a patient suffering an illness or has undergone surgery, and also taken to improve overall health (Mandel et al., 2005). The beneficial effects of nutraceuticals and functional foods have been attributed to their components, such as polyphenols, polyunsatured fatty acids (PUFAs), terpenes, chlorophyll, and accessory pigments of the photosynthetic apparatus in cyanobacteria such as *Spirullina*. In general these compounds are antioxidants that reduce intensity of oxidative stress or modulate intracellular communication

3. Nutraceutical effects of polyphenols, particularly flavonoids

The polyphenols are compounds characterized by a benzene ring bearing one or more hydroxyl groups attached to the ring. They are ubiquitous in the plants, vegetables, fruit, vines, tea, coffee and microalgae. The polyphenols in food originate from one of the main classes of secondary metabolites in plants. They are involved in the growth and reproduction and are produced as a response to defend injured plants against pathogens, and to participate in the defense mechanism against ultraviolet radiation (Biesalski, 2007). Polyphenols have different nutraceutical properties, such as an antioxidant, antiinflammatory (Biesalski, 2007), anticancer (Oz & Ebersole, 2010), antibacterial (Du et al.,

2011), antiatherogenic, and antiangiogenic (Rimbach et al., 2009). There are now polyphenols with therapeutic properties for which the mechanism of action at the molecular level has been discovered and they are used in clinical trials, e.g. flavonoids.

Flavonoids comprise the most common group of polyphenols and provide much of the flavor and color to fruit and vegetables. More than 6000 different flavonoids have been described and it is estimated that humans consume about 1 g/day.

The structure of flavonoids is C6-C3-C6 and they consist of two aromatic rings linked through three carbons usually forming an oxygenated heterocycle nucleus, named the flavan nucleus, and shown in figure 1. In general, the flavonoids are classified into six groups (Grassi et al., 2009).

1. **Flavones**: These kinds of flavonoids are used by angiosperms to color their flowers. Natural flavones include apigenin (4',5,7-trihydroxyflavone), (3',4',5,7-tetrahydroxyflavone), (4',5,6,7,8-pentamethoxyflavone), chrysin (5,7-dihydroxyflavone), baicalein (5,6,7-trihydroxyflavone), scutellarein (5,6,7,4'-tetrahydroxyflavone), wogonin (5,7-Dihydroxy-8-methoxyflavone). There are synthetic flavones such as diosmin and flavoxate.
2. **Flavonols**: These compounds are used by organisms to protect them from UV radiation. Their diversity stems from the different positions of the hydroxyl groups on the benzene rings (show figure 1). There are flavonols as kaempferol (3,4',5,7-tetrahydroxy-2-phenylchromen-4-one), quercetin (3,3',4',5,7-pentahydroxy-2-phenylchromen-4-one), myricetin (3,3',4',5',5,7-hexahydroxy-2-phenylchromen-4-one), galangin (3,5,7-trihydroxy-2-phenylchromen-4-one), and morin (2-(2,4-dihydroxyphenyl)-3,5,7-trihydroxychromen-4-one). **Flavanones**: These flavonoids are the direct precursors of the vast majority of flavonoids. Some examples of flavanones are: naringenin (4',5,7-trihydroxyflavanone) and butin (7,3',4'-trihydroxyflavanone).
3. **Catechin or flavanols**: These flavonoids have two chiral centers on the molecule on carbons 2 and 3, yielding four diastereoisomers. Two of the isomers are in the *trans* configuration and are called catechins and the other two are in the *cis* configuration and are called epicatechins. These flavonoids are present in food as a complexs or oligomerics and polymerics as procyanidins or proantocyanidins. The catechins are found in different fruits, i.e. apples, apricots, blackberries, and grapes. Catechins are also in red wine, but black tea and cocoa are the richest sources. The flavanols in finished food products depend on the cultivar type, geographical origin, agriculture practice, postharvesting handling, and food processing (Scalbert et al., 2005).
4. **Antocyanidins**: Antocyanidins are a large group of natural colorants. The color of most fruits, flowers, and berries are made from a combination of anthocyanins and anthocyanidins. Anthocyanins always contain a carbohydrate molecule, whereas anthocyanidins do not. Examples of antocyanidins are cyanidin (3,3',4',5,7-pentahydroxyflavylium chloride), pelargonidin (3,5,7-trihydroxy-2-(4-hydroxyphenyl) benzopyrylium chloride), and malvidin (3,5,7,4'-tetrahydroxy-3',5'-dimethoxyflavylium)
5. **Isoflavones**: This group is a class of organic compounds that sometimes act as phytoestrogens in mammals and are called antioxidants because of their ability to trap a singlet oxygen. Genistein (4',5,7-trihydroxyisoflavone) and daidzein (4',7-dihydroxyisoflavone) are two examples of isoflavones.

Some authors have proposed that aurones are another flavonoid group, however we consider that aurones are derived from chalcones (Fowler & Koffas, 2009).

The flavonoid synthesis is shown in figure 1. It begins when a cell transforms phenylananine or tyrosine into phenylpropanoic acid or cinnamic acid by phenylalanine-tyrosine ammonia lyase (PAL; EC 4.3.1.25/TAL; EC 4.3.1.25). Then cytochrome-P450 cinnamate 4-hydroxylase (C4H; EC 1.14.13.11) adds a 4′-hydroxyl group to form p-coumaric acid. The CoA esters are subsequently synthetized from cinnamic acid, caffeic acid, or *p*-coumaric acid by 4-coumaryl:CoA ligase (4CL; EC 6.2.1.12). The type III polyketide chalcone synthase (CHS; EC 2.3.1.74) catalyzes the sequential condensation of three malonyl-CoA moieties with one CoA-ester molecule to form chalcones. The flavanones are formed when chalcones are isomerized into (2S)-flavanones by chalcone isomerase (CHI; EC 5.5.1.6). Many enzymes can modify the flavanones. For example the flavanones could be reduced to form isoflavones by isoflavone synthase (IFS; EC 1.14.13.86). After that, isoflavones are modified by different enzymatic systems to produce hydroxylation, reduction, alkylation, oxidation, and glucosylation alone or in combination in the three-ring phenylpropanoid core. Enzymes such as O-methyltransferse (IOMT, EC 2.1.1.150), isoflavone 2′-reductase (I2′R; EC 1.3.1.45), andisoflavone reductase (IFR; EC 1.3.1.45) can yield over 8000 different chemical structures from isoflavone (Winkel-Shirley, 2001; Fowler & Koffas, 2009). Another branch of the biosynthetic pathway of flavonoids is the flavones that are synthesized from flavanones through the action of the flavone synthase type I and II (FSI; EC 1.14.11.22). Flavonones are hydroxylated and then with flavonol synthase (FLS; EC 1.14.11.23) form flavonols. These compounds are the precursors of anthocyanins.

The beneficial effects can be divided into

1. **Antioxidants**: Flavonoids suppress the formation of reactive oxygen species (ROS) either by inhibiting enzymes or chelating trace elements involved in free radical production. Thus flavonoids help maintain an ROS steady state in the case of physical and chemical injury of the cell (Corradini et al., 2011). Not all flavonoids are ROS scavengers because some flavonoids, as nucleophiles, trap electrons from the ROS and become a free radical themselves, which then propagate a chain reaction causing a deleterious effect in the cell (Grassi et al., 2009).
2. **Modulators of intracellular communication**: The flavonoids and their metabolites act in the phosphoinositide 3-kinase (PI3K), Akt-protein kinase B (Akt-PKB), tyrosine kinase, and protein kinase C (PKC) signalling cascade. The inhibition or activation of these cascades modifies cellular function by altering the phosphorylation state of target molecules that modulate the expression of genes. This can explain the anticancer and neuroprotector flavonoid activities (Williams et al., 2004).
3. **Enzyme activity modulator**: Flavonoids offer cardiovascular protection because of their indirect inhibition of the angiotensin-converting enzyme (ACE; EC 3.4.15.1) (Actis-Goretta et al., 2006). Other enzymes inhibited by flavonoids are aromatase (EC 1.14.14.1) and α–amylase (EC 3.2.2.1) (Hargrove et al., 2011). The inhibition of enzymes that have a Fe-S cluster has been demonstrated (Mena et al., 2011).

In general, flavonoids are molecules responsible of some of the beneficial effect of nutraceuticals and functional foods. The different effects of flavonoids are described in table 1.

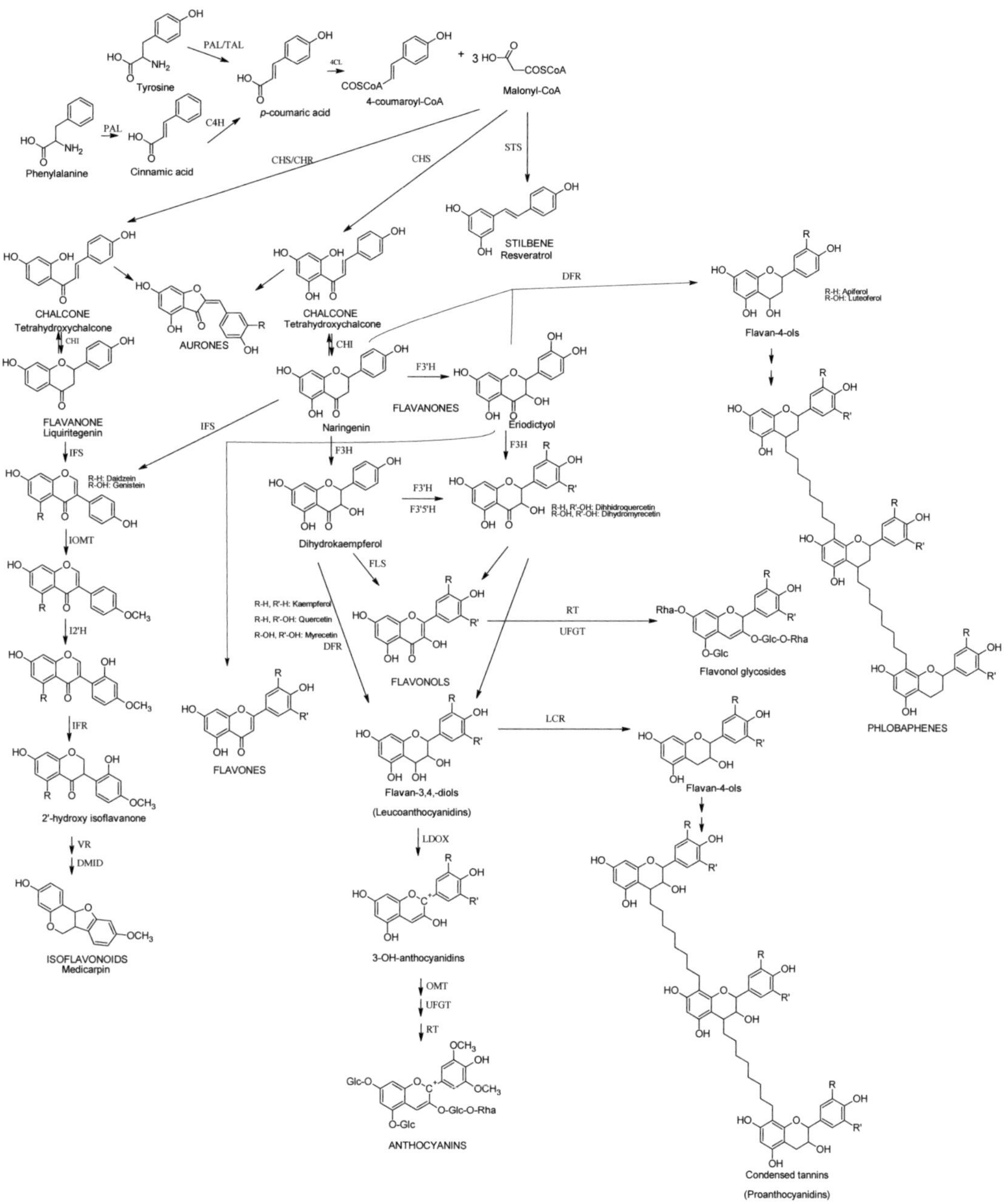

Fig. 1. Scheme of the major branch pathways of flavonoid biosynthesis, starting with general phenylpropanoid metabolism and leading to the nine major subgroups; chalcones, aurones, isoflavonoids, flavones, flavonols, flavandiols, anthocyanins, condensed tannins, and phlobaphene pigments

Flavonoid	Nutraceutic application	Reference
Flavanones	LDL oxidation (atherosclerosis) Cyclooxygenase inhibitory ability (cancer) Malaria chemotherapy (malaria) Inflammation response trigger (reduce inflammation) Antiangiogenic effect Reduce lung metastases Hepatoprotective action Antibacterial action Genoprotective action Inhibitors of NOS and COX in microglia Promote apoptosis in C6 glioma cells	(Miranda et al., 2000) (Kinghorn et al., 2004) (Kumar et al., 2003) (Kontogiorgis et al., 2008) (Mojzis et al., 2008) (Qin et al., 2011) (Prabu et al., 2011) (Celiz et al., 2011) (Orsolic et al., 2011) (Chao et al., 2010) (Sabarinathan et al., 2010)
Flavones	GLUT inhibitors (diabetes) Cyclooxygenase inhibitory ability (cancer) Antitumoral activity Pancreatic cholesterol esterase inhibitor Reduce neurodegeneration Produce apoptosis in melanoma cells Colitis treatment Antiinflammatory effect	(Kwon et al., 2007) (Kinghorn et al., 2004) (Balk, 2011; Polier et al., 2011) (Peng et al., 2011) (Gasiorowski et al., 2011) (Mohan et al., 2011) (Ganjare et al., 2011) (Funakoshi-Tago et al., 2011)
Flavonols	GLUT inhibitors (diabetes) Pancreatic lipase inhibitors (diabetes) Inhibitors of cell cycle control kinases (cancer) Regulate lipid profile in diabetic rats Regulate serum glucose Reduce apoptosis in cell culture Hepatoprotective action Promote new bone formation Anti-inflammatory effect Reduce neuronal damage	(Kwon et al., 2007; Park & Levine, 2000) (Nakai et al., 2005) (Hsu & Yen, 2006) (Liu et al., 2012) (Fontana Pereira et al., 2011) (Jang et al., 2011) (Singab et al., 2010) (Yang et al., 2010) (Mahat et al., 2010) (Lagoa et al., 2009) (Hirose et al., 2009)
Isoflavonoids	Alpha-glucosidase inhibitor (diabetes) GLUT inhibitor (diabetes) Improves cholesterol regulation (diabetes) Inhibitor of tyrosine kinase and antiinflammatory effect in kidney Induce apoptosis in leukemia Neuroprotective action Antiinflammatory action	(Kim et al., 2000) (Kwon et al., 2007; Song et al., 2002) (Lee, 2006) (Elmarakby et al., 2011) (Li et al., 2011a) (Xi et al., 2011) (Neelakandan et al., 2011)
Anthocyanins	Pancreatic lipase and glucosidase	(Kim et al., 2000)

Flavonoid	Nutraceutic application	Reference
	inhibitor (diabetes)	(Tsuda, 2008)
	Regulate adipocyte function (Obesity)	(Wolfram et al., 2006)
	Improves glucose and lipid metabolism	(Sternberg et al., 2008)
	(diabetes)	(Tokimitsu, 2004)
	Modulate blood hormone levels	(Mirshekar et al., 2010)
	(multiple sclerosis)	(Wang et al., 2010)
	Suppress body fat accumulation(obesity)	(Roghani et al., 2010)
	Reduce neuropathic hyperalgesia in	(Cvorovic et al., 2010)
	diabetic rats	
	Antioxidant effect	
	Neuroprotective action	
	produce cytotoxicity in colon cancer cells	

Table 1. Nutraceutical applications of flavonoids.

The mechanism of bioavailability and metabolism of particular flavonoids has been demonstrated in mammals. In general it has been shown that flavonoid absorption and metabolism occurs in a common pathway and it begins in the stomach and intestinal tract. In the small intestine flavonoids pass into the bloodstream in the form of glycosides, though esters or polymers cannot be absorbed. Some intestine cell enzymes or microorganisms of microflora hydrolyze them to be absorbed. In the bloodstream there are different thermodynamic pathways. They could interact with cells to modify intracellular communication. The polyphenols can be conjugated in the intestine or liver to form methylated, glucuronidated, or sulphated metabolites that reach the body via urinary and biliary excretion. The microflora also metabolizes some metabolized flavonoids that are secreted in the bile into the small intestine. Thus, there is a recycling of polyphenols that allow them more time in the plasma (Erdman et al., 2007; Manach et al., 2004). In general, the microalgae produce low quantities of polyphenols. For this reason, in the following parts of this chapter we give special attention to pigments and PUFAs.

4. Nutraceutical effects of terpenes

The terpenes are other secondary metabolites that have nutraceutical properties. The terpenes are not only the largest group of plant natural products, comprising at least 30,000 compounds, but also contain the widest assortment of structural types. Hundreds of different monoterpene (C10), sesquiterpene (C15), diterpene (C20), and triterpene (C30) carbon skeletons are known. The wealth of terpene carbon skeletons can be attributed to an enzyme class known as the terpene synthases (EC 4.2.3.20). These catalysts convert the acyclic prenyl diphosphates and squalene into a multitude of cyclic and acyclic forms. The chief causes of terpene diversity are the large number of different terpene synthases and that some terpene synthases produce multiple products. An excellent review of terpene synthase and the diversity of products were published by Degenhard and coworkers (Degenhardt et al., 2009). Microalgae produce terpenes in the form of carotenoids. These compounds offer therapeutic effects. Carotenoids are tetraterpenoid organic pigments that are naturally occurring in the chloroplasts and chromoplasts of photosynthetic organisms. The use of carotenoids by animals is because they cannot synthetize them. Animals obtain carotenoids in their diets, and they may employ them in various ways in their metabolism.

There are over 600 known carotenoids and they are divided into two classes, xanthophylls (that contain oxygen) and carotenes (that are purely hydrocarbons and contain no oxygen). Carotenoids in general absorb blue light. They serve two key roles in plants and algae; they absorb light energy for use in photosynthesis and they protect chlorophyll from photodamage (Armstrong & Hearst, 1996).

The biosynthesis of carotenes is explained in figure 2. The carotenogenesis differ somewhat among organisms and the current knowledge on the biosynthesis of carotenoids has been gained mainly from studies of bacteria and vascular plants (Armstrong & Hearst, 1996). In Figure 2, we proposed the model of Lohr for the carotenogenesis in *Chlamydomonas*. This is probably related to other microalgae of Chlorophyceae class (Lohr et al., 2005; Lohr, 2008). There are other major divisions in different organisms, such as diatoms (Bertrand, 2010) or plants (Cazzonelli & Pogson, 2010; Zhu et al., 2010), which references the readers can check to deepen their knowledge in this area.

There has been much interest in carotenoids, especially their effect on human health, because they have a market value of several hundred million Euros. Their chemical synthesis is still a demanding challenge for chemists. The major dietary source of vitamin A for mammals, including humans, is derived from carotenoids. Vitamin A is an essential micronutrient for cell growth, embryonic development, vision, and the function of the immune system (Jackson et al., 2008).

In general carotenoids exert their mechanism on health via an antioxidant pathway or by modulating intracellular communication.

1. **Antioxidant properties:** This property of carotenoids was characterized by the ability to quench singlet oxygen, the inhibition of peroxide formation, and the correlation of antioxidant dependency with oxygen partial pressures. The ketocarotenoids, such as astaxanthin and canthaxanthin, were the best radical scavengers that did not contain conjugated terminal carbonyl functions (see figure 2). These findings suggest that the keto function in conjugation with the polyene backbone is able to stabilize carbon-centered radicals more effectively than the polyene backbone alone (Jackson et al., 2008).
2. **Modulation of intracellular communication:** Carotenes modulate the intracellular communication because they or their metabolites interact with nuclear receptors like the pregnant-X-receptor (PXR) or retinoic acid receptor (RAR). For PXR it has been postulated that β-carotene activated the PXR more than its metabolites. Following this pathway, the β-carotene-PXR enhanced the metabolism of xenobiotics, bile acids, and retinoids (Ruhl, 2005). The carotenoids can be converted into two molecules of 9-*cis*-retinal, which is oxidized to 9-*cis*-retinoic acid. The RXR binds the 9-*cis*-retinoic acid with high affinity to modulate cell functions (Heyman et al., 1992). Carotenoids like lycopene modulate mevalonate and Ras pathways to modify cell growth inhibition of cancerous cells (Palozza et al., 2010), and it changes Wnt and hedgehog proteins in those cells (Sarkar et al., 2010). The PI3K-Akt and MAPK pathways are stimulated in kidney by lycopene (Chan et al., 2009).

In table 2, are some nutraceuticals of the most used carotenoids.

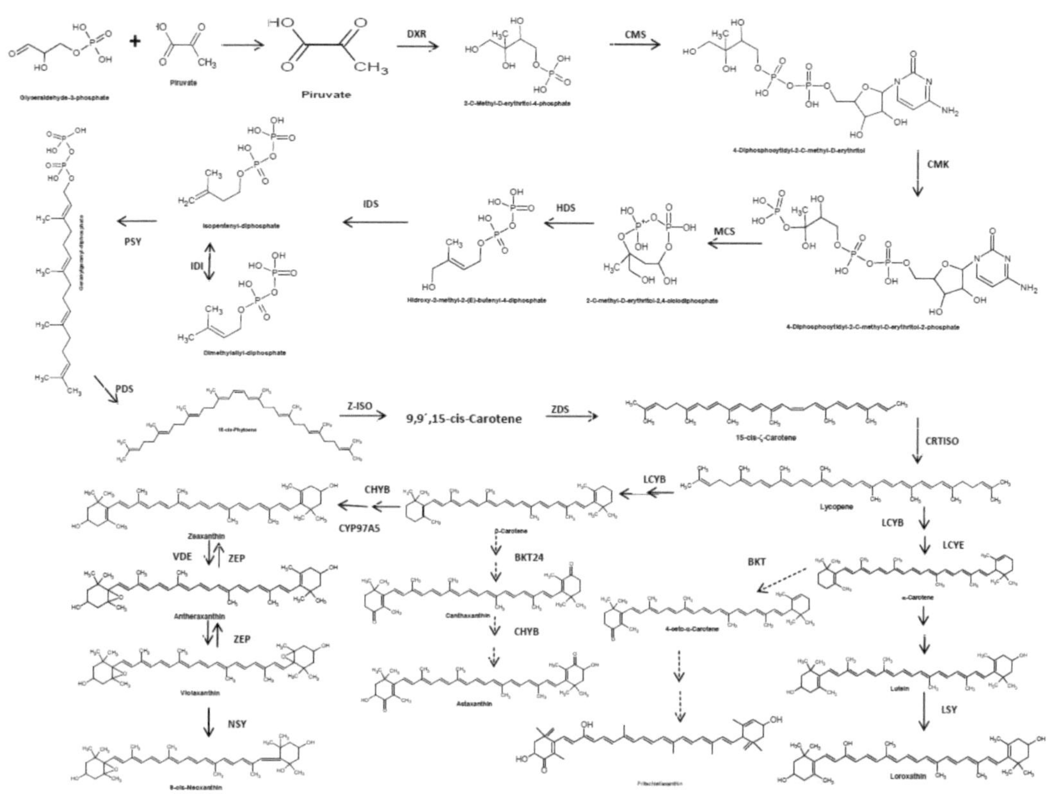

Fig. 2. Putative pathways of carotenoid biosynthesis in *Chlamydomonas*. Hypothetical zygospore-specific pathways are indicated by dotted arrows. For the enzymes of the pathways only abbreviations are given. DXS (1-deoxy-D-xylulose-5-phosphate synthetase, EC 2.2.1.7). DXR (1-deoxy-D-xylulose-5-phosphate reductoisomerase, EC 1.1.1.267). CMS (4-diphosphocytidil-2-C-methyl-D-erythriol synthase, EC 2.7.7.60). CMK (4-diphosphocytidil-2-C-methyl-D-erythriol kinase, EC 2.7.1.14.8). MCS (2-C-methyl-D-erythritol-2,4-cyclophosphate synthase, EC 4.6.1.12). HDS (4-hydroxy-3-methylbut-2-en-1-yl diphosphate synthase, EC 1.17.7.1). IDS (isopentenyl dimethylallyl diphosphate synthase, EC 1.17.1.2.3). IDI (isopentenyl-diphosphate delta-isomerase, EC 5.3.3.2). GGPPS (geranylgeranyl-diphosphate synthase, EC 2.5.1.81). PSY (phytoene synthase, EC 2.5.1.32). PDS (phytoene desaturase, EC 1.3.5.5). Z-ISO (ζ-Carotene isomerase); ZDS (ζ-carotene desaturase, EC 1.3.5.6). CRTISO (carotenoid isomerase, EC 5.2.1.13). LCYB (lycopene-β-cyclase). LCYE (lycopene-ε-cyclase), CHYB (carotene-β-hydroxylase, EC 1.14.13.-). CYP97A5 (carotene-β-hydroxylase, EC 1.14.13.129). CYP97C3 (carotene-ε-hydroxylase, EC 1.14.99.45). ZEP (zeaxanthin epoxidase, EC 1.14.13.90). VDE (violaxanthin epoxidase, EC 1.10.99.3). NSY (neoxanthin synthase, EC 5.3.99.9). LSY (loroxanthin synthase), and BKT (carotene-β-ketolase).

Carotenoid	Nutracetical effect	Reference
Lycopene	Antimutagenic effect	(Polivkova et al., 2010)
	Neuroprotective action	(Sandhir et al., 2010)
	Nephroprotective action	(Sahin et al., 2010)
	Prevent preclampsia	(Banerjee et al., 2009)
	Reduce risk of hip fracture	(Sahni et al., 2009)
	Antioxidant effect	(Erdman et al., 2009)
	Reduce eosinophil influx in asthma	(Wood et al., 2008)
	Cardioprotective effect against doxorubicin-caused damage	(Anjos Ferreira et al., 2007)
	Reduce inflammatory cytokines expression in pancreatitis	(Kim, 2011a; Kim, 2011b)
	Inhibit the growth and progression of colon cancer	(Tang et al., 2011)
	Enhanced antioxidant enzymes and immunity function in gastric cancer	(Luo & Wu, 2011)
	Inhibit NFκB-modulated IL-8 expression in macrophages-cigarette activated	(Simone et al., 2011)
	Reduced oxidative stress in allergic rhinitis	(Li et al., 2011b)
	Attenuated endothelial dysfunction in diabetes	(Zhu et al., 2011)
	Reduce cognitive decline in Parkinson's disease	(Kaur et al., 2011)
	Reduces LDC cholesterol and systolic blood pressure	(Ried & Fakler, 2011)
Asthaxanthin	Reduces endothelial dysfunction in diabetic rats	(Zhao et al., 2011)z
	Produces anxiolytic-like effects in mice	(Nishioka et al., 2011)
	Reduces oxidative stress and mitochondrial dysfunction in brain due MPTP/$MPTP^+$	(Lee et al., 2011)
	Reduce IL-6 microglia production	(Kim et al., 2010)
	Reduce blood pressure in hypertensive rats	(Monroy-Ruiz et al., 2011)
	Neuroprotective action against focal ischemia	(Lu et al., 2010)
	Attenuate thrombosis	(Khan et al., 2010)
	Reduce retinal injury in elevated intraocular pressure	(Cort et al., 2010)
	Reduce UVA - induced skins photoaging	(Suganuma et al., 2010)
	Hepatoprotective action	(Curek et al., 2010)

Table 2. Nutraceutical application of lycopene and astaxanthin.

Carotenoids are lipid soluble and in general they follow the same absorption pathway as lipids, however other mechanisms of absorption have been proposed. To learn more, read the review of Kotake-Nara and Nagao (Kotake-Nara & Nagao, 2011). Once in the bloodstream, carotenes are fundamentally ligated to low density lipoprotein (LDL) whereas the xanthophylls are more evenly distributed between high density lipoproteins (HDL) and low density lipoproteins (LDL). Nonpolar carotenoids (lycopene, α-carotene, β-carotene) are located in the hydrophobic core and the polar (xanthophylls) would be, at least in part, on the surface of lipoproteins (Furr & Clark, 1997). For the microalgae, carotenoids are synthesized in high concentrations under several different environmental conditions, and humans exploited these as nutraceuticals in food.

5. Nutraceutical effects of chlorophylls, PUFA and other vitamins

There are other components in microalgae that could modulate redox environment to prevent oxidative stress and can affect intracellular communication. These components are chlorophyll, PUFAs, and vitamins such as vitamin A, B, C, and E.

Microalgae, like all chloroplast-containing photosynthetic eukaryotes, synthesize chlorophyll pigments. In Chlorophyceae chorophylls a and b are the most predominant. The chlorophylls have a porphyrin ring structure similar to heme, but with a central nonreactive magnesium ion instead of iron. To review chlorophyll biosynthesis in microalgae, read the chapter of Beale (Beale, 2008). The information about the biological activities of chlorophyll as nutraceuticals is scarce. They do have antipoliferative (Wu et al., 2010) and antioxidant (Serpeloni et al., 2011) activities. The chlorophyllin-cooper complex, a water-soluble commercial version of chlorophyll, possesses antimutagenic (Chernomorsky et al., 1997) and anticancer activities (Chernomorsky et al., 1997). The other components of microalgae; PUFAs, and vitamins A, B, C, and E, could be a nutraceutical because there is much evidence of how they modulate intracellular signals and act as antioxidants.

6. *Chlorella* genus as nutraceutic

Chlorella species are encountered in all water habitats having cosmopolitan occurrences. The species of this genus have a simple form, a unicellular green alga belonging to the Chlorophyceae family. The *Chlorella* sp. is morphologically classified into four types; a) spherical cells (ratio of the two axes equals one), b) ellipsoidal cells (ratio of the longest axis to the shorter axis 1.45 to 1.60), spherical or ellipsoidal cells, and globular to subspherical cells. Their reproduction is asexual. Each mature cell divides usually producing four or eight (and more rarely 16) autospores, which are freed by rupture or dissolution of the parental walls.

Our research group has used *Chlorella vulgaris* as nutraceutical, particularly against mercury-caused oxidative stress and renal damage. For that we used male mice that were assigned into six groups; 1) a control group that received 100 mM phosphate buffer (PB) ig and 0.9% saline ip, 2) PB + $HgCl_2$ 5 mg/kg ip, 3) PB + 1000 mg/kg *Chlorella vulgaris* ig, and three groups receiving $HgCl_2$ + 250, 500, or 1000 mg/kg *Chlorella vulgaris* ig. The administration of the microalgae or PB was made 30 min before saline or $HgCl_2$ for 5 days. Our results demonstrated that $HgCl_2$ caused oxidative stress and cellular damage, whereas *Chlorella vulgaris* administration prevents oxidative stress (figure 3) and cellular damage (figure 4) in the kidney (Blas-Valdivia et al., 2011). We proposed that *Chlorella vulgaris's* carotenes play an important role in preventing $HgCl_2$-caused lipid peroxidation. Carotenes have a wide pharmacological spectrum of effects. The inhibition of lipid peroxidation may be caused by the free radical scavenging property of these compounds (Miranda et al., 2001). Carotenes can scavenge singlet oxygen and they terminate peroxides by their redox potential because of the hydroxyl group in its structure. Thus, the ROS-steady state is maintained in the kidney damage lower than in animals with mercury intoxication. The biochemical behavior of this microalgae against mercury-caused oxidative stress is similar to the purified component of cyanobacteria such as *Pseudoanabaena tenuis* (Cano-Europa et al., 2010) or *Spirulina maxima* (Sharma et al., 2007).

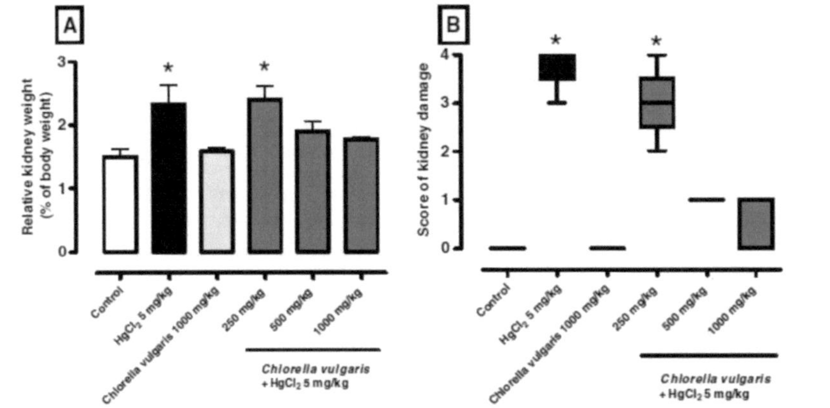

Fig. 3. Quantification of relative kidney weight (A) and the score of kidney damage (B) of mice treated with $HgCl_2$ and *Chlorella vulgaris*. In A each bar represents the mean ± S.E.M. In B each box represents the median ± intercuartilic space.* $P < 0.05$ vs. control. Author right permission. Springer ©.

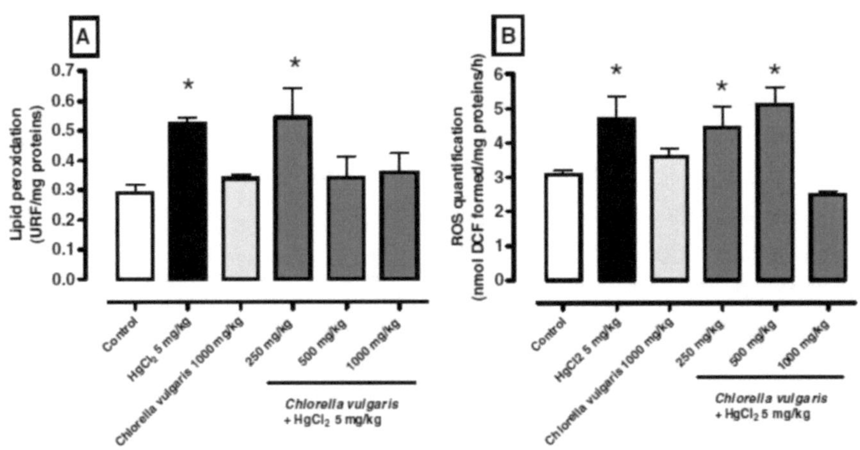

Fig. 4. Quantification of lipid peroxidation (A) and reactive oxygen species in the kidneys of mice treated with $HgCl_2$ and *Chlorella vulgaris*. Bar represents the mean ± S.E.M.* $P < 0.05$ vs. control. Author right permission. Springer ©.

Here are some experiments that demonstrated the nutraceutical use of *Chlorella (*Table 3*)*.

Study	Evidences
The administration of *Chlorella* sp. reduces endotoxemia, intestinal oxidative stress and bacterial traslocation in experimental biliary obstruction (Bedirli et al., 2009)	*Chlorella* administration inhibits bacterial culture and it avoids oxidative stress.
Hot water extract of *Chlorella vulgaris* induced DNA damage and apoptosis (Yusof et al., 2010)	The extract of *Chlorella vulgaris* inhibited DNA synthesis, causing apoptosis and it increases p53, caspase-3, and Bax expression in hepatoma cells (HEpG2)
Attenuating effect of *Chlorella* supplementation on oxidative stress and NFκB. Activation in peritoneal macrophages and liver of C57BL/6 mice fed on atherogenic diet (Lee et al., 2003)	*Chlorella* supplementation decreases the NFκB activation and superoxide anion production and because it increases SOD and catalase activity
Chlorella accelerates dioxin excretion in rats (Morita et al., 1999)	*Chlorella* enhanced dioxin metabolism and excretion by feces
Effect of *Chlorella* and its fractions on blood pressure, cerebral stroke lesions, and life-span in stroke-prone spontaneously hypertensive rats (Sansawa et al., 2006)	A *Chlorella* supplemented diet decreases blood pressure and the incidence rate of cerebral stroke in SHRSP.
Hypocholesterolemic mechanism of *Chlorella*: *Chlorella* and its indigestible fraction enhance hepatic cholesterol 7α-hydroxylase in rats (Shibata et al., 2007)	*Chlorella* powder increases the expression of CYP7A1, a limiting enzyme of the main pathway of the cholesterol catabolism, lowering the concentration of LDL in plasma
Chlorella vulgaris triggers apoptosis in hepatocarcinogenesis-induced rats (Mohd Azamai et al., 2009)	*Chlorella vulgaris* inhibits the anti-apoptotic protein Bcl-2
Effect of *Chlorella vulgaris* on lipid metabolism in Wistar rats fed high fat diet (Lee et al., 2008)	*Chlorella vulgaris* decreases HDL cholesterol concentration by a reduction in the intestinal absortion
Antioxidant effect of the marine algae *Chlorella vulgaris* against naphthalene-induced oxidative stress in the albino rats (Vijayavel et al., 2007)	*Chlorella vulgaris* inhibits production of free radicals, decreasing lipoperoxidation, and increasing the activity of antioxidant enzymes as SOD, catalase, GPX and reduced glutathione, preventing from the toxicity of naftalene
Six-week supplementation with *Chlorella* has favorable impact on antioxidant status in Korean male smokers (Lee et al., 2010)	*Chlorella* supplement exhibits antioxidant activity decreasing ROS and increasing the activity of SOD and catalase
Chlorella pyrenoidosa supplementation reduces the risk of anemia, proteinuria and edema in pregnant women (Nakano et al., 2010)	*Chlorella pyrenoidosa* exhibits an antiinflammatory activity regulated by cytokine. It increased the production of IL-10

Study	Evidences
Effect of *Chlorella* intake on cadmium metabolism in rats (Shim et al., 2009)	*Chlorella* inhibits cadmium absorption and it promotes the excretion through the feces. Also, it stimulates the production of metallothionein in the small intestine.
Isolation of phophorylated polysaccharides from algae: the inmmunostimulatory principle of *Chlorella pyrenoidosa* (Suarez et al., 2010)	The *Chlorella* polysaccharides increases the production of NO in macrophages enhancing the innate immune response, mediated by Toll-like receptors (TLR-4)
Influence of *Chlorella* powder intake during swimming stress in mice (Mizoguchi et al., 2011)	*Chlorella vulgaris* exhibits an antioxidant activity, reducing the lipoperoxidation, avoiding the DNA damage. However it does not show hypoglycemic activity

Table 3. Nutraceutical evidences of *Chlorella.*

7. *Chlamydomonas* genus as nutraceutic

Chlamydomonas spp. are unicellular algae with cell walls and with either two or four flagella. The genus *Chlamydomonas* is of worldwide distribution and is found in a diversity of habitats including temperate, tropical, and polar regions. *Chlamydomonas* species have been isolated from freshwater ponds and lakes, sewage ponds, marine and brackish waters, snow, garden and agricultural soil, forests, deserts, peat bogs, damp walls, sap on a wounded elm tree, an artificial pond on a volcanic island, mattress dust in the Netherlands, roof tiles in India, and a Nicaraguan hog wallow. These algae belong to the family *Chlamydomonadaceae* that consists of approximately 30 genera. DNA sequence analysis clearly demonstrates, however, that this family is composed of multiple phylogenetic lineages that do not correspond to the morphologically defined genera. Although the identities of the species are uncertain, it is noteworthy that the traits in which they differed included body shape, thickness of the cell wall, presence or absence of the apical papilla, lateral vs. basal position of the chloroplast, chloroplast position, and shape of the eyespot, all of which were later used as criteria to separate species. Although cell-body shape and size vary among *Chlamydomonas* species (as defined by morphological criteria), the overall polar structure, with paired apical flagella and basal chloroplast surrounding one or more pyrenoids, is constant. Cells are usually free-swimming in liquid media but on solid substrata may be nonflagellated, and are often seen in gelatinous masses similar to those of the algae *Palmella* or *Gloeocystis* in the order *Tetrasporales*. This condition has been referred to as a palmelloid state. Some species may also form asexual resting spores, or akinetes, in which the original vegetative cell wall becomes much thicker, and carotenoids, starch, and lipids may accumulate (Harris et al., 2008).

Our group has studied the nutraceutical properties of *Chlamydomonas gloeopara*, a microalgae collected from a eutrophic reservoir (La Piedad Lake) in Cuautitlan Izcalli, Mexico. That reservoir is located at 19°39′N (latitude) and 99°14′W (longitude). Our research group has used *Chlamydomonas gloeopara* as a nutraceutical, particularly against mercury-caused oxidative stress and renal damage. For that we used male mice that were assigned into six groups; 1) a control group that received 100 mM phosphate buffer (PB) ig and 0.9% saline ip, 2) PB + $HgCl_2$ 5 mg/kg ip, 3) PB + 1000 mg/kg *Chlamydomonas gloeopara* ig, and three groups receiving $HgCl_2$ + 250, 500, or 1000 mg/kg *Chlamydomonas gloeopara* ig. The administration of the microalgae or PB was made 30 min before saline or $HgCl_2$ for 5 days. Our results demonstrated that *Chlamydomonas gloeopara* as well as *Chlorella* prevents renal damage (figure 5, panel A-F) by reducing the oxidative stress of lipid peroxidation (figure 5, panel G).

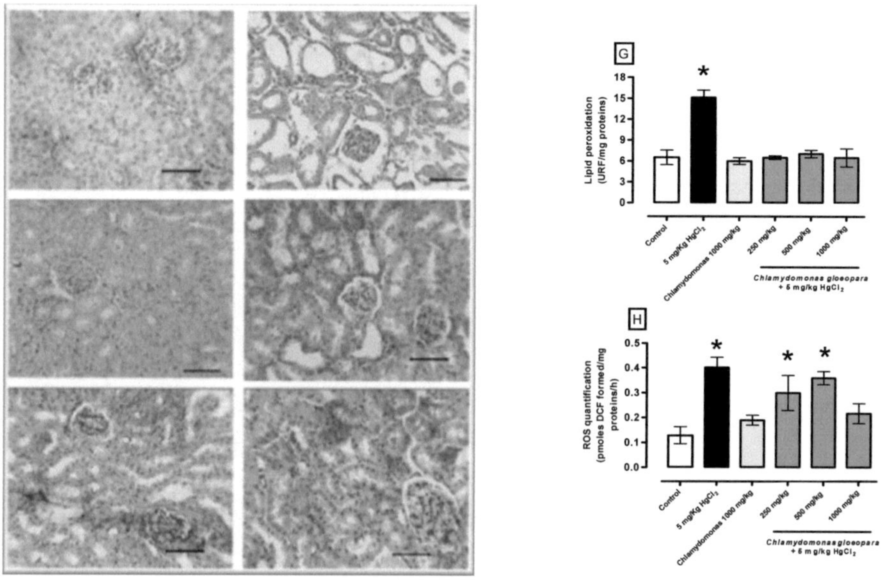

Fig. 5. Effect on *Chlamydomonas gloeopara* administation on $HgCl_2$-caused renal damage (panel A-F) and oxidative stress (panel G and H). Photomicrographs of renal cortex . Panel A shows control group. Panel B shows group treated with $HgCl_2$. Panel C shows group treated with *Chlamydomonas gloeopara* 1000 mg/kg . Panels D, E and F show groups treated with *Chlamydomonas gloeopara* 250, 500 and 1000 mg/kg plus $HgCl_2$. The tissue was stained by hematoxylin-eosin. Treatment with $HgCl_2$ causes cell atrophy, hyperchromatic nuclei, and edema. Histological alterations were partially ameliorated in groups treated with *Chlamydomonas gloeopara. Chlamydomonas gloeopara* administration reduced lipid peroxidation (G) and reactive oxygen species (H) in the kidneys of mice treated with $HgCl_2$ and *Chlorella vulgaris.* Bar is the mean ± SE * $P < 0.05$ vs. control.

8. *Haematococcus* genus as nutraceutic

Haematococcus are green microalgae; single-celled aquatic organisms. It is known that *Haematococcus* is the primarily source of astaxanthin, a ketocarotenoid that is a natural nutritional component. In the marine environment, astaxanthin is biosynthesized in the food chain, within the microalgae or phytoplankton, at the primary production level. When these algae are exposed to harsh environmental conditions and ultraviolet light, they accumulate the highest level of astaxanthin and in this process, the algae become blood red. Astaxanthin accumulates 2% to 3% of dry weight and constitutes 85% to 88% of the total carotenoids. Chemically it is a ketocarotenoid (3,3´-dihydroxy-β, β-carotene-4,4´dione) and is the principal pigment of salmonoids and shrimp. Astaxanthin has a higher antioxidant activity than lutein, lycopene, α or β-carotene, and α-tocopherol. Astaxanthin has 100 times and 10 times greater antioxidant activity than vitamin E and β-carotene (Guerin, 2003).

Morphological studies have shown that the algae have a life cycle. The, green vegetative cells with two flagellae grow autotrophycally in the light and heterotrophically in the dark. In culture, *H. pluvialis* has the typical characteristics of a motile stage, with biflagellate spherical cells. The growth in a bioreactor, with mechanical stirring, favors the occurrence of more or less mature aplanospores. This stage becomes dominant together with the evolution of growth. The aplanospore color turns gradually red, because of the accumulation of carotenoids in the chloroplast, and especially outside of them in lipid globules (astaxanthin). The red aplanospores are known as haematocysts. This stage may appear under stress conditions caused by light, high temperature, increased salinity, nutritional limitation, or change of carbon source. During the growth stage, the cells with a diameter of 30 μm were spherical to ellipsoid and enclosed by a cell wall. The cells had 2 flagellae of equal length emerging form an anterior papilla. As they age, the cells ceased to be mobile, yet the cellular structure remained the same without the flagellae. Under stress conditions, the volume of the cells increased to a diameter of > 40 μm and the cell wall became resistant. The maturation of the cyst cells was accompanied by enhanced carotenoid biosynthesis and a gradual change in cell color to red. When the cystic cells were transferred to optimal growth conditions, daughter cells were released from the cystic cells, and then vegetative cells regenerated from daughter cells (Cysewski & Todd Lorenz, 2004).

Haematococcus has the potential as a nutraceutical because there is various evidence of this. In table 4, we show some articles that employed *Haematococcus* or its astaxanthin.

Study	Evidences
Haematococcus astaxanthin: applications for human health and nutrition (Guerin, 2003)	This is a review about the uses of astaxantin from *Haematococcus* in health
Optimization of microwave-assisted extraction of astaxanthin from *Haematococcus pluvialis* by response surface methodology and antioxidant activities of the extracts (Zhao et al., 2009)	The extracts have a high antioxidant capacity, inhibit peroxidation of linoleic acid, and neutralize free radicals
Cardioprotection and myocardial salvage by a disodium disuccinate astaxanthin derivative (Cardax™) (Gross & Lockwood, 2004)	The astaxanthin is an antioxidant, antiinflammatory, and cardioprotective. reducer of levels of nitric oxide, tumor necrosis factor alpha, and prostaglandin E2
Ulcer preventive and antioxidative properties of astaxanthin from *Haematococcus pluvialis (Kamath et al., 2008)*	The astaxanthin exerts its gastroprotection of gastric ulceration by activation of antioxidant enzyme such as catalase, superoxide dismutase, and glutathione peroxidase. It inhibits the activity pump Na-K ATPase
Safety assessment of astaxanthin-rich microalgae biomass: acute and subchronic toxicity studies in	The administration of astaxanthin has no adverse effects

Study	Evidences
rats(Stewart et al., 2008)	
Astaxanthin, a carotenoid with potential in human health and nutrition (Hussein et al., 2006).	The antihypertensive and neuroprotective potentials of the compound
Protective effects of *Haematococcus* astaxanthin on oxidative stress in healthy smokers (Kim et al., 2011).	The results suggest that ASX supplementation might prevent oxidative damage in smokers by suppressing lipid peroxidation and stimulating the activity of the antioxidant system in smokers
Astaxanthin-rich extract from the green alga *Haematococcus pluvialis* lowers plasma lipid concentrations and enhances antioxidant defense in apolipoprotein E knockout mice (Yang et al., 2011)	It results suggest that supplementation of astaxanthin-rich *Haematococcus* extract improves cholesterol and lipid metabolism as well as antioxidant defense mechanisms, all of which could help mitigate the progression of atherosclerosis.

Table 4. Nutraceutical evidences of *Haematococcus.*

9. *Dunaliella* genus as nutreutic

Dunaliella salina is a unicelular green alga belonging to the Chlorophyceae family. *Dunaliella* cells are ovoid, spherical, pyriform, fusiform, or ellipsoid with sizes varying from 5 to 25 μm in length and from 3 to 13 μm in width. The cells also contain a single chloroplast, which mostly has a central pyrenoid surrounded by starch granules. *Dunaliella* multiplies by lengthwise division, but sexual reproduction does occur rarely by isogametes with a conjugation process. It proliferates in extremely varied salinities from 0.5 to 5.0 M NaCl. The alga cells do not contain a rigid cell wall; instead a thin elastic membrane surrounds them. It is known to accumulate carotenoids under various stress conditions. It possesses a remarkable degree of environmental adaptation by producing an excess of β-carotene and glycerol to maintain its osmotic balance. β-carotene occurs naturally as its isomers, namely, all-*trans*, 9-*cis*, 13-*cis*, and 15-*cis* forms and functions as an accessory light harvesting pigment, thereby protecting the photosynthetic apparatus against photo damage in all green plants including algae. β-carotene, a component of the photosynthetic reaction center is accumulated as lipid globules in the interthylakoid spaces of the chloroplasts of *Dunaliella.* They protect the algae from damage obtained during excessive irradiance by preventing the formation of reactive oxygen species, by quenching the triplet-state chlorophyll, or by reacting with singlet oxygen ($^1O_2$) and also act as a light filter (Ben-Amotz, 2004). *Dunaliella* nutraceutical properties are shown in table

Study	Conclusion
In vivo antioxidant activity of carotenoids from *Dunaliella salina* a green microalga (Chidambara-Murthy et al., 2005)	Carotenoids provide protection against CCl_4-caused hepatic damage by restoring the activity of hepatic enzymes like peroxidase, super oxide dismutase, and catalase, which reduce ROS and lipid peroxidation.

Study	Conclusion
9-*cis* β-carotene-rich powder of the alga *Dunaliella bardawil* increases plasma HDL-cholesterol in fibrate-treated patients (Shaish et al., 2006)	*Dunaliella* treatment increases plasma HDL-cholesterol and lower plasma triglyceride levels
Ethanol extract of *Dunaliella salina* induces cell cycle arrest and apoptosis in A545 human non-small cell lung cancer cells (Sheu et al., 2008)	Ethanol extract of *Dunaliella salina* inhibits cell proliferation and causes apoptosis possibly via p53 and p21 promoting the protein expression of Fas and FasL
Protective effects of *Dunaliella salina* against experimental induced fibrosarcoma on Wistar rats (Raja et al., 2007).	The *chlorophyta* has a protective effect against experimentally caused fibrosarcoma
Bioavailability of the isomer mixture of phytoene and phytofluene-rich alga *Dunaliella bardawil* in rat plasma and tissues (Werman et al., 2002).	9-*cis* phytoene has a stronger antioxidative effect than the all trans isomer
Hypercholesterolemia induced oxidative stress is reduced in rats with diets enriched with supplement from *Dunaliella salina* algae (Bansal & Sapna, 2011).	*Dunaliella salina* components inhibit lipid peroxidation and also increases Type1 5´-iodothyronine deiodinase (5´-DI) expression, which leads to a T_3 level increase
Evaluation of carotenoid extract from *Dunaliella salina* against cadmium-induced cytotoxicity and transforming growth factor β1 induced expression of smooth muscle α-actin with rat liver cell lines (Jau-Tien et al., 2011).	Carotenoid extract of *Dunaliella salina* contains abundant *cis* and *trans* β-carotenes. These antioxidants decrease the lipid peroxidation and also inhibit activation of hepatic stellate cells (HSCs).
Protective effects of *Dunaliella salina*- a carotenoids-rich alga, against carbon tetrachloride-induced hepatotoxicity in mice (Hsu et al., 2008).	Carotenoids of *D. salina* inhibit the lipid peroxidation and increases the antioxidant enzyme activity

Table 5. Nutraceutical evidences of *Dunaliella.*

10. Final remarks

The functional food and nutraceutical market is growing. However, to promote health the active compounds must be ingested in high concentration. This is a great problem because sometimes the components such as carotenoids, polyphenols, and chlorophylls are extracted from vegetables or plants. In their production, we are modifying the environment, thus the use of biotechnology of microalgae or other microorganisms like bacteria or fungus could be an alternative because they may be environmentally friendly. The sun can be used as energy source and the medium could be fresh or sea water, with the carbon source as CO_2 and other inorganic or organic sources. In this chapter we show the evidence of some genera, particularly of Chlorophyceae class as *Chlorella, Chlamydomonas, Haematococcus,* and *Dunaliella.* It is evident that their components modulate intracellular communication and they act as antioxidants.

There are many microalgae never used as nutraceuticals that could be used for human or animal health, such as the microalgae used in aquaculture to fed shrimp and fish. Examples of those kinds of microalgi are *Pavlova* and *Tetraselmis* that produce high concentration of PUFAs.

11. Acknowledgement

This study was partially supported by SIP-IPN 20110283 y 20110336. Thanks to Dr. Ellis Glazier for editing this English-language text.

12. References

Actis-Goretta,L., Ottaviani,J.I. & Fraga,C.G. (2006). Inhibition of angiotensin converting enzyme activity by flavanol-rich foods. *Journal Agriculture Food Chemestry* Vol.54, No. 1,(January 2006), pp. 229-234, ISNN 0021-8561

Anjos Ferreira,A.L., Russell,R.M., Rocha,N., Placido Ladeira,M.S., Favero Salvadori,D.M., Oliveira,N., Matsui,M., Carvalho,F.A., Tang,G., Matsubara, L.S. & Matsubara,B.B. (2007). Effect of lycopene on doxorubicin-induced cardiotoxicity: an echocardiographic, histological and morphometrical assessment. *Basic and Clinical Pharmacology and Toxicology* Vol.101, No.1,(July 2007) pp. 16-24, ISSN 1742-7843

Armstrong,G.A. & Hearst,J.E. (1996). Carotenoids 2: Genetics and molecular biology of carotenoid pigment biosynthesis. *FASEB Journal* Vol.10, No.2,(February 1996), pp. 228-237, ISSN 0950-9232

Balk,R. (2011). Roger C. Bone, MD and the evolving paradigms of sepsis. *Contributions to Microbioly* Vol.17, pp.1-11,(January 2011), ISSN 14209519

Banerjee,S., Jeyaseelan,S. & Guleria,R. (2009). Trial of lycopene to prevent pre-eclampsia in healthy primigravidas: results show some adverse effects. *Journal of Obstetrics and Gynaecology Research* Vol.35, No.2, pp.477-482,(June 2009), ISSN (printed).

Bansal,M. & Sapna,J. (2011). Hypercholesterolemia induced oxidative stress is reduced in rats with diets enriched with supplement from Dunaliella salina algae. *Americal Journal of Biomedical Science* Vol.1, pp.196-204, ISSN 14230127

Beale,S.I. (2008). Biosynthesis of chlorophylls and heme. In The *Chlamydomonas* Sourcebook, eds. Harris,E.H., Stern,D.B. & Witman,G.B., USA: Academic Press.

Bedirli,A., Kerem,M., Ofluoglu,E., Salman,B., Katircioglu,H., Bedirli,N., Ylmazer,D., Alper,M., and Pasaoglu,H. Administration of *Chlorella* sp. microalgae reduces endotoxemia, intestinal oxidative stress and bacterial translocation in experimental biliary obstruction. *Clinical nutrition* (Edinburgh, Scotland) Vol.28, No.6, pp.674-678,(December 2009), ISSN 0261-5614

Ben-Amotz,A. (2004). Industrial production of microalgal cell-mass and secondary products. Major industrial species: *Dunaliella. In Handbook of microalgal culture: Biotechnology and applied Phycology*, ed. Richmond Amos, pp. 273-280. Australia: Blackwell science.

Bernal,J., Mendiola,J.A., Ibanez,E. & Cifuentes,A. (2011). Advanced analysis of nutraceuticals. Journal of Pharmaceutical and Biomedical Analysis Vol.55, No.4, pp.758-774,(June 2011), ISNN 0731-7085

Bertrand,M. (2010). Carotenoid biosynthesis in diatoms. *Photosynthesis Research* Vol.106, No. 1-2, pp.89-102,(November 2010), ISNN 01668595

Biesalski,H.K. (2007). Polyphenols and inflammation: basic interactions. *Current Opinion in Clinical Nutrition and Metabolic Care* Vol.10, No.6, pp.724-728,(November 2007), ISNN 1473-6519.

Blas-Valdivia,V., Ortiz-Butron,R., Pineda-Reynoso,M., Hernandez-Garcia,A. & Cano-Europa,E. (2011). *Chlorella vulgaris* administration prevents $HgCl_2$-caused oxidative stress and cellular damage in the kidney. *Journal of Applied Phycology* Vol.23, No.1, pp.53-58,(February 2011), ISNN 1573-5176

Cano-Europa,E., Ortiz-Butron,R., Blas-Valdivia,V., Pineda-Reynoso,M., Olvera-Ramírez,R. & Franco-Colín,M. (2010). Phycobiliproteins from *Pseudanabaena tenuis* rich in c-phycoerythrin protect against $HgCl_2$-caused oxidative stress and cellular damage in the kidney. Journal of Applied Phycology Vol.22, No. 4, pp.495-501, ISSN 0921-8971

Cazzonelli,C.I. & Pogson,B.J. (2010). Source to sink: regulation of carotenoid biosynthesis in plants. *Trends in Plant Science* Vol.15, No.5, pp.266-274, (May 2010), ISSN 1360-1385

Celiz,G., Daz,M. & Audisio,M.C. (2011). Antibacterial activity of naringin derivatives against pathogenic strains. *Journal of Applied Microbiology* Vol.111, No.3, pp.731-738,(September 2011), ISSN 1364-5072

Chan,C.M., Fang,J.Y., Lin,H.H., Yang,C.Y. & Hung,C.F. (2009). Lycopene inhibits PDGF-BB-induced retinal pigment epithelial cell migration by suppression of PI3K/Akt and MAPK pathways. *Biochemical and Biophysical Research Communications* Vol.388, No.1, pp.172-176,(October 2009), ISSN 0006-291X

Chao,C.L., Weng,C.S., Chang,N.C., Lin,J.S., Kao,S.T. & Ho,F.M. (2010). Naringenin more effectively inhibits inducible nitric oxide synthase and cyclooxygenase-2 expression in macrophages than in microglia. *Nutrition Research* Vol.30, No.12, pp.858-864, (December 2010), ISSN 0271-5317

Chernomorsky,S., Rancourt,R., Virdi,K., Segelman,A. & Poretz,R.D. (1997). Antimutagenicity, cytotoxicity and composition of chlorophyllin copper complex. *Cancer Letters* Vol.120, No.2, pp.141-147, (December 1997), ISSN 0304-3835

Chidambara-Murthy,K., Vanitha,A., Rajesha,J., Mahadeva-Swamy,M., Sowmya,P. & Ravishankar,G. (2005). In vivo antioxidant activity of carotenoids from Dunaliella s salina--a green microalga. *Life Sciences* Vol.76, No.12, pp.1381-1390,(February 2005), ISSN 0024-3205.

Corradini,E., Foglia,P., Giansanti,P., Gubbiotti,R., Samperi,R. & Lagana,A. (2011). Flavonoids: chemical properties and analytical methodologies of identification and quantitation in foods and plants. *Natural Products Research* Vol.25, No.5, pp.469-495, (March 2011), ISNN 1478-6427

Cort,A., Ozturk,N., Akpinar,D., Unal,M., Yucel,G., Ciftcioglu,A., Yargicoglu,P. & Aslan,M. (2010). Suppressive effect of astaxanthin on retinal injury induced by elevated intraocular pressure. *Regulatory Toxicology and Pharmacology* Vol.58, No.1, pp.121-130,(October 2010), ISNN 0273-2300

Curek,G.D., Cort,A., Yucel,G., Demir,N., Ozturk,S., Elpek,G.O., Savas,B. & Aslan,M. (2010). Effect of astaxanthin on hepatocellular injury following ischemia/reperfusion. *Toxicology* Vol.267, No.1-3, pp.147-153, (January 2010), ISNN 0300-483X

Cvorovic,J., Tramer,F., Granzotto,M., Candussio,L., Decorti,G. & Passamonti,S. (2010). Oxidative stress-based cytotoxicity of delphinidin and cyanidin in colon cancer cells. *Archives of Biochemistry and Biophysics Vol.*501, No.1, pp.151-157, (October 2010), ISSN 0003-9861

Cysewski,G.R. & Todd Lorenz,R. (2004). Industrial production of microalgal cell-mass and secondary products. Species of high potential: Haematococcus. In Handbook of Microalgal Culture: Biotechnology and Applied Phycology, ed. Richmond Amos, pp. 281-288

Degenhardt,J., Kollner,T.G. & Gershenzon,J. (2009). Monoterpene and sesquiterpene synthases and the origin of terpene skeletal diversity in plants. Phytochemistry Vol.70, No.15-16, pp.1621-1637, (October 2010), ISNN 0031-9422

Du,W.X., Olsen,C.W., Avena-Bustillos,R.J., Friedman,M. & McHugh,T.H. (2011). Physical and antibacterial properties of edible films formulated with apple skin polyphenols. Journal of Food Science Vol.76, No.2, pp.M149-M155, (March 2011), ISNN 1750-3841

Elmarakby,A.A., Ibrahim,A.S., Faulkner,J., Mozaffari,M.S., Liou,G.I. & Abdelsayed,R. (2011). Tyrosine kinase inhibitor, genistein, reduces renal inflammation and injury in streptozotocin-induced diabetic mice. *Vascular Pharmacology*, (July 2011), In press, ISNN 1537-1891

Erdman,J.W., Balentine,D., Arab,L., Beecher,G., Dwyer,J.T., Folts,J., Harnly,J., Hollman,P., Keen,C.L., Mazza,G., Messina,M., Scalbert,A., Vita,J., illiamson,G. & urrowes,J. (2007). Flavonoids and heart health: Proceedings of the ILSI North America Flavonoids Workshop, May 31-June 1, 2005, Washington, DC. *The Journal of Nutrition* Vol.137, No. 3, pp.718S-7737,(March 2007), ISNN 1541-6100

Erdman,J.W., Ford,N.A. & Lindshield,B.L. (2009). Are the health attributes of lycopene related to its antioxidant function? *Archives of Biochemistry and Biophysics* Vol.483, No.2, pp.229-235, (March 2009), ISNN 003-9861.

Fontana Pereira,D., Cazarolli,L.H., Lavado,C., Mengatto,V., Figueiredo,M.S., Guedes,A., Pizzolatti,M.G. & Silva,F.R. (2011). Effects of flavonoids on α-glucosidase activity: Potential targets for glucose homeostasis. *Nutrition* Epv_ahead of print, (July 2011), ISNN 0899-9007

Fowler,Z.L. & Koffas,M.A. (2009). Biosynthesis and biotechnological production of flavanones: current state and perspectives. *Applied Microbioogyl and Biotechnology* Vol.83, No.5, pp.799-808, (July 2009), ISNN 1432-0614

Funakoshi-Tago,M., Nakamura,K., Tago,K., Mashino,T. & Kasahara,T. (2011). Anti-inflammatory activity of structurally related flavonoids, Apigenin, Luteolin and Fisetin. *International Immunopharmacology* Vol.11, No.9, pp.1150-1159, (September 2011), ISNN 1567-5769

Furr,H.C. & Clark,R.M. (1997). Intestinal absorption and tissue distribution of carotenoids. *Nutrional Biochemistry* Vol.8, pp.364-377, (1997), ISNN 0955-2863

Ganjare,A.B., Nirmal,S.A. & Patil,A.N. (2011). Use of apigenin from Cordia dichotoma in the treatment of colitis. *Fitoterapia* In press (June 2011), ISNN 0367-326X

Gasiorowski,K., Lamer-Zarawska,E., Leszek,J., Parvathaneni,K., Yendluri,B.B., Blach-Olszewska,Z. & Aliev,G. (2011). Flavones from root of Scutellaria baicalensis Georgi: drugs of the future in neurodegeneration? *CNS and Neurological Disorders-Drug Targets* Vol. 10, No.2, pp.184-191, (March 2011), ISNN 1871-5273

Grassi,D., Desideri,G., Croce,G., Tiberti,S., Aggio,A. & Ferri,C. (2009). Flavonoids, vascular function and cardiovascular protection. *Current Pharmaceutical Design* Vol. 15, No. 10, pp. 1072-1084 (January, 2009) ISSN 1381-6128

Gross,G.J. & Lockwood,S.F. (2004). Cardioprotection and myocardial salvage by a disodium disuccinate astaxanthin derivative (Cardax™). *Life Sciences* Vol. 75 No. 2 , pp 215-224 (May, 2004) ISSN 0024-3205

Guerin,M. (2003). Haematococcus astaxanthin: applications for human health and nutrition. *Trends in Biotechnology* Vol. 21, No. 5, pp 210-216, (May, 2003) ISSN 0167-7799

Hardy,G. (2000). Nutraceuticals and functional foods: introduction and meaning. *Nutrition* Vol. 16, No. 7-8,pp 688-689 (July, 2000) ISSN 0899-9007

Hargrove,J.L., Greenspan,P., Hartle,D.K. & Dowd,C. (2011). Inhibition of aromatase and α-amylase by flavonoids and proanthocyanidins from *Sorghum bicolor* bran extracts. *Journal Medical and Food* Vol. 14,No.7-8 , pp 799-807 (July,2011) ISSN 1557-7600

Harris,E.H., Stern,D.B. & Witman,G.B. (2008). The genus *Chlamydomonas*. In The *Chlamydomonas* Sourcebook, eds. Harris,E.H., Stern,D.B. & Witman,G.B., USA: Academic Press.

Heyman,R.A., Mangelsdorf,D.J., Dyck,J.A., Stein,R.B., Eichele,G., Evans,R.M. & Thaller,C. (1992). 9-cis retinoic acid is a high affinity ligand for the retinoid X receptor. *Cell* Vol. 68, No. 2, pp 397-406 (January, 1992) ISSN 0096-8674

Hirose,E., Matsushima,M., Takagi,K., Ota,Y., Ishigami,K., Hirayama,T., Hayashi,Y., Nakamura,T., Hashimoto,N., Imaizumi,K., Baba,K., Hasegawa,Y. & Kawabe,T. (2009). Involvement of heme oxygenase-1 in kaempferol-induced anti-allergic actions in RBL-2H3 cells. *Inflammation* Vol. 32, No. 2, pp 99-108 (April, 2009) ISSN 1466-1861

Hsu,C.L. & Yen,G.C. (2006). Induction of cell apoptosis in 3T3-L1 pre-adipocytes by flavonoids is associated with their antioxidant activity. Molecular *Nutrition & Food Research* Vol. 50, No. 11, pp 1072-1079 (November, 2006) ISSN 1613-4133

Hsu,Y., Tsai,C., Chang,W., Ho,Y., Chen,W. & Lu,F. (2008). Protective effects of *Dunaliella salina*--a carotenoids-rich alga, against carbon tetrachloride-induced hepatotoxicity in mice. *Food and Chemical Toxicology* Vol. 46, No. 10,pp 3311-3317 (October, 2008) ISSN 0278-6915

Hussein,G., Sankawa,U., Goto,H., Matsumoto,K. & Watanabe,H. (2006). Astaxanthin, a carotenoid with potential in human health and nutrition. *Journal Natural Products* Vol. 69, No. 3, pp 443-449 (March, 2003) ISSN 0970-129X

Jackson,H., Braun,C.L. & Ernst,H. (2008). The chemistry of novel xanthophyll carotenoids. *American Journal of Cardiology* Vol. 101, no 10A, pp 50D-57D (May, 2008) ISSN 0002-9149

Jang,Y.J., Kim,J., Shim,J., Kim,J., Byun,S., Oak,M.H., Lee,K.W. & Lee,H.J. (2011). Kaempferol Attenuates 4-hydroxynonenal-induced apoptosis in PC12 Cclls by directly inhibiting NADPH oxidase. *Journal of Pharmacology And Experimental Therapeutics* vol. 337, No. 3, pp 747-754 (June, 2011) ISSN 0022-3565

Jau-Tien,L., Ying-Chung,L., Chao-chin,H., You-Cheng,S., Fung-Jou,L. & Deng-Jye,Y. (2011). Evaluation of carotenoid extract from *Dunaliella salina* against cadmium-induced cytotoxicity and transforming qrowth factor b1 induced expression of smooth muscle a-actin with rat liver cell lines. *Journal of Food Science* Vol. 18, pp 301-306 (2011) ISSN 1750-3841

Kamath,B.S., Srikanta,B.M., Dharmesh,S.M., Sarada,R. & Ravishankar,G.A. (2008). Ulcer preventive and antioxidative properties of astaxanthin from *Haematococcus pluvialis*. *Europe Journal of Pharmacology* Vol. 590, No. 1-3, pp 387-395 (August, 2008) ISSN 0014-2999

Kaur,H., Chauhan,S. & Sandhir,R. (2011). Protective effect of lycopene on oxidative stress and cognitive decline in rotenone induced model of Parkinson's disease. *Neurochemical Reserch* Vol. 36, No.8, pp 1435-1443 (August ,2011) ISSN 1573-6903

Khan,S.K., Malinski,T., Mason,R.P., Kubant,R., Jacob,R.F., Fujioka,K., Denstaedt,S.J., King,T.J., Jackson,H.L., Hieber,A.D., Lockwood,S.F., Goodin,T.H., Pashkow,F.J. & Bodary,P.F. (2010). Novel astaxanthin prodrug (CDX-085) attenuates thrombosis in a mouse model. *Thrombosis Reserch* Vol. 126, No. 4, pp 299-305 (October, 2010) ISSN 0049-3848

Kim,H. (2011). Inhibitory mechanism of lycopene on cytokine expression in experimental pancreatitis. *Annals of the New York Academy of Sciences* Vol. 1229, No 1, pp 99-102 (July, 2011) ISSN 0077-8923

Kim,J.H., Chang,M.D., Choi,H.D., You,Y.K., Kim,J.T., Oh,J.M., and Shin,W.G. Protective effects of *Haematococcus* astaxanthin on oxidative stress in healthy smokers. *Journal of Medicinal Food* In press (2011) ISSN 1557-7600

Kim,J.S., Kwon,C.S. & Son,K.H. (2000). Inhibition of alpha-glucosidase and amylase by luteolin, a flavonoid. *Bioscience, Biotechnology, and Biochemistry* Vol. 64,No. 11, pp 2458-2461 (November, 2000) ISNN 0916-8451

Kim,Y.H., Koh,H.K. & Kim,D.S. (2010). Down-regulation of IL-6 production by astaxanthin via ERK-, MSK-, and NF-κB-mediated signals in activated microglia. *International Immunopharmacology* Vol. 10, No. 12, pp 1560-1572 (December, 2010) ISNN 1567-5769

Kinghorn,A.D., Su,B.N., Jang,D.S., Chang,L.C., Lee,D., Gu,J.Q., Carcache-Blanco,E.J., Pawlus,A.D., Lee,S.K., Park,E.J., Cuendet,M., Gills,J.J., Bhat,K., Park,H.S., Mata-Greenwood,E., Song,L.L., Jang,M. & Pezzuto,J.M. (2004). Natural inhibitors of carcinogenesis. *Planta Medica* Vol. 70, No. 8, pp 691-705 (August, 2004) ISNN 0032-0943

Kontogiorgis,C., Mantzanidou,M. & Hadjipavlou,L. (2008). Chalcones and their potential role in inflammation. *Mini-Reviews in Medicinal Chemistry* Vol. 8, No. 12, pp 1224-1242 (December, 2008) ISNN 1389-5575

Kotake-Nara,E. & Nagao,A. (2011). Absorption and metabolism of xanthophylls. *Marine Drugs* Vol. 9, No.6, pp 1024-1037 (January, 2011) ISSN 1660-3397

Kumar,A., Katiyar,S.B., Agarwal,A. & Chauhan,P.M. (2003). Perspective in antimalarial chemotherapy. *Current Medicinal Chemistry* Vol. 10, No. 13 , pp 1137-1150 (July, 2003) ISNN 1070-3632

Kwon,O., Eck,P., Chen,S., Corpe,C.P., Lee,J.H., Kruhlak,M. & Levine,M. (2007). Inhibition of the intestinal glucose transporter GLUT2 by flavonoids. *FASEB Journal* Vol. 21, No. 2, pp 366-377(February, 2007) ISNN 0717-7712

Lagoa,R., Lopez-Sanchez,C., Samhan-Arias,A.K., Ganan,C.M., Garcia-Martinez,V. & Gutierrez-Merino,C. (2009). Kaempferol protects against rat striatal degeneration induced by 3-nitropropionic acid. *Journal of Neurochemistry* Vol. 111, No. 2, pp 473-487(October, 2009) ISNN 1566-5240

Lee,D.H., Kim,C.S. & Lee,Y.J. (2011). Astaxanthin protects against MPTP/MPP+-induced mitochondrial dysfunction and ROS production in vivo and in vitro. *Food and Chemical Toxicology* Vol. 49, No. 1, pp 271-280 (January, 2011) ISSN 0278-6915

Lee,H.S., Choi,C.Y., Cho,C. & Song,Y. (2003). Attenuating effect of chlorella supplementation on oxidative stress and NFkappaB activation in peritoneal macrophages and liver of C57BL/6 mice fed on an atherogenic diet. *Bioscience, Biotechnology, and Biochemistry* Vol. 67, No. , pp 2083-2090 (October, 2003) ISSN 1347-6947

Lee,H.S., Park,H.J. & Kim,M.K. (2008). Effect of Chlorella vulgaris on lipid metabolism in Wistar rats fed high fat diet. *Nutrition Research and Practice* Vol. 2, No. 4, pp 204-210 (December, 2008) ISSN 0271-5317

Lee,J.S. (2006). Effects of soy protein and genistein on blood glucose, antioxidant enzyme activities, and lipid profile in streptozotocin-induced diabetic rats. *Life Sciences* Vol. 79, No. 16, pp 1578-1584 (September, 2006) ISSN 0024-3205

Lee,S.H., Kang,H.J., Lee,H.J., Kang,M.H. & Park,Y.K. (2010). Six-week supplementation with *Chlorella* has favorable impact on antioxidant status in Korean male smokers. *Nutrition* Vol. 26, No. 2, pp 175-183 (February, 2010) ISSN 0029-6643

Li,W., Frame,L.T., Hoo,K.A., Li,Y., D'Cunha,N. & Cobos,E. (2011a). Genistein inhibited proliferation and induced apoptosis in acute lymphoblastic leukemia, lymphoma and multiple myeloma cells in vitro. *Leukemia and Lymphoma* In press (July, 2011) ISSN 1029-2403

Li,X.L., Zhou,A.G., Zhang,L. & Chen,W.J. (2011b). Antioxidant status and immune activity of glycyrrhizin in allergic rhinitis mice. *International Journal of Molecular Sciences* Vol. 12, No. 2, pp 905-916 (January, 2011) ISSN 1422-0067

Liu,I.M., Tzeng,T.F., Liou,S.S. & Chang,C.J. (2012). Beneficial effect of traditional chinese medicinal formula danggui-shaoyao-san on advanced glycation end-product-mediated renal injury in streptozotocin-diabetic rats. *Evidence-based Complementary and Alternative Medicine* In press(January, 2012) ISSN 1741- 427X

Lohr,M., Im,C.S. & Grossman,A.R. (2005). Genome-based examination of chlorophyll and carotenoid biosynthesis in *Chlamydomonas reinhardtii*. Plant Physiology Vol. 138, No. 1, pp 490-515 (May, 2005) ISSN 1040-4651

Lohr,M. (2008). Carotenoids. In The *Chlamydomonas* Sourcebook, eds. Harris,E.H., Stern,D.B. & Witman,G.B., USA: Academic Press.

Lu,Y.P., Liu,S.Y., Sun,H., Wu,X.M., Li,J.J. & Zhu,L. (2010). Neuroprotective effect of astaxanthin on H_2O_2-induced neurotoxicity in vitro and on focal cerebral ischemia in vivo. *Brain Research* Vol. 1360, pp 40-48 (November, 2010) ISSN 0006-8993

Luo,C. & Wu,X.G. (2011). Lycopene enhances antioxidant enzyme activities and immunity function in N-Methyl-N'-nitro-N-nitrosoguanidine-induced gastric cancer rats. *International Journal of Molecular Sciences* Vol. 12, No. 5, pp 3340-3351 (January, 2011) ISSN 1422-0067

Mahat,M.Y., Kulkarni,N.M., Vishwakarma,S.L., Khan,F.R., Thippeswamy,B.S., Hebballi,V., Adhyapak,A.A., Benade,V.S., Ashfaque,S.M., Tubachi,S. & Patil,B.M. (2010). Modulation of the cyclooxygenase pathway via inhibition of nitric oxide production contributes to the anti-inflammatory activity of kaempferol. *European Journal of Pharmacology* Vol. 642, No.1-3, pp 169-176 (September, 2010) ISSN 0014-2999

Manach,C., Scalbert,A., Morand,C., Remesy,C. & Jimenez,L. (2004). Polyphenols: food sources and bioavailability. *American Journal of Clinical Nutrition* Vol. 79, No. 5, pp 727-747 (May, 2004) ISSN 0002-9165

Mandel,S., Packer,L., Youdim,M.B. & Weinreb,O. (2005). Proceedings from the "Third International Conference on Mechanism of Action of Nutraceuticals". *The Journal of | Nutritional Biochemistry* Vol. 16,No.9 , pp 513-520 (September, 2005) ISSN 0955-2863

Mena,N.P., Bulteau,A.L., Salazar,J., Hirsch,E.C. & Nunez,M.T. (2011). Effect of mitochondrial complex I inhibition on Fe-S cluster protein activity. *Biochemical and Biophysical Research Communications* Vol. 409, No. 2, pp 241-246 (June, 2011) ISSN 0006-291X

Miranda,C.L., Stevens,J.F., Ivanov,V., McCall,M., Frei,B., Deinzer,M.L. & Buhler,D.R. (2000). Antioxidant and prooxidant actions of prenylated and nonprenylated chalcones and flavanones in vitro. *Journal of Agricultural and Food Chemistry* Vol. 48, No.9 , pp 3876-3884 (September, 2000) ISSN 0021-8561

Miranda,M.S., Sato,S. & Mancini-Filho,J. (2001). Antioxidant activity ono.f the microalga *Chlorella vulgaris* cultered on special conditions. *Bollettino Chimico Farmaceutico* Vol. 140, No.3 , pp 165-168 (May,2001) ISSN 0006-6648

Mirshekar,M., Roghani,M., Khalili,M., Baluchnejadmojara...,T. & Arab Moazzen,S. (2010). Chronic oral pelargonidin alleviates streptozotocin-induced diabetic neuropathic hyperalgesia in rat: involvement of oxidative stress. *The Iranian Biomedical Journal* Vol. 14, No. 1-2, pp 33-39 (January, 2010) ISSN 1028-852X

Mizoguchi,T., Arakawa,Y., Kobayashi,M. & Fujishima,M. (2011). Influence of Chlorella powder intake during swimming stress in mice. *Biochemical and Biophysical Research Communications* Vol. 404, No. 1, pp 121-126 (January, 2011) ISSN 0006-291X

Mohan,N., Banik,N.L. & Ray,S.K. (2011). Combination of N-(4-hydroxyphenyl) retinamide and apigenin suppressed starvation-induced autophagy and promoted apoptosis in malignant neuroblastoma cells. *Neuroscience Letters* Vol. 502, No.1, pp 24-29 (September, 2011) ISSN 0304-3940

Mohd Azamai,E.S., Sulaiman,S., Mohd Habib,S.H., Looi,M.L., Das,S., Abdul Hamid,N.A., Wan Ngah,W.Z. & Mohd Yusof,Y.A. (2009). Chlorella vulgaris triggers apoptosis in hepatocarcinogenesis-induced rats. *Journal of Zheijang University SCIENCE B* Vol. 10, No. 1, pp 14-21 (January, 2009) ISSN 1862-1783

Mojzis,J., Varinska,L., Mojzisova,G., Kostova,I. & Mirossay,L. (2008). Antiangiogenic effects of flavonoids and chalcones. *Pharmacal Research* Vol. 57, No. 4, pp 259-265 (April, 2008) ISSN 1976-3786

Monroy-Ruiz,J., Sevilla,M., Carron,R. & Montero,M.J. (2011). Astaxanthin-enriched-diet reduces blood pressure and improves cardiovascular parameters in spontaneously hypertensive rats. *Pharmacal Research* Vol. 63, No.1, pp 44-50 (January, 2011) ISSN 1976-3786

Morita,K., Matsueda,T., Iida,T. & Hasegawa,T. (1999). Chlorella Accelerates Dioxin Excretion in Rats. *The Journal of Nutrition* Vol 129, No. 9, pp 1731-1736 (September, 1999) ISSN 0022-3166

Nakai,M., Fukui,Y., Asami,S., Toyoda-Ono,Y., Iwashita,T., Shibata,H., Mitsunaga,T., Hashimoto,F. & Kiso,Y. (2005). Inhibitory effects of oolong tea polyphenols on pancreatic lipase in vitro. *The Journal of Agricultural and Food Chemistry* Vol.53, No. 11, pp 4593-4598 (June, 2006) ISSN 0021-8561

Nakano,S., Takekoshi,H. & Nakano,M. (2010). Chlorella pyrenoidosa supplementation reduces the risk of anemia, proteinuria and edema in pregnant women. *Plant Foods for Human Nutrition* Vol. 65, No.1, pp 25-30 (March, 2010) ISSN 0921-9668

Neelakandan,C., Chang,T., Alexander,T., Define,L., Evancho-Chapman,M. & Kyu,T. (2011). In vitro evaluation of antioxidant and anti-inflammatory properties of genistein-modified hemodialysis membranes. *Biomacromolecules* Vol. 12, No. 7, pp 2447-2455 (July, 2011) ISSN 1525-7797

Nishioka,Y., Oyagi,A., Tsuruma,K., Shimazawa,M., Ishibashi,T. & Hara,H. (2011). The antianxiety-like effect of astaxanthin extracted from *Paracoccus carotinifaciens*. *Biofactors* Vol. 37, No. 1, pp 25-30 (January, 2011) ISSN 1872- 8081

Orsolic,N., Gajski,G., Garaj-Vrhovac,V., Dikic,D., Prskalo,Z. & Sirovina,D. (2011). DNA-protective effects of quercetin or naringenin in alloxan-induced diabetic mice. *European Journal of Pharmacology* Vol. 656, No. 1-3, pp 110-118 (April, 2011) ISSN 0014-2999

Oz,H.S. & Ebersole,J.L. (2010). Green tea polyphenols mediated apoptosis in intestinal epithelial cells by a FADD-dependent pathway. *Journal of Cancer Therapy* Vol. 1, No. 3, pp 105-113 (September, 2010) ISSN 2151-1934

Palozza,P., Colangelo,M., Simone,R., Catalano,A., Boninsegna,A., Lanza,P., Monego,G. & Ranelletti,F.O. (2010). Lycopene induces cell growth inhibition by altering mevalonate pathway and Ras signaling in cancer cell lines. *Carcinogenesis* Vol. 31, No. 7-8, pp 1813-1821 (October, 1999) ISSN 0143-3334

Park,J.B. & Levine,M. (2000). Intracellular Accumulation of Ascorbic Acid Is Inhibited by Flavonoids via Blocking of Dehydroascorbic Acid and Ascorbic Acid Uptakes in HL-60, U937 and Jurkat Cells. *The Journal of Nutrition* Vol. 130, No. 5, pp 1297-1302 (May, 2005) ISSN 0022-3166

Peng,G., Du,Y., Wei,Y., Tang,J., Peng,A.Y. & Rao,L. (2011). A new synthesis of fully phosphorylated flavones as potent pancreatic cholesterol esterase inhibitors. *Organic and Biomolecular Chemistry* Vol. 9, No.7, pp 2530-2534 (April, 2011) ISSN 1477-0520

Polier,G., Ding,J., Konkimalla,B.V., Eick,D., Ribeiro,N., Kohler,R., Giaisi,M., Efferth,T., Desaubry,L., Krammer,P.H. & Li-Weber,M. (2011). Wogonin and related natural flavones are inhibitors of CDK9 that induce apoptosis in cancer cells by transcriptional suppression of Mcl-1. Cell Death and Disease Vol. 2,pp e182 (January, 2011) ISSN 2041-4889

Polivkova,Z., merak,P., Demova,H. & Houska,M. (2010). Antimutagenic effects of lycopene and tomato puree. *Journal of Medicinal Food* Vol. 13, No. 6, pp 1443-1450 (December, 2010) ISSN 1096-620X

Prabu,S.M., Shagirtha,K. & Renugadevi,J. (2011). Naringenin in combination with vitamins C and e potentially protects oxidative stress-mediated hepatic injury in cadmium-intoxicated rats. *Journal of nutritional science and vitaminology* (Tokyo) Vol. 57, No. 2, pp 177-185 (January, 2011) ISSN 0301-4800

Qin,L., Jin,L., Lu,L., Lu,X., Zhang,C., Zhang,F. & Liang,W. (2011). Naringenin reduces lung metastasis in a breast cancer resection model. *Protein & Cell* Vol.2, No.6 (June 2011), pp.507-516, ISSN 1674-8018

Raja,R., Hemaiswarya,S., Balasubramanyam,D. & Rengasamy,R. (2007). Protective effect of *Dunaliella salina* (*Volvocales, Chlorophyta*) against experimentally induced fibrosarcoma on wistar rats. *Microbiological Research* Vol.162, No.2 (January 2007), pp.177-184, ISSN 0944-5013

Ried,K. & Fakler,P. (2011). Protective effect of lycopene on serum cholesterol and blood pressure: Meta-analyses of intervention trials. *Maturitas* Vol.68, No.4 (April 2011), pp.299-310, ISSN 0378-5122

Rimbach,G., Melchin,M., Moehring,J. & Wagner,A.E. (2009). Polyphenols from cocoa and vascular health-a critical review. *International ournal ofJ Molecular Science* Vol.10, No.10 (October 2009), pp.4290-4309, ISSN 1422-0057

Roghani,M., Niknam,A., Jalali-Nadoushan,M.R., Kiasalari,Z., Khalili,M. & Baluchnejadmojara...,T. (2010). Oral pelargonidin exerts dose-dependent neuroprotection in 6-hydroxydopamine rat model of hemi-parkinsonism. *Brain Research Bulletin* Vol.82, No.5-6 (July 2010), pp.279-283, ISSN 0361-9230

Ruhl,R. (2005). Induction of PXR-mediated metabolism by beta-carotene. *Biochimica et Biophysica Acta* Vol.1740, No.2 (May 2010), pp.162-169, ISSN 0006-3002

Sabarinathan,D., Mahalakshmi,P. & Vanisree,A.J. (2010). Naringenin promote apoptosis in cerebrally implanted C6 glioma cells. *Molecular and Cellular Biochemestry* Vol.345, No.1-2 (December 2010), pp.215-222, ISSN

Sahin,K., Tuzcu,M., Sahin,N., Ali,S. & Kucuk,O. (2010). Nrf2/HO-1 signaling pathway may be the prime target for chemoprevention of cisplatin-induced nephrotoxicity by lycopene. *Food and Chemical Toxicology* Vol.48, No.10 (October 2010), pp.2670-2674, ISSN 0278-6915

Sahni,S., Hannan,M.T., Blumberg,J., Cupples,L.A., Kiel,D.P. & Tucker,K.L. (2009). Protective effect of total carotenoid and lycopene intake on the risk of hip fracture: a 17-year follow-up from the Framingham Osteoporosis Study. *Neurochemical International* Vol.24, No.6 (Jun 2009), pp.1086-1094, ISSN 0197-0186

Sandhir,R., Mehrotra,A. & Kamboj,S.S. (2010). Lycopene prevents 3-nitropropionic acid-induced mitochondrial oxidative stress and dysfunctions in nervous system. *Neurochemestry International Vol.*57, No.5 (November 2010), pp.579-587, ISSN 0197-0186

Sansawa,H., Takahashi,M., Tsuchikura,S. & Endo,H. (2006). Effect of chlorella and its fractions on blood pressure, cerebral stroke lesions, and life-span in stroke-prone spontaneously hypertensive rats. *Journal of Nutritional Sciences and Vitaminology* (Tokyo) Vol.52, No.6 (December 2006), pp.457-466. ISSN 0301-4800

Sarkar,F.H., Li,Y., Wang,Z. & Kong,D. (2010). The role of nutraceuticals in the regulation of Wnt and Hedgehog signaling in cancer. *Cancer and Metastasis Review Vol.29,* No.3 (September 2010), pp.383-394, ISSN 0167-7659

Scalbert,A., Johnson,L.T. & Saltmarsh,M. (2005). Polyphenols: antioxidants and beyond. *American Journal of Clinical Nutrition* Vol.81, No.1 (January 2005), pp.215S-2217, ISSN 0002-9165

Serpeloni,J.M., Grotto,D., Aissa,A.F., Mercadante,A.Z., Bianchi,M.D. & Antunes,L.M. (2011). An evaluation, using the comet assay and the micronucleus test, of the antigenotoxic effects of chlorophyll b in mice. *Mutation Research,* ISSN 0027-5107

Shahidi,F. (2009). Nutraceutical and functional food: whole versus processed food. Trend *Food Science and Technology* Vol.20, pp. 376-387, ISSN 1365-2621

Shaish,A., Harari,A., Hananshvili,L., Cohen,H., Bitzur,R., Luvish,T., Ulman,E., Golan,M., Ben-Amotz,A., Gavish,D., Rotstein,Z. & Harats,D. (2006). 9-cis beta-carotene-rich powder of the alga Dunaliella bardawil increases plasma HDL-cholesterol in fibrate-treated patients. *Atherosclerosis* Vol.189, No.1 (November 2010), pp.215-221, ISSN

Sharma,M.K., Sharma,A., Kumar,A. & Kumar,M. (2007). Evaluation of protective efficacy of *Spirulina fusiformis* against mercury induced nephrotoxicity in Swiss albino mice. *Food and Chemical Toxicology* Vol.45, No.6 (June 2007), pp.879-887, ISSN 0278-6915

Sheu,M., Huang,G., Wu,C., Chen,J., Hang,H., Chang,S. & Chung,J. (2008). Ethanol Extract of *Dunaliella salina* induces cell cycle arrest and apoptosis in A549 human non- small cell lung cancer cells. *In Vivo* Vol.22, No.3 (May 2008), pp.369-378, ISSN 0258- 851X

Shibata,S., Hayakawa,K., Egashira,Y. & Sanada,H. (2007). Hypocholesterolemic mechanism of *Chlorella: Chlorella* and its indigestible fraction enhance hepatic cholesterol catabolism through up-regulation of cholesterol 7alpha-hydroxylase in rats. *Bioscience Biotechnology and Biochemestry* Vol.71, No.4(April 2007), pp.916-925, ISSN0916-8451

Shim,J.A., Son,Y.A., Park,J.M. & Kim,M.K. (2009). Effect of Chlorella intake on Cadmium metabolism in rats. *Nutrition Research and Practice* Vol.3, No.1 (March 2009), pp.15-22, ISSN 1976-1457

Simone,R.E., Russo,M., Catalano,A., Monego,G., Froehlich,K., Boehm,V. & Palozza,P. (2011). Lycopene inhibits NF-kB-mediated IL-8 expression and changes redox and PPAR? signalling in cigarette smoke-stimulated macrophages. *PLoS One* Vol.6, No.5 (January 2011), pp.e19652, ISSN 1932-6203

Singab,A.N., Ayoub,N.A., Ali,E.N. & Mostafa,N.M. (2010). Antioxidant and hepatoprotective activities of Egyptian moraceous plants against carbon tetrachloride-induced oxidative stress and liver damage in rats. *Pharmaceutical Biology* Vol.48, No.11 (November 2010), pp.1255-1264, ISSN 1388-0209

Song,J., Kwon,O., Chen,S., Daruwala,R., Eck,P., Park,J.B. & Levine,M. (2002). Flavonoid inhibition of sodium-dependent vitamin C transporter 1 (SVCT1) and glucose transporter isoform 2 (GLUT2), intestinal transporters for vitamin C and glucose. *Journal of Biological Chemistry* Vol.277, No.18 (may 2002), pp.15252-15260, ISSN 0021-9258

Sternberg,Z., Chadha,K., Lieberman,A., Hojnacki,D., Drake,A., Zamboni,P., Rocco,P., Grazioli,E., Weinstock-Guttman,B. & Munschauer,F. (2008). Quercetin and interferon-beta modulate immune response(s) in peripheral blood mononuclear cells isolated from multiple sclerosis patients. *Journal of Neuroimmunology* Vol.205, No.1-2 (December 2008), pp.142-147 ISSN 0165-5728

Stewart,J.S., Lignell,A., Pettersson,A., Elfving,E. & Soni,M.G. (2008). Safety assessment of astaxanthin-rich microalgae biomass: Acute and subchronic toxicity studies in rats. *Food and Chemical Toxicology* Vol.46, No.9 (September 2008), pp.3030-3036, ISSN 0278-6915

Suarez,E.R., Kralovec,J.A. & Grindley,T.B. (2010). Isolation of phosphorylated polysaccharides from algae: the immunostimulatory principle of Chlorella pyrenoidosa. *Carbohydrate Research* Vol.345 No.9 (June 2010), pp.1190-1204ISSN 0008-6215

Suganuma,K., Nakajima,H., Ohtsuki,M. & Imokawa,G. (2010). Astaxanthin attenuates the UVA-induced up-regulation of matrix-metalloproteinase-1 and skin fibroblast 2010), pp.136-142.

Tang,F.Y., Pai,M.H. & Wang,X.D. (2011). Consumption of lycopene inhibits the growth and progression of colon cancer in a mouse xenograft model. *Journal of Agricultural and Food Chemestry* Vol.59, No.16 (Agust 2011), pp.9011-9021, ISSN 0021-8561

Tokimitsu,I. (2004). Effects of tea catechins on lipid metabolism and body fat accumulation. *Biofactors* Vol.22, No.1-4 (January 2004), pp.141-143, ISSN 0951-6433

Tsuda,T. (2008). Regulation of adipocyte function by anthocyanins; possibility of preventing the metabolic syndrome. *Journal of Agricultural and Food Chemestry* Vol.56, No.3 (February 2008), pp.642-646, ISSN 0021-8561

Vijayavel,K., Anbuselvam,C. & Balasubramanian,M.P. (2007). Antioxidant effect of the marine algae Chlorella vulgaris against naphthalene-induced oxidative stress in the albino rats. *Molecular and Cellular Biochemestry* Vol.303, No.1-2 (September 2007), pp.39-44, ISSN 0300-8177

Wang,L.S., Sun,X.D., Cao,Y., Wang,L., Li,F.J. & Wang,Y.F. (2010). Antioxidant and pro-oxidant properties of acylated pelargonidin derivatives extracted from red radish (*Raphanus sativus* var. *niger, Brassicaceae*). *Food and Chemical Toxicology* Vol.48, No.10 (October 2010), pp.2712-2718, ISSN 0278-6915

Werman,M., Mokady,S. & Ben-Amotz,A. (2002). Bioavailability of the isomer mixture of phytoene and phytofluene-rich alga Dunaliella bardawil in rat plasma and tissues. *Journal of Nutrition and Biochemestry* Vol.13, No.10 (October 2010), pp.585-591, ISSN 0955-2863

Williams,R.J., Spencer,J.P. & Rice-Evans,C. (2004). Flavonoids: antioxidants or signalling molecules? *Free Radical Biology and Medical* Vol.36, No.7 (April 2004), pp.838-849, ISSN 8755-9668

Winkel-Shirley,B. (2001). Flavonoid biosynthesis. A colorful model for Genetics, Biochemistry, Cell Biology, and Biotechnology. *Plant Physiology* Vol.126, No.2 (June 2001), pp.485-493,ISSN 0032-0889

Wolfram,S., Raederstorff,D., Preller,M., Wang,Y., Teixeira,S.R., Riegger,C. & Weber,P. (2006). Epigallocatechin Gallate Supplementation Alleviates Diabetes in Rodents. The *Journal of Nutrition* Vol.136, No.10 (October 2010), pp.2512-2518, ISSN 0022-3166

Wood,L.G., Garg,M.L., Powell,H. & Gibson,P.G. (2008). Lycopene-rich treatments modify noneosinophilic airway inflammation in asthma: proof of concept. *Free Radical Reserch* Vol.42, No.1(January 2008), pp.94-102, ISSN 1029-2470

Wu,S.J., Ng,L.T., Wang,G.H., Huang,Y.J., Chen,J.L. & Sun,F.M. (2010). Chlorophyll a, an active anti-proliferative compound of *Ludwigia octovalvis*, activates the CD95 (APO-1/CD95) system and AMPK pathway in 3T3-L1 cells. *Food and Chemical Toxicology* Vol.48, No.2 (February 2010), pp. 716-721, ISSN 0278-6915

Xi,Y.D., Yu,H.L., Ma,W.W., Ding,B.J., Ding,J., Yuan,L.H., Feng,J.F. & Xiao,R. (2011). Genistein inhibits mitochondrial-targeted oxidative damage induced by beta-amyloid peptide 25-35 in PC12 cells. *Journal of Bioenergetics and Biomembranes* Vol.43, No.4 (Agust 2011), pp. 399-407, ISSN 0145-479X

Yang,L., Takai,H., Utsunomiya,T., Li,X., Li,Z., Wang,Z., Wang,S., Sasaki,Y., Yamamoto,H. & Ogata,Y. (2010). Kaempferol stimulates bone sialoprotein gene transcription and new bone formation. *Journal of Cellular Biochemestry* Vol.110, No.6 (Agust 2010), pp.1342-1355, ISSN 1097-4644

Yang,Y., Seo,J.M., Nguyen,A., Pham,T.X., Park,H.J., Park,Y., Kim,B., Bruno,R.S. & Lee,J. (2011). Astaxanthin-rich extract from the green alga *Haematococcus pluvialis* lowers plasma lipid concentrations and enhances antioxidant defense in apolipoprotein E knockout mice. *The Journal of Nutrition* Vol.141, No.9 (September 2011), pp. 1611-1617, ISSN 0022-3166

Yusof,Y.A., Saad,S.M., Makpol,S., Shamaan,N.A. & Ngah,W.Z. (2010). Hot water extract of *Chlorella vulgaris* induced DNA damage and apoptosis. *Clinics* (Sao Paulo) Vol.65, No.12 (January 2010), pp.1371-1377, ISSN 1807-5932

Zeisel,S.H. (1999). Regulation of "Nutraceuticals". *Science* Vol.285, No.5435 (September 1999), pp.1853-1855, ISSN 0036-8075

Zhao,L., Chen,G., Zhao,G. & Hu,X. (2009). Optimization of Microwave-Assisted Extraction of astaxanthin from Haematococcus pluvialis by response surface methodology and antioxidant activities of the extracts. *Separation Science and Technology* Vol.44, No.1 (January 2009), pp. 243-262, ISSN 0149-6395

Zhao,Z.W., Cai,W., Lin,Y.L., Lin,Q.F., Jiang,Q., Lin,Z. & Chen,L.L. (2011). Ameliorative effect of astaxanthin on endothelial dysfunction in streptozotocin-induced diabetes in male rats. *Arzneimittel-Forschung* Vol.61, No.4 (January 2011), pp. 61, 239-246. ISSN 0004-4172

Zhu,C., Bai,C., Sanahuja,G., Yuan,D., Farre,G., Naqvi,S., Shi,L., Capell,T. & Christou,P. (2010). The regulation of carotenoid pigmentation in flowers. *Archives of Biochemestry and Biophysics* Vol.504, No.1 (December 2010), pp. 132-141, ISSN 0003-9861

Zhu,J., Wang,C.G. & Xu,Y.G. (2011). Lycopene attenuates endothelial dysfunction in streptozotocin-induced diabetic rats by reducing oxidative stress. *Pharmaceutical Biology* (March 2011) ISSN 1388-0209